Introduction to
Critical Care
NURSING

SIXTH EDITION

Mary Lou Sole, PhD, RN, CCNS, CNL, FAAN, FCCM

Orlando Health Distinguished Professor
College of Nursing
University of Central Florida;
Research Scientist
Orlando Health
Orlando, Florida

Deborah G. Klein, MSN, RN, APRN-BC, CCRN, FAHA

Clinical Nurse Specialist
Coronary ICU and Heart Failure ICU
Cleveland Clinic;
Clinical Instructor
Frances Payne Bolton School of Nursing
Case Western Reserve University
Cleveland, Ohio;
Adjunct Faculty
College of Nursing
Kent State University
Kent, Ohio

Marthe J. Moseley, PhD, RN, CCNS

Associate Director Clinical Practice
Office of Nursing Services
Clinical Nurse Specialist, Critical Care
Veterans Healthcare Administration
Washington, DC;
Professor
Rocky Mountain University of Health Professions
Provo, Utah;
Adjunct Professor
University of Texas Health Science Center School of Nursing
San Antonio, Texas

With approximately 300 illustrations

ELSEVIER

3251 Riverport Lane
St. Louis, Missouri 63043

INTRODUCTION TO CRITICAL CARE NURSING, SIXTH EDITION ⬤ 978-0-323-08848-0

Notices

Knowledge and best practice in this field are constantly changing. As new research and experience broaden our understanding, changes in research methods, professional practices, or medical treatment may become necessary.

Practitioners and researchers must always rely on their own experience and knowledge in evaluating and using any information, methods, compounds, or experiments described herein. In using such information or methods they should be mindful of their own safety and the safety of others, including parties for whom they have a professional responsibility.

With respect to any drug or pharmaceutical products identified, readers are advised to check the most current information provided (i) on procedures featured or (ii) by the manufacturer of each product to be administered, to verify the recommended dose or formula, the method and duration of administration, and contraindications. It is the responsibility of practitioners, relying on their own experience and knowledge of their patients, to make diagnoses, to determine dosages and the best treatment for each individual patient, and to take all appropriate safety precautions.

To the fullest extent of the law, neither the Publisher nor the authors, contributors, or editors, assume any liability for any injury and/or damage to persons or property as a matter of products liability, negligence or otherwise, or from any use or operation of any methods, products, instructions, or ideas contained in the material herein.

Nursing Diagnoses – Definitions and Classification 2012-2014.
Copyright © 2012, 1994-2012 by NANDA International. Used by arrangement with Blackwell Publishing Limited, a company of John Wiley & Sons, Inc.

Library of Congress Cataloging-in-Publication Data
Introduction to critical care nursing / [edited by] Mary Lou Sole, Deborah G. Klein, Marthe J. Moseley.—
6th ed.
    p. ; cm.
 Critical care nursing
 Includes bibliographical references and index.
 ISBN 978-0-323-08848-0 (pbk. : alk. paper)
 I. Sole, Mary Lou. II. Klein, Deborah G. III. Moseley, Marthe J. IV. Title: Critical care nursing.
 [DNLM: 1. Critical Care. 2. Nursing Care. WY 154]

 616.02'8--dc23

                                                                      2012008134

Executive Content Strategist: Tamara Myers
Senior Content Development Specialist: Linda Thomas
Publishing Services Manager: Jeff Patterson
Senior Project Manager: Tracey Schriefer
Design Direction: Amy Buxton

Printed in China

Last digit is the print number: 9 8 7 6 5 4 3 2 1

A special dedication to my grandmother, Josephine Ferda, who has celebrated 100 years of health! To my husband, Bob, and daughter, Erin, for their encouragement and support of my many activities. To my parents, George and Margaret Ferda, who always encouraged me to shoot for the stars. Lastly, to my many students and colleagues, who inspire me and keep me grounded in clinical practice.

MLS

To the critical care nurses, patients, and their families, who guide the content of this book. To my husband, Ron, and my sons, David and Seth, for their support in all that I do. To my parents, Rena Sasson Goldenberg, RN, BSN, and Ira Goldenberg, MD, for their guidance and inspiration.

DGK

To my mom, sister, and son—Violet and Heidi Halvorson, and Nicholas—who are care receivers and givers both in and out of the hospital. For the Clinical Practice Portfolio—Chris Engstrom, Suzy Thorne-Odem, Evelyn Sommers, and Kelly Morrow—one of the best teams ever. For the lifelong influence and contributions of Marjory Olson. And to dear friends, Luann Mire and Lee White.

MJM

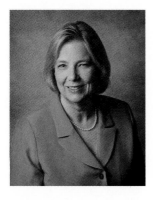

MARY LOU SOLE

Mary Lou Sole, PhD, RN, CCNS, CNL, FAAN, FCCM, has extensive experience in critical care practice, education, consultation, and research. She is the Orlando Health Distinguished Professor and a Pegasus Professor at the University of Central Florida (UCF) College of Nursing in Orlando, Florida. She coordinates the Clinical Nurse Specialist and Clinical Nurse Leader tracks at UCF, and regularly guest lectures during the undergraduate critical care course. She also holds a per diem appointment as a Research Scientist at Orlando Health. Her research focus is on airway management of the critically ill. She began her career as a diploma graduate from the Ohio Valley General Hospital School of Nursing in Wheeling, West Virginia. She received a BSN from Ohio University, a master's degree in nursing from The Ohio State University, and a PhD in nursing from The University of Texas at Austin. Dr. Sole has published extensively in peer-reviewed journals and serves on many editorial boards. Dr. Sole has been active locally and nationally in many professional organizations, including the American Association of Critical-Care Nurses (AACN), the Society of Critical Care Medicine, and the American Academy of Nursing. She has received numerous local, state, and national awards for clinical practice, teaching, and research. She has been inducted as a fellow in both the American Academy of Nursing and the American College of Critical Care Medicine. She has received two prestigious awards from AACN—the Flame of Excellence Award and the Distinguished Research Lecturer.

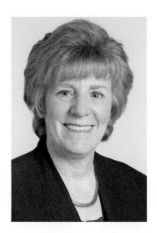

DEBORAH G. KLEIN

Deborah G. Klein, MSN, RN, APRN-BC, CCRN, FAHA, has more than 35 years of experience in critical care practice, education, consultation, and research. She is currently Clinical Nurse Specialist for the Coronary ICU, Heart Failure ICU, and Cardiac Short Stay/PACU/CARU at the Cleveland Clinic in Cleveland, Ohio. She is a Clinical Instructor at Frances Payne Bolton School of Nursing, Case Western Reserve University; and Adjunct Faculty at Kent State University College of Nursing. She received her BSN and MSN from Frances Payne Bolton School of Nursing, Case Western Reserve University, in Cleveland, Ohio. She is active both locally and nationally in professional organizations, including the American Association of Critical-Care Nurses and the American Heart Association. She has served on editorial boards of several critical care nursing journals and has published extensively on critical care topics in peer-reviewed journals. Mrs. Klein has received local and national awards for clinical practice and teaching.

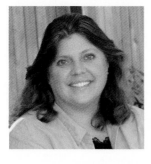

MARTHE J. MOSELEY

Marthe J. Moseley, PhD, RN, CCNS, has more than 28 years of experience in critical care practice, education, consultation, and research. She is currently the Associate Director of Clinical Practice in the Office of Nursing Service with the Veterans Healthcare Administration in Washington, DC, and a Clinical Nurse Specialist for Critical Care. She also holds faculty positions as a Professor at Rocky Mountain University of Health Professions in Provo, Utah, and an Adjunct Professor at The University of Texas Health Science Center San Antonio, Texas School of Nursing. Dr. Moseley received a bachelor of arts degree in nursing from Jamestown College in Jamestown, North Dakota, following the completion of a BA degree in health, physical education, and biology from Concordia College in Moorhead, Minnesota. She completed her MSN and PhD at The University of Texas Health Science Center San Antonio, Texas. She has been active locally and nationally in professional organizations, specifically the American Association of Critical-Care Nurses. She is on the editorial board for several critical care journals and has published in peer-reviewed journals on critical care topics. Dr. Moseley has received local and national awards for both clinical practice and teaching.

CONTRIBUTORS

Katherine F. Alford, MSN, RN, CCRN, PCCN
Acute Care Educator
South Texas Veterans Health Care System
San Antonio, Texas
Chapter 17, Gastrointestinal Alterations

David A. Allen, MSN, RN, CCRN, CCNS, CNS-BC
Clinical Nurse Specialist
Institute of Surgical Research Burn Center;
Major, United States Army Nurse Corps
Fort Sam Houston, Texas
Chapter 8, Hemodynamic Monitoring

Kathy Black, MSN, RN, NE-BC
Patient Care Administrator
Inpatient Surgery Units
Orlando Regional Medical Center
Orlando, Florida
Chapter 3, Ethical and Legal Issues in Critical Care Nursing

Jill T. Dickerson, MSN, RN, CNS-MS, FNP-BC, CWON
Clinical Nurse Specialist
South Texas Veterans Health Care System
Audie L. Murphy Memorial Veterans Hospital
San Antonio, Texas
Chapter 16, Hematological and Immune Disorders

Kathleen Hill, MSN, RN, CCNS-CSC
Clinical Nurse Specialist
Surgical Intensive Care Unit
Cleveland Clinic
Cleveland, Ohio
Chapter 11, Shock, Sepsis, and Multiple Organ Dysfunction Syndrome

Douglas Houghton, MSN, ARNP, ACNPC, CCRN, FAANP
Nurse Practitioner
Department of Trauma/Critical Care
Jackson Health System
Miami, Florida
Chapter 4, End-of-Life Care in the Critical Care Unit

Miranda Kelly, DNP, RN, ACNP-BC
Nurse Practitioner
Intensive Care Unit
Memorial Hermann Healthcare System
The Woodlands, Texas
Chapter 6, Nutritional Support

Kathleen Kerber, MSN, RN, ACNS-BC, CCRN
Clinical Nurse Specialist
Department of Nursing
MetroHealth Medical Center
Cleveland, Ohio
Chapter 15, Acute Kidney Injury

Karla S. Ahrns Klas, BSN, RN, CCRP
Injury Prevention Education Specialist
Trauma Burn Center
University of Michigan
Ann Arbor, Michigan
Chapter 20, Burns

Deborah G. Klein, MSN, RN, APRN-BC, CCRN, FAHA
Clinical Nurse Specialist
Cardiac ICU and Heart Failure ICU
Cleveland Clinic
Cleveland, Ohio;
Clinical Instructor
Frances Payne Bolton School of Nursing
Case Western Reserve University
Cleveland, Ohio;
Adjunct Faculty
College of Nursing
Kent State University
Kent, Ohio
Chapter 10, Rapid Response Teams and Code Management
Chapter 13, Nervous System Alterations
Chapter 21, Solid Organ Transplantation

Sandra J. Knapp, PhD, RN, CCRN, CNL
Clinical Assistant Professor
Adult and Elderly Department
College of Nursing
University of Florida
Gainesville, Florida
Chapter 2, Patient and Family Response to the Critical Care Experience

Jacqueline LaManna, MSN, ARNP-BC, ADM, CDE
Instructor
College of Nursing
University of Central Florida
Orlando, Florida
Chapter 18, Endocrine Alterations
QSEN Exemplars boxes

Mary Beth Flynn Makic, PhD, RN, CNS, CCNS, CCRN
Research Nurse Scientist, Critical Care
Professional Resources
University of Colorado Hospital;
Assistant Professor, Adjunct
College of Nursing
University of Colorado
Aurora, Colorado
Chapter 19, Trauma and Surgical Management

Julie Marcum, MS, APRN-BC, CCRN-CMC
Critical Care Clinical Nurse Specialist
Department of Nursing
Boise Veterans Administration Medical Center
Boise, Idaho
Chapter 7, Dysrhythmia Interpretation and Management

Maximino Martell, MSN, RN, CCRN, CCNS, CNS-BC
Critical Care Clinical Nurse Specialist
Department of Hospital Education
Brooke Army Medical Center
Fort Sam Houston, Texas
Chapter 8, Hemodynamic Monitoring

Marthe J. Moseley, PhD, RN, CCNS
Associate Director Clinical Practice
Office of Nursing Services
Clinical Nurse Specialist, Critical Care
Veterans Healthcare Administration
Washington, DC;
Professor
Rocky Mountain University of Health Professions
Provo, Utah;
Adjunct Professor
University of Texas Health Science Center School of Nursing
San Antonio, Texas
Chapter 16, Hematological and Immune Disorders

Linda Ohler, MSN, RN, CCTC, FAAN
Clinical Administrator
Transplant Institute
Georgetown University
Washington, DC
Chapter 21, Solid Organ Transplantation

Lynelle N.B. Pierce, MSN, RN, CCRN
Clinical Assistant Professor
University of Kansas School of Nursing;
Clinical Nurse Specialist, Critical Care
Nursing
The University of Kansas Hospital
Kansas City, Kansas
Chapter 9, Ventilatory Assistance

Mamoona Arif Rahu, PhD, RN, CCRN
School of Nursing
Virginia Commonwealth University Health
    System
Richmond, Virginia
Chapter 5, Comfort and Sedation

**Maureen A. Seckel, MSN, RN, APN,
    ACNS-BC, CCNS, CCRN**
Clinical Nurse Specialist
Medical Pulmonary Critical Care
Christiana Care Health System;
Adjunct Faculty, School of Nursing
University of Delaware
Newark, Delaware
Chapter 14, Acute Respiratory Failure

**Mary Lou Sole, PhD, RN, CCNS, CNL,
    FAAN, FCCM**
Orlando Health Distinguished Professor
College of Nursing
University of Central Florida;
Research Scientist
Orlando Health
Orlando, Florida
Chapter 1, Overview of Critical Care Nursing
*Chapter 2, Patient and Family Response to
    the Critical Care Experience*
QSEN Exemplars Boxes

**Christina Stewart-Amidei, PhD, RN,
    CNRN, CCRN, FAAN**
Instructor
College of Nursing
University of Central Florida
Orlando, Florida
Chapter 13, Nervous System Alterations
Chapter 18, Endocrine Alterations

**Tracy Evans Walker, MSN, RN, ANP-BC,
    CCTC**
Certified Nurse Practitioner
Transplant Center
Cleveland Clinic
Cleveland, Ohio
Chapter 21, Solid Organ Transplantation

**Colleen Walsh-Irwin, MS, RN, CCRN,
    ANP**
Nurse Practitioner, Division of Cardiology
Northport VA Medical Center
Northport, New York;
Clinical Instructor, School of Nursing
State University of New York
Stony Brook, New York
Chapter 12, Cardiovascular Alterations

Jayne M. Willis, MSN, RN, NEA-BC
Chief Nursing Officer
Orlando Regional Medical Center
Orlando, Florida
*Chapter 3, Ethical and Legal Issues in Critical
    Care Nursing*

**Chris Winkelman, PhD, RN, CCRN,
    ACNP**
Associate Professor
Frances Payne Bolton School of Nursing
Case Western Reserve University
Cleveland, Ohio
Genetics boxes

**Patricia B. Wolff, MSN, RN, ACNS-BC,
    AOCNS**
Clinical Nurse Specialist, Medical Oncology
South Texas Veterans Health Care System
Audie L. Murphy Division
San Antonio, Texas
*Chapter 16, Hematological and Immune
    Disorders*

Zara Brenner, MS, RN-BC, ACNS-BC
Assistant Professor
The College at Brockport
State University of New York
Clinical Nurse Specialist
Rochester General Hospital
Rochester, New York

Kenneth Brooks, BS, BSN, RN
Staff Nurse
Mayo Clinic;
Doctoral Student
University of Minnesota
Rochester, Minnesota

Janet E. Burton, MSN, BS, RN
Instructor
Department of Nursing
Ivy Tech Community College
Columbus, Indiana

Marilyn T. Caldwell, MS, RN, ANP
Assistant Professor
Department of Nursing
Morrisville State College
Morrisville, New York

Judy Crewell, PhD, RN, CNE
Associate Professor
Regis University
Denver, Colorado

Jane Haertlein, MS, RN, CNE
Division of Nursing and Health Science
Bob Jones University
Greenville, South Carolina

Rebecca Hickey, RN
Adjunct Instructor
University of Cincinnati-Raymond Walters
   Campus
Blue Ash, Ohio

Linda Howe, PhD, RN, CNS, CNE
Associate Professor
College of Nursing
University of Central Florida
Orlando, Florida

Ruthanne Kuiper, PhD, RN, CNE, ANEF
Associate Professor
Department Chair, Adult Health and
   Learning Technology
School of Nursing
University of North Carolina Wilmington
Wilmington, North Carolina

Robert Lamb, PharmD
REL & Associates, LLC
Downingtown, Pennsylvania

Kristine L'Ecuyer, MSN, RN, CCNS, CNL
Associate Professor
School of Nursing
St. Louis University
St. Louis, Missouri

Lynn Rowe, MSN, RN
Clinical Specialist
Florida Hospital
Critical Care Outcomes
Orlando, Florida

Jenny Sauls, DSN, RN, CNE
Professor
School of Nursing
Middle Tennessee State University
Murfreesboro, Tennessee

Scott Thigpen, DNP, RN, CCRN, CEN
Associate Professor of Nursing
South Georgia College
Douglas, Georgia;
Staff Nurse
Satilla Regional Medical Center
Waycross, Georgia

Jo Voss, PhD, RN
Associate Professor
College of Nursing
South Dakota State University
Rapid City, South Dakota

Kathleen Whalen, PhD, RN, CNE
Associate Professor
Loretto Heights School of Nursing
Regis University
Denver, Colorado

Critical care nursing deals with human responses to life-threatening health problems. Critically ill patients continue to have high levels of acuity and complex care needs. These patients are cared for in critical care units, intermediate care units, outpatient settings, and at home. The critical care nurse is challenged to provide comprehensive care for these patients and their family members. The demand for critical care nurses who can work across the continuum of care continues to increase.

A solid knowledge foundation in concepts of critical care nursing is essential for practice. Nurses must also learn the assessment and technical skills associated with management of the critically ill patient.

The goal of this sixth edition of *Introduction to Critical Care Nursing* is to facilitate attainment of this foundation for care of the acutely and critically ill patient. The book continues to provide essential information in an easy-to-learn format. The textbook is targeted to both undergraduate nursing students and experienced nurses who are new to critical care. Both groups have found past editions of the book beneficial. In fact, undergraduate students who have taken a critical care course based on this textbook have easily passed critical care courses offered in their first nursing position!

ORGANIZATION

Introduction to Critical Care Nursing is organized into three sections. Part 1, Fundamental Concepts, introduces the reader to critical care nursing; psychosocial concepts related to patients, families, and nurses; and legal, ethical, and end-of-life issues related to critical care nursing practice. Part 2, Tools for the Critical Care Nurse, remains a unique feature of this text. Chapters in this section provide vital information concerning comfort and sedation, nutrition, recognition of dysrhythmias, hemodynamic monitoring, airway management and mechanical ventilation, and management of life-threatening emergencies. These chapters provide information related to the many treatments and technologies that acutely and critically ill patients receive.

The final chapters of the book complete Part 3, Nursing Care during Critical Illness. The nursing process is used as an organizing framework for each chapter. Nursing care plans continue to be included so that nurses new to critical care become familiar with nursing diagnoses and interventions common to many critically ill patients. A summary of anatomy and physiology is provided, as are pathophysiology diagrams for common problems seen in critical care. Features of each chapter include pharmacology tables, evidence-based practice boxes, clinical and laboratory alerts, geriatric considerations, critical thinking exercises, case studies, genetics, and a new feature on bariatric considerations.

Another new feature is exemplars related to the Quality and Safety Education for Nurses (QSEN) competencies. Additions and revisions have been made based on reader feedback and current trends.

SPECIAL FEATURES

This edition features a full-color design with updated full-color figures to enhance reader understanding. Many new and revised learning aids appear in the sixth edition to highlight chapter content:

- **Evidence-Based Practice** boxes identify problems in patient care, ask pertinent questions related to the problems, supply evidence addressing the questions, and offer implications for nursing practice. Most boxes provide references to systematic reviews and meta-analyses that provide a greater synthesis of the research evidence related to a problem. New to this edition is the AACN's new system for Level of Evidence: A, B, C, D, E, and M.
- **QSEN Exemplars** present examples of quality and safety competencies in critical care.
- **Genetics** boxes discuss disorders with a genetic component, including diabetes, Marfan syndrome, and cystic fibrosis.
- **Clinical Alerts** highlight particular concerns, significance, and procedures in a variety of clinical settings to help students understand the potential problems encountered in that setting.
- **Laboratory Alerts** detail both common and cutting-edge tests and procedures to alert students to the importance of laboratory results.
- **Geriatric Considerations** alert the user to the special needs of the older patient in the critical care environment.
- **Bariatric Considerations** provide information related to the bariatric patient because these patients often present unique challenges in the delivery of care.
- Client-specific **Case Studies** with accompanying questions help students apply the chapter's content to real-life situations while also testing their critical-thinking abilities. Answers for these questions and the **Critical Thinking Exercises** found at the end of each chapter, are included in the Lesson Plan on the companion Evolve Web site, which is free to instructors upon adoption.
- **Nursing Care Plans** describe patient diagnoses, outcomes, nursing interventions, and rationales.
- **Pathophysiology Flow Charts** expand analysis of the course and outcomes of particular injuries and disorders.
- **Pharmacology Tables** reflect the most current and most commonly used critical care medications.
- A new **Appendix**, presents the QSEN pre-licensure knowledge, skills, and attitudes.

NEW CHAPTER

In addition to the new and updated special features, a new chapter on transplantation (Chapter 21, Solid Organ Transplantation) is found in this edition. Assessment and management of the organ donor and management of the patient after transplantation has become more common in critical care units. Concepts in this chapter tie in knowledge learned throughout the text; therefore it makes an excellent chapter to complete the textbook.

EVOLVE RESOURCES

We are pleased to offer additional content and learning aids to both instructors and students on our Evolve companion Web site, which has been customized for the new edition and is available at **http://evolve.elsevier.com/Sole/.**

For Students

Student resources on the Evolve site include the following:

- **Review Questions,** consisting of multiple-choice and multiple-response questions and answer rationales for each chapter.
- **Animations and Video Clips,** which feature innovative content from supplemental materials.
- **15 Procedures from the new edition of** *Mosby's Nursing Skills,* which demonstrate many of the primary procedures important in critical care nursing.

For Instructors

Instructor Resources on the Evolve site include the following materials:

- A **TEACH For Nurses Lesson Plan,** which provides the following for each chapter:
  - Objectives and teaching focus.
  - Nursing curriculum standards, including QSEN, concept-based curricula, BSN Essentials, Adult CCRN, and PCCN.

- Teaching and learning activities related to the chapter content outline.
- Brand new case study with questions and answers.
- Answers to the Case Study and Critical Thinking Exercises presented in the textbook.
- A **PowerPoint Presentation** collection of more than 1400 slides offers a presentation for every chapter. The presentation includes chapter images, lecture notes, and audience response questions, and a few select chapters include a progressive case study.
- An electronic **Test Bank** of more than 750 questions.
- An **Image Collection** including all of the images from the text.

Instructors have access to the student resources as well. Evolve can also be used to do the following:

- Publish your class syllabus, outline, and lecture notes.
- Set up "virtual office hours" and e-mail communication.
- Share important dates and information through the online class calendar.
  - Encourage student participation through chat rooms and discussion boards.

Critical care nursing is an exciting and challenging field. Healthcare organizations need critical care nurses who are knowledgeable about basic concepts as well as research-based practice, are technologically competent, and are caring toward patients and families. Our hope is that this edition of *Introduction to Critical Care Nursing* will provide the foundation for critical care nursing practice.

MLS

DGK

MJM

CONTENTS

PART 3 NURSING CARE DURING CRITICAL ILLNESS

Introduction to
Critical Care
NURSING

PART 1

Fundamental Concepts

1

Overview of Critical Care Nursing

Mary Lou Sole, PhD, RN, CCNS, CNL, FAAN, FCCM

⊖volve WEBSITE

Many additional resources, including self-assessment exercises, are located on the Evolve companion website at http://evolve.elsevier.com/Sole.

- Review Questions
- Mosby's Nursing Skills Procedures

- Animations
- Video Clips

Consider working in a care setting where the patients have life-threatening conditions and need intense, round-the-clock care by a team of multiprofessionals. The nurse/patient ratio is low, sometimes 1:1, to ensure that care is delivered timely and that response to treatment is continuously assessed. Technology is abundant and readily available to assist in managing these complex, acutely ill patients. Treatment varies, but often includes mechanical ventilation, multiple invasive lines, hemodynamic monitoring, and administration of many medications and fluids. This scenario depicts the essence of critical care. Many nurses choose to work in critical care settings because they enjoy working in a fast-paced environment that provides much contact with patients, families, and their multiprofessional colleagues. They constantly are learning new concepts in treatment and technology. Although not a career for every nurse, critical care nursing provides an exciting opportunity for those who thrive in working in such an environment.

DEFINITION OF CRITICAL CARE NURSING

Critical care nursing is concerned with human responses to life-threatening problems, such as trauma, major surgery, or complications of illness. The human response can be a physiological or psychological phenomenon. The focus of the critical care nurse includes both the patient's and family's responses to illness and involves prevention as well as cure. Because patients' medical needs have become increasingly complex, critical care nursing encompasses care of both acutely and critically ill patients.

EVOLUTION OF CRITICAL CARE

The specialty of critical care has its roots in the 1950s, when patients with polio were cared for in specialized units. In the 1960s, recovery rooms were established for the care of patients who had undergone surgery, and coronary care units were instituted for the care of patients with cardiac problems. The patients who received care in these units had improved outcomes. Figure 1-1 depicts an early cardiac surgical unit. Critical care nursing evolved as a specialty in the 1970s with the development of general intensive care units. Since that time, critical care nursing has become increasingly specialized. Examples of specialized critical care units are cardiovascular, surgical, neurological, trauma, transplantation, burn, pediatric, and neonatal units. Figure 1-2 shows a modern critical care unit.

Critical care nursing has expanded beyond the walls of traditional critical care units. For example, critically ill patients are cared for in emergency departments; postanesthesia units; step-down, intermediate care, and progressive care units; and interventional radiology and cardiology units. Critical care is also delivered during transport of critically ill patients from the field to the acute care hospital and during interfacility transport. With advances in technology, the electronic intensive care unit (eICU) has emerged as another setting for critical care nursing. In an eICU, patients are monitored remotely by critical care nurses and physicians.[37] Acutely ill patients with high-technology requirements or complex problems, such as patients who are ventilator dependent, may be cared for in medical-surgical units, in long-term acute care hospitals, or at home.

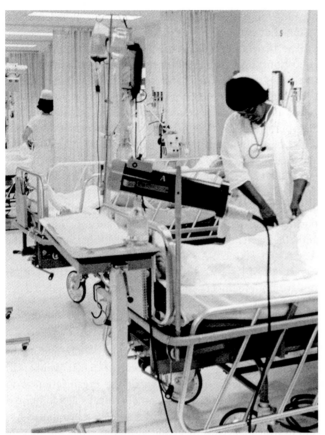

FIGURE 1-1 Early cardiac surgical critical care unit circa 1967, called the Cardiac Constant Care Unit. Note the open bay concept of care delivery, large cardiac monitor at foot of bed, and absence of multiple pumps. (Reprinted with permission, Cleveland Clinic Center for Medical Art & Photography © 2011-2012. All rights reserved.)

BOX 1-1   COMPETENCIES OF NURSES CARING FOR THE CRITICALLY ILL

- Clinical judgment and clinical reasoning skills
- Advocacy and moral agency in identifying and resolving ethical issues
- Caring practices that are tailored to the uniqueness of the patient and family
- Collaboration with patients, family members, and health-care team members
- Systems thinking that promotes holistic nursing care
- Response to diversity
- Facilitator of learning for patients and family members, team members, and the community
- Clinical inquiry and innovation to promote the best patient outcome

Data from American Association of Critical-Care Nurses. The AACN synergy model for patient care. www.aacn.org/wd/certifications/content/synmodel.pcms?pid=1&&menu=certification; 2011. Accessed May 30, 2011.

Acute and critical care nurses practice in varied settings to manage and coordinate care for patients who require in-depth assessment, high-intensity therapies and interventions, and continuous nursing vigilance. They also function in various roles and levels, such as staff nurse, educator, and advanced practice nurse. Competencies for critical care nursing practice are listed in Box 1-1.

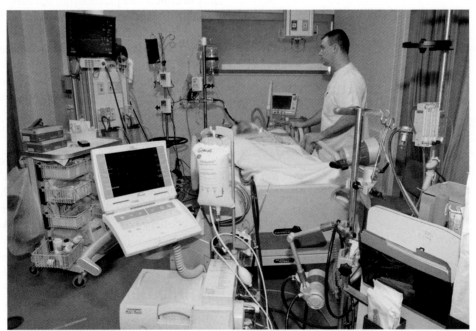

FIGURE 1-2 Modern Critical Care Unit. Note private room and abundance of electronic equipment supporting patient care management. (Reprinted with permission, Cleveland Clinic Center for Medical Art & Photography © 2011-2012. All rights reserved.)

PROFESSIONAL ORGANIZATIONS

Several professional organizations support critical care practice. These include the American Association of Critical-Care Nurses (AACN) and the Society of Critical Care Medicine (SCCM).

American Association of Critical-Care Nurses

The AACN is a professional organization that was established in 1969 to represent critical care nurses. The AACN is the largest nursing specialty organization in the world, with over 80,000 members, dedicated to providing knowledge and resources to those caring for acutely and critically ill patients.[6] In addition to the national organization, more than 240 chapters are in existence to support critical care nurses at the local level.[7] The mission of the organization focuses on assisting acute and critical care nurses to attain knowledge and influence to deliver excellent care. The vision of the organization supports creating a healthcare system driven by the needs of patients and families in which critical care nurses make their optimal contributions, which is described as synergy.[6] The synergy model is shown in Figure 1-3.

The association promotes the health and welfare of critically ill patients by advancing the art and science of critical care nursing and supporting work environments that promote professional nursing practice.[4,11] Values of the organization include accountability, advocacy, integrity, collaboration, leadership, stewardship, lifelong learning, quality, innovation, and commitment. These values are supported through education, research, and collaborative practice.[6] An ethic of care that focuses on compassion, collaboration,

accountability, and trust guides the organization's mission, vision, and values.

The benefits of AACN membership include continuing education offerings, educational advancement scholarships, research grants, awards, and several official publications: *Critical Care Nurse, American Journal of Critical Care, AACN News,* and *AACN Advanced Critical Care.* The organization also publishes *Practice Alerts,* which present succinct, evidence-based practices that are to be applied at the bedside. The organization also sponsors the Beacon Award for Excellence. Units apply for this honor, which is given for exceptional care, improved outcomes, and greater satisfaction with care. Nurses who work in a Beacon unit generally work in a positive and supportive setting. Membership information and other general information are available by contacting the AACN at 1-800-899-AACN or online at www.aacn.org. The website provides a wealth of information related to critical care for both members and nonmembers.

Society of Critical Care Medicine

The SCCM is a multiprofessional scientific and educational organization. The SCCM was founded in 1970 by a group of physicians, and it has grown to more than 15,000 members in over 100 countries. The mission of the organization is to secure the highest-quality care for all critically ill and injured patients. The vision of the SCCM is to have a healthcare system in which all critically ill and injured persons receive care from a multiprofessional team directed by an intensivist (physician who has education and training in the management of the critically ill patient and is board-certified). These teams use knowledge, technology, and compassion to provide timely, safe, effective, and efficient patient care.[41]

The SCCM is dedicated to ensuring excellence and consistency in critical care practice through education, research, and advocacy.[41] Membership in the SCCM is open to physicians and other healthcare providers in critical care, including nurses, respiratory therapists, and pharmacists. The SCCM publishes *Critical Care Medicine, New Horizons: The Science and Practice of Acute Medicine,* and *Pediatric Critical Care Medicine.* Membership and other information are available online at www.sccm.org.

Other Professional Organizations

Other professional organizations also focus on improving care of critically ill patients. Examples include the American College of Chest Physicians (www.chestnet.org), the American Thoracic Society (www.thoracic.org), and the professional scientific councils of the American Heart Association (www.americanheart.org). Nurses can apply for membership in these and other related professional organizations.

CERTIFICATION

Critical care nurses are eligible for certification. Certification validates knowledge of critical care nursing, promotes professional excellence, and helps nurses to maintain a current knowledge base.[8] The AACN Certification Corporation oversees the

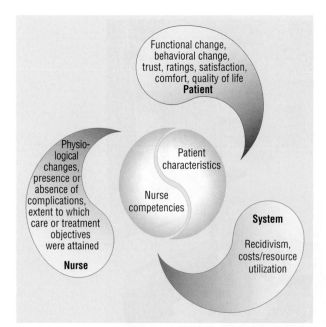

FIGURE 1-3 The American Association of Critical-Care Nurses Synergy Model for Patient Care. (From Curley M. Patient-nurse synergy: optimizing patients' outcomes. *American Journal of Critical Care.* 1998;7:69.)

critical care certification process. Its primary purpose is to protect the consumer by establishing high standards of professional practice.[5]

The certification for nurses in acute and critical care bedside practice is known as CCRN or PCCN. The CCRN certification is available for nurses who provide care of critically ill adult, pediatric, or neonatal populations. The CCRN-E credential is available for nurses working in eICUs. The PCCN is for nurses who provide acute care in progressive care, telemetry, and similar units. Once nurses achieve the CCRN or PCCN credential, they may be eligible to sit for additional subspecialty certification in cardiac medicine (CMC) or cardiac surgery (CSC).

Other certifications are available for managers and advanced practice nurses. AACN has partnered with the American Organization of Nurse Executives (AONE) to offer certification for critical care managers and leaders, the CNML. Advanced practice certification for critical care nurses is also available. Acute and critical care clinical nurse specialists can seek the CCNS credential. Acute care nurse practitioners can become certified as ACNPC.

All certifications have eligibility requirements to sit for the examination. Continuing education and ongoing care for acute or critically ill patients are required for recertification.

The AACN certification credentials are based on a synergy model of practice, which states that the needs of patients and families influence and drive competencies of nurses (see Figure 1-3 and Box 1-1). Each patient and family is unique, with a varying capacity for health and vulnerability to illness. Patients who are more severely compromised have more complex needs, and nursing practice is based on meeting these needs.[17]

STANDARDS

Standards serve as guidelines for clinical practice. They establish goals for patient care and provide mechanisms for nurses to assess the achievement of patient goals, regardless of the setting for practice. The *AACN Standards for Acute and Critical Care Nursing Practice* describe practice for nurses who care for critically ill patients.[12] The standards of practice delineate the nursing process: collect data, determine diagnoses, identify expected outcomes, develop a plan of care, implement interventions, and evaluate progress towards goals. The standards of professional performance (Box 1-2) describe expectations of the acute and critical care nurse.

CRITICAL CARE NURSE CHARACTERISTICS

Essential nursing practices include monitoring and assessment; reassessment, interpreting information, and problem solving; evaluation of progress to outcomes; development of sustainable evidence-based practice; coordination of team activities and the plan of care; patient and family education; and team skill development. The acuteness of patients' illnesses makes their care the top priority of critical care nurses. A missed detail in care could easily result in an adverse event

---

BOX 1-2 STANDARDS OF PROFESSIONAL PERFORMANCE

The Nurse Caring for Acute and Critically Ill Patients:

- Systematically evaluates the quality and effectiveness of nursing practice
- Evaluates own practice in relation to professional practice standards, guidelines, statutes, rules, and regulations
- Acquires and maintains current knowledge and competency in patient care
- Contributes to the professional development of peers and other healthcare providers
- Acts ethically in all areas of practice
- Uses skilled communication to collaborate with the healthcare team to provide care in a safe, healing, humane, and caring environment
- Uses clinical inquiry and integrates research findings into practice
- Considers factors related to safety, effectiveness, cost, and impact in planning and delivering care
- Provides leadership in the practice setting for the profession

Data from Bell, L. (2008). *AACN Scope and Standards for Acute and Critical Care Nursing Practice.* Aliso Viejo, CA: American Association of Critical-Care Nurses.

---

or even death. Critical care nurses are understandably very protective of their patients, wanting to make sure optimal outcomes are achieved. They typically are very busy and engrossed in their work. They are familiar with the noises, lights, and frequent interruptions of their patients' care. They know what to do and act quickly when doing so is indicated. A high level of organization is maintained to make sure everything is done.

In addition to technical competence, critical care nurses establish relationships with patients and families.[48] Relationships are an important part of critical care nursing practice. These relationships develop despite heavy workloads, and sometimes a lack of time to meet the psychosocial and spiritual needs when caring for an acutely ill patient.[32,49]

Juggling the patients' needs, the time available to care for them, and the nurse's needs make the job particularly challenging yet rewarding at the same time. Stress, burnout, and moral distress are issues that critical care nurses face because of the fast-paced environment, critical nature of illness, and issues surrounding life and death of patients. Well-educated and highly motivated critical care nurses may bring to the job perfectionist tendencies and unrealistic expectations of self, further contributing to high stress levels. Support groups and debriefing conducted by professionals are strategies to help reduce stress, anxiety, and moral distress.

QUALITY AND SAFETY EMPHASIS

Quality and safety are essential components of patient care. Patients are at risk for a myriad of harms, which increase morbidity, mortality, length of hospital stay, and costs for care. Since the publication of the Institute of Medicine (IOM) landmark report in 1999, *To Err is Human: Building a Safer Health System*, quality and safety initiatives have been forefront in health care delivery.[29] The Quality and Safety Education for Nurses (QSEN) project, sponsored by the American Association of Colleges of Nursing, provides a road map for integrating quality and safety principles into prelicensure nursing education.[15] The QSEN curriculum defines six core competencies that provide a foundation by which nurses may continuously deliver quality, safe nursing care in a variety of healthcare settings: *patient-centered care, teamwork and collaboration, evidence-based practice, quality improvement, informatics,* and *safety.* Specific knowledge, skills, and attitudes associated with each competency are defined (Appendix A) and will be incorporated into nursing program accreditation standards. Specific applications of QSEN competencies to critical care nursing topics are integrated throughout this text. Additional resources are related to the QSEN project (www.qsen.org). Many nursing programs have already implemented the QSEN standards into their curricula.

Nurses and other health care professionals have been challenged to reduce medical errors and promote an environment that facilitates safe practices. A 40% reduction in preventable hospital conditions over a 3-year period would result in 1.8 million fewer injuries and 60,000 fewer deaths.[47]

The Joint Commission has identified *National Patient Safety Goals* to be addressed in hospitals, long-term care facilities, and other agencies that it accredits.[26] Examples are shown in Box 1-3; however, because goals are updated annually, it is important to regularly review The Joint Commission website (www.jointcommission.org). Staff nurses are responsible for assisting in implementation of the goals.

Initiatives to promote a safe environment are being promoted by the government and other national groups, such as the Institute for Healthcare Improvement (IHI). The federal *Partnership for Patients* focus is on reducing all-cause harm to patients, such as preventing infection, falls, and pressure ulcers (Box 1-4), which are common complications of critical illness. An action plan for reducing healthcare-associated infections, and preventing infections with multidrug-resistant organisms has also been crafted by the federal government.[46]

The IHI *Protecting 5 Million Lives* campaign challenged hospitals to adopt changes in care to save lives and prevent patient injuries.[25] A component of many of the IHI recommendations is the concept of *bundles of care.* Bundles are described as evidence-based best practices that are done as a whole to improve outcomes.[31] Many bundles are described in the literature, such as the ventilator bundle. Bundles relevant to critical care are discussed throughout the textbook.

BOX 1-3   EXAMPLES OF PATIENT SAFETY GOALS

Improve Accuracy of Patient Identification
- Use at least two methods of patient identification
- Ensure correct patient identification for blood transfusions

Improve Communication among Healthcare Providers
- Report critical results of tests and diagnostic procedures on a timely basis

Improve Medication Safety
- Label all medications and containers, including syringes and medicine cups
- Reduce harm associated with administration of anticoagulants

Reduce Risk of Health Care–Associated Infection
- Comply with guidelines for hand hygiene
- Implement evidence-based guidelines for prevent infection with multidrug-resistant organisms
- Implement evidence-based guidelines to prevent central line–associated bloodstream infections
- Implement evidence-based guidelines to prevent surgical site infection

Reconcile Medications across the Continuum of Care
- Compare patient's current (home) medications with those ordered during hospitalization
- Communicate a complete list of medications to the next

provider when patients are transferred within an organization or to another setting
- Provide patient with a complete list of medications upon discharge
- Implement a modified medication reconciliation process in settings where medications are ordered in small amounts or for a short duration

Identify Safety Risks
- Assess patients for suicidal risk

Prevent Complications Associated with Surgery and Procedures
- Conduct a preprocedure verification process to ensure that surgery is done on the correct patient and site
- Mark the correct procedure site
- Perform a "time-out" before the procedure to ensure that the correct patient, site, and procedure are identified

Prevent Indwelling Catheter–Associated Urinary Tract Infection
- Insert indwelling catheters according to established guidelines
- Manage indwelling catheters according to established guidelines
- Measure and monitor prevention processes and outcomes in high-volume areas

Data from The Joint Commission. *National Patient Safety Goals.* www.jointcommission.org/PatientSafety/NationalPatientSafetyGoals; 2012. Accessed September 5, 2011.

BOX 1-4   REDUCING ALL-CAUSE HARM

- Adverse drug events
- Infections
  - Catheter-associated urinary tract infections (CAUTI)
  - Central line–associated bloodstream infections (CLABSI)
  - Surgical site infections
  - Ventilator-associated pneumonia (VAP)
- Injuries from falls and immobility
- Obstetric adverse events
- Pressure ulcers
- Venous thromboembolism (VTE)
- Other hospital-acquired conditions

Data from U.S. Department of Health and Human Services. Partnership for patients: better care, lower costs. http://www.healthcare.gov/compare/partnership-for-patients/index.html. Accessed May 29, 2011.

Another strategy to improve patient safety is the implementation of rapid response teams or medical emergency teams to address changes in patients' conditions.[13,14,21] These teams bring critical care expertise to the bedside to assess and manage patients whose conditions are deteriorating. Although the majority of rapid response calls are initiated by healthcare team members, patients and families should also be empowered to activate the team if needed. The goal of a rapid response team is to identify and manage both unstable patients and those at high risk for cardiopulmonary arrest to prevent unnecessary deaths. Critical care nurses are often the leaders on such teams. Data show implementation of rapid response teams reduces episodes of cardiac arrest but not mortality.[14]

EVIDENCE-BASED PRACTICE

Clinical practice guidelines are being implemented to ensure that care is appropriate and based on research. Examples of guidelines include management of sedation and nutritional support of critically ill patients. These and other relevant guidelines are discussed throughout the textbook.

The National Guideline Clearinghouse provides a compendium of guidelines published by various professional organizations and health care agencies (www.guidelines.gov). Advanced practice nurses often assist the staff in developing and implementing evidence-based practice guidelines.

Nurses are encouraged to implement care that is evidence-based and to challenge practices that have "always been done" but are not supported by clinical evidence. Research studies are graded by the quality of evidence, with many different schemes used by professional organizations and individuals to rate the quality of research. Meta-analysis of many related research studies is considered to be the highest level of evidence; the next highest is derived from the randomized controlled trial (RCT). After rating the evidence, recommendations for practice are provided. The AACN scale for rating evidence (Table 1-1) is a simple-to-use method for evaluating research studies.[9] Nurses can get involved in research in many ways, including participating in unit-based journal clubs to review studies and rate their quality.

HEALTHY WORK ENVIRONMENT

The culture of a critical care unit includes its shared values, attitudes, and beliefs, which in turn reflect behavioral norms that guide the functional dynamics of staff interactions. Interactions among providers, especially nurses and physicians, affect patient safety, clinical outcomes, and the recruitment and retention of nurses.

The AACN initiated a campaign to create work environments that are safe, healing, and humane.[3] Essential components of healthy work environments include respect, responsibility, and acknowledgment of the unique contributions of patients, families, nurses, and healthcare team members (Figure 1-4). Other aspects of a healthy work environment include effective decision making, appropriate staffing, meaningful recognition, and authentic leadership. Communication and collaboration warrant additional discussion because they provide the foundation for achieving a healthy work environment.

TABLE 1-1   AMERICAN ASSOCIATION OF CRITICAL-CARE NURSES' LEVELS OF RESEARCH EVIDENCE

LEVEL	DESCRIPTION
A	Meta-analysis of multiple controlled studies or metasynthesis of qualitative studies with results that consistently support a specific action, intervention, or treatment
B	Well-designed controlled studies, both randomized and nonrandomized, with results that consistently support a specific action, intervention, or treatment
C	Qualitative, descriptive, or correlational studies; integrative reviews; systematic reviews; or randomized controlled trials with inconsistent results
D	Peer-reviewed professional organizational standards, with clinical studies to support recommendations
E	Theory-based evidence from expert opinion or multiple case reports
M	Manufacturer's recommendation only

From Armola RR, Bourgault AM, Halm MA, Board RM, Bucher L, Harrington L, Heafey C, Lee RK, Shellner PK, Medina J: Upgrading the American Association of Critical-Care Nurses' evidence-leveling hierarchy. *American Journal of Critical Care.* 2009; 18:405-409.

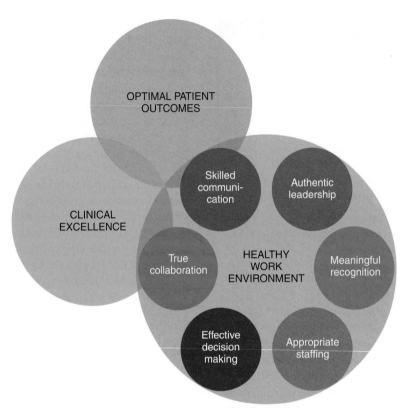

FIGURE 1-4 Essential components of a healthy work environment. Interdependence of healthy work environment, clinical excellence, and optimal patient outcomes. (From AACN. AACN standards for establishing and sustaining healthy work environments: a journey to excellence. *American Journal of Critical Care.* 2005;14[3]:189.)

Communication

Effective communication is essential for delivering safe patient care. Many adverse events are directly attributable to faulty communication. At least half of all communication breakdowns occur during *handoff* situations, when patient information is being transferred or exchanged.[42] Common handoff situations include nursing shift reports, transcription of verbal orders, and interfacility patient transfers. Barriers to effective handoffs are noted in Box 1-5.[10]

Standardized approaches can improve communication and are easily learned. Approaches include *Ask-Tell-Ask*, a strategy for encouraging nurses to assess concerns before providing more information, especially when discussing stressful issues with patients and families. *Tell Me More* is a tool that encourages information sharing in challenging situations, and the SBAR approach—*Situation, Background, Assessment, Recommendation*—is useful in communication, especially with physicians (Box 1-6).[22,38] The SBAR technique delivers information in a way that is brief and action oriented. One researcher modified the SBAR for nurse-to-nurse reporting to SBAP—*Situation, Background, Assessment, Plan*.[43] The box, "QSEN Exemplar," illustrates an example of SBAR communication for a patient handoff. Other strategies

---

BOX 1-5 BARRIERS TO EFFECTIVE HANDOFF COMMUNICATION

- **Physical setting:** background noise, lack of privacy, interruptions
- **Social setting:** organizational hierarchy and status issues
- **Language:** differences between people of varying racial and ethnic backgrounds or geographical areas
- **Communication medium:** limitations of communications via telephone, e-mail, paper, or computerized records versus face-to-face

---

BOX 1-6 SBAR APPROACH

S—Situation: State what is happening at the present time that has warranted the SBAR communication.

B—Background: Explain circumstances leading up to this situation. Put the situation into context for the reader/listener.

A—Assessment: State what you think is the problem.

R—Recommendation: State your recommendation to correct the problem.

QSEN EXEMPLAR

SBAR for Teamwork and Collaboration

Best Practice Tool: The Situation-Background-Assessment-Recommendation (SBAR) report methodology may be particularly helpful in the critical care setting as a method of improving interdepartmental and shift-to-shift information transfer. A sample transfer SBAR report is illustrated:

Situation: My name is (caregiver): Mary Smith, RN from the (unit) emergency department. I will be transferring (patient name) John Jones, a (age) 34-year-old (gender) male admitted (time/date) 3 hours ago with (diagnosis) diabetic ketoacidosis, to (receiving department) medical ICU. Attending physician is Dr. Michael Miller.

Background: Pertinent history – type 1 diabetes for 20 years; on insulin pump; managed pump failure 24 hours ago inappropriately; renal insufficiency. Summary of episode of care:

- Admitting glucose 648 mg/dL; positive ketones; pH 7.27; PaO_2 90 mm Hg; $PaCO_2$ 20 mm Hg; HCO_3^- 12 mEq/L; K^+ 3.4 mEq/L; BUN 40 mg/dL; creatinine 1.8 mg/dL; admitting weight 65 kg; lethargic
- Received 1 L normal saline in field. Normal saline now infusing at 200 mL/hr.
- Received IV bolus of 6.5 units regular insulin at 1300. Insulin infusion of 100 units regular in 100 mL normal saline infusing at 7.5 units per hour (7.5 mL/hr). 1500 repeat glucose 502 mg/dL.
- 20 mEq potassium chloride infused in emergency department
- 200 mL urine output last hour – hourly intake and output
- Hemoglobin A1c level 6 weeks ago was 9.2% (patient report)

Assessment:

- Vital signs: B/P 102/60 mm Hg; Pulse 106 beats/min; Respirations 30 breaths/min; Temperature 37.5° C
- Intake: 1400 mL Output: 450 mL
- Pain level: 0/10
- Neurological: Lethargic; but responsive to stimuli
- Respirations: Deep with acetone odor noted. Lungs clear.
- Cardiac: S1/S2; no murmurs
- Cardiac rhythm: Sinus tachycardia
- Code Status: Full
- GI: Abdomen soft/slightly distended, hypoactive bowel sounds
- GU: Voiding frequently. Urine concentrated.
- Skin: Skin dry with poor turgor; intact
- IV: (location) right forearm (catheter size) 18 g (condition) no redness/edema
- Assessment: Diabetic ketoacidosis secondary to poorly managed insulin pump failure with gradual improvement of glucose over past 2 hours

Recommendation:

- Hourly vital signs
- Repeat glucose, K^+, arterial blood gas due at 1600 today.
- Continue normal saline at 200 mL/hour for 4 hours
- IV insulin infusion at 6.5 units (6.5 mL) per hour – bedside glucose monitoring hourly and adjust per protocol
- Monitor urine output hourly
- Contact Dr. Miller with 1600 lab work for further orders
- Refer to diabetes educator and clinical dietitian
- Repeat renal profile in AM

to improve handoff communication include standardizing processes for the handoff situation, using checklists to prompt and document essential information, and training all personnel in effective communication techniques.

Communication techniques and protocols from other high-risk industries have been implemented in healthcare settings to improve patient safety.[33,34,44] One technique comes from the aviation industry crew resource management (CRM). Flight crews depend on precise communication to ensure passenger safety. CRM was developed to promote communication and accountability among team members. In a CRM environment, everyone from the captain of the aircraft to the baggage handlers on the ground shares responsibility for safe flight operations. Differences in training are acknowledged and respected, but each member of the team is empowered and has the autonomy to address problems without fear of retaliation or ridicule. Several components that underpin the effectiveness of CRM are pertinent to critical care nursing. One CRM principle is to monitor others' actions by double-checking, verifying, and when necessary, correcting inaccurate or ambiguous information.[18] A comparable situation in nursing is administration of blood products and high risk medications, where an additional independent double verification is required. Situational awareness is a second component of CRM and means being aware of one's surroundings. The expectation is that if something seems wrong, individuals should trust their "gut instinct" and speak up to correct the situation.[18]

Collaboration

The ultimate goal of true collaboration in critical care is to create a *culture of safety,* defined as a nonhierarchical culture where all members have the opportunity, as well as the duty, to ensure safe and effective care.[40] As with effective communication, collaboration is founded on mutual respect and the recognition that each discipline involved in patient care brings distinct skills and perspectives to the table.

One strategy for collaboration is the implementation of multiprofessional bedside rounds one to two times per shift. Intensivist-led rounds and daily goal setting are recommended to address patient care issues and adherence to recommended guidelines and bundles of care.[35,39] Examples of daily goals to be addressed are noted in Box 1-7. In addition, patients and families are continually updated about the patient's condition with this increased frequency of communication. In some instances, families are actually included in the team rounds, facilitating communication and involvement.

Conducting morning briefings before interdisciplinary rounds is another strategy to improve communication, collaboration, and patient safety. Suggested content of the morning briefings include answers to three questions: (1) *What happened during the night that the team needs to know* (e.g., adverse events, admissions)? (2) *Where should rounds begin* (e.g., the sickest patient who needs the most attention)? and (3) *What potential problems have been identified for the day* (e.g., staffing, procedures)?[45]

BOX 1-7   ITEMS TO CONSIDER IN DAILY MULTIPROFESSIONAL ROUNDS

- Discharge needs
- Greatest safety risk
- Implementation of ventilator "bundle"
  - Head-of-bed elevation
  - Titration of sedation for assessing readiness to extubate
  - Prophylaxis for peptic ulcer disease
  - Prophylaxis for venous thromboembolism
- Assessment and recommended follow-up
  - Cardiac and hemodynamic status
  - Volume status
  - Neurological status
  - Pain management
  - Sedation needs
  - Gastrointestinal status, including bowel management
  - Nutrition
  - Skin issues

- Activity
- Infection status (culture results/therapeutic levels of antibiotics)
- Laboratory results
- Radiological test results
- Assess need for all ordered medications
- Identify whether central lines and invasive catheters/tubes can be removed
- Identify whether indwelling urinary catheter can be removed
- Issues that need to be addressed
  - Family needs—educational, psychosocial, spiritual
  - Code status
  - Advanced directives
  - Parameters for calling the physician
- Treatment goals and strategies to achieve them
- Plans for discussing care and needs with families

OTHER TRENDS AND ISSUES

As changes in health care delivery evolve, critical care nursing continues to expand and develop to meet patients' needs. Critical care nurses must be aware of current and emerging trends that impact their practice and patient care. Reading professional journals, participating in journal clubs, becoming involved in unit-based nurse practice councils, and attending local and national professional meetings are strategies for nurses to maintain currency in the ever-changing critical care environment.

Critical illnesses have increased complexity, and critically ill patients are sicker than ever before. The critical care nurse is challenged to provide care for patients who have multisystem organ dysfunction and complex needs. Contributing to this trend is the increasingly aging population. The elderly have more chronic illnesses that contribute to the complexity of their care than do younger patients. They also tend to develop multisystem organ failure, which requires longer hospital stays, increases cost, and increases the need for intensive nursing care.

A current healthcare goal of institutions is to reduce hospital readmission rates. Both aging and chronic illness increase the likelihood of hospital readmissions. One strategy to achieve this goal is to improve care transitions. Collaboration among hospitals, community organizations, caregivers, and patients is essential to achieve seamless care among multiple providers and sites.[47]

Healthcare costs continue to escalate while reimbursement rates are reduced. Delivery of critical care services account for a large portion of an institution's budget. Hospitals are often reimbursed based on performance and do not receive reimbursement to treat complications that may result from treatment. Critical care nurses are thus challenged to provide comprehensive services while reducing costs and lengths of stay. Protocol-based care is being implemented to standardize care and reduce complications and their associated costs. Changing nurse/patient ratios and employing unlicensed assistive personnel are also strategies being implemented to reduce costs. However, outcomes associated with changes in staffing need to be monitored and evaluated to ensure that outcomes and patient safety are not compromised.

Technology that assists in patient care continues to grow rapidly. Invasive and noninvasive monitoring systems are used to facilitate patient assessment and to evaluate responses to treatment. Many technological interventions have been introduced to improve patient safety. Point-of-care laboratory testing is done at the bedside to provide immediate values to expedite treatment. Computerized physician order entry and nursing documentation are commonplace. In many institutions, data from monitoring equipment are automatically downloaded into the computerized medical record. Sophisticated computer programs are being developed to analyze physiological data for signs of patient deterioration, such as sepsis, and provide earlier alerts to caregivers. Nurses must become increasingly comfortable with applying the technology, troubleshooting equipment, and evaluating the accuracy of values. The use of technology must be balanced with delivering compassionate care.

As more technological advances become available to sustain and support life, ethical issues have skyrocketed. Termination of life support, organ and cell transplantation, and quality of life are just a few issues that nurses must address in everyday practice. Decisions are regularly made regarding applying technology to sustain life or withdrawing technology in futile situations. Nurses must be comfortable addressing ethical issues as they arise in the critical care setting. Increased attention to end-of-life care in the critical care unit is also needed. Palliative care that includes spiritual care is an important intervention that must be embraced by those working in critical care units (see Chapters 3 and 4).

Using telemedicine or eICUs to manage critically ill patients is another emerging trend. Technology allows experts to provide consultation and evaluation of patients who may be a great distance from a tertiary critical care hospital. Data from monitors and robotics are transferred for evaluation, and the expert conducts an assessment from a distant location.[1,16,50] These virtual critical care consultations have improved patient outcomes. Nurses consult with those providing the telemedicine service based on established protocols and parameters, and then they identify changes in a patient's condition that need to be addressed. These telemedicine strategies do not replace the high-touch, hands-on care delivered by nurses in the critical care unit, but they assist healthcare workers at remote sites in decision making and treatment.

The critical care environment itself is changing. Units are being redesigned with the interests of both patients and nurses in mind. Equipment is becoming more portable, thus making the transfer of patients for diagnostic testing or to other units easier and safer. Additionally, portable equipment can be brought to the bedside for diagnostic testing, preventing the need to transfer unstable patients from the critical care unit. Some institutions have adopted a universal care model, or *acuity-adaptable* rooms. In this setting, patients remain in one unit throughout their hospitalization. The level of nursing care is adjusted to meet the needs of the patient. The universal care model eliminates the need to transfer patients to other units and promotes continuity of care.[23]

Patients are being transferred from critical care units much earlier than before and are discharged from the hospital often while they are still acutely ill. Nurses must ensure that patients and their family members are able to provide care in the home setting, which may be challenging given the reduced length of hospital stays.

Like the population in general, critical care nurses are growing older. To accommodate this growing workforce, hospitals are focusing attention on redesigning the environment with a focus on ergonomics, ease of use, and safety.[19] Innovative staffing models are being developed to continue tapping into the wealth of clinical knowledge and expertise of older nurses who may no longer desire or be able to work full time or 12-hour shifts. Having adequate staffing with paraprofessionals who can assume responsibility for nonnursing tasks is another strategy to facilitate practice.

The last and most important trend is that the United States will soon face a shortage of critical care nurses. Many factors contribute to the shortage: (1) decreased supply and higher demand for critical care nursing services, (2) an increased number of acute and critical care beds in hospitals, (3) issues related to retention in the workplace, and (4) greater availability of other career choices. Priorities for recruiting, educating, and retaining more nurses to work in critical care settings are essential. A related issue is hiring new graduates to work in critical care settings. Before the nursing shortage, many believed that every nurse should have at least 1 year of medical-surgical experience before working in critical care. That belief has been challenged by many who recognize the need to increase the critical care workforce. In addition, many new graduates want to specialize in critical care. New graduates can be successful in the critical care setting with adequate supervision, orientation, and mentorship.[24,30,36] A critical care course, which often includes simulation, is an important strategy to ensure successful orientation.[2,28] Orientation courses are being offered in both traditional and online formats.[20,27] Adequate time in orientation, under the guidance of a supportive preceptor to develop and learn the critical care nursing role, is also essential.

These and other trends will continue to shape the future of critical care practice. Many challenges and opportunities exist in critical care delivery. New diagnostic tests, therapies, and technology will continue to be developed to enhance patient care management. Each nurse must continue to monitor trends, issues, and evidence. One of the best ways to influence practice in an ever-changing environment is through participation in nursing organizations. Regularly reading print and online journals and attending continuing education offerings are also essential.

SUMMARY

Because the boundaries of critical care have expanded, all nurses will be providing care for critically ill patients. Knowledge of professional organizations and of the scope and standards of practice is important for the nurse entering critical care practice. The purpose of this textbook is to provide fundamental information essential to the care of critically ill patients. The reader is challenged to apply the concepts discussed throughout this book to daily practice.

CRITICAL THINKING EXERCISES

1. Compare perceptions of critical care from the viewpoints of student, nurse, multiprofessional healthcare team, patient, and family. What are the similarities and differences?
2. Provide examples of strategies to improve communication and collaboration among the multiprofessional team members in critical care.
3. Debate the pros and cons of hiring new graduates to work in a critical care unit.
4. Identify and debate strategies for reducing stress and anxiety of critical care nurses.
5. Envision the critical care unit of the future. Describe the environment and how care could be delivered.

REFERENCES

1. Ackerman MJ, Filart R, Burgess LP, et al. Developing next-generation telehealth tools and technologies: patients, systems, and data perspectives. *Telemedicine Journal of E Health.* 2010;16(1):93-95.

2. Ackermann AD, Kenny G, Walker C. Simulator programs for new nurses' orientation: a retention strategy. *Journal of Nurses in Staff Development.* 2007;23(3):136-139.

3. American Association of Critical-Care Nurses. AACN standards for establishing and sustaining healthy work environments: a journey to excellence. *American Journal of Critical Care.* 2005;14(3):187-197.

4. American Association of Critical-Care Nurses. *AACN Standards for Establishing and Sustaining Healthy Work Environments.* Aliso Viejo, CA: 2005.

5. American Association of Critical-Care Nurses. *The AACN Synergy Model for Patient Care.* http://www.aacn.org/wd/certifications/content/synmodel.pcms?pid=1&&menu=certification; 2011a. Accessed May 30, 2011.

6. American Association of Critical-Care Nurses. *About AACN.* http://www.aacn.org/wd/mainpages/content/aboutus.pcms?menu=aboutus&lastmenu=; 2011b. Accessed May 29, 2011.

7. American Association of Critical-Care Nurses. *Chapters.* http://www.aacn.org/ChaptersHome.aspx?pageid=315&menu=Chapters; 2011c. Accessed May 27, 2011.

8. American Association of Critical-Care Nurses. *Value of Certification.* http://www.aacn.org/wd/certifications/content/benefitsofcert.pcms?menu=certification&lastmenu=; 2011d. Accessed May 29, 2011.

9. Armola RR, Bourgault AM, Halm MA, et al. Upgrading the American Association of Critical-Care Nurses' evidence-leveling hierarchy. *American Journal of Critical Care.* 2009;18(5):405-409.

10. Arora V, Johnson J. A model for building a standardized hand-off protocol. *Joint Commission Journal of Quality and Patient Safety.* 2006;32(11):646-655.

11. Barden C, Distrito C. Toward a healthy work environment. *Health Progress.* 2005;86(6):16-20.

12. Bell L. *AACN Scope and Standards for Acute and Critical Care Nursing Practice.* Aliso Viejo, CA: American Association of Critical-Care Nurses; 2008.

13. Calzavacca P, Licari E, Tee A, et al. The impact of Rapid Response System on delayed emergency team activation patient characteristics and outcomes—a follow-up study. *Resuscitation.* 2010;81(1):31-35.

14. Chan PS, Jain R, Nallmothu BK, et al. Rapid response teams: a systematic review and meta-analysis. *Archives of Internal Medicine.* 2010;170(1):18-26.

15. Cronenwett L, Sherwood G, Gelmon SB. Improving quality and safety education: the QSEN Learning Collaborative. *Nursing Outlook.* 2009;57(6):304-312.

16. Cummings J, Krsek C, Vermoch K, et al. Intensive care unit telemedicine: review and consensus recommendations. *American Journal of Medical Quality.* 2007;22(4):239-250.

17. Curley MA. Patient-nurse synergy: optimizing patients' outcomes. *American Journal of Critical Care.* 1998;7(1):64-72.

18. Doucette JN. View from the cockpit: what the airline industry can teach us about patient safety. *Nursing.* 2006;36(11):50-53.

19. Eaton-Spiva L, Buitrago P, Trotter L, et al. Assessing and redesigning the nursing practice environment. *Journal of Nursing Administration.* 2010;40(1):36-42.

20. Graham P. Critical care education: experience with a community-based consortium approach. *Critical Care Nursing Quarterly.* 2006;29(3):207-217.

21. Grimes C, Thornell B, Clark AP, et al. Developing rapid response teams: best practices through collaboration. *Clinical Nurse Specialist.* 2007;21(2):85-92; quiz 93-84.

22. Haig KM, Sutton S, Whittington J. SBAR: a shared mental model for improving communication between clinicians. *Joint Commission Journal of Quality and Patient Safety.* 2006;32(3):167-175.

23. Hendrich AL, Lee N. Intra-unit patient transports: time, motion, and cost impact on hospital efficiency. *Nursing Economics.* 2005;23(4):157-164.

24. Ihlenfeld JT. Hiring and mentoring graduate nurses in the intensive care unit. *Dimensions of Critical Care Nursing.* 2005;24(4):175-178.

25. Institute for Healthcare Improvement. *Protecting 5 Million Lives from Harm Campaign.* http://www.ihi.org/offerings/Initiatives/PastStrategicInitiatives/5MillionLivesCampaign/Pages/default.aspx; 2007. Accessed June 25, 2011.

26. The Joint Commission. *National Patient Safety Goals.* http://www.jointcommission.org/PatientSafety/NationalPatientSafetyGoals; 2011. Accessed June 25, 2011.

27. Kaddoura MA. Effect of the essentials of critical care orientation (ECCO) program on the development of nurses' critical thinking skills. *Journal of Continuing Education in Nursing.* 2010a;41(9):424-432.

28. Kaddoura MA. New graduate nurses' perceptions of the effects of clinical simulation on their critical thinking, learning, and confidence. *Journal of Continuing Education in Nursing.* 2010b;41(11):506-516.

29. Kohn LT, Corrigan JM, Donaldson MS, eds. *To Err is Human: Building a Safer Health System.* Washington, D.C.: National Academy Press; 1999.

30. Lindsey G, Kleiner B. Nurse residency program: an effective tool for recruitment and retention. *Journal of Health Care Finance.* 2005;31(3):25-32.

31. Litch B. How the use of bundles improves reliability, quality and safety. *Healthcare Executive.* 2007;22(2):12-14, 16, 18.

32. McKnight M. Hospital nurses: no time to read on duty. *Journal of Electronic Resources in Medical Libraries.* 2004;1(3):13-23.

33. Oriol MD. Crew resource management: applications in healthcare organizations. *Journal of Nursing Administration.* 2006;36(9):402-406.

34. Powell SM, Hill RK. My copilot is a nurse—using crew resource management in the OR. *AORN Journal.* 2006;83(1):179-180, 183-190, 193-178 passim; quiz 203-176.

35. Pronovost P, Berenholtz S, Dorman T, et al. Improving communication in the ICU using daily goals. *Journal of Critical Care.* 2003;18(2):71-75.

36. Reddish MV, Kaplan LJ. When are new graduate nurses competent in the intensive care unit? *Critical Care Nursing Quarterly.* 2007;30(3):199-205.

37. Rosenfeld B. eICU: more data are now available. *Health Affairs.* 2009;28(6):1859; author reply 1860.

38. Shannon SE, Long-Sutehall T, Coombs M. Conversations in end-of-life care: communication tools for critical care practitioners. *Nursing in Critical Care.* 2011;16(3):124-130.

39. Simpson SQ, Peterson DA, O'Brien-Ladner AR. Development and implementation of an ICU quality improvement checklist. *AACN Advanced Critical Care.* 2007;18(2):183-189.

40. Smith AP. Partners at the bedside: the importance of nurse-physician relationships. *Nursing Economics.* 2004;22(3):161-164.

41. Society of Critical Care Medicine. *About SCCM.* http://www.sccm.org/SCCM/About+SCCM/; 2011. Accessed May 30, 2011.

42. Solet DJ, Norvell JM, Rutan GH, et al. Lost in translation: challenges and opportunities in physician-to-physician communication during patient handoffs. *Academic Medicine.* 2005;80(12):1094-1099.

43. Stevens JD, Bader MK, Luna MA, et al. Implementing standardized reporting and safety checklists. *American Journal of Nursing.* 2011;111(5):48-53.

44. Sundar E, Sundar S, Pawlowski J, et al. Crew resource management and team training. *Anesthesiology Clinics.* 2007;25(2):283-300.

45. Thompson D, Holzmueller C, Hunt D, et al. A morning briefing: setting the stage for a clinically and operationally good day. *Joint Commission Journal of Quality and Patient Safety.* 2005;31(8):476-479.

46. U.S. Department of Health and Human Services. *Partnership for Patients: Better Care, Lower Costs.* http://www.healthcare.gov/compare/partnership-for-patients/index.html; 2011. Accessed June 25, 2011.

47. U.S. Department of Health and Human Services. *HHS Action Plan to Prevent Healthcare-Associated Infections.* http://www.hhs.gov/ash/initiatives/hai/actionplan/index.html; 2009. Accessed June 25, 2011.

48. Vouzavali FJD, Papathanassoglou EDE, Karanikola MNK, et al. 'The patient is my space': hermeneutic investigation of the nurse-patient relationship in critical care. *Nursing in Critical Care.* 2011;16(3):140-151.

49. Walters AJ. A Heideggerian hermeneutic study of the practice of critical care nurses. *Journal of Advanced Nursing.* 1995;21(3):492-497.

50. Young LB, Chan PS, Cram P. Staff acceptance of tele-ICU coverage: a systematic review. *Chest.* 2010;139(2):279-288.

2

Patient and Family Response to the Critical Care Experience

Sandra J. Knapp, PhD, RN, CCRN, CNL
Mary Lou Sole, PhD, RN, CCNS, CNL, FAAN, FCCM

evolve WEBSITE

Many additional resources, including self-assessment exercises, are located on the Evolve companion website at http://evolve.elsevier.com/Sole.
- Review Questions
- Mosby's Nursing Skills Procedures
- Animations
- Video Clips

INTRODUCTION

Although any hospitalization is stressful, the critical care experience is especially challenging. This situation presents patients and families with issues beyond those that are directly related to the illness. Personal lives of the patients and those who care about them are affected in many ways. Being in an environment that is foreign to most, and dealing with an undesirable health state create feelings of helplessness and powerlessness for patients and family members.[26] Lack of sleep, poor nutrition, and economic concerns are just a few of the many problems frequently faced by both patients and families when one is hospitalized in a critical care setting.[32,61] Healthcare team members, especially nurses, are often so involved with the care of the patients that they may neglect the concerns of families and even consider family care to be a burden.

Ongoing research into the experiences of critically ill patients and their families consistently supports the premise that care of the patient and the patient's family must be considered holistically.[42] Nurses play a unique role in addressing needs of both patients and their families in a busy and complex environment. Constant presence at the bedside facilitates nurses' interaction with patients and their families and facilitates their ability to serve as patient and family advocates.[42]

Advances in life-sustaining procedures and treatments present complicated ethical considerations in caring for the most seriously ill, and it is often family members who weigh the efficacy and ethics of extending life versus the potential loss of quality of life (see Chapter 3). In addition, social and demographic changes, such as an aging population, and changes in family structure have altered the traditional definition of what constitutes *family.* Critical care nurses assume an advocacy role in caring for patients and their family members who have life-threatening illnesses and problems. The purpose of this chapter is to describe the critical illness experience and its effects on patients and their families.

THE CRITICAL CARE ENVIRONMENT

The *built environment,* or physical layout, of a critical care unit has a subtle but profound effect on patients, families, and the critical care team. Amid an apparent confusion of wires, tubes, and machinery, a critical care unit is designed for efficient and expeditious life-sustaining interventions. Patients and their family members are cared for in this environment with little or no advance preparation, often causing stress and anxiety. The resultant high stress levels are compounded by the often unrelenting sensory stimulation from light and noise, loss of privacy, lack of nonclinical physical contact, and emotional and physical pain. Issues related to the environment include sensory overload, noise, and sensory deprivation.

Many studies have documented the detrimental effects of the sensory overload found in a typical critical care unit.[15,35] The noise level alone is sufficient to cause discomfort and sleep deprivation, and it is a major factor contributing to sensory overload. The World Health Organization established guidelines for hospital noise levels that recommend daytime levels no greater than 35 dB, and nighttime levels of 30 dB.[36] Yet noise levels in hospitals routinely exceed those recommended, with sounds higher during the day than at night.[23] High levels of noise are associated with many deleterious effects—sleep disruption, decreased oxygen saturation, elevated blood pressure, and delayed wound healing. Noise also affects the critical care team, often leading to increased stress, emotional exhaustion and burnout, and increased fatigue.[21] Excessive noise can also lead to difficult communication, distractions, or both, and may contribute to medical errors.[36] In addition, loud conversations may compromise patient confidentiality if communication with patients and family members, or between healthcare providers, is heard throughout the unit. Table 2-1 provides a list of noise levels associated with patient care and discloses just how much noise is emitted with each device or activity.

Several strategies have been identified to reduce noise within the acute care environment: placing patients in private rooms, installing sound-absorbing ceiling tiles, modifying overhead paging systems, and initiating programs to raise awareness among staff about their role in reducing noise.[36] Providing "sedative" music is another strategy to reduce anxiety and discomfort associated with increased noise levels.[14,19,30] Such music has no accented beats, no percussion, a slow tempo, and a smooth melody. Confidentiality can be improved by designating a private place for communication with family members and closing the door during conversations that may be overheard by others. Staff can also help minimize the noise level by avoiding excessive or loud talking, responding to phones quickly, and readily assessing alarms on intravenous and feeding pumps, mechanical ventilation, and monitors.

Despite the potential for sensory overload, patients can also experience sensory deprivation in an environment that is very different from their usual surroundings. Sensory deprivation has been connected to an increase in perceptual disturbances such as hallucinations, especially in older adults.[45] Providing stimulation by interacting with the patient and encouraging visitation of family and friends can decrease its occurrence. Posting family photos and providing music or television that the patient usually enjoys are other strategies to reduce sensory deprivation.

Lighting is another issue in the critical care environment. Adequate and appropriate exposure to light is a therapeutic modality for the health of both patients and staff.[34] Inadequate or poorly placed lighting makes it more difficult to read medical records and medication labels and complicates adequate physical assessment of patients. In addition, the constant artificial lighting present in most critical care units tends to override patients' natural circadian rhythms, which increases disorientation and agitation.[34] Simple measures, such as designing rooms to take advantage of natural light, can have a number of positive effects, including decreased episodes of depression, improved sleep quality, and more effective pain management.[34]

The design of the critical care unit can affect delivery of care as well as responses of patients and their families. New hospital construction, or renovation of existing facilities, provides an opportunity to design hospitals to best meet the needs of patients, families, and staff members. It is important for members of the healthcare team to work with architects and other planners to design a safe and healing environment. Best practices for design of critical care units include private rooms that promote safety, privacy, and comfort; easy access to patients and monitoring devices from all sides of the bed; accessible sinks and waste disposal; and natural lighting.[56] Characteristics of recent award-winning critical care design trends are described in Table 2-2.[8]

TABLE 2-1 NOISE LEVELS ASSOCIATED WITH PATIENT CARE DEVICES AND ACTIVITIES

ACTIVITY	SOUND LEVEL [dB(A)]
Call-bell activation	48-63
Oxygen/chest tube bubbling	49-70
Conversations (staff, patients, and family)	59-90
Voice over intercom	60-70
Telephone ringing	60-75
Television (normal volume at 12 feet)	65
Raising/lowering head of bed	68-78
Cardiac monitor	72-77
Infusion pump	73-78
Ventilator sounds	76
Pneumatic tube arrival	88

TABLE 2-2 BEST PRACTICES IN AWARD-WINNING CRITICAL CARE DESIGNS

DESIGN	TRENDS
Larger units	Units with more beds and increased space
Patient rooms	Private rooms of about 250 sq ft; increased space if accommodating space for family members
Family zone	Designated family/visitor space in the unit, and often in the patient room
Technology	Redesigned for functionality; increased use of ceiling mounted equipment rather than headwall systems
Team space	Designated staff work stations
Proximity to diagnostics and treatment	Ready access to diagnostic testing equipment; more portable equipment that can be brought to the bedside
Administrative space	Increased space for administrative staff and education
Unit geometry	Varied; pod concept has been popular
Access to nature	Access to natural elements for patients, family, and staff members increasing

Modified from Cadenhead CD, Anderson DC. Critical care design: trends in award winning designs. http://www.worldhealthdesign.com/Critical-Care-Design-Trends-in-Award-Winning-Designs.aspx; 2011. Accessed September 11, 2011.

Adequate ventilation and noise abatement must also be addressed. It is also important when designing or adapting a unit to meet the comfort needs of family members and promote rest should they wish to remain in a patient's room.[28]

THE CRITICALLY ILL PATIENT

Many factors influence an individual's response to critical illness. Factors include age and developmental stage, experiences with illness and hospitalization, family relationships and social support, other stressful experiences and coping mechanisms, and personal philosophies about life, death, and spirituality.

Stressors related to both treatment and the critical care environment affect patients. In one study, patients identified many different stressors: the need for nursing presence, nightmares, delusions, confusion, fear of transfer from the critical care unit, inability to remember, disorientation, and lack of preparation for the critical care experience.[54] Many individuals suffer from posttraumatic stress disorder (PTSD) after treatment in a critical care setting.[6,29]

Pain is a major issue for all critically ill patients, whether conscious or not. It may be induced directly by disease, through invasive procedures, or from routine interventions such as suctioning, turning, and bathing.[55] The experience of mechanical ventilation, along with difficulty communicating, pain, dyspnea, fatigue, and the need for endotracheal suctioning, creates a common stressful scenario for the critically ill patient.

Stressors that have been identified by patients when recalling their critical care experience are listed in Box 2-1. The cumulative effect of these stressors can promote anxiety and agitation, and in some cases it leads to the development of delirium and PTSD. Nursing interventions to reduce stress are to ensure safety, reduce sleep deprivation, and minimize noxious sensory overload. One effective intervention is to

---

BOX 2-1 **PATIENTS' RECOLLECTION OF THE CRITICAL CARE EXPERIENCE**

- Difficulty communicating
- Pain
- Thirst
- Difficulty swallowing
- Anxiety
- Lack of control
- Depression
- Fear
- Lack of family or friends
- Physical restraint
- Feelings of dread
- Inability to get comfortable
- Difficulty sleeping
- Loneliness
- Thoughts of death and dying

---

group nursing activities and medical procedures together to maximize patients' resting periods. Chapter 5 further discusses interventions to promote comfort and reduce anxiety.

Even if patients are sedated or unconscious, it is important to remember that many patients can still hear, understand, and respond emotionally to what is being said. Thus nurses as well as family members should make every effort to simply talk to patients, regardless of the patients' ability to interact. Conversation topics include reorienting patients to time and place, updating them on their progress, and reminding them that they are safe and have family and people nearby who care about their well-being.

It is important to increase pleasant sensory input, so the family should be encouraged to speak to and touch the patient. In addition, day-night cycles can be reestablished by positioning the patient near natural light during the day and reducing light levels in the patient's room at night. Reorienting the patient every 2 to 4 hours and addressing the patient directly helps to minimize disorientation. Instead of repeatedly questioning the patient (e.g., "Do you know what day it is? Do you know where you are?"), a less demeaning and less frustrating way to reorient the patient is to incorporate this content into normal conversation (e.g., "It's 8 o'clock in the morning on the fifth of September. You are still in the critical care unit. Your family will be here to see you in about 10 minutes."). Conversations about other patients and personal issues are conducted outside the patient's hearing range because such information can increase confusion on the part of the patient and can contribute to sensory overload. It is also very helpful to have objects that facilitate orientation, such as a clock, a calendar, and windows, within the patient's visual field. Personal and meaningful items brought from home by the family assist in reorienting the patient. These items also humanize the patient and help staff to recognize that the patient has a unique personality and should be treated accordingly.

Promoting rest and sleep are other important nursing interventions. Sleep is frequently interrupted by such activities as blood draws, physician visits, medication administration, and frequent assessment. A retrospective analysis of interactions that potentially disrupt sleep documented an average of 43 interactions during the 12-hour night shift, peaking at midnight. Uninterrupted periods lasting 2 to 3 hours were documented only 6% of the time.[59] Multiple health care providers are involved in patient care, and their interventions are often determined by when staff can be present rather than when it is ideal for the patients. Developing a plan of care that promotes uninterrupted periods for sleep and rest is thus important.

Anxiety for the critical care patient can be caused by pain, discomfort, and many other factors. The provision of high-quality nursing care, offered with humanity and delivered professionally, decreases the anxiety experienced by critically ill patients.[24] Patients have indicated they have a need for nursing presence and being prepared for what they experience.[54] Many small changes in delivery of care are helpful in reducing anxiety: explaining procedures or interventions before they are performed, planning care so the patient can have quality time with family members, encouraging decision making when possible, and facilitating communication.

Discharge from Critical Care and Quality of Life after Critical Care

Many critically ill patients survive critical illnesses and injuries. Although discharge from a critical care area represents progress toward recovery, many patients are discharged "quicker and sicker," either to units that care for patients with lesser acuity, long-term acute care hospitals, or to home. Transfer or discharge from the critical care unit often results in stress for both patients and families.[10] As a result of transfer from the critical care unit to another unit or area, patients may experience physiological or psychological disturbances, referred to as *relocation stress*. They may also perceive a sense of abandonment and fear losing the security of the higher level of care afforded in the critical care unit.[9,16,47,50,57]

Survivors of critical illness report a variety of concerns including fatigue, muscle weakness, sleep disturbance, pain, poor concentration, memory impairment, and poor appetite.[25] Despite these complaints, in most cases former critically ill patients and their family members identify their willingness to undergo critical care treatment to prolong survival.[48] Both patients and family members have an increased risk of developing PTSD after a critical care experience.[3] Once home, the demands of follow-up care can place an enormous burden on family members, who may be ill-prepared or unwilling to shoulder such a burden.

Discharge planning and teaching patients and their families are essential nursing interventions to improve patient and family outcomes. Ongoing family involvement and teaching, beginning at admission and continuing throughout the hospital stay, are crucial interventions to ensure optimal patient outcomes. One technique used to facilitate teaching and learning is the *teach-back method,* in which patients and family members are asked to repeat the information and instructions they have been given.[35]

Geriatric Concerns

Each patient's response to critical illness is influenced by various factors, including age and developmental stage, prior experiences with illness and hospitalization, family relationships and social support, prior stressful experiences and coping mechanisms, and personal philosophies about life, death, and spirituality. Some elderly patients have a diminished ability to adapt and cope with the major physical and psychosocial stressors of critical illness. This is often the result of multiple losses over the years, including loss of physical function, loss of family members, and loss of resources, such as homes and income. Yet some elderly patients with chronic illnesses who have endured multiple critical illnesses demonstrate amazing resilience. Patients who have survived a prior critical illness generally have less anxiety during subsequent admissions. For other patients, their only prior experience with critical illness may have

ended with the death of a family member. This scenario can add considerably to the patient's fears and anxiety.

Although the fears and concerns of the geriatric patient are similar to those of younger critically ill patients, the elderly patient is at greater risk of negative outcomes. In a large sample of critically ill patients over the age of 65 years, one third died within 6 months after discharge from a critical care unit. Among survivors, health-related quality of life (HRQOL) worsened significantly in the oldest patients and improved in the youngest ones.[38] An extensive review of the literature related to HRQOL and functional outcomes in elderly survivors of critical illness reported mixed results. Some elderly patients were satisfied with their experiences. However, increased mortality, functional decline, and a decrease in HRQOL were noted in many studies, especially after a prolonged stay in critical care and in the very elderly (>85 years).[3]

FAMILY MEMBERS OF THE CRITICALLY ILL PATIENT

The critical care hospitalization of a loved one is considered a crisis situation that affects both patient and family.[7] The stress experienced by the family may be detected by the patient, and the patient can suffer as a result of a family member's stress.[1] The family is an integral part of the healing process of the critically ill patient, and critical care nursing interventions must also focus on the family. Family-centered care is the concept of treating the patient and family as an inseparable entity, recognizing that illness or injury of one family member invariably affects all other family members.[31]

Families are in a vulnerable state due to the stress they are experiencing and the fact they are in foreign surroundings. For many families, both the hospital and the critical care unit are "alien" environments. Most family members have never or only rarely seen a critical care unit. The machines and monitors that are commonplace can be frightening and overwhelming to them. Figure 2-1 depicts what a family member sees when entering the room of a critically ill loved one. Imagine your thoughts and feelings if you encounter this situation.

Family Assessment

Once the patient has been admitted to the critical care unit, an assessment of the family provides valuable information for developing the plan of care. Essential information is gathered during the admission assessment, and additional information is obtained as available, often during visitation. Structured tools are available to assess the family, but are not consistently used in every-day practice. However, concepts incorporated into tools can guide the nursing assessment. The structural, developmental, and functional categories described in the Calgary Family Assessment Model provide a useful way to gather information about the family. *Structural assessment* is done upon admission, and it identifies immediate family, extended family, and the decision maker(s). Other aspects of family structure include ethnicity, race, religion,

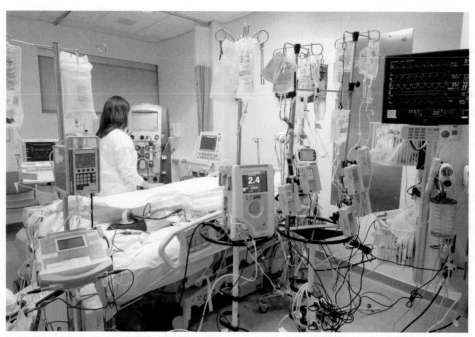

FIGURE 2-1 If you were the family member and your loved one was this patient, how would you feel when you saw this situation? (Reprinted with permission, Cleveland Clinic Center for Medical Art & Photography © 2011-2012. All rights reserved.)

and spirituality.[62] Designating a spokesperson for primary communication with the family members is beneficial. The *developmental assessment* includes information related to the family's developmental stages, tasks, and attachments. The *functional assessment* reveals how family members function and behave in relation to one another.[62]

In today's diverse society, it is important to assess the influence of culture and spirituality on both the patient and family. Especially important are beliefs about health and healing, cultural and spiritual practices, personal space and touch preferences, social organization, and the role of the family. Identification of primary language used for verbal and written communication is essential. Language interpreters who also help to serve as cultural guides are needed to facilitate communication and understanding of the critical care experience when communicating with non-English speakers.

A simple approach to cultural and spiritual assessment has been described as effective when addressing family needs at the end of life.[63] It includes three questions that can easily be adapted for most situations: (1) What are your specific religious and spiritual practices? (2) What are your beliefs about illness (and death)? and (3) What is most important to you and your family at this time?

An early, proactive approach is advised when assessing a patient's family. This may be easily accomplished by observing the family, interacting with them, and making note of significant facts such as the patient's role, family coping strategies, and socioeconomic issues. The family assessment may reveal whether the family members are angry, feeling guilty, or have unaddressed concerns regarding the patient's condition and care. An illness within the family may also uncover underlying conflicts among family members, especially when family members are estranged or have other unresolved issues. Although assessment data can be challenging to gather for complex family units, concisely recording the collected data can be even more daunting. It is important to identify key information related to family assessment that is shared among all nurses caring for the patient.

Family Needs

Molter conducted a groundbreaking study of family needs, which was published in 1979; 6 of the top 10 needs of relatives of the critically ill were directly related to receiving information.[51] Many researchers have conducted follow-up studies using the Critical Care Family Needs Inventory[52] and have identified a predictable set of needs of family members of critically ill patients: receiving information, receiving assurance, remaining near the patient, being comfortable, and having support available.[2,7,12,13,43,44] Table 2-3 compares the top 10 needs as perceived by family members in 1979 and in recent studies conducted in the United States and abroad. Family members also report feelings of uncertainty and a loss of control or sense of powerlessness when a loved one is critically ill.[11]

Addressing stress and coping of family members is important. If family members perceive stress, it may increase the workload of the nurse to address the stress. Knowledge of interventions that are proven to be effective in reducing stress and promoting coping of family members enables the critical care nurse to create a plan of care that will assist patients and their families.

Some family members may be demanding or disruptive, or they may insist on constant vigilance from the nursing staff. These behaviors may reflect a sense of loss of control

TABLE 2-3	COMPARISON OF NEEDS OF FAMILY MEMBERS FROM SELECTED STUDIES		
MOLTER, 1979, UNITED STATES[51]	**BIJTTEBIER ET AL, 2001, BELGIUM**[7]	**CHIEN ET AL, 2005, HONG KONG**[13]	**MAXWELL, 2008, UNITED STATES**[46]
1. To feel there is hope	1. Have questions answered honestly	1. To know specific facts concerning the patient's progress	1. To have questions answered honestly
2. To feel that hospital personnel care about the patient	2. Be assured that the best possible care is being given	2. To know the expected outcome	2. To know the prognosis
3. To have the waiting room near the patient	3. Know the expected outcome	3. To talk about negative feelings such as guilt or anger	3. To talk with the nurse each day
4. To be called at home about changes in the condition of the patient	4. Be given understandable explanations	4. To know exactly what is being done for the patient	4. To know how the patient is being treated
5. To know the prognosis	5. Be called at home about changes in the condition	5. To have directions as to what to do at the bedside	5. To know why things were done for the patient
6. To have questions answered honestly	6. Know specific facts concerning patient's progress	6. To know how the patient is being treated medically	6. To be called at home about changes in the patient's condition
7. To know specific facts concerning the patients progress	7. Feel that hospital personnel care about patient	7. To know about the types of staff members taking care of the patient	7. To receive information about the patient once per day
8. To receive information about the patient once a day	8. Know why things were done for patient	8. To have explanations of the environment before going into the critical care unit for the first time	8. To be assured that the best possible care was being given to the patient
9. To have explanations given in terms that are understandable	9. Receive information once a day	9. To know why specific things were done for the patient	9. To have explanations given in terms that are understandable
10. To see the patient frequently	10. Be told about transfer plans	10. To talk about the possibility of the patient's death	10. To feel there was hope

or possibly memories of an adverse outcome during a previous hospitalization. Recognition of the likely cause of the behavior can assist the nurse in determining how to best communicate and intervene. It is important to reassure the family member that everything is being done for the patient and to communicate that standards of critical care practice are being followed.

Some nurses have difficulty interacting with family members who want confirmation that everything is being done for the patient. It is important for the nurse to establish a partnership with the family built on mutual respect as well as credibility, competence, and compassion. One strategy is to encourage family members to assist in patient assessment (e.g., identify changes) and participate in selected aspects of the patient's care. Depending on institutional policy, it may be possible to enlist family members to help with tasks such as oral care, hygiene, range-of-motion exercises, or repositioning the patient. These activities give family members a sense of purpose and control, as well as potentially provide an additional layer of safety when the nurse is unavailable.

Simple acts of helping can also facilitate patient-family bonding and togetherness, promote patient healing and comfort, decrease a family member's sense of helplessness and anxiety, and assist family members in grasping their loved one's condition.[4]

A few structured methods for providing family assistance have been developed. However, a single and standardized method to ensure families receive the care they need has not been accepted into everyday critical care practice. The CHEST Critical Care Family Assistance Program was established to provide education and family support in response to unmet family needs.[60] *The Clinical Practice Guidelines for Support of the Family in the Patient-Centered Intensive Care Unit* were developed by a multiprofessional group of the American College of Critical Care Medicine. Recommendations that received a grade of C (based on some evidence) or better are listed in Box 2-2.[17]

Another researcher developed a "family bundle" to provide structure for planning and carrying out family care (Figure 2-2). The family bundle is based on five

BOX 2-2 EVIDENCE-BASED RECOMMENDATIONS FOR SUPPORTING FAMILY MEMBERS OF CRITICALLY ILL PATIENTS

Decision Making
- Make decisions based on a partnership between the patient, family, and the healthcare team.
- Communicate the patient's status and prognosis to family members and explain options for treatment.
- Hold family meetings with the healthcare team within 24 to 48 hours after intensive care unit (ICU) admission and repeat as often as needed.
- Train ICU staff in communication, conflict management, and facilitation skills.

Family Coping
- Train ICU staff in assessment of family needs, stress, and anxiety levels.
- Assign consistent nursing and physician staff to each patient if possible. Update family members in language they can understand. Keep the number of staff members who provide information to a minimum.
- Provide information to family members in a variety of formats.
- Provide family support using a team effort, including social workers, clergy, nursing and medical staff, and support groups.

Staff Stress
- Keep all healthcare team members informed of treatment goals to ensure that messages given to the family are consistent.
- Develop a mechanism for staff members to request a debriefing to voice concerns with the treatment plan, decompress, share feelings, or grieve.

Cultural Support of Family
- If possible, match the provider's culture to that of the patient.
- Educate staff on culturally competent care.

Spiritual and Religious Support
- Assess spiritual needs and incorporate into plan of care.
- Educate staff in spiritual and religious issues that facilitate patient assessment.

Family Visitation
- Facilitate open visitation in the adult intensive care environment if possible.
- Determine visitation schedules in collaboration with the patient, family, and nurse; consider the best interest of the patient.
- Provide open visitation in the pediatric ICU and neonatal ICU, 24 hours a day.
- Allow siblings to visit in the pediatric ICU and neonatal ICU (with parental approval) after participation in a previsit education program.
- Do not restrict pets that are clean and properly immunized from visiting the ICU. Develop guidelines for animal-assisted therapy.

Family Environment of Care
- Build new ICUs with single-bed rooms to improve patient confidentiality, privacy, and social support.
- Develop signage (e.g., easy-to-follow directions) to reduce stress on visitors.

Family Presence During Rounds
- Allow parents or guardians of children in the ICU to participate in rounds.
- Allow adult patients and family members to participate in rounds.

Family Presence During Resuscitation
- Develop a process to allow the presence of family members during cardiopulmonary resuscitation.

Palliative Care
- Educate staff in palliative care during formal critical care education.

From Davidson JE, Powers K, Hedayat KM, et al. Clinical practice guidelines for support of the family in the patient-centered intensive care unit: American College of Critical Care Medicine Task Force 2004-2005. *Critical Care Medicine.* 2007;35(2):605-622.

concepts: *evaluate, plan, involve, communicate, and support* (EPICS).[40] By basing family care on these five concepts, the nurse is able to tailor nursing interventions based on what is needed (*evaluate*). It is possible to determine how to provide the care (*plan*) on an individual basis. The family is *involved* in care to the extent and in the ways the evaluation determines is appropriate. *Communication* remains at the forefront of providing family care, and *support* is based on the evaluation and provided as is appropriate. Because no standardized approach for family-centered care has been adopted, it is the responsibility of nurses to be aware of the tools that are available, assess what their families need, and determine how they best can provide care for family members to meet their needs, reduce stress, and enhance coping.

Communication

Receiving information and feeling safe are predominant, complementary needs of critically ill patients and their family members. Of all the members of the critical care team, nurses spend the most time at the bedside and as such are usually the first to hear about any perceived unmet needs of family members. Frequent updates on the patient's condition, anticipated therapies or procedures, and goals of the critical care team are an easy and effective way to allay anxiety while building a relationship of mutual trust.

Lack of communication is a principal complaint when families are dissatisfied with care.[17,20] Nurses can facilitate better communication by providing a simple, honest report of the patient's condition, free of medical jargon. A follow-up

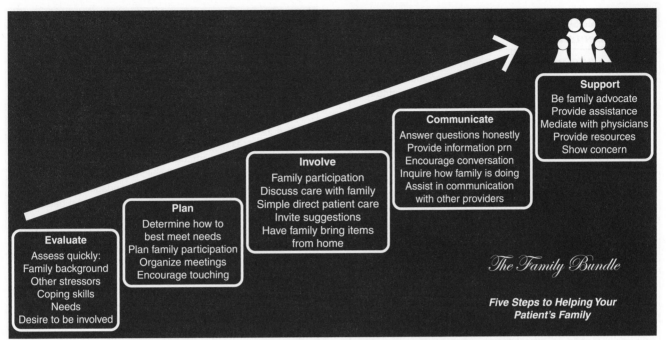

FIGURE 2-2 EPICS family bundle. (From Knapp S. Effects of an Evidence-based Intervention on Stress and Coping of Family Members of Critically Ill Trauma Patients. Unpublished Dissertation, University of Central Florida, Orlando, Florida; 2009.)

assessment to gauge the family's level of understanding helps to tailor the care plan accordingly.

Scheduled rounds between the healthcare team and the family assist in maintaining open communication. A predetermined routine for these rounds provides an opportunity for the team to update the family on the patient's condition and answer questions posed by the family. It also provides the time to identify goals for care and treatment to facilitate shared decision making. Scheduled family conferences provide a similar opportunity to facilitate communication. Family conferences may be held at the bedside or in a conference room, depending on space available and family needs. Holding a preconference among team members ensures that consistent messages are delivered during the conference.

Empathetic communication is important during rounds and family conferences. The VALUE mnemonic (Box 2-3) is a useful tool to enhance communication with family members of critically ill patients.[41]

Visitation

Visitation is among the most contentious and widely researched issues in nursing. Some critical care units still maintain rigid visiting hours, despite research that has repeatedly indicated this is not in the best interest of the patients or their family members.[58] A national study on visitation practices in critical care units found that 44% still have restricted visitation policies. However, 45% of units had policies that were open at all times or restricted only during rounds and change of shift.[39] Critical care units have operated under their own set of rules regarding visitation, often enacting strict controls

---

BOX 2-3   ENHANCING COMMUNICATION WITH FAMILY MEMBERS: VALUE PRINCIPLES

V—Value what the family tells you
A—Acknowledge family emotions
L—Listen to the family members
U—Understand the patient as a person
E—Elicit (ask) questions of family members

From Lautrette A, Darmon M, Megarbane B, et al. A communication strategy and brochure for relatives of patients dying in the ICU. *New England Journal of Medicine*. 2007;356(5):469-478.

---

on both the timing and the length of visits. Proposals to liberalize visitation rules often meet resistance from critical care staff. Reasons cited for opposition to liberal visitation include the presumed increased physiological stress for the patient, family interference with the provision of care, and physical and mental exhaustion of family and friends.[5] An additional concern is that family members will be intrusive or overly critical of the nurse's performance. However, concerns about negative outcomes of liberalized visitation are unfounded. Contrary to traditional thinking, family presence often has a positive effect on the patient's condition.[22] The box, "QSEN Exemplar," illustrates an example of family-centered care.

Although many institutions prohibit visitation by children, research to support this policy is limited. Decisions regarding allowing children in critical care units should be based on factors such as developmental stage of the child and

Mr. K. is a 34-year-old male who suffered a C7 spinal cord injury 10 years ago as a result of a diving accident. His primary caregiver is his mother. Mr. K. has been admitted to the medical intensive care unit with respiratory failure secondary to pneumonia three times in the past year. A unit nurse reports that his mother obstructs care and has been uncooperative with unit visitation policies. During the admission process, Mr. K.'s mother requests permission to stay with him while he is in the critical care unit. She states that he developed a stage IV pressure ulcer during his last admission, and she feels the need to oversee his physical care. The ulcer took months to heal and significantly limited Mr. K.'s activities. Citing concerns related to the privacy of other patients and prior poor family relations, the staff ask management to deny the family's request. The clinical nurse specialist is consulted and meets with unit management and nursing staff to formalize a plan that will promote family involvement. Mr. K.'s mother is permitted to spend the night but is told that she will be asked to leave the unit during physician rounds or emergencies. After several days, the staff becomes comfortable with her presence, and team members actively engage her in tasks such as bathing, turning, and feeding. During a follow-up unit meeting, the staff suggest establishment of a facility-wide policy that provides specific guidelines to promote inclusion of family members as active partners in care.

CASE STUDY

Mr. D., a 40-year-old male, was involved in a head-on motor vehicle crash. His main injuries are a closed head injury with fractures to the right femur and left tibia and fibula. He also has a minor liver laceration. He was unresponsive and hemodynamically unstable on arrival to the Emergency Department, and was admitted to the surgical intensive care unit after a ventriculostomy was placed to reduce and monitor intracranial pressure (ICP). Surgery on the femur fracture is delayed until Mr. D.'s intracranial pressure is under control. He is married and has two small children: a 5-year-old boy and a 3-year-old girl. Mr. D. has multiple bandages, casts on his legs, and an ICP monitoring device. He is intubated and dependent on a ventilator.

His wife is at the bedside and expresses a feeling of "helplessness." She cries frequently and expresses great concern every time one of the alarms in the room sounds. She watches the monitor almost constantly and repeatedly asks what each waveform and number means. The nurses notice that she asks the same questions repeatedly as if she does not remember having asked them before.

She states she wants to be able to help in any way she can. She says Mr. D. is a hard worker and he loves his children very much. She also mentions that she does not work outside of the home, because the cost of daycare is more than the income she would produce if she did have a job. A friend who comes to visit tells Mrs. D. to "be strong for the children."

Questions

1. Mr. D.'s ICP increases to unsatisfactory levels when Mrs. D. enters the room and talks to him. Should she be discouraged from talking to him? Should visitation be suspended? Why or why not?
2. Are Mrs. D.'s concerns about the monitor and alarms appropriate? What measures would likely help her to manage her fears regarding them?
3. What are some things Mrs. D. could be encouraged to do to make her feel less helpless?
4. Should the children be allowed to visit their father? Why or why not?

adequate preparation of the child for the visit.[33] Visitation provides children with an opportunity to access information about their loved one and provides support during times of uncertainty.[37] Visitation by children may also assist in meeting the patient's emotional needs.[53]

Animal-assisted therapy may also be beneficial to a patient's recovery. Some critical care units have extended visitation to include pet therapy. These institutions have policies that permit the family pet or designated therapy animals to visit the patient.[18,49]

Nurses can assist in promoting policy changes to affect open visitation policies.[5] Unit based councils and staff-led research are helpful to create change in the visitation policies. A significant benefit of a liberal visitation policy is its positive impact on the opinions of both patients and families regarding the quality of nursing care. When combined with family support, as demonstrated by the nurses' caring behaviors and interactions, liberal visitation is influential in shaping the critical care experience for both patients and families.

Family Presence During Procedures and Resuscitation

In conjunction with more liberal visitation policies, many institutions have implemented policies to allow families to be present during invasive procedures and cardiopulmonary resuscitation (CPR). (See Chapter 10 for an in-depth discussion of family presence during CPR.) Factors cited for limiting family members' presence include limited space at

the bedside, violations of patient confidentiality, not enough staff members available to assist family members, increased stress on healthcare staff members (e.g., performance anxiety and risk for litigation), and increased stress and anxiety for family members.[3,27] However, these factors have not been substantiated by research. Research studies have found that allowing family members to observe invasive procedures and resuscitation efforts promotes increased knowledge of the patient's condition. Observation also allows the family to witness that everything was done, reduces fear and anxiety, and promotes adaptation.[27] Box 2-4 presents the benefits of family presence.

Practice Alerts

The AACN has issued Practice Alerts to guide the critical care nurse in implementing open visitation and family presence during procedures and resuscitation. Expected nursing practices are highlighted in Box 2-5.

BOX 2-4   BENEFITS OF FAMILY PRESENCE

Being Present Helps Family Members to:
- Remove doubt about the patient's condition
- Witness that everything possible was done
- Decrease their anxiety and fear about what was happening to their loved one

Being Present Facilitates Family Members':
- Need to be together with their loved one
- Need to help and support their loved one
- Sense of closure and grieving should death occur

BOX 2-5   EXPECTED PRACTICES TO SUPPORT FAMILY PRESENCE

- Facilitate unrestricted access (24 hours/day) of a chosen support person according to patient preference, unless support person infringes on the rights and safety of others, or visitation is medically contraindicated.
- Allow family members the option of remaining present at the bedside during resuscitation and invasive procedures.
- Develop written practice documents for facilitating unrestricted access of the support person during the patient's hospitalization, according to patient preference.
  - Ensure that policies are non-discriminatory
  - Ensure that policies include practices for limiting visitors when contraindicated and/or their presence impinges upon the rights and safety of others

- Develop written practice document for permitting family presence during resuscitation and invasive procedures.
  - Identify strategies for ensuring family presence, such as use of trained family facilitators
  - Ensure that policies include practices for restricting family presence during resuscitation and procedures when indicated: combative or violent behavior, uncontrolled outbursts, altered/impaired mental status, or suspicion of abuse

From American Association of Critical-Care Nurses. Family presence: Visitation in the adult ICU. http://www.aacn.org/WD/practice/docs/practicealerts/family-visitation-adult-icu-practicealert.pdf; 2010 and American Association of Critical-Care Nurses. Family presence during resuscitation and invasive procedures. http://www.aacn.org/WD/practice/docs/practicealerts/family-visitation-adult-icu-practicealert.pdf; 2011. Accessed April 20, 2012.

SUMMARY

This chapter has provided an overview of the critical care environment and the experience of critical illness from the perspective of the patient, family, and nurse. As key players among equals on the critical care team, nurses are ideally positioned to shape the future of critical care by ensuring that the patient remains the focus of that care. By understanding the critical care experience from a variety of perspectives, critical care nurses are better able to tailor their responses and interventions to meet what is both desired and required by critically ill patients and their family members. The resulting synergy is essential to achieving optimal patient, family, and critical care nurse outcomes.

CRITICAL THINKING EXERCISES

1. You are bringing family members to the critical care unit to see the patient for the first time. The patient has been involved in a motor vehicle crash and the environment is similar to that depicted in Figure 2-1. What strategies do you use to explain the patient and the environment to the family members?

2. You are in charge of coordinating a family conference to discuss a patient's condition and goals for care and treatment. All family members speak Creole. What strategies do you incorporate when planning the conference?

3. You are leading a work group charged with revising the critical care visitation policy, specifically with regard to open visitation. The majority of the staff members are skeptical. What are some of the objections you might encounter, and how would you address them?

4. You are caring for a patient whose family members include other medical professionals (e.g., staff nurse, nurse practitioner, physician). The family is frequently critical of the patient's management and is constantly making suggestions regarding nursing care. How do you respond?

REFERENCES

1. Ahrens T, Yancey V, Kollef M. Improving family communications at the end of life: implications for length of stay in the intensive care unit and resource use. *American Journal of Critical Care.* 2003;12(4):317-323.
2. Auerbach S, Kiesler D, Wartella J, et al. Optimism, satisfaction with needs met, interpersonal perceptions of the healthcare team, and emotional distress in patients' family members during critical care hospitalization. *American Journal of Critical Care.* 2005;14(3):202-210.
3. Azoulay E, Pochard F, Chevret S, et al. Family participation in care to the critically ill: opinions of families and staff. *Intensive Care Medicine.* 2003;29(9):1498-1504.
4. Benner P, Hooper-Kyriakidis P, Stannard D. *Clinical Wisdom and Interventions in Critical Care: a Thinking-in-action Approach.* Philadelphia: Saunders; 1999.
5. Berwick DM, Kotagal M. Restricted visiting hours in ICUs: time to change. *Journal of the American Medical Association.* 2004;292(6):736-737.

6. Bienvenu OJ, Neufeld KJ. Post-traumatic stress disorder in medical settings: focus on the critically ill. *Current Psychiatry Report.* 2010;13(1):3-9.

7. Bijttebier P, Vanoost S, Delva D, et al. Needs of relatives of critical care patients: perceptions of relatives, physicians and nurses. *Intensive Care Medicine.* 2001;27(1):160-165.

8. Cadenhead CD, Anderson DC. Critical care design: trends in award winning designs. http://www.worldhealthdesign.com/Critical-Care-Design-Trends-in-Award-Winning-Designs.aspx; 2011. Accessed September 11, 2011.

9. Chaboyer W. Intensive care and beyond: improving the transitional experiences for critically ill patients and their families. *Intensive and Critical Care Nursing.* 2006;22(4):187-193.

10. Chaboyer W, Kendall E, Kendall M, et al. Transfer out of intensive care: an exploration of patient and family perceptions. *Australian Critical Care.* 2005;18(4):138-145.

11. Chan K.-S, Twinn S. An analysis of the stressors and coping strategies of Chinese adults with a partner admitted to an intensive care unit in Hong Kong: an exploratory study. *Journal of Clinical Nursing.* 2007;16(1):185-193.

12. Chartier L, Coutu-Wakulczyk G. Families in ICU: their needs and anxiety level. *Intensive Care Nursing.* 1989;5(1):11-18.

13. Chien W-T, Chiu YL, Lam L-W, et al. Effects of a needs-based education programme for family carers with a relative in an intensive care unit: a quasi-experimental study. *International Journal of Nursing Studies.* 2006;43(1):39-50.

14. Chlan L. A review of the evidence for music intervention to manage anxiety in critically ill patients receiving mechanical ventilatory support. *Archives of Psychiatric Nursing.* 2009;23(2):177-179.

15. Cmiel CA, Karr DM, Gasser DM, et al. Noise control: a nursing team's approach to sleep promotion. *American Journal of Nursing.* 2004;104(2):40-49.

16. Coyle MA. Transfer anxiety: preparing to leave intensive care. *Intensive and Critical Care Nursing.* 2001;17(3):138-143.

17. Davidson JE, Powers K, Hedayat KM, et al. Clinical practice guidelines for support of the family in the patient-centered intensive care unit: American College of Critical Care Medicine Task Force 2004-2005. *Critical Care Medicine.* 2007;35(2):605-622.

18. DeCourcey M, Russell AC, Keister KJ. Animal-assisted therapy: evaluation and implementation of a complementary therapy to improve the psychological and physiological health of critically ill patients. *Dimensions of Critical Care Nursing.* 2010;29(5):211-214.

19. Dijkstra BM, Gamel C, van der Bijl JJ, et al. The effects of music on physiological responses and sedation scores in sedated, mechanically ventilated patients. *Journal of Clinical Nursing.* 2010;19(7-8):1030-1039.

20. Downey L, Engelberg RA, Shannon SE, et al. Measuring intensive care nurses' perspectives on family-centered end-of-life care: evaluation of 3 questionnaires. *American Journal of Critical Care.* 2006;15(6):568-579.

21. Dracup K. Are critical care units hazardous to health? *Applied Nursing Research.* 1988;1(1):14-21.

22. Duran CR, Oman KS, Abel JJ, et al. Attitudes toward and beliefs about family presence: a survey of healthcare providers, patients' families, and patients. *American Journal of Critical Care.* 2007;16(3):270-279; quiz 280; discussion 281-282.

23. Elliott RM, McKinley SM, Eager D. A pilot study of sound levels in an Australian adult general intensive care unit. *Noise Health.* 2010;12(46):26-36.

24. Ferns T. Factors that influence aggressive behaviour in acute care settings. *Nursing Standard.* 2007;21(33):41-45.

25. Fletcher SN, Kennedy DD, Ghosh IR, et al. Persistent neuromuscular and neurophysiologic abnormalities in long-term survivors of prolonged critical illness. *Critical Care Medicine.* 2003;31(4):1012-1016.

26. Fontana JS. A sudden, life-threatening medical crisis: the family's perspective. *Advances in Nursing Science.* 2006;29(3):222-231.

27. Halm MA. Family presence during resuscitation: a critical review of the literature. *American Journal of Critical Care.* 2005;14(6):494-512.

28. Hardin SR, Bernhardt-Tindal K, Hart A, et al. Critical-care visitation: the patients' perspective. *Dimensions of Critical Care Nursing.* 2011;30(1):53-61.

29. Hatch R, McKechnie S, Griffiths J. Psychological intervention to prevent ICU-related PTSD: who, when and for how long? *Critical Care.* 2011;15(2):141.

30. Hellstrom A, Willman A. Promoting sleep by nursing interventions in health care settings: a systematic review. *Worldviews on Evidence Based Nursing;* 2011.

31. Hennessy D, Juzwishin K, Yergens D, et al. Outcomes of elderly survivors of intensive care: a review of the literature. *Chest.* 2005;127(5):1764-1774.

32. Hweidi IM. Jordanian patients' perception of stressors in critical care units: a questionnaire survey. *International Journal of Nursing Studies.* 2007;44(2):227-235.

33. Ihlenfeld JT. Should we allow children to visit ill parents in intensive care units? *Dimensions of Critical Care Nursing.* 2006;25(6):269-271.

34. Joseph A. *The Impact of Light on Outcomes in Healthcare Settings.* (Issue Paper No. 2). Concord, CA: The Center for Health Design; 2006.

35. Joseph A. *The Role of the Physical Environment in Promoting Health, Safety, and Effectiveness in the Healthcare Workplace.* (Issue Paper No. 3). Concord, CA: The Center for Health Design; 2006.

36. Joseph A, Ulrich R. *Sound Control for Improved Outcomes in Healthcare Settings.* (Issue Paper No. 4). Concord, CA: The Center for Health Design and the Robert Wood Johnson Foundation; 2007.

37. Kean S. Children and young people's strategies to access information during a family member's critical illness. *Journal of Clinical Nursing.* 2009;19(1-2):266-274.

38. Khouli H, Astua A, Dombrowski W, et al. Changes in health-related quality of life and factors predicting long-term outcomes in older adults admitted to intensive care units. *Critical Care Medicine.* 2011;39(4):731-737.

39. Kirchhoff KT, Dahl N. American Association of Critical-Care Nurses' national survey of facilities and units providing critical care. *American Journal of Critical Care.* 2006;15(1):13-27.

40. Knapp S. *Effects of an Evidence-based Intervention on Stress and Coping of Family Members of Critically Ill Trauma Patients.* Unpublished Dissertation, University of Central Florida, Orlando; 2009.

41. Lautrette A, Darmon M, Megarbane B, et al. A communication strategy and brochure for relatives of patients dying in the ICU. *New England Journal of Medicine.* 2007;356(5):469-478.

42. Leon A, Knapp S. Involving family systems in critical care nursing: challenges and opportunities. *Dimensions of Critical Care Nursing.* 2008;27(6):255-262.

43. Leske JS. Overview of family needs after critical illness: from assessment to intervention. *AACN Clinical Issues in Critical Care Nursing.* 1991;2(2):220-229.

44. Leske JS. Needs of adult family members after critical illness: prescriptions for interventions. *Critical Care Nursing Clinics of North America.* 1992;4(4):587-596.

45. Mason OJ, Brady F. The psychotomimetic effects of short-term sensory deprivation. *Journal of Nervous & Mental Disease.* 2009;197(10):783-785.

46. Maxwell KE, Stuenkel D, Saylor C. Needs of family members of critically ill patients: a comparison of nurse and family perceptions. *Heart & Lung: The Journal of Acute and Critical Care.* 2007;36(5):367-376.

47. McKinney AA, Melby V. Relocation stress in critical care: a review of the literature. *Journal of Clinical Nursing.* 2002;11(2):149-157.

48. Mendelsohn AB, Belle SH, Fischhoff B, et al. How patients feel about prolonged mechanical ventilation 1 year later. *Critical Care Medicine.* 2002;30(7):1439-1445.

49. Miracle VA. Pet visitation. *Dimensions of Critical Care Nursing.* 2009;28(2):93-94.

50. Mitchell ML, Courtney M, Coyer F. Understanding uncertainty and minimizing families' anxiety at the time of transfer from intensive care. *Nursing and Health Sciences.* 2003;5(3):207-217.

51. Molter N. Needs of relatives of critically ill patients: a descriptive study. *Heart & Lung.* 1979;8:332-339.

52. Molter N, Leske J. Critical care family needs inventory. 1986. Available from authors. Molter@texas.net or Jsl@jwm.edu.

53. Nicholson AC, Titler M, Montgomery LA, et al. Effects of child visitation in adult critical care units: a pilot study. *Heart & Lung.* 1993;22(1):36-45.

54. Pattison NA, Dolan S, Townsend P, et al. After critical care: a study to explore patients' experiences of a follow-up service. *Journal of Clinical Nursing.* 2007;16(11):2122-2131.

55. Puntillo KA, White C, Morris AB, et al. Patients' perceptions and responses to procedural pain: results from Thunder Project II. *American Journal of Critical Care.* 2001;10(4):238-251.

56. Rashid M. A decade of adult intensive care unit design: a study of the physical design features of the best-practice examples. *Critical Care Nursing Quarterly.* 2006;29(4):282-311.

57. Roberts BL, Rickard CM, Rajbhandari D, et al. Factual memories of ICU: recall at two years post-discharge and comparison with delirium status during ICU admission—a multicentre cohort study. *Journal of Clinical Nursing.* 2007;16(9):1669-1677.

58. Roland P, Russell J, Richards KC, et al. Visitation in critical care: processes and outcomes of a performance improvement initiative. *Journal of Nursing Care Quality.* 2001;15(2):18-26.

59. Tamburri LM, DiBrienza R, Zozula R, et al. Nocturnal care interactions with patients in critical care units. *American Journal of Critical Care.* 2004;13(2):102-112; quiz 114-105.

60. The Chest Foundation. *The Chest Foundation critical care family assistance program.* http://www.chestfoundation.org/foundation/critical/ccfap/index.php; 2011. Accessed April 12, 2011.

61. Van Horn E, Tesh A. The effect of critical care hospitalization on family members: stress and responses. *Dimensions of Critical Care Nursing.* 2000;19(4):40-49.

62. Wright LM, Leahey M. *Nurses and Families: A Guide to Family Assessment and Intervention.* 5th ed. Philadelphia, PA: FA Davis; 2009.

63. Yeager S, Doust C, Epting S, et al. Embrace hope: an end-of-life intervention to support neurological critical care patients and their families. *Critical Care Nurse.* 2010;30(1):47-58.

3

Ethical and Legal Issues in Critical Care Nursing

Jayne M. Willis, MSN, RN, NEA-BC
Kathy Black, MSN, RN, NE-BC

⊖volve WEBSITE

Many additional resources, including self-assessment exercises, are located on the Evolve companion website at http://evolve.elsevier.com/Sole.

- Review Questions
- Mosby's Nursing Skills Procedures

- Animations
- Video Clips

INTRODUCTION

Critical care nurses are often confronted with ethical and legal dilemmas related to informed consent, withholding or withdrawing life-sustaining treatment, organ and tissue transplantation, confidentiality, and increasingly, justice in the distribution of healthcare resources. Many dilemmas are by-products of advanced medical technologies and therapies developed over the past several decades. Although technology provides substantial benefits to critically ill patients, extensive public and professional debate occurs over the appropriate use of these technologies, especially those that are life sustaining. One of the primary concerns in critical care is whether a patient's values and beliefs about treatment can be overridden by the technological imperative, or the strong tendency to use technology because it is available.

Although many ethical dilemmas are not unique to critical care, they occur with greater frequency in critical care settings. Therefore it is crucial that critical care nurses examine the nature and scope of their ethical and legal obligations to patients.

The ethical and legal issues that frequently arise in the nursing care of acute and critically ill patients are examined in this chapter. The discussion includes problems that surround patients' rights and nurses' obligations, informed consent, and withholding and withdrawing treatment. The elements of ethical decision making and the involvement of the nurse are discussed.

ETHICAL OBLIGATIONS AND NURSE ADVOCACY

Critical care nurses' ethical and legal responsibilities for patient care have increased dramatically since the early 1990s. Evolving case law and current concepts of nurse advocacy and accountability indicate that nurses have substantial ethical and legal obligations to promote and protect the welfare of their patients.

The duty to practice ethically and to serve as an ethical agent on behalf of patients is an integral part of nurses' professional practice. The nurse's duty is stated in the *Code of Ethics for Nurses with Interpretive Statements,* which was adopted by the American Nurses Association (ANA) in 1976 and was last revised in 2001.[6] The document describes the moral principles that guide professional nursing practice, and serves the following purposes: (1) it delineates the ethical obligations and duties of every individual who enters the profession; (2) it is the profession's nonnegotiable ethical standard; and (3) it is the expression of nursing's own understanding of its commitment to society.[6] The *Code of Ethics* consists of nine provision statements. The first three describe fundamental values and commitments of the nurse, the next three describe the boundaries of duty and loyalty, and the last three describe duties beyond individual patient encounters. Nurses in all practice arenas, including critical care, must be knowledgeable about the provisions of the code and must incorporate its basic tenets into their clinical practice.[10] The code is a powerful tool that shapes and evaluates individual practice as well as the nursing profession. However, situations may arise in which the code provides only limited direction. Critical care nurses must remain knowledgeable and abreast of ethical issues and changes in the literature so they may make appropriate decisions when difficult situations arise in practice. Additional ANA position statements related to human rights and ethics are available from the ANA website (www.nursingworld.org).

Nurses' ethical obligation to serve as advocates for their patients is derived from the unique nature of the nurse-patient relationship. Critical care nurses assume a significant caregiving role that is characterized by intimate, extended contact with persons who are often the most physiologically and psychologically vulnerable and with their families. Critical care nurses have a moral and professional responsibility to act as advocates on their patients' behalf because of their unique relationship with their patients and their specialized nursing knowledge. The American Association of Critical-Care Nurses (AACN) published *An Ethic of Care*,[1] which illustrates the ethical foundations for critical care practice. Ethics involves the interrelatedness and interdependence of individuals, systems, and society. When ethical care is practiced, individual uniqueness, personal relationships, and the dynamic nature of life are respected. Compassion, collaboration, accountability, and trust are essential characteristics of ethical nursing practice.[1] The AACN *Ethic of Care* statement is available from the organization's website (www.aacn.org).

ETHICAL DECISION MAKING

As reflected in the ANA code of ethics, one of the primary ethical obligations of professional nurses is protection of their patients' basic rights. This obligation requires nurses to recognize ethical dilemmas that actually or potentially threaten patients' rights and to participate in the resolution of those dilemmas.[6]

An ethical dilemma is a difficult problem or situation in which conflicts arise during the process of making morally justifiable decisions. In identifying a situation as an ethical dilemma, certain criteria must be met. More than one solution must exist, and there is no clear "right" or "wrong." Each solution must carry equal weight and must be ethically defensible. Whether to give the one available critical care bed to a patient with cancer who is experiencing hypotension after chemotherapy or to a patient in the emergency department who has an acute myocardial infarction is an example of an ethical dilemma. The conflicting issue in this example is which patient should be given the bed, based on the moral allocation of limited resources.

Several warning signs can assist the critical care nurse in recognizing an ethical dilemma. If these warning signs occur, the critical care nurse must reassess the situation and determine whether an ethical dilemma exists and what additional actions are needed[16]:

- Is the situation emotionally charged?
- Has the patient's condition changed significantly?

- Is there confusion or conflict about the facts?
- Is there increased hesitancy about the right course of action?
- Is the proposed action a deviation from customary practice?
- Is there a perceived need for secrecy around the proposed action?

Arriving at a morally justifiable decision when an ethical dilemma exists can be difficult for patients, families, and health professionals. Critical care nurses must be careful not to impose their own value system on that of the patient. Each patient and family has a set of personal values that are influenced by their environment and culture.

One helpful way to approach ethical decision making is to use a systematic, structured process, such as the one depicted in Figure 3-1. This model provides a framework for evaluating the related ethical principles and the potential outcomes, as well as relevant facts concerning the contextual factors and the patient's physiological and personal factors. Using this approach, the patient, family, and healthcare team members evaluate choices and identify the option that promotes the patient's best interests.

Ethical decision making includes implementing the decision and evaluating the short-term and long-term outcomes. Evaluation provides meaningful feedback about decisions and actions in specific instances, as well as the effectiveness of the decision-making process. The final stage in the decision-making process is assessing whether the decision in a specific case can be applied to other dilemmas in similar circumstances. In other words, is this decision useful in similar cases? A systematic approach to decision making does not guarantee that morally justifiable decisions are reached or that the outcome is beneficial to the patient. However, it ensures that all applicable information is considered in the decision.

ETHICAL PRINCIPLES

As reflected in the decision-making model, relevant ethical principles should be considered when a moral dilemma exists. Principles facilitate moral decisions by guiding the decision-making process, but they may conflict with each other and may force a choice among the competing principles based on their relative weight in the situation. Several ethical principles are pertinent in the critical care setting. These principles are intended to provide respect and dignity for all persons (Box 3-1).

Principlism is a widely applied ethical approach based on four fundamental moral principles to contemporary ethical dilemmas: respect for autonomy, beneficence, nonmaleficence, and justice.[8] The principle of *autonomy* states that all persons should be free to govern their lives to the greatest degree possible. The autonomy principle implies a strong sense of self-determination and an acceptance of responsibility for one's own choices and actions. To respect autonomy of others means to respect their freedom of choice and to allow them to make their own decisions.

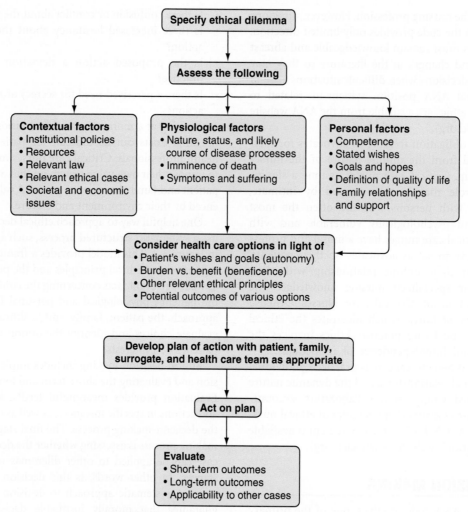

FIGURE 3-1 The process of ethical decision making.

BOX 3-1   ETHICAL PRINCIPLES

- **Autonomy:** Respect for the individual and the ability of individuals to make decisions with regard to their own health and future (the basis for the practice of informed consent)
- **Beneficence:** Actions intended to benefit the patients or others
- **Nonmaleficence:** Actions intended not to harm or bring harm to others
- **Justice:** Being fair or just to the wider community in terms of the consequences of an action. In health care, justice is described as the fair allocation or distribution of healthcare resources
- **Veracity:** The obligation to tell the truth
- **Fidelity:** The moral duty to be faithful to the commitments that one makes to others
- **Confidentiality:** Respect for an individual's autonomy and the right of individuals to control the information relating to their own health

---

The principle of *beneficence* is the duty to provide benefits to others when in a position to do so, and to help balance harms and benefits. In other words, the benefits of an action should outweigh the burdens. A related concept is *futility*. Care should not be given if it is futile in terms of improving comfort or the medical outcome. The principle of *nonmaleficence* is the explicit duty not to inflict harm on others intentionally.

The principle of *justice* requires that health care resources be distributed fairly and equitably among groups of people. The principle of justice is particularly relevant to critical care because most healthcare resources, including technology and pharmaceuticals, are expended in this practice setting.

In addition to the four principles described previously, the following principles are relevant. The principle of *veracity* states that persons are obligated to tell the truth in their communication with others. The principle of *fidelity* requires that one has a moral duty to be faithful to the commitments made to others. These two principles, along with *confidentiality,* are the key to the nurse-patient relationship.

Creating an Ethical Environment

In the quest for excellence, critical care nurses and their leadership focus on nursing initiatives at the unit, service line, and organizational levels to improve quality, patient satisfaction, and nursing retention. AACN's Healthy Work Environment Initiative and American Nurses Credentialing Center (ANCC) Magnet Recognition Program assist critical care nursing teams to create a positive and fulfilling organizational culture through engagement and empowerment.[2,7] Both programs allow nurses to promote, plan, and develop an ethical environment in which to practice.

Addressing ethical problems and participating in ethical decision making are key to improving quality of care. Interdisciplinary collaboration and collegial working relationships that generate mutual respect are important elements of a successful critical care team. Hospitals that are pursuing or achieve Magnet certification must demonstrate evidence of creating ethical work environments by meeting specific criteria. Box 3-2 lists examples of evidence required to support ANCC Magnet criteria related to ethical work environments.[7]

INCREASING NURSES' INVOLVEMENT IN ETHICAL DECISION MAKING

Although nurses play a significant role in the care of patients, they often report limited involvement in the formal processes of ethical decision making. Nurses' perception of this limited involvement may be related to many factors, such as lack of formal education in ethics, lack of institutional mechanisms for review of dilemmas, perceived lack of administrative or peer support for involvement in decision making, concern about reprisals, and perceived lack of decision-making authority. Research has shown that ethics education has a significant positive influence on moral confidence, moral action, and use of ethics resources by nurses.[11]

If nurses are to fulfill their advocacy obligations to patients, they must become active in the process of ethical decision making at all levels. Ethical dilemmas are among the many issues that can lead to *moral distress* for critical care nurses. Moral distress occurs when the nurse knows the ethically appropriate action to take but is unable to act upon it, or when the nurse acts in a manner contrary to personal and professional values. Moral distress is one of the key issues affecting the workplace environment.[4] Moral distress contributes to the loss of nurses from the workforce and threatens the quality of patient care. Ways for nurses to address moral distress and increase their participation in ethical decision making starts with open communication with the healthcare team, the patient, and the family regarding the patient's wishes and ethical concerns.

A critical element for true collaboration is that healthcare organizations ensure unrestricted access to structured forums such as ethics committees, and allow time to resolve disputes among critical participants, including patients, families, and the healthcare team.[2] Actively addressing ethical dilemmas and avoiding moral distress are crucial factors to creating a healthy workplace where critical care nurses can make optimal contributions to patients and their families.

The Joint Commission requires that a formal mechanism be in place to address patients' ethical concerns. Bioethics committees are one way to address this need. Typical membership of a bioethics committee includes physicians, nurses, chaplains, social workers, and, if available, bioethicists. A multiprofessional committee can serve as an education and policy-making body and, in some cases, provide ethics consultation on a case-by-case basis. The purpose of ethics consultation is to improve the process and outcomes of patient care by helping to identify, analyze, and resolve ethical problems. This service should be used when the issues cannot be resolved among the healthcare team, patient, and family. Box 3-3 lists examples of situations where an ethics consultation may be considered.

BOX 3-4   ETHICS CONSULTATION SERVICES

AMERICAN NURSES ASSOCIATION CENTER FOR ETHICS AND HUMAN RIGHTS
8515 Georgia Avenue, Suite 400
Silver Springs, MD 20910
Telephone: (301) 628-5000
E-mail: ethics@ana.org
http://nursingworld.org/ethics/

KENNEDY INSTITUTE OF ETHICS
Georgetown University
P.O. Box 571212
Washington, DC 20057-1212
Telephone: (202) 687-8089
www.georgetown.edu/research/kie

BOX 3-5   INTERNET RESOURCES FOR BIOETHICS

- *American Journal of Bioethics:* http://bioethics.net
- *American Society for Bioethics and Humanities:* www.asbh.org
- *University of Pennsylvania Center for Bioethics:* http://bioethics.upenn.edu
- *National Institutes of Health Bioethics Resources on the Web:* http://bioethics.od.nih.gov/

Nurses can become more involved with ethical decision making through participation in institutional ethics committees, multiprofessional ethics forums and roundtables, peer review and quality assurance committees, and institutional research review boards. Nurses can also improve and update their knowledge through formal and continuing education courses on bioethics, as well as through telephone and computerized electronic consultation and reference services. Educational programs and ethics consultation services are available through several ethics and law centers in the United States. Two important ethical consultation services are listed in Box 3-4. Additional Internet educational resources are listed in Box 3-5.

SELECTED ETHICAL TOPICS IN CRITICAL CARE

Informed Consent

Many complex dilemmas in critical care nursing concern informed consent. Consent problems arise because patients are experiencing acute, life-threatening illnesses that interfere with their ability to make decisions about treatment or participation in a clinical research study. The doctrine of informed consent is based on the principle of autonomy; competent adults have the right to self-determination or to make decisions regarding their acceptance or rejection of treatment.

Elements of Informed Consent

Three primary elements must be present for a person's consent or decline of medical treatment or research participation to be considered valid: competence, voluntariness, and disclosure of information. Competence (or capacity) refers to a person's ability to understand information regarding a proposed medical or nursing treatment. Competence is a legal term and is determined in court. Healthcare providers evaluate mental capacity. The ability of patients to understand relevant information is an essential prerequisite to their participation in the decision-making process and should be carefully evaluated as part of the informed consent process. Patients providing informed consent should be free from severe pain and depression. Critically ill patients usually do not have the mental capacity to provide informed consent because of the severe nature of their illness or their treatment (e.g., sedation). If the patient is not mentally capable of providing consent, informed consent is obtained from the designated healthcare surrogate or legal next of kin. State law governs consent issues, and legal counsel should be consulted for specific questions.

Consent must be given voluntarily, without coercion or fraud, for the consent to be legally binding. This includes freedom from pressure from family members, healthcare providers, and payers. Persons who consent should base their decision on sufficient knowledge. Basic information considered necessary for decision making includes the following:

- A diagnosis of the patient's specific health problem and condition
- The nature, duration, and purpose of the proposed treatment or procedures
- The probable outcome of any medical or nursing intervention
- The benefits of medical or nursing interventions
- The potential risks that are generally considered common or hazardous
- Alternative treatments and their feasibility
- Short-term and long-term prognoses if the proposed treatment or treatments are not provided

Informed consent is not a form. It is a process that entails the exchange of information between the health care provider and the patient or patient's proxy. Frequently, critical care nurses are asked to witness the consent process for procedures and tests. Critical care nurses should serve as advocates for the patient and ensure that the informed consent process has been completed per legal standards and institutional policy. Critical care nurses may provide additional patient education to support decision making, but the process of obtaining informed consent is a physician obligation.

Decisions Regarding Life-Sustaining Treatment

Care of persons who are terminally ill or in a persistent vegetative state raises profound questions about the constitutional

TABLE 3-1	LANDMARK LEGAL CASES IN THE RIGHT-TO-DIE DEBATE	
CASE	**EVENTS**	**IMPACT**
Karen Quinlan	Karen Ann Quinlan was the first modern icon of the right-to-die debate. The 21-year-old Quinlan collapsed at a party after swallowing alcohol and the tranquilizer diazepam (Valium) on April 14, 1975. Doctors saved her life, but she suffered brain damage and lapsed into a "persistent vegetative state." Her family waged a much-publicized legal battle for the right to remove her life-support machinery. They succeeded, but in a final twist, Quinlan kept breathing after the respirator was unplugged. She remained in a coma for almost 10 years in a New Jersey nursing home until her 1985 death.	In finding for the Quinlan family, the courts identified a right to decline lifesaving medical treatment under the general right of privacy. According to the court, her right to privacy outweighed the state's interest in preserving her life, and her father, as her surrogate, could exercise that right for her.
Nancy Cruzan	Nancy Cruzan became a public figure after a 1983 auto accident left her permanently unconscious and without any higher brain function. She was kept alive only by a feeding tube and steady medical care. Cruzan's family waged a legal battle to have her feeding tube removed. The case went all the way to the U.S. Supreme Court, which ruled that the Cruzans had not provided "clear and convincing evidence" that Nancy Cruzan did not wish to have her life artificially preserved. The Cruzans later presented such evidence to the Missouri courts, which ruled in their favor in late 1990. The Cruzans stopped feeding Nancy in December of 1990, and she died later the same month.	The Cruzan case had a significant impact on end-of-life decision making across the country. After the Cruzan decision, the Patient Self-Determination Act was passed by Congress to allow individuals to make their own decisions about end-of-life care and/or routine care, should they be unable to make decisions for themselves. The case prompted the development of hospital ethics councils and increased the number of advance directives.
Theresa Schiavo	Theresa Marie "Terri" Schiavo was a Florida woman who sustained brain damage and became dependent on a feeding tube. She collapsed in her home in 1990, experienced respiratory and cardiac arrest, leading to 15 years of institutionalization and a diagnosis of persistent vegetative state. In 1998, her husband, who was her guardian, petitioned the court to remove her feeding tube. Terri Schiavo's parents opposed the removal, arguing that Terri was conscious. The court determined that Terri would not wish to continue life-prolonging measures. Subsequently a 7-year battle occurred that included involvement by politicians and advocacy groups. Before the court's decision was carried out on March 18, 2005, the Florida legislature and the United States Congress had passed laws to prevent removal of Schiavo's feeding tube. These laws were later overturned by the Supreme Courts of Florida and the United States. On March 31, 2005, after a complex legal history in the courts, Terri Schiavo died at a Florida hospice at the age of 41.	This case received national and international media attention with very public debate regarding the moral consequences of withdrawing life support. The movement to challenge the decisions made for Terri Schiavo threatened to destabilize end-of-life law that had developed principally through the cases of Quinlan and Cruzan. Although the Schiavo case had little effect on right-to-die jurisprudence, it illustrated the range of difficulties that can complicate decision making concerning the termination of treatment in incapacitated persons and the importance of having written advance directives.

rights of persons or surrogates to make decisions related to death or life-sustaining care, as well as the rights of the state to intervene in treatment decisions. Table 3-1 reviews three landmark legal cases—Quinlan, Cruzan, and Schiavo—that have influenced legal and ethical precedents in the right-to-die debate. Table 3-2 lists definitions for some terms pertinent to these issues.

The issue of treatment for persons whose quality of life is severely compromised, as in irreversible coma or brain death, is often a result of advanced biomedical technology. Technology frequently sustains life in persons who would have previously died of their illnesses. The widespread use of advanced life-support systems and cardiopulmonary resuscitation (CPR) has changed the nature and context of dying. A "natural death" in the traditional sense is rare; most patients who die in healthcare facilities undergo resuscitation efforts.

The benefits derived from aggressive technological management often outweigh the negative effects, but the use of life-sustaining technologies for persons with severely impaired quality of life, or for those who are terminally ill, has stimulated intensive debate and litigation. Two key issues in this debate are the appropriate use of technology and the ability of the seriously ill person to retain decision-making rights. These issues are based on the ethical principles of beneficence and autonomy.

At the heart of the technology controversy are conflicting beliefs about the morality and legality of allowing persons who are terminally ill or severely debilitated to request withdrawing or withholding medical treatment. In these situations, two levels of treatment must be considered: ordinary care and extraordinary care. These levels of care are at two ends of a continuum of potential treatment options.

TABLE 3-2	DEFINITIONS IN CRITICAL CARE DECISION MAKING
CONCEPT	**DEFINITION**
Advance directive	Witnessed written document or oral statement in which instructions are given by a person to express desires related to healthcare decisions. The directive may include, but is not limited to, the designation of a healthcare surrogate, a living will, or an anatomical gift.
Living will	A witnessed written document or oral statement voluntarily executed by a person that expresses the person's instructions concerning life-prolonging procedures.
Healthcare decision	Informed consent, refusal of consent, or withdrawal of consent for health care, unless stated in the advance directive.
Incapacity or incompetent decision	Patient is physically or mentally unable to communicate a willful and knowing health care.
Informed consent	Consent voluntarily given after a sufficient explanation and disclosure of information.
Proxy	A competent adult who has not been expressly designated to make health care decisions for an incapacitated person, but is authorized by state statute to make healthcare decisions for the person.
Surrogate	A competent adult designated by a person to make health care decisions should that person become incapacitated.
Terminal condition	A condition in which there is no reasonable medical probability of recovery and can be expected to cause death without treatment.
Persistent vegetative state	A permanent, irreversible unconsciousness condition that demonstrates an absence of voluntary action or cognitive behavior, or an inability to communicate or interact purposefully with the environment.
Brain death	Complete and irreversible cessation of brain function.
Clinical death or cardiac death	Irreversible cessation of spontaneous ventilation and circulation.
Life-prolonging procedure	Any medical procedure or treatment, including sustenance and hydration, that sustains, restores, or supplants a spontaneous vital function. Does not include the administration of medication or treatments deemed necessary to provide comfort care or to alleviate pain.
Resuscitation	Intervention with the intent of preserving life, restoring health, or reversing clinical death.
Do not resuscitate (DNR) order	A medical order that prohibits the use of cardiopulmonary resuscitation and emergency cardiac care to reverse signs of clinical death. The DNR order may or may not be specified in patients' advance directives.
Allow natural death	An alternate term with less negative connotations, but essentially meaning DNR.

Adapted from Florida Statutes Chapter 765.101 definitions. www.flsenate.gov/statutes; 2011. Accessed July 24, 2011.

Although, based on one's beliefs, some therapies could be put in either category; this distinction is still helpful from a legal and ethical perspective. However, ethicists believe that any treatment can become extraordinary whenever the patient decides that the burdens outweigh the benefits.

Patient and family expectations have changed over time. Although not new, the concept of medical futility is moving to the forefront of the end-of-life debate. Judgment regarding futility in the critical care setting is difficult because it differs greatly among cultures and disciplines. Each goal is then evaluated based on what is achievable or deemed "futile." Debate over futility of specific treatments is essentially a debate on quality of life and which treatments are worthwhile to assist patients in achieving their goals. The cost of health care and the push toward major healthcare reform are generating public discussion regarding the financial impact of medical treatments at the end of life. Discussion on the economics of treatments is as uncomfortable in the United States as talking about death. This topic has not played a major role in

end-of-life decision making in the past, but experts agree it is moving up the line of priorities in medical futility debates.[13]

Traditionally, extraordinary care includes complex, invasive, and experimental treatments such as resuscitation efforts by CPR or emergency cardiac care, maintenance of life support through invasive means, or renal dialysis. Experimental treatments such as gene therapy also are extraordinary therapies.

Ordinary care usually involves common, noninvasive, to tested treatments such as providing nutrition, hydration, or antibiotic therapy. In the critical care setting the noninvasive criterion does not apply; ordinary care is defined as usual and customary for the patient's condition. Maintenance of hydration and nutrition through a tube feeding is an example of a treatment that falls somewhere between ordinary and extraordinary care and is a highly debatable issue. Therefore it is important for individuals to document their wishes rather than relying on the members of the healthcare team to assist in the decision-making process related to nutrition and hydration.

Cardiopulmonary Resuscitation Decisions

The goals of emergency cardiovascular care are to preserve life, restore health, relieve suffering, limit disability, and reverse clinical death.[5] Frequently, ethical questions arise about the use of CPR and emergency cardiac care because such treatment may conflict with a patient's desires or best interests. The critical care nurse should be guided by scientifically proven data, patient preferences, and ethical and cultural norms.

The American Heart Association has developed guidelines to assist practitioners in making the difficult decision to provide or withhold emergency cardiovascular care.[5] The generally accepted position is that resuscitation should cease if the physician determines that efforts are futile or hopeless. Futility constitutes sufficient reason for either withholding or ceasing extraordinary treatments.

Withholding or stopping extraordinary resuscitation efforts is ethically and legally appropriate if patients or surrogates have previously made their preferences known through advance directives. It is also acceptable if the physician determines that resuscitation is futile or has discussed the situation with the patient, family, and/or surrogate as appropriate, and there is mutual agreement not to resuscitate in the event of cardiopulmonary arrest. For the nurse not to initiate the resuscitation, a *do not resuscitate* (DNR) order must be written. Most physicians also write supporting documentation regarding the order in the progress notes, such as conversations held with the patient and family members.

Family presence during resuscitation and invasive procedures has been a debated topic for the last decade. There is growing evidence that family presence during resuscitation and invasive procedures helps not only families but also the healthcare team.[3] Family presence during resuscitation and invasive procedures is now supported by multiple entities including the Emergency Nurses Association and the American Association of Critical-Care Nurses.[14] The topic has been added to the American Heart Association's Guidelines for Cardiopulmonary Resuscitation and Emergency Cardiovascular Care.[5] Even with this growing support, only 5% of critical care units in the United States have written policies allowing families to be present during resuscitation and invasive procedures.[14] Current recommendations are for institutions to establish a process for allowing families who wish to be present to do so. This includes designating a trained clinician or chaplain to support the family throughout the process

Withholding or Withdrawing Life Support

Withholding life support, withdrawing life support, or both, can range from not initiating hemodialysis (withholding) to terminal weaning from mechanical ventilation (withdrawing). Decisions are made based on consideration of all factors in the ethical decision-making model. In all instances of withholding and withdrawing life support, comfort measures are maintained, including management of pain, pulmonary secretions, and other symptoms as needed.

Most decisions regarding withdrawing and withholding of life support are not made in the courts. They are made based on open communication with the patient, family, and surrogate, as appropriate. An ethical decision-making approach is used to decide on the best actions to take or not take in the situation. If ethical or legal questions arise, ethics consultation services, ethics committees, and risk managers can provide assistance. The value of clearly stating in writing one's end-of-life issues before becoming critically ill (advance directive) is key to avoiding having treatment given or not given against one's wishes.

End-of-Life Issues
Patient Self-Determination Act

In response to public concern about end-of-life decisions and the overall lack of consistent hospital policies, the United States Congress enacted the Patient Self-Determination Act.[15] This act requires that all healthcare facilities that receive Medicare and Medicaid funding inform their patients about their right to initiate an advance directive and the right to consent to or refuse medical treatment.

Discussions regarding advance directives and end-of-life wishes should be made as early as possible, preferably before death is imminent. The ideal time to discuss advance directives is when a person is relatively healthy, not in the critical care or hospital setting. This allows more time for discussion, processing, and decision making. Nurses in every practice setting should assess patients regarding their perceptions of quality of life and end-of-life wishes in a caring and culturally sensitive way, and should document the patient's wishes. Patients should be strongly encouraged to complete advance directives, including living wills and durable power of attorney, to ensure that their wishes will be followed if they are terminally ill or in a persistent vegetative state.

Advance Directives

An *advance directive* is a communication that specifies a person's preference about medical treatment should that person become incapacitated. Several types of advance directives exist, including DNR orders, allow-a-natural-death orders, living wills, health care proxies, and other types of legal documents (Table 3-2). It is important for nurses to know whether a patient has an advance directive and that the directive be followed.

The *living will* provides a mechanism by which individuals can authorize the withholding of specific treatments if they become incapacitated. Although living wills provide direction to caregivers, in some states, living wills are not legally binding and are seen as advisory. When completing a living will, individuals can add special instructions about end-of-life wishes. Individuals can change their directive at any time.

The *durable power of attorney for health care* is more protective of patients' interests regarding medical treatment than is the living will. With a durable power of attorney for health care, patients legally designate an agent whom they trust, such as a family member or friend, to make decisions on their behalf should they become incapacitated. This person is called the *health care surrogate* or proxy. A durable power of attorney for health care allows the surrogate to make decisions whenever the patient is incapacitated, not just at the time of terminal illness. Some legal commentators recommend the joint use of a living will and a durable power of attorney to give added protection to a person's preferences about medical treatment.

Ultimately, if self-determination and informed consent are to have real value, patients or their surrogates must be given an opportunity to consider options and to shape decisions that affect their life or death. Communication and shared decision making among the patient, family, and healthcare team regarding end-of-life issues are key.[12] Unfortunately, this frequently does not happen before admission to a critical care unit. The critical care nurse must be part of the team that educates the patient and family, so they can determine and communicate end-of-life wishes.

Some situations may result in moral distress for the nurse. A nurse who is unable to follow these legal documents because of personal or religious beliefs must ask to have the client reassigned to another nurse. For instance, some advance directives may call for withdrawing life support when certain conditions are met, and this may conflict with the nurse's personal or religious beliefs. Nurses who frequently ask to be reassigned to another client may need to think about another nursing specialty where their beliefs do not conflict with advance directives.

The nurse must also be cognizant of the facility's policies regarding advance directives. For example, if a DNR order is on the chart, does it meet all the requirements for a legal document per facility policy? Is it signed by the physician? Is the chart notated properly? Is there a health care proxy? Are the forms proper? Is there a living will? All critical care nurses should review key policies and documents related to DNR and withdrawing and withholding of life support, because these situations occur frequently. Knowledge of institutional policies will facilitate honoring of patients' and families' wishes in a compassionate and caring environment.

Organ and Tissue Transplantation

Improved surgical methods and increasingly effective immunosuppressive drug therapy have increased the number and the types of successfully transplanted organs and tissues.

Despite the successes in transplantation, there is a severe shortage of organs to meet the growing demand. Under the National Organ Transplant Act of 1984, the United States Congress established the Organ Procurement and Transplantation Network to facilitate fair allocation of organs and tissues for transplantation. This system is administered by the United Network for Organ Sharing, a group that maintains a list of patients who are awaiting organ and tissue transplantation and helps to coordinate the procurement of organs. In 2011, more than 111,000 people were on the organ transplantation waiting list for the United States.[18] This shortage has motivated multiple efforts to increase the organ supply.

These efforts include creating registries for donors and designating organ donor status on driver's licenses. There are legal mandates for *required request* and mandatory organ procurement organization notification when a patient's death is imminent. In some situations, removal of the organ to be transplanted is not life threatening and can be accomplished without causing significant harm to a living donor (e.g., kidney and bone marrow). Other types of organ and tissue removal (e.g., heart) are performed only in donors who meet the legal definition for brain death.

Since the 1968 Harvard Medical School Ad Hoc Committee's brain death definition, organs have primarily been removed from patients with cardiac function who have been pronounced dead on the basis of neurological criteria but continue to receive mechanical ventilation. The concept of *brain death* is distinct from the concept of persistent vegetative state or irreversible coma. In brain death, complete and irreversible cessation of brain function occurs, whereas in irreversible coma or persistent vegetative state, some brain function remains intact. If a patient is a designated organ donor and brain death is determined, the patient is pronounced to be dead; however, perfusion and oxygenation of organs are maintained until the organs can be removed in the operating room. Even with optimal artificial perfusion and oxygenation, organs intended for transplantation must be removed and transplanted quickly.

The most rapid increase in the rate of organ recovery from deceased persons has occurred in the category of donation after cardiac death—that is, a death declared on the basis of cardiopulmonary criteria (irreversible cessation of circulatory and respiratory function) rather than brain death.[17] Most commonly, the kidneys, liver, and pancreas are recovered after cardiac death because of the length of time in which these organs can be deprived of oxygen and still be transplanted successfully. In 2005 a conference on donation after cardiac death concluded that it is an ethically acceptable practice to retrieve organs after cardiac death to increase the number of organs available for transplantation.[9] Nonetheless, the practice remains controversial because of the complexities required during the transition from end-of-life care to organ donation.

Critical care professionals must ensure that the decision to withdraw care is made separately from the decision to donate organs. In addition, donation after cardiac death is often performed in the operating room. Critical care personnel need to create a plan of care should the patient not die as expected. Donors must be dead according to specified hospital policy before organ procurement. The process of organ procurement cannot be the proximate cause of death.

Everyone in the United States has the legal right to donate organs. To uphold that right, family members or significant others must be given the opportunity to donate organs or tissues on behalf of their loved ones if there is no advance directive. Local organ procurement organizations have *designated requestors* whose role is to seek consent for organ donation. The role of the critical care nurse is to refer potential organ donors to the organ procurement organization. Because the consent rate for organ donation is only about 50%, it is important to approach potential donors sensitively and with awareness of cultural and religious implications. The designated requestors are trained to address donation with regard to such issues.

Ethical Concerns Surrounding Organ and Tissue Transplantation

Organ and tissue transplantation involve numerous and complex ethical issues. The first consideration is given to the rights and privileges of all moral agents involved: the donor, the recipient, the family or surrogate, and all other recipients and donors. Important ethical principles that are useful in ethical decision making regarding transplantation include respect for persons and their autonomous choices, beneficence and nonmaleficence, justice, and fidelity. Three of the most controversial issues in transplantation are the moral value that should be placed on the human body part, the just distribution of a human body part, and the complex problems inherent in applying the concept of brain death to clinical situations.

CASE STUDY

Mr. W. is a 67-year-old patient in the coronary care unit who has severe heart failure and chronic obstructive pulmonary disease. Mr. W. has been in and out of the hospital for 3 years and requires oxygen therapy at night. He has severe, chronic chest pain and dyspnea. He had a respiratory arrest and was put on the ventilator last night. He awakens after the resuscitation and communicates that the breathing tube be removed and that he be allowed to die. He is tired of the pain and dyspnea. He asks for medication to make him comfortable after the tube is removed. His family agrees with the plan of care.

Mr. W.'s wishes are followed. He is extubated and is given morphine for sedation and comfort. Mr. W.'s family members all remain at the bedside, taking turns holding his hand and talking to him.

Questions

1. Apply the ethical decision-making model discussed in this chapter to this case. What are the relevant ethical principles? Are there other areas that must be assessed before proceeding?
2. As the critical care nurse caring for Mr. W., what are your priorities at this point? On what ethical principles are these priorities based?
3. Suppose that you have strong religious beliefs about withdrawal of life support. If you were assigned to Mr. W., what actions should you take?

SUMMARY

The ethical responsibilities of nurses who work in acute care settings have increased dramatically since the early 1990s. Based on evolving case law, state statutes, and state nurse practice acts, nurses are held to a high standard of care and are also held directly accountable for their individual nursing actions. Nurses who care for critically ill patients are challenged by ethical dilemmas on a daily basis. In their role of patient advocate, ethical decision making and open communication must be facilitated. Numerous resources are available to assist with developing the knowledge and skill to do this well. There are no easy answers to ethical dilemmas. A formal decision-making model assists the nurse, but some situations may still remain very ambiguous. Appropriate ethical nursing responses are based on wanting to do the right thing for the patients and families that you care for and initiating the steps to advocate for the patient.

CRITICAL THINKING EXERCISES

1. You are taking care of Mrs. H., a 90-year-old patient with gastrointestinal bleeding. She has developed numerous complications and requires mechanical ventilation. She is unresponsive to nurses and family members. She has been in the hospital for 2 weeks and requires a transfusion nearly every day to sustain adequate hemoglobin and hematocrit levels. Her prognosis is poor. Before this hospitalization, she lived independently at her own home. Her children tell you they are tired of seeing their mother suffer. How do you respond to the family, and what follow-up do you perform?

2. You are taking care of Mr. J., a 23-year-old man with a closed head injury. During the night shift, you note a change in the level of consciousness at 3:00 AM. You call the physician, who tells you to watch Mr. J. until the physician attends rounds the next morning. He tells you not to call him back. Mr. J.'s neurological status continues to deteriorate. What actions do you take? What is the rationale for your actions?

Continued

▌CRITICAL THINKING EXERCISES—cont'd

3. It is 2 days later, and Mr. J., as described earlier, now has a herniated brainstem and is declared brain dead but remains on life support. His wife is at the bedside and is fully aware of the situation. You do not know whether Mr. J. signed an organ donor card. What are your ethical and legal obligations regarding organ donation at this point? How would you approach the situation?

4. You are caring for Mrs. M., a 68-year-old woman with an acute myocardial infarction. She is in the critical care unit after a successful angioplasty. Her husband brought in her living will, which states that Mrs. M. does not desire resuscitation. Mrs. M. is pain free and alert. As you start your beginning-of-shift assessment, Mrs. M. says, "You know, now that I've made it through the angioplasty, I realize that tubes and machines may not be so bad after all. I haven't made it this far to give up now. If I go into cardiac arrest, I want you to do all that you can for me." What ethical principle is Mrs. M. using? As her nurse, what actions should you take and why?

5. You are the charge nurse of a nine-bed critical care unit. You have one open bed. The house supervisor calls and tells you that there are two patients who need a critical care bed. The first is a 23-year-old woman currently in the operating room after multiple trauma. The second patient is a 78-year-old man who is in the emergency department with severe septic shock. According to the supervisor, both patients are going to need mechanical ventilation and inotropic therapy. What are your decisions and actions at this point? What ethical principles are your actions based on?

REFERENCES

1. American Association of Critical-Care Nurses. *An Ethic of Care.* www.aacn.org; 2002. Accessed July 24, 2011.
2. American Association of Critical-Care Nurses. *AACN Standards for Establishing and Sustaining Healthy Work Environments.* www.aacn.org/hwe; 2005. Accessed June 3, 2011.
3. American Association of Critical-Care Nurses. *AACN Practice Alert, Family Presence During Resuscitation and Invasive Procedures.* www.aacn.org; 2010. Accessed July 24, 2011.
4. American Association of Critical-Care Nurses. *Position Statement, Moral Distress.* www.aacn.org; 2006. Accessed July 24, 2011.
5. American Heart Association. *American Heart Association 2010 Guidelines for Cardiopulmonary Resuscitation and Emergency Cardiopulmonary Care.* www.heart.org; 2010. Accessed July 24, 2011.
6. American Nurses Association. *Code of Ethics for Nurses with Interpretive Statements.* Silver Springs, MD; 2001.
7. American Nurses Credentialing Center. *Magnet Recognition Program: Application Manual.* Silver Springs, MD; 2008.
8. Beauchamp T, Childress J. *Principles of Biomedical Ethics.* 5th ed. Oxford, England: Oxford University Press; 2001.
9. Bernat JL, D'Alessandro AM, Port FK, et al. Report of a national conference on donation after cardiac death. *American Journal of Transplantation.* 2006;6:281-291.
10. Fowler DM. *Guide to the Code of Ethics for Nurses.* 4th ed. Silver Springs, MD: American Nurses Association; 2008.
11. Grady C, Danis M, Soeken KL, et al. Does ethics education influence the moral action of practicing nurses and social workers? *American Journal of Bioethics.* 2008;8(4):2-14.
12. Heyland DK, Tranmer J, Feldman-Steward D. End-of-life decision making in the seriously ill hospitalized patient: an organizing framework and results of a preliminary study. *Journal of Palliative Care.* 2000;16:S31-S39.
13. Kummer HB, Thompson DR. *Critical Care Ethics: A Practice Guide.* 2nd ed. Mount Prospect, IL: Society of Critical Care Medicine; 2009.
14. Maclean SL, Guzzetta CE, White C, et al. Family presence during cardiopulmonary resuscitation and invasive procedures: practices of critical care and emergency nurses. *American Journal of Critical Care.* 2003;12(3):246-257.
15. Public Law No. 101-508, 4206, 104 Stat. 291. The Self-Determination Act amends the Social Security Act's provisions on Medicare and Medicaid. Social Security Act 1927, 42 U.S.C. 1396; 1990.
16. Rushton CH, Scanlon C. A road map for negotiating end-of-life care. *Medsurg Nursing.* 1998;6(1):59-62.
17. Steinbrook R. Organ donation after cardiac death. *New England Journal of Medicine.* 2007;357(3):209-213.
18. United Network for Organ Sharing. *Data.* www.unos.org/; 2011. Accessed June 7, 2011.

End-of-Life Care in the Critical Care Unit

Douglas Houghton, MSN, ARNP, ACNPC, CCRN, FAANP

Evolve WEBSITE

Many additional resources, including self-assessment exercises, are located on the Evolve companion website at http://evolve.elsevier.com/Sole.

- Review Questions
- Mosby's Nursing Skills Procedures

- Animations
- Video Clips

INTRODUCTION

Advances in technology during the past several decades have vastly improved the ability of healthcare providers to care for the sickest patients and have led to increasingly successful outcomes. However, the appropriate use of these often invasive and frequently expensive resources is still a matter of debate, leading to complex ethical issues in the care of persons with a critical illness. One epidemiological study found that approximately 38% of all deaths in the United States occur in an acute care setting, with 22% of the deaths occurring after admission to a critical care unit.[2] This finding is disturbing, because research evidence has shown that the vast majority of Americans would like to die in the comfort of their home environment.[17] However, most critical care units remain a relatively hostile, often uncomfortable and impersonal place for dying patients and their families.[14] The landmark Study to Understand Prognoses and Preferences for Outcomes and Risks of Treatment (SUPPORT) revealed many disparities between patients' care preferences and the care they received. The most significant findings from the study included a lack of clear communication between patients and healthcare providers, a high frequency of aggressive care, and widespread pain and suffering among inpatients.[51] Although some improvements have been made, these study findings have subsequently been confirmed by additional research during the past decade.[60,67] Increasing national attention to the issue has stimulated the growth of funding for research and development of medical and nursing care guidelines for the care of the dying person in the critical care unit (see online resources in Box 4-5).

The majority of deaths in the critical care unit are preceded by decisions to withhold or withdraw aggressive support.[32,49,60] Up to 95% of patients in the critical care unit are unable to make decisions about their own care; thus they rely on surrogates to decide for them.[61] Surrogate decision makers frequently rely on factors other than the prognosis relayed to them by the physician, increasing the likelihood of conflict situations.[6,31,47] Multiple factors influence the continuation of aggressive care in the face of a poor or futile prognosis, including religious beliefs and ethnicity.[41] The failure of clinicians, family members, and patients to openly and honestly discuss prognoses, end-of-life issues, and preferences is one of the most significant factors preventing early identification of patients unlikely to benefit from aggressive care. Patients and surrogates often do not understand the ramifications of their choices, and nurses play a key role in ensuring that choices are understood.[46]

The fact that no valid assessment tools exist to accurately predict when care is medically futile is another major contributing factor to many conflicts at the end of life (Box 4-1).[26,32] The identification of the dying patient is often subjective and based on the healthcare providers' opinions and interpretations of patient response and results. This makes the determination of the appropriate intensity of care for patients near the end of life extremely difficult.[13] Mounting evidence demonstrates that high-intensity or aggressive care near the end of life is associated with a *decreased* quality of life and little to no improvement in duration of life.[3,67]

Societal values and those of healthcare providers also play a significant role in how end-of-life care in the United States

---

BOX 4-1	**DEFINITION OF MEDICAL FUTILITY**

Medical futility: Situation in which therapy or interventions will not provide a foreseeable possibility of improvement in the patient's health condition. Legal and organizational definitions may vary, and much controversy exists.

From Lewis CL, Hanson LC, Golin C, et al. Surrogates' perceptions about feeding tube placement decisions. *Patient Education and Counseling.* 2006;61:246-252.

---

is provided. These values include a commonly held belief that patients die of distinct illnesses, which implies that such illnesses are potentially curable.[10] Dying is often viewed as failure on the part of the system or providers. The purpose of the healthcare system in the United States is to treat illness, disease, and injury, and this "lifesaving" culture continues to drive aggressive care even when it becomes obvious that the ultimate outcome will be the death of the individual.[14,23]

Effects on Nurses and the Healthcare Team

Many clinicians experience personal ethical conflicts when providing painful interventions and aggressive care to patients when they believe the situation is futile, causing significant moral distress that can lead to burnout.[15,21,45] Care choices made by patients or surrogates often differ from those that clinicians might personally make, causing further strain in remaining nonjudgmental in such situations. Experiencing recurrent moral distress was cited as the cause of leaving a job by 45% of nurses in one recent study.[21] Whereas moral distress is most common among nurses, it is reported in physicians and other care providers as well.[15,21]

Patients' dignity is often impaired during a critical care unit stay, and their preferences and wishes may be ignored, dictated for them by providers and surrogates. Such situations contradict basic nursing ethical principles, causing further moral distress.[15,66] At times, healthcare providers do not clearly communicate a futile prognosis to patients or the family members, denying them the ability to make informed choices.[64,65] When care is withdrawn and patients die, caregivers often experience a sense of loss or grief, especially if the patient's stay was lengthy. Attendance at funerals or unit debriefing sessions after a death may help to resolve emotional strain, but finding a balance between maintaining a professional, healthy distance and being authentic and humane in our care is a difficult task.

DIMENSIONS OF END-OF-LIFE CARE

Nursing care in the critical care setting at the end of life is focused on five dimensions. These dimensions of nursing care consist of alleviation of distressing symptoms (palliation); communication and conflict resolution; withdrawing, limiting, or withholding of therapy; emotional and psychological care of the patient and family; and caregiver organizational support.

Palliative Care

Palliation is the provision of care interventions that are designed to relieve symptoms of illness or injury that negatively impact the quality of life of the patient or family.[9,34,39] Common distressing symptoms that may occur with multiple disease states include pain, anxiety, hunger, thirst, dyspnea, diarrhea, nausea, confusion, agitation, and disturbance in sleep patterns.[34,51] Palliative care should be viewed as an integral part of every ill or injured patient's care and should not be reserved only for the dying patient. Relief of distressing symptoms should always be provided whenever possible, even when the primary focus of care is lifesaving or aggressive treatment. An important part of palliative care consists of "simple" nursing interventions, such as frequent repositioning, good hygiene and skin care, and creation of a peaceful environment to the extent possible in the critical care setting.

For those patients with recognized life-limiting illness or injury, palliative care consultations with experts in symptom management can provide significant benefits to the patients and their families. The use of palliative care experts to assist in managing patients' care decreases hospital lengths of stay and resource utilization. Improved communication with patients and families, and better management of pain and other symptoms, are additional benefits noted.[9,12,34,55] Palliative care may be provided through a consultative model or via an integrative approach, in which palliative care principles are integrated into the daily medical and nursing practice in the critical care unit.[3,36,39] Some institutions have implemented pathways to assist in patient care management at the end of life. Although there have not been randomized trials to evaluate their outcomes, these pathways promote increased accessibility to palliative care (see box, "Evidence-Based Practice").[42]

Earlier identification of patients who are unlikely to benefit from further aggressive care, and improved management of pain and other symptoms, are effective strategies to improve end-of-life care.[4,37,56] Pain is considered the "fifth vital sign," so frequent nursing assessment for symptoms of pain is necessary. Additionally, people express pain in different ways, which may vary among cultural groups and individuals; knowledge of these differences is required for proper pain assessment.[34] Medications to control pain and relieve anxiety in the critically ill patient are described in Chapter 5.

Communication and Conflict Resolution

Clear, ongoing, and honest communication between the members of the healthcare team, the patient, and the family is a key factor in improving the quality of care for the dying patient in the critical care unit.[29,35,40] Interventions testing various communication strategies when dealing with end-of-life issues have had positive results.[29] Guidelines for effective communication are described in Box 4-2.

EVIDENCE-BASED PRACTICE

Implementing End-of-Life Care Pathways

Problem

End-of-life care pathways are being implemented at facilities to better manage end-of-life care in a variety of settings, including acute care. It is not known if adoption of these pathways improves implementation of palliative and end-of-life care.

Clinical Question

What has been the impact of implementing end-of-life care pathways in the acute care setting?

Evidence

An integrative review of the literature was conducted to answer the clinical question. After an extensive search, 26 articles met inclusion criteria and were reviewed by two researchers. The majority of studies (58%) were conducted in the United Kingdom. Only three were conducted in the United States. No randomized clinical trials have been conducted to compare implementation of a pathway with the standard of care. The majority of findings were extrapolated from retrospective chart audits conducted before and after implementation of a pathway. Several positive findings were reported for using an end-of-life pathway, including the following:

- Increases accessibility to palliative care, regardless of unit or service
- Addresses patient comfort issues proactively
- Improves goal setting and communication among patient, family, and the multiprofessional team
- Engages both patient and family in decision making

Limitations of implementing a pathway included issues in properly identifying patients who might benefit from a palliative care service and the challenge of integrating it with a healthcare culture focused on "cure" versus "care."

Implications for Nursing

The opportunity to develop and implement end-of-life pathways in critical care units exists. Facilities in the United States could model pathways that have been developed in the United Kingdom. The pathway must be designed with input from the multiprofessional team. Strong leadership is needed for successful implementation of pathways; a critical care clinical nurse specialist could provide such leadership and engage staff nurses on the unit in identifying and implementing best practices. Computer decision support triggers from the electronic medical record may alert the nurse and identify patients who might benefit from palliative care services. Randomized trials with clearly defined outcome measures are needed to evaluate these pathways.

Level of Evidence

C—Review of descriptive studies

Reference

Phillips JL, Halcomb EJ, Davidson PM. End-of-life care pathways in acute and hospice care: an integrative review. *Journal of Pain and Symptom Management.* 2011;41(5): 940-950.

BOX 4-2   GUIDELINES FOR EFFECTIVE COMMUNICATION TO FACILITATE END-OF-LIFE CARE

- **Present a clear and consistent message** to the family. Mixed messages confuse families and patients, as do unfamiliar medical terms. The multiprofessional team needs to communicate and strive to reach agreement on goals of care and prognosis.[4,11]
- **Allow ample time** for family members to express themselves during family conferences.[28,32,54] This increases their level of satisfaction and decreases dysfunctional bereavement patterns after the patient's death.
- Aim for all (healthcare providers, patients, and families) to **agree on the plan of treatment.** The plan should be based on the known or perceived preferences of the patient.[11,31,54] Arriving at such a plan through communication minimizes legal actions against providers, relieves patient and family

anxiety, and provides an environment in which the patient is the focus of concern.

- **Emphasize that the patient will not be abandoned** if the goals of care shift from aggressive therapy to "comfort" care (palliation) only.[62] Let the patient and family know who is responsible for their care and that they can rely on those individuals to be present and available when needed.
- **Facilitate continuity of care.**[33,54] If a transfer to an alternative level of care, such as a hospice unit or ventilator unit, is required, ensure that all pertinent information is conveyed to the new providers. Details of the history, prognosis, care requirements, palliative interventions, and psychosocial needs should be part of the information transfer.

BOX 4-3 ETHICAL PRINCIPLES FOR WITHHOLDING AND WITHDRAWING LIFE-SUSTAINING TREATMENT

1. Death occurs as a consequence of the underlying disease. The goals of care are to relieve suffering and not to hasten death.
2. Withholding life-sustaining treatment is morally and legally equivalent to withdrawing treatment. Both actions require the same degree of active participation by multiprofessional team members as any other procedure.
3. Any treatment can be withdrawn or withheld, including nutrition, fluids, antibiotics, or blood products.
4. Any dose of analgesic or anxiolytic medication may reasonably be used to relieve suffering, even if the medication has the potential to hasten death. Signs of suffering include dyspnea, tachypnea, diaphoresis, grimacing, accessory muscle use, nasal flaring, and restlessness.
5. Life-sustaining treatment should not be withdrawn while a patient is receiving paralytic agents. After discontinuation of such drugs, the patient must demonstrate sufficient motor activity to allow thorough clinical assessment before withdrawal of support.
6. Cultural and religious views influence the perspectives of patients and family members regarding life-sustaining treatment. These issues should be openly discussed and an effort made to accommodate various perspectives. Pastoral or spiritual care providers may assist in this process.

Adapted from University of Washington/Harborview Medical Center. Physician orders. http://depts.washington.edu/eolcare/instruments/wls-orders2.pdf. Accessed May 30, 2011.

Withholding, Limiting, or Withdrawing Therapy

The majority of deaths in the critical care unit are preceded by some manner of withholding, withdrawing, or limiting medical treatments.[24,64] Such a decision should be made with input and agreement in a shared decision-making model.[56,63] Appropriate withdrawal, limiting, or withholding of therapy does not constitute euthanasia or assisted suicide, both of which are illegal in the United States (with the exception of Oregon, Washington, and Montana, where assisted suicide is permitted in select instances). Minimal moral distress on the part of the healthcare team, patients, and families should result if generally accepted ethical and legal principles are followed during this process (Box 4-3).[18,44]

Preparing patients (if conscious) and families for what will likely occur during the withdrawal process is key to alleviating anxiety and undue distress.[7,12,34] A nursing care priority should be anticipating patient symptoms such as dyspnea during ventilator withdrawal, and medicating to alleviate such symptoms, even if high doses of medications are required. Assessment of patient response (e.g., comfort) is the sole means of deciding how much medication is appropriate in a given situation, and therapy should be titrated to relieve emotional and physical distress even if such dosing hastens the death of the patient as a secondary effect.[8,56] Commonly used

medication regimens include morphine sulfate and intravenous benzodiazepines for anxiolysis (Figure 4-1). Recent data have supported the perception that most patients die in comfort during the withdrawal process.[43,60]

Ventilator Withdrawal

The most commonly withheld or withdrawn medical intervention in the critical care setting is mechanical ventilation. Some debate and regional practice variations exist, but excellent practice guidelines for end-of-life care and ventilator withdrawal are available from the American Association

⚠ CLINICAL ALERT

Ventilator Withdrawal

During terminal weaning of ventilatory support, patients may exhibit symptoms of respiratory distress, such as tachypnea, dyspnea, or use of accessory muscles. Pain medication and sedation should be titrated as needed to relieve such symptoms.

of Critical-Care Nurses website.[57,64] This process is known as "terminal weaning" (see box, "Clinical Alert") and can consist of titration of ventilator support to minimal levels, removal of the ventilator but not the artificial airway, or complete extubation.[9] Nurses should consult their institution's policy and procedure manual for specific requirements or variation.

Other Commonly Withheld Therapies

Vasopressors, antibiotics, blood and blood products, dialysis, and nutritional support are other common therapies that may be ethically withheld when goals of treatment shift to palliation instead of cure. Because of the rapid increase in the use of cardiovascular implantable electronic devices such as cardioverter-defibrillators, it is important to address the deactivation of these devices as appropriate before withdrawing or withholding ventilation or other therapies, which may result in cardiac arrest.[27] Again, the primary nursing responsibility is to assess and ensure patient comfort during the withdrawal or withholding process.

Hospice Referral

When it has been determined that aggressive medical care interventions will be withheld or withdrawn, it may be appropriate to initiate a referral to a hospice care provider for transfer of the patient.[35] Hospice is a model of care that emphasizes comfort rather than cure, and views dying as a normal human process. It is a philosophy of care rather than a specific place, and can be provided in various care settings, as dictated by patient needs. Although referrals for hospice care are common in oncology, referrals are increasingly made to improve quality of end-of-life care regardless of diagnosis. Individuals in end-stage chronic obstructive pulmonary disease or heart failure may benefit from hospice care (see box, "QSEN Exemplar").

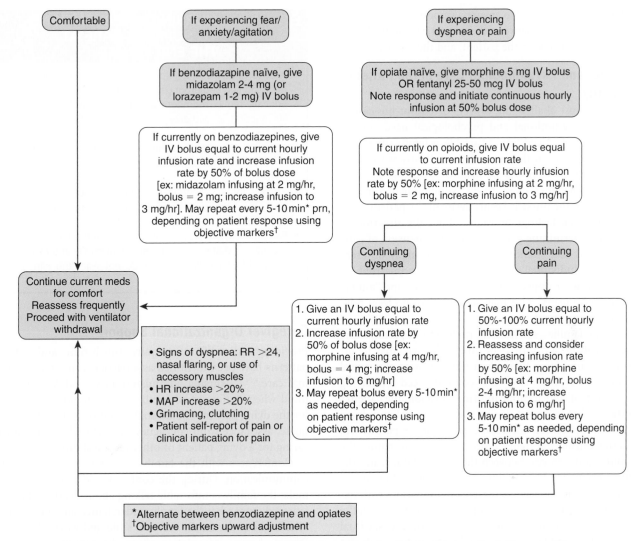

FIGURE 4-1 Guidelines for pharmacological interventions during withdrawal of life support. (From Virginia Commonwealth University Hospital, Richmond, Virginia.) *IV, Intravenous.*

QSEN EXEMPLAR

Patient Centered Care, Teamwork, and Collaboration

Mr. J., a 68-year-old man with end-stage chronic obstructive pulmonary disease, was hospitalized for exacerbation of his condition. He was hypoxemic and dyspneic and was being treated with bilevel positive airway pressure (BiPap). He was alert, oriented, and able to make his own decisions. His wife, Mrs. J., was at the bedside and stated she did not like to see her husband suffer. She also noted how uncomfortable Mr. J. was with the BiPap treatment. Mr. J. acknowledged his discomfort. During multiprofessional rounds led by the intensivist, Mrs. J. was in the room. The nurse conveyed to the physician Mr. J's discomfort and low oxygen saturation (85%) despite the BiPap. This communication created the opportunity for shared decision making and goal setting. The physician noted that the BiPap was not effective and asked, "What are the goals of care—comfort or more aggressive treatment?" Both Mr. and Mrs. J. acknowledged that comfort was most important. A shared decision was made to place Mr. J. on high-flow oxygen rather than the BiPap. The respiratory therapist replaced the BiPap with the high-flow oxygen. Mr. J. immediately noted increased comfort. His oxygen saturation improved, and he was able to clear his airway better. This example demonstrates the importance of multiprofessional rounds, family participation during such rounds, and the complementary roles of team members.

Hospice care for the critically ill patient is usually provided in an inpatient setting and can include withdrawal of ventilator support or other therapies.[28] For patients who are less dependent upon technologies for survival, the dying process may occasionally be managed in the patient's home with multiprofessional team support. Referral to hospice may provide a more supportive and tranquil environment for the patient during the dying process. Should such a transfer occur, it is crucial to ensure a smooth transition and good communication between the critical care staff, the receiving hospice provider, the patient, and the family.

Emotional and Psychological Care of the Patient and Family

One of the most challenging aspects of end-of-life care is addressing the emotional and psychological needs of the patient and family. Needs are as variable as family situations, and it is important for the nurse to carefully assess what the patient's and family's needs *are* instead of making assumptions about what they *ought* to be. Nonjudgmental assessment, in which the nurse is keenly aware of the patient's and family's personal feelings or values about the situation, is essential in determining priorities in this dimension of care. Keep in mind that "family" can consist of many different persons in an individual's life; it may include unmarried life partners (same or opposite sex), close friends, and "aunts," "uncles," or "cousins" who may actually have no legal relationship to the patient.

For some families, spiritual counseling from pastoral care services might be a priority. For others, the need may be for statistics documenting their loved one's chances of survival with a particular diagnosis.[59] One common need is receiving clear, consistent, and accurate information about the patient's condition, what to expect during the withdrawal and dying process (if applicable), and reassurance that the patient will not suffer during the dying process.[5,11,56] Coordinating the communication process between the patient, family, and the healthcare team is a key nursing action in end-of-life care.

Many institutions have bereavement counselors with extensive training in assisting patients and families through the dying process and its aftermath. Social workers, spiritual care providers, and licensed mental health professionals can frequently assist in meeting the needs of families. Cultural sensitivity is essential to accurately determine situational priorities, meanings, and perceptions, which may vary widely across cultures.

Maintaining the patient's dignity during the dying process is of the utmost importance. The nurse should make time to listen to family accounts of the patient's life before the illness or injury and acknowledge the patient's individuality and humanity. A calm manner and voice, a quiet and private environment, and unrestricted family presence with the patient are key nursing interventions before, during, and after the patient's death.[4,30] It is important to provide items for family comfort, such as tissues, refreshments, and chairs. When no words seem appropriate, maintaining a respectful conscious presence can speak volumes. The patient's death may be a relatively routine part of the nurse's day, but it is important to keep in mind that family members will likely remember the situation and the actions of the nurse and healthcare team for many years. Nursing interventions to support the family at the end of life are summarized in Box 4-4.

BOX 4-4 **NURSING INTERVENTIONS TO SUPPORT CARE AT THE END OF LIFE**

- Assess patient's and family members' understanding of the condition and prognosis to address educational needs.
- Educate family members about what will happen when life support is withdrawn to decrease their fear of the unknown.
- Assure family members that the patient will not suffer.
- Assure family members that the patient will not be abandoned.
- Provide for any needed emotional support and spiritual care resources, such as grief counselors and spiritual care providers.
- Facilitate physician communication with the family.
- Provide for visitation and presence of family and extended family. Most family members do not want the patient to die alone.

Caregiver Organizational Support

Providing end-of-life care requires much time, and staffing patterns have been identified as a barrier to providing optimal care.[4,11,38] Nursing administrators should keep this in mind when staffing to allow nurses time to adequately care for the dying patient. Should staffing ratios be less than adequate, assistance from colleagues can help relieve the nurse caring for a dying patient of other responsibilities.[53]

Conferences with the family are often held to facilitate communication. During the conference, it is important to make the family comfortable talking about death and dying issues, discuss what the family understands, and allow them to talk about the family member's life and medical history. Provide honest information about the patient's prognosis. Discuss goals for palliative care, emphasizing that patient comfort will be maintained. Use skills of effective communication such as reflection, empathy, and silence. Conclude with a plan and follow-up communication.

In addition to providing adequate staffing resources, helpful organizational behaviors include bereavement programs for families and assistance or guidance in making funeral arrangements. For situations in which the nurse and the patient or family do not speak the same language, interpreter services are essential to providing excellent end-of-life care. Debriefing or support sessions for staff members may be helpful in easing the stress of caring for dying patients.[15,34]

Critical care nurses have expressed the need for provider and public education concerning end-of-life issues.[4,20] Efforts to educate the public on a variety of end-of-life issues are vital to improving care through promotion of advance directives and conversations with loved ones concerning life-support options.

Nurses have also identified the need for professional end-of-life education.[4,20,66] The American Association of Colleges

BOX 4-5	**END-OF-LIFE ONLINE RESOURCES**

- http://depts.washington.edu/eolcare/ (University of Washington/ Harborview Medical Center)
- www.aacn.nche.edu/elnec (American Association of Colleges of Nursing)
- http://www.aacn.org/WD/Palliative/Content/PalAnd EOLInfo.pcms?menu=Practice (American Association of Critical-Care Nurses)
- www.nationalconsensusproject.org (National Consensus Project for Quality Palliative Care)
- www.nlm.nih.gov/medlineplus/endoflifeissues.html (National Library of Medicine – resources for the general public)
- www.eperc.mcw.edu (Medical College of Wisconsin)
- http://www.capc.org/ipal-icu/ (Center to Advance Palliative Care)
- www.endoflife.northwestern.edu (Northwestern University)

of Nursing first developed the *End-of-Life Competency Statements for a Peaceful Death,* which has spurred the improvement of end-of-life education in undergraduate nursing curricula.[1] Training is also available to prepare nurse educators to educate nurses in bedside practice about delivering competent and compassionate care to the dying patient.[34] Additional online resources can be found in Box 4-5.

CULTURALLY COMPETENT END-OF-LIFE CARE

Many clinicians believe that they lack the skills and preparation to tackle difficult end-of-life issues with patients and families of critically ill patients.[11,40] This discomfort may be magnified when clinicians deal with patients and families from a cultural or ethnic background that differs from their own.[5,11,25] Cultural influences on care at the end of life are highly variable, even by region.[16]

The United States is well recognized as a nation of people from increasingly diverse cultural backgrounds and ethnicities.[58] Therefore it is necessary to understand how cultural and ethnic differences affect crucial end-of-life decision-making processes and communication preferences in diverse groups and how these may vary during stressful situations.[48,50] Caring for persons of diverse cultural backgrounds can be difficult and frustrating for nurses, especially when institutional resources to support culturally diverse care is lacking.[52] Better understanding and institutional support of these cultural differences in end-of-life care preferences will lead to more effective and satisfying care and communication with patients and families.

Religious doctrine and beliefs profoundly influence patients' and families' choices for end-of-life care.[41] Significant differences in perspective may exist between and *within* many major religious groups, and these values are often deeply and subtly ingrained in belief systems underpinning care choices, including those of healthcare providers.[25,40]

Research on end-of-life care preferences in various cultural, ethnic, and religious groups has grown rapidly, although it is scarce in smaller cultural groups. In general, whites prefer less invasive and aggressive options near the end of life, whereas blacks and Hispanic ethnic groups tend to choose more aggressive care options.[19,22] Nurses are encouraged to become familiar with the values and beliefs of common cultural groups in their practice setting, as well as to recognize the influences of personal religious and cultural contexts.

CASE STUDY

Mr. M. is a 26-year-old Hispanic man who sustained severe injuries in a high-speed motorcycle accident, requiring admission to the critical care unit. According to his mother, he had previously been in perfect health other than having mild asthma as a child. His most significant injuries are a cervical spine fracture and quadriplegia at the C2 level, and a devastating traumatic brain injury consisting of a subarachnoid hemorrhage and diffuse axonal injury. He has subsequently developed acute respiratory distress syndrome (ARDS), requiring high levels of mechanical ventilation support during the first 3 days of his hospitalization. His prognosis for functional recovery from his brain injury is deemed "poor" by the neurosurgeon, and because of his high quadriplegia, he will remain ventilator dependent for life. Mr. M's family is Cuban, very close-knit, and religious (Catholic), and it consists of two sisters, his father and mother, and a grandmother who lives with them. Many of them do not speak English well, including his mother who is his designated legal surrogate. All are very tearful and devastated by

his injuries but remain hopeful that "God will help him recover and move again." His 20-year-old sister, in a private conversation with the nurse, states that her brother had told her before that he would prefer to die if he was ever paralyzed "from the neck down." She is afraid to verbalize these feelings with the rest of the family, because she thinks her mother will accuse her of not loving her brother or of wanting to kill him.

Questions

1. What should the nurse say to Mr. M's sister? What course of action could the nurse recommend?
2. What resources in the institution would be most helpful to this family at this time? Why?
3. How does the family's cultural and religious background influence its perspective on this situation?
4. What learning needs does this family have? How could these be most appropriately met?

SUMMARY

End-of-life care is challenging, but many nurses find it to be an extremely rewarding element of their practice. Making a positive difference in a person's life at this critical time requires skill, compassion, education, and self-awareness. Key dimensions of end-of-life care include alleviation of distressing symptoms (palliation); communication and conflict resolution; withdrawing, limiting, or withholding therapy; emotional and psychological care of the patient and family; and caregiver organizational support.

CRITICAL THINKING EXERCISES

1. When educating a family about the process of withdrawal of life support such as mechanical ventilation, what concepts are important to convey?
2. What is palliative care, and does it apply only to patients with a terminal illness?
3. The nurse assesses that there is significant disagreement among family members about what course of treatment is best for the patient. What action would be most effective in improving the situation?

REFERENCES

1. American Association of Colleges of Nursing. *End-of-Life Competency Statements for a Peaceful Death*. Washington, DC: Author; 2002.
2. Angus DC, Barnato AE, Linde-Zwirble WT, et al. Use of intensive care at the end of life in the United States: an epidemiologic study. *Critical Care Medicine*. 2004;32:638-643.
3. Barnato AE, Chang CC, Farrell MH, et al. Is survival better at hospitals with higher "end-of-life" treatment intensity? *Medical Care*. 2010;48:125-132.
4. Beckstrand RL, Callister LC, Kirchhoff KT. Providing a "good death:" critical care nurses' suggestions for improving end-of-life care. *American Journal of Critical Care*. 2006;15(1):38-46.
5. Beckstrand RL, Rawle NL, Callister L, et al. Pediatric nurses' perceptions of obstacles and supportive behaviours in end-of-life care. *American Journal of Critical Care*. 2010;19(6):543-552.
6. Boyd EA, Lo B, Evans LR, et al. "It's not just what the doctor tells me:" factors that influence surrogate decision-makers' perceptions of prognosis. *Critical Care Medicine*. 2010;38(5):1270-1275.
7. Boyle DK, Miller PA, Forbes-Thompson SA. Communication and end-of-life care in the intensive care unit. *Critical Care Nursing Quarterly*. 2005;28(4):302-316.
8. Campbell ML. Terminal dyspnea and respiratory distress. *Critical Care Clinics*, 2004;20(3):403-417.
9. Campbell ML. Palliative care consultation in the intensive care unit. *Critical Care Medicine*. 2006;34(11):S355-S358.
10. Cook D, Rocker G, Giacomini M, et al. Understanding and changing attitudes toward withdrawal and withholding of life support in the intensive care unit. *Critical Care Medicine*. 2006;34(11):S317-S323.
11. Crump SK, Schaffer MA, Schulte E. Critical care nurses' perceptions of obstacles, supports, and knowledge needed in providing quality end-of-life care. *Dimensions in Critical Care Nursing*. 2010;29(6):297-306.
12. Curtis JR. Interventions to improve care during withdrawal of life-sustaining treatments. *Journal of Palliative Medicine*. 2005;8(1):S116-S131.
13. Curtis JR, Engelberg RA. What is the "right" intensity of care at the end of life and how do we get there? *Annals of Internal Medicine*. 2011;154(4):283-285.
14. Dracup K, Bryan-Brown CW. Dying in the intensive care unit. *American Journal of Critical Care*. 2006;14:456-458.
15. Epstein EG, Delgado S. Understanding and addressing moral distress. *The Online Journal of Issues in Nursing*. 2010;15(3):Manuscript 1.
16. Fassier T, Lautrette A, Ciroldi M. Care at the end of life in critically ill patients: the European perspective. *Current Opinion in Critical Care*. 2005;11(6):616-623.
17. Field MJ, Cassel CK, eds. *Approaching death: improving care at the end of life*. Washington, D.C.: National Academy Press (Institute of Medicine); 1997.
18. Gavrin JR. Ethical considerations at the end of life in the intensive care unit. *Critical Care Medicine*. 2007;35(2):S85-S94.
19. Hanchate A, Kronman AC, Young-Xu Y, et al. Racial and ethnic differences in end-of-life costs: why do minorities cost more than whites? *Archives of Internal Medicine*. 2011;169(5):493-501.
20. Hansen L, Goodell TT, DeHaven J. Nurses' perceptions of end-of-life care after multiple interventions for improvement. *American Journal of Critical Care*. 2009;18(3):263-271.
21. Hamric AB, Blackhall LJ. Nurse-physician perspectives on the care of dying patients in intensive care units: collaboration, moral distress, and ethical climate. *Critical Care Medicine*. 2007;35(2):422-429.
22. Johnson RW, Newby LK, Granger CB, et al. Differences in level of care at the end of life according to race. *American Journal of Critical Care*. 2010;19(4):335-342.
23. Kaufman SR. *And a Time to Die: How American Hospitals Shape the End of Life*. New York: Simon & Schuster; 2005.
24. Kirchhoff KT, Kowalkowski JA. Current practices for withdrawal of life support in intensive care units. *American Journal of Critical Care*. 2010;19(6):532-541.
25. Kwak J, Haley WE. Current research findings on end-of-life decision making among racially or ethnically diverse groups. *The Gerontologist*. 2005;45(5):634-641.

26. Lamont EB. A demographic and prognostic approach to defining the end of life. *Journal of Palliative Medicine.* 2005;8(1):S12-S21.

27. Lampert R, Hayes DL, Annas GJ, et al. HRS expert consensus statement on the management of cardiovascular implantable electronic devices (CIEDs) in patients nearing end of life or requesting withdrawal of therapy. *Heart Rhythm.* 2010;7(7): 1008-1026.

28. Lanken P, Terry P, DeLisser H, et al. An official American Thoracic Society Clinical Policy Statement: Palliative Care for Patients with Respiratory Diseases and Critical Illnesses. *American Journal of Respiratory and Critical Care Medicine.* 2008;177:912-927.

29. Lautrette A, Darmon M, Megarbane B, et al. A communication strategy and brochure for relatives of patients dying in the ICU. *New England Journal of Medicine.* 2007;365(5):469-478.

30. Levy ML, McBride DL. End-of-life care in the intensive care unit: state of the art in 2006. S306-S308.

31. Lewis CL, Hanson LC, Golin C, et al. Surrogates' perceptions about feeding tube placement decisions. *Patient Education and Counseling.* 2006;61:246-252.

32. Luce JM. A history of resolving conflicts over end-of-life care in intensive care units in the United States. *Critical Care Medicine.* 2010;38(8):1623-1629.

33. McDonagh JR, Elliott TB, Engleberg RA, et al. Family satisfaction with family conferences about end-of-life care in the intensive care unit: increased proportion of family speech is associated with increased satisfaction. *Critical Care Medicine.* 2004;32(7):1484-1488.

34. Medina J, Puntillo K, eds. *AACN Protocols for Practice: Palliative Care and End-of-Life Issues in Critical Care.* Sudbury, MA: Jones and Bartlett; 2006.

35. Moore S, von Gunten C. Pulmonary/critical care physicians and hospice patients: billing specialty care for patients enrolled in a hospice program. *Chest.* 2010;137:1427-1431.

36. Mosenthal AC, Murphy PA. Interdisciplinary model for palliative care in the trauma and surgical intensive care unit: Robert Wood Johnson Foundation demonstration project for improving palliative care in the intensive care unit. *Critical Care Medicine.* 2006; 34(11):S399-S403.

37. Mularski RA, Curtis JR, Billings JA, et al. Proposed quality measures for palliative care in the critically ill: a consensus from the Robert Wood Johnson Foundation Critical Care Workgroup. *Critical Care Medicine.* 2006;34(11):S404-S411.

38. Nelson JE. Identifying and overcoming the barriers to high-quality palliative care in the intensive care unit. *Critical Care Medicine.* 2006;34(11):S324-S331.

39. Nelson JE, Bassett R, Boss RD, et al. Models for structuring a clinical initiative to enhance palliative care in the intensive care unit: a report from the IPAL-ICU Project (Improving Palliative Care in the ICU). *Critical Care Medicine.* 2006;38(9): 1765-1771.

40. Nelson JE, Angus DC, Weissfeld LA, et al. End-of-life care for the critically ill: a national intensive care unit survey. *Critical Care Medicine.* 2006;34:2547-2553.

41. Phelps AC, Jaciejewski PK, Nilsson M, et al. Religious coping and use of intensive life-prolonging care near death in patients with advanced cancer. *Journal of the American Medical Association.* 2009;301(11):1140-1147.

42. Phillips JL, Halcomb EJ, Davidson PM. End-of-life care pathways in acute and hospice care: an integrative review. *Journal of Pain and Symptom Management.* 2011;41(5):940-950.

43. Rocker GM, Heyland DK, Cook DJ, et al. Most critically ill patients are perceived to die in comfort during withdrawal of life support: a Canadian multicentre study. *Canadian Journal of Anaesthesia.* 2004;51:623-630.

44. Rubenfeld GD, Elliott M. Evidence-based ethics? *Current Opinion in Critical Care.* 2005;11:598-599.

45. Rushton CH. Defining and addressing moral distress. *AACN Advanced Critical Care.* 2006;17(2):161-168.

46. Scott SA. Life-support interventions at the end-of-life: unintended consequences. *The American Journal of Nursing.* 2010; 110(1):32-39.

47. Shalowitz DI, Garrett-Mayer E, Wendler D. The accuracy of surrogate decision makers. *Archives of Internal Medicine.* 2006; 166:493-497.

48. Shrank WH, Kutner JS, Richardson T, et al. Focus group findings about the influence of culture on communication preferences in end-of-life care. *Journal of General Internal Medicine.* 2005;20:703-709.

49. Siegel MD. Do you see what I see? Families, physicians, and prognostic dissonance in the intensive care unit. *Critical Care Medicine.* 2010;38(5):1381-1382.

50. Siriwardena AN, Clark DH. End-of-life care for ethnic minority groups. *Clinical Cornerstone.* 2004;6(1):43-48.

51. SUPPORT Principal Investigators. A controlled trial to improve care for seriously ill hospitalized patients: The Study to Understand Prognoses and Preferences for Outcomes and Risks of Treatments (SUPPORT). *Journal of the American Medical Association,* 2005;274(20):1591-1598.

52. Taylor RA, Alfred MV. Nurses' perceptions of the organizational supports needed for the delivery of culturally competent care. *Western Journal of Nursing Research.* 2010;32(5):591-609.

53. Thompson DR. Principles of ethics: in managing a critical care unit. *Critical Care Medicine.* 2007;35(2):S2-S10.

54. Tonelli MR. Waking the dying: must we always attempt to involve critically ill patients in end-of-life decisions? *Chest.* 2005; 127(2):637-642.

55. Treece PD, Engleberg RA, Shannon SE, et al. Integrating palliative and critical care: Description of an intervention. *Critical Care Medicine.* 2006;34(11):S380-S387.

56. Truog RD, Campbell ML, Curtis JR, et al. American Academy of Critical Care Medicine. Recommendations for end-of-life care in the intensive care unit: a consensus statement by the American College of Critical Care Medicine. *Critical Care Medicine.* 2006;36(3):953-963.

57. Truog RD, Meyer EC, Burns JP. Toward interventions to improve end-of-life care in the pediatric intensive care unit. *Critical Care Medicine.* 2006;34(11):S373-S379.

58. U.S. Census Bureau. *Overview of Race and Hispanic Origin: 2010.* http://www.census.gov/prod/cen2010/briefs/c2010br-02.pdf; 2010. Accessed May 30, 2011.

59. Wall RJ, Engelberg RA, Gries CJ, et al Spiritual care of families in the intensive care unit. *Critical Care Medicine.* 2007;35(4): 1084-1090.

60. Walling AM, Asch SM, Lorenz KA, et al. the quality of care provided to hospitalized patients at the end of life. *Archives of Internal Medicine.* 2010;170(12):1057-1063.

61. Wendler D, Rid A. Systematic review: the effect on surrogates of making treatment decisions for others. *Annals of Internal Medicine.* 2011;154(5):336-346.

62. West HR, Engleberg RA, Wenrich MD. Expressions of non-abandonment during the intensive care unit family conference. *Journal of Palliative Medicine.* 2005;8(4):797-807.

63. White DB, Curtis JR. Establishing an evidence base for physician-family communication and shared decision making in the intensive care unit. *Critical Care Medicine.* 2006;34(9):2500-2501.

64. White DB, Curtis JR, Lo B, et al. Decisions to limit life-sustaining treatment for critically ill patients who lack both decision-making capacity and surrogate decision-makers. *Critical Care Medicine.* 2006;34(8):2053-2059.

65. White DB, Engelberg RA, Wenrich MD, et al. Prognostica-tion during physician-family discussions about limiting life support in intensive care units. *Critical Care Medicine.* 2007;35(2):442-448.

66. Wlody GS. Nursing management and organizational ethics in the intensive care unit. *Critical Care Medicine.* 2007;35(2):S29-S35.

67. Wright AA, Zhang B, Ray A, et al. Associations between end-of-life discussions, patient mental health, medical care near death, and caregiver bereavement adjustment. *Journal of the American Medical Association.* 2008;300(14):1665-1673.

PART 2

Tools for the Critical Care Nurse

Comfort and Sedation

Mamoona Arif Rahu, PhD, RN, CCRN

evolve WEBSITE

Many additional resources, including self-assessment exercises, are located on the Evolve companion website at http://evolve.elsevier.com/Sole.

- Review Questions
- Mosby's Nursing Skills Procedures

- Animations
- Video Clips

INTRODUCTION

Maintaining an optimal level of comfort for the critically ill patient is a universal goal for physicians and nurses.[50] Patients in the critical care unit experience pain from preexisting diseases, invasive procedures, or trauma. Pain can also be caused by monitoring devices (catheters, drains), noninvasive ventilating devices, endotracheal tubes, routine nursing care (airway suctioning, dressing changes, and patient positioning), and prolonged immobility. It has been reported that 64% of patients recall having pain as a stressful experience during their critical care unit stay.[38]

Unrelieved pain may contribute to inadequate sleep, which may lead to exhaustion, anxiety, disorientation, and agitation. Patients who have recollections of their stay in the critical care unit cite pain (46%) and noise (40%) most frequently as concerns, and 22% complained of not getting enough pain medication. In addition, patients complain of sleeping problems (48%) related to noise (54%), fear (5%), and pain (21%).[46] Furthermore, 26% of critically ill patients experienced delusional memories such as dreams, hallucinations, nightmares, and the illusion that people were trying to hurt them.[100] Patients with memory of the critical care experience report development of posttraumatic stress disorder (PTSD) related to delusions, pain, and anxiety,[52] delirium,[103] sleep disturbance,[46] and uninterrupted sedative infusions.[59]

The patient's perception, expression, and tolerance of pain and anxiety may vary because of different psychological and social influences.[78] Evidence of ethnic differences in pain perception has also been reported.[73,95] Therefore it is important for healthcare providers to assess and manage pain and anxiety appropriately. Hospitals and healthcare accrediting agencies have recognized that pain and anxiety are major contributors to patient morbidity and length of stay. According to a National Patient Safety Goals Survey, pain assessment remains one of the top standards of noncompliance among hospitals (19%).[51] The Joint Commission requires that pain be assessed in "all patients" and that it be considered the "fifth vital sign." The Joint Commission also recommends that tools to evaluate pain should be specific to the age and disease state of the patient and to the site of pain.[51]

Promoting rest, comfort, and frequent reorientation are important nursing interventions to reduce pain and anxiety for a critically ill patient. The treatment of pain and anxiety should be individualized to the patient's needs for analgesia and sedation. Many critically ill patients have underlying chronic pain, thus making assessment and management more challenging. This chapter focuses on the assessment and management strategies for the critically ill patient experiencing acute pain, anxiety, or both.

DEFINITIONS OF PAIN AND ANXIETY

The International Association for the Study of Pain defines pain as an unpleasant sensory and emotional experience associated with actual or potential tissue damage, or described in terms of such damage.[48,76] McCartney[70] defines pain as "whatever the experiencing person says it is, existing whenever he says it does." Applying this definition, the patient becomes the true authority on the pain that is being experienced, and the patient's pain should be managed accordingly.

GATE CONTROL THEORY OF PAIN

Innocuous (nonpainful) stimuli transmitted by large afferent nerve fibers may prevent the transmission of painful stimuli. Stimulation of larger nerve fibers causes synapses in the dorsal horn of the spinal cord to cease firing, thus creating a "closed gate." A closed gate decreases the stimulation of trigger cells, decreases transmission of impulses, and diminishes pain perception. Persistent stimulation of the large fibers may allow for adaptation, allowing pain signals to reach the spinal cord and brain.

Modified from Huether SE. Pain, temperature regulation, sleep, and sensory function. In McCance KL & Huether SE, eds. *Pathophysiology: The Pathologic Basis for Disease in Adults and Children.* 6th ed. 481-521. St. Louis: Mosby; 2010.

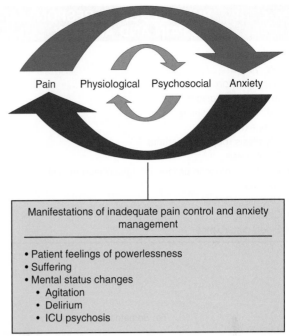

FIGURE 5-1 The anxiety-pain cycle. (From Cullen L, Greiner J, Titler MG. Pain management in the culture of critical care. *Critical Care Nursing Clinics of North America.* 2001;13[2]: 151-166.)

Many theoretical bases for the development of pain have been proposed. The gate control theory is the most widely used in research and therapy (Box 5-1).[47]

Anxiety is a state marked by apprehension, agitation, autonomic arousal, fearful withdrawal, or any combination of these.[70] It is a prolonged state of apprehension in response to a real or perceived fear. Anxiety must be assessed in the same way used to assess pain: the patient's level of anxiety is whatever the patient reports.

Pain and anxiety are often interrelated and may be difficult to differentiate because the physiological and behavioral findings are similar for each. The relationship between pain and anxiety is cyclical (Figure 5-1), with each exacerbating the other.[20] Inadequately treated pain leads to greater anxiety, and anxiety is associated with higher pain intensity. Anxiety may contribute to pain perception by activating pain pathways, altering the cognitive evaluation of pain, increasing aversion to pain, and increasing the report of pain.[20] If pain and anxiety are unresolved and escalate, the patient may experience feelings of powerlessness, suffering, and psychological changes, such as agitation and delirium. Anxiety is not a benign state, and unrelieved anxiety may lead to greater morbidity and mortality, especially in patients with cardiovascular disease. PTSD may occur after discharge from the critical care unit.[21,52,53]

Because interventions to manage pain may differ from those used to manage anxiety, the nurse must be astute about the patient's precipitating problem. If pain is being treated in a patient who is experiencing anxiety only, the anxiety may worsen while potentially ineffective management strategies are used. For example, the pharmacological agents used to treat pain have very different properties compared with those used to treat anxiety. Pain is managed with antiinflammatory and analgesic medications, whereas anxiety is treated with sedative medications.

PREDISPOSING FACTORS TO PAIN AND ANXIETY

Many factors inherent to the critical care environment place patients at risk of developing pain and anxiety. Pain perception may occur as a result of preexisting diseases, invasive procedures, monitoring devices, nursing care, or trauma. The perception of pain is also influenced by the expectation of pain, prior pain experiences, a patient's emotional state, and the cognitive processes of the patient.[14] Although pain perception involves conscious experience, new evidence shows a higher prevalence of pain in adult patients with impaired cortical function or cortical immaturity during early development in children.[12,75] Yet, these vulnerable populations receive fewer analgesics as compared with patients with intact cognitive function.[17,58]

Anxiety is likely to result from the inability to communicate; the continuous noise of alarms, equipment, and personnel; bright ambient lighting; and excessive stimulation from inadequate analgesia, frequent assessments, repositioning, lack of mobility, and uncomfortable room temperature. Sleep deprivation and the circumstances that resulted in an admission to the critical care unit may also increase patient anxiety. Intubated patients receiving mechanical ventilation experience moderate levels of anxiety.[16]

PHYSIOLOGY OF PAIN AND ANXIETY

Pain

All pain results from a signal cascade within the body's neurological network. Pain is initiated by signals that travel through the peripheral nervous system to the central nervous system for processing.[23] Pain can be classified as acute or chronic, malignant or nonmalignant, and nociceptive or neuropathic. In all forms of acute pain, the sympathetic nervous

BOX 5-2	PHYSIOLOGICAL RESPONSES TO PAIN AND ANXIETY

- Tachycardia
- Tachypnea
- Hypertension
- Increased cardiac output
- Pallor and/or flushing
- Cool extremities
- Mydriasis (pupillary dilation)
- Diaphoresis
- Increased glucose production (gluconeogenesis)
- Nausea
- Urinary retention
- Constipation
- Sleep disturbance

system (SNS) is usually activated quickly, and several physiological responses typically occur (Box 5-2). In contrast, some forms of chronic pain may result in less activation of the SNS and a different clinical presentation.

The sensation of pain is carried to the central nervous system by activation of two separate pathways (Figure 5-2). The fast (sharp) pain signals are transmitted to the spinal cord by slowly conducting, thinly myelinated A-delta afferent fibers. A-delta fibers are activated by high-intensity physical (hot and cold) stimuli that are important in initiating rapid reactions. Conversely, slow (burning; chronic) pain is transmitted by the unmyelinated, polymodal C fibers, which are activated by a variety of high-intensity mechanical, chemical, hot, and cold stimuli.[56]

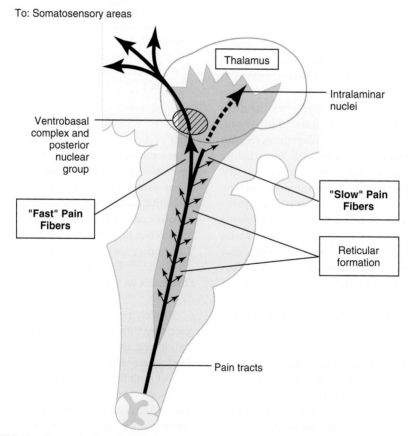

FIGURE 5-2 Transmission of pain signals into the brainstem, thalamus, and cerebral cortex by way of the "fast" pain pathway and "slow" pain pathway. (From Guyton A, Hall J. *Textbook of Medical Physiology.* 12th ed. Philadelphia: Saunders; 2011.)

The most abundant receptors in the nervous system for pain recognition are nociceptors whose cell bodies are located in the dorsal root ganglia.[56] The sensation of pain received by peripheral endings of sensory neurons is called *nociception.* The nociceptive pain is divided into somatic and visceral. Nociceptive pain is detected by specialized transducers attached to A-delta and C fibers. *Somatic pain* results from irritation or damage to the nervous system. *Visceral pain* is diffuse, poorly localized, and often referred.[56]

Mechanical, chemical, and thermal stimuli activate nociceptors to produce a painful sensation. Examples of mechanical stimuli include a crushing injury or a surgical wound. A chemical stimulus is any substance that produces skin irritation, and burn injury is a thermal stimulus for pain. Identifying the correct pain-inducing stimulus is important in the effective management of pain. Removal of the stimulus should always precede other treatment measures in managing pain.[41]

Nociceptors differ from other nerve receptors in the body in that they adapt very little to the pain response. If the stimulus for pain is not removed, the body continues to experience pain until the stimulus is discontinued, or other interventions (e.g., analgesic agents) are initiated. This is a protective mechanism so the body tissues being damaged will be removed from harm.

Nociceptors usually lie near capillary beds and mast cells. When tissue injury occurs, the nociceptor initiates an inflammatory response near the injured capillary.[32,72,79] The mast cells in the damaged tissues degranulate, releasing histamine and chemotactic agents that promote infiltration of injured tissues with neutrophils and eosinophils. As neutrophils move into the site of injury, more neurotransmitter-like substances (acetylcholine, bradykinins, substance P, and enkephalins) are released from the neutrophils into the surrounding tissue. These substances act as mediators and may induce or suppress pain. Endogenous cytokines that suppress pain induction are commonly referred to as the *endorphins.*

Advances in neuroimaging studies have identified a more complex level of processing of pain in the human cerebral cortex. The neuroimaging studies have identified multiple nociceptive pathways that deliver parallel inputs to somatosensory, limbic, and associative structures.[4,63] These techniques (Table 5-1) allow noninvasive examination of brain mechanisms involved in acute and chronic pain processing.

Anxiety

The physiology of anxiety is less clearly understood in comparison with pain and is a more complex process because no actual tissue injury is thought to occur. Anxiety stimulates the SNS response.

Anxiety has been linked to the reward and punishment centers within the limbic system of the brain. Stimulation in the punishment centers frequently inhibits the reward centers completely.[41] The punishment center is also responsible for helping a person escape from potentially harmful situations. The punishment center has dominance over the reward center for the person to escape harm.

POSITIVE EFFECTS OF PAIN AND ANXIETY

In the healthy person, pain and anxiety are adaptive mechanisms used to increase mental and physical performance levels to allow a person to move away from potential harm. When the SNS is activated, the person usually becomes more vigilant of the environment, especially to potential dangers. Once dangers are recognized, the person makes a choice whether to flee the situation or combat the possible threat. For this reason, SNS activation is known as the "fight-or-flight" response.

TABLE 5-1	NEUROIMAGING STUDIES	
METHOD	**APPLICATION IN PAIN STUDIES**
Functional magnetic resonance imaging (fMRI)	Localizing brain activity
Electroencephalography (EEG); Magnetoencephalography (MEG)	Detecting temporal sequences and measuring neuronal activity
Single photon emission computed tomography (SPECT) Positron emission tomography (PET)	Identifying neurotransmitter systems and drug uptake
Magnetic resonance (MR) spectroscopy	Detecting long-term changes in brain chemistry

Data from Apkarian AV, Bushnell MC, Treede RD, et al. Human brain mechanisms of pain perception and regulation in health and disease. *European Journal of Pain.* 2005;9:463-484.

NEGATIVE EFFECTS OF PAIN AND ANXIETY

Physical Effects

Both pain and anxiety activate the SNS. Catecholamine levels increase, which may place a significant burden on the cardiovascular system, especially in a critically ill patient. Activation of the SNS results in tachycardia and hypertension, which leads to increased myocardial oxygen demand. In patients with a history of cardiovascular disease, anxiety is associated with recurrent cardiac events and increased mortality. Patients with silent myocardial infarction do not experience chest pain and therefore do not seek immediate medical treatment.[39] These patients are also at high risk for increased morbidity and mortality.

The physiological response to stress also interferes with the healing process and impairs perfusion and oxygen delivery to tissue.[10] Hemodynamic instability, immunosuppression, and tissue catabolism may also occur.[117] Any large organ that experiences an increase in oxygen consumption places the critically ill patient at risk of increased rates of complications related to end organ ischemia.[67]

Hyperventilation (tachypnea) secondary to pain and anxiety can be stressful to the patient because rapid breathing requires significant effort with the use of accessory muscles. Hyperventilation may cause respiratory alkalosis. Respiratory alkalosis may result in impaired tissue perfusion, and many vasoactive medications become less effective.

If the patient is mechanically ventilated, an increased respiratory rate leads to feelings of breathlessness. As the patient "fights" the mechanical ventilator (dyssynchrony), further alveolar damage ensues, and the endotracheal or tracheostomy tube creates a "choking" sensation and increased anxiety. Anxiety has been linked to dyspnea and delayed ventilator weaning.[105]

Psychological Effects

Many patients in the critical care unit report feelings of panic and fear. Pain and anxiety exacerbate reports of lack of sleep, nightmares, and feelings of bewilderment, isolation, and loneliness. The effects of a critical care unit stay may persist long after discharge, and many patients develop PTSD as a result of their critical care unit experience.[52]

Extreme anxiety, pain, and adverse effects of medications can also lead to agitation, which is commonly seen in the critically ill patient. Agitation is associated with inappropriate verbal behavior, physical aggression, increased movement (head or extremities), and ventilator dyssynchrony, any of which may harm the patient or caregiver.[30,49,113] The failure to manage agitation may have severe consequences, such as a higher rate of self-extubation and self-removal of catheters and invasive lines, a higher rate of nosocomial infections, and a longer duration of stay; agitated patients also require extra resources for their care.[49]

ASSESSMENT

Quality pain management begins with a thorough assessment, ongoing reassessment, and documentation to facilitate treatment and communication among health care providers.[37] The American Pain Society guidelines recommend a five-step hierarchy approach to pain measures[37,88]:

- Pain should be assessed and treated promptly in all patients. Pain assessment and documentation should be clearly communicated with other healthcare providers.
- The patient should be actively engaged in the pain management plan.
- Healthcare providers need to preemptively treat patients with analgesics to safely, effectively, and equitably manage pain.
- Pain should be reassessed and treatment adjusted to meet the patient's needs.
- Healthcare facilities need to establish a comprehensive quality improvement program that monitors both healthcare provider practice and patient outcomes.

Pain assessment is challenging in patients who cannot communicate; these patients represent the majority of critically ill patients. Factors that alter verbal communication in critically ill patients include endotracheal intubation, altered level of consciousness, restraints, sedation, and therapeutic paralysis[6] (see box, "Evidence-Based Practice").

The American Pain Society guidelines mandate evaluation of both physiological and behavioral response to pain in patients who are unable to communicate.[45] At present, no universally accepted pain scale for use in the noncommunicative (cognitively impaired, sedated, paralyzed, or mechanically ventilated) patient exists.[50] Optimal pain assessment in adult critical care settings is essential because it has been reported that nurses underrate the patient's pain.[1,2,43,92] Nurses often undermedicate the critically ill patient as well. One study reported that more than 60% of critically ill patients did not receive any medications before and/or during painful procedures such as central line insertions, wound dressing changes, and suctioning.[94] Inaccurate pain assessments and resulting inadequate treatment of pain in critically ill adults can lead to significant physiological consequences.

Assessment involves the collection of the patient's self-report of the pain experience as well as behavioral markers. If a patient is able to respond, nurses can ask the patient to describe the pain or anxiety being experienced, or to provide a numerical score to indicate the level of pain or anxiety. In addition, behavioral or physiological cues of pain can be observed. For example, increased blood pressure or a facial grimace or frown may indicate pain or anxiety. Typical physiological responses related to pain are detailed in Box 5-2. In the healthy person, these responses are adaptive mechanisms and result from activation of the SNS to prepare the individual for the fight-or-flight response. In the critically ill patient, these changes may induce further stress in an already compromised individual.

EVIDENCE-BASED PRACTICE
Are Facial Expressions a Reliable Indicator of Pain?

Problem
Assessing pain in critically ill patients who are unable to communicate is challenging. Nurses rely on objective assessment of the patient's expressions, responses to painful stimuli, and physiological parameters, such as heart rate and blood pressure.

Clinical Question
Does nursing assessment of facial expressions in patients who are unable to communicate provide a reliable indicator of pain?

Evidence
The authors conducted an extensive review of the literature to examine the study of facial expression and its application as a pain assessment tool in critically ill patients who are unable to communicate. They summarized the reliability and validity of various pain assessment tools that incorporate assessment of facial expression. The tools include a variety of facial behaviors—wincing, frowning, and grimacing—but scoring of these behaviors varies widely. The Facial Action Coding System (FACS) identifies facial muscle movement during a response, such as pain. It is a reliable method for assessing pain in adults, but its utility has not been tested in critically ill patients. No single tool was identified as a superior method of assessing pain responses.

Implications for Nursing
Many critically ill patients are unable to communicate because of intubation, a decreased level of consciousness, or both. Assessment of pain in these individuals is an important yet challenging component of nursing care. Evaluating facial expressions that may indicate pain is one component of a comprehensive pain assessment, but cannot be used as the sole indicator of presence or absence of pain. Assessment of wincing, frowning, and grimacing are included in many critical care pain assessment tools. Additional knowledge gained by studying FACS in critically ill patients who are unable to communicate is needed.

Level of Evidence
C—Descriptive studies

Reference
Arif-Rahu M, Grap MJ. Facial expression and pain in the critically ill non-communicative patient: state of science review. *Intensive and Critical Care Nursing.* 2010;26:343-352.

As part of the assessment of pain and anxiety, the nurse must be aware of what procedures may cause pain, and evaluate the effectiveness of interventions to prevent or relieve pain and anxiety.[93] When patients exhibit signs of anxiety or agitation, the assessment also includes identification and treatment of the potential cause, such as hypoxemia, hypoglycemia, hypotension, pain, and withdrawal from alcohol and drugs. When possible, patients should be asked about any herbal remedies used as complementary and alternative medical therapies and whether they take them along with prescription or over-the-counter medications.[13,112] These products may lead to adverse herb-drug interactions, especially in the elderly who are more likely to be taking multiple drugs.[13,68,125]

Pain Measurement Tools

In the assessment of pain, the nurse asks the patient to identify several characteristics associated with the pain. These characteristics include the precipitating cause, severity, location (including radiation to other sites), duration, and any alleviating or aggravating factors. Any pain assessment should address these pain characteristics or the assessment is incomplete. Patients with chronic pain conditions, such as arthritis, may be able to provide a detailed list of effective pain remedies that may be useful to implement.

Several tools are available to ensure that the appropriate pain assessment questions are asked. One tool used in assessing the patient with chest pain is the PQRST method. The PQRST method is a mnemonic the nurse can use to ensure that all chest pain characteristics are documented.

P—*Provocation or position.* What precipitated the chest pain symptoms, and where in the chest area is the pain located?

Q—*Quality.* Is the pain sharp, dull, crushing?

R—*Radiation.* Does the pain travel to other parts of the body?

S—*Severity or symptoms associated with the pain.* The patient is asked to rate the pain on a numerical scale and to describe what other symptoms are present.

T—*Timing or triggers* for the pain. Is the pain constant or intermittent, and does it occur with certain activities?

One of the most common methods to determine pain severity is to ask for a pain score. Patients are asked to rate their pain on a numbered scale such as 0 to 10. A score of 0 indicates no pain, and a score of 10 indicates the worst pain the patient could possibly imagine. The pain score is reassessed after medications or other pain-relieving measures have been provided. Institutional policy provides guidelines for the method and frequency of pain assessment. Some institutions require nurses to intervene for a pain score greater than a predesignated number. The pain score method should be used only with patients who are cognitively aware of their surroundings and are able to follow simple commands. It is possible for patients with mild to moderate dementia to self-report pain, but this ability decreases with progression of the disease.[45] Numeric rating is not an appropriate method to assess pain in patients who are disoriented or have severe cognitive impairment.

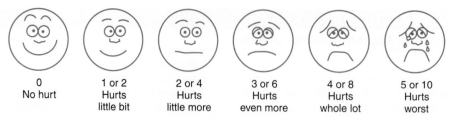

| 0 No hurt | 1 or 2 Hurts little bit | 2 or 4 Hurts little more | 3 or 6 Hurts even more | 4 or 8 Hurts whole lot | 5 or 10 Hurts worst |

FIGURE 5-3 A version of the FACES scale. (From Hockenberry M, Wilson D. *Wong's Essentials of Pediatric Nursing.* 8th ed. St. Louis: Mosby; 2009.)

A second tool is known as the FACES Pain Scale. Patients are asked to describe how they feel by pointing to a series of faces ranging from happy to distressed (Figure 5-3). The FACES method involves a higher level of emotional intellect because the patient must be able to accurately process different yet similar visual stimuli.[64] The most common versions of the FACES scale use between five and seven different images.

Another widely used subjective pain measurement tool is the visual analog scale (VAS). The VAS is a 10-cm line that looks similar to a timeline. The scale may be drawn horizontally or vertically, and it may or may not be numbered. If numbered, 0 indicates no pain, whereas 10 indicate the most pain (Figure 5-4). When using the VAS, the nurse holds up the scale, and the patient points to the level of pain on the line. If the patient is able to communicate in writing, the patient can place an "X" on the VAS with a pencil. The VAS can also be used to evaluate a patient's level of anxiety, with 0 representing no anxiety and 10 the most anxiety. The VAS must only be used with patients who are alert and able to follow directions.

Pain Measurement Tools for Nonverbal Patients

Identification of the optimal pain scales for noncommunicative patients has been the focus of several studies. To date, no one tool is universally accepted for use in this patient population.[44] Assessment of pain intensity may be quantified by using the behavioral-physiological scales.

Several behavioral pain tools are available to assess critically ill adult patients. Widely used and validated, the behavioral pain scale was developed to assess pain in the critically ill adult who is nonverbal and unable to communicate (Table 5-2).[90] The Behavioral Pain Scale provides critical care nurses with an objective and reliable pain measurement tool.[90,91] It is designed to be used for the mechanically ventilated patient and therefore may not be appropriate in other patients.

Another behavioral pain tool is the Critical-Care Pain Observation Tool (Table 5-3). It was initially validated in cardiac surgery patients and most recently in other critically ill patients.[33-35,126] The Critical-Care Pain Observation Tool is appropriate for the assessment of patients with or without an endotracheal tube.

The Checklist of Nonverbal Pain Indicators[27,29,84] provides a good indicator of the patient's distress by looking for pain-related behaviors. The tool was initially developed because of concerns that some of the cognitively impaired patients are not able to respond reliably to the yes/no questions about pain. This tool showed no significant differences in observed pain behaviors between the cognitively impaired group and the cognitively intact group. The Checklist of Nonverbal Pain Indicators has been tested in acute and long-term care settings to assess acute and chronic pain in elderly patients.[29,84]

The Faces, Legs, Activity, Cry, Consolability (FLACC) Behavioral Scale has been widely used in the pediatric setting. Researchers have recently tested the applicability of the FLACC in the adult population and suggest that it may be useful in the critically ill patient[127] (see box, "QSEN Exemplar").

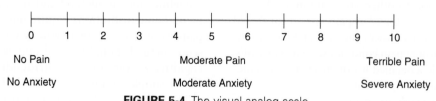

| 0 | 1 | 2 | 3 | 4 | 5 | 6 | 7 | 8 | 9 | 10 |

No Pain   Moderate Pain   Terrible Pain

No Anxiety   Moderate Anxiety   Severe Anxiety

FIGURE 5-4 The visual analog scale.

TABLE 5-2   THE BEHAVIORAL PAIN SCALE*

ITEM	DESCRIPTION	SCORE
Facial expression	Relaxed	1
	Partially tightened (e.g., brow lowering)	2
	Fully tightened (e.g., eyelid closing)	3
	Grimacing	4
Upper limbs	No movement	1
	Partially bent	2
	Fully bent with finger flexion	3
	Permanently retracted	4
Compliance with ventilation	Tolerating movement	1
	Coughing but tolerating ventilation most of the time	2
	Fighting ventilator	3
	Unable to control ventilation	4

*Each of the categories—facial expression, upper limbs, and compliance with ventilation—is scored from 1 to 4. The values are added together for a total score between 3 and 12.
From Payen JF, Bru O, Bosson JL, et al. Assessing pain in critically ill sedated patients by using a behavioral pain scale. *Critical Care Medicine*. 2001;29(12):2258-2263.

TABLE 5-3   CRITICAL-CARE PAIN OBSERVATION TOOL

INDICATOR	SCORE
Facial Expression	
• Relaxed, no muscle tension	0
• Tense facial muscles (brow lowering, orbit tightening, and levator contraction)	1
• Grimacing with tense facial muscles	2
Body Movements	
• Absence of movements	0
• Protection	1
• Restlessness	2
Muscle Tension in Upper Extremities	
• Relaxed	0
• Tense, rigid	1
• Very tense or rigid	2
Compliance with the Ventilator	
• Tolerating ventilator or movement	0
• Coughing but tolerating ventilator	1
• Fighting ventilator	2
Nonventilator, Vocalization	
• No sound	0
• Sighing, moaning	1
• Crying out, sobbing	2
Total Score	—

Data from Gelinas C, Fillion L, Puntillo KA, et al. Validation of the critical-care pain observation tool in adult patients. *American Journal of Critical Care*. 2006;15:420-427.

QSEN EXEMPLAR

Patient Centered Care, Evidence-Based Practice

Pain assessment is challenging in the critical care setting because of the physical and cognitive impairments of many critically ill patients, and impediments to communication such as intubation.[1] Critical care nurses commonly use behavioral observations and vital signs as primary assessment data when developing pain relief strategies and comfort-promoting interventions. The Face, Legs, Activity, Cry, Consolability (FLACC) behavioral scale is a five-item instrument that may be useful for assessing pain in critically ill patients. The tool is simple to score and provides a pain rating on a traditional 0 to 10 scale. The instrument includes items that have been previously validated as pain indicators in children, cognitively impaired adults, and critically ill adults. A prospective, observational study was conducted to evaluate the validity and reliability of the FLACC scale in a sample of critically ill adults and children. Criterion validity, construct validity, internal consistency reliability, and interrater reliability were reported. The authors suggest that the FLACC scale may be useful in a variety of patient populations, and it generates an easy-to-use pain assessment score. Further study of easy-to-use pain assessment instruments remains a priority in critical care nursing.

Reference
Voepel-Lewis T, Zanotti J, Dammeyer JA, et al. Reliability and validity of the Face, Legs, Activity, Cry, Consolability (FLACC) behavioral tool in assessing acute pain in critically ill patients. *American Journal of Critical Care*. 2010;19:55-61.

Anxiety and Sedation Measurement Tools
Sedation Scales

No objective tool is considered the gold standard for determining a patient's level of anxiety. Anxiety typically produces hyperactive psychomotor functions including tachycardia, hypertension, and movement. Patients are typically sedated to limit this hyperactivity. The level of sedation can be measured by using objective tools or scales. An ideal sedation scale provides data that are simple to compute and record, accurately describe the degree of sedation or agitation within well-defined categories, guide the titration of therapy, and are valid and reliable in critically ill patients.[50]

When administering medications to sedate a patient, the goal is to achieve a level of sedation with the lowest dose. By using lower doses of medications, the patient is less likely to experience drug accumulation or adverse effects. These adverse effects include increased hospital stay, delayed ventilator weaning, immobility, and increased rates of ventilator-associated pneumonia. Conversely, not enough sedation may lead to agitation, inappropriate use of paralytics, increased metabolic demand, and an increased risk of myocardial ischemia.[71] Sedation scales assist in the accurate identification and communication of sedation level. The most frequently used sedation scales are the Richmond Agitation-Sedation Scale (RASS),[108] the Ramsay Sedation Scale,[96] and the Sedation-Agitation Scale.[99]

The RASS is a 10-point scale, from 4 (combative) through 0 (calm, alert) to −5 (unarousable). The patient is assessed for 30 to 60 seconds in three steps, using discreet criteria (Table 5-4). The RASS has strong interrater reliability, is useful in detecting changes in sedation status over consecutive days of critical care unit care, and correlates with the administered dose of sedative and analgesic medications.[26,109]

The Ramsay Sedation Scale was developed for evaluation of postoperative patients emerging from general anesthesia.[96] The scale includes three levels of wakefulness and three levels of sedation (Table 5-5). The nurse makes a visual and cognitive assessment of the patient. Scores range from 1 (awake) to 6 (asleep/unarousable).

The Sedation-Agitation Scale (Table 5-6) describes patient behaviors seen in the continuum of sedation to agitation.[99] Scores range from 1 (unarousable) to 7 (dangerously agitated).

The appropriate target level of sedation depends on the patient's disease process and therapeutic or support interventions required. A common target level of sedation is a calm patient who is easily aroused; however, deeper levels of sedation may be needed to facilitate mechanical ventilation. To optimize patient comfort and minimize distress, a structured approach to sedation management includes: frequent assessments for pain, anxiety, and agitation using a reproducible scale; combination therapy coupling opioids and sedatives that is best suited to patient characteristics, including the presence of organ dysfunction that may influence drug metabolism or excessive risk for side effects; and careful communication between multiprofessional team members, including physician, nurse, and pharmacist, with a particular recognition that the bedside nurse must be empowered to pair assessments with drug manipulation.[106,110,111]

TABLE 5-4	RICHMOND AGITATION-SEDATION SCALE (RASS)	
TERM		**SCORE**
Combative		+4
Very agitated		+3
Agitated		+2
Restless		+1
Alert and calm		0
Drowsy—sustains (>10 sec) awakening, with eye contact to voice*		−1
Light sedation—sustains (<10 sec) awakening with eye contact to voice*		−2
Moderate sedation—any movement (but no eye contact) to voice*		−3
Deep sedation—no response to voice, but any movement to physical stimulation*		−4
Unarousable		−5

*In a loud voice, state patient's name and direct patient to open eyes and look at speaker.
From Sessler CN, Gosnell MS, Grap MJ, et al. The Richmond Agitation-Sedation Scale: Validity and reliability in adult intensive care unit patients. *American Journal of Respiratory and Critical Care Medicine.* 2002;166:1338-1344.

TABLE 5-5	THE RAMSAY SEDATION SCALE
LEVEL	**SCALE**
1	Patient awake, anxious and agitated or restless, or both
2	Patient awake, cooperative, oriented, and tranquil
3	Patient awake; response to commands only
4	Patient asleep; brisk response to light glabellar tap or loud auditory stimulus
5	Patient asleep; sluggish response to light glabellar tap or loud auditory stimulus
6	Patient asleep; no response to light glabellar tap or loud auditory stimulus

From Ramsay MA, Savege TM, Simpson BR, et al. Controlled sedation with alphaxalone-alphadolone. *British Medical Journal.* 1974;2(90):656-659.

TABLE 5-6	SEDATION-AGITATION SCALE	
SCORE	CHARACTERISTIC	EXAMPLES OF PATIENT'S BEHAVIOR
7	Dangerously agitated	Pulls at endotracheal tube, tries to remove catheters, climbs over bed rail, strikes at staff, thrashes from side to side
6	Very agitated	Does not calm despite frequent verbal reminding of limits, requires physical restraints, bites endotracheal tube
5	Agitated	Anxious or mildly agitated, attempts to sit up, calms down in response to verbal instructions
4	Calm and cooperative	Calm, awakens easily, follows commands
3	Sedated	Difficult to arouse, awakens to verbal stimuli or gentle shaking but drifts off again, follows simple commands
2	Very sedated	Arouses to physical stimuli but does not communicate or follow commands, may move spontaneously
1	Unarousable	Minimal or no response to noxious stimuli, does not communicate or follow commands

From Riker RR, Fraser GL, Simmons LE, et al. Validating the Sedation-Agitation Scale with the Bispectral Index and Visual Analog Scale in adult ICU patients after cardiac surgery. *Intensive Care Medicine.* 2001;27(5):853-858.

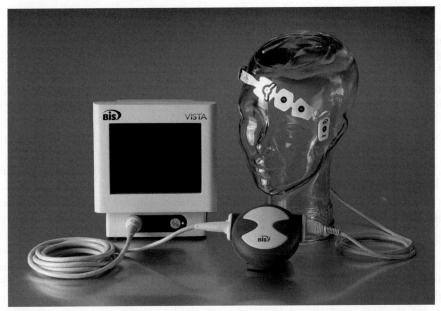

FIGURE 5-5 The Bispectral Index (BIS) monitor and electrode. (Image used by permission of Nellcor Puritan Bennett LLC, Boulder, Colorado, doing business as Covidien.)

Continuous Monitoring of Sedation

No technological device provides the bedside nurse with an absolute measurement of the patient's pain or anxiety. Various devices may be used to measure a patient's level of consciousness by assessing the patient's brain activity.

The electroencephalogram (EEG) records spontaneous brain activity that originates from the cortical pyramidal cells on the surface of the brain by placing electrodes on patient's head. Any major brain activity produces a peak in activity on the EEG monitor. In the critical care unit, the EEG is used infrequently to assess levels of sedation because it takes significant time (up to 60 minutes) to properly place electrodes, and a high level of skill is required to interpret the EEG recording.

However, devices that monitor continuous EEG signals without using the traditional 21-electrode system are frequently used to assess levels of sedation in the critically ill patient. These devices digitize the raw EEG signal and apply a complex algorithm that results in a numeric score ranging from 0 (iso-electric EEG) to 100 (fully awake).[31] The EEG generally changes from a low-amplitude, high-frequency signal while the patient is awake to a high-amplitude, low-frequency signal when the patient is deeply anesthetized.[7] Examples of such devices are the Bispectral Index Score (BIS) monitor (Aspect Medical Systems, Newton, MA) and the Patient State Index (PSI) Analyzer (Physiometrix, North Billerica, MA). The resulting score provides an objective analysis of the level of wakefulness resulting from agitation or pain.[35,60]

To obtain a signal, an electrode is placed across the patient's forehead and is attached to a monitor. The monitor displays the raw EEG and the BIS or PSI value. The BIS monitor and electrode are shown in Figure 5-5. A value greater than 90 typically indicates full consciousness, a score of 40 to 60 represents deep sedation, and a score of 0 represents complete EEG suppression. A BIS value of greater than 60 is associated with patient awareness and recollection. A BIS value of less than 60 should be the goal in critically ill patients who require sedation.[31,55] Several studies have found strong correlation with BIS in assessment of sedation level and the RASS in the ICU.[55,121] For adequate sedation (RASS value of 0 to −3), the median BIS value was found to be 56.[55,121]

A score is usually documented with each set of vital signs. When using BIS or PSI monitoring, results must be correlated with the patient's clinical assessment and correct electrode placement. All muscle activity may not be completely filtered, which may affect the value. These devices are especially useful for critically ill patients who are treated with medications that produce deep sedation or neuromuscular blockade. They provide a continuous evaluation of sedation that may also be less affected by rater bias. When used with standardized sedation protocols, BIS is highly correlated with sedation scale (RASS)[55] and pain scale (Critical-Care Pain Observation Tool).[35] However, care must be taken when evaluating the BIS scores, as some patients with greater facial muscle activities during routine care or procedures may overestimate BIS scores.[35] Therefore BIS may not be ideal as a single method of sedation assessment in the critically ill.

Pain and Anxiety Assessment Challenges

Many situations may lead to an incomplete assessment and/or management of pain or anxiety. These include delirium and the administration of neuromuscular blocking (NMB) agents.

Delirium

A relationship exists among acute delirium, pain, and anxiety. Delirium (acute brain dysfunction) is characterized by an acutely changing or fluctuating mental status, inattention, disorganized thinking, and altered levels of consciousness as defined by the Diagnostic and Statistical Manual of Mental Disorders-IV.[81] Acute delirium is common in critically ill patients; more than 70% to 80% of patients develop some form of delirium, resulting in longer duration of mechanical ventilation and longer ICU stay than those without delirium.[86,116]

Delirium is categorized according to the level of alertness and level of psychomotor activity. It is divided into three clinical subtypes: hyperactive, hypoactive, and mixed (Table 5-7). Patients with *hyperactive delirium* are agitated, combative, and disoriented.[81,86,120] These patients place themselves or others at risk for injury because of their altered thought processes and resultant behaviors.[4] Psychotic features such as hallucinations, delusions, and paranoia may be seen. Patients may believe that members of the nursing or medical staff are attempting to harm them.

Hypoactive delirium is often referred to as quiet delirium and often goes undiagnosed and underestimated when there is no active monitoring with a validated clinical instrument; it is also the most prevalent, occurring in more than 60% of patients.[86] The *mixed subtype* describes the fluctuating

TABLE 5-7	**CLINICAL SUBTYPES OF DELIRIUM**
SUBTYPE	**CHARACTERISTICS**
Hyperactive	Agitation Restlessness Attempts to remove catheters or tubes Hitting Biting Emotional lability
Hypoactive	Withdrawal Flat affect Apathy Lethargy Decreased responsiveness
Mixed	Concurrent or sequential appearance of some features of both hyperactive and hypoactive delirium

From Truman B, Ely EW. Monitoring delirium in critically ill patients: using the confusion assessment method for the intensive care unit. *Critical Care Nurse.* 2003;23(2):25-36.

nature of delirium. Some agitated patients with hyperactive delirium may receive sedatives to calm them, and then may emerge from sedation in a hypoactive state; this subtype occurs in about 6% of patients. Pure hyperactive delirium is rare, occurring in less than 1% of patients.[86]

The exact pathophysiological mechanisms involved with the development and progression of delirium are unknown. However, they may be related to imbalances in the neurotransmitters that modulate the control of cognitive function, behavior, and mood.[120] Risk factors for the development of delirium include hypoxemia, metabolic disturbances, electrolyte imbalances, head trauma, the presence of catheters and drains, and certain medications. Neurotransmitter levels are affected by medications with anticholinergic properties. Benzodiazepines, opioids, and other psychotropic medications are associated with an increased risk of developing delirium (Box 5-3), yet these medications are commonly given to critically ill patients.

Since delirium occurs in many patients receiving mechanical ventilation and is independently associated with more deaths, longer hospital stays, and higher costs, all critically ill patients should be assessed for delirium.[25,50,118] Older patients are especially at risk for delirium.[8] Delirium may be assessed in critical care settings by nonpsychiatrists. Two of the most frequently used validated instruments are the Confusion Assessment Method for the ICU (CAM-ICU)[20] and the Intensive Care Delirium Screening Checklist (ICDSC).[9] The CAM-ICU (Box 5-4) is designed to be a serial assessment tool for use by bedside nurses and physicians. It is easy to use, takes only 2 minutes to complete, and requires minimal training.[120] A patient is considered delirium positive in CAM-ICU if the following are present: criteria 1 (acute mental status change) and 2 (inattention), and either 3 (disorganized thinking) or 4 (altered level of consciousness).

Similarly, the ICDSC is a screening checklist of eight items based on Diagnostic and Statistical Manual of Mental Disorders (DSM) criteria (Table 5-8). After consciousness is

BOX 5-3 RISK FACTORS FOR DELIRIUM

- Older than 70 years
- Transfer from a nursing home
- History of depression, dementia, stroke
- Alcohol or substance abuse
- Electrolyte imbalance
- Hypothermia or fever
- Renal failure
- Liver disease
- Cardiogenic or septic shock
- Human immunodeficiency virus infection
- Rectal or bladder catheters
- Tube feedings
- Central venous catheters
- Malnutrition
- Presence of physical restraints
- Visual or hearing impairment

Modified from Truman B, Ely EW. Monitoring delirium in critically ill patients: using the confusion assessment method for the intensive care unit. *Critical Care Nurse.* 2003;23(2):25-36.

assessed and rated on a scale of A through E, the patient is assessed for seven indicators of delirium. One point is given for each positive sign of delirium that is identified. The scores range from 0 to 8 points, and a patient with more than 4 points is defined as delirium positive.

Management of delirium focuses on keeping the patient safe. The least restrictive measures are used because unnecessary use of restraints or medication may precipitate or exacerbate delirium. Splints or binders may be needed to restrict movement if the patient is pulling at catheters, drains, or dressings. Any type of tubing should be removed as soon as possible, particularly nasogastric tubes, which are irritating to agitated patients.[54] If these measures are not successful, medication may be necessary to improve cognition, not to sedate the patient. Haloperidol, a neuroleptic agent, is the recommended medication for delirium because it produces mild sedation without analgesia or amnesia, and it has few anticholinergic and hypotensive effects. In the critically ill patient, the intermittent intravenous route of delivery is preferred because it results in better absorption and fewer side effects than the oral or intramuscular routes. Prolongation of the QT interval on the electrocardiogram may be seen and can result in torsades de pointes. Patients with cardiac disease are at higher risk for this dysrhythmia. Other side effects include neuroleptic syndrome, as evidenced by extreme anxiety, tachycardia, tachypnea, diaphoresis, fever, muscle rigidity, increased creatine phosphokinase levels, and hyperglycemia.[36,50] The ABCDE bundle associated with preventing delirium associated with critical care illness is presented in a QSEN Exemplar box.

BOX 5-4 THE CONFUSION ASSESSMENT METHOD FOR THE CRITICAL CARE UNIT

Delirium is diagnosed when both Features 1 and 2 are positive, along with either Feature 3 or Feature 4.

Feature 1. Acute Onset of Mental Status Changes or Fluctuating Course
- Is there evidence of an acute change in mental status from the baseline?
- Did the (abnormal) behavior fluctuate during the past 24 hours, that is, did it tend to come and go or increase and decrease in severity?

Sources of information: Serial Glasgow Coma Scale or sedation score ratings over 24 hours as well as readily available input from the patient's nurse or family.

Feature 2. Inattention
- Did the patient have difficulty focusing attention?
- Is there a reduced ability to maintain and shift attention?

Sources of information: Attention screening examinations by using either simple picture recognition or random letter test. These tests don't require verbal response, and thus they are ideally suited for mechanically ventilated patients.

Feature 3. Altered Level of Consciousness: Any Level of Consciousness Other Than "Alert"
- **Alert:** normal, spontaneously fully aware of environment and interacts appropriately
- **Vigilant:** hyperalert

Feature 3—cont'd
- **Lethargic:** drowsy but easily aroused, unaware of some elements in the environment, or not spontaneously interacting appropriately with the interviewer; becomes fully aware and appropriately interactive when prodded minimally
- **Stupor:** difficult to arouse, unaware of some or all elements in the environment, or not spontaneously interacting with the interviewer; becomes incompletely aware and inappropriately interactive when prodded strongly
- **Coma:** unarousable, unaware of all elements in the environment, with no spontaneous interaction or awareness of the interviewer, so that the interview is difficult or impossible even with maximal prodding

Feature 4. Disorganized Thinking
- Was the patient's thinking disorganized or incoherent, such as rambling or irrelevant conversation, unclear or illogical flow of ideas, or unpredictable switching from subject to subject?
- Was the patient able to follow questions and commands throughout the assessment?
  1. "Are you having any unclear thinking?"
  2. "Hold up this many fingers."
  3. "Now, do the same thing with the other hand." (not repeating the number of fingers)

Sources of information: Present if RASS score anything other than zero.

TABLE 5-8	INTENSIVE CARE DELIRIUM SCREENING CHECKLIST (ICDSC)				
Patient evaluation	**Day 1**	**Day 2**	**Day 3**	**Day 4**	**Day 5**
Altered level of consciousness* (A–E)					
If A or B do not complete patient evaluation for the period					
Inattention					
Disorientation					
Hallucination-delusion-psychosis					
Psychomotor agitation or retardation					
Inappropriate speech or mood					
Sleep/wake cycle disturbance					
Symptom fluctuation					
Total score (0-8)					

*Level of consciousness:
A: No response, score: None
B: Response to intense and repeated stimulation (loud voice and pain), score: None
C: Response to mild or moderation stimulation, score: 1
D: Normal wakefulness, score: 0
E: Exaggerated response to normal stimulation, score: 1

From Bergeron N, Dubois MJ, Dumont M, Dial S, & Skrobik Y. (2001). Intensive Care Delirium Screening Checklist: evaluation of a new screening tool. *Intensive Care Medicine. 2001;27,* 859-864.

QSEN EXEMPLAR

Patient Centered Care, Evidence-Based Practice

Recent emphasis on preventing delirium and weakness associated with critical illness has resulted in the development of the **Awakening and Breathing Coordination, Delirium Monitoring and Management, and Early Mobility** (ABCDE) bundle. Implementation of the ABCDE bundle focuses on improving communication among team members, standardizing care of the critically ill patient, and avoiding oversedation, which can lead to prolonged mechanical ventilation, delirium, and weakness. The authors described roles of team members in implementing the ABCDE bundle. Nurses lead protocol-driven sedation management, including regular assessment of sedation and agitation. They also communicate with team members to coordinate spontaneous breathing trials, early mobility, and extubation. Ongoing implementation of the ABCDE bundle as part of the management of the critically ill patient results in improved outcomes.

Reference

Balas MC, Vasilevskis EE, Burke WJ, et al. Critical care nurses' role in implementing the "ABCDE Bundle" into practice. *Critical Care Nurse.* 2012;32:35-47.

Neuromuscular Blockade

NMB agents, historically used in the operating room, are used in critically ill patients to facilitate endotracheal intubation and mechanical ventilation, to control increases in intracranial pressure (ICP), and to facilitate procedures at the bedside (e.g., bronchoscopy, tracheostomy). The goal of neuromuscular blockade is complete chemical paralysis.

During a difficult endotracheal intubation, the use of a rapidly acting NMB agent allows the airway to be secured quickly and without trauma. Some patients are unable to tolerate mechanical ventilation despite adequate sedation, especially nontraditional modes such as inverse ratio and pressure control.[69] Long-acting NMB agents may improve chest wall compliance, reduce peak airway pressures, and prevent the patient from ventilator dyssynchrony. The result is improved gas exchange with increased oxygen delivery and decreased oxygen consumption. In patients with elevated ICP, suctioning, coughing, and agitation can provoke dangerous elevations in ICP. NMB agents diminish ICP elevations during these activities. In some patients, complete immobility may be required for a short period for minor surgical and diagnostic procedures performed at the bedside.

NMB agents do not possess any sedative or analgesic properties. Any patient who receives effective neuromuscular blockade is not able to communicate or to produce any voluntary muscle movement, including breathing. Therefore any patient receiving these agents must also be sedated. Many institutions start continuous infusions of sedative medications before they administer an NMB agent.

Patients receiving NMB therapy are closely monitored for respiratory problems, skin breakdown, corneal abrasions, and the development of venous thrombi. If a patient experiences pain or anxiety while receiving an NMB agent, an increase in heart rate or blood pressure may be noted. Nursing care for patients receiving NMB therapy is presented in Box 5-5.

One important nursing intervention is assessing the level or degree of paralysis by using a peripheral nerve stimulator to determine a *train-of-four* (TOF) response. The TOF evaluates the level of neuromuscular blockade to ensure that the greatest amount of neuromuscular blockade is achieved with the lowest dose of NMB medication. The ulnar nerve and the facial nerve are the most frequently used sites for peripheral nerve stimulation. The peripheral nerve stimulator delivers four low-energy impulses, and the

BOX 5-5	NURSING CARE OF THE PATIENT RECEIVING NEUROMUSCULAR BLOCKADE

- Perform train-of-four testing before initiation, 15 minutes after dosage change, then every 4 hours, to monitor the degree of paralysis.
- Ensure appropriate sedation.
- Lubricate eyes to prevent corneal abrasions.
- Ensure prophylaxis for deep vein thrombosis.
- Reposition the patient every 2 hours as tolerated.
- Monitor skin integrity.
- Provide oral hygiene.
- Maintain mechanical ventilation.
- Monitor breath sounds; suction airway as needed.
- Provide passive range of motion.
- Monitor heart rate, respiratory rate, blood pressure, and oxygen saturation.
- Place indwelling urinary catheter to monitor urine output.
- Monitor bowel sounds; monitor for abdominal distention.

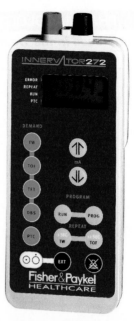

FIGURE 5-6 A train-of-four peripheral nerve stimulator. (Courtesy Fisher & Paykel Healthcare, Auckland, New Zealand.)

number of muscular twitches is assessed. Four twitches of the thumb or facial muscle indicate incomplete neuromuscular blockade. The absence of twitches indicates complete neuromuscular blockade. The TOF goal is two out of four twitches. An example of a peripheral nerve stimulator is shown in Figure 5-6.

No tools or devices can adequately assess pain and sedation in patients receiving NMB agents. The patient is monitored for physiological changes (see Box 5-2), and if changes occur, the nurse must determine whether pain or anxiety is the potential cause. The BIS or PSI system may assist in monitoring in these patients.

Although several NMB agents are available, the most frequently used are outlined in Pharmacology Table 5-9.

TABLE 5-9	PHARMACOLOGY

*Drugs Frequently Used in the Treatment of Anxiety, Pain, or for Neuromuscular Blockade**

MEDICATION	ACTION/USES	DOSE/ROUTE	SIDE EFFECTS	NURSING IMPLICATIONS
Treatment of Anxiety				
Midazolam (Versed)	Benzodiazepine; anxiety/sedation	*IV loading dose:* 0.5-4 mg; may repeat in 10-15 min *Infusion:* 1-7 mg/hr	CNS depression Hypotension Respiratory depression Paradoxical agitation	Titrate infusion up or down by 25% to 50% of the initial infusion rate to ensure adequate titration of sedation level and to prevent tolerance development. Monitor blood pressure and respiratory status. Administer fluids as indicated. Slowly wean drug after prolonged therapy (decrease by 10% to 25% every few hours).
Diazepam (Valium)	Benzodiazepine; anxiety/sedation	*PO:* 2-10 mg bid-qid *Elderly* 2-2.5 mg 1-2 times/day; increase gradually PRN *IM/IV:* 30 mg, depending on assessment; may repeat in 1 hr *Moderate anxiety:* 2-5 mg IM or IV, repeat 3-4 hr PRN	Hypotension Respiratory depression Paradoxical agitation	Monitor blood pressure and respiratory status. Inject slowly over 1 min (5 mg/mL). Unstable in plastic (PVC) infusion bags; possibility of precipitation.

Continued

TABLE 5-9 **PHARMACOLOGY**

Drugs Frequently Used in the Treatment of Anxiety, Pain, or for Neuromuscular Blockade—cont'd

MEDICATION	ACTION/USES	DOSE/ROUTE	SIDE EFFECTS	NURSING IMPLICATIONS
Diazepam (Valium)—cont'd		*Severe anxiety:* 5-10 mg IM or IV, repeat 3-4 hr PRN *IV:* inject no faster than 5 mg/min		
Lorazepam (Ativan)	Benzodiazepine; anxiety/sedation	*PO:* 2-6 mg/day given bid-tid *IM:* 0.05 mg/kg; 4 mg maximum *IV:* 2 mg initially; may repeat 1-2 mg in 10 min *Mild anxiety:* 0.5-1 mg *Moderate-severe anxiety:* 2-4 mg; inject no faster than 2 mg/min *Elderly* 1-2 mg/day, PRN *IV, continuous infusion:* 0.01-0.1 mg/kg/hr IV to maintain desired level of sedation.	Hypotension (less than midazolam) Respiratory depression Paradoxical agitation Hyperosmolar metabolic acidosis (IV prolonged infusion)	Monitor blood pressure and respiratory status. Assess acid-base status with prolonged infusion. Avoid smaller veins to prevent thrombophlebitis. High-dose infusions (greater than 18 mg/hr for more than 4 weeks, or greater than 25 mg/hr for several hours or days) have been associated with tubular necrosis, lactic acidosis, and hyperosmolality states due to the polyethylene glycol and propylene glycol solvents.
Propofol (Diprivan)	Nonbenzodiazepine; sedative/anesthetic	*Initial infusion:* 5 mcg/kg/min for 5 min; increase dose in 5-10 mcg/kg/min increments over 5-10-min until sedation target achieved *Maintenance:* infusion rate of 5-50 mcg/kg/min (or higher)	Hypotension Fever, sepsis Hyperlipidemia Respiratory depression CNS depression	Patient should be intubated and mechanically ventilated. Monitor blood pressure and hemodynamic status. Change infusion set every 12 hr. Monitor plasma lipid levels.
Dexmedetomidine (Precedex)	Selective alpha$_2$-adrenoreceptor agonist; anesthetic; sedative	*IV: loading dose:* 1 mcg/kg over 10 min (must dilute) *Infusion:* 0.2-0.7 mcg/kg/hr	Hypotension Nausea Bradycardia	Give only by continuous infusion. It is recommended not to exceed 24 hr, but in several studies prolonged use of the drug did not increase adverse-event.[40,62,98] Evaluate hepatic and renal function. Observe for bradycardia.
Management of Pain				
Fentanyl (Sublimaze [IV]/ Duragesic [patch])	Opioid; treat pain	Dosage varies depending on desired effect *Infusion:* general pain relief (1-3 mcg/kg/hr); sedation (up to 20 mcg/kg/hr); or amnesia (20-50 mcg/kg/hr) *TD:* 25 mcg/hr, titrate as needed	Hypotension Muscle rigidity Decreased gastric motility Respiratory depression Bradycardia Itching	Titrate infusion slowly in increments. Monitor blood pressure, heart rate, and respiratory status. Administer fluids as indicated. Give as an infusion for extended therapy. Patch: avoid direct heat (e.g., heating blanket), which accelerates fentanyl release. Change patch every 72 hr.
Hydromorphone (Dilaudid)	Opioid; treat pain	*PO:* 2-4 mg every 4-6 hr *SC/IM:* 1-2 mg every 4-6 hr PRN *IV:* 1-2 mg every 4-6 hr slowly over 2-3 min	Hypotension Decreased gastric motility; constipation Respiratory depression	Titrate infusion slowly in increments. Monitor blood pressure, heart rate, and respiratory status. Administer fluids as indicated.

TABLE 5-9   PHARMACOLOGY

Drugs Frequently Used in the Treatment of Anxiety, Pain, or for Neuromuscular Blockade—cont'd

MEDICATION	ACTION/USES	DOSE/ROUTE	SIDE EFFECTS	NURSING IMPLICATIONS
Morphine (Duramorph/MS Contin/Roxanol)	Opioid; treat pain	*SC/IM:* 2.5-20 mg every 3-4 hr PRN. Give very slowly over 4-5 min. *PO:* 5-30 mg every 4 hr PRN *Extended release:* 15-60 mg every 8 to 12 hr *Rectal:* 10-30 mg every 4 hr PRN *Chest pain:* 2-4 mg repeat as necessary *IV:* 10 mg every 4 hr *Continuous IV:* 0.8-10 mg/hr *Maintenance dose:* 0.8-80 mg/hr; rates up to 440 mg/hr have been used *IV patient-controlled analgesia or subcutaneous patient-controlled analgesia:* 1-2 mg injected 30 min after a standard IV dose of 5-20 mg. The lockout period is 6-15 minutes. The 4-hr limit is 30 mg. *Continuous subcutaneous:* 1 mg/hr after a standard dose of 5-20 mg *Epidural:* initial injection of 5 mg in lumbar region may provide relief for up to 24 hr; may give 1-2 mg more after 1 hr to a maximum of 10 mg. *Intrathecal:* 0.2-1 mg one time *Intrathecal continuous:* 0.2 mg/24 hr. May be increased up to 20 mg/24 hr. *Intracerebroventricular:* 0.25 mg via an Ommaya reservoir	Hypotension Decreased gastric motility; constipation Urinary retention Respiratory depression Nausea and vomiting Itching or rash	Titrate infusion slowly in increments. Monitor blood pressure, heart rate, and respiratory status. Administer fluids as indicated.
Acetaminophen (Tylenol) IV (Ofirmev)	Nonnarcotic analgesic	*PO/PR:* 325-1000 mg every 4-6 hours PRN, not to exceed 4 g/day *IV:* patient 50 kg or greater: 650 mg IV every 4hr OR 1000 mg IV every 6hr; not to exceed 4 g/day *Patient less than 50 kg:* 12.5 mg/kg IV every 4hr OR 15 mg/kg IV every 6hr; not to exceed 750 mg/dose or 3.75 g/day Infuse IV over at least 15 min	Renal failure with chronic overdosage Blood dyscrasias Hepatic toxicity	Monitor renal and liver function. Assess other drugs for acetaminophen content (e.g., Percocet).
Aspirin (Ecotrin/Bayer)	Nonsteroidal antiin-flammatory drug (NSAID)	*PO:* 325-1000 mg every 4-6 hr PRN, not to exceed 4 g/day (analgesic) *Rectal:* 1 suppository every 4 hr for no more than 10 days or as directed	Bleeding Gastrointestinal ulcers Tinnitus Thrombocyto-penia	Administer with food if taking PO. Do not exceed recommended doses. Monitor complete blood count and renal function.

Continued

TABLE 5-9 **PHARMACOLOGY**

Drugs Frequently Used in the Treatment of Anxiety, Pain, or for Neuromuscular Blockade—cont'd

MEDICATION	ACTION/USES	DOSE/ROUTE	SIDE EFFECTS	NURSING IMPLICATIONS
Ibuprofen (Advil, Motrin) (IV: Caldolor)	NSAID	*PO:* Mild to moderate pain: 200-400 mg orally every 4-6 hr as needed. Doses greater than 400 mg have not been proven to provide greater efficacy. Do not exceed 3200 mg total daily dose. *IV-Pain:* 400-800 mg intravenously over 30 min every 6 hr as needed. Do not exceed 3200 mg total daily dose.	Bleeding Gastrointestinal ulcers Tinnitus Thrombocyto-penia	Do not exceed recommended doses. Monitor complete blood count. Monitor renal and liver function. Patients should be well hydrated before IV ibuprofen administration.
Ketorolac (Toradol)	NSAID	*IV/IM:* 30 mg every 6 hr (max 120 mg); duration should not exceed 5 days *Patients greater than or equal to 65 years of age, renal impair-ment, or patient less than 50 kg:* the recommended dose is 15 mg IV/IM every 6 hr (max daily dose not to exceed 60 mg)	Headache Dyspepsia Nausea Acute renal failure	Monitor complete blood count. Monitor renal and liver function.
Epidural Analgesia				
Bupivacaine	Local anesthetics/ analgesic	Concentration of 0.1% to 0.75% (25-150 mg) provides partial to complete motor block	Hypotension, respiratory paralysis, nausea, itching, urinary retention, or vomiting	Assess dermatomes for sen-sation and movement. Moni-tor renal and liver function.
Levobupivacaine		Concentration of 0.125% (0.1 mL/kg/hr-0.3 mL/kg/hr)	Urinary retention, hypotension, hypokinesia, respiratory paralysis, nausea, itch-ing, urinary retention, or vomiting	Assess dermatomes. Monitor renal and liver function.
Ropivacaine	Postoperative pain management	Dosing varies based on location. Concentration of 0.2% (2-5 mg/mL). Lumbar/thoracic epidural for con-tinuous infusion (12-28 mg/hr)	Hypotension, bradycardia, paresthesia, pruritus, rigors	Assess dermatomes. Monitor renal and liver function.
Therapeutic Paralysis				
Atracurium (Tracrium)	Neuromuscular blockade	*IV:* loading dose: 0.4-0.5 mg/kg *Maintenance infusion:* 5-10 mcg/kg/min to a maximum of 17.5 mcg/kg/min	Hypotension Tachycardia Rash	Ensure adequate airway. Safer than other paralytic agents in patients with hepatic or renal failure.

TABLE 5-9 PHARMACOLOGY

Drugs Frequently Used in the Treatment of Anxiety, Pain, or for Neuromuscular Blockade—cont'd

MEDICATION	ACTION/USES	DOSE/ROUTE	SIDE EFFECTS	NURSING IMPLICATIONS
Succinylcholine	Neuromuscular blockade; short-term use	*IV:* loading dose: 1-1.5 mg/kg; maximum 2 mg/kg	Hyperkalemia	Secure airway. Avoid in patients with elevated serum potassium.
Delirium				
Haloperidol (Haldol)	Neuroleptic; used to treat delirium and alcohol withdrawal	*PO:* 0.5-5 mg bid or tid; maximum 30 mg/day *IM:* 2-5 mg every 1-8 hr PRN *IV, intermittent:* 0.03-0.15 mg/kg IV (2-10 mg) every 30 min to 6 hr. Mild agitation: 0.5-2 mg Moderate agitation: 5 mg Severe agitation: 10 mg; may require dosing every 30 min (maximum single dose, 40 mg) *IV, infusion:* 3-25 mg/hr by continuous IV infusion has been used for ventilator patients with agitation and delirium.	Drowsiness Prolonged QT interval Extrapyramidal symptoms Euphoria/ agitation Paradoxical agitation Neuroleptic malignant syndrome Tachycardia	Measure QT interval at start of therapy and periodically. Monitor blood pressure with initial treatment or change in the dose. Use with caution when patient is receiving other proarrhythmic agents. Administer anticholinergic for extrapyramidal symptoms.

Data from *Drug Facts and Comparisons*. St. Louis: Wolters Kluwer Health; 2010; McKenry L, Tessier E, Hogan M. *Mosby's Pharmacology in Nursing*. 22nd ed. St. Louis; 2006; OFIRMEV™ (acetaminophen) injection prescribing information. Cadence Pharmaceuticals, Inc. http://www.ofirmev.com/Dosing.aspx. Accessed September 23, 2011; Drugs.com, 2000-11 [Updated: Aug 11th, 2011], http://www.drugs.com. Accessed September 23, 2011.

*All dosages are for adult patients; this table does not account for typical dose adjustments used with the geriatric population (or those undergoing alcohol withdrawal).

bid, Two times per day; *CNS,* central nervous system; *g,* gram; *IM,* intramuscular; *IV,* intravenous; *PO,* by mouth; *PR,* per rectum; *PRN,* as needed; *qid,* four times per day; *SC,* subcutaneous; *tid,* three times per day; *TD,* transdermal.

Succinylcholine (paralytic), when administered with etomidate (sedative), is frequently used for rapid sequence intubation because of its short half-life. However, succinylcholine should not be used in the presence of hyperkalemia because ventricular dysrhythmias and cardiac arrest may occur. Pancuronium is a long-acting NMB agent. When it is given in bolus doses, tachycardia and hypertension may result. The effects of pancuronium are prolonged in patients with liver disease and renal failure. Newer NMB agents such as atracurium and cisatracurium are used in critically ill patients because they are associated with fewer side effects and can be used safely in patients with liver or renal failure.[74]

MANAGEMENT OF PAIN AND ANXIETY

Nonpharmacological Management

Nonpharmacological approaches to manage pain and anxiety are early strategies because many medications used for analgesia or sedation have potentially negative hemodynamic effects. Efforts to reduce anxiety include frequent reorientation, providing patient comfort, and optimizing the environment. For example, a nurse's explanation to the patient and family of the different types of alarms heard in the critical care unit may lessen anxiety levels. Many nonpharmacological approaches are categorized as complementary and alternative therapies. The most commonly used complementary therapies in the critical care unit are environmental manipulation, guided imagery, and music therapy.

Environmental Manipulation

The nurse may decrease patient anxiety and pain by changing the environment so it appears less hostile. The presence of calendars and clocks is helpful. For a patient experiencing delirium, continual reorientation and repetition of explanations and information is helpful.

Family involvement is one of the most important strategies to decrease the patient's anxiety or pain. Family members often benefit from role modeling, as nursing staff members offer support and reassurance to patients while avoiding arguments with patients who have irrational ideas or misperceptions (see Chapter 2).

Another effective strategy is altering the patient's room. Pictures of family members and other small keepsakes provide diversions from the stressful critical care environment. In some critical care units, it may be possible to move the patient's bed so it faces a window. Some patients may benefit from being moved to a different room. Physically moving the patient to a different location prevents the patient from becoming tired of the surroundings, and it may provide some sense of clinical improvement for the patient and family. There are also critical care units in which the monitoring equipment is concealed behind cabinetry to provide a homelike atmosphere.

The patient's family is often able to interpret patient behaviors to the nursing staff, especially those associated with pain or anxiety. Families should be asked to participate in the care whenever the patient's condition allows it. Examples of family participation include coaching during breathing exercises, assisting with passive range of motion, and providing hygiene measures.

Complementary and Alternative Therapy
Guided Imagery

Guided imagery is a mind-body intervention intended to relieve stress and to promote a sense of peace and tranquility.[122] It involves a form of directed daydreaming. It is a way of purposefully diverting and focusing thoughts. Critically ill patients may be instructed in the use of guided imagery during painful procedures or weaning from mechanical ventilation. For example, when performing a needlestick puncture, the nurse may instruct a patient to imagine walking on a beach.

Relaxation and guided imagery have been found to reduce anxiety and depression in cancer patients.[66] Guided imagery with gentle touch or light massage has shown to decrease pain and tension in critically ill patients.[61] Benefits of the guided imagery program included reduced stress and anxiety, decreased pain and narcotic consumption, decreased complications, decreased length of stay, enhanced sleep, and increased patient satisfaction.[61,87,97] Guided imagery is a simple and inexpensive strategy that all nurses can easily incorporate into their daily practice during most procedures and interventions.

Music Therapy

Similar to guided imagery, a music therapy program offers patients a diversionary technique for pain and anxiety relief. Some medical institutions have staff members dedicated solely to music therapy. When appropriate, a music therapist comes to the patient's bedside in the critical care unit and offers one-on-one therapy.[101]

Music therapy may be effective in reducing pain and anxiety if patients are able to participate. Its effect on patients who are heavily sedated, chemically paralyzed, or physically restrained needs further study. Music therapy is an ideal intervention for patients with low energy states who fatigue easily, such as those who require ventilatory support, because it does not require the focused concentration necessary for guided imagery.

Musical selections without lyrics that contain slow, flowing rhythms that duplicate pulses of 60 to 80 beats per minute decrease anxiety in the listener.[15] Music can also provide an alternative focus on a pleasant, comforting stimulus, rather than on stressful environmental stimuli or thoughts. Music therapy can reduce anxiety, and some studies show a shorter duration of intubation.[65,123] Careful scrutiny of musical selections and of personal preferences of what is considered relaxing is important for success.

Animal-Assisted Therapy

Animal-assisted therapy (AAT) involves interaction between patients and trained animals (as therapist) accompanied by human owners or handlers. Commonly used animals are dogs and cats, but use of fish and guinea pigs in the hospital setting has been reported.[22,42] AAT has shown to improve patient's physiological and emotional well-being, lowering cardiopulmonary pressures, decreasing neurohormone levels, and reducing anxiety levels.[18,42]

Pharmacological Management

Even with the most aggressive nonpharmacological therapies, many critically ill patients require medications to relieve pain, anxiety, or both. The appropriate management of pain may result in improved pulmonary function, earlier ambulation and mobilization, decreased stress response with lower catecholamine concentrations, and lower oxygen consumption, leading to improved outcomes.[11,19,117] Pharmacology Table 5-9 summarizes pharmacological therapies used in managing pain and anxiety.

Opioids

Medications for managing pain include opioids and nonsteroidal antiinflammatory drugs (NSAIDs) (see box, "Clinical Alert"). The most commonly used opioids in the critically ill are fentanyl, morphine, and hydromorphone. The selection

---

! CLINICAL ALERT

Intravenous Administration of NSAIDs

Intravenous (IV) preparations of acetaminophen (Ofirmev) and ibuprofen (Caldolor) are now available to treat mild to moderate pain, providing more options for the critically ill patient. These drugs are active ingredients in many other preparations; therefore it is important to ensure that the maximum daily dosage is not exceeded. When these drugs are given, patients are at an increased risk for liver damage (acetaminophen) or renal damage (ibuprofen). Laboratory results must be used to guide therapy and monitor effects of treatment. Results will also assist in determining the most appropriate NSAID for the patient. Collaboration with the clinical pharmacist is essential.

of an opioid is based on its pharmacology and potential for adverse effects. The benefits of opioids include rapid onset, ease of titration, lack of accumulation, and low cost. Fentanyl has the fastest onset and the shortest duration, but repeated dosing may cause accumulation and prolonged effects. Morphine has a longer duration of action, and intermittent dosing may be given. However, hypotension may result from vasodilation, and its active metabolite may cause prolonged sedation in patients with renal insufficiency. Hydromorphone is similar to morphine in its duration of action.

Fentanyl may also be administered by a transdermal patch in hemodynamically stable patients with chronic pain. The patch provides consistent drug delivery, but the extent of absorption varies depending on permeability, temperature, perfusion, and thickness of the skin. Fentanyl patches are not recommended for acute analgesia because it takes 12 to 24 hours to achieve peak effect and, once the patch is removed, another 12 to 24 hours until the medication is no longer present in the body.

Adverse effects of opioids are common in critically ill patients. Respiratory depression is a concern in nonintubated patients. Hypotension may occur in hemodynamically unstable patients or in hypovolemic patients. A depressed level of consciousness and hallucinations leading to increased agitation may be seen in some patients. Gastric retention and ileus may occur as well.

Renal or hepatic insufficiency may alter opioid and metabolite elimination. Titration to the desired response and assessment of prolonged effects are necessary. Elderly patients may have reduced opioid requirements. Administration of a reversal agent such as naloxone is not recommended after prolonged analgesia. It can induce withdrawal and may cause nausea, cardiac stress, and dysrhythmias.[50]

Preventing pain is more effective than treating established pain. When patients are administered opioids on an "as needed" basis, they may receive less than the prescribed dose, and delays in treatment may occur. Analgesics should be administered on a continuous or scheduled intermittent basis, with supplemental bolus doses as required.[50] Intravenous administration usually requires lower and more frequent doses than intramuscular administration to achieve patient comfort. Intramuscular administration is not recommended in hemodynamically unstable patients because of altered perfusion and variable absorption.[50] A pain management plan should be established for each patient and reevaluated as the patient's clinical condition changes.

Patient-Controlled Analgesia

Patient-controlled analgesia (PCA) is a medication delivery system in which the patient is able to control when medication is given. PCA involves a special type of infusion pump (Figure 5-7) that has a "locked" supply of opioid medication. When the patient feels pain or just before any pain-inducing therapy, the patient can depress a button on the

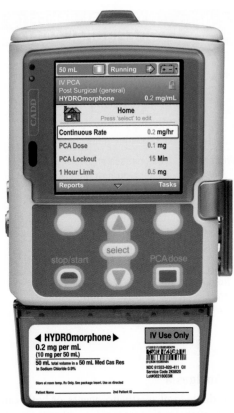

FIGURE 5-7 A patient-controlled analgesia infusion pump. (Courtesy Smiths Medical ASD, Inc., St. Paul, Minnesota.)

BOX 5-6	TYPICAL PATIENT CRITERIA FOR PATIENT-CONTROLLED ANALGESIA THERAPY

- An elective surgical procedure
- Large surgical wounds likely to result in pain (e.g., thoracotomy incisions)
- Large traumatic wounds
- Normal cognitive function
- Normal motor skills (able to depress the medication delivery button)

pump that will deliver a prescribed bolus of medication. Opioids delivered by PCA pump result in stable drug concentrations, good quality of analgesia, less sedation, less opioid consumption, and potentially fewer side effects. PCA is a safe and effective method of pain management.[89]

PCA management is rarely appropriate for critically ill patients because most are unable to depress the button, or they are too ill to manage their pain effectively.[89] However, some critically ill patients may benefit from PCA therapy to manage postoperative incisional pain. Typical patient criteria for PCA therapy are listed in Box 5-6.

TABLE 5-10	POTENTIAL BENEFITS OF EPIDURAL ANALGESIA
SYSTEM	RESPONSE
Pulmonary	↑ Vital capacity ↑ Functional residual capacity Improved airway resistance
Cardiac	Coronary artery vasodilation ↓ Blood pressure, heart rate
Gastrointestinal	Less nausea and vomiting Faster return of gastrointestinal function
Neurological	↓ Total opioid requirement ↓ Sedation
Activity	Earlier extubation Earlier mobilization Decreased length of stay

Modified from Alpen MA, Morse C. Managing the pain of traumatic injury. *Critical Care Nursing Clinics of North America.* 2001;13(2):243-257.

Epidural Analgesia

Opioids or dilute local anesthetics agents, or both, can also be delivered through a catheter placed in either the epidural, intrathecal caudal space, or via nerve blockade to interrupt the transmission of pain. The discovery of opioid receptors in the spinal cord is considered a major breakthrough in the management of pain associated with traumatic injury of the chest and abdomen. Patients with such injuries do not want to cough, breathe deeply, ambulate, or participate in pulmonary exercises because these activities are too painful. Eventually, atelectasis, hypoxemia, respiratory failure, and pneumonia result.

The administration of epidural agents has many benefits in addition to pain relief (Table 5-10). Some of the most commonly used epidural local anesthetics include bupivacaine, levobupivacaine, and ropivacaine. A recent advancement in epidural analgesia is the combination of magnesium sulfate ($MgSO_4$) with epidural or intrathecal analgesia.[5] $MgSO_4$ blocks the N-methyl-D-aspartate (NMDA) receptor in the spinal cord, which decreases the induction and maintenance of central sensitization, thereby decreasing pain.

Patients receiving epidural analgesia are carefully assessed to determine the appropriateness of spinal analgesia. Contraindications include coagulopathies, cardiovascular instability, sepsis, spine injury, infection or injury to the skin at the proposed insertion site, patient refusal, inability to lie still during catheter insertion, and alcohol or drug intoxication.[3] In addition, it is difficult to place an epidural catheter in patients who are obese or have compression fractures of the lumbar spine. Because of issues associated with spinal analgesia, research is being conducted to assess outcomes of caudal epidural analgesia or paravertebral blockade as an alternative to spinal epidural analgesia.[57,77,104]

Potential side effects of spinal analgesia with opioids include respiratory depression, sedation, nausea and vomiting, and urinary retention. Potential side effects of spinal analgesia with local anesthetics include sympathetic blockade (hypotension, venous pooling), motor weakness, sensory block, and urinary retention.

Nonsteroidal Antiinflammatory Drugs

NSAIDs provide analgesia by inhibiting cyclooxygenase, a critical enzyme in the inflammatory cascade. NSAIDs have the potential to cause significant adverse effects including gastrointestinal bleeding, bleeding secondary to platelet inhibition, and renal insufficiency. The risk of developing NSAID-induced renal insufficiency is higher in patients with hypovolemia or renal hypoperfusion, in the elderly, and in patients with preexisting renal impairment. NSAIDs should not be administered to patients with asthma and aspirin sensitivity.

NSAIDs are available in oral, liquid, and intravenous forms. NSAIDs such as ibuprofen have been used to treat the hypermetabolic response and fever. More recently, demonstrated effects of ibuprofen that is administered intravenously include significant reductions in opioid requirements and decrease in pain levels.[114]

Other Pain Relievers

Acetaminophen is used to treat mild to moderate pain, such as pain associated with prolonged bed rest. In combination with an opioid, acetaminophen has a greater analgesic effect than higher doses of an opioid alone. Acetaminophen is administered cautiously in patients with hepatic dysfunction.

Sedative Agents

Anxiety in the critical care setting is typically treated with benzodiazepines, propofol, or dexmedetomidine. Both pain and anxiety may exist with evidence of psychotic features (as manifested in delirium). In this situation, neuroleptic agents, antidepressants, and anesthetic agents are administered.

Benzodiazepines are sedatives and hypnotics that block new information and potentially unpleasant experiences at that moment. Although they are not considered analgesics, they do moderate the anticipatory pain response. Benzodiazepines vary in their potency, onset and duration of action, distribution, and metabolism. The patient's age, prior alcohol abuse, concurrent drug therapy, and current medical condition affect the intensity and duration of drug activity. Elderly patients and patients with renal or hepatic insufficiency may exhibit slower clearance of benzodiazepines, which may contribute to a significant delay in elimination.

Benzodiazepines should be titrated to a predefined end point, for example, a specific level of sedation using a standard sedation scale. Sedation may be maintained with intermittent doses of lorazepam, diazepam, or midazolam; however, patients requiring frequent doses to maintain the desired effect may benefit from a continuous infusion by using the lowest effective dose. Patients receiving continuous infusions must be monitored for the effects of oversedation.

Additionally, patients who are hemodynamically unstable may become hypotensive with the initiation of sedation; the nurse must be cautious when administering medication to these patients.

Propofol is an intravenous general anesthetic; however, sedative and hypnotic effects are achieved at lower doses. Propofol has no analgesic properties. It has a rapid onset and short duration of sedation once it is discontinued. Adverse effects include hypotension, bradycardia, and pain when the drug is infused through a peripheral intravenous site. Propofol is available as an emulsion in a phospholipid substance, which provides 1.1 kcal/mL from fat, and it should be counted as a caloric source.[50] Long-term or high-dose infusions may result in high triglyceride levels, metabolic acidosis, or dysrhythmias. Propofol requires a dedicated intravenous catheter for continuous infusion because of the risk of incompatibility and infection. The infusion should not hang for more than 12 hours.

Dexmedetomidine is an anesthetic agent with selective alpha-2 agonist properties that is approved for short-term use as a sedative (less than 24 hours) in patients receiving mechanical ventilation. It reduces concurrent analgesic and sedative requirements and produces anxiolytic effects comparable to those of the benzodiazepines. Transient elevations in blood pressure may be seen with rapid administration.

Bradycardia and hypotension may develop, especially in the presence of hypovolemia, in patients with severe ventricular dysfunction and in the elderly. The role of this medication in the sedation of critically ill patients is being determined.

Implementation of sedation guidelines have been shown to reduce the cost of sedation medication, the number of hours patients require mechanical ventilation, and the length of time patients spend in the critical care unit.[50] The use of an algorithm assists in this process (Figure 5-8).

Tolerance and Withdrawal

Patients who require high-dose opioid or sedative therapy to maintain sedation may develop physiological dependence and tolerance to the drug. Drugs should be tapered slowly and another drug selected. Stopping these medications abruptly may lead to withdrawal symptoms. Opioid withdrawal symptoms include pupillary dilation, sweating, rhinorrhea, tachycardia, hypertension, tachypnea, vomiting, diarrhea, increased sensitivity to pain, restlessness, and anxiety. Signs of benzodiazepine withdrawal include tremor, headache, nausea, sweating, fatigue, anxiety, agitation, increased sensitivity to light and sound, muscle cramps, sleep disturbances, and seizures. Doses should be tapered slowly and systematically.

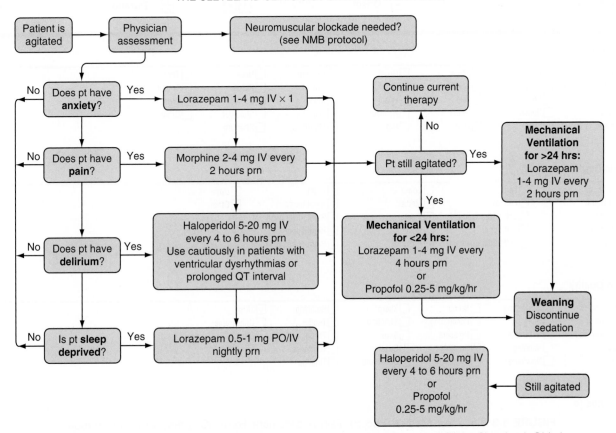

FIGURE 5-8 Sample algorithm of sedation guidelines. (Courtesy Cleveland Clinic, Cleveland, Ohio.)

MANAGEMENT CHALLENGES

Invasive Procedures

Many invasive procedures, including nasogastric tube insertion, tracheal suctioning, central venous catheter insertion, chest tube insertion, wound care, and removal of tubes, lines, and sheaths, take place in the critical care unit. All these invasive procedures have the likelihood of inducing pain or anxiety.[93] If pain or anxiety occurs during a procedure, the length and difficulty of the procedure may be increased, inaccurate data may be obtained, and physical harm can result.[80] To avoid negative outcomes, the patient's comfort and anxiety must be appropriately assessed and managed. Many times, the patient is kept in a conscious state during the procedure to avoid the risk of complications such as respiratory depression and hypotension. Therefore sedative or analgesic agents, or both, are given in a way that the patient appears sedate yet is able to verbalize. This type of sedation has been referred to as *procedural sedation* or *conscious sedation.*

Typical nursing care during these procedures involves monitoring vital signs including pulse oximetry, ensuring a patent airway, and observing for the adverse effects of medications. With the advent of the electronic medical record (EMR), customized pain assessment forms can be developed to improve clinical efficiency and documentation (Figures 5-9 and 5-10). Many institutions use specialized flow sheets in which assessment findings are documented during invasive procedures (Figure 5-11).

Substance Abuse

Critically ill patients who have a history of substance abuse or drug use disorders pose special challenges. Drug use disorder combined with alcohol has been associated with increased need for mechanical ventilation, increased risk of developing pneumonia and sepsis, and a longer critical care stay.[102] A history of alcoholism alone also increases hospital length of stay and mortality secondary to complications such as higher infection rates, sepsis, septic shock, acute respiratory distress syndrome, and acute delirium.[82,83,85,124] The pharmacological management of patients in the critical care unit typically involves the administration of sedative and hypnotic medications. Patients with a history of substance abuse may have a higher-than-normal dosage threshold to achieve therapeutic actions with many of these pharmacological agents. If alcoholism or drug abuse is suspected, it may be beneficial

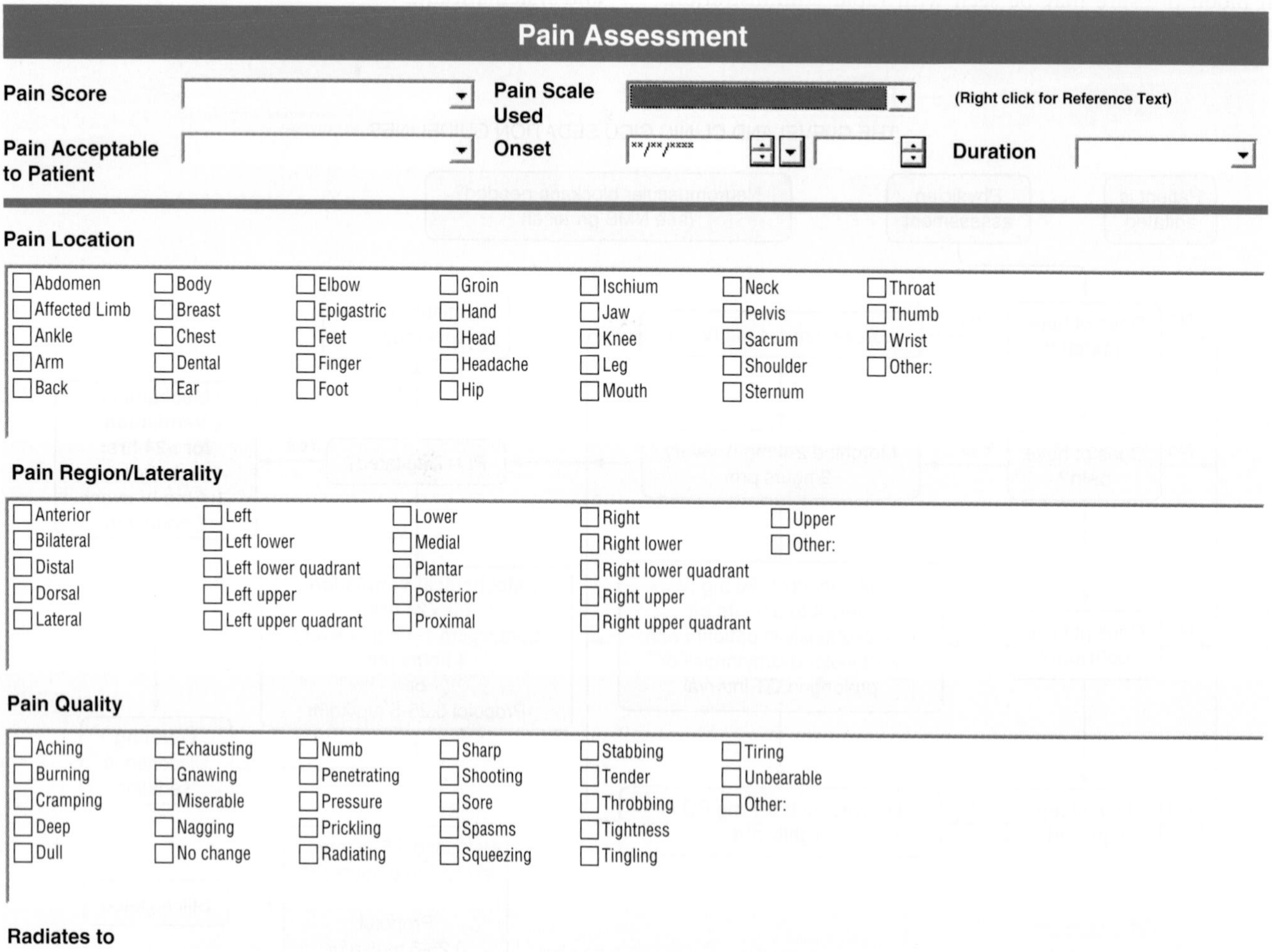
Pain Assessment

Pain Score | Pain Scale Used | (Right click for Reference Text)

Pain Acceptable to Patient | Onset | Duration

Pain Location

Abdomen, Affected Limb, Ankle, Arm, Back, Body, Breast, Chest, Dental, Ear, Elbow, Epigastric, Feet, Finger, Foot, Groin, Hand, Head, Headache, Hip, Ischium, Jaw, Knee, Leg, Mouth, Neck, Pelvis, Sacrum, Shoulder, Sternum, Throat, Thumb, Wrist, Other:

Pain Region/Laterality

Anterior, Bilateral, Distal, Dorsal, Lateral, Left, Left lower, Left lower quadrant, Left upper, Left upper quadrant, Lower, Medial, Plantar, Posterior, Proximal, Right, Right lower, Right lower quadrant, Right upper, Right upper quadrant, Upper, Other:

Pain Quality

Aching, Burning, Cramping, Deep, Dull, Exhausting, Gnawing, Miserable, Nagging, No change, Numb, Penetrating, Pressure, Prickling, Radiating, Sharp, Shooting, Sore, Spasms, Squeezing, Stabbing, Tender, Throbbing, Tightness, Tingling, Tiring, Unbearable, Other:

Radiates to

FIGURE 5-9 Electronic Medical Record: Pain Assessment Form. (Courtesy Virginia Commonwealth University Health System, Richmond, Virginia.)

Pain Management Instruction

*Indicates Required Field

*Which Type/Therapy		*Ready to learn ☐ No ☐ Yes, alert and oriented
Individualized pt exceptions		

*Person taught: ☐ Patient ☐ Family Member ☐ Parent ☐ Guardian ☐ Significant Other ☐ Other:

Learning Barriers encountered
☐ None
☐ Cognitive Limitations (Unable to grasp concepts and/or respond to questions)
☐ Cultural/Religious (Culture/religious beliefs conflict with treatment plan)
☐ Language (Does not speak/understand English)
☐ Physical Impairment (Visual/auditory/psychomotor deficits)
☐ Psychosocial (Anger, denial, powerlessness, etc.)
☐ Family/Significant Other not available for teaching
☐ Other:

Interventions used
☐ Adapt learning/teaching methods
☐ Education of family member/caretaker
☐ Telephone Interpreter
☐ On-site interpreter
☐ Interpretation services waived
☐ Other:

Language Telephone Operator ID Number		**Interpreter Name (Last, First)**	
Language Used		**Relationship to Patient**	☐ Family Member ☐ Friend ☐ Staff member ☐ Other:

*Teaching Method Used:
☐ Audiovisual/Printed materials ☐ Explanation ☐ Unable to teach at this time
☐ Demonstration ☐ Nurse Diane

Teaching Materials Used

*Behavioral Response:
☐ Not ready to learn ☐ Needs reinstruction ☐ Verbalizes knowledge
☐ No evidence of learning ☐ Demonstrates skill ☐ Other:

Specific details to reinstruct		**Future Topics to instruct**	

FIGURE 5-10 Electronic Medical Record: Pain Management Patient Education Form. (Courtesy Virginia Commonwealth University Health System, Richmond, Virginia.)

to start with higher-than-normal doses of sedative and analgesic medications. Based on the patient's response, it may be necessary to exceed the recommended maximum dosage of a medication.

Patients with a history of alcohol use must be assessed for symptoms of alcohol withdrawal syndrome (AWS), which usually present within 72 to 96 hours after the patient's last alcohol intake. The initial symptoms, such as disorientation, agitation, and tachycardia, and delirium tremens (shaking of the extremities or digits), may be mild. If untreated, symptoms can progress to severe confusion, paranoid-like behavior, seizures, convulsions, and even death. The most important treatment of AWS is prevention, which has been shown to improve morbidity and mortality and decrease hospital and critical care unit lengths of stay. Continuous infusion of ethanol as prophylaxis decreases the rate of withdrawal symptoms.[24] In addition, thiamine is frequently given to patients with a history of alcoholism to prevent Wernicke encephalopathy.[107,119] Research shows that surgical patients who received symptom-oriented bolus titration of intravenous flunitrazepam (agitation), intravenous clonidine (sympathetic hyperactivity), or intravenous haloperidol (productive psychotic symptoms) required fewer days of mechanical ventilation, had a lower incidence of pneumonia, and had shorter ICU stays.[115] Flunitrazepam is not approved in the United States.

Restraining Devices

Restraining or immobilizing devices are commonly used in the critical care setting to ensure that the patient is unable to disrupt invasive lines or pull at lifesaving devices. The purpose of restraints is to promote patient safety; however, restraints can be dangerous if the patient is disoriented.[28] Use of physical restraint without sedation has been associated with PTSD after critical care unit discharge.[52] The goal of applying restraints is to use the least restrictive device so the patient still has some movement. Commonly used restraining devices are listed in Table 5-11.

A common adverse event associated with restraints involves complications associated with immobility. Patients with restraining devices must be repositioned, and the areas where the restraints are applied are assessed for perfusion and sensation at least every hour. This assessment is documented on the critical care flow sheet.

Effects of Aging

As the population ages, the number of elderly patients admitted to a critical care unit continues to increase. Elderly patients have a high prevalence of pain, and they might experience a multitude of painful conditions (neoplasms, injuries and other external causes, and diseases of the musculoskeletal and connective tissues systems). Patients older than 65 years pose special concerns because of their physiology, many comorbidities, use of multiple medications, physical frailty, and

Cleveland Clinic
PROCEDURAL SEDATION RECORD
Page 2 of 4

For scanning accuracy, affix patient label within this outlined box.

Transportation home verified? ☐ Yes ☐ No ☐ Not applicable
Support person: _____ Phone Number: _____
Nothing by mouth since: _____
Identification Band check: _____

Dentures: ☐ Yes ☐ No ☐ Not applicable

Glasses: ☐ Yes ☐ No ☐ Not applicable

Other: _____

Initials: _____ Time: _____

Prep: _____
Intravenous site/gauge: _____
Initials: _____ Date: _____ Time: _____

Nursing Assessment:

Patient Education re: procedure ☐ Yes ☐ No ☐ Not applicable

Nursing Plan of care initiated: ☐ Yes ☐ No ☐ Not applicable

INTAKE

TIME	SOLUTION - ml's/hour	ABSORBED	CREDIT	INITIALS

Patient Assessment Score	pre	post
Moves 4 extremities voluntarily on command	2	2
Moves 2 extremities voluntarily on command	1	1
Moves 0 extremities voluntarily on command	0	0
Able to breathe deeply & cough freely	2	2
Dyspnea or limited breathing	1	1
Apneic	0	0
Fully awake	2	2
Arousable on calling	1	1
Not responding	0	0
Able to maintain oxygen saturation greater than 90 percent on RA	2	2
Needs oxygen to maintain oxygen sat greater than 90 percent	1	1
Oxygen sat less than 90 percent with oxygen	0	0
Able to stand up and walk upright	2	2
Vertigo when erect	1	1
Dizziness when supine	0	0
Non-ambulatory	0	0
TOTAL		
Initials		
Time		

OUTPUT

TIME	URINE			INITIALS

NOTES: _____
_____
_____
_____
_____
_____
_____
_____

PRE-PROCEDURAL VASCULAR ASSESSMENT ☐ No deferred/not indicated
ASSESSMENT OF EXTREMITY ACCESSED: PALPABLE: 4+= BOUNDING 3+= normal 2+= decreased 1+= weak 0= absent
CHECK APPROPRIATE BOX

Pulses: Post Check Appropriate Box	F	P	DP	PT	AXILLARY	BRACHIAL	ULNAR	RADIAL
Right ☐ Leg ☐ Arm								
Left ☐ Leg ☐ Arm								

Procedure Information

Procedure Start Time: _____
Procedure Finish Time: _____
Endoscope Size: _____
Total fluoroscopy time: _____
Electrosurgical Unit #: _____ Pad #: _____
Pad Location: _____
Site Condition after removal: _____
Specimens Collected: _____
_____
Specimens sent to: _____

Initials _____ Time _____

Sign in Communication: ☐ Completed ☐ Emergent Case N / A
Initials: _____
Time Out–Team Agrees:
Correct Patient   Correct Side / Site Marking
Correct Procedure   Correct Position (if applicable)
Initials: _____ Time: _____
complete (if applicable):
Affirmation of time out
Initials: _____

Procedural Activities completed Initials: _____ Time: _____

102708 Rev. 7/11

FIGURE 5-11 The Cleveland Clinic Procedural Sedation Record: Nursing Assessment Page. (Courtesy Cleveland Clinic, Cleveland, Ohio.)

Cleveland Clinic

PROCEDURAL SEDATION RECORD

Page 3 of 4

Vital Signs

***Airway Manipulation:** Intervention required to assist in maintaining adequate airway:
CL=chin lift, JT=jaw thrust, OA=oral airway, NA=nasal airway, MV=mask ventilation,
LMA=laryngeal mask airway, ETT=endotracheal tube

Modified Ramsay Score LOC 1=Anxious, 2=Awake, tranquil, 3=Drowsy, responds
easily to verbal commands, 4=Asleep, brisk response to tactile or loud auditory stimulus,
5=Asleep, minimal but purposeful response to painful or loud auditory stimulus,
6=Asleep, no response even to painful stimuli (pure reflex)

Pain Key
Pain Level: 0=None, 10=Extreme
Pain Quality: <u>Type:</u> Cramping (CR) Burning (B) Aching (A)
Throbbing (T) Dull (D) Sharp <u>Consistency:</u> Intermittent (I) Consistent (C)

TIME	BP	P	R	O₂ SAT	Airway Manip.	LOC	PAIN LEVEL	PAIN QUALITY	MEDS/O₂	NOTES	INITIALS
										Immediate Pre-Sedation Vital Signs	

POCT Stickers

Sign Out Discussion ☐ Completed   Initials: _____

Brief Post Procedural Note
List Proceduralist and assistants: _____

☐ **Please check if Brief Post Procedural Note is in EPIC, if not complete below.**

Pre-Procedural Diagnosis: _____ Post-Procedural Diagnosis: _____

Procedure performed if different from the planned procedure: _____

Findings: _____

_____

No specimens collected unless noted here: _____

Discharge / Transfer when discharge assessment criteria are met. Estimated Blood Loss if greater than minimal: _____

Physician / Licensed Independent Practitioner Signature: _____
     (For Procedural/Medication Orders)

Print Name: _____   Date: _____ Time: _____

102708 Rev. 7/11

FIGURE 5-11, cont'd

TABLE 5-11　COMMON RESTRAINING DEVICES

RESTRAINT TYPE	DESCRIPTION
Soft wrist restraints	Constructed from padded foam with Velcro or tie straps. Typically applied around the wrist and tied to the bed frame. Prevents the patient from pulling at items on the upper torso or near the face.
Soft mitts	Constructed from a padded foam material with mesh. Slipped over the hand so the palm rests on a pillow foam. Allows the patient full range of motion with the upper extremities but does not allow a grasping motion with the fingers. Ideal for patients who are "picking" at items such as dressings, intravenous infusion sites, or feeding tubes.
Elbow immobilizer	Large plastic sheath that is soft but does not have any flexion. Slipped over the forearm and placed over the elbow joint. Allows full range of motion at the shoulder and wrist but does not allow the elbow to bend. The patient cannot bring the forearm towards the head. Works well for patients who are attempting to remove an endotracheal tube.
Vest	Made from a Teflon mesh material with straps that can be tied. Typically worn around the upper torso and can be tied to a bed frame or a chair. Keeps the patient bound to the bed or chair. Full range of motion in the lower extremities is possible. Ideal for patients who are sitting in chairs. Prevents the patient from standing unassisted.

GERIATRIC CONSIDERATIONS

Strategies for Managing Pain and Anxiety
- Speak slowly and clearly.
- Verify any underlying cognitive deficits (e.g., dementia, Alzheimer's disease, cerebrovascular accident).
- Ensure that scales or other assessment tools have a large font/text.
- Stoic behavior may be the patient's normal baseline; therefore, assess for nonverbal cues to pain (facial grimace or withdrawal).
- Observe for changes in behavior, such as confusion or agitation. Elderly patients are at risk of developing delirium.
- Elderly patients may be resistant to taking additional medications; therefore, offer nonpharmacological strategies to manage anxiety or pain.
- Elderly patients may not ask for as-needed medications in a timely fashion. Pain medications should be routinely scheduled.
- Medication dosages may be reduced because of decreased renal and liver clearance.
- Certain medications may have paradoxical effects in the elderly (e.g., benzodiazepines causing agitation).

cognitive and sensory deficits. Elderly patients are also more vulnerable to alcohol abuse and substance abuse, and they may be more vulnerable to toxicity from analgesics. Elderly patients often have decreased renal function with a reduced creatinine clearance rate, resulting in a longer elimination half-life of analgesic drugs.

Older patients generally receive less analgesia or sedation compared with younger adults, perhaps because of elderly patients' beliefs about their pain and anxiety. Some elderly patients believe that pain is a normal process of aging and is something that they must learn to accept as normal. Elderly patients often believe that complaining of pain to nursing staff will label them as "problem" patients. Finally, elderly patients may comment to their family and friends that the nurse is too busy to listen to their complaints, and they do not want to be a "bother." Refer to the box titled "Geriatric Considerations" for strategies to manage pain and anxiety in the elderly patient.

CASE STUDY

Mr. B. is a 52-year-old man in the surgical intensive care unit after liver transplantation the previous day. He has a 15-year history of hepatic cirrhosis secondary to alcohol abuse. He is intubated and is receiving multiple vasopressor medications for hypotension. At 6:30 AM, he follows simple commands and denies pain or anxiety with simple head nods. At 7:00 AM, Mr. B. is kicking his legs and places his arms outside the side rails. Attempts by the nurse to reorient him result in his pulling at his endotracheal tube. His wrists are restrained with soft restraints. At this time, he does not follow any simple commands. He continually shakes his head back and forth. Facial grimacing is noted, and he is biting down on the endotracheal tube, which is causing the ventilator to sound the high-pressure alarm. His blood pressure is 185/110 mm Hg, with a mean arterial pressure of 135 mm Hg. The monitor displays sinus tachycardia at a rate of 140 beats per minute. Medication infusions include epinephrine (3 mcg/min), norepinephrine (15 mcg/min), dopamine (2 mcg/kg/min), and fentanyl (100 mcg/hr). His only other medications are his immunosuppressive drug regimen.

Questions

1. Score Mr. B.'s pain and/or anxiety using the objective tools listed below:

TOOL	SCORE
Behavioral Pain Scale (BPS):	_____
Critical-Care Pain Observation Tool (CPOT):	_____
Richmond Agitation Sedation Scale (RASS):	_____
Ramsay Sedation Scale (RSS):	_____
Sedation-Agitation Scale (SAS):	_____
The Confusion Assessment Method for the Intensive Care Unit (CAM-ICU)	_____

2. Would complementary or alternative medicine therapies be appropriate at this time? If not, what therapies would be appropriate?
3. What type of medication is Mr. B. receiving for pain?
4. Is this an appropriate dose of pain medication for Mr. B.?
5. What other medications could be given to manage his agitated state?

SUMMARY

Patients admitted to the critical care unit are at an increased risk of developing pain and anxiety. The critical care environment and medical interventions may be the greatest contributing factors in the development of pain and anxiety. The assessment of both is a challenge for the critical care nurse because patients may not be able to communicate. The use of assessment tools designed to recognize pain and anxiety is helpful. Nonpharmacological and pharmacological strategies to relieve pain and anxiety should be used so that critical care patients have the best possible outcomes.

CRITICAL THINKING EXERCISES

1. Describe factors that increase the risk for pain and anxiety in critically ill patients.
2. Differentiate between subjective and objective tools when assessing pain, and provide examples of each.
3. What is delirium? What are some of the behaviors seen in the hyperacute subtype?

REFERENCES

1. Ahlers SJ, van d V, van DM, et al. The use of the Behavioral Pain Scale to assess pain in conscious sedated patients. *Anesthesia Analgesia.* 2010;110:127-133.
2. Ahlers SJ, van GL, van d V, et al. Comparison of different pain scoring systems in critically ill patients in a general ICU. *Critical Care.* 2008;12:R15.
3. Alpen MA, Morse C. Managing the pain of traumatic injury. *Critical Care Nursing Clinics of North America.* 2001; 13:243-257.
4. Apkarian AV, Bushnell MC, Treede RD, et al. Human brain mechanisms of pain perception and regulation in health and disease. *European Journal of Pain.* 2005;9:463-484.
5. Arcioni R, Palmisani S, Tigano S, et al. Combined intrathecal and epidural magnesium sulfate supplementation of spinal anesthesia to reduce post-operative analgesic requirements: a prospective, randomized, double-blind, controlled trial in patients undergoing major orthopedic surgery. *Acta Anaesthesiology Scandinavia.* 2007;51:482-489.
6. Arif-Rahu M. Grap MJ. Facial expression and pain in the critically ill non-communicative patient: state of science review. *Intensive and Critical Care Nursing.* 2010;26: 343-352.
7. Aspect Medical Systems. Overview: the effects of electromyography (EMG) and other high-frequency signals on the Bispectral Index (BIS) [pamphlet]. Newton, MA, Aspect Medical Systems, Inc.; 1999.

8. Balas MC, Deutschman CS, Sullivan-Marx EM. Delirium in older patients in surgical intensive care units. *Journal of Nursing Scholarship*. 2007;39:147-154.

9. Bergeron N, Dubois MJ, Dumont M, et al. Intensive Care Delirium Screening Checklist: evaluation of a new screening tool. *Intensive Care Medicine*. 2001;27:859-864.

10. Birka A. New perspectives on the use of propofol [commentary]. *Critical Care Nurse*. 1999;19:18-19.

11. Bonnet F, Marret E. Postoperative pain management and outcome after surgery. *Best Practice & Research Clinical Anaesthesiology*. 2007;21:99-107.

12. Breau LM, Camfield CS, McGrath PJ, et al. Risk factors for pain in children with severe cognitive impairments. *Developmental Medicine & Child Neurology*. 2004;46:364-371.

13. Bush TM, Rayburn KS, Holloway SW, et al. Adverse interactions between herbal and dietary substances and prescription medications: a clinical survey. *Alternative Therapies in Health and Medicine*. 2007;13:30-35.

14. Carroll KC, Atkins PJ, Herold GR, et al. Pain assessment and management in critically ill postoperative and trauma patients: a multisite study. *American Journal of Critical Care*. 1999;8:105-117.

15. Chlan LL. Music therapy as a nursing intervention for patients supported by mechanical ventilation. *AACN Clinical Issues*. 2000;11:128-138.

16. Chlan LL. Relationship between two anxiety instruments in patients receiving mechanical ventilatory support. *Journal of Advanced Nursing*. 2004;48:493-499.

17. Closs SJ, Barr B, Briggs M. Cognitive status and analgesic provision in nursing home residents. *British Journal of General Practice*. 2004;54:919-921.

18. Cole KM, Gawlinski A, Steers N, et al. Animal-assisted therapy in patients hospitalized with heart failure. *American Journal of Critical Care*. 2007;16:575-585.

19. Costa MG, Chiarandini P, Della RG. Sedation in the critically ill patient. *Transplantation Proceedings*. 2006;38:803-804.

20. Cullen L, Greiner J, Titler MG. Pain management in the culture of critical care. *Critical Care Nursing Clinics of North America*. 2001;13:151-166.

21. De Jong MM, Burns SM, Campbell ML, et al. Development of the American association of critical-care nurses' sedation assessment scale for critically ill patients. *American Journal of Critical Care*. 2005;14:531-544.

22. DeCourcey M, Russell AC, Keister KJ. Animal-assisted therapy: evaluation and implementation of a complementary therapy to improve the psychological and physiological health of critically ill patients. *Dimensions of Critical Care Nursing*. 2010;29:211-214.

23. DeLeo JA. Basic science of pain. *Journal of Bone and Joint Surgery*. 2006;88(2):58-62.

24. Dissanaike S, Halldorsson A, Frezza EE, et al. An ethanol protocol to prevent alcohol withdrawal syndrome. *Journal of the American College of Surgeons*. 2006;203:186-191.

25. Ely EW, Shintani A, Truman B, et al. Delirium as a predictor of mortality in mechanically ventilated patients in the intensive care unit. *Journal of the American Medical Association*. 2004;291:1753-1762.

26. Ely EW, Truman B, Shintani A, et al. Monitoring sedation status over time in ICU patients: reliability and validity of the Richmond Agitation-Sedation Scale (RASS). *Journal of the American Medical Association*. 2003;289:2983-2991.

27. Ersek M, Herr K, Neradilek MB, et al. Comparing the psychometric properties of the Checklist of Nonverbal Pain Behaviors (CNPI) and the Pain Assessment in Advanced Dementia (PAIN-AD) instruments. *Pain Medicine*. 2010;11:395-404.

28. Evans D, Wood J, Lange P. Patient injury and physical restraint devices: A systematic review. *Journal of Advanced Nursing*. 2003;413:282.

29. Feldt KS. The checklist of nonverbal pain indicators (CNPI). *Pain Management Nursing*. 2000;1:13-21.

30. Fraser GL, Prato BS, Riker RR, et al. Frequency, severity, and treatment of agitation in young versus elderly patients in the ICU. *Pharmacotherapy*. 2000;20:75-82.

31. Fraser GL, Riker RR. Bispectral index monitoring in the intensive care unit provides more signal than noise. *Pharmacotherapy*. 2005;25:19S-27S.

32. Galli SJ, Nakae S, Tsai M. Mast cells in the development of adaptive immune responses. *Nature Immunology*. 2005;6:135-142.

33. Gelinas C, Fillion L, Puntillo KA, et al. Validation of the critical-care pain observation tool in adult patients. *American Journal of Critical Care*. 2006;15:420-427.

34. Gelinas C, Johnston C. Pain assessment in the critically ill ventilated adult: validation of the Critical-Care Pain Observation Tool and physiologic indicators. *Clinical Journal of Pain*. 2007;23:497-505.

35. Gelinas C, Tousignant-Laflamme Y, Tanguay A, et al. Exploring the validity of the bispectral index, the Critical-Care Pain Observation Tool and vital signs for the detection of pain in sedated and mechanically ventilated critically ill adults: a pilot study. *Intensive and Critical Care Nursing*. 2011;27:46-52.

36. Girard TD, Pandharipande PP, Carson SS, et al. Feasibility, efficacy, and safety of antipsychotics for intensive care unit delirium: the MIND randomized, placebo-controlled trial. *Critical Care Medicine*. 2010;38:428-437.

37. Gordon DB, Dahl JL, Miaskowski C, et al. American pain society recommendations for improving the quality of acute and cancer pain management: American Pain Society Quality of Care Task Force. *Archives of Internal Medicine*. 2005;165:1574-1580.

38. Granja C, Lopes A, Moreira S, et al. Patients' recollections of experiences in the intensive care unit may affect their quality of life. *Critical Care*. 2005;9:R96-R109.

39. Granot M, Khoury R, Berger G, et al. Clinical and experimental pain perception is attenuated in patients with painless myocardial infarction. *Pain*. 2007;133:120-127.

40. Guinter JR, Kristeller JL. Prolonged infusions of dexmedetomidine in critically ill patients. *American Journal of Health-System Pharmacy*. 2010;67:1246-1253.

41. Guyton AC, Hall JE. *Textbook of Medical Physiology*. 12th ed. Philadelphia: Saunders; 2011.

42. Halm MA. The healing power of the human-animal connection. *American Journal of Critical Care*. 2008;17:373-376.

43. Hamill-Ruth RJ, Marohn ML. Evaluation of pain in the critically ill patient. *Critical Care Clinics*. 1999;15:35-54, v-vi.

44. Herr K, Bjoro K, Decker S. Tools for assessment of pain in nonverbal older adults with dementia: a state-of-the-science review. *Journal of Pain and Symptom Management*. 2006;31:170-192.

45. Herr K, Coyne PJ, Key T, et al. Pain assessment in the nonverbal patient: position statement with clinical practice recommendations. *Pain Management Nursing*. 2006b;7:44-52.

46. Hofhuis JG, Spronk PE, van Stel HF, et al. Experiences of critically ill patients in the ICU. *Intensive and Critical Care Nursing.* 2008;24:300-313.

47. Huether SE. Pain, temperature regulation, sleep, and sensory function. In McCance KL, & Huether SE, eds. *Pathophysiology: The Biologic Basis for Disease in Adults and Children.* 6th ed. St. Louis, MO: Mosby; 2010.

48. International Association for the Study of Pain (IASP). Pain Terminology updated 2011 from "Part III: Pain Terms, A Current List with Definitions and Notes on Usage" (pp 209-214) *Classification of Chronic Pain, Second Edition* IASP Task Force on Taxonomy, edited by H. Merskey and N. Bogduk, IASP Press, Seattle, 1994. www.iasp-pain.org; 2011. Accessed August 10, 2011.

49. Jaber S, Chanques G, Altairac C, et al. A prospective study of agitation in a medical-surgical ICU: incidence, risk factors, and outcomes. *Chest.* 2005;128:2749-2757.

50. Jacobi J, Fraser GL, Coursin DB, et al. Clinical practice guidelines for the sustained use of sedatives and analgesics in the critically ill adult. *Critical Care Medicine.* 2002;30:119-141.

51. Joint Commission. Top compliance issues for 2006. *Joint Commission: The Source.* 2007;5(December):4-5.

52. Jones C, Backman C, Capuzzo M, et al. Precipitants of posttraumatic stress disorder following intensive care: a hypothesis generating study of diversity in care. *Intensive Care Medicine.* 2007;33:978-985.

53. Jones C, Griffiths RD, Humphris G, et al. Memory, delusions, and the development of acute posttraumatic stress disorder-related symptoms after intensive care. *Critical Care Medicine.* 2001;29:573-580.

54. Justic M. Does "ICU psychosis" really exist? *Critical Care Nurse.* 2000;20:28-39.

55. Karamchandani K, Rewari V, Trikha A, et al. Bispectral index correlates well with Richmond agitation sedation scale in mechanically ventilated critically ill patients. *Journal of Anesthesia.* 2010;24:394-398.

56. Katz WA, Rothenberg R. Section 3: the nature of pain: pathophysiology. *Journal of Clinical Rheumatology.* 2005;11:S11-S15.

57. Kita T, Maki N, Song YS, et al. Caudal epidural anesthesia administered intraoperatively provides for effective postoperative analgesia after total hip arthroplasty. *Journal of Clinical Anesthesiology.* 2007;19:204-208.

58. Koh JL, Fanurik D, Harrison RD, et al. Analgesia following surgery in children with and without cognitive impairment. *Pain.* 2004;111:239-244.

59. Kress JP, Gehlbach B, Lacy M, et al. The long-term psychological effects of daily sedative interruption on critically ill patients. *American Journal of Respiratory Critical Care Medicine.* 2003;168:1457-1461.

60. Kruskamp T. The changing face of sedation: goal-directed care. *AACN News.* 2003;20(11):12-16.

61. Kshettry VR, Carole LF, Henly SJ, et al. Complementary alternative medical therapies for heart surgery patients: feasibility, safety, and impact. *Annals of Thoracic Surgery.* 2006;81:201-205.

62. Kunisawa T. Dexmedetomidine hydrochloride as a long-term sedative. *Journal of Therapeutics and Clinical Risk Management.* 2011;7:291-299.

63. Kupers R, Kehlet H. Brain imaging of clinical pain states: a critical review and strategies for future studies. *Lancet Neurology.* 2006;5:1033-1044.

64. Kwekkeboom KL, Herr K. Assessment of pain in the critically ill. *Critical Care Nursing Clinics of North America.* 2001;13:181-194.

65. Lee OK, Chung YF, Chan MF, et al. Music and its effect on the physiological responses and anxiety levels of patients receiving mechanical ventilation: a pilot study. *Journal of Clinical Nursing.* 2005;14:609-620.

66. Leon-Pizarro C, Gich I, Barthe E, et al. A randomized trial of the effect of training in relaxation and guided imagery techniques in improving psychological and quality-of-life indices for gynecologic and breast brachytherapy patients. *Psychooncology.* 2007;16:971-979.

67. Lighthall GK, Pearl RG. Volume resuscitation in the critically ill: choosing the best solution: how do crystalloid solutions compare with colloids? *The Journal of Critical Illness.* 2003;18:252-260.

68. Liu CX, Yi XL, Si DY, et al. Herb-drug interactions involving drug metabolizing enzymes and transporters. *Current Drug Metabolism.* May 27, 2011; Epub ahead of print.

69. Luer JM. Sedation and neuromuscular blockade in patients with acute respiratory failure: protocols for practice. *Critical Care Nurse.* 2002;22:70-75.

70. McCartney JBR. Anxiety and delirium in the intensive care unit. *Critical Care Clinics.* 1994;10:673-680.

71. McGaffigan P. Advancing sedation assessment to promote patient comfort. *Critical Care Nurse.* 2002;(suppl):29-36.

72. McHugh JM, McHuch WB. Pain: neuroanatomy, chemical mediators, and clinical implications. *AACN Clinical Issues.* 2000;11:168-178.

73. Mechlin MB, Maixner W, Light KC, et al. African Americans show alterations in endogenous pain regulatory mechanisms and reduced pain tolerance to experimental pain procedures. *Psychosomatic Medicine.* 2005;67:948-956.

74. Melloni C, Devivo P, Launo C, et al. Cisatracurium versus vecuronium: a comparative, double blind, randomized, multicenter study in adult patients under propofol/fentanyl/N_2O anesthesia. *Minerva Anesthesiologica.* 2006;72:299-308.

75. Merker B. Consciousness without a cerebral cortex: a challenge for neuroscience and medicine. *Behavioral and Brain Science.* 2007;30:63-81.

76. Merskey H, Bogduk N. *Classification of Chronic Pain: Descriptions of Chronic Pain Syndromes and Definitions of Pain Terms. Task Force on Taxonomy of the International Association for the Study of Pain.* 2nd ed. Seattle: IASP Press; 1994.

77. Messina M, Boroli F, Landoni G, et al. A comparison of epidural vs. paravertebral blockade in thoracic surgery. *Minerva Anesthesiologica.* 2009;75:616-621.

78. Miller C, Newton SE. Pain perception and expression: the influence of gender, personal self-efficacy, and lifespan socialization. *Pain Management Nursing.* 2006;7:148-152.

79. Moalem G, Tracey DJ. Immune and inflammatory mechanisms in neuropathic pain. *Brain Research Reviews.* 2006;51:240-264.

80. Moline LR. Patient psychologic preparation for invasive procedures: an integrative review. *Journal of Vascular Nursing.* 2000;18:117-122.

81. Morandi A, Pandharipande P, Trabucchi M, et al. Understanding international differences in terminology for delirium and other types of acute brain dysfunction in critically ill patients. *Intensive Care Medicine.* 2008;34:1907-1915.

82. Moss M, Burnham EL. Alcohol abuse in the critically ill patient. *Lancet.* 2006;368:2231-2242.

83. Moss M, Parsons PE, Steinberg KP, et al. Chronic alcohol abuse is associated with an increased incidence of acute respiratory distress syndrome and severity of multiple organ dysfunction in patients with septic shock. *Critical Care Medicine.* 2003;31:869-877.

84. Nygaard HA, Jarland M. The Checklist of Nonverbal Pain Indicators (CNPI): testing of reliability and validity in Norwegian nursing homes. *Age Ageing.* 2006;35:79-81.

85. O'Brien JM Jr, Lu B, Ali NA, et al. Alcohol dependence is independently associated with sepsis, septic shock, and hospital mortality among adult intensive care unit patients. *Critical Care Medicine.* 2007;35:345-350.

86. Pandharipande P, Cotton BA, Shintani A, et al. Motoric subtypes of delirium in mechanically ventilated surgical and trauma intensive care unit patients. *Intensive Care Medicine.* 2007;33:1726-1731.

87. Papathanassoglou ED. Psychological support and outcomes for ICU patients. *Nursing in Critical Care.* 2010;15:118-128.

88. Pasero C. Challenges in pain assessment. *Journal of Peri Anesthesia Nursing.* 2009;24:50-54.

89. Pasero C, McCaffery M. Multimodal balanced analgesia in the critically ill. *Critical Care Nursing Clinics of North America.* 2001;13:195-206.

90. Payen JF, Bru O, Bosson JL, et al. Assessing pain in critically ill sedated patients by using a behavioral pain scale. *Critical Care Medicine.* 2001;29:2258-2263.

91. Payen JF, Chanques G, Mantz J, et al. Current practices in sedation and analgesia for mechanically ventilated critically ill patients: a prospective multicenter patient-based study. *Anesthesiology.* 2007;106:687-695.

92. Puntillo K. Stitch, stitch ... creating an effective pain management program for critically ill patients. *American Journal of Care.* 1997;6:259-260.

93. Puntillo KA, Morris AB, Thompson CL, et al. Pain behaviors observed during six common procedures: results from Thunder Project II. *Critical Care Medicine.* 2004;32:421-427.

94. Puntillo KA, Wild LR, Morris AB, et al. Practices and predictors of analgesic interventions for adults undergoing painful procedures. *American Journal of Critical Care.* 2002; 11:415-429.

95. Rahim-Williams FB, Riley JL III, Herrera D, et al. Ethnic identity predicts experimental pain sensitivity in African Americans and Hispanics. *Pain.* 2007;129:177-184.

96. Ramsay MA, Savege TM, Simpson BR, et al. Controlled sedation with alphaxalone-alphadolone. *British Medical Journal.* 1974;2:656-659.

97. Richardson S. Effects of relaxation and imagery on the sleep of critically ill adults. *Dimens Crit Care Nurs.* 2003;22: 182-190.

98. Riker RR, Shehabi Y, Bokesch PM, et al. Dexmedetomidine vs midazolam for sedation of critically ill patients: a randomized trial. *Journal of the American Medical Association.* 2009;301:489-499.

99. Riker RR, Fraser GL, Simmons LE, et al. Validating the Sedation-Agitation Scale with the Bispectral Index and Visual Analog Scale in adult ICU patients after cardiac surgery. *Intensive Care Medicine.* 2001;27:853-858.

100. Ringdal M, Johansson L, Lundberg D, et al. Delusional memories from the intensive care unit—experienced by patients with physical trauma. *Intensive & Critical Care Nursing.* 2006;22:346-354.

101. Robillard D, Shim S, Irwin R, et al. Support services perspective: the Critical Care Family Assistance Program. *Chest.* 2005; 128:124S-127S.

102. Rootman DB, Mustard R, Kalia V, et al. Increased incidence of complications in trauma patients cointoxicated with alcohol and other drugs. *The Journal of Trauma.* 2007;62:755-758.

103. Salluh JI, Soares M, Teles JM, et al. Delirium epidemiology in critical care (DECCA): an international study. *Critical Care.* 2010;14:R210.

104. Scarci M, Joshi A, Attia R. In patients undergoing thoracic surgery is paravertebral block as effective as epidural analgesia for pain management? *Interactive Cardiovascular and Thoracic Surgery.* 2010;10:92-96.

105. Schmidt M, Demoule A, Polito A, et al. Dyspnea in mechanically ventilated critically ill patients. *Critical Care Medicine.* 2011;39:2059-2065.

106. Schweickert WD, Kress JP. Strategies to optimize analgesia and sedation. *Critical Care.* 2008;12(suppl 3):S6.

107. Sechi G, Serra A. Wernicke's encephalopathy: new clinical settings and recent advances in diagnosis and management. *Lancet Neurology.* 2007;6:442-455.

108. Sessler CN, Gosnell MS, Grap MJ, et al. The Richmond Agitation-Sedation Scale: validity and reliability in adult intensive care unit patients. *American Journal of Respiratory and Critical Care Medicine.* 2002;166:1338-1344.

109. Sessler CN, Grap MJ, Ramsay MA. Evaluating and monitoring analgesia and sedation in the intensive care unit. *Critical Care.* 2008;12(suppl 3):S2.

110. Sessler CN, Pedram S. Protocolized and target-based sedation and analgesia in the ICU. *Critical Care Clinics.* 2009;25: 489-513, viii.

111. Sessler CN, Varney K. Patient-focused sedation and analgesia in the ICU. *Chest.* 2008;133:552-565.

112. Setty AR, Sigal LH. Herbal medications commonly used in the practice of rheumatology: mechanisms of action, efficacy, and side effects. *Seminars in Arthritis and Rheumatism.* 2005; 34:773-784.

113. Siegel MD. Management of agitation in the intensive care unit. *Clinics in Chest Medicine.* 2003;24:713-725.

114. Southworth S, Peters J, Rock A, et al. A multicenter, randomized, double-blind, placebo-controlled trial of intravenous ibuprofen 400 and 800 mg every 6 hours in the management of postoperative pain. *Clinical Therapeutics.* 2009;31:1922-1935.

115. Spies CD, Otter HE, Huske B, et al. Alcohol withdrawal severity is decreased by symptom-orientated adjusted bolus therapy in the ICU. *Intensive Care Medicine* 2003;29:2230-2238.

116. Spronk PE, Riekerk B, Hofhuis J. Occurrence of delirium is severely underestimated in the ICU during daily care. *Intensive Care Medicine.* 2009;35:1276-1280.

117. Szokol JW, Vender JS. Anxiety, delirium, and pain in the intensive care unit. *Critical Care Clinics.* 2001;17:821-842.

118. Thomason JW, Shintani A, Peterson JF, et al. Intensive care unit delirium is an independent predictor of longer hospital stay: a prospective analysis of 261 non-ventilated patients. *Critical Care.* 2005;9:R375-R381.

119. Thomson AD, Marshall EJ. The treatment of patients at risk of developing Wernicke's encephalopathy in the community. *Alcohol and Alcoholism.* 2006;41:159-167.

120. Truman B, Ely EW.. Monitoring delirium in critically ill patients: using the confusion assessment method for the intensive care unit. *Critical Care Nurse.* 2003;23:25-36.

121. Turkmen A, Altan A, Turgut N, et al. The correlation between the Richmond agitation-sedation scale and bispectral index during dexmedetomidine sedation. *European Journal of Anaesthesiology*. 2006;23:300-304.

122. Tusek DL, Cynar RE. Strategies for implementing a guided imagery program to enhance patient experience. *AACN Clinical Issues*. 2000;11(1):68-76.

123. Twiss E, Seaver J, McCaffrey R. The effect of music listening on older adults undergoing cardiovascular surgery. *Nursing in Critical Care*. 2006;11:224-231.

124. Uusaro A, Parviainen I, Tenhunen JJ. The proportion of intensive care unit admissions related to alcohol use: a prospective cohort study. *Acta Anaesthesiologica Scandinavica*, 2005;49:1236-1240.

125. Valente G, Sanges M, Campione S, et al. Herbal hepatotoxicity: a case of difficult interpretation. *European Review for Medical and Pharmacological Sciences*. 2010;14:865-870.

126. Vazquez M, Pardavila MI, Lucia M, et al. Pain assessment in turning procedures for patients with invasive mechanical ventilation. *Nursing in Critical Care*. 2011;16:178-185.

127. Voepel-Lewis T, Zanotti J, Dammeyer JA, et al. Reliability and validity of the Face, Legs, Activity, Cry, Consolability (FLACC) behavioral tool in assessing acute pain in critically ill patients. *American Journal of Critical Care*. 2010;19:55-61.

CHAPTER

6

Nutritional Support

Miranda Kelly, DNP, RN, ACNP-BC

⊖volve WEBSITE

Many additional resources, including self-assessment exercises, are located on the Evolve companion website at http://evolve.elsevier.com/Sole.

- Review Questions
- Mosby's Nursing Skills Procedures

- Animations
- Video Clips

INTRODUCTION

"Let food be thy medicine, and medicine be thy food." The father of medical science, Hippocrates, made this statement around the fifth century BC. Adequate nutrition remains an important part of comprehensive patient care management. Rates of malnutrition in hospitalized patients range from 20% to 50%, and nutritional status typically worsens during the hospital stay.[17] The components of nutrition—proteins, carbohydrates, and fats—are the body's building blocks for maintaining both mental and physical health. Without appropriate nutrition, individuals are at a higher risk for complications during recovery and increased rates of mortality and morbidity.[17]

This chapter reviews the gastrointestinal (GI) system's function related to nutrition and the basic assessment of a patient's nutritional status. Nutrient additives and formulas, goals of therapy, practice guidelines for enteral and parenteral nutrition, drug-nutrient interactions, and complications related to nutritional therapy are also discussed.

GASTROINTESTINAL TRACT

A functioning GI tract, or gut, is essential to the health and well-being of a critically ill patient. The gut has protective mechanisms that include intestinal permeability and intestinal mucosal defense. Intestinal permeability is controlled by junctions of epithelial cells lining the intestinal mucosa, which prevent passage of molecules into or out of the GI tract. Failure of the junctions related to inflammation or lack of nutrition allows volatile bacteria to escape, which can result in systemic infection. The mucosal defense, regulated

by the gut-associated lymphoid tissue, is designed to protect the GI tract from toxic invaders and inflammatory mediators, and prevents passage of these harmful particles into the systemic circulation. When the gut's defense mechanisms are suboptimal, the functional structures (the villi, which absorb and process nutrients) can atrophy. The villi are replenished every 3 to 4 days, and without adequate nutritional stimulation, the cells are not available to absorb nutrients. Dysfunction of the GI tract, or an extended period of hypoperfusion in critical illness, can impair a critically ill patient's recovery by disrupting the epithelial cells lining the mucosa and lymphoid tissue. Providing and maintaining adequate nutrition is essential to protecting the continuity and function of the GI tract.

UTILIZATION OF NUTRIENTS

The body uses nutrients in a variety of ways. Each cell requires carbohydrates, proteins, fats, water, electrolytes, vitamins, and trace elements to provide the energy necessary to maintain bodily functions. The proper combination of nutrients necessary to meet energy requirements is acquired through metabolism. When nutrients are ingested, they are broken down to form a food bolus through the mixture of salts and enzymes (salivary amylase, which digests starch) secreted by the salivary glands to create saliva. Saliva is rich in mucus and helps to coat the food bolus. The food bolus stimulates peristalsis, the contraction and relaxation of esophageal muscles, which continues until the bolus reaches the esophageal sphincter. Peristalsis causes the esophageal sphincter to relax so the bolus can pass into the stomach. The

80

function of the stomach is to break down larger molecules into smaller ones and to store food before delivery to the duodenum. The stomach produces both acidic and basic secretions. Acidic secretions, produced at a rate of 2 to 3 liters per day, assist in the breakdown of proteins to facilitate digestion. Chyme, which is the mixture of the gastric secretions and the food bolus formed by the stomach is very acidic with a pH of around 2. The gastric mucosal cells provide a protective coating to lubricate the stomach lining and shield it from erosion by the harsh acidic secretions. The stomach also secretes intrinsic factor, which is necessary for the absorption of vitamin B_{12} in the ileum. Vitamin B_{12} is critical for the formation of red blood cells. The stomach secretes fluid that is high in sodium, potassium, and other electrolytes. If excessive fluid is lost from the stomach, either from vomiting or from gastric suction, the patient is at risk for fluid and electrolyte imbalances.

The first part of the small intestine is the duodenum, the area where the pancreatic juices and the bile from the liver empty, and minerals such as chloride, sulfate, iron, calcium, and magnesium are absorbed. The duodenum contains mucus-secreting glands called Brunner glands that produce an alkaline compound. The glands' secretions protect the duodenal wall from the acidic chyme and raise the pH of the chyme to around 7.0 before it reaches the ileum. The next segment is the jejunum; monosaccharides (sugars), glucose, galactose, and fructose are absorbed in the first part of the jejunum along with the water-soluble vitamins: thiamine, riboflavin, pyridoxine, folic acid, and vitamin C. At the end of the jejunum is the ileum. Protein is broken down into amino acids and absorbed in the first part of the ileum. The fat-soluble vitamins (A, D, E, and K), fat, cholesterol, bile salts, and vitamin B_{12} are absorbed at the end of the ileum. The ileocecal valve located at the end of the ileum helps to prevent reflux of colonic contents from the large intestine into the ileum.

The colon is next and is divided into the ascending, transverse, and descending colons and the rectum. Sodium and potassium are absorbed in the first part of the colon. Vitamin K and some B vitamins are synthesized by bacterial action and absorbed toward the distal portion of the colon. Water is reabsorbed at the end of the colon. The colon is also a major site for generation and absorption of short-chain fatty acids. These fatty acids are the products of bacterial metabolism of undigested complex carbohydrates such as fruits and vegetables.

The pancreas aids in digestion, has both exocrine and endocrine functions, and secretes bicarbonate and enzymes into the first part of the duodenum. Exocrine digestive enzymes (trypsinogen and chymotrypsinogen) are secreted in an inactive form to prevent autodigestion of the pancreas. Bicarbonate is also secreted by the pancreas and aids in neutralizing the pH of gastric chyme. The endocrine function produces insulin, glucagon, and somastatin.

The contraction of the gallbladder and the relaxation of the sphincter of Oddi control the bile flow that is secreted into the duodenum. The body produces anywhere from 400 to 800 mL of bile per day. Bile helps to emulsify and absorb fats and provides the primary route for the breakdown and elimination of cholesterol.

The largest solid organ in the body is the liver. It aids in digestion by filtering out bacteria and foreign material, and also secretes bile. The liver detoxifies ammonia (a by-product of the breakdown of amino acids) by combining it with carbon dioxide, producing urea, and releasing it into the bloodstream. The liver is also responsible for more than half of the body's lymph production. It is important to note this lymph production because liver dysfunction may force lymph into the abdominal cavity, thus decreasing liver blood flow and increasing hepatic pressure.

Metabolism is a key function of the liver. The liver is important in lipid and vitamin A metabolism, synthesis of clotting factors, and synthesis of most circulating proteins and albumin. Protein metabolism occurs through amino acid synthesis, which converts glycogen, fat, and protein to glucose. Fatty acids are synthesized from carbohydrate precursors and are generally stored in the form of triglycerides to be metabolized later by other tissues. Carbohydrate metabolism helps maintain normal blood glucose concentrations. When serum glucose levels fall, glucose stored as glycogen is readily transported back to the cells as needed for energy. Another pathway that generates glucose is gluconeogenesis, carried out only in the liver and the renal cortex. Gluconeogenesis creates glucose from other substrates (amino acids) when glycogen reserves are depleted.

ASSESSMENT OF NUTRITIONAL STATUS

Nutritional screening identifies patients who are malnourished or nutritionally at risk, and should be completed by the nurse within 24 hours of hospital admission.[20] All patients identified by screening to be at nutritional risk receive a comprehensive nutritional assessment. Evaluating nutritional status is essential to determine whether a hypermetabolic or catabolic state exists.

Nutritional status is the balance between a patient's current nutritional supply and demand. A comprehensive approach to determine nutritional status evaluates several criteria: medical history and examination, nutrition and medication histories, physical assessment, anthropometric measurements, and laboratory data.[15] The data are organized and evaluated to form a professional consult regarding the patient's nutritional status and needs during hospitalization. The purposes of a nutritional assessment in the critically ill patient are to document baseline subjective and objective nutritional parameters, determine nutritional risk factors, identify nutritional deficits, establish nutritional needs for patients, and identify medical, psychosocial, and socioeconomic factors that may influence the administration of nutrition support therapy (see box, "Geriatric Considerations").[15]

Nutritional assessment of the critically ill patient begins with the collection of subjective and objective data. The nurse determines whether the patient is alert and oriented, has an adequate gag reflex, and is able to swallow without difficulty.

GERIATRIC CONSIDERATIONS

- Elderly patients (older than 65 years) are at a higher risk for altered nutrition due to:
  - Chronic diseases that affect the appetite or the ability to obtain and prepare appropriate and adequate caloric intake—dementia, chronic obstructive pulmonary disease, osteoarthritis, heart failure, and impaired mobility.
  - Decreased intake due to poorly fitting dentures or missing teeth.
  - Decreased income levels, which may lead to food choices based on cost rather than nutritional value.
  - Social isolation. Older adults living alone are more likely to experience hunger.
  - Inability to obtain food because of lack of transportation or minimal access to a home delivery food service such as Meals on Wheels.
- Potential drug-nutrient interactions are assessed in all elderly patients. A person who takes multiple daily medications is at a higher risk for nutritional alterations due to medication side effects, which may alter appetite. Medications may change flavor, taste, and odor perceptions affecting nutritional intake.

From Rourke KM. Nutrition. In Meiner SE, ed. *Gerontologic Nursing.* St. Louis: Mosby; 2011:177-193.

A speech pathologist can perform a bedside assessment of patient's ability to swallow. Based on that assessment, patients may require a more comprehensive study such as a modified barium swallow completed in radiology. Overly sedated or intubated patients are not candidates for oral feedings; overly sedated patients must wait until their mental or respiratory status improves before receiving an oral feeding and an intubated patient must be extubated and have met the criteria to feed prior to offering oral feedings. If an oral diet is appropriate, the ability to tolerate a variety of textures is determined in part by adequate dentition and also by sufficient saliva production, which is determined through assessment of the mouth looking for a pink, moist oral mucosa. Extra fluids may be required to facilitate easier swallowing if dryness is apparent.

Additional assessments that assist in determining nutritional deficits include muscle or adipose tissue loss, the appearance of wasting associated with chronic disease (e.g., cancer, multiple sclerosis), and whether the patient is retaining fluid, which could be related to a protein deficit. Critically ill obese patients may also have nutritional deficits despite their physical appearance (see box, "Bariatric Considerations"). The patient's medical history also identifies the

BARIATRIC CONSIDERATIONS

Assessment
- Assessment of an obese patient's nutritional status includes body mass index (BMI), actual and ideal body weight, waist circumference, history of weight gain, health-related conditions, and family history of obesity.
- BMI is calculated using the formula: weight (kg)/height (m²).
- BMI is a reflection of body fat and correlates with morbidity and mortality.

BMI Classification:

CLASSIFICATION	BMI
Normal	18.5-24.9
Overweight	25.0-29.9
Obese	30.0-39.9
Extreme obesity	≥40.0

- Waist circumference greater than 35 inches in woman and greater than 40 inches in men is an indication of abdominal obesity. Abdominal obesity increases a patient's risk for coronary artery disease and type 2 diabetes.

Evidence-Based Recommendations
- Permissive underfeeding or hypocaloric feeding
- Recommendations for caloric intake:
  If BMI is greater than 30, the caloric goal of nutrition should not exceed 60% to 70% of targeted requirements for patients (22-25 kcal/kg ideal body weight [IBW])
- Recommendations for protein intake:
  If BMI is 30-40, the protein goal of nutrition is at least 2.0 g/kg IBW
  If BMI is greater than 40, the protein goal of nutrition is at least 2.5 g/kg IBW

Implications for Nursing
- Nurses must be aware of their personal beliefs and biases about obesity.
- Provide education about nutritional recommendations, weight loss, comorbid conditions related to obesity, and available community resources.
- Use small bowel feeding tubes to decrease the risk of aspiration, because abdominal weight increases intraabdominal pressure.
- Bariatric surgery is an ever growing field, providing options for the morbidly obese patient.
- Meticulous skin care is necessary because obese patients are at high risk for skin breakdown.

Data from Kushner RF, Drover JW. Current strategies of critical care assessment and therapy of the obese patient (hypocaloric feeding): what are we doing and what do we need to do? *Journal of Parenteral and Enteral Nutrition.* 2011;35(suppl 5):365-435. Rollinson D, Shikora SA, Saltzman E. Obesity. In Gottschlich MM, eds. *The ASPEN Nutrition Support Core Curriculum: A Case-based Approach the Adult Patient.* Silver Spring, MD: American Society for Parenteral and Enteral Nutrition (ASPEN); 2007:695-721. U.S. Department of Health and Human Services, National Institutes of Health, National Heart, Lung, and Blood Institute. How are overweight and obesity diagnosed? http://www.nhlbi.nih.gov/health/health-topics/topics/obe/diagnosis.html; 2010.

presence of malabsorptive syndromes that can impair the patient's ability to utilize nutrients. These conditions include short bowel syndrome, a history of radiation to the bowel, a history of bariatric surgery, the presence of an ileus, intestinal pseudo-obstruction, persistent vomiting, Crohn's disease, diverticulosis, or gastroparesis.

OVERVIEW OF NUTRITIONAL SUPPORT

Enteral Nutrition

Patients who are not able to meet their needs orally are started on enteral nutrition in the first 24 to 48 hours.[14] Enteral nutrition (EN) refers to the delivery of nutrients into the GI tract, which is the preferred route of nutrient administration unless contraindicated. Decisions regarding access for enteral nutrition take into account the effectiveness of gastric emptying, GI anatomy, and aspiration risk. In addition, enteral nutrition depends on an intact bowel that is able to absorb nutrients. All feeding tubes require radiological confirmation of placement prior to use (see box, "Clinical Alert"). Large-bore nasogastric (NG) tubes can be used for administration of enteral nutrition, medication administration, or decompression of the gut. A flexible small-bore tube (usually 5 to 12 French) may be inserted in place of large-bore tubes for feedings when a patient does not tolerate gastric feeding tube placement. The small-bore tube is better tolerated because of its size, flexibility, and location in the duodenum; it also reduces the risk of nasal tissue necrosis. Nasally inserted, small-bore tubes (nasojejunal) can be used in short-term situations, usually no more than 6 weeks. Many studies have compared outcomes of nutritional support administered through an NG tube and a small-bore feeding tube, with no significant difference noted in pneumonia rates, length of stay, or mortality.[9] Feeding tubes directly inserted into the stomach or jejunum (e.g., gastrojejunostomy or jejunostomy) are chosen for long-term access, especially for patients at high risk of aspiration pneumonia. A percutaneous endoscopic gastrostomy (PEG) tube is often inserted because placement does not require general anesthesia, and it allows feedings to begin soon after placement. A jejunostomy tube can only be placed during a laparotomy.

Parenteral Nutrition

Parenteral nutrition refers to the infusion of nutrient solutions into the bloodstream by some form of central intravenous access catheter. A central catheter (or central line) is defined as a line placed into the vascular system with the distal tip in the superior vena cava, right atrium, or inferior vena cava. The central catheter options include a peripherally inserted central catheter (PICC), an external tunneled catheter, or a subcutaneous port. Placement of these lines is verified by chest radiograph immediately after insertion. There are two options for parenteral nutrition administration available: peripheral parenteral nutrition (PPN) or total parenteral nutrition (TPN) solutions. Solution concentration is the main determinant of administration site, specifically the carbohydrate concentration. Isotonic parenteral solutions, such as PPN, are appropriate for peripheral administration, whereas hypertonic parenteral solutions, such as TPN, can only be administered centrally because of the risk of phlebitis and the potential for vascular damage.[20]

Parenteral nutrition is a successful method to provide nutrients to patients who are unable to tolerate enteral therapy because of a GI obstruction, intractable vomiting or diarrhea, or because they must have *nothing by mouth* for an extended period, usually for longer than 1 week. One exception is the patient who is admitted to the hospital malnourished. Parenteral nutrition should be initiated immediately for those patients who are unable to tolerate enteral nutrition.[14] Parenteral nutrition may also be used if patients are unable to meet their nutritional needs with EN alone. Both the timing of initiation of parenteral nutrition and the clinical benefit are controversial. Current findings by researchers recommend each patient be assessed individually.[7,13] Factors for deciding which therapy to use are based on the length of time the patient will receive parenteral nutrition, as well as the patient's vascular access history, venous anatomy, and coagulation status related to central line site selection. See the Evidence-Based Practice box about the use of parenteral nutrition to supplement enteral nutrition.

> **! CLINICAL ALERT**
>
> ### Assessment of Feeding Tube Placement
>
> Misplacement of feeding tubes increases the risk of complications including nutrition delays, aspiration pneumonia, and pneumothorax. Radiographic confirmation of correct tube placement is expected before initiation of tube feedings or administration of medications. Tube placement must also be verified if the tube becomes dislodged and requires reinsertion. Auscultatory methods for assessing tube placement are unreliable. Patients with the highest risk of placement complications are intubated patients and those with an altered level of consciousness or an impaired gag reflex.[9]

EVIDENCE-BASED PRACTICE

Parenteral Nutrition Supplementation with Enteral Nutrition

Problem

Early initiation of enteral nutrition (EN) is the recommended form of nutritional support for critically ill patients. Some patients do not receive adequate nutrition from EN because of high gastric residual volumes (GRV), abdominal distention, nausea, or vomiting. Patients may also have contraindications due to bowel obstruction or ischemia, GI perforation, or short gut syndrome. Parenteral nutrition (PN) can be used for nutritional support in select patients, but the recommendations are controversial.

Clinical Question

Does the addition of PN to supplement early EN improve nutritional intake and clinical outcomes?

Evidence

The authors conducted two international, prospective, observational studies, one in 2007 and one in 2008. The study included 2920 mechanically ventilated patients from 260 intensive care units (ICU) in 28 countries. The authors compared three groups of patients that received (1) early EN only, (2) early EN and early PN (less than 48 hours after admission), or (3) early EN and late PN (more than 48 hours after admission). The authors found that patients receiving late PN experienced early GI dysfunction for 2 or more days when compared to the EN group. The 60-day mortality rate, days on mechanical ventilation, ICU

length of stay, and hospital length of stay were significantly lower in the EN group. Overall the EN-only group had the best outcomes. The authors concluded that patients receiving supplemental PN may have improved nutritional intake, but there was no demonstrated clinical benefit, and outcomes were worse than the EN-only group. The authors determined that further randomized studies are required before recommendations can be implemented.

Implications for Nursing

Implementation of early EN is a current ASPEN recommendation for critically ill patients. Nurses are instrumental in the implementation of the recommendations by promoting early initiation and management of EN. Implementation of the ASPEN recommendations emphasizing initiation of EN within 24 to 48 hours and management of GRV contribute to patients receiving early and adequate nutritional support.

Level of Evidence

C—Descriptive study

Reference

Kutsogiannis J, Alberda C, Gramlich L, et al. Early use of supplemental parenteral nutrition in critically ill patients: results of an international multicenter observation study. *Critical Care Medicine.* 2011;39(12):2691-2699.

Nutritional Additives

Specialized nutritional formulas, specifically immune-enhancing formulas, are recommended for specific patient populations, including patients with burns on more than 30% of the body, head and neck cancer, trauma injuries, major elective gastrointestinal surgery, and a need for mechanical ventilation without severe sepsis.

Several immune-enhancing formulas are available and are listed in Table 6-1. Immune-enhancing formulas have been demonstrated to decrease length of stay, duration of mechanical ventilation, hospital costs, and infection risk, and they improve wound healing in specified patient populations. Research on the effectiveness of the various additives and supplements is ongoing.[2]

QSEN EXEMPLAR

Evidence-Based Practice

Cahill and colleagues conducted an international study to identify adherence to evidence-based guidelines for nutritional support. The study included 158 ICUs from 20 countries with a total of 2946 patients and 27,944 patient days. The current practice of enteral nutrition administration was compared to the evidence-based practice guidelines to determine opportunities for achieving best practice. Gaps were identified between the clinical guidelines and current practice related to delivery of enteral nutrition across sites. The authors found that patients only received 60% of the recommended goal and the average time for enteral nutrition to start was 46.5 hours from admission. Use of enteral nutrition protocols, glycemic control, and standardized management of gastric residuals were all found to improve the patient's nutritional status. Several barriers to implementation of evidence-based guidelines were identified, including implementation strategies, providers' knowledge and attitudes, and institutional factors. Facilities engaged in

performance improvement activities were found to be high achievers, and these efforts contributed to reductions in mortality and morbidity. By participating in multiprofessional performance improvement processes, nursing can promote implementation of enteral nutrition protocols and the latest clinical guidelines. Early implementation of enteral nutrition and consistent management of gastric residual volumes are two areas in which nursing can make an impact. Monitoring of patient outcomes related to nutritional support can provide facilities data for benchmarking and developing the best achievable practice implementing clinical guidelines.

References

Cahill NE, Dhaliwal R, Day AG, et al. Nutrition therapy in the critical care setting: what is "best achievable" practice? An international multicenter observational study. *Critical Care Medicine.* 2010;38(2):395-401.

TABLE 6-1	COMPONENTS OF IMMUNE-ENHANCING FORMULAS		
COMPONENT	**ACTION**	**POPULATION BENEFITED**	**EXAMPLES**
Arginine	• Decreases T-suppressor cells • Increases T-helper cells • Improves wound healing • Substrate used for nitric oxide production	• Postoperative patients especially abdominal surgery • Mild sepsis • Trauma • ARDS	• Juven • Vivonex Plus
Glutamine	• Essential acid at times of stress and hypercatabolism • May diminish atrophy of GI tract mucosa and bacterial translocation • Stimulates protein synthesis and inhibits protein breakdown • Acts as fuel for antiinflammatory cells such as colonocytes, enterocytes, and macrophages	• Burn injury • Trauma • Wound healing	• AlitraQ • Juven • Vivonex Plus
Omega-3 fatty acids	• Important for cell membrane stabilization • Improves immune function • Antiinflammatory properties especially to the lungs • Reduces the hypermetabolic response	• Postoperative patients, especially abdominal surgery • Mild sepsis • Trauma • ARDS	• Oxcepa • Impact Extra
Branched-chain amino acids	• Supplies fuel to skeletal muscle during times of stress • Important defense mechanism for infection, especially for patients with hepatic dysfunction • Improves protein synthesis • Improves nitrogen balance	• Stressed patients with hepatic dysfunction • ARDS	• Oxcepa • Impact
Nucleotides	• Increases protein synthesis • Aids in the immune function and helps fight infection • Aids in preventing immunosuppression • Essential for protein, carbohydrate, and fat synthesis	• Mild sepsis • Trauma • ARDS • Lactose-free • Kosher • Malabsorption	• Impact • Vivonex Plus
Vitamin A	• Improves immune response, particularly in conjunction with arginine	• Wound healing • Critical illness	• Replete • Vivonex Plus
Vitamin C	• Traps free radicals • Increases antibody production and lymphocyte response • Promotes collagen formation and improves wound healing	• Wound healing • Critical illness	• Vivonex Plus
Vitamin E	• Antioxidant properties • Cytoprotective, protects red blood cells from destruction	• Wound healing • Critical illness	• Vivonex Plus

ARDS, Acute respiratory distress syndrome.
Abbott Nutrition. *Brands.* http://abbottnutrition.com/our-Products/brands.aspx; 2012; Hall JE. Dietary balances; regulation of feeding; obesity and starvation; vitamins and minerals. In *Guyton and Hall Textbook of Medical Physiology.* Philadelphia, PA: Saunders; 2011:843-858; Nestle Nutrition. *Products & Applications.* www.nestle-nutrition.com/Products/Default.aspx; 2012. Accessed April 2, 2012.

NUTRITIONAL THERAPY GOALS

The goals of nutritional therapy are to provide nutritional support consistent with specific metabolic needs and disease processes, to avoid complications of feedings, and ultimately to improve patient outcomes. This is accomplished by creating a *nutrition care plan*. A multiprofessional approach, which includes a registered dietitian, is used to analyze the patient's information, including energy and nutrient requirements and intake targets, the route of nutritional support administration, and measurable short- and long-term goals of care. Patients and families are educated and included in decisions about nutritional support. Discussions address therapy, goals, expectations, and the patient and family wishes. The first step in formulating the nutrition care plan is to estimate the patient's calorie and protein requirements (Table 6-2).

Parenteral nutrition (PN) support is usually individualized, and a pharmacist or dietician often assists in determining

TABLE 6-2   ESTIMATION OF NUTRIENT NEEDS

CALORIC REQUIREMENTS	PROTEIN REQUIREMENTS	PATIENT APPEARANCE/CONSIDERATIONS
Normal Nonstressed 25 kcal/kg/day	0.8 g/kg/day	Normal
Mildly Stressed 25-30 kcal/kg/day	0.8-1.0 g/kg/day	May appear malnourished Postoperative or acutely ill
Moderately Stressed 30-35 kcal/kg/day	1.0-1.5 g/kg/day	May appear malnourished May have trouble with absorption Signs of sepsis Recent major surgery
Severely Stressed 35 kcal/kg/day	1.0-2.0 g/kg/day	Likely to be underweight Major procedure with a septic event Catabolic state Unable to meet nutritional needs by oral intake alone
Obese (BMI >30) 22-25 kcal/kg/day (ideal body weight)	≥2.0 g/kg/day (BMI 30-40) ≥2.5 g/kg/day (BMI >40)	Critically ill obese patient

the prescription that best meets the patient's nutritional needs. Although the prescription is individualized, the process for PN preparation should be standardized in facilities. The standard dosing ranges for parenteral electrolytes and minerals assume normal organ function without abnormal losses and follow the recommended dietary allowance (RDA) and dietary reference intake (DRI). Lipids are often given concurrently with PN. However, current guidelines recommend that PN formulas *without* soy-based lipids be given during the first week of critical illness. This recommendation is based largely on one study in which researchers reported a decrease in infection, length of stay, and mechanical ventilation days when lipid-free PN was administered. More research is needed in this area because most currently available lipids are soy-based.[14]

Enteral nutrition is preferred to parenteral nutrition in most cases to preserve gut integrity and modulate the systemic immune response and stress.[14] It is commonly selected for patients with neuromuscular impairment, patients who cannot meet their nutritional needs by oral intake alone, patients who are hypercatabolic, or patients who are unable to eat as a result of their underlying illness, such as those receiving mechanical ventilation or those with hypoperfusion states. Enteral feeding is associated with a significantly lower risk for infection; it is relatively inexpensive; and placement of a feeding tube in the correct site is relatively easy.[14] An enteral formula is selected that most closely meets the patient's current requirements.

Consideration of how the gut is functioning is weighed along with other underlying medical problems, such as gastroparesis. Administration of enteral feedings, even if the gut cannot tolerate a full enteral feeding schedule, is advantageous because it prevents bacterial overgrowth and potential bacterial migration across the intestinal wall and into the bloodstream. These benefits are crucial in critically ill patients. Enteral feedings have been used successfully in almost all situations, including the presence of ileus and pancreatitis.[14] TPN can be used in combination with enteral nutrition to meet the nutritional needs of the patient whose GI tract cannot tolerate the full caloric load of enteral feeding.

Various enteral formulas are marketed (Table 6-3). Standard formulas are typically 1 kcal/mL and are not designed for any specific disease state (e.g., Osmolite). Complete protein sources include soy protein isolate, calcium caseinate, sodium caseinate, and milk protein concentrate. The protein may be prepared as a form of hydrolyzed protein, which is broken down into smaller components to aid in digestion. In addition, the protein can be in the form of an elemental protein (e.g., Criticare HN), which is completely broken down and ready for absorption. Patients with short bowel syndromes or malabsorption may benefit from elemental protein formulas. Fat sources include canola oil, a medium-chain triglyceride oil, sunflower oil, safflower oil, soy, and lecithin. Lipids provide 30% to 50% of the total kilocalories. Carbohydrates are the most easily digested and absorbed component of enteral formulas. Sources include corn syrup, hydrolyzed cornstarch, and maltodextrin. The carbohydrates are not usually from lactose to minimize complications related to lactose intolerance. Fiber can also be added to improve blood glucose control, reduce hyperlipidemia, and improve diarrhea symptoms (e.g., Jevity).

Vitamins and trace elements are essential nutrients that act as coenzymes and cofactors in metabolism. For enteral nutrition, recommendations are based on the RDA and DRI levels with the exception of immune-modulating formulas (e.g., Oxepa). These formulas, used in patients with sepsis, adult respiratory distress syndrome, and acute lung injury,

TABLE 6-3 ENTERAL FORMULAS

GENERIC DESCRIPTION	SAMPLE PRODUCT	INDICATIONS
Elemental/Predigested 1 kcal/mL 45 g pro/L Free amino acids	Perative Criticare HN	GI dysfunction: short bowel syndrome, impaired digestion
Standard Isotonic 1 kcal/mL 37 g pro/L	Osmolite Nutren 1.0 Isosource	Normal GI function
High Protein 1 kcal/mL 62.5 g pro/L	Promote	Normal GI function with need for increased protein because of catabolism—burns, critical illness
1 kcal/mL 93.2 g pro/L	Peptamen Bariatric	Patients requiring high protein needs, including critically ill obese patients Antioxidants, prebiotic fiber, low carbohydrates
Fiber Enriched 1 kcal/mL 44 g pro/L	Jevity	Normal GI function Need for increased fiber for diarrhea or constipation
Calorie Dense 2 kcal/mL 70 g pro/L	Two Cal HN	Heart failure Liver disease
Wound Healing 1 kcal/mL 62.4 g pro/L Vitamins, some with arginine, glutamine, and/or omega-3 fatty acids	Replete with Fiber Juven Promote with Fiber	Wounds, trauma, burns
Immune Modulating 1.5 kcal/mL 62.7 g pro/L	Oxepa	Acute lung injury Adult Respiratory Distress Syndrome Sepsis
Oral Supplements 1 kcal/mL 37.5 g pro/L	Ensure	Inability to consume enough calories and protein
1 kcal/mL 41.7 g pro/L	Boost	

Kcal, Kilocalorie; *Pro,* protein.

provide vitamins and minerals above the RDA and DRI values. The dosing guidelines for parenteral vitamins and trace elements are considered as approximations of need during critical illness.

PRACTICE GUIDELINES

Enteral Nutrition

Nursing care of the patient receiving enteral nutrition involves administering feedings and assessing the patient's tolerance. EN in the critical care area is typically administered continuously via a feeding pump. The feedings can also be administered intermittently, in which the amount prescribed is infused via gravity administration. The intermittent feeding is ordered at intervals, for example every 4 hours, based on the patient's needs. Feeding tubes are routinely flushed with 30 mL of water every 4 hours during the continuous feedings, and before and after intermittent feedings and medication administration.[3]

When patients receive enteral feedings via gastric feeding tubes, the gastric residual volume (GRV) is checked every 4 hours. It is easier to assess GRV in large-bore gastric tubes, and sometimes small bore tubes collapse when assessing GRV. However, GRV should be assessed in all types of feeding tubes to assess for intolerance of feedings. Although recommendations vary, GRVs of 200 to 250 mL should be of concern, and a promotility agent may be ordered. If GRV is greater than

500 mL, the feedings should be held and patient assessed for other signs of intolerance.[5] Tolerance of feedings includes the presence of bowel sounds in four quadrants, as determined by auscultation; the presence of bowel motility or bowel movements; palpation of a soft abdomen; and percussion of the abdomen revealing tympanic findings. Signs of intolerance include the presence of nausea or vomiting, absent bowel sounds, abdominal distension, or cramping.

Patients may require more fluid intake than provided by enteral nutrition, and it is given in the form of free water. The water is administered via the feeding tube as ordered and is based on the patient's total fluid intake requirements. In general, patients require 30 mL/kg of total fluid intake daily, but considerations for the patient's disease process must also be considered.[8] Complications of enteral feedings are summarized in Table 6-4. Tube-fed patients are at a high

TABLE 6-4   TUBE FEEDING COMPLICATIONS AND NURSING INTERVENTIONS

COMPLICATIONS	NURSING INTERVENTIONS
Mechanical	
Tube obstruction	• Flush feeding tube with at least 30 mL of water every 4 hours during continuous feeding, after medications, after intermittent feedings, and before and after gastric residuals are checked. • Administer medications in elixir diluted with water whenever possible. • Irrigate tube with warm water or pancreatic enzymes to relieve obstruction.
Pulmonary	
Improper tube placement	• Verify the position of all feeding tubes by x-ray before initiating feedings; auscultatory methods of assessment are inaccurate. • Identify patients at risk for malposition of the tube, such as those with impaired gag/cough reflex, those who are obtunded or heavily sedated, and those receiving neuromuscular blocking agents.
Aspiration	• Mark feeding tube at exit site to monitor for proper tube placement; assess placement every 4 hours. • Monitor gastric residual volume (GRV) every 4 hours. • Attempting to aspirate gastric contents may be difficult because small-bore tubes collapse easily; it may be helpful to inject 30 mL of air into tube before assessing residuals. It may also be helpful to reposition the patient when assessing GRV. • If gastric residual volume >200 to 250 mL consider a promotility agent. • If gastric residual volume >500 mL hold feeding and assess patient for other signs of intolerance; consider small bowel feedings. • Do not use blue dye in enteral formulas to assess for aspiration; it is an unreliable indicator and may cause death. • To prevent reflux, keep head of bed elevated at least 30 degrees (preferably 45 degrees) during feedings. • Monitor abdominal girth measurements for signs of distention. • Assess bowel sounds.
Gastrointestinal	

Diarrhea	• Review medications that may increase the likelihood of diarrhea: sorbitol, laxatives, digitalis, antibiotics.
	• Assess for *Clostridium difficile*; obtain order for stool sample culture.
	• If infection is not the cause of the diarrhea, administer fiber-enriched formulas or bulking agents to normalize stool consistency (e.g., psyllium).
	• Prevent bacterial contamination:
	  • When possible, use full-strength, ready-to-use formula.
	  • Use meticulous hand-washing techniques before handling formulas and supplies.
	  • Avoid touching the inside of delivery sets.
	  • Rinse delivery sets with warm (preferably soapy) water after feedings.
	  • Change administration sets every 24 hours.
	  • Limit hanging time of formulas at room temperature to 8 hours; hang time for closed system and pre-filled sets of enteral formulas is 24-48 hours per manufacturer's recommendations.
	• Administer feedings at room or body temperature.
	• Limit bolus feedings to <300 mL.

Dumping syndrome	• Slow the rate and frequency of feeding bolus if abdominal distention or cramping occurs.
Metabolic	
Hyperglycemia	• Administer insulin as ordered, usually per sliding scale. • Monitor fluid status closely.
Electrolyte imbalance	• Monitor electrolytes for changes.

Prevention of Aspiration

Problem

Critically ill patients are at high risk for aspiration of both oropharyngeal secretions and gastric contents. Tube-fed patients are at especially high risk.

Clinical Question

What are expected nursing practices for preventing aspiration?

Evidence

The AACN reviewed available data and identified several factors associated with aspiration: supine positioning, displacement of feeding tubes, intolerance to feeding, and bolus feedings. Impaired swallowing after extubation and low endotracheal tube cuff pressures were also identified as risks.

Implications for Nursing

AACN identified several expected actions for practice.

- Maintain head of bed elevation at 30 to 45 degrees, unless contraindicated.
- Administer sedatives sparingly.
- Assess feeding tube placement every 4 hours
- Assess for feeding intolerance every 4 hours: gastric residual volume, abdominal discomfort or distention, and nausea or vomiting.
- Avoid bolus tube feedings.
- Obtain order for swallowing assessment prior to oral feedings after extubation.
- Maintain pressure in endotracheal tube cuff between 20 and 30 cm H_2O.

Level of Evidence

D—Professional standards developed from evidence

Reference

American Association of Critical-Care Nurses. Practice Alert: Prevention of Aspiration. http://www.aacn.org/WD/practice/docs/practicealerts/aacn-aspiration-practice-alert.pdf; 2011. Accessed April 24, 2012.

---

risk for aspiration. AACN has issued a practice alert to prevent aspiration (see "Evidence-Based Practice: Prevention of Aspiration").

Parenteral Nutrition

Each parenteral nutrition formulation that is compounded is inspected for signs of gross particulate contamination, discoloration, particulate formation, and phase separation at the time of compounding.[14] Maintaining the sterility of the setup is essential. All tubing is changed every 24 hours. The TPN or PPN line is a dedicated line for only parenteral nutrition; no intravenous push or infusion medications are given in this line except lipid infusions. Intravenous site care must be meticulous because of the infection risk related to the administration of high glucose content of TPN and use of an invasive line.[20] Monitoring for fluid and electrolyte imbalance, including chemistry panels and glucose levels, and monitoring for early signs of infection or signs of thrombosis are important aspects of nursing care because of the potential for adverse outcomes. Patients receiving parenteral nutrition have blood glucose monitoring at least every 6 hours. Insulin is also added to the TPN solution; the amount of insulin is adjusted daily based on the patient's glucose values over the previous 24 hours. Additional insulin therapy is usually administered subcutaneously according to a sliding scale.

Drug-Nutrient Interactions

Medication profiles of patients receiving nutritional support therapy are reviewed for potential effects on nutritional and metabolic status. Medications that are coadministered with enteral nutrition are reviewed periodically for potential incompatibilities. Whenever medications are administered via an enteral feeding tube, the tube should be flushed with 30 mL of water before and after each medication is administered.[4] Patients requiring a fluid restriction may receive 15 mL for flush.

Bioavailability of some medications (e.g., phenytoin) is reduced when administered with enteral feedings. Enteral nutrition may require temporary discontinuation before and after medication administration. For example, current recommendations for administration of phenytoin are to stop enteral feedings 1 to 2 hours before and after dosing.[22] This method may not always be optimal, especially for malnourished patients. Another option is to monitor and adjust phenytoin dosages based on serum drug levels while the patient is receiving enteral nutrition. Once enteral nutrition is discontinued, the drug dosage is readjusted.

Liquid medication formulations are preferred for administration via the enteral feeding tube. Pharmacists can often order and prepare many medications in liquid form upon request. Sustained-release medications must not be crushed and given via a feeding tube because of the potential for overdose.

The coadministration of an admixture of medications known to be incompatible with parenteral nutrition must also be prevented.

MONITORING NUTRITIONAL STATUS AND COMPLICATIONS OF NUTRITIONAL SUPPORT

Malnourished patients are at risk for refeeding syndrome, which leads to sudden electrolyte abnormalities and fluid shifts. Glucose and electrolytes (sodium, chloride, potassium, magnesium, and phosphorus) are monitored regularly until stable. This is especially important in patients with diabetes or in those who have risk factors for glucose intolerance. Nurses must be diligent in managing glucose levels in patients receiving TPN. Administration of insulin when TPN is temporarily discontinued can lead to hypoglycemia.[19] Patients receiving intravenous fat emulsion require evaluation and monitoring of serum triglyceride levels until they are stable. Additional monitoring may be needed when changes are made to the lipid content, such as administration of propofol, a lipid-based sedative-anesthetic agent.

Monitoring and Evaluating the Nutrition Care Plan

Documentation of daily weights, tolerance to eating or feeding, and evaluation of enteral or parenteral intake is important. Tests commonly ordered to assess nutritional status include complete blood count, chemistry panels, and liver function tests (triglycerides, albumin, and prealbumin levels). Any changes in medications are reviewed, and decisions are made regarding whether the patient is meeting intermediate outcomes toward the goals of nutritional support (see box, "Laboratory Alert"). If goals are not being met, reassessment of the plan is necessary to help the patient to achieve optimal nutritional goals. Assessment of weight loss, elevated glucose levels, or the appearance of dehydration or fluid overload are indicators that the nutritional care plan may need to be adjusted.

❗ LABORATORY ALERT

LAB TEST	GENERAL CRITICAL VALUES*	SIGNIFICANCE
Prealbumin	<6.0 mg/dL	• 2-day half-life makes it a sensitive indicator of protein synthesis and catabolism • Decreased in inflammatory process • Decreased in response to increased catabolism
Albumin	<3.5 g/dL	• Half-life of 20-22 days makes it a poor indicator of acute changes • Decreased in protein deficiency
Triglycerides	>400 mg/dL	• If elevated, evaluate feeding route and formula • Dosages of propofol and/or lipids may need to be adjusted
Sodium	<120 mEq/L >150 mEq/L	• Low levels can affect neurological status • Elevated level indicates free water excess, which can exacerbate heart failure
Potassium	<3.0 mEq/L >6.0 mEq/L	• Hypokalemia; can cause dysrhythmias • Hyperkalemia; can cause dysrhythmias, may be due to dehydration or renal impairment
Magnesium	<1.9 mEq/L	• May indicate malnutrition and/or malabsorption
Phosphate	<1.0 mg/dL	• Can be due to malnutrition, sepsis, increased calcium delivery (calcium and phosphate are inversely related)
Glucose	>200 mg/dL	• Indicates inability to tolerate glucose in parenteral nutrition and/or carbohydrate load in enteral nutrition formulas • Additional administration of insulin required to achieve glycemic control

*Depends on facility laboratory ranges.

◎ NURSING CARE PLAN

for Nutritional Status of Patients

NURSING DIAGNOSIS

Imbalanced Nutrition: Less Than Body Requirements

PATIENT OUTCOMES

Achieve adequate nutritional status

- Stable or gradual weight gain
- Increase in physical strength
- Improved wound healing

NURSING INTERVENTIONS	RATIONALES
• Determine, with dietician, patient caloric and nutritional needs	• Meet patient nutritional requirements
• Use BMI and ideal body weight in the obese patient to determine needs	• Using actual body weight will lead to overfeeding
• Monitor daily weight	• Used to make adjustments in caloric intake
• Monitor bowel sounds and assess abdomen	• Indication of bowel function
• Discard enteral feeding container and administration set every 24 hours	• Prevent contamination

NURSING DIAGNOSIS

Risk for Aspiration Related to Presence of Feeding Tube

PATIENT OUTCOMES

Patent airway with no signs or symptoms of aspiration

- Normal breath sounds
- Absence of cough
- No shortness of breath
- Absence of infection

NURSING INTERVENTIONS	RATIONALES
• Obtain x-ray after placement of nasoenteral tube	• Confirms placement prior to using tube
• Assess tube placement and gastric residual volumes every 4 hours	• Reaffirm placement and assess tolerance to feedings; feedings should be held if residual volume is 500 mL or greater
• Keep head of bed 30-45 degrees at all times	• Facilitates gravity flow of feedings through gastrointestinal tract and prevents aspiration; reduces gastric regurgitation
• In case of aspiration:	• Immediate action is required to maintain a patent airway
• Stop feeding	
• Keep head of bed elevated	
• Suction airway as needed	
• Document patient's appearance and adventitious breath sound	

Based on data from Ecklund MM. Small-bore Feeding Tube Insertion and Care. In Wiegand D, ed. *AACN Procedure Manual for Critical Care.* St. Louis: Saunders; 2011:1206-1210; Gulanick M, Myers J. Gastrointestinal and Digestive Care Plans. In *Nursing Care Plans: Diagnoses, Interventions, and Outcomes.* St. Louis: Mosby; 2011:550-619.

CASE STUDY

Mr. H. is at postoperative day 7 after coronary artery bypass graft surgery. He has not eaten any significant calories since the operation. He does not like hospital food and has trouble chewing because of poor dentition. Objective data include the following: height, 6 feet; weight, 135 pounds; and a history of a 20-pound weight loss in the last month. Laboratory data include a prealbumin level of less than 7.4 g/dL (normal values, 16.4-38 g/dL) and an albumin level of 1.6 g/dL (normal values, 3.5-5 g/dL); urine output has been adequate, and he has hypoactive bowel sounds.

Estimation of the patient's calorie and protein needs are noted using data in Table 6-2. Based on the subjective and objective data presented, Mr. H. is a combination of moderately

stressed to severely stressed. His kilocalorie intake requirements are 35 kcal/kg/day, and his protein requirements are approximately 1.5 to 2.0 g/kg/day.

Questions

1. What combination of assessment findings determines the patient's nutritional status in this case study?
2. How do you justify the preferred route of intake in the critically ill patient?
3. What laboratory data best determine the patient's state within a nutritional context?
4. What is the overall goal of nutritional therapy?

SUMMARY

Patients with critical illness are at high risk for nutritional deficits. Nutritional support therapy is initiated based on the nutritional needs of patients, which are identified upon admission. Enteral nutrition is the preferred route for nutritional support therapy and is typically initiated within 24 to 48 hours following a determination that a patient is unable to meet nutritional needs. Parenteral nutrition is reserved for patients in whom enteral nutrition is not possible; the initiation time is based on the patient's condition.[14] Nutritional

support is critical for optimal outcomes and successful management of critically ill patients. Adequate nutrition provides for the basic metabolic needs of the critically ill patient and aids in wound healing, tissue repair, and immune function, while minimizing muscle wasting. Assessment of patients' nutritional status by the critical care nurse and timely intervention by the interdisciplinary healthcare team can optimize and improve patients' outcomes.

CRITICAL THINKING EXERCISES

1. What factors are considered when selecting a type of enteral tube for feedings?
2. What assessment findings are indicative of a patient's intolerance to feedings, both enteral and parenteral?
3. What factors would you consider in selecting an enteral formula?
4. What types of drug interactions can cause potential complications with either enteral or parenteral formulas?

REFERENCES

1. Abbott Nutrition. Brands. http://abbottnutrition.com/Our-Products/brands.aspx; 2012. Accessed April 2, 2012.
2. Andrews PJ, Avenell A, Noble DW, et al. Randomized trial of glutamine, selenium, or both, to supplement parenteral nutrition for critically ill patients. *BMJ.* 2011;17:342:d1542.
3. Bankhead R, Boullata J, Brantley S, et al. Section VI: Enteral nutrition administration. Enteral nutrition practice recommendations. *Journal of Parenteral and Enteral Nutrition.* 2009;33(2):28-35.
4. Bankhead R, Boullata J, Brantley S, et al. Section VII: Medication administration. Enteral nutrition practice recommendations. *Journal of Parenteral and Enteral Nutrition.* 2009;33(2):37-39.
5. Bankhead R, Boullata J, Brantley S, et al. Section VIII: Monitoring enteral nutrition administration. Enteral nutrition practice recommendations. *Journal of Parenteral and Enteral Nutrition.* 2009;33(2):41-44.
6. Cahill NE, Dhaliwal R, Day AG, et al. Nutrition therapy in the critical care setting: what is "best achievable" practice? An international multicenter observational study. *Critical Care Medicine.* 2010;38(2):395-401.
7. Casaer MP, Mesotten D, Hermans G, et al. Early versus late parenteral nutrition in critically ill adults. *New England Journal of Medicine.* 2011;365(6):506-517.
8. DiMaria-Ghalili RA, Guenter P. Nursing management: nutritional problems. In Lewis S, Dirkson S, Heitkemper M, Bucher L, Camera I, eds. *Medical-surgical Nursing Assessment and Management of Clinical Problems.* St. Louis, MO: Elsevier; 2011: 920-943.
9. Ecklund MM. Small-bore feeding tube insertion and care. In Wiegand D, ed. *AACN Procedure Manual for Critical Care.* St Louis, MO: Saunders; 2011: 1206-1210.
10. Gulanick M, Myers J. Gastrointestinal and digestive care plans. In *Nursing Care Plans Diagnosis, Interventions, and Outcomes.* St Louis, MO: Mosby; 2011: 550-619.

11. Hall JE. Dietary balances; regulation of feeding; obesity and starvation; vitamins and minerals. In *Guyton and Hall Textbook of Medical Physiology*. Philadelphia, PA: Saunders; 2011: 843-858.

12. Kushner RF, Drover JW. Current strategies of critical care assessment and therapy of the obese patient (hypocaloric feeding): what are we doing and what do we need to do? *Journal of Parenteral and Enteral Nutrition*. 2011;35(suppl 5):365-435.

13. Kutsogiannis J, Alberda C, Gramlich L, et al. Early use of supplemental parenteral nutrition in critically ill patients: results of an international multicenter observation study. *Critical Care Medicine*. 2011;39(12):2691-2699.

14. McClave SA, Martindale RG, Vanek VW, et al. Guidelines for the provision and assessment of nutrition support therapy in the adult critically ill patient: Society of Critical Care Medicine (SCCM) and American Society for Parenteral and Enteral Nutrition (ASPEN). *Journal of Parenteral and Enteral Nutrition*. 2009;33(3):277-316.

15. Mueller C, Compher C, Ellen DM, American Society for Parenteral and Enteral Nutrition Board of Directors. ASPEN clinical guidelines: nutrition screening, assessment, and intervention in adults. *Journal of Parenteral and Enteral Nutrition*. 2011;35(16):16-24.

16. Nestle Nutrition. Products & applications. www.nestle-nutrition.com/Products/Default.aspx; 2012. Accessed April 2, 2012.

17. Norman K, Pichard C, Lochs H, et al. Prognostic impact of disease-related malnutrition. *Clinical Nutrition*. 2008;27(1): 5-15.

18. Rollinson D, Shikora SA, Saltzman E. Obesity. In Gottschlich MM, eds. *The ASPEN Nutrition Support Core Curriculum: A Case-based Approach-the Adult Patient*. Silver Spring, MD: American Society for Parenteral and Enteral Nutrition; 2007: 695-721.

19. Rourke KM. Nutrition. In Meiner SE, ed. *Gerontologic nursing*. St Louis, MO: Mosby; 2011: 177-193.

20. Ukleja A, Freeman KL, Gilbert K, et al. Standards for nutrition support: adult hospitalized patients. *Nutrition in Clinical Practice*. 2010;25(4):403-414,

21. U.S. Department of Health and Human Services, National Institutes of Health, National Heart, Lung, and Blood Institute. *How are Overweight and Obesity Diagnosed?* http://www.nhlbi.nih.gov/health/health-topics/topics/obe/diagnosis.html; 2010. Accessed April 2, 2012.

22. Williams NT. Medication administration through enteral feeding tubes. *American Journal of Health-System Pharmacy*. 2008; 65(24):2347-2357.

Dysrhythmia Interpretation and Management

Julie Marcum, MS, APRN-BC, CCRN-CMC

evolve WEBSITE

Many additional resources, including self-assessment exercises, are located on the Evolve companion website at
http://evolve.elsevier.com/Sole.

- Review Questions
- Mosby's Nursing Skills Procedures

- Animations
- Video Clips

INTRODUCTION

The interpretation of cardiac rhythm disturbances or dysrhythmias is an essential skill for nurses employed in patient care areas where electrocardiographic monitoring occurs. The ability to rapidly analyze a rhythm disturbance as well as initiate appropriate treatment improves patient safety and optimizes successful outcomes. The critical care nurse is often the healthcare professional responsible for the continuous monitoring of the patient's cardiac rhythm, and has the opportunity to provide early intervention that can prevent an adverse clinical situation. This responsibility requires not only a mastery of interpreting dysrhythmias but also the ability to critically identify the unique monitoring needs of each patient. This chapter presents a review of basic cardiac dysrhythmias, etiology, clinical significance, and appropriate treatments to aid the novice critical care nurse in mastering dysrhythmia recognition.

The word *dysrhythmia* refers to an abnormal cardiac rhythm. People also speak of cardiac arrhythmias. Either term may be used to describe deviations from normal sinus rhythm. The term *dysrhythmia* is used throughout this text.

The goal of this chapter is to provide a basic understanding of electrocardiography for analyzing and interpreting cardiac dysrhythmias. Electrocardiography is the process of creating a visual tracing of the electrical activity of the cells in the heart. This tracing is called the *electrocardiogram* (ECG). The critical care nurse must have a clear understanding of cardiac monitoring, lead selection, and rhythm interpretation. Part of the difficulty in learning rhythm interpretation is that many of the terms used are synonymous. Throughout

this chapter, those terms are clarified. This chapter discusses general concepts of dysrhythmia interpretation.

OVERVIEW OF ELECTROCARDIOGRAM MONITORING

The first ECG was recorded in 1887 by British physiologist Augustus Waller via a capillary electrometer.[9] The electrocardiogram was subsequently named, and the P Q R S T complex was described by Dr. Willem Einthoven, who proceeded to commercially produce a string galvanometer that became popularized in the early 1900s. Dr. Einthoven won the Nobel Peace prize in 1924 for inventing the electrocardiograph. The first electrical electrocardiogram machine weighed 50 pounds and was powered by a 6-volt automobile battery. Today, the 12-lead ECG machine is an essential element or mainstay of health care as a diagnostic tool.

Continuous ECG monitoring did not become common practice until the 1960s, when the first coronary care units were developed. Early cardiac monitoring consisted of monitoring for a heart rate that was too fast or too slow, and for identifying life-threatening dysrhythmias, including ventricular tachycardia, ventricular fibrillation, and asystole.[9] Today, cardiac monitoring is increasingly sophisticated. Technologies have been developed that allow continuous monitoring of 12 leads, and trending of a variety of physiological variables can be performed for any time frame. Cardiac monitoring is also performed in a variety of clinical areas outside the critical care unit. Nurse researchers have contributed a wealth of new knowledge about best practices for cardiac monitoring and

- Resuscitated from cardiac arrest
- Early phase of acute coronary syndromes
- Newly diagnosed high-risk coronary lesions
- After cardiac surgery
- After nonurgent percutaneous coronary intervention
- After implantation of automatic defibrillator or pacemaker leads
- Temporary or transcutaneous pacemaker
- Heart block
- Dysrhythmias complicating Wolff-Parkinson-White syndrome
- Drug-induced long QT syndrome
- Intraaortic balloon counterpulsation
- Acute heart failure, pulmonary edema
- Conditions requiring critical care admission
- Procedures that require conscious sedation or anesthesia

Adapted from American Heart Association (AHA). (2011). *2010 Handbook of Emergency Cardiovascular Care for Healthcare Providers.* Dallas, Texas.

have published comprehensive standards for cardiac monitoring in hospital settings.[4,5] Box 7-1 lists priority patient populations for dysrhythmia monitoring.

CARDIAC PHYSIOLOGY REVIEW

The electrocardiogram detects a summation of electrical signals generated by specialized cells of the heart called pacemaker cells. Pacemaker cells have the property of *automaticity,* meaning these cells can generate a stimulus or an action potential without outside stimulation. This electrical signal is conducted through specialized fibers of the conduction system to the mechanical or muscle cells of the heart where a cardiac contraction is generated. Thus there must be an electrical signal for the mechanical event of contraction to occur. The coordinated electrical activity followed by a synchronous mechanical event constitutes the *cardiac cycle.*

The *cardiac cycle* (Figure 7-1) begins with an impulse that is generated from a small concentrated area of pacemaker cells high in the right atria called the sinoatrial node (SA or sinus node). The SA node has the fastest rate of discharge and thus is the dominant pacemaker of the heart. The sinus impulse quickly passes through the internodal conduction tracts and the Bachmann bundle, conductive fibers in the right and left atria. The impulse quickly reaches the atrioventricular (AV) node located in the area called the AV junction, between the atria and the ventricles. Here the impulse is slowed to allow time for ventricular filling during relaxation or ventricular *diastole.* The AV node has pacemaker properties and can discharge an impulse if the SA node fails. The electrical impulse is then rapidly conducted through the bundle of His to the ventricles via the left and right bundle branches. The left bundle branch further divides into the left anterior fascicle and the left posterior fascicle. The bundle branches divide into smaller and smaller branches, finally terminating in tiny fibers called Purkinje fibers that reach the myocardial muscle cells or myocytes. The bundle of His, the right and left bundle branches, and the Purkinje fibers are also known as the His-Purkinje system. The ventricles have pacemaker capabilities if the sinus or AV nodes cease to generate impulses.

The electrical signal stimulates the atrial muscle, called *atrial systole,* and causes the atria to contract simultaneously and eject their blood volume into the ventricles. Simultaneously, the ventricles fill with blood during *ventricular systole.* During atrial systole, a bolus of atrial blood is ejected into the ventricles. This step is called the *atrial kick,* and it contributes approximately 30% more blood to the cardiac output of the

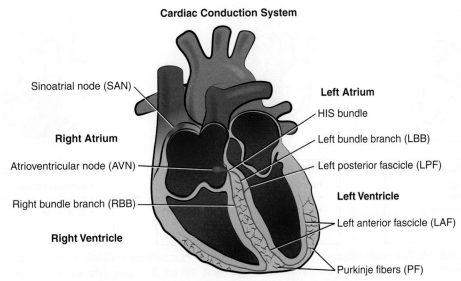

Cardiac Conduction System

Sinoatrial node (SAN)

Left Atrium

HIS bundle

Left bundle branch (LBB)

Right Atrium

Left posterior fascicle (LPF)

Atrioventricular node (AVN)

Left Ventricle

Right bundle branch (RBB)

Left anterior fascicle (LAF)

Right Ventricle

Purkinje fibers (PF)

FIGURE 7-1 The electrical conduction system of the heart.

ventricles. The inflow or atrioventricular valves (tricuspid and mitral) close because of the increasing pressure of the blood volume in the ventricles. By this time the electrical impulse reaches the Purkinje fibers, and the muscle cells have become stimulated and cause ventricular contraction. The outflow valves open (aortic and pulmonic) because of increased pressure and volume in the ventricles, allowing for ejection of the ventricular blood, called ventricular systole. At the same time ventricular systole is occurring, *atrial diastole* or filling is occurring. The atria are relaxed and filling with blood from the periphery (deoxygenated) and the lungs (oxygenated). Then because of the rhythmic pacing of the heart, the muscle cells are again stimulated, the atria contract, and atrial blood is ejected once again into the ventricles. This process of electrical stimulation and mechanical response occurs rhythmically 60 to 100 times per minute in the normal heart. The coordination of the electrical and mechanical

events in the upper and lower chambers of the heart result in the emptying and filling of these chambers, and the valves open and close because of pressure changes. These physiological actions result in what is known as cardiac output, which continually adjusts to the needs of the body's tissues (Figure 7-2).

Cardiac Electrophysiology

Specialized cardiac pacemaker cells possess the property of automaticity and can generate an electrical impulse on their own. Nonpacemaker or muscle cells must receive an outside stimulus in normal circumstances to generate a response. The response generated either by the pacemaker or muscle cells once stimulated is called the *action potential*. The cardiac action potential consists of phases related to depolarization, repolarization and the resting or polarized state of the cell. While this summary describes the action potential of a single

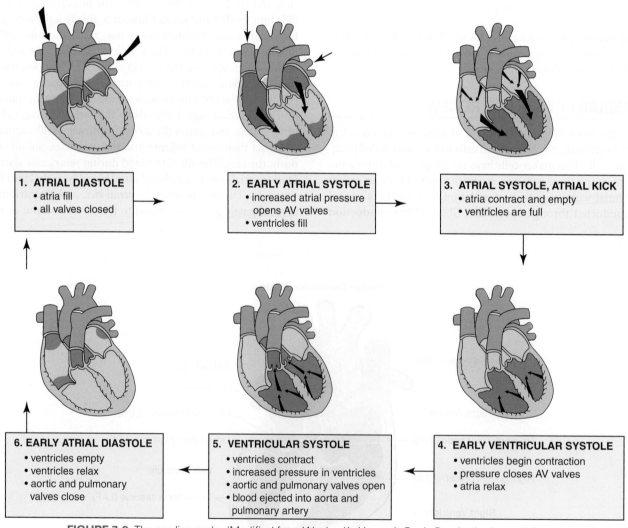

FIGURE 7-2 The cardiac cycle. (Modified from Wesley K. *Huszar's Basic Dysrhythmias and Acute Coronary Syndromes: Interpretation and Management.* 4th ed. St. Louis: Mosby JEMS; 2010.)

cell, imagine that this is occurring in millions of cardiac cells almost simultaneously resulting in a coordinated contraction of the atria and ventricles.

During the resting state of the cell, there is a difference in polarity, or charge, between the extracellular and intracellular environments that is maintained by the cell membrane. Specialized pumps prevent ions from passing through the cell membrane by diffusion. The inside of the cell is predominately negatively charged, whereas the outside is positively charged. The resting membrane potential occurs when the cell is in the polarized or resting state. The polarized cell has a higher concentration of positive ions including sodium outside the cell, causing the extracellular environment to be positive. The interior of the cell is more negative and the concentration of potassium is higher (Figure 7-3). The voltage in the interior of the cardiac muscle cell during resting membrane potential is −90 mV, whereas that of the pacemaker cells in the SA and AV nodes is −65 mV.

The stimulation of a cardiac muscle cell by an electrical impulse changes the permeability of the myocardial cell membrane. Sodium ions rush into the cell via sodium channels in the cell membrane, and potassium ions flow out of the cell, resulting in a more positively charged cell interior. The action potential describes the flow of ions inside and outside the cell as well as the voltage changes that occur. The first phase of the action potential occurs when the cell membrane becomes permeable to sodium molecules. When the membrane potential reaches −65 mV, also known as threshold, more channels in the cell membrane open up and allow sodium ions to rush into the cell; the cell interior quickly reaches +30 mV, resulting in depolarization. Following this fast phase in sodium influx, the plateau phase of the action potential occurs when calcium channels open and calcium flows into the cell. This slower phase allows for a longer period of depolarization, resulting in sustained muscle contraction. The next event of the action potential occurs when the cell returns to resting state. This process is called *repolarization* and results from ions returning to the outside (calcium and sodium) and the interior of the cell (potassium). Sodium and potassium pumps within the cell membrane maintain this concentration gradient across the cell membrane when the cell is polarized. These pumps require energy in the form of adenosine triphosphate (ATP). Now the cell has returned to its resting state with a polarity of −90 mV once again. *Depolarization* of adjacent cells occurs simultaneously as the stimulus moves across the cardiac muscle allowing for almost instantaneous depolarization of the entire muscle mass and resultant contraction (Figure 7-4).

Pacemaker cells exhibit the property of automaticity, enabling these cells to reach threshold and depolarize without an outside stimulus. The cell membrane becomes suddenly permeable to sodium during the resting state and reaches threshold, resulting in spontaneous depolarization. Resting membrane potential for these automatic cells is −65 mV, and threshold is reached at approximately −50 mV.[13] The sinus node reaches threshold at a rate of 60 to 100 times per minute. Because this is the fastest pacemaker in the heart, the SA node is the dominant pacemaker of the heart. The AV node and His-Purkinje pacemakers are latent pacemakers that reach threshold at a slower rate but can take over if the SA node fails or if sinus impulse conduction is blocked. The AV node has an inherent rate of 40 to 60 beats per minute and the His-Purkinje system can fire at a rate of 20 to 40 beats per minute.

Autonomic Nervous System

The rate of spontaneous depolarization of the pacemaker cells is influenced by the autonomic nervous system. The

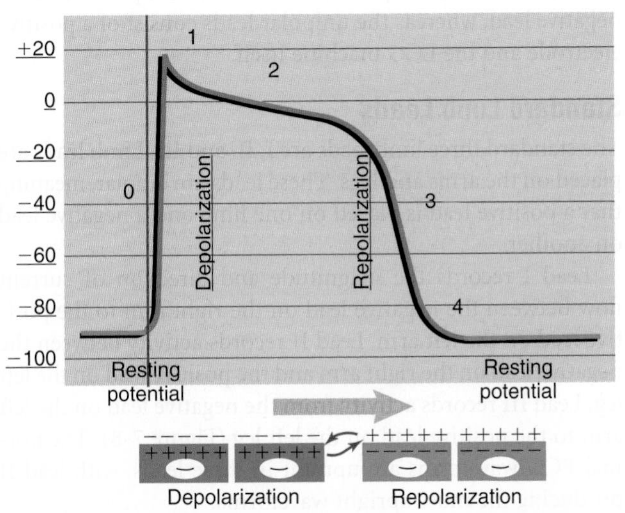

FIGURE 7-3 Cardiac action potential. (From Association of Critical-Care Nurses: *Essentials of Critical Care Orientation 2.0.*)

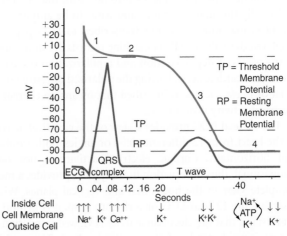

FIGURE 7-4 Cardiac action potential with the electrocardiogram and movement of electrolytes. *ATP,* Adenosine triphosphate; *Ca,* calcium; *K,* potassium; *Na,* sodium. (From American Heart Association. *Advanced Cardiac Life Support Textbook.* Dallas: Author; 1997.)

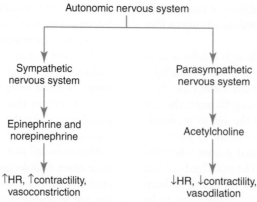

FIGURE 7-5 Autonomic nervous system.

sympathetic nervous system releases catecholamines, causing the SA node to fire more quickly in response to epinephrine and norepinephrine. The parasympathetic nervous system releases acetylcholine, which slows the heart rate. During normal circumstances these substances modulate each other, and the cardiac response allows for appropriate changes in cardiac output to meet the varying demands of the body (Figure 7-5).

THE 12-LEAD ELECTROCARDIOGRAM

The 12-lead ECG is an important diagnostic tool that provides information about myocardial ischemia, injury, cell necrosis, electrolyte disturbances, increased cardiac muscle mass (hypertrophy), conduction abnormalities, and abnormal heart rhythms.

Electrodes applied to the skin transmit the electrical signals of the movement of the cardiac impulse through the conduction system. This signal passes through skin, muscle, bone, and finally through electrodes and wires to be amplified by the ECG machine and either transcribed to ECG paper or displayed digitally. The ECG machine records the summation of the waves of depolarization and repolarization occurring during the cardiac cycle. During the polarized or resting state, a flat or *isoelectric* line is inscribed that means no current or electrical activity is occurring.

The 12-lead ECG provides a view of the electrical activity of the heart from 12 different views or angles, both frontally and horizontally. Cardiac electrical activity is not one-dimensional; thus observation in two planes provides a more complete view in the horizontal and vertical planes. When assessing the 12-lead ECG or a rhythm strip, it is helpful to understand that the electrical activity is viewed in relation to the positive electrode of that particular lead. The positive electrode is the "viewing eye" of the camera. When an electrical signal is aimed directly at the positive electrode, an upright inflection is visualized. If the impulse is going away from the positive electrode, a negative deflection is seen; and if the signal is perpendicular to the imaginary line between

the positive and negative poles of the lead, the tracing is equiphasic, with equally positive and negative deflection (Figure 7-6). A tracing may be observed on a monitor, displayed digitally on a computer screen, or recorded on paper.

The electrical activity of normal conduction occurs downward between the left arm and the left leg, called the *mean cardiac vector* or direction of current flow. Thus the positive electrode reflects this electrical activity by an upright inflection if the flow of current is directed at that positive electrode, or negative deflection if moving away from that positive electrode. The vector of a lead is an imaginary line between the positive and negative electrodes. The wave of current flow of the cardiac cycle or the vector is inscribed on the ECG paper in relation to the lead vector that is being viewed. The lead reflects the magnitude and the direction of current flow (Figure 7-7).

The 12-lead ECG consists of three standard bipolar limb leads (I, II, and III), three augmented unipolar limb leads (aV_R, aV_L, and aV_F), and six precordial unipolar leads (V_1, V_2, V_3, V_4, V_5, and V_6). Bipolar leads consist of a positive and a negative lead, whereas the unipolar leads consist of a positive electrode and the ECG machine itself.

Standard Limb Leads

The standard three limb leads are I, II, and III. Limb leads are placed on the arms and legs. These leads are bipolar, meaning that a positive lead is placed on one limb and a negative lead on another.

Lead I records the magnitude and direction of current flow between the negative lead on the right arm to the positive lead on the left arm. Lead II records activity between the negative lead on the right arm and the positive lead on the left leg. Lead III records activity from the negative lead on the left arm to the positive lead on the left leg (Figure 7-8). The normal ECG waveforms are upright in these leads, with lead II producing the most upright waveforms.

The bipolar limb leads form Einthoven's triangle (Figure 7-9). This is an equilateral upside-down triangle with the heart in the center.

Three Basic Laws of Electrocardiography

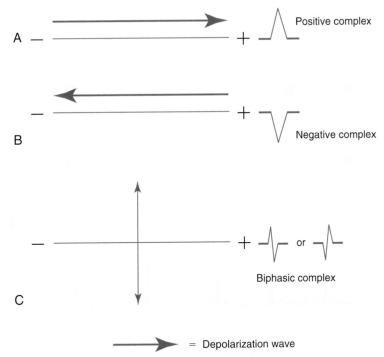

FIGURE 7-6 **A,** A positive complex is seen in any lead if the wave of depolarization spreads toward the positive pole of the lead. **B,** A negative complex is seen if the depolarization wave spreads toward the negative pole (away from the positive pole) of the lead. **C,** A biphasic (partly positive, partly negative) complex is seen if the mean direction of the wave is at right angles. These apply to the P wave, QRS complex, and T wave. (From Goldberger AL. *Clinical Electrocardiography: A Simplified Approach.* 7th ed., St. Louis: Mosby; 2006.)

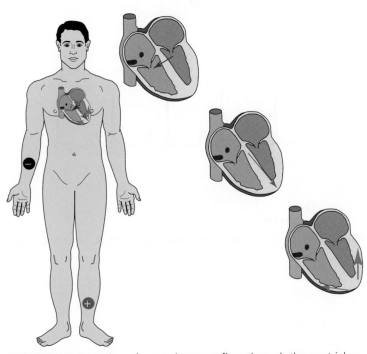

FIGURE 7-7 Direction of normal current flow through the ventricles.

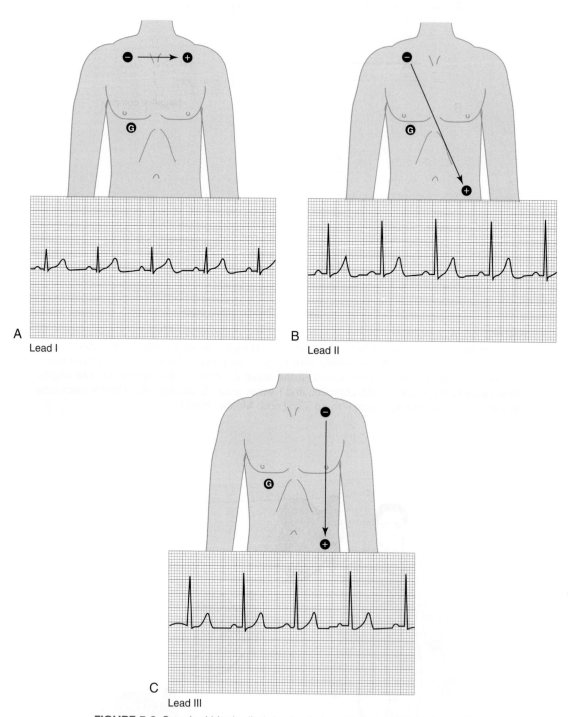

A
Lead I

B
Lead II

C
Lead III

FIGURE 7-8 Standard bipolar limb leads. **A,** Lead I. **B,** Lead II. **C,** Lead III.

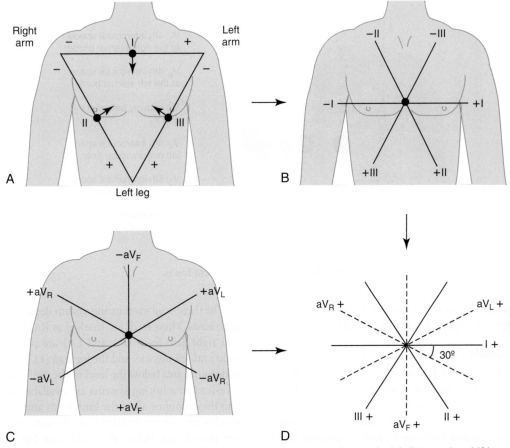

FIGURE 7-9 A, Einthoven's triangle. **B,** The triangle is converted to a triaxial diagram by shifting leads I, II, and III so that they intersect at a common point. **C,** Triaxial lead diagram showing the relationship of the three augmented (unipolar) leads, aV_R, aV_L, and aV_F. Notice that each lead is represented by an axis with a positive and negative pole. **D,** The hexaxial reference figure

Augmented Limb Leads

The augmented limb leads are unipolar, meaning that they record electrical flow in only one direction. A reference point is established in the ECG machine, and electrical flow is recorded from that reference point toward the right arm (aV_R), the left arm (aV_L), and the left foot (aV_F) (see Figure 7-9, *A-C*). The *a* in the names of these leads means augmented; because these leads produce small ECG complexes, they must be augmented or enlarged. The *V* means voltage and the subscripts *R*, *L*, and *F* stand for right arm, left arm, and left foot, where the positive electrode is located. The augmented limb leads are displayed by using the electrodes already in place for the limb leads.

The addition of the augmented limb leads to Einthoven triangle form a hexaxial reference figure when the six frontal plane leads are intersected in the center of each lead (see Figure 7-9, *D*). The figure is used to determine the exact direction of current flow called axis determination, a requisite skill of 12-lead ECG analysis. Assessment of axis deviation is an advanced skill and not addressed in this chapter. Figure 7-9 demonstrates that leads I and aV_L are close in proximity, as are leads II, III, and aV_F. Therefore the QRS patterns of leads that are close together

appear similar. Because current flow is directed between the left arm and left foot, leads I, II, III, aV_L, and aV_F are usually positive if conduction is normal.

Precordial Leads

The six *precordial leads* (also called chest leads) are positioned on the chest wall directly over the heart. These leads provide a view of cardiac electrical activity from a horizontal plane rather than the frontal plane view of the limb leads. Precise placement of these leads is crucial for providing an accurate representation and for comparing with previous and future ECGs. A misplaced V lead can result in erroneous or missed diagnoses of acute coronary syndrome and lethal dysrhythmias. The precordial leads are unipolar, with a positive electrode and the AV node as a center reference (Figure 7-10). Landmarks for placement of these leads are the intercostal spaces, the sternum, and the clavicular and axillary lines. Positions for these six leads are as follows:

V_1: Fourth intercostal space, right sternal border
V_2: Fourth intercostal space, left sternal border
V_3: Halfway between V_2 and V_4
V_4: Fifth intercostal space, left midclavicular line

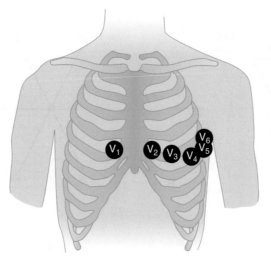

V₁: 4th intercostal space at the right sternal border

V₂: 4th intercostal space at the left sternal border

V₃: midway between V₂ and V₄

V₄: 5th intercostal space, left midclavicular line

V₅: 5th intercostal space, left anterior axillary line

V₆: 5th intercostal space, left midaxillary line

FIGURE 7-10 Precordial chest leads.

V_5: Fifth intercostal space, left anterior axillary line
V_6: Fifth intercostal space, left midaxillary line

Grouping of Leads

Each lead provides a view of the electrical activity of the heart from a different angle. Leads that view the current flow in the heart from the same angle can be grouped together. Anatomical regions are described as septal, anterior, lateral, inferior, and posterior. Septal leads are V_1 and V_2; anterior leads are V_3 and V_4; lateral leads are V_5, V_6, I, and aV_L; and inferior leads are II, III, and aV_F.[3] Assessing leads that localize these regions of the heart assists in identifying the location of myocardial ischemia, injury, and infarct. Posterior and right ventricular electrodes are not commonly part of the standard 12-lead ECG; however, if indicated, newer ECG machines can record tracings from these areas. The 15-lead ECG is an essential additional assessment that is made if the patient is suspected of having an inferior myocardial infarction, because right ventricular and posterior infarctions are common with this type of infarct (Figure 7-11).

Continuous Cardiac Monitoring

Continuous cardiac monitoring is conducted in a variety of patient care settings, including the emergency department, ambulances, high-risk obstetrical units, cardiac catheterization and electrophysiology laboratories, critical care units, operating rooms, postanesthesia care units, endoscopy suites, and progressive care units. Depending upon the sophistication of the monitoring system, any of the 12 leads can be monitored continuously. The most critical initial elements of cardiac monitoring are in skin preparation, lead placement, and appropriate lead selection.

Skin Preparation and Lead Placement

Adequate skin preparation of electrode sites requires clipping the hair, cleansing the skin, and drying vigorously. Cleansing includes washing with soap and water, or alcohol, to remove skin debris and oils.

The three-lead monitoring system depicts only the standard limb leads. These leads are marked as RA, LA, and LL. The left and right arm leads (RA and LA) are placed just below the right and left clavicle, and the leg lead (LL) is placed on the left abdominal area below the level of the umbilicus (Figure 7-12). Five-lead monitoring systems are available on many systems, and they monitor all of the limb leads and one chest lead. Instead of placing the limb leads on the arms and legs, these leads are placed just below the right and left clavicles and on the right and left abdomen below the level of the umbilicus. The precordial or chest lead is placed in the selected V lead position, usually V_1 (see Figure 7-12) Some five-lead systems have the ability to derive a 12-lead tracing (Figure 7-13).

Before application, the electrodes are checked to ensure that the gel is moist. The electrode is attached to the lead wire and placed in the designated location. Following electrode placement, the signal is assessed to insure that the waveform is clear and not disrupted by artifact. The frequency of changing electrodes is based on institutional policy. Nursing assessment must include that electrodes are placed in the correct anatomical positions at the beginning of each shift.

Lead selection is determined by the patient's diagnosis and based on risk for an ischemic cardiac event, dysrhythmia, or other factors. Typically the first lead selected is V_1 for dysrhythmia monitoring. If the system is able to simultaneously monitor a second lead, selection of this lead is based on the patient's diagnosis and individual needs. A limb lead is usually selected, such as III or II, because of the easy visualization of P waves; however, if the patient has a history of ischemia, the second lead can be based on the patient's 12-lead ECG, identifying the lead showing the greatest ischemic change. For dysrhythmia monitoring in a system allowing for continuous monitoring of two leads, V_1 and III are the standard recommendations.[1,4,5]

In most settings a 6-second strip of the patient's rhythm is obtained and documented in the patient's chart at intervals from every 4 hours to 8 hours, based on the patient acuity level and institutional policy. In addition to scheduled times, a rhythm strip is documented any time there is a change in

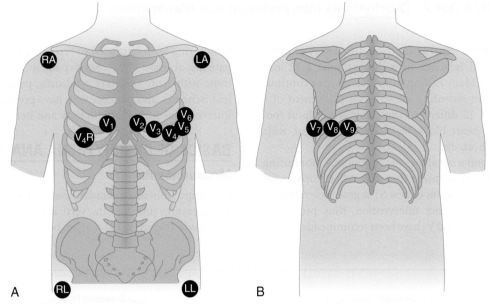

FIGURE 7-11 Lead placement for a 15-lead ECG. **A,** Anterior leads. **B,** Posterior leads.

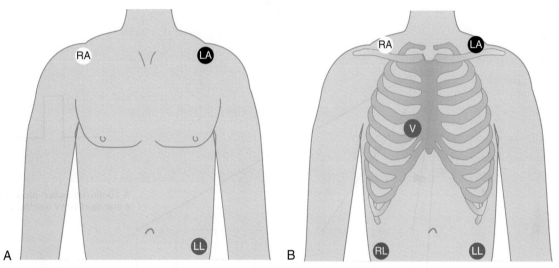

FIGURE 7-12 A, Three-lead ECG monitoring system. **B,** Five-lead monitoring system with V lead placed in V$_1$ position.

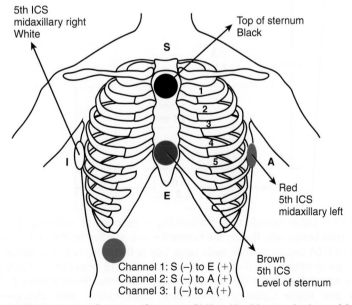

5th ICS
midaxillary right
White

Top of sternum
Black

S

1
2
3
4
5

I

A

Red
5th ICS
midaxillary left

E

Brown
5th ICS
Level of sternum

Channel 1: S (−) to E (+)
Channel 2: S (−) to A (+)
Channel 3: I (−) to A (+)

FIGURE 7-13 EASI Monitoring System. (Courtesy Philips Healthcare, Andover, Massachusetts.)

rhythm. If the patient experiences chest discomfort or other signs of myocardial ischemia or a dysrhythmia, a 12-lead ECG is performed. Many ECG machines can print a continuous 12-lead rhythm recording, allowing for assessment of a dysrhythmia from 12 different views. This is a helpful tool when diagnosing heart block, atrial dysrhythmia, or wide QRS complex tachycardia.

ST-segment monitoring allows for continuous monitoring for changes in the ST segment that may reflect myocardial ischemia.[11] Early recognition of new ST segment elevation or depression facilitates earlier intervention, thus preserving myocardium. Leads III and V_3 have been recommended as the monitoring leads best used to recognize ischemic changes in patients at risk.[2,4,6,11,12] Such patient populations include those with acute coronary syndrome, patients at risk for silent ischemia, and patients who have previously had cardiac interventions such as angioplasty and stent placement.

BASICS OF DYSRHYTHMIA ANALYSIS

Measurements

ECG paper contains a standardized grid where the horizontal axis measures time and the vertical axis measures voltage or amplitude (Figure 7-14). Larger boxes are circumscribed by

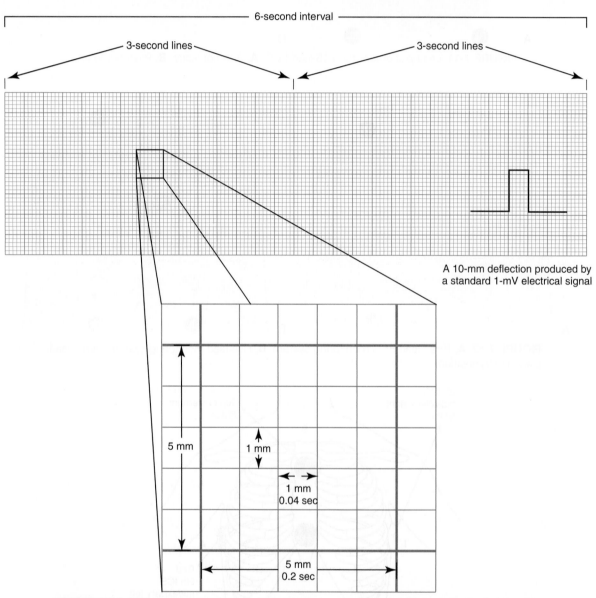

FIGURE 7-14 ECG paper records time horizontally in seconds or milliseconds. Each large box contains 25 smaller boxes with five on the horizontal axis and five on the vertical axis. Each small horizontal box is 0.04 seconds while each large box is 0.20 seconds in duration. Vertically, the graph depicts size or voltage in millivolts and in millimeters. 15 large boxes equals 3 seconds and 30 large boxes equals 6 seconds used in calculating heart rate. (From Wesley K. *Huszar's Basic Dysrhythmias and Acute Coronary Syndromes: Interpretation and Management.* 4th ed. St. Louis: Mosby JEMS; 2010.)

darker lines and the smaller boxes by lighter lines. The larger boxes contain 5 smaller boxes on the horizontal line and 5 on the vertical line for a total of 25 per large box. Horizontally, the smaller boxes denote 0.04 seconds each or 40 milliseconds; the larger box contains five smaller horizontal boxes and thus equals 0.20 seconds or 200 milliseconds. Along the uppermost aspect of the ECG paper are vertical hatch marks that occur every 15 large boxes. The area between these marks equals 3 seconds. Some ECG paper has markings every second.

The monitoring standard is to use 6-second rhythm strips for analysis and documentation of cardiac rhythms. A 6-second strip consists of two 3-second intervals or a span of three hatch marks. The measurement of time on the ECG tracing represents the speed of depolarization and repolarization in the atria and ventricles and is printed at 25 mm/sec.

Amplitude is measured on the vertical axis of the ECG paper (see Figure 7-14). Each small box is equal to 0.1 mV in amplitude. Waveform amplitude indicates the amount of electrical voltage generated in the various areas of the heart. Low-voltage and small waveforms are expected from the small muscle mass of the atria. Large-voltage and large waveforms are expected from the larger muscle mass of the ventricles.

Waveforms and Intervals

The normal ECG tracing is composed of P, Q, R, S, and T waves (Figure 7-15). These waveforms rise from a flat baseline called the *isoelectric line.*

P Wave

The P wave represents atrial depolarization. It is usually upright in leads I and II and has a rounded, symmetrical shape. The amplitude of the P wave is measured at the center of the waveform and normally does not exceed three boxes, or 3 mm, in height.

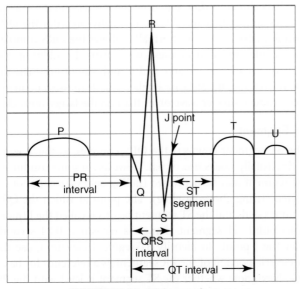

FIGURE 7-15 ECG waveforms.

Normally a P wave indicates that the SA node initiated the impulse that depolarized the atrium. However, a change in the shape of the P wave may indicate that the impulse arose from a site in the atria other than the SA node.

PR Interval

The downslope of the P wave returns to the isoelectric line for a short time before the beginning of the QRS complex. The interval from the beginning of the P wave to the next deflection from the baseline is called the PR interval. The PR interval measures the time it takes for the impulse to depolarize the atria, travel to the AV node, and dwell there briefly before entering the bundle of His. The normal PR interval is 0.12 to 0.20 seconds, three to five small boxes wide (see Figure 7-15). When the PR interval is longer than normal, the speed of conduction is delayed in the AV node. When the PR interval is shorter than normal, the speed of conduction is abnormally fast.

QRS Complex

The QRS complex represents ventricular depolarization (see Figure 7-15). Atrial repolarization also occurs simultaneously to ventricular depolarization, but because of the larger muscle mass of the ventricles, visualization of atrial repolarization is obscured by the QRS complex. The classic QRS complex begins with a negative, or downward, deflection immediately after the PR interval. The first negative deflection after the P wave is called the Q wave.

A Q wave may or may not be present before the R wave. If the first deflection from the isoelectric line is positive, or upright, the waveform is called an R wave. The size of the R wave varies across leads. The R wave is positive and tall in those leads where the direction of current is going towards the positive electrode lead. All the limb leads, with the exception of aV$_R$, normally have tall R waves. In the precordial leads, the R wave begins small and progressively becomes larger and more positive, going from small in V$_1$ to a maximal size in V$_5$. This change in size is termed R wave progression and occurs because the direction of current flow is moving more directly toward the positive electrode of V$_4$. (Figure 7-16).

The S wave is a negative waveform that follows the R wave. The S wave deflects below the isoelectric line. Some patients may have a second positive waveform in their QRS complex. If so, then that second positive waveform is called *R prime (R′).*

The term *QRS complex* is a generic term designating the waveforms representing ventricular depolarization. In reality, the complex may be an R wave, a QS wave, or other wave, depending on the lead viewed or any abnormalities that are present. Figure 7-17 depicts the various shapes of the QRS complex and their nomenclature.

If a Q wave is present on the 12-lead ECG (not the cardiac monitor), it must be determined if it is pathological or normal. A pathological Q wave has a width of 0.04 seconds and a depth that is greater than one fourth of the R wave amplitude. Pathological Q waves are found on ECGs of individuals

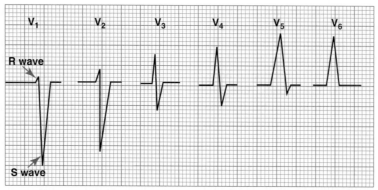

FIGURE 7-16 The normal 12-lead precordial R wave progression.

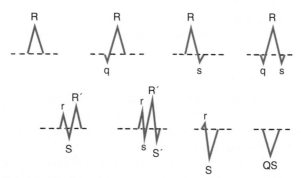

FIGURE 7-17 Nomenclature for QRS Complexes of Various Shapes. Different types of QRS complexes. An R wave is a positive waveform. A negative deflection before the R wave is a Q wave. The S wave is a negative deflection after the R wave. If the waveform is tall or deep, the letter naming the waveform is a capital letter. If the waveform is small in either direction, the waveform is labeled with a lowercase letter.

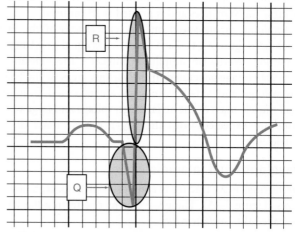

FIGURE 7-18 Pathological Q wave is greater than one fourth the height of the R wave.

who have had myocardial infarctions, and they represent myocardial muscle death (Figure 7-18).

QRS Interval

The QRS interval is measured from where it leaves the iso-electric line of the PR interval to the end of the QRS complex (see Figure 7-15). The waveform that initiates the QRS complex (whether it is a Q wave or an R wave) marks the beginning of the interval. The normal width of the QRS complex is 0.06 to 0.10 seconds. This width equals 1.5 to 2.5 small boxes.

A QRS width greater than 0.10 seconds may signify a delay in conduction through the ventricles due to a variety of factors, including myocardial infarction, atherosclerosis of the aging conduction system, or cardiomyopathy.

T Wave

The T wave represents ventricular repolarization (see Figure 7-15). T-wave amplitude is measured at the center of the waveform and is usually no higher than five small boxes, or 5 mm. In contrast to P waves, which are usually symmetrical, T waves are usually asymmetrical. Changes in T-wave amplitude or direction can indicate electrical

disturbances resulting from an electrolyte imbalance, or myocardial ischemia or injury. For example, hyperkalemia can cause tall, peaked T waves, and ischemia may cause an inverted or upside-down T wave.

Some students who are novices in dysrhythmia interpretation have difficulty differentiating the P wave and the T wave. Understanding that the P wave normally precedes the QRS complex and the T wave normally follows the QRS complex aids in identification of these waveforms. In addition, the T wave usually has greater width and amplitude than the P wave, because the atria are smaller muscle masses and therefore produce smaller waveforms than do the larger ventricles.

ST Segment

The ST segment connects the QRS complex to the T wave, and is usually isoelectric, or flat. However, in some conditions the segment may be depressed (falling below baseline) or elevated (rising above baseline). The point at which the QRS complex ends and the ST segment begins is called the J (junction) point. ST-segment change is measured 0.04 seconds after the J point. To identify ST-segment elevation, use the isoelectric portion of the PR segment as a reference for baseline. Next, note whether the ST segment is level with the PR segment (see Figure 7-15). If the ST segment is above or

EVIDENCE-BASED PRACTICE

Should QT Interval Monitoring be Part of Nursing Care?

Problem

QT-interval monitoring is recommended by the American Heart Association (AHA) for several conditions: administration of medications that prolong the QT interval, overdose of medications that prolong the QT interval, electrolyte disturbances (K^+, Mg^+), and bradycardia. It is not known what proportion of patients meet these criteria and would benefit from QT interval monitoring.

Clinical Question

What proportion of critically ill patients meet the AHA criteria for QT interval monitoring?

Evidence

The researchers collected data on 1039 critically ill patients who were monitored with a system that provided continuous QT interval monitoring. A QT interval greater than 500 milliseconds for 15 minutes or longer was considered to be prolonged. All electronic data were validated by the investigators. They found that 69% of patients had at least one of the AHA criteria for monitoring. They also found that the odds for QT interval prolongation increased with the number of AHA conditions present.

Implications for Nursing

Findings of this study reinforce the need for QT interval monitoring in critically ill patients, because the majority of patients had at least one risk factor for prolonged QT intervals. As monitoring systems include more features such as QT interval monitoring, it is also important for nurses to be aware of the features available and to use them as part of routine patient monitoring.

Level of Evidence

C—Descriptive Study

Reference

Pickham, D., Helfenbein, E., Shinn, J.A., Chan, G., Funk, M., & Drew, B.J. (2010). How many patients need QT interval monitoring in critical care units? Preliminary report of the QT in practice study. *Journal of Electrocardiology*, 43, 572-576.

---

below the baseline, count the number of small boxes above or below at 0.04 seconds after the J point. A displacement in the ST segment can indicate myocardial ischemia or injury.[2,5,11,12] If ST displacement is noted and is a new finding, a 12-lead ECG is performed and the provider notified. The patient is assessed for signs and symptoms of myocardial ischemia.

QT Interval

The QT interval is measured from the beginning of the QRS complex to the end of the T wave (see Figure 7-15). This interval measures the total time taken for ventricular depolarization and repolarization. Abnormal prolongation of the QT interval increases vulnerability to lethal dysrhythmias, such as ventricular tachycardia and fibrillation. Normally, the QT interval becomes longer with slower heart rates and shortens with faster heart rates, thus requiring a correction of the value. Generally, the QT interval is less than half the RR interval (see Figure 7-15).

A preferred calculation that corrects for varying heart rates is a calculated QT interval, or QTc, based on the QT divided by the square root of the R to R interval. QT and QTc are routinely measured when analyzing a rhythm strip. Normal QTc is less than 0.47 seconds in males and 0.48 seconds in females. Many monitoring systems can calculate the QTc if the R to R interval is measured. QTc accuracy is based on a regular rhythm. In irregular rhythms such as atrial fibrillation, an average QTc may be necessary because the QT varies beat to beat.

Risk of a lethal heart rhythm called *torsades de pointes* occurs if QTc is prolonged greater than 0.50 seconds.[5,6] Many medications may precipitate prolonged QT, thus it is important to be vigilant about monitoring for a prolonged QT interval (see box, Evidence-Based Practice).

U Wave

A final waveform that is occasionally noted on the ECG is the U wave. If present, this waveform follows the T wave, and it represents repolarization of a small segment of the ventricles. The U wave is usually small, rounded, and less than 2 mm in height (see Figure 7-15).[13] Larger U waves may be present in patients with hypokalemia, cardiomyopathy, and digoxin toxicity.

CAUSES OF DYSRHYTHMIAS

Dysrhythmias may occur when automaticity of the normal pacemaker cells of the heart is either stimulated or suppressed. For example, if the SA node fails to fire, latent pacemakers from the AV node or ventricles may fire as a backup safety mechanism. The SA node may fire more rapidly because of the influence of circulating catecholamines. Cells either within or outside the normal conduction system may take on characteristics of pacemaker cells and begin firing because of electrolyte imbalances, ischemia, injury, necrosis, and myocardial stretch due to hypertrophy. *Ectopic beats* or *ectopic rhythms* arise from cells that normally do not have pacemaker capabilities. Slowed conduction can create alternative conductive pathways that produce abnormally fast heart rhythms. If conduction is sufficiently decreased, latent pacemakers may take over this function. Table 7-1 presents a list of antidysrhythmic drugs and their effects on changes in heart rate and rhythm.

TABLE 7-1 PHARMACOLOGY

Antidysrhythmic Drug Classifications

CLASS*	DESCRIPTION	EXAMPLES
IA	Inhibits the fast sodium channel Prolongs repolarization time Used to treat atrial and ventricular dysrhythmias	Quinidine, disopyramide, procainamide
IB	Inhibits the fast sodium channel Shortens the action potential duration Used to treat ventricular dysrhythmias only	Lidocaine, phenytoin, mexiletine, tocainide
IC	Inhibits the fast sodium channel Shortens the action potential duration of only Purkinje fibers Controls ventricular tachydysrhythmias resistant to other drug therapies Has proarrhythmic effects	Flecainide, propafenone
II	Causes beta-adrenergic blockade	Esmolol, propranolol, sotalol
III	Lengthens the action potential Acts on the repolarization phase	Amiodarone, sotalol, dofetilide; ibutilide
IV	Blocks the slow inward movement of calcium to slow impulse conduction, especially in the atrioventricular node Used for treatment of supraventricular tachycardias	Diltiazem, verapamil
IVb-like	Opens the potassium channel	Adenosine, ATP

*Class I, sodium channel blockers; Class II, beta-adrenergic blockers; Class III, potassium channel blockers; Class IV, calcium channel blockers.
Adapted from Skidmore-Roth, L. (2011). *Mosby's Nursing Drug Reference.* (24th ed.). St. Louis: Elsevier Mosby.

DYSRHYTHMIA ANALYSIS

Analysis of a cardiac rhythm must be conducted systematically to correctly interpret the rhythm. Proper dysrhythmia analysis includes assessment of the following:

- Atrial and ventricular rates
- Regularity of rhythm
- Measurement of PR, QRS, and QT/QTc intervals
- Shape or morphology of waveforms and their consistency
- Identification of underlying rhythm and any noted dysrhythmia
- Patient tolerance of rhythm
- Clinical implication of the rhythm

Rate

The rate represents how fast the heart is depolarizing. Under normal conditions, the atria and the ventricles depolarize in a regular sequence. However, each can depolarize at a different rate. P waves are used to calculate the atrial rate, and QRS waves or R waves are used to calculate the ventricular rate. Rate can be assessed in various ways that are described as follows.

Six-second method: A quick and easy estimate of heart rate can be accomplished by counting the number of P waves or QRS waves within a 6-second strip to obtain atrial and ventricular heart rates per minute. This is the optimal method for irregular rhythms. Identify the lines above the ECG paper that represent 6 seconds, and count the number of P waves within the lines; then add a zero to identify the atrial heart rate estimate for 1 minute. Next, identify the number of QRS waves in the 6-second strip and again add a zero to identify the ventricular rate (Figure 7-19).

Large box method: In this method, two consecutive P and QRS waves are located. The number of large boxes between the highest points of two consecutive P waves is counted, and that number of large boxes is divided into 300 to determine the atrial rate. The number of large boxes between the highest points of two consecutive QRS waves is counted, and that number of large boxes is divided into 300 to determine the ventricular rate (Figure 7-20). This method is accurate only if the rhythm is regular. If one large box is between the two QRS waves, the rate is 300 beats per minute ($300 \div 1 = 300$); if there are two large boxes, the heart rate is 150 beats per minute ($300 \div 2 = 150$); if there are three large boxes, the heart rate is 100 beats per minute ($300 \div 3 = 100$); if there are four large boxes, the heart rate is 75 beats per minute ($300 \div 4 = 75$), and so on. A simple mnemonic can be used to simplify this method. Memorize 300-150-100-75-60-50-42-38.

Small box method: The small box method is used to calculate the *exact* rate of a regular rhythm. In this method, two consecutive P and QRS waves are located. The number of small boxes between the highest points of these consecutive P waves is counted, and that number is divided into 1500 to determine the atrial rate. The number of small boxes between the highest points of two consecutive QRS waves is counted, and that number is divided into 1500 to determine the ventricular rate (Figure 7-21). This method is accurate only if the rhythm is regular. Charts are available to calculate heart rate based on the rule of 1500.

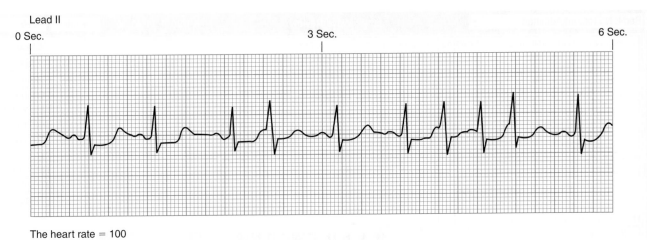

The heart rate = 100

FIGURE 7-19 Six-second method of rate calculation.

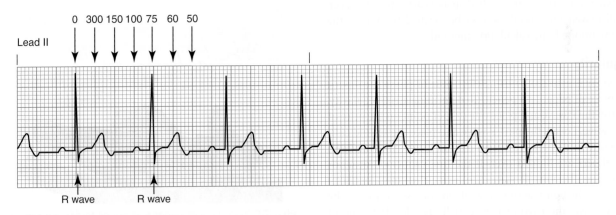

Big Box Method of Heart Rate Calculation

- Identify an R wave on a solid vertical line.
- Count the number of big boxes between the first and the following R waves.
- Divide 300 by the number of big boxes between R waves or count the cadence (300...150...100...75...60) representing the big boxes between R waves.

NOTE: Since the position of the second R wave occurs with the arrow reading 75, the heart rate in this example is approximately 75 beats per minute.

FIGURE 7-20 Big box method of heart rate calculation.

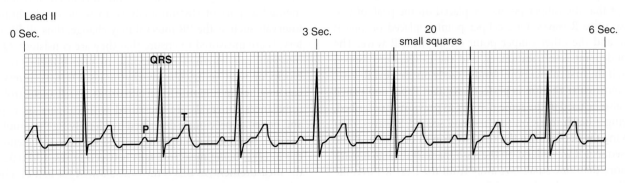

The heart rate = 75

FIGURE 7-21 Small box method of heart rate calculation. (Modified from Wesley K. *Huszar's Basic Dysrhythmias and Acute Coronary Syndromes: Interpretation and Management.* 4th ed. St. Louis: Mosby JEMS; 2010.)

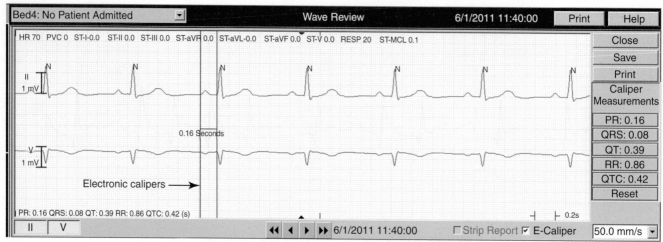

FIGURE 7-22 Electronic calipers. (Courtesy Philips Healthcare, Andover, Massachusetts.)

Cardiac monitors continuously display heart rates. However, the displayed rate should always be verified by one of the aforementioned rate calculation methods.

Regularity

Regularity is assessed by using electronic or physical calipers, or a piece of paper and pencil. To determine atrial regularity, identify the P wave and place one caliper point on the peak of the P wave. Locate the next P wave and place the second caliper point on its peak. The second point is left stationary, and the calipers are flipped over. If the first caliper point lands exactly on the next P wave, the atrial rhythm is perfectly regular. If the point lands one small box or less away from the next P wave, the rhythm is essentially regular. If the point lands more than one small box away, the rhythm is considered irregular. Electronic calipers on some monitoring systems are used the same way (Figure 7-22).

The same process can be performed with a simple piece of paper. Place the paper parallel and below the rhythm line, make a hatch mark below the first and second P waves, then move the paper over to determine if the distance between the second and third P waves is equal to the first and second. When an atrial rhythm is perfectly regular, each P wave is an equal distance from the next P wave.

This process is also used to assess ventricular regularity, except that the caliper points are placed on the peak of two consecutive R waves. One caliper point is placed on one R wave and the other caliper point on the next R wave. The second point is left stationary, and the calipers are flipped over. If the first caliper point lands exactly on the next R wave, the ventricular rhythm is perfectly regular. Paper and pencil can also be used in the same manner as previously described, placing a hatch mark on the first and second R waves, then moving the paper down the rhythm strip to determine if the subsequent R waves land on the hash mark. If the hatch mark is more than one small box away from the next R wave, the rhythm is irregular (Figure 7-23).

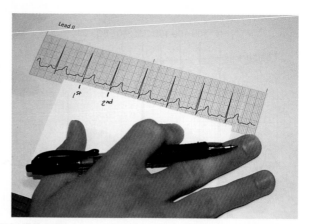

FIGURE 7-23 Use of paper and pencil to assess regularity.

Irregular rhythms can be regularly irregular or irregularly irregular. Regularly irregular rhythms have a pattern. Irregularly irregular rhythms have no pattern and no predictability. Atrial fibrillation is an example of an irregularly irregular rhythm.

Measurement of PR, QRS, QT/QTc Intervals

PR, QRS, and QT/QTc intervals are measured and documented as part of rhythm analysis. In some dysrhythmias, intervals such as the PR interval may change; thus all PR intervals are measured to ensure that they are consistent. QRS intervals can lengthen in response to new bundle branch blocks or with ventricular dysrhythmias. QT/QTc intervals can lengthen in response to certain drugs as well as electrolyte imbalances. Intervals are measured with calipers or paper and pencil as previously described by identifying the number of small boxes and multiplying by 0.04 seconds. If the end of the interval being measured falls between boxes, add 0.02 to the measurement, as this is the time allowed for half of a box of measurement.

Shape or Morphology of Waveforms

The P, QRS, and T waves of the rhythm strip are assessed for shape and consistency. All waveforms should look alike in the normal ECG. Abnormal shapes may indicate that the stimulus that caused the waveform came from an ectopic focus, or that there is a delay or block in conduction creating a bundle branch block. It is important to also confirm that a P wave precedes the QRS complex and that the T wave follows the QRS complex. Several dysrhythmias are characterized by abnormal location or sequencing of waveforms, such as the P waves in complete heart block.

Identification of Underlying Rhythm and Any Noted Dysrhythmia

The underlying rhythm is identified first. Following this step, the dysrhythmia that disrupts the underlying rhythm is determined.

Patient Tolerance of the Rhythm and Clinical Implication of the Rhythm

Once an abnormal heart rhythm is identified, the priority is to assess the patient for any symptoms that may be related to the dysrhythmia (Box 7-2). Assessment for hemodynamic deterioration includes obtaining vital signs, assessing for alterations in level of consciousness, auscultating lung sounds, and asking the patient if there are any complaints of dyspnea or chest discomfort. Instability is manifested by any of the following: hypotension, acutely altered mental status, signs of shock, ischemic chest discomfort, or acute heart failure.[3] Additionally, a 12-lead ECG is obtained to aid in identification of the dysrhythmia.

The next step is to determine if there are causes of the dysrhythmia that can be treated immediately. An example is a patient with a fast, wide complex tachycardia who has a pulse but low blood pressure. The immediate priority is to treat the patient's fast heart rhythm with a therapy such as emergent cardioversion, but the next critical step is to identify potential causes of the dysrhythmia, such as hypokalemia, hypomagnesemia, hypoxemia, or ischemia.

BASIC DYSRHYTHMIAS

The basic dysrhythmias are classified based on their site of origin, including:

- SA node
- Atrial
- AV node or junctional
- Ventricular
- Heart blocks of the AV node

The following discussion reviews the ECG characteristics and provides examples of each dysrhythmia. Specific criteria that can be used to recognize and identify dysrhythmias are presented systematically for each one. The discussion includes typical causes, patient responses, and appropriate treatment. Medications used to treat common dysrhythmias are described in Table 7-1.

The learner who is new to identification of dysrhythmias will benefit from extensive practice reading rhythm strips and collaborating with seasoned colleagues who are adept at rhythm interpretation. Maintaining a pocket notebook (or using handheld devices with cardiac rhythm applications) with ECG criteria for each rhythm helps the learner memorize the criteria specific to common dysrhythmias. Other suggested learning aids are to complete a course in basic rhythm interpretation, either in the classroom or by computerized instruction. Finally, mastering the identification of dysrhythmias requires practice, practice, and more practice. Another essential assessment skill is recognition of hemodynamic instability related to decreased cardiac output because of the cardiac dysrhythmia (see Box 7-2).

Normal Sinus Rhythm

Normal sinus rhythm (NSR) reflects normal conduction of the sinus impulse through the atria and ventricles. Any deviation from sinus rhythm is a dysrhythmia, thus it is critical to remember and understand the criteria that determine NSR.

Sinus rhythm is initiated by an impulse in the sinus node. The generated impulse propagates through the conductive fibers of the atria, reaches the AV node where there is a slight pause, and then spreads throughout the ventricles, causing depolarization and resultant cardiac contraction in a timely and organized manner (Figure 7-24).

Rhythm Analysis

- *Rate:* Atrial and ventricular rates are the same and range from 60 to 100 beats per minute.
- *Regularity:* Rhythm is regular or essentially regular.
- *Interval measurements:* PR interval is 0.12 to 0.20 seconds. QRS interval is 0.06 to 0.10 seconds.
- *Shape and sequence:* P and QRS waves are consistent in shape. P waves are small and rounded. A P wave precedes every QRS complex, which is followed by a T wave.
- *Hemodynamic effect:* Patient is hemodynamically stable.

BOX 7-2	SYMPTOMS OF DECREASED CARDIAC OUTPUT

- Change in level of consciousness
- Chest discomfort
- Hypotension
- Shortness of breath; respiratory distress
- Pulmonary congestion; crackles
- Rapid, slow, or weak pulse
- Dizziness
- Syncope
- Fatigue
- Restlessness

Lead II

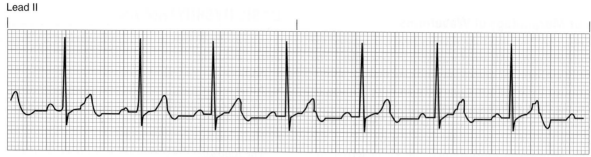

FIGURE 7-24 Normal sinus rhythm.

Lead II

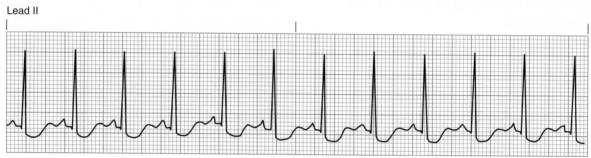

FIGURE 7-25 Sinus tachycardia.

Dysrhythmias of the Sinoatrial Node
Sinus Tachycardia

Tachycardia is defined as a heart rate greater than 100 beats per minute. Sinus tachycardia results when the SA node fires faster than 100 beats per minute (Figure 7-25). Sinus tachycardia is a normal response to stimulation of the sympathetic nervous system. Sinus tachycardia is also a normal finding in children younger than 6 years.

Rhythm analysis
- *Rate:* Both atrial and ventricular rates are greater than 100 beats per minute, up to 160 beats per minute, but may be as high as 180 beats per minute.[13]
- *Regularity:* Onset is gradual rather than abrupt. Sinus tachycardia is regular or essentially regular.
- *Interval measurements:* PR interval is 0.12 to 0.20 seconds (at higher rates, the P wave may not be readily visible). QRS interval is 0.06 to 0.10 seconds. QT may shorten.
- *Shape and sequence:* P and QRS waves are consistent in shape. P waves are small and rounded. A P wave precedes every QRS complex, which is then followed by a T wave.
- *Patient response:* The fast heart rhythm may cause a decrease in cardiac output because of the shorter filling time for the ventricles. Vulnerable populations are those with ischemic heart disease who are adversely affected by the shorter time for coronary filling during diastole.
- *Causes:* Hyperthyroidism, hypovolemia, heart failure, anemia, exercise, use of stimulants, fever, and sympathetic response to fear or pain and anxiety may cause sinus tachycardia.

- *Care and treatment:* The dysrhythmia itself is not treated, but the cause is identified and treated appropriately. For example, pain medications are administered to treat pain or antipyretics are given to treat fever.

Sinus Bradycardia

Bradycardia is defined as a heart rate less than 60 beats per minute. Sinus bradycardia may be a normal heart rhythm for some individuals such as athletes, or it may occur during sleep. Although sinus bradycardia may be asymptomatic, it may cause instability in some individuals if it results in a decrease in cardiac output. The key is to assess the patient and determine if the bradycardia is accompanied by signs of instability (Figure 7-26).

Rhythm analysis
- *Rate:* Both atrial and ventricular rates are less than 60 beats per minute.
- *Regularity:* Rhythm is regular or essentially regular.
- *Interval measurements:* Measurements are normal, but QT may be prolonged.
- *Shape and sequence:* P and QRS waves are consistent in shape. P waves are small and rounded. A P wave precedes every QRS complex, which is followed by a T wave.
- *Patient response:* The slowed heart rhythm may cause a decrease in cardiac output, resulting in hypotension and decreased organ perfusion.
- *Causes:* Vasovagal response; medications such as digoxin or AV nodal blocking agents, including calcium channel blockers and beta blockers; myocardial infarction; normal

Lead II

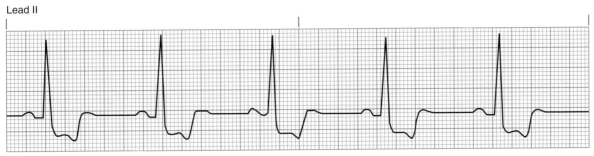

FIGURE 7-26 Sinus bradycardia.

Lead V1

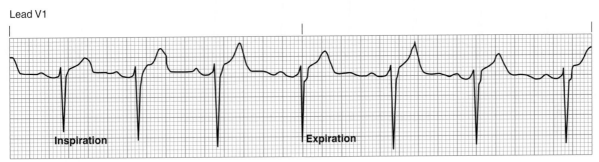

Inspiration   Expiration

FIGURE 7-27 Sinus arrhythmia. The heart rate increases slightly with inspiration and decreases slightly with expiration.

physiological variant in the athlete; disease of the sinus node; increased intracranial pressure; hypoxemia; and hypothermia may cause sinus bradycardia.

- *Care and treatment:* Assess for hemodynamic instability related to the bradycardia. If the patient is symptomatic, interventions include administration of atropine. If atropine is not effective in increasing heart rate, then transcutaneous pacing, dopamine infusion, or epinephrine infusion may be administered.[3] Atropine is avoided for treatment of bradycardia associated with hypothermia.

Sinus Arrhythmia

Sinus arrhythmia is a cyclical change in heart rate that is associated with respiration. The heart rate slightly increases during inspiration and slightly slows during exhalation because of changes in vagal tone.[13] The ECG tracing demonstrates an alternating pattern of faster and slower heart rate that changes with the respiratory cycle (Figure 7-27).

Rhythm analysis
- *Rate:* Atrial and ventricular rates are between 60 and 100 beats per minute.
- *Regularity:* This rhythm is cyclically irregular, slowing with exhalation and increasing with inspiration.
- *Interval measurements:* Measurements are normal.
- *Shape and sequence:* P and QRS waves are consistent in shape. P waves are small and rounded. A P wave precedes every QRS complex, which is then followed by a T wave.
- *Patient response:* This rhythm is tolerated well.
- *Care and treatment:* No treatment is required.

Sinus Pauses

Sinus pauses occur when the SA node either fails to generate an impulse (sinus arrest) or the impulse is blocked and does not exit from the SA node (sinus exit block). The result of the sinus node not firing is a pause without any electrical activity.

Sinus arrest. Failure of the SA node to generate an impulse is called *sinus arrest.* The arrest results from a lack of stimulus from the SA node. The sinus beat following the arrest is not on time because the sinus node has been reset and the next sinus impulse begins a new rhythm. The end result is that no atrial or ventricular depolarization occurs for one heartbeat or more (Figure 7-28, *A*).

If the pause is long enough, the AV node or ventricular backup pacemaker may fire, resulting in *escape beats.* These beats are called junctional escape or ventricular escape beats. Typically, the sinus node resumes normal generation of impulses following the pause.

Sinus exit block. Sinus exit block also results in a pause, but the P wave following the pause in rhythm is on time or regular because the sinus node does not reset. The sinus impulse simply fails to "exit" the sinus node (Figure 7-28, *B*).

Rhythm analysis
- *Rate:* Atrial and ventricular rates are usually between 60 and 100 beats per minute, but any pause may result in a heart rate less than 60 beats per minute.
- *Regularity:* The rhythm is irregular for the period of the pause but regular when sinus rhythm resumes. In SA exit

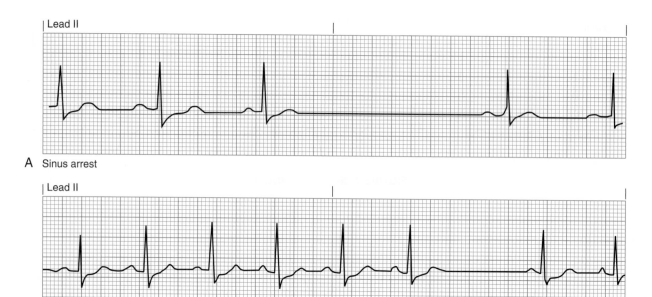

A Sinus arrest

B Sinus exit block

FIGURE 7-28 A, Sinus arrest. **B,** Sinus exit block.

block, the P wave following the pause occurs on time. In sinus arrest, the P wave following the pause is not on time.
- *Interval measurements:* Measurements of conducted beats are normal.
- *Shape and sequence:* P and QRS waves are consistent in shape. P waves are small and rounded. A P wave precedes every QRS complex, which is followed by a T wave.
- *Patient response:* Single pauses in rhythm may not be significant, but frequent pauses may result in a severe bradycardia. The patient with multiple pauses may experience signs and symptoms of decreased cardiac output (see Box 7-2).
- *Causes:* Hypoxemia; ischemia or damage of the sinus node related to myocardial infarction; AV nodal blocking medications such as beta blockers, calcium channel blockers, and digoxin; and increased vagal tone may cause sinus exit block.
- *Care and treatment:* If the patient is symptomatic, significant numbers of pauses may require treatment, including temporary and permanent implantation of a pacemaker. Causes are explored, and prescribed medications may need to be adjusted or discontinued.

Dysrhythmias of the Atria

Normally, the SA node is the dominant pacemaker initiating the heart rhythm; however, cells outside the SA node within the atria can create an ectopic focus that can cause a dysrhythmia. An ectopic focus is an abnormal beat or a rhythm that occurs outside the normal conduction system. In this case, atrial dysrhythmias arise in the atrial tissue.

Premature Atrial Contractions

A premature atrial contraction (PAC) is a single ectopic beat arising from atrial tissue, not the sinus node. The PAC occurs earlier than the next normal beat and interrupts the regularity of the underlying rhythm. The P wave of the PAC has a different shape than the sinus P wave because it arises from a different area in the atria; it may follow or be in the T wave of the preceding normal beat. If the early P wave is in the T wave, this T wave will look different from the T wave of a normal beat. Following the PAC, a pause occurs and then the underlying rhythm typically resumes. The pause is noncompensatory, which means that when measuring the P-P intervals for atrial regularity, the P wave following the pause does not occur on time. Box 7-3 discusses how to distinguish compensatory and noncompensatory pauses. PACs are common but denote an irritable area in the atria that has developed the property of automaticity (Figure 7-29).

Nonconducted PACs are beats that create an early P wave but are not followed by a QRS complex. The ventricles are unable to depolarize in response to this early stimulus because they are not fully repolarized from the normally conducted beat preceding the PAC (see Figure 7-29). This creates a pause, but a P wave occurs either in or after

BOX 7-3   COMPENSATORY VERSUS NONCOMPENSATORY PAUSE

- A rhythm strip with a premature beat is analysed using calipers or paper and pencil.
- Two consecutive normal beats are located just before the premature beat, and the caliper points or pencil marks are placed on the R wave of each normal beat.
- The calipers are flipped over, or the paper is slid over, to where the next normal beat should have occurred. The premature beat occurs early.

- Now, with care taken not to lose placement, the calipers are flipped or the paper is slid over one more time. If the point of the calipers or the mark on the paper lands exactly on the next normal beat's R wave, the sinus node compensated for the one premature beat and kept its normal rhythm (see figure).
- If the caliper point or pencil mark does not land on the next normal beat's R wave, then the sinus node did not compensate and had to establish a new rhythm, resulting in a noncompensatory pause.

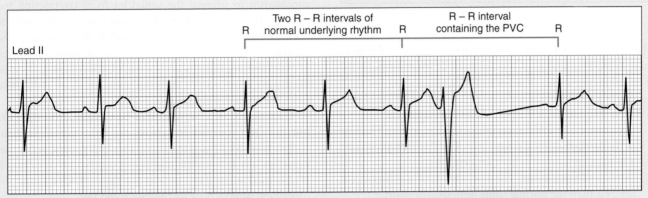

Compensatory pause; sinus rhythm with premature ventricular contraction (PVC). The pause following the PVC is compensatory. (From Paul S, Hebra JD. *The Nurse's Guide to Cardiac Rhythm Interpretation: Implications for Patient Care*. Philadelphia, Saunders; 1998.)

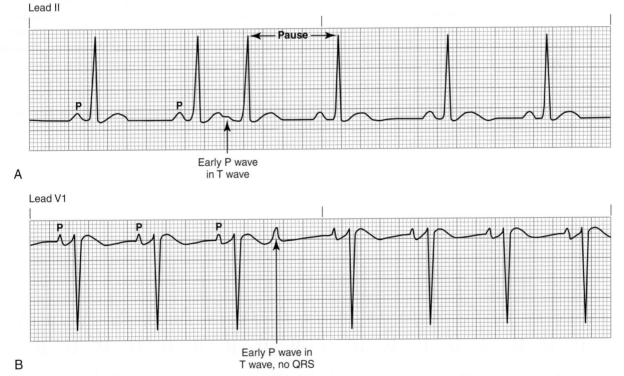

FIGURE 7-29 A, Premature atrial contractions (PAC) shown in the third beat. **B,** A nonconducted PAC. (Modified from Association of Critical-Care Nurses: *Essentials of Critical Care Orientation*.)

the T wave. This is why comparing the shapes of the normal PQRST is a critical requirement in rhythm analysis. The frequency of occurrence of PACs varies (Box 7-4).

Rhythm analysis

- *Rate:* The rate matches that of the underlying rhythm.
- *Regularity:* The PAC interrupts the regularity of the underlying rhythm for a single beat. The PAC is followed by a noncompensatory pause (see Box 7-3).
- *Interval measurements:* The PAC may have a different PR interval than the normal sinus beat, usually shorter.
- *Shape and sequence:* The P wave of the PAC is typically a different shape than the sinus P wave. The T wave of the preceding beat may be distorted if the P wave of the PAC lies within it.
- *Patient response:* PACs are usually well-tolerated, although the patient may complain of palpitations.
- *Causes:* Stimulants such as caffeine or tobacco, myocardial hypertrophy or dilatation, ischemia, lung disease, hypokalemia, and hypomagnesemia may cause PACs. It may also be a normal variant.
- *Care and treatment:* Increasing numbers of PACs may occur before atrial fibrillation or atrial flutter. No treatment is indicated for PACs.

Atrial Tachycardia

Atrial tachycardia is a rapid rhythm that arises from an ectopic focus in the atria. Because of the fast rate, atrial tachycardia can be a life-threatening dysrhythmia. The ectopic atrial focus generates impulses more rapidly than the AV node can conduct while still in the refractory phase from the previous impulse, and these impulses are not transmitted to the ventricles. Therefore more P waves may be seen than QRS complexes and T waves. This refractoriness serves as a safety mechanism to prevent the ventricles from contracting too rapidly. The AV node may block impulses in a set pattern, such as every second, third, or fourth beat. However, if the ventricles respond to every ectopic atrial impulse, it is called 1:1 conduction, one P wave for each QRS complex. Because the P wave arises outside the sinus node, the shape is different from the sinus P wave (Figure 7-30).

If an abnormal P wave cannot be visualized on the ECG but the QRS complex is narrow, the term *supraventricular tachycardia* (SVT) is often used. This is a generic term that describes any tachycardia that is not ventricular in origin; it is also used when the source above the ventricles cannot be identified, usually because the rate is too fast.

Rhythm analysis

- *Rate:* The rate ranges from 150 to 250 beats per minute.
- *Regularity:* The rhythm is regular if all P waves are conducted.
- *Interval measurements:* The PR interval is different from the sinus PR interval. If the ectopic P wave arises near the junction, the PR interval may be shortened. If close to the sinus node, it is nearer the normal PR interval in duration.
- *Shape and sequence:* The P wave shape is different from that of the sinus P wave. The QRS complex is narrow unless there is a bundle branch block. If the P wave of the ectopic rhythm occurs in the T wave, this may alter the shape.

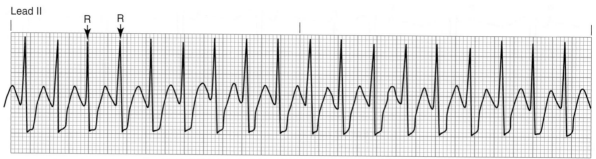

FIGURE 7-30 Atrial tachycardia with 1:1 conduction.

- *Patient response:* The faster the tachycardia, the more symptomatic the patient may become. This arises from decreased cardiac output (see Box 7-2) and resultant decreased organ perfusion.
- *Causes:* Atrial tachycardia can occur in patients with normal hearts as well as those with cardiac disease. Causes include digitalis toxicity, electrolyte imbalances, lung disease, ischemic heart disease, and cardiac valvular abnormalities.
- *Care and treatment:* Treatment is directed at assessing the patient's tolerance of the tachycardia. If the rate is over 150 beats per minute and the patient is symptomatic, emergent cardioversion is considered. Cardioversion is the delivery of a synchronized electrical shock to the heart by an external defibrillator (see Chapter 10). Medications that may be used include adenosine, beta-blockers, calcium channel blockers, and amiodarone.[3]

Wandering Atrial Pacemaker

Wandering atrial pacemaker is a dysrhythmia characterized by at least three different ectopic atrial foci followed by a QRS complex at a rate less than 100 beats per minute. At least three different P wave shapes are noted. P waves in wandering atrial pacemaker can be upright, inverted, flat, pointed, notched, and/or slanted in different directions. The PR interval varies because the impulses originate from different locations within the atria, taking various times to reach the AV node (Figure 7-31).

Rhythm analysis
- *Rate:* Rate is less than 100 beats per minute.
- *Regularity:* The rate may be slightly irregular.
- *Interval measurements:* PR intervals vary based on the sites of the ectopic foci.
- *Shape and sequence:* At least three different P shapes are noted. The QRS complex is narrow and followed by a T wave.
- *Patient response:* Patients usually tolerate this rhythm unless the rate increases.
- *Causes:* Lung disease such as chronic obstructive pulmonary diseases may cause wandering atrial pacemaker. It may also be a normal variant in the young and the elderly.
- *Care and treatment:* No treatment is usually indicated.

Multifocal Atrial Tachycardia

Multifocal atrial tachycardia is essentially the same as wandering atrial pacemaker, except the heart rate exceeds 100 beats per minute (Figure 7-32). At least three ectopic P waves are noted. This dysrhythmia is almost exclusively found in the patient with chronic obstructive pulmonary disease. Pulmonary hypertension occurs and results in increased atrial pressure and dilatation, creating irritable atrial foci.

Rhythm analysis
- *Rate:* The heart rate is greater than 100 beats per minute.
- *Regularity:* The rhythm is slightly irregular.
- *Interval measurements:* PR intervals vary.

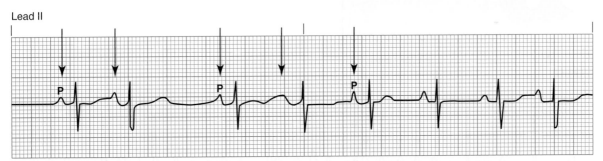

FIGURE 7-31 Wandering atrial pacemaker. Arrows indicate different shapes of P waves.

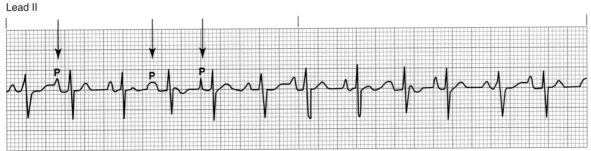

FIGURE 7-32 Multifocal atrial tachycardia. Arrows indicate different shapes of P waves.

- *Shape and sequence:* P waves differ in shape. A P wave precedes every QRS complex, which is followed by a T wave.
- *Patient response:* The response varies and is determined by the patient's tolerance of the tachycardia.
- *Causes:* Chronic obstructive pulmonary disease causes dilatation of the atria with resultant ectopic foci from the stretched tissue.
- *Care and treatment:* The treatment goal is to optimize the patient's pulmonary status.

Atrial Flutter

Atrial flutter arises from a single irritable focus in the atria. The atrial focus fires at an extremely rapid, regular rate, between 240 and 320 beats per minute.[8] The P waves are called flutter waves and have a sawtooth appearance (Figure 7-33, *A*). The ventricular response may be regular or irregular based on how many flutter waves are conducted through the AV node. The number of flutter waves to each QRS complex is called the *conduction ratio.* The conduction ratio may remain the same or vary depending on the number of flutter waves that are conducted to the ventricles. The description of atrial flutter might be constant at 2:1, 3:1, 4:1, 5:1, and so forth, or it may be variable. Flutter waves occur through the QRS complex and the T wave, and often alter their appearance (Figure 7-33). It is helpful to identify the best lead for visualizing the flutter waves in atrial flutter and use this as the second monitor lead.

Rhythm analysis

- *Rate:* Atrial rate is between 240 and 320 beats per minute but is typically 300 beats per minute (one large box between flutter waves, Figure 7-33, *B*. Ventricular rate is determined by the conduction ratio of the flutter waves.
- *Regularity:* Flutter waves are regular but the QRS complex and T waves may not be regular depending on the conduction ratio of the atrial flutter.
- *Interval measurements:* No PR interval is present. QRS and QT intervals are normal unless distorted by a flutter wave.
- *Shape and sequence:* P or flutter waves are consistent in shape and look like tines on a sawtooth blade. QRST waves are altered in shape by the flutter waves.

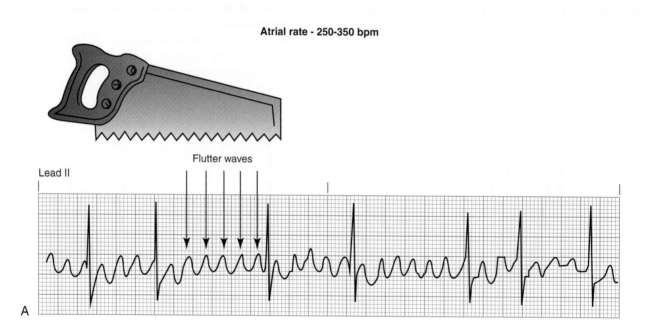

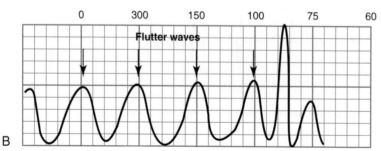

FIGURE 7-33 Atrial flutter. **A,** Flutter waves show sawtooth pattern. **B,** Enlarged view shows one large box between flutter waves.

- *Patient response:* Usually the patient is asymptomatic unless atrial flutter results in a tachycardia called rapid ventricular response (RVR). Atrial flutter with RVR occurs when atrial impulses cause a ventricular response greater than 100 beats per minute.
- *Causes:* Lung disease, ischemic heart disease, hyperthyroidism, hypoxemia, heart failure, and alcoholism can cause atrial flutter.
- *Care and treatment:* Alterations in atrial blood flow leading to blood stasis can cause clot formation. Patients identified with atrial flutter usually receive chronic antithrombotic therapy unless contraindicated. Rate control is accomplished with medications that block the AV node. Elective cardioversion may be performed once the patient has been taking anticoagulants for approximately 6 weeks. Interventional electrophysiological treatments including ablation of the irritable focus may be done in the electrophysiology lab.[8]

Atrial Fibrillation

Atrial fibrillation is the most common dysrhythmia observed in clinical practice.[8] Atrial fibrillation arises from multiple ectopic foci in the atria, causing chaotic quivering of the atria and ineffectual atrial contraction. The AV node is bombarded with hundreds of atrial impulses and conducts these impulses in an unpredictable manner to the ventricles. The atrial rate may be as high 700 and no discernible P waves can be identified, resulting in a wavy baseline and an extremely irregular ventricular response. This irregularity is called *irregularly irregular* (Figure 7-34). The ineffectual contraction of the atria results in loss of *atrial kick.* If too many impulses conduct to the ventricles, atrial fibrillation with rapid ventricular response may result and compromise cardiac output. When atrial fibrillation occurs sporadically it is called paroxysmal atrial fibrillation.

If the atrial impulse is conducted through the ventricles in a normal fashion, the QRS complex is narrow and appears normal although irregularly irregular. But if the impulse reaches one of the bundle branches before full repolarization, the QRS complex is widened in classic bundle branch

block morphology. The widened QRS is due to the delay caused by the bundle branch block, and results in slowed conduction through either the right or left ventricle, depending on which bundle branch has not fully repolarized. When this event occurs, the impulse is said to be *aberrantly conducted* (Figure 7-35).

In atrial fibrillation, aberrantly conducted beats are referred to as *Ashman beats.* Ashman beats are more likely to occur when an atrial impulse arrives at the AV node just after a previously conducted impulse (see Figure 7-35). Ashman beats are often seen when the rate changes from slower to faster, referred to as a long-short cycle. Ashman beats are not clinically significant.

One complication of atrial fibrillation is thromboembolism. The blood that collects in the atria is agitated by fibrillation, and normal clotting is accelerated. Small thrombi, called *mural* thrombi, begin to form along the walls of the atria. These clots may dislodge, resulting in pulmonary embolism or stroke.

Rhythm analysis

- *Rate:* Atrial rate is uncountable; ventricular rate may vary widely.
- *Regularity:* Ventricular response is irregularly irregular, unless the patient has complete heart block. In complete heart block, the ventricular response is regular, widened, and between 20 and 40 beats per minute.
- *Interval measurements:* PR interval is absent. The QRS complex and QT interval are normal in duration unless a bundle branch block exists.
- *Shape and sequence:* No recognizable or discernible P waves are present. The isoelectric line is wavy. QRS waves are consistent in shape unless aberrantly conducted. The QRS complex is followed by a T wave.
- *Patient response:* The patient may or may not be aware of the atrial fibrillation. If the ventricular response is rapid, the patient may show signs of decreased cardiac output, or worsening of heart failure symptoms.
- *Causes:* Ischemic heart disease, valvular heart disease, hyperthyroidism, lung disease, heart failure, and aging may cause atrial fibrillation.

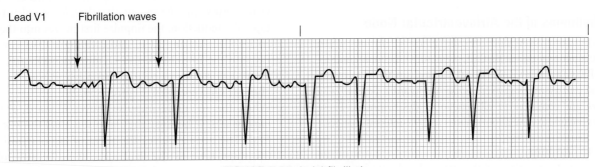

Lead V1   Fibrillation waves

FIGURE 7-34 Atrial fibrillation.

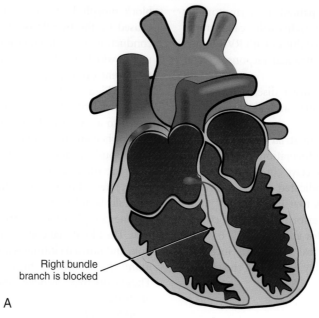

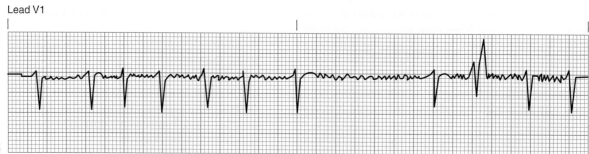

FIGURE 7-35 Atrial fibrillation with single aberrantly conducted beat (9th beat) due to right bundle branch block.

- *Care and treatment:* As with atrial flutter, alterations in blood flow and hemostasis may predispose the patient to clot formation. If there are no contraindications, the patient is prescribed anticoagulants. After at least 4 to 6 weeks of antithrombotic therapy, elective cardioversion can be considered. Amiodarone may be administered to enhance success of cardioversion. Ventricular rate control is attained by administration of AV nodal blocking agents. As with atrial flutter, ablation may be attempted. Symptomatic tachycardia is usually treated with medications because of the risk of thromboembolism. Emergent cardioversion is considered if the tachycardia is associated with hemodynamic instability.[8]

Dysrhythmias of the Atrioventricular Node

Dysrhythmias of the AV node are called *junctional rhythms,* which include junctional escape rhythm, premature junctional contractions (PJCs), accelerated junctional rhythm, junctional tachycardia, and paroxysmal supraventricular tachycardia. Several ECG changes are common to all junctional dysrhythmias. These changes include P-wave abnormalities and PR-interval changes.

P-Wave Changes

Because of the location of the AV node—in the center of the heart—impulses generated may be conducted forward, backward, or both. With the potential of forward, backward, or bidirectional impulse conduction, three different P wave-forms may be associated with junctional rhythms:

1. When the AV node impulse is conducted backward, the impulse enters the atria first. Conduction back toward the atria allows for at least partial depolarization of the atria. When depolarization occurs backward, an inverted P wave is created. Once the atria have been depolarized, the impulse then moves down the bundle of His and depolarizes both ventricles normally (Figure 7-36, *A*). A short PR interval (<0.12 second) is noted.

2. When the impulse is conducted both forward and backward, *P waves may be present after the QRS complex.* In this type of conduction, the impulse first moves into the ventricles, depolarizing them and creating a QRS complex. Because the impulse is also conducted backward, some atrial depolarization occurs, and a late P wave is noted after the QRS complex (Figure 7-36, *B*).

3. When the AV node impulse moves forward, *P waves may be absent* because the impulse enters the ventricle first. The atria receives the wave of depolarization at the same time as the ventricles; thus, because of the larger muscle mass of the ventricles, there is no P wave (Figure 7-36, *C*).

Lead III

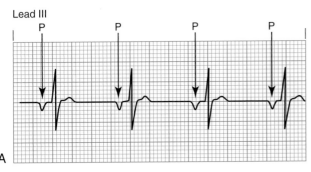

A

Lead II

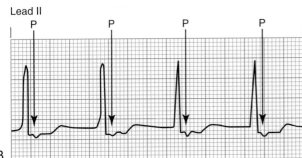

B

Lead V3

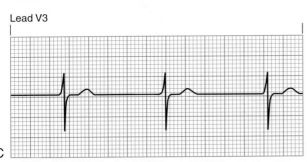

C

FIGURE 7-36 P waves in junctional dysrhythmias. **A,** Backward conduction with inverted P wave. **B,** Forward and backward conduction with retrograde P wave. **C,** Forward conduction with absent P wave.

Junctional Escape Rhythm

Junctional escape rhythms occur when the dominant pacemaker, the SA node, fails to fire. A junctional escape rhythm has either an inverted P wave and short PR interval preceding the QRS complex, a P wave that follows the QRS complex (retrograde), or no visible P wave. The escape rhythm may consist of many successive beats (Figure 7-37, A) or it may occur as a single escape beat that follows a pause, such as a sinus pause (Figure 7-37, B).

Rhythm analysis

- *Rate:* Heart rate is 40 to 60 beats per minute.
- *Regularity:* The rhythm is regular.
- *Interval measurements:* If a P wave is present before the QRS complex, the PR interval is shortened less than 0.12 milliseconds. QRS complex is normal.
- *Shape and sequence:* P waves may be inverted, follow the QRS complex, or be absent.
- *Patient response:* The patient is assessed for tolerance of the bradycardia.
- *Causes:* The escape rhythm results from loss of sinus node activity.

- *Care and treatment:* Determine the patient's tolerance of the bradycardia. Alert the provider of the change in rhythm. If symptomatic, administer atropine; consider transcutaneous pacing, dopamine infusion, or epinephrine infusion.[3]

Accelerated Junctional Rhythm and Junctional Tachycardia

The normal intrinsic rate for the AV node and junctional tissue is 40 to 60 beats per minute, but rates can accelerate. An accelerated junctional rhythm has a rate between 60 and 100 beats per minute (Figure 7-38, A) and the rate for junctional tachycardia is greater than 100 beats per minute (Figure 7-38, B).

Rhythm analysis

- *Rate:* Accelerated junctional rhythm is 60 to 100 beats per minute. Junctional tachycardia rhythm is greater than 100 beats per minute.
- *Regularity:* Regular
- *Interval measurements:* If a P wave is present before the QRS, the PR interval is shortened less than 0.12 ms. QRS is followed by T wave and both are normal in shape.
- *Shape and sequence:* If P wave precedes QRS, it is inverted or upside down, the P wave may not be visible or may follow the QRS.
- *Patient response:* Patient may have a decrease in cardiac output and hemodynamic instability, depending on the rate.
- *Causes:* SA node disease, ischemic heart disease, electrolyte imbalances, digitalis toxicity, and hypoxemia can be causes.
- *Care and treatment:* Assess and treat the tachycardia if the patient is hemodynamically unstable. Alert the provider of the change in rhythm.

Premature Junctional Contractions

Irritable areas in the AV node and junctional tissue can generate premature beats that are earlier than the next expected beat (Figure 7-39). These premature beats are similar to PACs but with characteristics of a junctional beat. The regularity of the underlying rhythm is interrupted by the premature junctional beat. The premature junctional contraction (PJC) is followed by a noncompensatory pause.

Rhythm analysis

- *Rate:* That of the underlying rhythm.
- *Regularity:* Underlying rhythm is interrupted by a premature beat that momentarily disrupts regularity.
- *Interval measurements:* The PJC is early, thus next to the T wave.
- *Shape and sequence:* If P wave precedes QRS, it is inverted, may not be visible, or follows the QRS. QRS is followed by T wave and both are normal in shape.
- *Patient response:* Well tolerated but patient may experience palpitations if the PJCs occur frequently.
- *Causes:* Normal variant; digitalis toxicity; ischemic or valvular heart disease; heart failure; response to endogenous or exogenous catecholamines, such as epinephrine.
- *Care and treatment:* No treatment indicated.

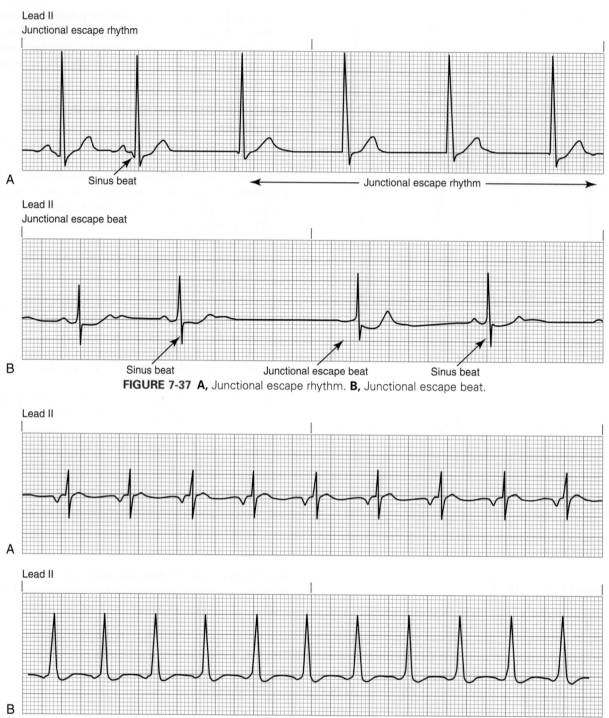

FIGURE 7-37 **A,** Junctional escape rhythm. **B,** Junctional escape beat.

FIGURE 7-38 **A,** Accelerated junctional rhythm. **B,** Junctional tachycardia.

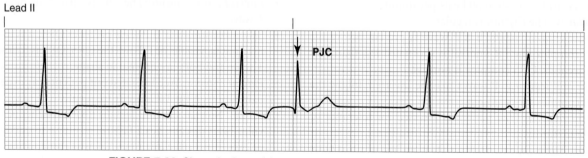

FIGURE 7-39 Sinus rhythm with premature junctional contraction (PJC).

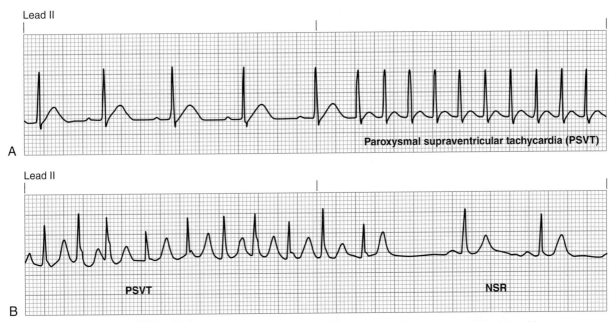

FIGURE 7-40 Paroxysmal supraventricular tachycardia (PSVT). **A,** The abrupt onset initiated by a PJC. **B,** The abrupt cessation of the PSVT.

Paroxysmal Supraventricular Tachycardia

Paroxysmal supraventricular tachycardia (PSVT) occurs above the ventricles, and it has an abrupt onset and cessation. It is initiated by either a PAC or a PJC. An abnormal conduction pathway through the AV node or an accessory pathway around the AV node results in extreme tachycardia. The QRS complex is typically narrow and a P wave may or may not be present. The primary criteria are those of the abrupt onset and cessation of the dysrhythmia (Figure 7-40, A-B).

Rhythm analysis

- *Rate:* Heart rate is 150 to 250 beats per minute.
- *Regularity:* The rhythm is regular.
- *Interval measurements:* If the P wave is present, the PR interval is shortened. Other intervals are normal.
- *Shape and sequence:* P wave (if present) and QRS complex are consistent in shape. The QRS complex is narrow and followed by a T wave.
- *Patient response:* The patient may be asymptomatic or symptomatic.
- *Causes:* PSVT often occurs in healthy, young adults without structural heart disease. It may be precipitated by increased catecholamines, stimulants, heart disease, electrolyte imbalances, and anatomical abnormality.
- *Care and treatment:* If the patient is asymptomatic, vagal maneuvers may be attempted. If the patient is symptomatic and the heart rate is over 150 beats per minute, emergent cardioversion is considered. Adenosine or AV nodal blocking agents are usually administered. Once stabilized, the patient is referred for further evaluation by an electrophysiologist.

Dysrhythmias of the Ventricle

Ventricular dysrhythmias arise from ectopic foci in the ventricles. Because the stimulus depolarizes the ventricles in a slower, abnormal way, the QRS complex appears widened and has a bizarre shape. The QRS complex is wider than 0.12 seconds and often wider than 0.16 seconds. The polarity of the T wave is opposite that of the QRS complex.

Depolarization from abnormal ventricular beats rarely activates the atria in a retrograde fashion. Therefore most ventricular dysrhythmias have no apparent P waves. However, if a P wave is present, it is usually seen in the T wave of the following beat; or it has no relationship to the QRS complex and is dissociated from the ventricular rhythm. Ventricular dysrhythmias can be life-threatening, thus fast recognition and intervention is imperative.

Premature Ventricular Contractions

Premature ventricular contractions (PVCs) are a common ventricular dysrhythmia. PVCs are early beats that interrupt the underlying rhythm; they can arise from a single ectopic focus or from multiple foci within the ventricles. A single ectopic focus produces PVC waveforms that look alike, called *unifocal PVCs* ((Figure 7-41, A, C). Waveforms of PVCs arising from multiple foci are not identical and are called *multifocal PVCs* (Figure 7-41, B). PVCs do not generally reset the sinus node, so the next sinus beat following the pause occurs on time. This is called a compensatory pause.

PVCs may occur in a predictable pattern, such as every other beat, every third beat, or every fourth beat. Box 7-4 lists the nomenclature for early beats. *Bigeminal* PVCs are noted in Figure 7-41, A. PVCs can also occur sequentially. Two PVCs in

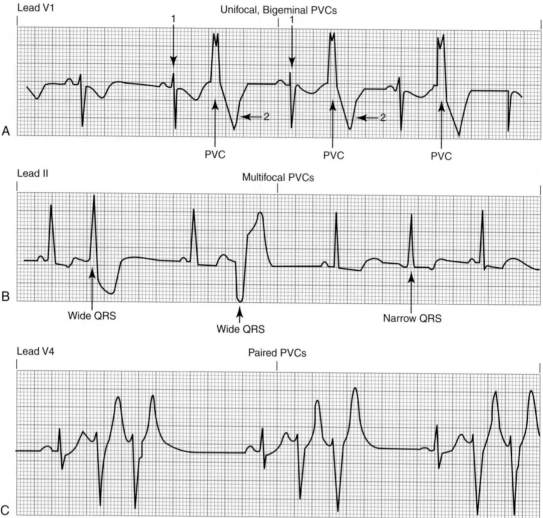

FIGURE 7-41 Premature ventricular contractions (PVCs). **A,** Sinus rhythm with unifocal PVCs. 1 is the sinus beat; 2 points to the presence of an inverted T wave. **B,** Sinus rhythm with multifocal PVCs; note the different configuration of the PVCs, indicating generation from more than one focus. **C,** The PVCs are in pairs and look the same, indicating that they are from the same foci.

a row are called a pair (Figure 7-41, *C*), and three or more in a row are called nonsustained ventricular tachycardia.

The peak of the T wave through the downslope of the T wave is considered the *vulnerable period,* which coincides with partial repolarization of the ventricles. If a PVC occurs during the T wave, ventricular tachycardia may occur. When the R wave of PVC falls on the T wave of a normal beat, it is referred to as the *R-on-T phenomenon* (Figure 7-42, *A, B*).

PVCs may occur in healthy individuals and usually do not require treatment. The nurse must determine if PVCs are increasing in number by evaluating the trend. If PVCs are increasing, the nurse should evaluate for potential causes such as electrolyte imbalances, myocardial ischemia or injury, and hypoxemia. Runs of nonsustained ventricular tachycardia may be a precursor to development of sustained ventricular tachycardia.

Rhythm analysis

- *Rate:* The rate matches the underlying rhythm.
- *Regularity:* The rhythm is interrupted by the premature beat.

- *Interval measurements:* There is no PR interval and the QRS complex is greater than 0.12 seconds.
- *Shape and sequence:* The QRS complex of the PVC is wide and bizarre looking. The T wave may be oriented opposite to the direction of the QRS complex of the PVC.
- *Patient response:* PVCs may be experienced as palpitations. Patients may become symptomatic if the PVCs occur frequently.
- *Causes:* Hypoxemia, ischemic heart disease, hypokalemia, hypomagnesemia, acid-base imbalances, and increased catecholamine levels can cause PVCs.
- *Care and treatment:* Treat the cause if PVCs are increasing in frequency.

Ventricular Tachycardia

Ventricular tachycardia (VT) is a rapid, life-threatening dysrhythmia originating from a single ectopic focus in the ventricles. It is characterized by at least three PVCs in a row. VT occurs at a rate greater than 100 beats per minute, but the rate is usually around 150 beats per minute and may be up to

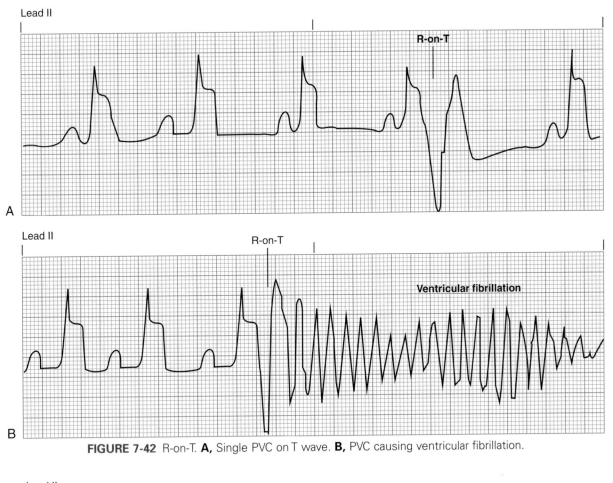

Lead II

R-on-T

A

Lead II

R-on-T

Ventricular fibrillation

B

FIGURE 7-42 R-on-T. **A,** Single PVC on T wave. **B,** PVC causing ventricular fibrillation.

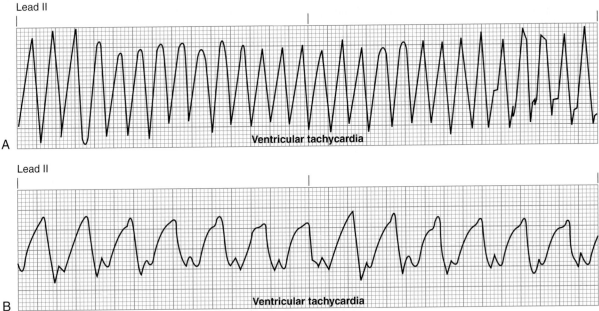

Lead II

Ventricular tachycardia

A

Lead II

Ventricular tachycardia

B

FIGURE 7-43 Ventricular tachycardia.

250 beats per minute. Depolarization of the ventricles is abnormal and produces a widened QRS complex (Figure 7-43). The patient may or may not have a pulse.

The wave of depolarization associated with ventricular tachycardia rarely reaches the atria. Therefore P waves are usually absent. If P waves are present, they have no association with the QRS complex. The sinus node may continue to depolarize at its normal rate, independent of the ventricular ectopic focus. P waves may appear to be randomly scattered throughout the rhythm, but the P waves are actually fired at a consistent rate from the sinus node. This is called *AV dissociation,* another clue that the rhythm is VT. Occasionally a P wave will "capture" the ventricle because of the timing of atrial depolarization, interrupting the VT with a single capture beat that appears normal and narrow. Then the VT reoccurs. Capture beats are a diagnostic clue to differentiating wide complex tachycardias.

Torsades de pointes ("twisting about the point") is a type of VT that is caused by a prolonged QT interval. Unlike VT, where the QRS complex waveforms have similar shapes, torsades de pointes is characterized by the presence of both positive and negative complexes that move above and below the isoelectric line. This lethal dysrhythmia is treated as pulseless VT.[3] Magnesium deficiency is often a cause of this dysrhythmia.[3] The dysrhythmia can often be prevented by routine measurement of the QT/QTc intervals, especially if the patient is receiving drugs that prolong the QT interval. Increases in QT/QTc interval are reported to the provider, potential drug-related causes are explored, and magnesium levels are monitored and corrected (Figure 7-44).[6]

Rhythm analysis

- *Rate:* The heart rate is 110 to 250 beats per minute.
- *Regularity:* The rhythm is regular unless capture beats occur and momentarily interrupt the VT.
- *Interval measurements:* There is no PR interval. The QRS complex is greater than 0.12 seconds and often wider than 0.16 seconds
- *Shape and sequence:* QRS waves are consistent in shape but appear wide and bizarre. The polarity of the T wave is opposite to that seen in the QRS complex.
- *Patient response:* If enough cardiac output is generated by the VT, a pulse and blood pressure are present. If cardiac output is impaired, the patient has signs and symptoms of low cardiac output; the patient may experience a cardiac arrest.
- *Causes:* Hypoxemia, acid-base imbalance, exacerbation of heart failure, ischemic heart disease, cardiomyopathy, hypokalemia, hypomagnesemia, valvular heart disease, genetic abnormalities, and QT prolongation are all possible causes of VT.

- *Care and treatment:* Determine whether the patient has a pulse. If no pulse is present, provide emergent basic and advanced life support interventions, including defibrillation.[3] If a pulse is present and the blood pressure is stable, the patient can be treated with intravenous amiodarone or lidocaine. Cardioversion is used as an emergency measure in patients who become hemodynamically unstable but continue to have a pulse.

Ventricular Fibrillation

Ventricular fibrillation (VF) is a chaotic rhythm characterized by a quivering of the ventricles, which results in total loss of cardiac output and pulse. VF is a life-threatening emergency, and the more immediate the treatment, the better the survival will be. VF produces a wavy baseline without a PQRST complex (Figure 7-45).

Because a loose lead or electrical interference can produce a waveform similar to VF, it is always important to immediately assess the patient for pulse and consciousness.

Rhythm analysis

- *Rate:* Heart rate is not discernible.
- *Regularity:* Heart rhythm is not discernible.
- *Interval measurements:* There are no waveforms.
- *Shape and sequence:* The baseline is wavy and chaotic, with no PQRST complexes.
- *Patient response:* The patient is in cardiac arrest.
- *Causes:* VF can be caused by ischemic and valvular heart disease, electrolyte and acid-base imbalances, and QT prolongation.
- *Care and treatment:* Immediate BLS and ACLS interventions are required.

Idioventricular Rhythm or Ventricular Escape Rhythm

Idioventricular rhythm is an escape rhythm that is generated by the Purkinje fibers. This rhythm emerges only when the SA and AV nodes fail to initiate an impulse. The Purkinje fibers are capable of an intrinsic rate of 20 to 40 beats per minute. Because this last pacemaker is located in the

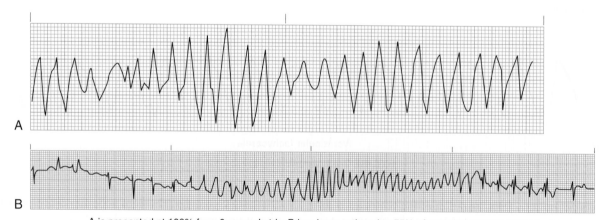

A is presented at 100% for a 6-second strip. B has been reduced to 55% of actual size to be able to see a longer waveform over 12 seconds, showing how a patient goes into and comes out of rhythm.

FIGURE 7-44 Torsades de pointes.

Lead II

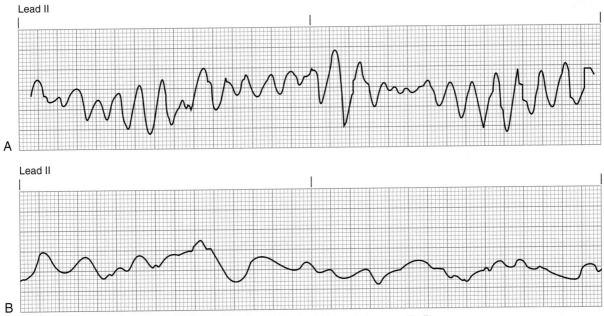

FIGURE 7-45 Ventricular fibrillation. **A,** Course. **B,** Fine.

Lead V1

Lead II

Sinus beat

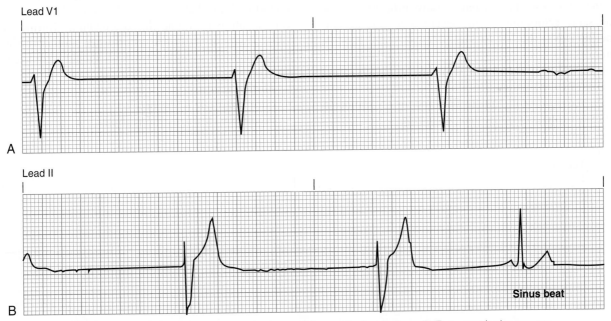

FIGURE 7-46 A, Ventricular escape rhythm or idioventricular rhythm. **B,** Two ventricular escape beats followed by sinus rhythm.

ventricles, the QRS complex appears wide and bizarre with a slow rate (Figure 7-46, *A-B*).

An idioventricular rhythm is considered a lethal dysrhythmia because the Purkinje fiber pacemakers may cease to fire, resulting in asystole. A single ventricular escape beat may occur following a pause if the junctional escape pacemaker does not fire (see Figure 7-46, *A-B*).

If the rate is between 40 and 100 beats per minute, this rhythm is called accelerated idioventricular rhythm (AIVR). This wide complex rhythm is often seen following reperfusion of a coronary artery by thrombolytics; percutaneous coronary interventions, such as angioplasty or stent placement; and cardiac surgery (Figure 7-47).

Lead V1

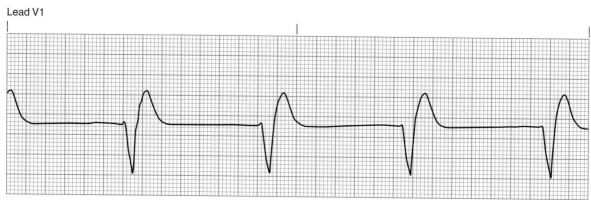

FIGURE 7-47 Accelerated idioventricular rhythm (AIVR).

Rhythm analysis

- *Rate:* The rate of idioventricular rhythm is 20 to 40 beats per minute, and the rate of AIVR is 40 to 100 beats per minute.
- *Regularity:* The rhythm is regular.
- *Interval measurements:* No P waves are present, and the QRS complex is greater than 0.12 seconds.
- *Shape and sequence:* QRS waves are wide and bizarre in shape. The QRS complex is followed by a T wave of opposite polarity.
- *Patient response:* The extreme bradycardia may cause the same symptoms as any severe bradycardia. This mechanism is the last backup pacemaker and asystole may occur.
- *Causes:* Failure of the SA and AV nodal pacemakers causes idioventricular rhythm.
- *Care and treatment:* Initiate BLS and ACLS protocols. Consider emergent transcutaneous pacing.

Asystole

Asystole is characterized by complete cessation of electrical activity. A flat baseline is seen, without any evidence of P, QRS, or T waveforms. A pulse is absent and there is no cardiac output; cardiac arrest has occurred (Figure 7-48, *A*).

Asystole often occurs following VF or ventricular escape rhythm. Following a ventricular escape rhythm this rhythm is referred to as *ventricular standstill* (Figure 7-48, *B*). Pulse should be immediately assessed because a lead or electrode coming off may mimic this dysrhythmia. During cardiac arrest situations, if asystole occurs when another rhythm has been monitored, a check of two leads should occur to confirm asystole.

Rhythm analysis

- *Rate:* Heart rate is absent.
- *Regularity:* Heart rhythm is absent.

Lead II

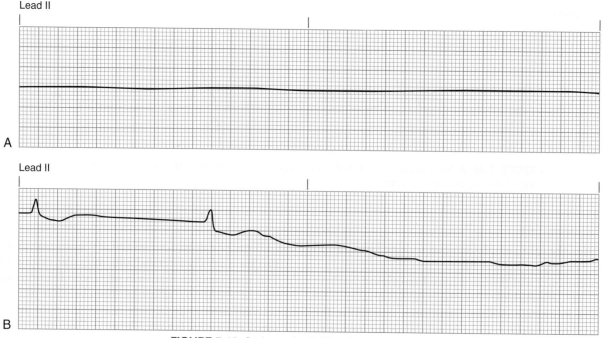

A

Lead II

B

FIGURE 7-48 A, Asystole. **B,** Ventricular standstill.

- *Interval measurements:* PQRST waveforms are absent.
- *Shape and sequence:* Waveform is a flat or undulating line on the monitor.
- *Patient response:* The patient is in cardiac arrest.
- *Causes:* Asystole is usually preceded by another dysrhythmia such as VF or ventricular escape rhythm.
- *Care and treatment:* BLS and ACLS protocols are initiated for asystole.

Atrioventricular Blocks

AV block, which is also known as heart block, refers to an inability of the AV node to conduct sinus impulses to the ventricles in a normal manner. AV blocks can cause a delay in conduction from the SA node through the AV node, or completely block conduction intermittently or continuously. AV blocks may arise from normal aging of the conduction system or be caused by damage to the conduction system from ischemic heart disease.

Four types of AV block exist, each categorized in terms of degree. The four types of block are first-degree, second-degree type I, second-degree type II, and third-degree. The greater the degree of block, the more severe are the consequences. First-degree block has minimal consequences, whereas third-degree block may be life-threatening.

First-Degree AV Block

First-degree AV block describes consistent delayed conduction through the AV node or the atrial conductive tissue. It is represented on the ECG as a prolonged PR interval. It is a common dysrhythmia in the elderly and in patients with cardiac disease. As the normal conduction pathway ages or becomes diseased, impulse conduction becomes slower than normal (Figure 7-49).

Rhythm analysis

- *Rate:* Heart rate is determined by the underlying rhythm.
- *Regularity:* The underlying rhythm determines regularity.
- *Interval measurements:* PR interval is prolonged and is greater than 0.20 seconds. QRS complex and QT/QT$_c$ measurements are normal.
- *Shape and sequence:* P and QRS waves are consistent in shape. P waves are small and rounded. A P wave precedes every QRS complex, which is followed by a T wave.
- *Patient response:* AV block is well tolerated.

- *Causes:* Aging and ischemic and valvular heart disease can cause AV block.
- *Care and treatment:* No treatment is required.

Second-Degree Heart Block

Second-degree heart block refers to AV conduction that is intermittently blocked. Two types of second-degree block may occur, and each has specific diagnostic criteria for accurate diagnosis.

Second-degree AV block type I. Also called Mobitz I or Wenckebach phenomenon, second-degree AV block type I is represented on the ECG as a progressive lengthening of the PR interval until there is a P wave without a QRS complex. The AV node progressively delays conduction to the ventricles resulting in a longer PR intervals until finally a QRS complex is dropped. The PR interval following the dropped QRS complex is shorter than the PR interval preceding the dropped beat. By not conducting this one beat, the AV node recovers and is able to conduct the next atrial impulse (Figure 7-50). If dropped beats occur frequently, it is useful to describe the conduction ratio, such as 2:1, 3:1, or 4:1.

Rhythm analysis

- *Rate:* The rate is slower than the underlying rhythm because of the dropped beat.
- *Regularity:* P-P intervals stay the same but the R-R intervals shorten until the dropped beat.
- *Interval measurements:* The PR interval becomes progressively longer until a QRS complex is dropped. The PR interval before the dropped QRS is longer than the PR interval of the next conducted PQRST waveforms.
- *Shape and sequence:* P and QRS waves are consistent in shape. P waves are small and rounded. A P wave precedes every QRS complex, which is followed by a T wave.
- *Patient response:* This rhythm is usually well tolerated unless there is an underlying bradycardia, or frequent dropped beats.
- *Causes:* Aging, AV nodal blocking drugs, acute inferior wall myocardial infarction or right ventricular infarction, ischemic heart disease, digitalis toxicity, and excess vagal response are all possible causes of second-degree AV block type I.
- *Care and treatment:* This type of block is usually well tolerated and no treatment is indicated unless the dropped beats occur frequently. If the patient is symptomatic,

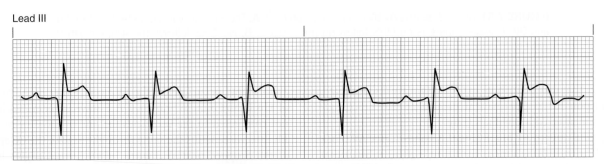

Lead III

FIGURE 7-49 First-degree AV block.

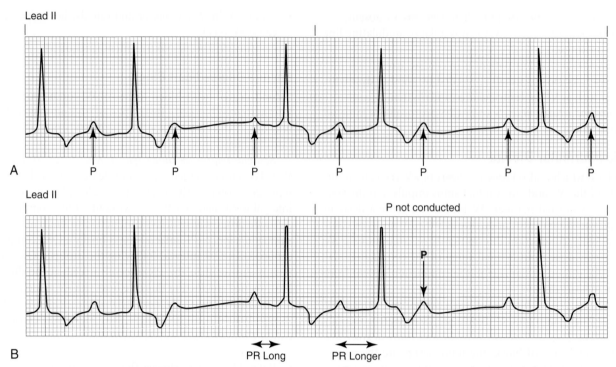

FIGURE 7-50 Second-degree AV block type I (Mobitz I, Wenckebach).

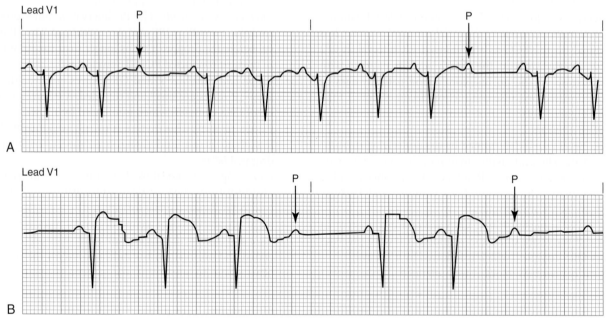

FIGURE 7-51 Second-degree AV block type II (Mobitz II). **A,** The PR interval is constant; at the 3rd and 9th P waves, there is no QRS following the P wave. **B,** No QRS follows the 4th and 7th P waves.

drugs that may contribute to the rhythm are discontinued, and potentially a permanent pacemaker may be considered in selected individuals (rare).

Second-degree AV block type II. Second-degree AV block type II (Mobitz II) is a more critical type of heart block that requires early recognition and intervention. The conduction abnormality occurs below the AV node, either in the bundle of His or the bundle branches. A P wave is generated but is not conducted to the ventricles for one or more beats. The PR interval remains the same throughout with the exception of the dropped beat(s) (Figure 7-51). Second-degree block type II is often associated with a bundle branch block and a corresponding widened QRS complex; however, narrow QRS complexes may be observed. Second-degree block type II can progress to the more clinically significant third-degree block and may cause the patient to be symptomatic.

Rhythm analysis

- *Rate:* Heart rate is slower than the underlying rhythm because of the dropped beats.
- *Regularity:* P waves are regular, but QRS complexes are occasionally absent.
- *Interval measurements:* Intervals are constant for the underlying rhythm. PR intervals of the conducted beats do not change. QRS complexes may be widened because of a bundle branch block.
- *Shape and sequence:* P and QRS waves are consistent in shape. P waves are small and rounded. QRS complexes are missing.
- *Patient response:* The patient may tolerate one missed beat, but symptoms may occur if frequent beats are missed.
- *Causes:* Heart disease, increased vagal tone, conduction system disease, ablation of the AV node, and inferior and right ventricular myocardial infarctions are possible causes of second-degree AV block type II.
- *Care and treatment:* Patient may require a pacemaker, administration of atropine, and transcutaneous or transvenous pacing for emergent treatment.[3]

Third-Degree Block

Third-degree block is often called *complete heart block* because no atrial impulses are conducted through the AV node to the ventricles. The block in conduction can occur at the level of the AV node, the bundle of His, or the bundle branches.

In complete heart block, the atria and ventricles beat independently of each other because the AV node is completely blocked to the sinus impulse and it is not conducted to the ventricles. An escape rhythm arises from the junctional tissue or the ventricles. The atria beat at one rate, and the ventricles beat at a different rate. The atrial rate is dictated by the sinus node. The ventricular rate is slow, and usually only a ventricular or junctional escape rhythm is present. No communication exists between the atria and ventricles. Third-degree block is a type of AV dissociation (Figure 7-52).

One hallmark of third-degree heart block is that the P waves have no association with the QRS complexes and appear throughout the QRS waveform. Both the P-P and R-R intervals are regular, but the rates for each are different because they have no relationship to each other. Whenever a rhythm strip appears to have no consistent, predictable relationship between P waves and QRS complexes, third-degree block is considered.

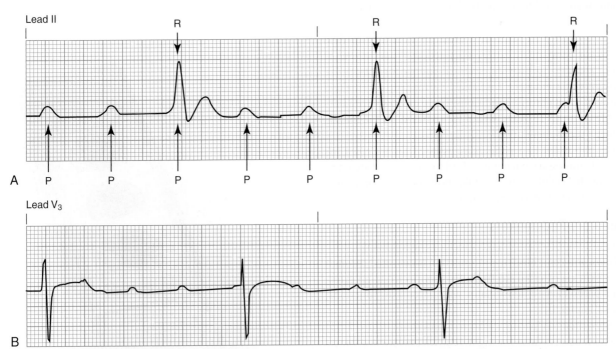

FIGURE 7-52 Third-degree AV block (complete heart block). **A,** P waves regular and present throughout at an atrial rate of 94 beats per minute and ventricular rhythm of 30 beats per minute. The P waves are not associated with the QRS complexes. **B,** Similar tracing; atrial rate 100 and ventricular rate of 30.

Rhythm analysis
- *Rate:* The atrial rate is greater than the ventricular rate.
- *Regularity:* P-P intervals are regular and R-R intervals are regular, but they not associated with each other.
- *Interval measurements:* There is no PR interval in the absence of conduction. The QRS complex is often widened greater than 0.12 seconds with a ventricular escape rhythm.
- *Shape and sequence:* P and QRS waves are consistent in shape. P waves are small and rounded. The QRS complex is followed by a T wave. There is no relationship between the P waves and QRS complexes.
- *Patient response:* Patients may become symptomatic because of the bradycardia of the escape rhythm.
- *Causes:* Ischemic heart disease, acute myocardial infarction, and conduction system disease are possible causes of third-degree heart block.
- *Care and treatment:* Treatments include transcutaneous or transvenous pacing and implanting a permanent pacemaker.

CARDIAC PACEMAKERS

A cardiac pacemaker delivers electrical current to the myocardium to stimulate depolarization when the heart rate is too slow or the heart is unable to initiate and/or conduct a native beat. A pacemaker is often implanted to treat symptomatic bradycardia, which may occur from a number of different pathophysiological conditions. These include second-degree AV block type II, third-degree AV block, and sick sinus syndrome. The need for a pacemaker may be temporary (e.g., after an acute myocardial infarction or cardiac surgery) or permanent. Battery-operated, external pulse generators are used to provide electrical energy for temporary transvenous pacemakers. Implanted permanent pacemakers are used to treat chronic conditions. These devices have a battery life of up to 10 years, which varies based on the manufacturer's recommendations.

It is important that patients be assessed for the need for pacing. Unnecessary pacing may lead to worsened outcomes, including heart failure, rehospitalization, increased mortality, and new onset of atrial fibrillation.[7]

Temporary Pacemakers

Types of temporary pacemakers include the following:
- *Transcutaneous:* Electrical stimulation is delivered through the skin via external electrode pads connected to an external pacemaker (a defibrillator with pacemaker functions; see Chapter 10).
- *Transvenous:* A pacing catheter is inserted (Figure 7-53) percutaneously into the right ventricle, where it contacts the endocardium near the ventricular septum. It is connected to a small external pulse generator (Figure 7-54) by electrode wires. Note the electrical ports on the pacing catheter which are covered by black caps (see Figure 7-53). These are connected to the pulse generator (see Figure 7-54) whereupon pacing thresholds are set for each specific patient.

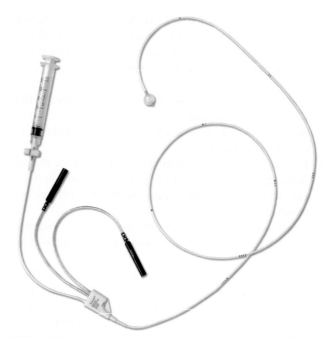

FIGURE 7-53 Balloon-tipped bipolar lead wire for transvenous pacing. (From Wiegand DLM: *AACN Procedure Manual for Critical Care.* 6th ed. St. Louis: Elsevier, 2011.)

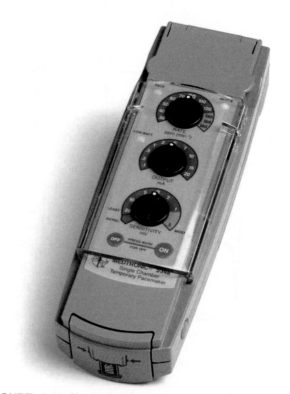

FIGURE 7-54 Single-chamber temporary pulse generator. (Courtesy Medtronic USA, Inc. Minneapolis, Minnesota).

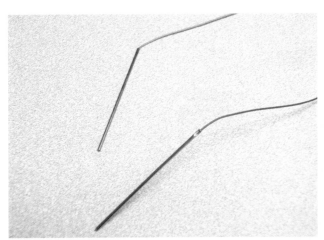

FIGURE 7-55 Epicardial wires. (From Wiegand DLM: *AACN Procedure Manual for Critical Care*. 6th ed. St. Louis: Elsevier, 2011.)

- *Epicardial:* Pacing wires are inserted into the epicardial wall of the heart during cardiac surgery (Figure 7-55); wires are brought through the chest wall and can be connected to a pulse generator if needed (Figure 7-56). Note that there are only two pacing wires shown in Figure 7-55; however, in cardiac bypass surgery patients, there are often four wires placed through the chest wall of the patient, two wires from the atrium and two wires from the ventricles. These four

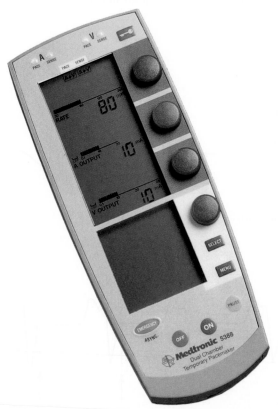

FIGURE 7-56 Dual-chamber temporary pulse generator. (Courtesy Medtronic USA, Inc. Minneapolis, Minnesota).

wires are connected to the temporary pacemaker (see Figure 7-56), and pacing thresholds are set for each patient.

Permanent Pacemakers

Permanent pacemakers have electrode wires that are typically placed transvenously through the cephalic or subclavian vein into the heart chambers (Figure 7-57). The leads are attached to the pulse generator, placed in a surgically created pocket just below the left clavicle.

Pacemakers may be used to stimulate the atrium, ventricle, or both chambers (dual-chamber pacemakers). Atrial pacing is used to mimic normal conduction and to produce atrial contraction, thus providing atrial kick. Ventricular pacing stimulates ventricular depolarization and is commonly used in emergency situations or when pacing is required infrequently. Dual-chamber pacing allows for stimulation of both atria and ventricles as needed to synchronize the chambers and mimic the normal cardiac cycle.

Permanent pacemakers may be programmed in a variety of ways, and a standardized code is used to determine the pacing mode that is programmed. The North American Society of Pacing and Electrophysiology (NASPE) and the British Pacing and Electrophysiology Group have revised the standardized generic code for pacemakers; it is described in Chapter 12. It is important to know the programming information for the pacemaker to assess proper functioning on the rhythm strip.

Terms for Pacemaker Function

Other terms used in describing pacemaker function are *mode, rate, electrical output, sensitivity, sense-pace indicator,* and *AV interval.*

Mode. Pacemakers can be operated in a *demand* mode or *fixed rate (asynchronous)* mode. The demand mode paces the heart when no intrinsic or native beat is sensed. For example, if the rate control is set at 60 beats per minute, the pacemaker will only pace if the patient's heart rate drops to less than 60. The fixed rate mode paces the heart at a set rate, independent of any activity the patient's heart generates. The fixed rate mode may compete with the patient's own rhythm and deliver an impulse on the T wave (R on T), with the potential for producing ventricular tachycardia or fibrillation. The demand mode is safer and is the mode of choice.

Rate. The rate control determines the number of impulses delivered per minute to the atrium, the ventricle, or both. The rate is set to produce effective cardiac output and to reduce symptoms.

Electrical output. The electrical output is the amount of electrical energy needed to stimulate depolarization. The output is measured in *milliamperes (mA)*, of which it varies depending on the type of pacing. Transcutaneous pacing requires higher milliamperes than transvenous or epicardial pacing, because the electrical energy must be delivered through the chest wall.

Sensitivity. The sensitivity is the ability of the pacemaker to recognize the body's intrinsic or native electrical activity. It is measured in *millivolts (mV)*. Some temporary pacemakers

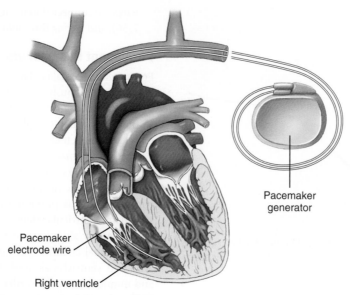

FIGURE 7-57 Permanent dual chamber (A-V) pacemaker. (From Wesley K. *Huszar's Basic Dysrhythmias and Acute Coronary Syndromes: Interpretation and Management.* 4th ed. St. Louis: Mosby JEMS; 2010.)

have a *sense-pace indicator.* If the generator detects the patient's own beat, the "sense" indicator lights. When the generator delivers a paced beat, the "pace" light comes on. Temporary pacemakers have dials or key pads for adjusting sensitivity.

AV interval indicator. The AV interval indicator is used to determine the interval between atrial and ventricular stimulation. It is used only in dual-chamber pacemakers.

Pacemaker Rhythms

Pacemaker rhythms are usually easy to identify on the cardiac monitor or rhythm strip. The electrical stimulation is noted by an electrical artifact called the *pacer spike.* If the atrium is paced, the spike appears before the P wave (Figure 7-58). If the ventricle is paced, the spike appears before the QRS complex (Figure 7-59). If both the atrium and ventricle are paced,

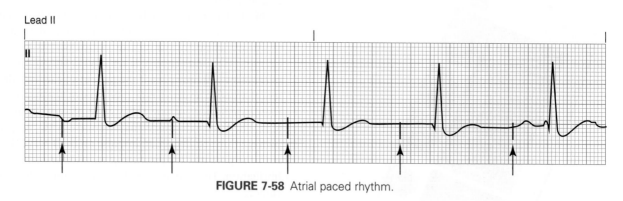

FIGURE 7-58 Atrial paced rhythm.

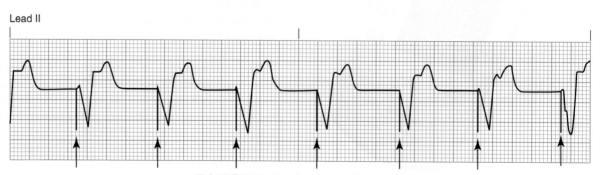

FIGURE 7-59 Ventricular paced rhythm.

Lead II

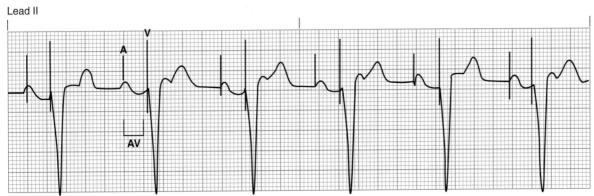

FIGURE 7-60 Dual-chamber (AV) paced rhythm. *A,* Atrial pacer spike; *AV,* AV pager spike interval; *V,* Ventricular paced spike.

spikes are noted before both the P wave and the QRS complex (Figure 7-60). The heart rate is carefully assessed on the rhythm strip. The heart rate should not be lower than the rate set on the pacemaker.

The pacemaker spike is usually followed by a larger-than-normal P wave in atrial pacing or a widened QRS complex in ventricular pacing. Sometimes the P wave is not seen even though an atrial pacer spike is present. Because the heart is paced in an artificial or abnormal fashion, the path of depolarization is altered, resulting in waveforms and intervals that are also altered.

Pacemaker Malfunction

Three primary problems can occur with a pacemaker. These problems include *failure to pace* (also called failure to fire), *failure to capture,* and *failure to sense.* If troubleshooting does

not resolve pacemaker malfunction, emergency transcutaneous pacing may be needed to ensure an adequate cardiac output.

Failure to pace. Failure to pace or fire occurs when the pacemaker fails to initiate an electrical stimulus when it should fire. The problem is noted by absence of pacer spikes on the rhythm strip. Causes of failure to pace include battery or pulse generator failure, fracture or displacement of a pacemaker wire, or loose connections (Figure 7-61).

Failure to capture. When the pacemaker generates an electrical impulse (pacer spike) and no depolarization is noted, it is described as *failure to capture.* On the ECG, a pacer spike is noted, but it is not followed by a P wave (atrial pacemaker) or a QRS complex (ventricular pacemaker) (Figure 7-62). Common causes of failure to capture include output (milliamperes) set too low, or displacement of the

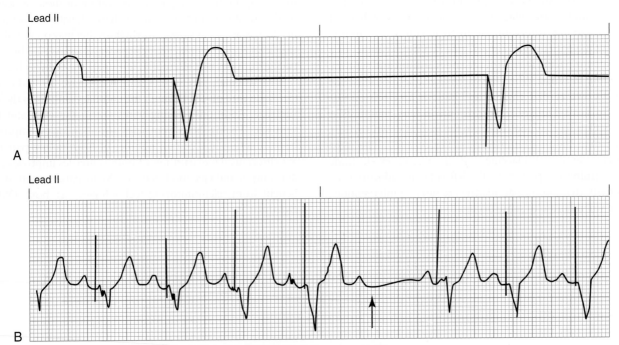

FIGURE 7-61 Failure to pace/fire.

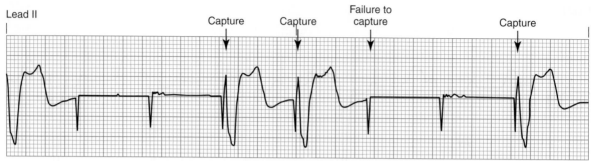

FIGURE 7-62 Failure to capture: ventricular pacemaker.

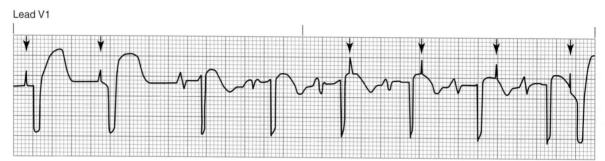

FIGURE 7-63 Failure to sense.

pacing lead wire from the myocardium (transvenous or epicardial leads). Other causes of failure to capture include battery failure, fracture of the pacemaker wire, or increased pacing threshold as a result of medication or electrolyte imbalance. Adjusting the output if the patient has a temporary pacemaker, and placing the patient on his or her left side are nursing interventions to treat failure to capture. Turning the patient onto the left side facilitates contact of a transvenous pacing wire with the endocardium and septum.

Failure to sense. When the pacemaker does not sense the patient's own cardiac rhythm and initiates an electrical impulse, it is called *failure to sense.* Failure to sense manifests as pacer spikes that fall too closely to the patient's own rhythm, earlier than the programmed rate (Figure 7-63). The most common cause is displacement of the pacemaker electrode wire. Turning the patient to the left side and adjusting the sensitivity (temporary pacemaker) are nursing interventions to use when failure to sense occurs.

OTHER DEVICES WITH PACEMAKER CAPABILITIES

All implantable cardioverter-defibrillators (ICDs) have pacemaker capabilities. The pacemaker feature of these devices is used to treat fast heart rhythms, such as VT, with antitachycardia pacing, as well as slow heart rhythms that may occur following defibrillation. Antitachycardia pacing is a short, fast burst of pacing impulses that attempt to terminate the tachycardia.[10]

Biventricular pacemakers and ICDs have an additional electrode wire placed through the coronary sinus into the left ventricle. Additional pacing wires are in the atria and the ventricle. Pacing both ventricles simultaneously improves heart function in a certain number of heart failure patients. Synchronous depolarization of both ventricles improves cardiac output and ejection fraction.[10] Many patients with ICDs benefit from telemonitoring technologies (see box, "QSEN Exemplar").

QSEN EXEMPLAR

Informatics

Integrating Clinical Informatics with Emerging Critical Care Technologies

Use of internal cardioverter-defibrillators (ICDs) is becoming more commonplace in the primary and secondary prevention of sudden cardiac death. Patients who receive these devices require evaluation during the immediate postimplantation period and frequent ongoing assessment for the duration of the implantation. Remote patient-oriented telemonitoring using a team approach may augment the clinical management and safety of patients with ICDs. Remote monitoring has the potential to diagnose dysrhythmias and device-related performance issues in real time. Shirato presented an overview of remote ICD telemonitoring methods, advantages and disadvantages of this form of telehealth, and legal and ethical concerns related to this emerging technology.

Reference

Shirato, S. (2009). The use of remote monitoring for internal cardioverter defibrillators (ICDs): The infusion of information technology and medicine. *Online Journal of Nursing Informatics, 13*(3), 1-16.

CASE STUDY

Mr. P. is a 56-year-old man who was successfully extubated (endotracheal tube removed) 4 hours after coronary artery bypass graft surgery. However, 2 hours later, the patient complains of his heart racing, and it is determined that he has palpitations. The heart rate on the bedside monitor is 168 beats per minute, blood pressure is 100/60 mm Hg, and respiratory rate is 26 breaths per minute. The ECG shows an irregularly irregular rhythm, a change from the sinus rhythm noted at the last assessment.

Questions

1. Based on this description, what is your interpretation of the rhythm?
2. What complications could occur as a result of this rhythm?
3. What clinical data would lead you to believe this complication could occur?
4. What data are you going to give to the provider?
5. What orders do you expect to get?
6. What nursing actions do you need to take and why?
7. What are some of the etiologies of this dysrhythmia?

▌ S U M M A R Y

Interpretation of cardiac rhythms is an essential skill that is developed through practice and clinical experience. For the beginning student, the critical criteria for diagnosis provide the structure by which rhythms are analyzed. The initial effort is focused on learning these criteria. It is hoped that this chapter is a valuable reference in the delivery of high-quality care to patients with cardiac dysrhythmias and to their families. Care for a patient with dysrhythmias is summarized in the nursing care plan.

◎ NURSING CARE PLAN

Patient with Dysrhythmias

NURSING DIAGNOSIS

Risk for Decreased Cardiac Tissue Perfusion related to altered perfusion.

PATIENT OUTCOMES

Adequate tissue perfusion

- Strong peripheral pulses
- Blood pressure within normal limits for patient
- Skin warm and dry
- Lungs clear bilaterally
- Urine output greater than 30 mL/hr
- Regular cardiac rhythm

NURSING INTERVENTIONS	RATIONALES
• Assess patient for tachycardia, bradycardia and/or irregularity of cardiac rhythm; monitor vital signs for change from baseline	• Early recognition and treatment will prevent further deterioration of patient condition and end organ damage
• Assess for signs of reduced cardiac output: rapid, slow, or weak pulse; hypotension; dizziness; syncope; shortness of breath; chest discomfort; fatigue; change in level of consciousness or restlessness	• Detect subtle signs of decreased cardiac output because many dysrhythmias affect cardiac output
• Determine if dysrhythmia is acute or chronic	• Assess and guide treatment
• Review history and assess for causative factors	• Identify factors causing dysrhythmias that can be eliminated or corrected, such as cardiac ischemia, hypoxemia, and electrolyte imbalance
• Determine specific type of dysrhythmia	• Guide assessment and treatment according to current guidelines
• Determine appropriate lead selection(s) based on current monitoring standards and individualized to patient's diagnosis	• Differentiate atrial from ventricular and lethal from nonlethal dysrhythmias; detect changes in ST segment that may indicate ischemia, injury, or infarct
• Obtain baseline QT/QTc measurements and regularly monitor with other intervals	• Many current medications can cause QT prolongation, placing the patient at risk for torsades de pointes
• Provide psychological support to the patient and family; provide education as to the purpose of ECG monitoring	• Decrease stressors of the hospitalized patient
• Provide oxygen therapy	• Relieve dysrhythmias associated with hypoxemia and myocardial ischemia
• If the patient has a new-onset acute dysrhythmia, assess the patient immediately, then obtain a 12-lead ECG to document the rhythm; use rhythm recording of all 12 leads if available on bedside monitor	• Capture elusive dysrhythmias that are intermittent, or disclose P waves in SVTs, which will guide diagnosis and treatment
• Assess urine output hourly	• Assess adequacy of perfusion to kidneys

ECG, Electrocardiogram.

Based on data from Gulanick M and Myers JL. *Nursing Care Plans: Diagnoses, Interventions, and Outcomes,* 7th ed. St. Louis; Mosby; 2011.

▌CRITICAL THINKING EXERCISES

1. You are working in the critical care unit and your patient's heart rate suddenly decreases from 88 to 50 beats per minute. What may be some of the reasons for the decreased heart rate? What assessments will you make?
2. Discuss why patients with pulmonary disease are prone to atrial dysrhythmias.
3. A 65-year-old woman with type 2 diabetes presents to the emergency department; she is short of breath and complaining of neck and shoulder pain. Her blood pressure is 185/95 mm Hg, and her heart rate is 155 beats per minute. How will you initially manage this patient? What medical intervention would you anticipate? List serious signs and symptoms of hemodynamic instability in a patient with a tachydysrhythmia.
4. Why does tachycardia sometimes lead to heart failure?

REFERENCES

1. American Association of Critical-Care Nurses. Nursing practice alert: dysrhythmia monitoring. Available at http://www.aacn.org/WD/Practice/Docs/PracticeAlerts/Dysrhythmia_Monitoring_04-2008.pdf; 2008. Accessed May 27, 2011.
2. American Association of Critical-Care Nurses. Nursing practice alert: ST segment monitoring. Available at http://www.aacn.org/WD/Practice/Docs/PracticeAlerts/ST_Segment_Monitoring_05-2009.pdf; 2008. Accessed May 27, 2011.
3. American Heart Association (AHA). *2010 Handbook of Emergency Cardiovascular Care for Healthcare Providers*. Dallas, TX; 2011.
4. Drew BJ, Funk M. Practice standards for ECG monitoring in hospital settings: executive summary and guide for implementation. *Critical Care Nursing Clinics of North America*. 2006;18(2):157-168.
5. Drew BJ, Califf RM, Funk M, et al. Practice standards for electrocardiographic monitoring in hospital settings. *Circulation*. 2004;110:2721-2746.
6. Drew BJ, Ackerman MJ, Funk M, et al. Prevention of torsades de pointes in hospital settings: a scientific statement from the American Heart Association and the American College of Cardiology foundation. *Journal of the American College of Cardiology*. 2010;55(9):934-947.
7. Epstein AE, DiMarco JP, Ellenbogen KA, et al. ACC/AHA/HRS 2008. Guidelines for Device-Based Therapy of Cardiac Rhythm Abnormalities: a report of the American College of Cardiology/American Heart Association Task Force on Practice Guidelines. *Circulation*. 2008;117(21):e350.
8. Fuster V, Ryden LE, Cannom DS, et al. 2011 ACCF/AHA/HRS Focused Updates Incorporated Into the ACC/AHA/ESC 2006 Guidelines for the Management of Patients With Atrial Fibrillation: a Report of the American College of Cardiology Foundation/American Heart Association Task Force on Practice Guidelines. *Circulation*. 2011;123(10):e269-e367.
9. Hannibal G. It started with Einthoven: the history of the ECG and cardiac monitoring. *AACN Advanced Critical Care*. 2011;22:93-96.
10. Hayes DL, Friedman PA, eds. *Cardiac Pacing, Defibrillation and Resynchronization: a Clinical Approach*. Oxford, UK: Wiley-Blackwell; 2008.
11. Sandau KE, Smith M. Continuous ST-segment monitoring: protocol for practice. *Critical Care Nurse*. 2009;29(4):39-49.
12. Webner C. Applying evidence at the bedside. *Dimensions of Critical Care Nursing*. 2011;30(1):8-18.
13. Wesley K. *Huszar's Basic Dysrhythmias and Acute Coronary Syndromes: Interpretation and Management*. 4th ed. St. Louis: Mosby JEMS; 2010.

8

Hemodynamic Monitoring

Maximino Martell, MSN, RN, CCRN, CCNS, CNS-BC
David A. Allen, MSN, RN, CCRN, CCNS, CNS-BC

⊖volve WEBSITE

Many additional resources, including self-assessment exercises, are located on the Evolve companion website at
http://evolve.elsevier.com/Sole.

- Review Questions
- Mosby's Nursing Skills Procedures

- Animations
- Video Clips

INTRODUCTION

The use of invasive devices coupled with advances in technology has had a profound effect on critical care nursing practice. Therefore hemodynamic monitoring is an essential competency that all critical nurses must possess. The goal of hemodynamic monitoring is to maintain adequate tissue perfusion. This can be accomplished by monitoring the dynamic physiological relationship between several variables, including heart rate, blood flow, and oxygen delivery. Although gathering the physiological data is straightforward, ensuring that the data are accurate and analyzing and interpreting the data are more complex skills. The interpretation requires that clinicians have a broad theoretical understanding of hemodynamic monitoring and the ability to apply that knowledge to clinical situations. This chapter reviews the basics of cardiovascular anatomy and physiology, the fundamentals of hemodynamic monitoring, and various modalities available to the clinician to assess hemodynamic status.

REVIEW OF ANATOMY AND PHYSIOLOGY

Cardiovascular System Structure

The cardiovascular system is a closed network of arteries, capillaries, and veins through which blood, oxygen, hormones, and nutrients are delivered to the tissues by the pumping action of the heart (Figure 8-1). Metabolic wastes are removed from the circulating blood via the liver and kidneys. The major components of the cardiovascular system are described.[22]

Heart

The heart is a four-chambered organ that weighs approximately 1 pound and lies obliquely in the thoracic cavity. The heart is responsible for pumping oxygenated blood forward through the arterial vasculature and receiving deoxygenated blood via the venous vasculature. Blood flow through the heart itself is regulated by four one-way valves. Two atrioventricular (AV) valves (tricuspid and mitral) open during ventricular diastole, allowing blood to flow from the atria into the ventricles. As the ventricles begin to contract in systole, the AV valves close and the semilunar valves (pulmonic and aortic) open, allowing blood to flow into the pulmonary and systemic vasculature. At the end of ventricular systole, the semilunar valves close and the cycle begins again (Figure 8-2).

Arteries

Arteries are the tough, elastic vessels that carry blood away from the heart. Arteries consist of three layers: the adventitia, the media, and the intima. The adventitia is composed chiefly of longitudinally arranged collagen fibers, which make up the tough outer lining. The media consists of concentrically arranged smooth muscle. The intima consists of endothelial connective tissue that is continuous with that of the heart. The elasticity of the vessels allows them to expand to accommodate volumetric changes that result with the contraction and relaxation of the heart. When the artery diameter is less than 0.5 mm, it is termed an arteriole. The arterial system is a high-pressure, low-volume, high-resistance circuit responsible for delivering oxygen and nutrient rich blood to the

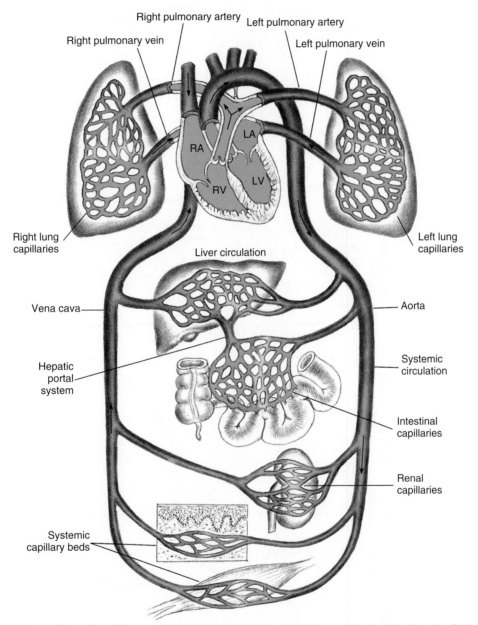

FIGURE 8-1 Diagram of the cardiovascular system. (From McCance KL, Huether S, eds. *Pathophysiology: the Biologic Basis for Disease in Adults and Children*, 6th ed. St. Louis: Mosby; 2010.)

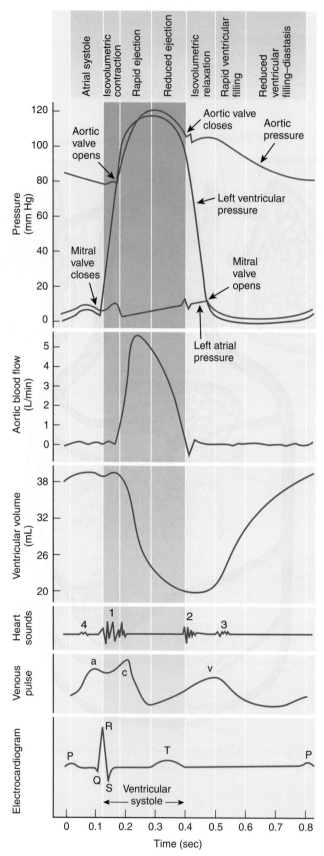

FIGURE 8-2 Cardiac cycle. (From McCance KL, Huether S, eds. *Pathophysiology: the Biologic Basis for Disease in Adults and Children*, 6th ed. St. Louis: Mosby; 2010.)

capillary system. Furthermore, arteries have the ability to dilate or constrict in response to metabolic demand.

Capillaries

The capillaries, which are exchange vessels, are composed of a network of low-pressure, thin-walled microscopic vessels allowing for easy passage of hormones, nutrients, and oxygen to the target tissues. They also receive metabolic wastes from the tissues and begin the process of returning deoxygenated blood to the venous portion of the cardiovascular system.

Veins

Compared with the arterial system, veins are thin-walled, less elastic, fibrous, larger in diameter, and are known as high capacity, low resistance vessels. Veins of the extremities contain valves to assist with maintaining a one-way flow of deoxygenated blood returning to the heart. Eventually the veins connect and become the coronary sinus, which empties into the right atrium. The venous system has the ability to respond to metabolic needs by vasodilatation or vasoconstriction, thereby increasing or decreasing venous return. Venous return is the flow of blood back to the heart. Approximately 70% of the circulating blood volume is located in the venous system at any given time. Several factors influence venous return, including muscle contraction, breathing, venous compliance, and gravity.

Blood

Blood accounts for approximately 7% of our body weight, which is about 5 liters of blood. The fluid component, or plasma, makes up approximately 60% of the blood volume. The remaining 40% consists of the cellular components—erythrocytes (red blood cells), leukocytes (white blood cells), and platelets. The more viscous the blood, the greater the turbulence in blood flow, resulting in a reduction in flow in the microcirculation. The red blood cell component of blood is essential for oxygen delivery to the tissues. A reduction in oxygen delivery or an increase in oxygen consumption directly impacts the hemodynamic responses of the body.

Principles of Physics

According to Poiseuille's law, the rate of fluid flow through a vessel is determined by the pressure difference between the two ends of the vessel and the resistance within the lumen. Mathematically, this is represented as:

$$\text{Flow}(Q) = \frac{\text{Pressure difference }(\Delta P)}{\text{Resistance (R)}}$$

For any fluid to flow within a circuit, a difference in pressures within the circuit must exist. In the cardiovascular system, the driving pressure is generated by the contractile force of the heart. There is a continuous drop in pressure from the left ventricle to the tissues, and further reduction in pressure from the tissue bed to the right atrium. Without these pressure gradients, no flow occurs.

Resistance is a measure of the ease with which the fluid flows through the lumen of a vessel. It is essentially a measure of friction, which is dependent upon *viscosity* of the fluid and the radius and length of the vessel. A vessel with a small diameter has a greater resistance than one with a larger diameter (Figure 8-3). Longer vessels have greater resistance to the flow of fluid within the vessel. Increased viscosity of a fluid results in increased friction within the fluid; rate of flow is inversely proportional to the fluid viscosity.

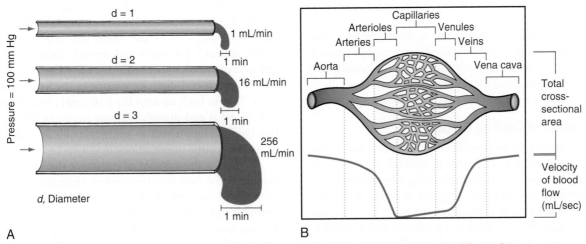

FIGURE 8-3 Relationship between vessel diameter, flow, and resistance. **A,** Effect of lumen diameter on flow through vessel. **B,** Blood flows with great speed in the large arteries. However, branching of arterial vessels increases the total cross-sectional areas of the arterioles and capillaries, thus reducing the flow rate. (**A** from McCance KL, Huether S, eds. *Pathophysiology: the Biologic Basis for Disease in Adults and Children*, 6th ed. St. Louis: Mosby; **B** from Thibodeau G, Patton K. *Anatomy and Physiology*, 8th ed. St. Louis: Mosby; 2013.)

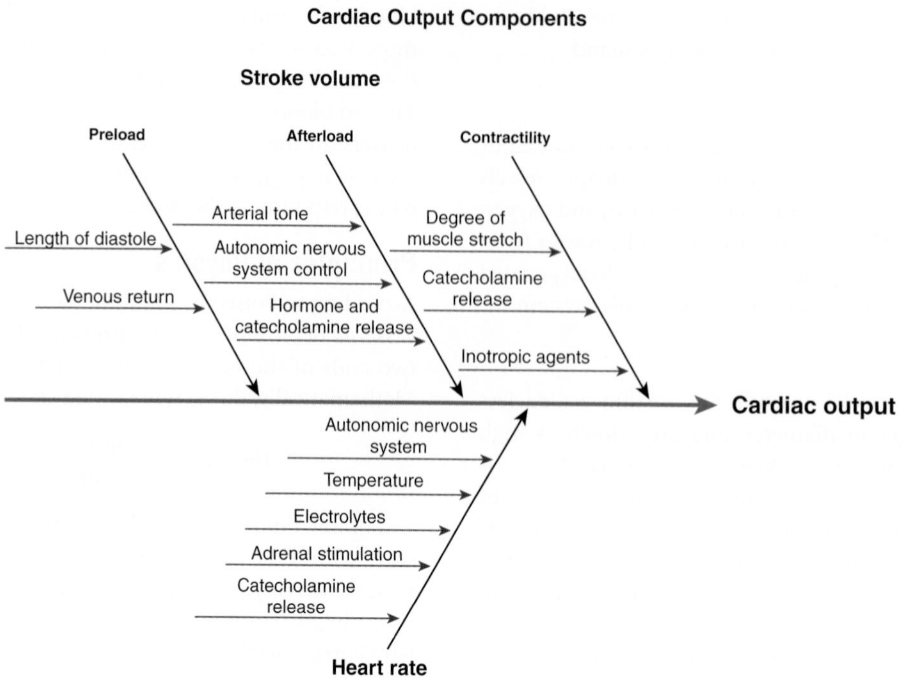

Cardiac Output Components

Stroke volume

FIGURE 8-4 Cardiac output components. Cardiac output is determined by heart rate and stroke volume.

Highly compliant systems have low resistance; therefore, if resistance increases, compliance decreases. For example, an atherosclerotic vessel, which causes narrowing of the intima, has a reduced capacitance and compliance, leading to increased resistance and hypertension.

The body's response to metabolic demands alters the flow of blood to and from the target tissues. In response to increased metabolic demands, the circulatory system increases the volume of blood flow to the target tissues by increasing the diameter of the vessel, thereby reducing the resistance within the vessel.

Another determinant of flow rate is the degree of turbulence within a vessel. The rate of fluid movement in laminar flow is greater than the rate in turbulent flow. A vessel lining that has excess plaque accumulation or calcification results in more turbulence, reduced flow, and reduced tissue perfusion.

Components of Cardiac Output

Cardiac output (CO) is determined by heart rate and stroke volume. Stroke volume is affected by preload, afterload, and contractility (Figure 8-4). Comprehending hemodynamics requires having a working knowledge of normal intracardiac pressures, because each chamber of the heart has a unique pressure (Figure 8-5). In addition, a familiarity with the cardiac cycle (see Figure 8-2) assists in understanding hemodynamic concepts. Relevant concepts are defined next.

Systole is the contraction or pumping portion of the cardiac cycle. Left ventricular systole usually occurs slightly before right ventricular systole.

Diastole is the relaxation or filling part of the cardiac cycle. The majority of ventricular diastole is a passive event that occurs as the AV valves open. However, as the atria contract,

they force the remaining atrial blood into the ventricles—this is commonly referred to as the "atrial kick" and contributes up to 30% of the CO.

Preload is the degree of ventricular stretch before the next contraction. The degree of stretch is directly impacted by the amount of blood volume present in the ventricles at end-diastole. In hemodynamic monitoring, preload is quantified by measuring ventricular end-diastolic pressures. Based on the Frank-Starling mechanism, when ventricular fibers are at maximal stretch, maximal CO results. Another way of explaining the mechanism is that within physiological limits, the heart pumps all of the blood that is returned by the venous system.[16] Too much end-diastolic volume in the right ventricle can result in congestion of the systemic vasculature, and too much end-diastolic volume in the left ventricle can cause fluid to back up into the pulmonary vasculature. Too little blood at end-diastolic volume results in a reduction in CO. Optimizing preload or ventricular filling is the goal of many therapeutic interventions in critical care.

Afterload is the amount of resistance the ventricles must overcome to deliver the stroke volume into the receiving vasculature (pulmonary via the pulmonary artery for the right ventricle and systemic via the aorta for the left ventricle). Arterial systemic tone, blood viscosity, flow patterns (laminar versus turbulent), and valve competency all affect the degree of afterload the ventricle must overcome.

Contractility is the strength of myocardial muscle fiber shortening during the systolic phase of the cardiac cycle. It is the force with which the heart propels the stroke volume forward into the vasculature. The preload influences contractility, because optimizing the preload ensures maximal stretch of the myocardial fibers according to the Frank-Starling law.

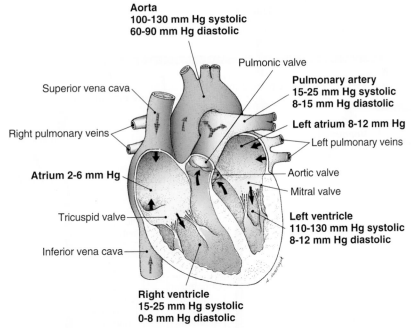

FIGURE 8-5 Normal blood flow through the heart and intrachamber pressures; arrows indicate the normal direction of blood flow. This schematic representation of the heart shows all four chambers and valves visible in the anterior view to facilitate conceptualization of blood flow. (Modified from Darovic, G. *Hemodynamic Monitoring: Invasive and Noninvasive Clinical Application.* Philadelphia: Saunders; 2002.)

Contractility is not directly measured; however, it can be expressed by the calculated values of right or left ventricular stroke work index.

Regulation of Cardiovascular Function

Cardiovascular anatomy and physiology were described in Chapter 7. Sympathetic nervous system activity enhances myocardial performance by shortening the conduction time through the AV node and enhancing rhythmicity of the AV pacemaker cells. Parasympathetic nervous system activity via the vagus nerve results in blocking of cardiac action potentials initiated by the atria, thus decreasing heart rate.

The cardiac system has hormonal influences that also assist in regulation of cardiovascular function. Norepinephrine increases the heart rate and myocardial contractility, and causes vasoconstriction. Epinephrine produces its effects by stimulating the alpha-adrenergic receptors located in the walls of the arteriole. Additionally, epinephrine is a beta-adrenergic stimulator and may cause vasodilatation of arterioles in skeletal muscle.

The hormonal influence on blood pressure and CO regulation is complex and not completely understood. Adrenocortical hormones potentiate the effects of catecholamines. Thyroid hormones influence sympathetic activity by an as yet undefined mechanism, which promotes an increase in CO. Intravascular fluid balance is affected by antidiuretic hormone and aldosterone balance. Several hormones (i.e., endothelin-1, serotonin, and thromboxane A_2) are released at the local tissue level and result in vasoconstriction of the vascular bed. Other hormones have vasodilatory properties such as nitric oxide, prostaglandins, bradykinin, and kallidin.[22] Figure 8-6 depicts the many factors that regulate blood flow and relate to the concepts of hemodynamic monitoring.

Effects of Aging

As the human body ages, normal physiological changes and changes associated with disease processes occur.[22] Differentiating between normal and pathological changes is difficult and poses a challenge in the management of the elderly patient. As elasticity and compliance decrease, the pressure within the arterial system increases, resulting in systemic hypertension. The increase in impedance to the left ventricular ejection often leads to left ventricular hypertrophy. As the left ventricle stiffens, diastolic filling is impaired, leading to diastolic heart failure. The number and sensitivity of β-adrenergic receptors in the sinoatrial node decreases, resulting in a decreased intrinsic and maximal heart rate. Fibrosis of the cardiac structures and conduction system can lead to heart block and valvular dysfunction. All of these changes significantly impact hemodynamic functioning. Figure 8-7 highlights the age-related changes on the cardiac system.

HEMODYNAMIC MONITORING MODALITIES

Invasive and noninvasive hemodynamic monitoring is a major part of a comprehensive assessment of the critically ill patient. Hemodynamic assessment aids in detecting an im-

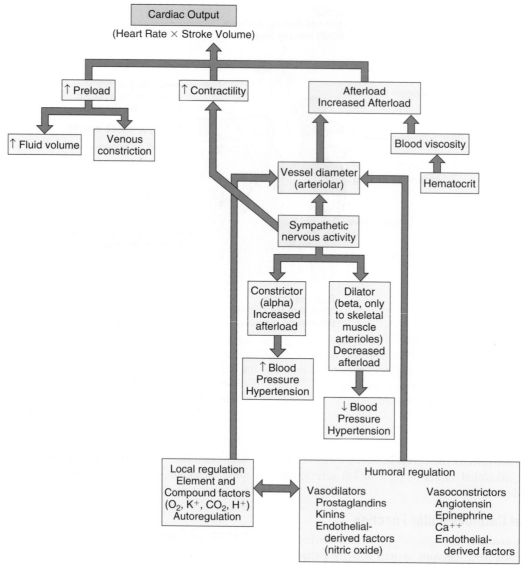

FIGURE 8-6 Factors regulating blood flow. (Modified from McCance KL, Huether S, eds. *Pathophysiology: the Biologic Basis for Disease in Adults and Children*, 6th ed. St. Louis: Mosby; 2009.)

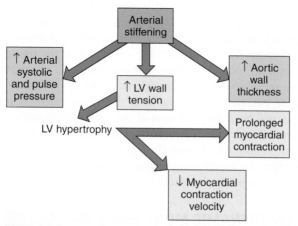

FIGURE 8-7 Impact of age-related changes on cardiac function. (Adapted from McCance KL, Huether S, eds. *Pathophysiology: the Biologic Basis for Disease in Adults and Children*, 5th ed. St. Louis: Mosby; 2005.)

pending cardiovascular crisis before any end organ damage occurs. The information gathered is used to titrate therapies to a specific end point (e.g., mean arterial pressure, CO), detect inadequate tissue perfusion, quantify severity of disease, and guide therapy. Normal hemodynamic values are described in Table 8-1; however, these values only provide a guideline to assist interpretation of assessment findings. The primary goal of hemodynamic monitoring is to assess and trend adequacy of tissue perfusion, rather than to compare a patient's values to so-called normal parameters.

Noninvasive Monitoring

Many critically ill patients can be adequately assessed and managed with noninvasive hemodynamic monitoring. Two frequently applied noninvasive technologies are noninvasive blood pressure (NIBP) measurement and assessment of jugular venous pressure.

TABLE 8-1   NORMAL HEMODYNAMIC VALUES

HEMODYNAMIC PARAMETER	SIGNIFICANCE	NORMAL RANGE
Cardiac output (CO)	Amount of blood pumped out by a ventricle every minute	4-8 L/min
Cardiac index (CI)	CO individualized to patient body surface area (size)	2.5-4.2 L/min/m^2
Central venous pressure (CVP)	Pressure created by volume of blood in right heart; used to guide assessment of fluid balance and responsiveness	2-6 mm Hg
Right atrial pressure (RAP)	Used interchangeably with CVP	2-6 mm Hg
Left atrial pressure (LAP)	Pressure created by volume of blood in left heart; used after open heart surgery to evaluate ability of left ventricle to eject blood volume ($\uparrow$ LAP = $\downarrow$ Ejection fraction)	8-12 mm Hg
Pulmonary artery occlusion pressure (PAOP)	Pressure created by volume of blood in left heart	8-12 mm Hg
Pulmonary artery pressure (PAP) (systole [PAS] and diastole [PAD])	Pressure created by the pulmonary system on the pulmonary pressures	Pulmonary artery systolic 15-25 mm Hg Pulmonary artery diastolic 8-15 mm Hg
Stroke volume (SV)	Amount of blood ejected from the ventricle with each contraction	60-130 mL/beat
Stroke volume index (SI)	SV individualized to patient size	30-65 mL/beat/m^2
Systemic vascular resistance (SVR)	Resistance that the left ventricle must overcome to eject a volume of blood; generally as SVR increases, CO falls	770-1500 dynes/sec/cm^{-5}
Stroke volume variation (SVV)	Parameter and indicator for preload responsiveness in mechanically ventilated patients (SVmax − SVmin/SVmean × 100)	10%-15%
Systemic vascular resistance index (SVRI)	SVR individualized to patient size	1680-2580 dynes/sec/cm^{-5}/m^2
Pulmonary vascular resistance (PVR)	Resistance that the right ventricle must overcome to eject a volume of blood, normally one sixth of SVR	20-120 dynes/sec/cm^{-5}
Pulmonary vascular resistance index (PVRI)	PVR individualized to patient size	69-177 dynes/sec/cm^{-5}/m^2
Right cardiac work index (RCWI)	Amount of work the right ventricle performs each minute when ejecting blood; increases or decreases depending upon changes in volume (CO) or pressure (PA mean)	0.54-0.66 kg-m/m^2
Right ventricular stroke work index (RVSWI)	Amount of work the right ventricle performs with each heartbeat; increases or decreases depending upon changes in volume (SV) or pressure (PA mean); quantifies contractility	7.9-9.7 g-m/beat/m^2
Left cardiac work index (LCWI)	Amount of work the left ventricle performs each minute when ejecting blood; increases or decreases depending upon changes in volume (CO) or pressure (MAP)	3.4-4.2 kg-m/m^2
Left ventricular stroke work index (LVSWI)	Amount of work the left ventricle performs with each heartbeat; increases or decreases depending upon changes in volume (SV) or pressure (MAP); quantifies contractility	50-62 g-m/beat/m^2
Right ventricular end diastolic volume (RVEDV) and pressure (RVEDP)	Measures right ventricular preload	0-8 mm Hg (RVEDP)
Left ventricular end diastolic volume (LVEDV) and pressure (LVEDP)	Measures left ventricular preload	4-12 mm Hg (LVEDP)

Continued

TABLE 8-1	NORMAL HEMODYNAMIC VALUES—cont'd	
HEMODYNAMIC PARAMETER	SIGNIFICANCE	NORMAL RANGE
Mixed venous oxygen saturation (SvO_2)	Provides an assessment of balance between oxygen supply and demand. Measured in the pulmonary artery; increased values indicate ↑ supply and ↓ demand, or ↓ ability to extract oxygen from blood. Decreased values indicate ↓ oxygen supply from low hemoglobin, low CO, low SaO_2 and/or ↑ consumption	60%-75%
Central venous oxygen saturation ($ScvO_2$)	Similar to SvO_2 but measured in the distal portion of the subclavian vein before right atrium and before the point where the cardiac sinus returns deoxygenated blood from the myocardium, thus the reason for the discrepancy between SvO_2 and $ScvO_2$ normal ranges	65%-85%

Noninvasive Blood Pressure

For decades, clinicians have used NIBP monitoring to assess patients. Typically NIBP is used for routine examinations and monitoring. Benefits of NIBP monitoring are ease of use, quick availability, and minimal patient complications.[36] To obtain accurate and reliable readings an understanding of the science of pressure measurement is required. It is critical that the proper size cuff be selected. If the cuff size is too small for the patient, the pressures recorded will be falsely elevated; if the cuff size is too large, the resulting pressures will be falsely low. In addition, the patient's arm should be positioned at the level of the heart. Patients who are hemodynamically unstable—either profoundly hypotensive or hypertensive—cannot be adequately assessed using NIBP measurement.[36] In the profoundly obese patient with conically shaped upper arms, it is also technically difficult to measure an NIBP because the cuff often does not fit appropriately or stay positioned. Blood pressure readings are also affected by the presence of cardiac dysrhythmias, respiratory variation, shivering, seizures, external cuff compression, decreased peripheral perfusion, and patient talking or movement during the measurement. Routine calibration of the NIBP equipment is required to ensure accurate measurement. The nurse must also understand that isolated blood pressure readings are not used to guide patient management; trending of values over time and assessing the response to interventions are crucial to maximize patient outcomes.

Jugular Venous Pressure

Assessment of the jugular veins provides an estimate of intravascular volume, and it is an indirect measure of central venous pressure (CVP). Because the internal jugular vein directly communicates with the right atrium, it can serve as a manometer to provide an estimate of the CVP. Jugular venous distention occurs when the CVP is elevated, which can occur with fluid overload, right ventricular dysfunction, superior vena cava obstruction, and right heart failure. The technique for assessing jugular venous pressure is pictured in Figure 8-8.

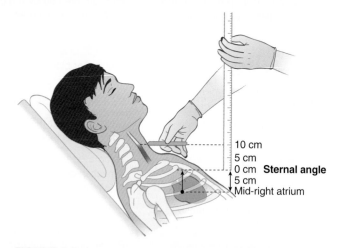

10 cm
5 cm
0 cm **Sternal angle**
5 cm
Mid-right atrium

FIGURE 8-8 Assessment of jugular venous pressure:
1. Place the patient in a supine position with the head of bed elevated 30 to 45 degrees.
2. Position yourself at the patient's right side.
3. Have the patient turn head slightly to the left.
4. If you cannot readily identify the jugular vein, place light pressure with your fingertips across the sternocleidomastoid muscle just superior and parallel to the clavicle. This pressure obstructs the external jugular vein and allows it to fill. Shine a pen light tangentially across the neck to accentuate the pulsations.
5. Assess for jugular venous distention at end exhalation.
6. Any fullness in the vein extending >3 cm above the sternal angle or angle of Louis is considered elevated jugular venous pressure. The higher the degree of elevation, the higher the central venous pressure.
7. Observe the highest point of pulsation in the internal jugular vein at end exhalation.
8. Measure the vertical distance between this pulsation and the angle of Louis in centimeters.
9. Add 5 cm to this number for an estimation of central venous pressure.
10. Normal is 7 to 9 cm.

Lactate

Anything that deprives the tissues of oxygen disrupts the Krebs cycle, resulting in anaerobic metabolism and increased production of lactic acid. Normal arterial lactate levels range from 0.5 to 1.6 mEq/L.[7] In lactic acidosis the lactate level is elevated, commonly 10 to 30 mEq/L. Lactate levels may be measured to determine tissue hypoperfusion in circulatory shock, to establish adequacy of resuscitation, and to assist in diagnosis of patients who have metabolic acidosis of unknown etiology.[18] Although lactate levels are not a specific marker for assessing hemodynamic status, they may be useful in determining end-organ perfusion.

Invasive Hemodynamic Monitoring
Indications

Invasive methods of hemodynamic monitoring are used to obtain more detailed physiological information. Common indications for invasive monitoring are outlined in Box 8-1. Cardiogenic shock, hypovolemic shock, cardiac tamponade, ruptured ventricular septum, low cardiac output syndrome, and right ventricular infarction are a few of the diagnoses that treatment may be guided with hemodynamic assessment.

The majority of these medical diagnoses can be summarized by three nursing diagnoses:
- Ineffective tissue perfusion
- Decreased CO
- Fluid volume excess or deficit

Understanding these three major indications assists the critical care nurse in identifying the rationale for interventions and anticipating potential complications (Box 8-2).

Equipment Common to All Intravascular Monitoring

The basic hemodynamic monitoring system has five major components: (1) the invasive catheter, (2) high-pressure noncompliant tubing, (3) the transducer (and stopcocks), (4) a pressurized flush system, and (5) the bedside monitoring system (Figure 8-9).

BOX 8-1 INDICATIONS FOR INVASIVE HEMODYNAMIC MONITORING

Arterial Line
- Hemodynamic instability
- Assess efficacy of vasoactive medications
- Frequent arterial blood gas analysis

Central Venous Catheter
- Measure right heart filling pressures
- Estimate fluid status
- Guide volume resuscitation
- Assess central venous oxygen saturation—$ScvO_2$
- Administer large-volume fluid resuscitation or irritant medications
- Access to place transvenous pacemaker

Pulmonary Artery Catheter
- Indentify and treat cause of hemodynamic instability
- Assess pulmonary artery pressures
- Assess mixed venous oxygen saturation—SvO_2
- Directly measure cardiac output

BOX 8-2 POTENTIAL COMPLICATIONS OF INVASIVE HEMODYNAMIC MONITORING DEVICES

- Vascular complications
  - Thrombosis
  - Hematoma
- Infection
- Bleeding
- Pneumothorax and/or hemothorax
- Cardiac dysrhythmias
- Pericardial tamponade

The *invasive catheter* varies depending upon the type of catheter, purpose, and location of insertion. The catheter can be placed into an artery, a vein, or the heart. An arterial catheter consists of a relatively small-gauge, short, pliable catheter that is placed over a guidewire or in a catheter-over-needle system. CVP or central venous oxygen saturation ($ScvO_2$) monitoring is obtained through a central venous catheter (CVC), most commonly placed in the subclavian or internal jugular veins (Figure 8-10). The femoral vein may be used when the thoracic veins are not available, or in a trauma situation. If inserted, femoral catheters should be removed as soon as possible to avoid catheter-associated complications. Pulmonary artery (PA) pressure and mixed venous oxygen saturation (SvO_2) monitoring requires a longer catheter that is placed into the PA (Figure 8-11).

Noncompliant pressure tubing designed specifically for hemodynamic monitoring is used to minimize artifact and increase the accuracy of the data transmission. Noncompliant tubing allows for the efficient and accurate transfer of intravascular pressure changes to the transducer and the monitoring system. In order to maintain the most accurate pressure readings the tubing should be no longer than 36 to 48 inches, with a minimum number of additional stopcocks.

The *transducer* (Figure 8-12) translates intravascular pressure changes into waveforms and numeric data. To ensure that the data are accurate, the system must be calibrated to atmospheric pressure by zeroing the transducer. A three-way stopcock attached to the transducer is generally used as the reference point for zeroing and leveling the system. This is referred to as the *air-fluid interface* or the *zeroing stopcock*. Discussion of these concepts follows.

The *flush system* maintains patency of the pressure tubing and catheter. A solution of 0.9% normal saline is recommended for the flush system. The flush solution is placed in a pressure bag that is inflated to 300 mm Hg to ensure a constant flow of fluid through the pressure tubing. The rate of fluid administration varies from 2 to 5 mL/hr per lumen. A clinical review concluded that flush systems using heparin prolongs catheter patency.[17] However, the use of heparin carries additional risks including the development of heparin-induced thrombocytopenia. A risk-to-benefit ratio should be considered before determining whether to use heparin or nonheparin flush solutions.

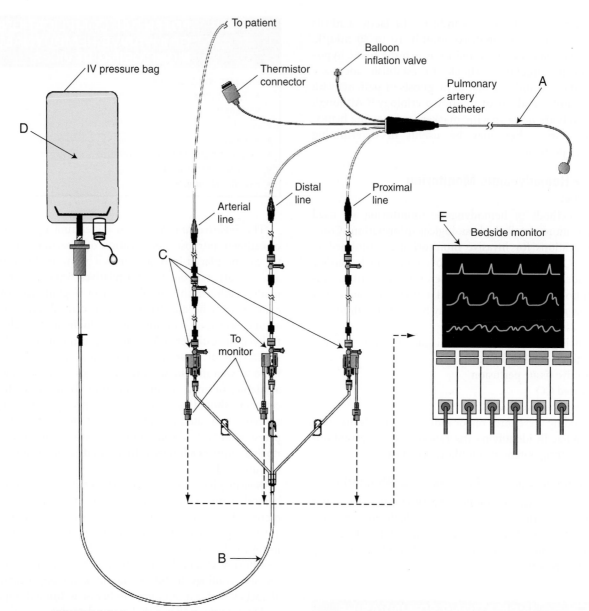

FIGURE 8-9 Components of an invasive monitoring system (pulmonary artery catheter and designated arterial line) connected to one flush solution. **A,** Invasive catheter. **B,** Noncompliant pressure tubing. **C,** Transducer and zeroing stopcock. **D,** Pressurized flush system. **E,** Bedside monitoring system. (Not to scale.)

Bedside *monitoring systems* vary in accessories and capabilities, but all have the same general function and purpose. They provide the visual display of the signal information generated by the transducer and have the ability to store and record the data. Interpretation of the data is the responsibility of the clinician.

Nursing Implications

Accuracy in hemodynamic monitoring is essential for ensuring clinically relevant decision making and proper patient management (see box, "Clinical Alert"). Four major components for validating the accuracy of hemodynamic monitoring systems are (1) patient positioning, (2) zeroing the transducer, (3) leveling the air-fluid interface (zeroing stopcock) to the phlebostatic axis, and (4) assessing dynamic responsiveness (performing the *square wave test*).[29] Prevention of infection is another key nursing intervention for patients with invasive hemodynamic monitoring catheters.

Patient Position

Assessment of hemodynamic status would be easier if patients remained in the supine, flat position all the time. However, most patients are more comfortable with the head of the bed (HOB) elevated, and elevation of the HOB is a key factor in the prevention of complications, such as ventilator-associated pneumonia. Hemodynamic parameters can be accurately measured and trended with the HOB elevated up to 45 degrees as long as the zeroing stopcock is properly leveled to the phlebostatic axis.[29,30]

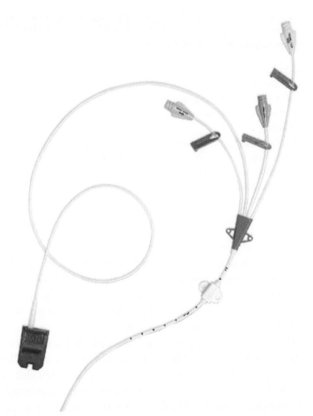

FIGURE 8-10 Example of a triple-lumen central line to measure central venous pressure and oxygen saturation. (Courtesy Edwards Lifesciences, Irvine, CA.)

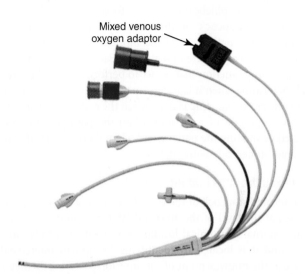

FIGURE 8-11 Example of a pulmonary artery catheter with capability of monitoring mixed venous oxygenation. (Courtesy Edwards Lifesciences, Irvine, CA.)

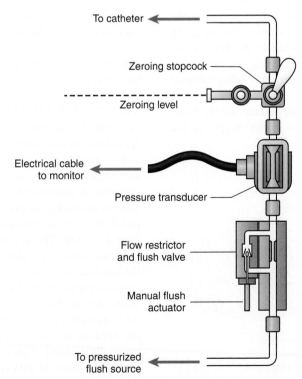

FIGURE 8-12 A schematic of a typical pressure transducer. (From Kruse JA. Fast flush test. In: Kruse JA, Fink MP, Carlson RW, eds. *Saunders Manual of Critical Care*. Philadelphia: Saunders; 2003.)

Zero Referencing

The effects of atmospheric pressure on the fluid-filled hemodynamic monitoring system must be negated for accurate measurements. At sea level the atmospheric pressure exerts a force of 760 mm Hg on any object on the earth's surface. To eliminate the impact of the atmospheric pressure on the physiological variables, the transducer system is "zeroed" at the level of the phlebostatic axis.[29] To accomplish this task, the zeroing stopcock of the transducer is opened to air (closed to the patient), and the monitoring system is calibrated to read a pressure of 0 mm Hg. Each computer system has a zeroing function that is easy to perform. Clinical protocols determine when it is necessary to zero the system, but in general zero referencing is done when the catheter is inserted, at the beginning of each shift, when the patient is disconnected or moving the patient, and when there are significant changes in hemodynamic status.

Leveling the Air-Fluid Interface

The zeroing stopcock of the transducer system must be positioned at the level of the atria and PA for accurate readings. This external anatomical location is termed the *phlebostatic axis,* and it is located by identifying the fourth intercostal space at the midway point of the anterior-posterior diameter of the chest wall (Figure 8-13).[29] Once the level of the phlebostatic axis is identified, the transducer and zeroing stopcock can be secured to the chest wall or to a standard intravenous pole positioned near the patient. However, the relationship of the air-fluid interface to the phlebostatic axis must be maintained so that the numerical readings transmitted to the monitor are accurate. When the transducer is affixed to the patient's chest wall, it is important to assess skin integrity to prevent skin breakdown. An indelible marker can be used to mark the location of the phlebostatic axis on the patient to ensure future measurements are done using the same reference point.[28]

Because of the effects of hydrostatic pressure on the fluid-filled monitoring system, variations in the height of the

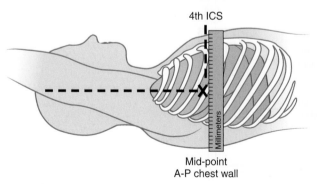

4th ICS

Millimeters

Mid-point
A-P chest wall

FIGURE 8-13 Locating the phlebostatic axis in the supine position.

---

transducer system by as little as 1 cm below the phlebostatic axis can result in a false elevation by as much as 0.73 mm Hg. Conversely, if the transducer is above the phlebostatic axis, a false low reading results. Therefore the location of the zeroing stopcock must be regularly monitored and releveled with each change in the patient's position.

The American Association of Critical-Care Nurses (AACN) 2009 Practice Alert summarized results of studies and determined that accurate hemodynamic data can also be obtained in lateral positions from 30 to 90 degrees, although it is technically more difficult to level the transducer to the atria.[1] In the 30-degree lateral position, the transducer is placed half the distance from the surface of the bed to the left sternal border. The patient must be positioned *exactly* at a 30-degree lateral position for this method to be accurate. If the patient is in a 90-degree right lateral position, the transducer is leveled to the fourth intercostal space, midsternum. If the patient is in a 90-degree left lateral position, the transducer is leveled to the fourth intercostal space, left parasternal border.[1,27] The clinician should document patient position (e.g., HOB angle, lateral rotation) with each hemodynamic measurement.

Dynamic Response Testing

Fluid-filled monitoring systems rely on the ability of the transducer to translate the vascular pressure into waveforms and numeric data. To verify that the transducer system can accurately represent cardiovascular pressures, the dynamic response or *square wave* test must be performed. This test is done by recording the pressure waveform while activating the fast flush valve/actuator on the pressure tubing system for at least 1 second. The resulting graph should depict a rapid upstroke from the baseline with a plateau before returning to the baseline (i.e., *square wave*).[32] Upon the return of the pressure tracing to the baseline, a small undershoot should occur below the baseline, along with one or two oscillations, within 0.12 seconds before resuming the pressure waveform. If the dynamic response test meets these criteria, the system is optimally damped (Figure 8-14, *A*), and the resulting waveforms and numeric data can be interpreted as accurate. The dynamic response test should be performed after catheter insertion, at least once per shift, and after opening the system.

Square wave test configuration

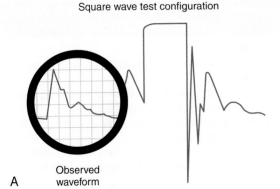

A Observed waveform

Square wave test configuration

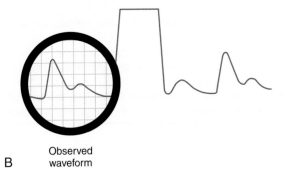

B Observed waveform

Square wave test configuration

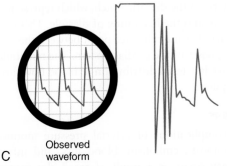

C Observed waveform

FIGURE 8-14 A, Optimal dynamic response test. **B,** Overdamped dynamic response test. **C,** Underdamped dynamic response test.

BOX 8-3 ABNORMAL DYNAMIC RESPONSE TEST: CAUSES AND INTERVENTIONS

Overdamped System
- Blood clots, blood left in the catheter after obtaining a blood sample, air bubbles at any point between the catheter tip and transducer
  - Flush the system or aspirate, disconnecting from the patient if needed to adequately flush the system to remove clots or air bubbles
- Compliant tubing
  - Change to noncompliant tubing or commercially available tubing system
- Loose connections
  - Ensure all connections are secure
- Kinks in the tubing system
  - Straighten tubing

Underdamped System
- Excessive tubing length (<36 to 48 inches)
  - Remove extraneous tubing, stopcocks, or extensions
- Small bore tubing
  - Replace small bore tubing with a larger bore set
- Cause unknown
  - Add a damping device into the system to reduce artifact

It is a simple but crucial test that must be incorporated into routine hemodynamic assessment to ensure accuracy.[32]

The system is overdamped if the dynamic response test results in no oscillations, the upstroke is slurred, or a small undershoot is not produced (Figure 8-14, B). An overdamped system can result in a systolic pressure that is falsely low and a diastolic pressure that is falsely elevated.

Conversely, the system is underdamped if the dynamic response test results in excessive oscillations (Figure 8-14, C). The displayed pressure waveform and numeric data will show erroneously high systolic pressures and low diastolic pressures. Box 8-3 describes causes of abnormal dynamic response test results and interventions for troubleshooting systems that are overdamped or underdamped.

Infection Control

The U.S. Centers for Disease Control and Prevention estimate that 250,000 catheter-related bloodstream infection (CRBSI) occur annually in the United States.[6] Invasive catheters are direct portals into the circulating blood volume; strict infection control measures must be implemented to reduce catheter-related bloodstream infections, sometimes referred to as central line–associated bloodstream infections (CLABSI). To help reduce the risk for CRBSI, a central line bundle was developed that emphasizes strict hand washing, strict sterile technique with maximal barrier precautions during placement, chlorhexidine skin antisepsis, optimal catheter site selection, and daily review of line necessity.[6] Duration of catheterization is an independent risk factor for CRBSI, and removal of the catheter when not needed to guide treatment is associated with a reduction in mortality.[24] Additionally, maintaining the site properly and minimizing the number of times the system is opened by changing the tubing system and flush bag no more frequently than every 72 to 96 hours is recommended.[6] Institutional policies dictate the frequency of tubing change with consideration of CVC location. A decreased rate of infection is associated with use of the subclavian vein site, although it has the highest rate of complications of pneumothorax and phrenic nerve damage. In comparison, use of the internal jugular site has a lower complication rate than the subclavian. The femoral site is the least preferred for cannulation among adult patients.[24] Box 8-4 describes general strategies for managing hemodynamic monitoring systems.

BOX 8-4 **GENERAL NURSING STRATEGIES FOR MANAGING HEMODYNAMIC MONITORING SYSTEMS**

- Document insertion date
- Change dressings according to institutional policy
  - Assess for signs of infection
  - Date dressing changes
- Maintain patency of the flush system
  - Flush the system after each use of a port
  - Clear any blood from the tubing, ports, and/or stopcocks
  - Maintain a pressure of 300 mm Hg on the flush solution using a pressure bag
  - Ensure adequate amount of flush solution in the intravenous bag
- Ensure tightened connections in the tubing and flush system
- Keep tubing free of kinks
- Minimize excess tubing and the number of stopcocks
- Limit disconnecting or opening the system
- Ensure that alarm limits are set on the monitor and alarms are turned on

---

BOX 8-5 **ALLEN AND MODIFIED ALLEN TEST PROCEDURE**

Allen Test
- The patient forms a tight fist with the wrist in a neutral position
- The clinician occludes the radial artery by applying pressure with the thumb for approximately 10 seconds
- Patient opens fist while the clinician maintains thumb pressure on radial artery
- Ulnar circulation is adequate if blanching resolves within 5 seconds, inadequate if hand remains pale for >10 seconds

Modified Allen Test
- The patient forms a tight fist with the wrist in a neutral position
- Clinician occludes radial and ulnar arteries for approximately 10 seconds
- Patient opens fist, revealing a blanched hand
- Clinician releases pressure on ulnar artery, maintaining pressure on radial artery
- Ulnar circulation is adequate if blanching resolves within 5 seconds, inadequate if hand remains pale for >10 seconds

---

Arterial Pressure Monitoring

Arterial pressure monitoring is indicated for patients who are at risk for compromised tissue perfusion and volume status. Other indications include patients that need frequent lab work including arterial blood gas sampling, patients with either hypotension or hypertension, and patients whose treatment includes vasoactive agents. This common procedure involves cannulating an artery and recording pressures via the fluid-filled monitoring system. Radial artery placement remains the site of choice because of its ready accessibility, collateral perfusion to the hand via the ulnar artery, and compressibility of the location. Alternative sites include the femoral and brachial arteries. Before cannulation of the radial artery, it is necessary to assess collateral circulation.[3] This can be accomplished by Doppler ultrasonography or by performing an Allen test or a modified Allen test (Box 8-5).

Invasive arterial pressure monitoring is considered to be the most accurate method of obtaining the systemic blood pressure because it allows for continuous, beat-to-beat analysis of the arterial pressure. As a result of its real-time blood pressure reading, arterial pressure monitoring is the method of choice in assessing blood pressure in the hemodynamically unstable patient.[34]

The normal arterial waveform (Figure 8-15) consists of a sharp upstroke, the peak of which represents the systolic pressure. This pressure is a direct reflection of left ventricular function. Normal values for systolic pressures are less than 140 mm Hg. The lowest point on the arterial waveform represents the end-diastolic pressure value and reflects systemic resistance. Normal values for diastolic pressure are less than 90 mm Hg.[32]

The downstroke of the arterial waveform consists of a small notch termed the dicrotic notch, which represents aortic valve closure and the beginning of diastole. This is commonly considered as the reference point between the systolic and diastolic phases of the cardiac system. The remainder of the downstroke is arterial distribution of blood flow through the arterial system.

Complications

The major complications of arterial pressure monitoring include thrombosis, embolism, blood loss, and infection. Embolism may occur as a result of small clot formation around the tip of the catheter or from air entering the system. Thrombosis (clot) may occur if a continuous flush solution is not properly maintained. Blood loss results from sudden dislodgment of the catheter from the artery or from a disconnection in the tubing. Rapid blood loss may occur (because this is in an artery, not a vein) if either of these events is not promptly recognized. Infection may occur if the catheter is left in place for a prolonged period; however, routine replacement of the catheter is not recommended unless an infection is suspected.[32]

Clinical Considerations

The invasive method of obtaining blood pressure is considered to be more accurate than noninvasive methods because it gives beat-by-beat information instead of measuring vibrations (Korotkoff sounds) of the arterial wall over several beats. In patients who are hypotensive, a serious discrepancy may exist between the blood pressures obtained by invasive and noninvasive means.[34] The cuff pressure may be significantly

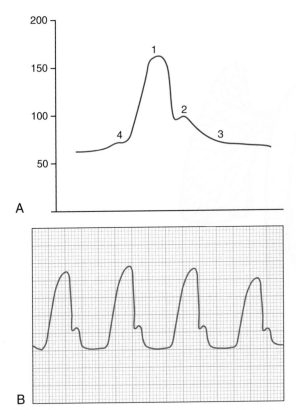

A

B

FIGURE 8-15 A, Normal arterial pressure tracing; *1,* peak systolic pressure; *2,* dicrotic notch; *3,* diastolic pressure; *4,* anacrotic notch. **B,** Arterial pressure waveform obtained from arterial line.

BOX 8-6 CAUSES OF HIGHER NONINVASIVE VERSUS INVASIVE BLOOD PRESSURE

- Air bubbles in the catheter system
- Failure to *zero* the transducer air-fluid interface
- Blood in the catheter system
- Blood clot at the catheter tip
- Kinking of the tubing system
- Catheter tip lodging against the arterial wall
- Soft, compliant tubing
- Long tubing (>48 inches)
- Too many stopcocks (>3)
- Improper cuff size
- Improper cuff placement

lower, leading to dangerous mistakes in the treatment of such a patient. Under normal circumstances, a difference of 10 to 20 mm Hg or more between invasive and noninvasive blood pressure is expected, with the invasive blood pressure generally higher than the noninvasive value.[4] This difference may vary substantially from the invasive blood pressure determination, and, for this reason, treatment should never be based on the measurement of a single determination of NIBP. When the noninvasive value is higher than the invasive number, one must suspect equipment malfunction or technical error. Box 8-6 lists the possible causes.

Nursing Implications

Standard management of all invasive hemodynamic systems is described in Box 8-4. Additional interventions specific to management of the intraarterial catheter include the following:

- Document assessment of the extremity every 2 hours for perfusion: color, temperature, sensation, pulse, and capillary refill (normal time to refill is less than 3 seconds).
- Keep the patient's wrist in a neutral position and/or place it on an armboard (radial artery catheters).
- When the catheter is removed, ensure that adequate pressure is applied to the site of insertion until hemostasis is obtained (for a minimum of 5 minutes for radial artery

catheters). The time required varies, depending on the type, size, and location of the catheter and the patient's coagulation status.
- Medications should never be administered via an arterial line because of potential harmful complications.

Right Atrial Pressure/Central Venous Pressure Monitoring

In critically ill patients, the right atrial pressure (RAP) or central venous pressure (CVP) has been used to estimate central venous blood volume and right heart function. The pressure is obtained from the right atrial port of a pulmonary artery catheter (PA catheter or PAC), and is also called the RAP. Because no valves are present between the venae cavae and right atrium, both the CVP and RAP are essentially equal pressures. This measurement assesses "preload" of the right side of the heart. The term RAP is used most of the time in this textbook. Normal CVP/RAP ranges from 2 to 6 mm Hg.

The RAP is obtained from a central line inserted into the superior or inferior venae cavae. The thoracic central veins (subclavian and internal jugular veins) are the most common insertion sites. Catheters used for RAP measurement are generally stiff and radiopaque, and they vary in length and diameter depending on the vein that is used. Shorter catheters are inserted into the subclavian and internal jugular veins, and longer catheters are used for insertion into the upper extremities or femoral vein. CVCs often have multiple lumens that facilitate pressure monitoring, administration of several types of fluids, and blood sampling. Insertion is similar to that for a PA catheter, which is described later in the chapter.

Figure 8-16 shows a position of a CVC in the right atrium along with the corresponding waveform. During right ventricular diastole, the tricuspid valve is open, thereby allowing a clear passage for blood to flow from the right atrium to the right ventricle. Therefore, RAP provides a reliable measurement of right ventricular preload.

RAP, along with other measurements, is used to assess and guide fluid resuscitation and estimate right-sided cardiac

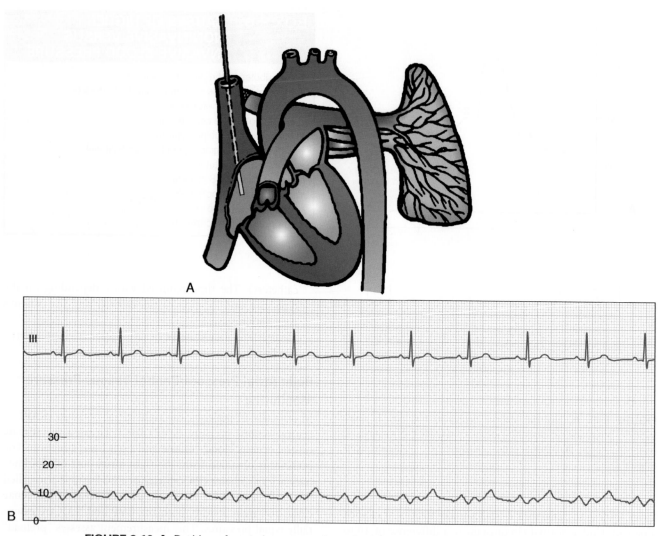

FIGURE 8-16 A, Position of central venous catheter in right atrium **B,** along with cardiac rhythm and associated waveforms.

function. The interpretation of the RAP should be compared with the stroke index (SI).[25] If both the RAP and SI are low, hypovolemia is likely. If RAP is high and SI is low, RV dysfunction is likely.

Because the normal RAP value is low and within a narrow range, it is important to obtain an accurate reading of the RAP; this requires the nurse to properly zero and level the system at the phlebostatic axis and verify an optimal dynamic response test.

The RAP must be measured at end expiration and at the end of ventricular diastole. Simultaneous graphing of the cardiac rhythm (electrocardiogram [ECG]), RAP, and respiratory tracing (if available) is done in obtaining an accurate measurement of RAP. The RAP tracing is composed of three major waveforms: *a, c,* and *v* waves (see Figure 8-17). The *a* wave is produced by atrial contraction and follows the P wave on the ECG tracing. The *c* wave is produced by closure of the tricuspid valve and follows the R wave. Finally, the *v* wave correlates with right atrial filling; it follows the T wave on the ECG.[25]

To measure the RAP, the *a, c,* and *v* waves of the RAP tracing at end expiration are identified (Figure 8-17). The RAP is measured at end expiration to ensure that pleural pressure changes do not skew the numeric value. True RAP is best measured by locating the *c* wave and identifying the value immediately preceding the *c* wave (termed the pre-*c* measurement). Alternatively, the average of the *a* waves may be computed, or the z-point method may be determined. The z-point method consists of identifying the RAP by locating the end of the QRS complex and using that as the reference point on the tracing. Box 8-7 outlines circumstances for using the different methods for determining RAP.

Complications

Nurses assist in inserting and maintaining central lines. Maximum sterile barrier precautions must be observed during insertion because catheter-related bloodstream infections are common with a central line, which increases the risk of sepsis.[12] Other complications may occur during insertion, including carotid puncture, pneumothorax, hemothorax,

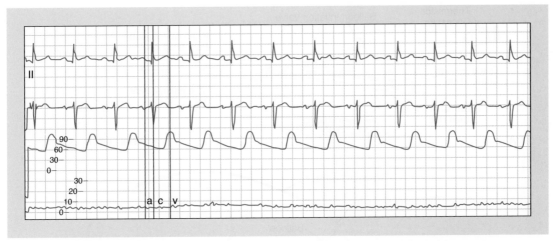

FIGURE 8-17 Identifying the *a, c,* and *v* waveforms to determine right atrial pressure.

BOX 8-7	METHODS FOR DETERMINING ACCURATE RIGHT ATRIAL PRESSURE

Pre-*c* Method
- Most accurate measure of right-sided preload; method of choice for numeric assessment
- Represents the last atrial pressure before ventricular contraction
- Difficult to use because the *c* wave is often unidentifiable

Mean of the *a* Wave
- Clinically significant because the *a* wave results from atrial contraction
- Used if the *c* wave cannot be identified
- Obtain the numeric for the top and bottom of the *a* wave. Calculate the sum and divide by 2.

Z-Point Method
- Used when *atrial-ventricular* synchrony is not present; atrial fibrillation, 3rd degree heart block
- Standardized approach results in the most reproducible value between clinicians
- Does not account for hemodynamic effects on kidneys or liver that result from the prominent *a* or *v* waves
- Locate the end of the QRS complex; use the numeric associated with the exact point of intersection of the RA wave.

perforation of the right atrium or ventricle, and cardiac dysrhythmias. A chest x-ray is obtained after insertion to confirm placement and detect complications.

Clinical Considerations

Abnormalities in RAP are generally caused by any condition that alters venous tone, blood volume, or right ventricular contractility. For example, a patient with a low RAP may be hypovolemic because of dehydration or traumatic blood loss. Low pressures are also seen in relative hypovolemia as a result of vasodilation from rewarming, medications, or sepsis. In all of these conditions, RAP reflects blood return to the heart that is insufficient to meet the body's requirements. Confounding the interpretation of a low RAP, is that the value may be negative in an individual in the upright position, even if cardiac function and volume status are normal.

A high RAP measurement indicates conditions that reduce the right ventricle's ability to eject blood, thereby increasing right ventricular pressure and RAP. Such conditions include hypervolemia (seen with aggressive administration of intravenous fluids), severe vasoconstriction, and mechanical ventilation (additional positive pressure increases RAP). Conditions causing RAP increase include pulmonary hypertension and right-sided heart failure (often seen in cardiac ischemia of the right heart, causing a backup of blood into the right side of the heart).

Nursing Implications

The critical care nurse is responsible for collecting and recording patient data, ensuring the accuracy of the data, and reporting abnormal findings and trends to the provider. Analyzing the various hemodynamic parameters is a collaborative responsibility between clinical and nursing staff to ensure prompt and appropriate treatments occur. Measurements of RAP are essential to compare with other physiological parameters and physical assessment.

Pulmonary Artery Pressure Monitoring

PACs are used to diagnose and manage a variety of conditions in critically ill patients. The ability to measure pressures in the pulmonary artery (PA) and the left side of the heart became reality after a flow-directed PA catheter was invented by Drs. Jeremy Swan and William Ganz in 1970.[35] Thermodilution PA catheters with ability to obtain PA pressures and CO measurement became the *gold standard* to which all new hemodynamic monitors are compared.[33] In the last 30 years, the PA catheter has been redesigned to obtain a variety of hemodynamic parameters, including continuous CO (CCO)

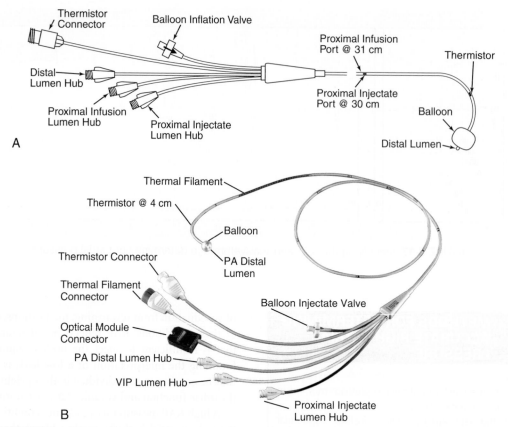

FIGURE 8-18 A, A five-lumen pulmonary artery (PA) catheter containing the four-lumen components in addition to a second proximal lumen for infusion of fluid or medications. **B,** CCOmbo 777 catheter. (Courtesy of Edwards Lifesciences, Irvine, CA.)

measurement rather than intermittent CO readings, continuous right ventricular end diastolic volume (RVEDV), right ventricular ejection fraction (RVEF), and continuous mixed venous oxygen saturation SvO_2.

To determine PA pressure (PAP) a specialized catheter is placed directly into the PA (Figure 8-18). The PA catheter is a long, flexible, multilumen balloon-tipped catheter that enables measurement of a variety of hemodynamic parameters. The proximal port lies in the right atrium and measures RAP; it is also used to administer fluids and electrolytes and to obtain intermittent thermodilution CO measurements. The distal port measures PAP and PA occlusion pressure (PAOP); mixed venous blood samples are also drawn from this port. The thermistor port incorporates a temperature sensitive wire that allows computer calculation of CO with the thermodilution method. Many catheters have an additional proximal infusion port for fluid and medication administration. The balloon inflation lumen provides the ability to inflate and deflate the small-volume (approximately 1.5 mL) balloon at the distal tip of the catheter. The balloon is inflated to facilitate insertion of the catheter and to measure PAOP, which provides information about the function of the left side of the heart.[28] The concept of PAOP is discussed later in the chapter.

Several specialized PA catheters are available. One PA catheter enables transvenous pacing. This technique involves the insertion of pacemaker wires through additional lumina in the PA catheter, which exit the catheter into the right ventricle to provide ventricular pacing. Other PA catheters have CCO capabilities. This type of catheter was developed to provide continuous monitoring of CO. For assessing continuous mixed venous oxygenation (SvO_2), a PA catheter with a fiberoptic lumen at the tip of the catheter was developed. The concepts of CCO and SvO_2 are discussed later in this chapter.

Nurses assist providers during PA catheter insertion. The nursing interventions include patient education and advocacy. Though it is the provider's responsibility to obtain the informed consent for catheter insertion, the critical care nurse provides much of the education regarding patient positioning and what the patient may feel or experience during the procedure. An additional nursing goal is to alleviate the patient's anxiety before and during the procedure.

The method of PA catheter insertion is similar to that of the CVC.[11] The patient's bed is placed in Trendelenburg position to promote venous filling in the upper body for easier insertion of the catheter, unless the patient has respiratory distress or increased intracranial pressure. This position can also prevent air embolism during insertion. If Trendelenburg position is contraindicated, a blanket roll can be placed between the patient's shoulder blades to facilitate insertion. The skin is cleaned and draped and is then injected with a local anaesthetic. A needled syringe is used to puncture the vessel and to confirm placement by backward flow of blood into the syringe. The syringe is removed, and a guidewire is threaded through the needle into the vessel. The needle is then removed so a hollow tube, called an introducer, may be passed over the guidewire. The wire is then removed, and the PA catheter is passed freely into the vessel through the introducer. The provider inserting the catheter will instruct the nurse (or other professional helping during insertion) to inflate and deflate the balloon during the procedure to facilitate flow from the right atrium to the PA. The insertion technique may vary according to provider preference, brand of equipment used, and the patient's anatomy.[11,28]

During the PA catheter insertion, the critical care nurse is responsible for monitoring and recording heart rate and rhythm, recognizing dysrhythmias, monitoring blood pressure, and visualizing waveforms while the catheter is advanced. Ventricular dysrhythmias may occur as the catheter passes through the right ventricle into the PA. The nurse may assist with balloon inflation during the procedure. As the catheter passes through each chamber, the nurse observes the waveform characteristics and records pressure values: RAP, right ventricular pressure, PAP, and PAOP (Figure 8-19, *A* and *B*). The PAOP waveform signals the end of insertion, at which time the balloon is deflated. Once the balloon is deflated, the tip of the catheter falls back into position in the PA. After the catheter is

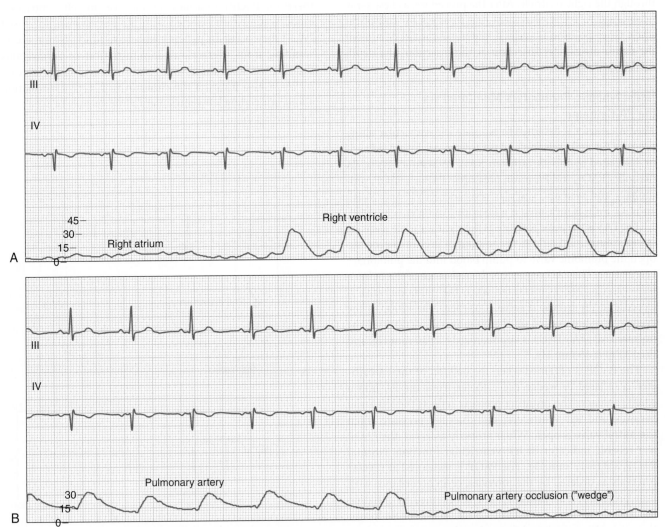

FIGURE 8-19 Position of pulmonary artery (PA) catheter and associated waveforms. **A,** Dual-channel tracing of cardiac rhythm with pressure waveforms obtained as the PA catheter is inserted into the right atrium (RA) and right ventricle (RV). **B,** Dual-channel tracing of cardiac rhythm with PA, and pulmonary artery occlusion pressure (PAOP) waveforms as the catheter is floated into proper position.

inserted and placement verified, the balloon is only inflated to obtain periodic PAOP measurements; otherwise it remains deflated to prevent complications (e.g., pulmonary infarction, PA rupture). Nursing priorities are to accurately interpret PA catheter waveforms, recognize effect of respiratory variations, prevent complications, and document hemodynamic values. Graphing the pressure waveforms and ECG tracing is also recommended.[28]

As a patient advocate, the critical care nurse is responsible for promoting patient safety throughout the procedure. This includes ensuring that sterility is maintained, monitoring the patient, and assisting with balloon inflation and deflation. Because PA catheter insertion involves certain risks, emergency medications and equipment must be readily available. Complications of insertion include hemothorax, pneumothorax, perforation of the vein or cardiac chamber, and cardiac dysrhythmias—especially as the PA catheter passes through the right ventricle. After the procedure, a chest x-ray is obtained to verify placement and to assess for complications. Once position is verified, the nurse should document the depth of catheter insertion at the insertion site; depth markings are noted on the PA catheter.

Hemodynamic Parameters Monitored via the PA Catheter

The PA catheter is designed to estimate left ventricular filling pressure. Several pressures and parameters are measured and/or calculated by the PA catheter: RAP; PA systolic (PAS), PA diastolic (PAD), and PA mean pressures (PAPm); PAOP; pulmonary and systemic vascular resistance (PVR and SVR); and CO. SvO_2 is measured if a fiberoptic catheter is inserted.

The PAS is the peak pressure as the right ventricle ejects its stroke volume, and reflects the amount of pressure needed to open the pulmonic valve to pump blood into the pulmonary vasculature. The PAD represents the resistance of the pulmonary vascular bed as measured when the pulmonic valve is closed and the tricuspid valve is opened. The PAPm is the average pressure exerted on the pulmonary vasculature. The normal PAP (PAS/PAD) is approximately 25/10 mm Hg, and the PAPm is 15 mm Hg.[10]

The PAOP is obtained when the balloon of the PA catheter is inflated to wedge the catheter from the PA into a small capillary. The resulting pressure reflects the left atrial pressure and left ventricular end-diastolic pressure when the mitral valve is open. When properly assessed, the PAOP is a reliable indicator of left ventricular function. Normal PAOP is 8 to 12 mm Hg. The PAOP is measured at regular intervals as ordered by the provider, or in accordance with unit protocols. The measurement is obtained by inflating the balloon with no more than 1.5 mL of air, for no longer than 8 to 10 seconds, while noting the waveform change from the PAP to the PAOP (see Figure 8-19, B).[10] To obtain accurate measurement of the PAOP, the critical care nurse must print the PAOP waveform simultaneously with the ECG waveform and respiratory patterns. Similar to RAP, PAP and PAOP measurements must be obtained at end expiration. In the patient who is spontaneously breathing, pressures are highest at end expiration and decline with

inhalation (Figure 8-20, A). Measurements are obtained from the waveform just before pressures decline. In the mechanically ventilated patient, pressures increase with inhalation and decrease with exhalation (see Figure 8-20, B). Measurements are obtained just before the increase in pressures during inhalation.

Clinical Considerations

Trending of PAP provides an indirect measure of left ventricular function. The PAOP is a reliable indirect measurement of left ventricular function, and it provides data to guide treatment and monitor the patient's response. In the absence of valvular disease and pulmonary vascular congestion, the PAD also closely approximates left ventricle function because the mitral valve is open during end-diastole. The PAD is often used as an indirect measurement of PAOP.

An increase in left ventricular end-diastolic pressure (and therefore PAOP) indicates an increase in left ventricular blood volume to be ejected with the next systole. Increased PAOP may occur in patients who have fluid volume excess resulting from overzealous administration of intravenous fluid, as well as in those with renal dysfunction. An increase in PAOP also provides the clinician with early information about impending left ventricular failure, as may be seen with myocardial infarction.

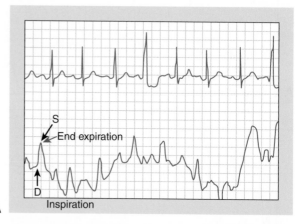

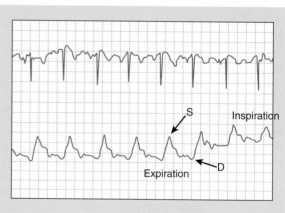

FIGURE 8-20 Effect of respiration on pulmonary artery waveforms in patients with spontaneous breathing **(A)** and mechanical ventilation **(B)**. *D,* Diastolic pressure; *S,* systolic pressure.

A decrease in left ventricular end-diastolic pressure (and a subsequently low PAOP) signals a reduction in left ventricular blood volume available for the next contraction. Conditions causing a low PAOP include those that cause fluid volume deficit, such as dehydration, excessive diuretic therapy, and hemorrhage. Through monitoring of changes and trends, the PAOP can be invaluable in determining appropriate therapy as well as the effectiveness of that therapy.

Nursing Implications

Patients with prolonged PA catheterization must be carefully examined for signs or symptoms of infection. Nurses routinely monitor RAP, PAP, and PAOP to identify trends and the clinical significance of the values. The catheter position must be maintained in the PA; the nurse assesses placement and will review results of chest x-rays, monitor for normal PA waveforms, and ensure that the balloon is deflated except during PAOP measurements.

It is helpful to know how much air is needed to obtain the PAOP (≤1.5 mL). If the PAOP is obtained with a much smaller amount of air, the catheter may have migrated further into the PA. The nurse should never force the balloon to inflate if resistance is met. If the PAOP is not noted with inflation of 1.5 mL of air, the catheter may have been pulled out of position, or the balloon may have ruptured. In both of these situations, verification of proper positioning by a chest x-ray and observation of the PAP waveform are important interventions. The nurse should also make periodic comparisons of the PAD and PAOP to assess the accuracy of the PAOP measurement, especially in patients experiencing acute hemodynamic changes. When it is determined that the PA catheter is no longer needed, nurses who are specially trained in withdrawing the catheter often perform the procedure and have a validated and documented clinical competency outlined in the policy and procedure manual for the unit.

A standardized, Web-based education program, the Pulmonary Artery Catheter Education Project (www.pacep.org), is available to educate multiprofessional team members on hemodynamic concepts. Nurses can take advantage of this free program.

Controversy Surrounding the PA Catheter

The risk versus benefit of the pulmonary artery catheter has been debated since the catheter's inception. Outcomes of using a PA catheter to guide treatment vary from study to study. A recent meta-analysis found use of the PA catheter to implement a hemodynamic protocol was beneficial in high-risk surgical patients,[13] yet other studies have reported a higher mortality in patients treated with a PA catheter.[17,33] Therefore the decision to insert a PA catheter should be based on clinical circumstances of the patient and risk versus benefit determination. The present practice is focused on targeting hemodynamic and oxygen delivery goals to optimize tissue perfusion. Less invasive methods of measuring hemodynamic status are often preferred (see box, "Evidence-Based Practice").

EVIDENCE-BASED PRACTICE

Usefulness of Stroke Volume Variation Monitoring

Problem
Newer technologies that use pulse contour analysis are providing additional hemodynamic data on which to guide treatments. One measurement that is available is stroke volume variation (SVV).

Clinical Question
How useful is SVV is predicting fluid responsiveness in critically ill patients?

Evidence
The authors conducted a meta-analysis of 23 studies that tested outcomes of SVV in 568 critically ill patients. In this sample of patients the PiCCO or FloTrac/Vigileo was studied in patients on mechanical ventilation at a tidal volume of 8 mL/kg or higher. The authors reported both high sensitivity (0.81) and specificity (0.80) for predicting fluid responsiveness. The odds ratio for diagnosing fluid responsiveness was 18.4. They concluded that SVV was a useful tool for measuring fluid responsiveness.

Implications for Nursing
As less invasive measures (than the pulmonary artery catheter) of hemodynamic monitoring are developed and implemented in critical care practice, it is important to assess their clinical application and utility. This meta-analysis showed a strong predictive ability of SVV to assess response to fluid administration. Nurses will be responsible for learning and using the technology in patient care management.

Level of Evidence
A—Meta analysis

Cardiac Output Monitoring

The CO is the amount of blood ejected by the heart each minute and is calculated from the heart rate and stroke volume. Cardiac index (CI) is the CO adjusted for an individual's size or body surface area. Monitoring of CO and CI is done to assess the heart's ability to pump oxygenated blood to the tissues. Causes of low and high COs are outlined in Box 8-8. Two methods are commonly used to evaluate CO via the PA catheter: thermodilution cardiac output (TdCO) and CCO.

Thermodilution Cardiac Output

To measure the CO via the TdCO method, the thermistor connector on the PA catheter is attached to a CO module on the cardiac monitor. A set volume (5 to 10 mL) of room temperature solution of 0.9% normal saline is injected quickly and smoothly via the proximal port. Many institutions use a closed injectate delivery system to facilitate the procedure (Figure 8-21). As the fluid bolus passes into the right ventricle and subsequently the PA, the difference in temperature is sensed by the thermistor located at the distal portion of the catheter (Figure 8-22). The TdCO is calculated as the difference in temperature over time washout curve. Normal CO is represented by a smooth curve with a rapid upstroke and slow return to the baseline. The CO module calculates the

BOX 8-8   INTERPRETATION OF ABNORMAL CARDIAC OUTPUT/INDEX VALUES

Low Cardiac Output/Index
- Heart rate that is too fast or too slow leading to inadequate ventricular filling
- Stroke volume reduction as a result of:
  - **Decreased preload**
    Hemorrhage
    Hypovolemia from diuresis, dehydration, etc.
    Vasodilatation
    Fluid shifts (i.e., third spacing) outside the intravascular space
  - **Increased afterload**
    Vasoconstriction
    Increased blood viscosity
  - **Decreased contractility**
    Myocardial infarction or ischemia
    Heart failure
    Cardiomyopathy
    Cardiogenic shock
    Cardiac tamponade

High Cardiac Output/Index
- Heart rate elevation secondary to:
  - Increased activity
  - Anemia
  - Metabolic demands
  - Adrenal disorders
  - Fever
  - Anxiety
- Stroke volume increase as a result of:
  - **Increased preload**
    Fluid resuscitation
    Alteration in ventricular compliance
  - **Decreased afterload**
    Vasodilatation in sepsis
    Decreased blood viscosity (anemia)
    Increased contractility
    Hypermetabolic states
    Medication therapy

BOX 8-9   STEPS TO ENSURE ACCURATE THERMODILUTION CARDIAC OUTPUT MEASUREMENTS

- Before the procedure, assess the correct position of the PAC by verifying the waveform or measuring the PAOP.
- Enter the appropriate computation or calibration constant (per manufacturer's instruction) into the CO computer. The type and size of the PAC and the volume and temperature of the injectate solution are factors that determine this value.
- Assess the proximal port for the patency.
- Do not infuse vasoactive drugs through the port used to obtain TdCO measurements. Rapid infusion of the injectate solution for the TdCO will result in delivery of these medications beyond the recommended dosage and cause potentially harmful side effects.
- Position the patient in the supine position with the backrest elevation 0 to 30 degrees.
- Room temperature injectate is acceptable as long as there is at least a 10° F difference between the temperature of the injectate and the patient's temperature.
- Inject the solution smoothly and rapidly (within 4 seconds) at the end of expiration to reduce the impact of chest wall motion and intrathoracic pressure changes.
- Obtain three CO measurements, and calculate the average CO (a feature on the CO computer averages the measurements). Values should be within 10% of each other. Measurements outside of 10% agreement should be discarded and repeated before averaging the results.
- The first CO is usually the most variable.

PAC, Pulmonary artery catheter; *PAOP,* pulmonary artery occlusion pressure; *CO,* cardiac output; *TdCO,* thermodilution cardiac output.

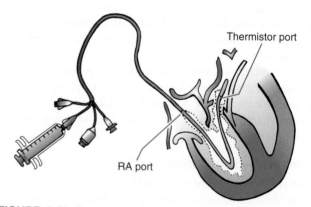

FIGURE 8-22 Illustration of injection of fluid into the right atrium (RA) for cardiac output measurement.

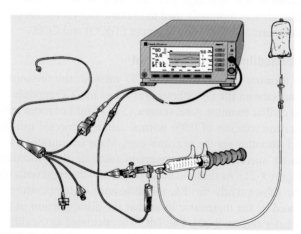

FIGURE 8-21 Illustration of the closed injectate delivery system (room temperature fluids) for thermodilution cardiac output measurement.

area under this curve. The CO is inversely proportional to the area under the curve—patients with a high CO have a low calculated area under the curve.[19] Therefore, the TdCO measurement is least accurate in patients with a low CO state and most accurate in a high CO state. Several steps must be taken to obtain accurate TdCO measurements. Box 8-9 describes these important points.

Continuous Cardiac Output

Measurement of CCO is based on the same principles as TdCO. The CCO system uses a modified PA catheter and a CO computer specific to the device. The specialized catheter has a copper filament near the distal end that delivers pulses of energy at prescribed time intervals and warms the blood in the right ventricle. This temperature change is detected by the thermistor at the tip of the catheter about every 3 to 6 seconds. The computer interprets the temperature change and averages the CO measurements over the last 60 seconds. Figure 8-23 shows an example of a computer interface for CCO and other hemodynamic parameters. CCO removes the potential for operator error associated with intermittent TdCO measurement. Other advantages of CCO are that no extra fluid is administered to the patient, data are available for trending throughout the shift, and there is no need to change the computation constant in the CO module. Patients with a CCO device can be positioned supine with the HOB elevated up to 45 degrees. Drawbacks to CCO include that the device may not accurately sense the CCO in the patient whose body temperature is greater than 40° C to 43° C, because the thermal filament heats to a maximum of 44° C. CCO does not reflect acute changes in CO. Because the measurements provide an average of CO over time, a delay may be common in detecting acute changes in CO of 1 L/min.[19]

Oxygen Delivery and Consumption

One of the key indices of adequate CO is the ability of the cardiovascular system to meet the metabolic needs of the tissues. Venous oxygen saturation is the percent of hemoglobin saturation in the central venous circulation, and provides an assessment of the amount of oxygen extracted by the tissues. Oxygenated arterial blood passes through the capillary network to deliver oxygen and nutrients to the tissues; however, not all the oxygen is used, and residual oxygen bound to the hemoglobin is returned to the central circulation to be reoxygenated. The oxygen saturation of this *mixed venous* blood from various

organs and tissues that have different metabolic needs provides a global picture of oxygen delivery and oxygen consumption. Factors that affect venous oxygen saturation include CO, hemoglobin, arterial oxygen saturation, and tissue metabolism.

Oxygen delivery and consumption can be calculated by a variety of formulas (Table 8-2). Two invasive techniques are also available for clinical determination of venous oxygen saturation: SvO_2 and central venous oxygen saturation ($ScvO_2$). SvO_2 is measured in the PA, and $ScvO_2$ is measured in the central venous system, usually the superior vena cava. Both SvO_2 and $ScvO_2$ methods use fiberoptic catheters that are connected to monitors and computers with an optical module (see Figure 8-11). Calibration of the system is done upon insertion, and if the system becomes disconnected from the optical module. To calibrate the equipment, a blood sample is obtained from either the PA (SvO_2) or central venous catheter ($ScvO_2$), and a blood gas analysis is done. Oxygen saturation results are used for calibration. Figure 8-23 shows an example of the clinical information provided by one monitoring device.

Monitoring of SvO_2 and $ScvO_2$ is indicated for any critically ill or injured patient who has the potential to develop an imbalance between oxygen delivery and demand by the tissues. Patients with trauma, acute respiratory distress syndrome, and septic shock and those undergoing complex cardiac surgery may benefit from venous oxygen saturation monitoring (SvO_2).[5]

A SvO_2 between 60% and 75% indicates an adequate balance between supply and demand. The normal range for $ScvO_2$ (65% to 85%) is slightly higher because the measurement is from the blood in the central venous circulation versus the PA.

Many nursing interventions and clinical conditions affect the SvO_2 and $ScvO_2$. Table 8-3 highlights causes for alterations

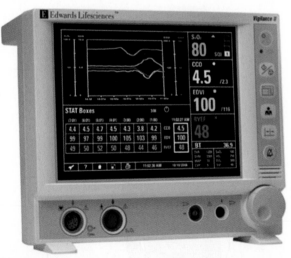

FIGURE 8-23 A sample monitor interface displaying hemodynamic parameters and trends, including continuous cardiac output (CCO) and mixed venous oxygen saturation (SvO_2). (Courtesy Edwards Lifesciences, Irvine, CA.)

TABLE 8-2	HEMODYNAMIC CALCULATIONS	
PARAMETER	**CALCULATION**	**NORMAL VALUES**
Mean arterial pressure	[Systolic BP + (2 × DBP)] ÷ 3	70-105 mm Hg
Arterial oxygen content (CaO_2)	[1.34 × Hgb (g/dL) × SaO_2] + [0.003 × PaO_2]	19-20 mL/dL
Venous oxygen content (CvO_2)	[1.34 × Hgb (g/dL) × SvO_2] + [0.003 × PvO_2]	12-15 mL/dL
Oxygen delivery (DO_2)	CO × CaO_2 × 10	900-1100 mL/min
Oxygen consumption (VO_2)	C(a-v)O_2 × CO × 10	200-250 mL/min
Oxygen extraction ratio (O_2ER)	[(CaO_2 − CvO_2)/ CaO_2] × 100	22%-30%

BP, Blood pressure; *CO*, cardiac output; *Hgb*, hemoglobin; *PaO_2*, partial pressure of arterial oxygen; *PvO_2*, partial pressure of venous oxygen; *SaO_2*, arterial oxygen saturation; *SvO_2*, mixed venous oxygen saturation.

TABLE 8-3		ALTERATIONS IN MIXED VENOUS OXYGEN SATURATION
ALTERATION	**CAUSE**	**POSSIBLE ETIOLOGY**
Low SvO₂ (<60%)	↓ O₂ delivery	Hypoxia or hemorrhage, anemic states, hypovolemia, cardiogenic shock, dysrhythmias, myocardial infarction, congestive heart failure, cardiac tamponade, massive transfusions of stored blood, restrictive lung disease, ventilation/perfusion abnormalities
	↑ O₂ consumption	Strenuous activity, fever, pain, anxiety or stress, hormonal imbalances, increased work of breathing, bathing, septic shock (late), seizures, shivering
High SvO₂ (>75%)	↑ O₂ delivery	Increase in FiO₂, hyperoxygenation
	↓ O₂ consumption	Hypothermia, anesthesia, hypothyroidism, neuromuscular blockade, early stages of sepsis
High SvO₂ (>80%)	Technical error	PA catheter in wedged position, fibrin clot at end of catheter, computer needs to be recalibrated

FiO₂, Fractional concentration of oxygen in inspired gas; *O₂*, oxygen; *PA*, pulmonary artery; *SvO₂*, mixed venous oxygen saturation.

in SvO_2 values. Any changes in arterial oxygen saturation, tissue metabolism, hemoglobin, or CO affect the values. For example, endotracheal suctioning may cause a transient decrease in the SvO_2 and $ScvO_2$ values if arterial oxygen saturation decreases during the procedure. Factors that increase the metabolic rate, such as shivering, can also lead to a dramatic decrease in SvO_2 and $ScvO_2$.

SvO_2 and $ScvO_2$ values in the normal range can be misleading to clinicians, and like all other hemodynamic parameters, they should not be assessed in isolation. Integration of clinical data is crucial to ensure good clinical decision-making. Decreased SvO_2/$ScvO_2$ values result from a failure to deliver adequate oxygen to the tissues or increased oxygen consumption. Elevated SvO_2 and $ScvO_2$ values indicate that the tissues are not using the oxygen delivered, which is related to four physiological reasons:

1. Shunting, either intravascular or intracardiac, does not allow the tissues to be exposed to the oxygen being delivered to the tissue bed.
2. A shift of the oxyhemoglobin dissociation curve to the left results in an increased affinity of hemoglobin for oxygen.
3. An increased diffusion distance between the capillaries and cells is present because of interstitial edema.
4. Inability of cells to take up or use the oxygen being delivered, or both, a frequent phenomenon in sepsis.

ADDITIONAL TECHNIQUES AND TECHNOLOGIES

Several less invasive techniques for assessment of hemodynamic status and tissue perfusion have emerged as alternatives to PA catheters. It is imperative to understand the science as well as the ability of the new technology to assist in guiding therapies to improve patient outcomes. This is an active area of research in critical care.

Esophageal Doppler Monitoring

Optimization of intravenous fluid replacement (colloid or crystalloid solutions) is essential to achieve and maintain adequate organ perfusion. Ideally, this requires measurement of blood pressure and flow. Blood pressure must be sufficient to maintain a patent vessel lumen, and blood flow must be sufficient to deliver adequate oxygen and metabolites to every cell (as well as

remove metabolic by-products such as carbon dioxide and lactate). If fluid volume is inadequate, hypovolemia, hypotension, and inadequate perfusion of end-organs such as kidneys, mesentery, and skin may occur. Conversely, excess administration of fluids may precipitate heart failure, especially in patients with underlying cardiac disease. Clinicians have struggled to find a method to evaluate and assess a patient's clinical volume status.[31]

Doppler techniques for assessing CO and function have been used extensively by cardiologists for years. The technology for bedside assessment of CO and fluid responsiveness in critically ill patients is rapidly evolving. Esophageal Doppler Monitoring (EDM) uses a thin silicone probe placed in the distal esophagus, allowing the clinician to evaluate descending aortic blood flow, which provides an immediate assessment of left ventricular performance (Figure 8-24). EDM provides real-time hemodynamic assessment. The probe is easily placed in a manner similar to an orogastric or nasogastric tube. Some patients may require a small amount of sedation to tolerate the procedure. The probe is lubricated and inserted either orally or nasally with the bevel facing upward until the depth of the catheter is approximately 35 to 40 cm. Focusing the probe entails rotating, advancing, and/or withdrawing the probe until the

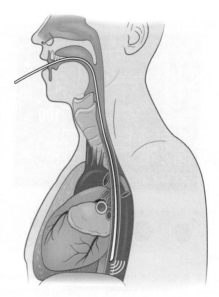

FIGURE 8-24 Esophageal Doppler probe placement. (Courtesy Deltex Medical, Inc., Branford, CT.)

BOX 8-10   ESOPHAGEAL DOPPLER MONITORING INDICATIONS AND CONTRAINDICATIONS

Indications

- States of hypoperfusion (hypovolemia, hemorrhagic shock, septic shock)
- Hemodynamic monitoring and evaluation of major end-organ dysfunction
- Differential diagnosis of hypotensive states
- As an adjunct for diagnosis and management of heart failure, cardiogenic shock, valvular dysfunction, ventricular septal rupture, cardiac rupture with tamponade
- Preoperative, intraoperative, and postoperative management of high-risk cardiac patients undergoing surgical procedures

Contraindications

- Local disease
  - Esophageal stent
  - Carcinoma of the esophagus or pharynx
  - Previous esophageal surgery
  - Esophageal stricture
  - Esophageal varices
  - Pharyngeal pouch
- Aortic abnormalities
  - Intraaortic balloon pump
  - Coarctation of the aorta
- Systemic
  - Severe coagulopathy

---

loudest sound is heard from the monitor. Box 8-10 outlines indications and contraindications for the EDM.

The EDM monitor interface (Figure 8-25) provides a variety of clinical parameters including CO and stroke volume derived from a proprietary algorithm. The corrected flow time (FTc), peak velocity (PV) and minute distance are obtained from the Doppler velocity measurements.[2,14] The base of the waveform depicts the FTc and is indicative of left ventricular preload. The height of the waveform represents peak velocity and reflects contractility. Normal FTc is 330 to 360 milliseconds. Normal peak velocity varies by age: 90 to 120 cm/sec for a 20-year-old person, 70 to 100 cm/sec for a 50-year-old person, and 50 to 80 cm/sec for a 70-year-old person.[23] An FTc of less than 330 milliseconds almost always represents an underfilled left ventricle. Critically ill patients often have maximum ventricular filling with an FTc near 400 milliseconds. Normal values are relative and do not replace physiological targets for optimization of fluid administration. Table 8-4 provides interpretation guidelines for waveform and numeric variations. Box 8-11 provides an example of a nurse-driven protocol to guide therapy and optimize ventricular filling.

The EDM technology has been demonstrated to reduce intensive care unit length of stay, hospital length of stay, and infectious complications when compared with those patients managed by invasive technologies.[8] Because EDM is minimally invasive, risks to the patient are significantly lower than those with invasive monitoring. In addition, EDM is simple to use and provides a vast amount of clinical information to guide therapy in the critical care environment.

Pulse Contour Cardiac Output Monitoring

Several devices are available that use pulse contour analysis to determine CO, stroke volume, and other hemodynamic

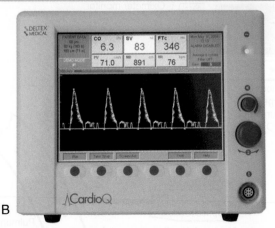

FIGURE 8-25 A, CardioQ monitoring system for assessing cardiac output and function via the esophageal Doppler probe. **B,** Numeric and graphic data provided by the CardioQ device. (Courtesy Deltex Medical, Inc., Branford, CT.)

TABLE 8-4	INTERPRETATION GUIDELINES FOR ESOPHAGEAL DOPPLER MONITORING	
WAVEFORM ALTERATION	**NUMERIC CORRELATION**	**INTERPRETATION**
↓ Base width	↓ FTc	Hypovolemia
↑ Base width	↑ FTc	Euvolemia
↓ Waveform height	↓ PV or SV	Left ventricular failure
↑ Waveform height	↑ PV or SV	Hyperdynamic state (i.e., sepsis)
↓ Waveform height + ↓ base width	↓ FTc ↓ PV or SV	Elevated systemic vascular resistance

FTc, Corrected flow time; *PV,* peak velocity; *SV,* stroke volume.

parameters. The CO derived from arterial pulse contour analysis is comparable to that obtained via PA catheter methods.[31] Current devices that use the pulse contour analysis for assessing CO include the PiCCO (PULSION Medical Systems), FloTrac (Edwards Lifesciences), and LiDCO plus systems (LiDCO Cardiac Sensor Systems).[15] These devices provide data for hemodynamic assessment and involve less risk than the PA catheter. The systems, with the exception of the PiCCO system, are generally fast to set up. They can provide stroke volume variation (SVV) and pulse pressure variation (PPV) data and are better predictors of fluid responsiveness in mechanically ventilated patients than a static measurement of RAP or PAOP[26]. The pulse contour analysis provides an alternative to the PA catheter for measuring CO, even in patients who are hemodynamically unstable. Pulse contour analysis is inaccurate in patients with significant aortic insufficiency and those with peripheral vascular disease. The use of an intra aortic balloon counterpulsation also excludes the use of this technique at present. For illustration purposes (Figure 8-26), the Vigileo system (Edwards Lifesciences) provides CCO, stroke volume (SV), SVV, and SVR data through an existing arterial line. The technology requires no manual calibration since the FloTrac algorithm automatically compensates for the continuously changing effects of vascular tone on hemodynamic parameters.[9]

The continuous measurement of SVV and PPV is only possible under full mechanical ventilation. Application of the pulse contour analysis and the derived cardiac preload parameters are limited when cardiac dysrhythmias are present. SVV and PPV are superior to the RAP and PAOP for predicting volume responsiveness.

Assessing Effect of Respiratory Variation on Hemodynamic Parameters
Right Atrial Pressure Variation
While the RAP is less predictive of responsiveness to fluid resuscitation, assessing the degree of change with respiration has the potential to be a useful indicator of responsiveness. A

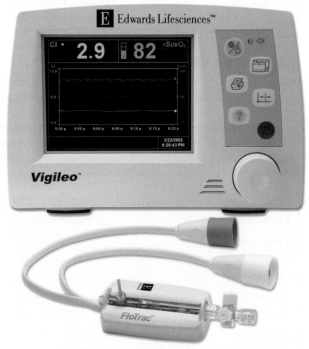

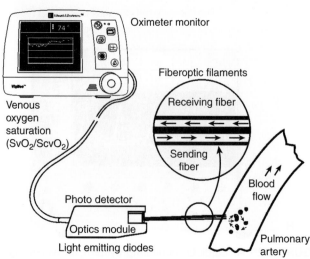

FIGURE 8-26 Vigileo. This monitor allows for the continuous monitoring of essential hemodynamic information, providing rapid insight on a minimally invasive, easy-to-use platform. (Courtesy Edwards Lifesciences, Irvine, CA.)

change (Δ) of RAP greater than 1 mm Hg with inspiration is indicative of a positive responder, whereas a Δ of RAP of less than 1 mm Hg is likely to be a nonresponder.[20,21] Assessment of variation does not require specialized equipment to evaluate (other than a central line connected to a pressure transducer) and can be used on the spontaneously breathing patient.

Systolic Pressure Variation

Patients receiving positive pressure ventilation have a decrease in stroke volume with inspiration that ultimately leads to a decrease in systolic blood pressure. The normal systolic pressure variation (ΔP) is 8 to 10 mm Hg. A ΔP of greater than 10 mm Hg is indicative of a patient who would respond to fluid resuscitation and improve tissue perfusion.[5] The limitation to this strategy is that it requires the patient to be mechanically ventilated in a strict volume control mode. In addition, the predictive capability may be affected if a patient has an alteration of the compliance in the lung or chest wall.

Arterial Pulse Pressure Variation

Arterial pulse pressure is defined as the difference between arterial systolic and diastolic pressure measurements. The arterial pulse pressure is affected by three variables: stroke volume, resistance, and compliance. Since arterial resistance and compliance do not change significantly with each breath, the variation in pulse pressure is likely due to variations in stroke volume. A pulse pressure variation of 13% or greater is believed to be predictive of a patient's ability to respond to fluid resuscitation. To be predictive, the patient must be mechanically ventilated in a controlled mode, possibly requiring deep sedation, chemical paralysis, or both. The limited studies that have been conducted used tidal volumes of 10 mL/kg, which may not be feasible or recommended for optimal mechanical ventilation. Efficacy of this strategy with lower tidal volumes (currently used in clinical practice) has not yet been demonstrated.

Stroke Volume Variation

Another potential modality for assessing volume status is analysis of the degree of variation in stroke volume. The dividing line between responders and nonresponders with regards to fluid resuscitation is a stroke volume variability of 9.5%.[5,20,21] Assessment of stroke volume variability requires the use of proprietary pulse contour analysis via an arterial line with a specialized transducer. Again, this is only predictive in the patient who is mechanically ventilated in a controlled mode. Also, dysrhythmias affect the ability to consistently quantify the degree of variability, as the dysrhythmia itself can lead to a decreased stroke volume independent of respiratory variability.

CASE STUDY

Mr. J, a 44-year-old man with no previous medical history, presents to the emergency department with a chief complaint of severe abdominal pain, fever, and chills. He is subsequently admitted to the critical care unit after an open exploratory laparotomy where it was found that he had a perforated appendix and diffuse peritonitis. Intraoperatively he had an estimated blood loss of 200 mL, and he received 2.5 L of crystalloid solution. He arrives at the critical care unit intubated and sedated with an arterial line, subclavian triple-lumen catheter, indwelling urinary catheter, and esophageal Doppler monitor in place. He is placed on mechanical ventilation with the following settings: assist/control mode at 12 breaths/min; tidal volume, 700 mL; fraction of inspired oxygen, 1.0 (100%); and positive end-expiratory pressure, 5 cm H_2O. His initial vital signs are:

Heart rate	133 beats/min
Blood pressure	88/49 mm Hg
Mean arterial pressure	62 mm Hg
Respiratory rate	12 breaths/min
Right atrial pressure	3 mm Hg
Temperature	39.2° C (102.6° F)
Flow time corrected (FTc)	250 milliseconds
Peak velocity (PV)	130 cm/sec

The provider orders administration of a 250-mL infusion of 5% albumin and to prepare to replace the triple-lumen catheter with an $ScvO_2$ catheter. You administer the albumin and assist with the placement of the $ScvO_2$ catheter. After these interventions, his vital signs are now:

Heart rate	120 beats/min
Blood pressure	94/50 mm Hg
Mean arterial pressure	65 mm Hg
Right atrial pressure	5 mm Hg
Flow time corrected (FTc)	277 milliseconds
Peak velocity (PV)	120 cm/sec
$ScvO_2$	65%

Questions

1. The 2.5 L of crystalloid solution the patient received during surgery should have provided adequate volume resuscitation. What was the rationale for the albumin bolus?
2. Discuss which hemodynamic parameters you would monitor to assess efficacy of the bolus and why.
3. What advantage would the $ScvO_2$ catheter provide over the traditional triple-lumen catheter?
4. What technical factors would you need to consider to ensure accuracy in the hemodynamic parameters that you are monitoring?
5. Discuss the significance of the $ScvO_2$ value.
6. Recently, you attended an in-service workshop on the esophageal Doppler monitoring device that your unit uses. The representative stated that the best way to evaluate preload optimization was to assess FTc before and after each intervention. He provided a journal article outlining a study that suggested that you should continue to administer boluses of albumin to the patient until you no longer see an increase in the FTc by 10% after each intervention. Given that information, what would you suggest to the provider?

SUMMARY

Hemodynamic monitoring of the critically ill patient is exciting yet challenging. It is important that the clinician remember that no single hemodynamic parameter can be used to determine volume status, contractility, or tissue perfusion. A holistic approach to patient evaluation, assessment, and treatment is vital to ensuring patient outcomes. Understanding the fundamentals of hemodynamic assessment, cardiac anatomy and physiology, and equipment function are critical in accurately evaluating and managing the critically ill or injured patient. The critical care nurse also needs to understand that although there are established normal values for the various hemodynamic parameters, it is more important to optimize a patient's tissue perfusion and clinical stability than to try to attain a normal numeric value for a particular parameter.

The development of new devices to assist in determining hemodynamic function is just the beginning of a revolution in methods for managing critically ill patients. Each new product needs to be critically reviewed and evaluated for efficacy and the ability to impact length of stay and patient outcomes before being applied to the general population. No single instrument will ever replace the vigilant clinician with strong assessment skills and the ability to critically think and put the clinical puzzle pieces together at the bedside.

CRITICAL THINKING EXERCISES

1. How does stroke volume affect CO?
2. Describe how CO affects the delivery of oxygen to tissues. What parameters would be the best to monitor in a patient to assess this influence?
3. If a patient's mean arterial pressure continues to rise significantly, indicating an increase in resistance and an altered ability of the heart to eject blood, what parameters would also be affected as a result?
4. A patient who has undergone surgery has received a bed bath with back care and then undergoes suctioning and is turned. During these care activities, the patient experiences pain. What consequences does this pain have on the patient's SvO_2 status?
5. A patient is bleeding significantly and receives a transfusion of packed red blood cells. You note that the PAOP remains low, and the CI drops again. What is the significance of these alterations? What additional interventions would you expect?

REFERENCES

1. American Association of Critical-Care Nurses. *Practice alert: pulmonary artery/central venous pressure measurement.* Available at http://www.aacn.org/WD/Practice/Docs/PracticeAlerts/PAP_Measurement_05-2004.pdf; 2009. Accessed December 5, 2011.
2. Archer TL, Funk DJ, Moretti E, et al. Stroke volume calculation by esophageal Doppler integrates velocity over time and multiplies this "area under the curve" by the cross sectional area of the aorta. *Anesthesia Analgesia.* 2009;109(3):996.
3. Barone JE, Madlinger RV. Should an Allen test be performed before radial artery cannulation? *Journal of Trauma.* 2006; 61(2):468-470.
4. Becker DE. Arterial catheter insertion (perform). In: Wiegand DLM, ed. *AACN Procedure Manual for Critical Care*, 6th ed, pp. 527-533. Philadelphia: Elsevier/Saunders; 2011.
5. Bridges EJ. Pulmonary artery pressure monitoring: when, how, and what else to use. *AACN Advanced Critical Care.* 2006; 17(3):286-303.
6. Centers for Disease Control and Prevention. Vital signs: central line-associated bloodstream infections-United States, 2001, 2008, and 2009. *Annals of Emergency Medicine.* 2011;58(5): 447-450.
7. Chernecky CC, Berger BJ. *Laboratory Tests and Diagnostic Procedures*, 5th ed. Philadelphia: Saunders; 2008.
8. Chytra I, Pradl R, Bosman R, et al. Esophageal Doppler-guided fluid management decreases blood lactate levels in multiple-trauma patients: a randomized controlled trial. *Critical Care.* 2007;11(1):R24.
9. Compton FD, Zukunft B, Hoffmann C, et al. Performance of a minimally invasive uncalibrated cardiac output monitoring system (Flotrac/Vigileo) in haemodynamically unstable patients. *British Journal of Anaesthesia.* 2008;100(4):451-456.
10. Darovic GO. *Handbook of hemodynamic monitoring*, 2nd ed. Philadelphia: Saunders; 2004.
11. Fleck DA. Pulmonary artery catheter insertion (perform). In: Wiegand DLM, ed. *AACN Procedure Manual for Critical Care*, 6th ed., pp. 617-625). Philadelphia: Elsevier/Saunders; 2011.
12. Garnacho-Montero J, Aldabó-Pallás T, Palomar-Martínez M, et al. Risk factors and prognosis of catheter-related bloodstream infection in critically ill patients: a multicenter study. *Intensive Care Medicine.* 2008;34(12):2185-2193.
13. Gurgel ST, do Nascimento P Jr. Maintaining tissue perfusion in high-risk surgical patients: a systematic review of randomized clinical trials. *Anesthesia Analgesia.* 2010;112(6):1384-1391.
14. Hadian M, Angus DC. Protocolized resuscitation with esophageal Doppler monitoring may improve outcome in post-cardiac surgery patients. *Critical Care.* 2005;9(4):E7.
15. Hadian M, Kim HK, Severyn DA, et al. Cross-comparison of cardiac output trending accuracy of LiDCO, PiCCO, FloTrac and pulmonary artery catheters. *Critical Care.* 2006;14(6):R212.
16. Hall JE. *Guyton and Hall Textbook of Medical Physiology*, 12th ed. Philadelphia: Saunders; 2011.
17. Harvey S, Young D, Brampton W, et al. Pulmonary artery catheters for adult patients in intensive care. *Cochrane Database of Systematic Reviews.* 2006;3:CD003408.

18. Jansen TC, van Bommel J, Schoonderbeek FJ, et al. Early lactate-guided therapy in intensive care unit patients: a multi-center, open-label, randomized controlled trial. *American Journal of Respiratory and Critical Care Medicine.* 2010;182(6):752-761.

19. Klein DG. Cardiac output measurement techniques (invasive). In: Wiegand DLM, ed. *AACN Procedure Manual for Critical Care*, 6th ed., pp. 577-594. Philadelphia: Elsevier/Saunders; 2011.

20. Marik PE, Baram M, Vahid B. Does central venous pressure predict fluid responsiveness? A systematic review of the literature and the tale of seven mares. *Chest.* 2008;134(1):172-178.

21. Marik PE, Cavallazzi R, Vasu T, et al. Dynamic changes in arterial waveform derived variables and fluid responsiveness in mechanically ventilated patients: a systematic review of the literature. *Critical Care Medicine.* 2009;37(9):2642-2647.

22. McCance KL, Huether SE. *Pathophysiology: the Biological Basis for Disease in Adults and Children*, 6th ed. St. Louis: Mosby; 2010.

23. McKendry M, McGloin H, Saberi D, et al. Randomised controlled trial assessing the impact of a nurse delivered, flow monitored protocol for optimisation of circulatory status after cardiac surgery. *British Medical Journal.* 2004;329(7460):258.

24. Meyer J. A broad-spectrum look at catheter-related bloodstream infections: many aspects, many populations. *Journal of Infusion Nursing.* 2009;32(2):80-86.

25. Pasion E, Good L, Tizon J, et al. Evaluation of the monitor cursor-line method for measuring pulmonary artery and central venous pressures. *American Journal of Critical Care.* 2010;19(6):511-521.

26. Peyton PJ, Chong SW. Minimally invasive measurement of cardiac output during surgery and critical care: a meta-analysis of accuracy and precision. *Anesthesiology.* 2010;113(5):1220-1235.

27. Preuss T, Wiegand DLM. Pulmonary artery catheter and pressure lines, troubleshooting. In: Wiegand DLM, ed. *AACN Procedure Manual for Critical Care*, 6th ed., pp. 655-669. Philadelphia: Elsevier/Saunders; 2011a.

28. Preuss T, Wiegand DLM. Pulmonary artery catheter insertion (assist) and pressure monitoring. In: Wiegand DLM, ed. *AACN Procedure Manual for Critical Care*, 6th ed., pp. 626-647. Philadelphia: Elsevier/Saunders; 2011b.

29. Preuss T, Wiegand DLM. Single-pressure and multiple-pressure transducer systems. In: Wiegand DLM, ed. *AACN Procedure Manual for Critical Care*, 6th ed. Philadelphia: Elsevier/Saunders; 2011.

30. Rauen CA, Makic MB, Bridges E. Evidence-based practice habits: transforming research into bedside practice. *Critical Care Nurse.* 2009;29(2):46-59.

31. Rhodes A, Grounds RM, Bennett ED. Hemodynamic monitoring. In: Vincent JL, Abraham E, Moore FA, Kochanek PM, Fink M, eds. *Textbook of Critical Care*, 6th ed., pp. 533-537. Philadelphia: Elsevier/Saunders; 2011.

32. Shaffer R. Arterial catheter insertion (assist), care, and removal. In: Wiegand DLM, ed. *AACN Procedure Manual for Critical Care*, 6th ed., pp. 534-546. Philadelphia: Elsevier/Saunders; 2011.

33. Shah MR, Hasselblad V, Stevenson LW, et al. Impact of the pulmonary artery catheter in critically ill patients: meta-analysis of randomized clinical trials. *Journal of the American Medical Association.* 2005;294(13):1664-1670.

34. Stover JF, Stocker R, Lenherr R, et al. Noninvasive cardiac output and blood pressure monitoring cannot replace an invasive monitoring system in critically ill patients. *BMC Anesthesiology.* 2009;9:6.

35. Swan HJ, Ganz W, Forrester J, et al. Catheterization of the heart in man with use of a flow-directed balloon-tipped catheter. *New England Journal of Medicine.* 1970;283(9):447-451.

36. Westhrope RB. Blood pressure monitoring: automated non-invasive blood pressure monitors. *Anaesthesia and Intensive Care.* 2009;37(3):343.

Ventilatory Assistance

Lynelle N. B. Pierce, MSN, RN, CCRN

Evolve WEBSITE

Many additional resources, including self-assessment exercises, are located on the Evolve companion website at http://evolve.elsevier.com/Sole.

- Review Questions
- Mosby's Nursing Skills Procedures
- Animations
- Video Clips

INTRODUCTION

Essential nursing interventions for all patients include maintaining an adequate airway, and ensuring adequate breathing (ventilation) and oxygenation. These nursing interventions provide the framework for this chapter. Respiratory anatomy and physiology are reviewed to provide a basis for discussing ventilatory assistance. Assessment of the respiratory system includes physical examination, arterial blood gas (ABG) interpretation, and noninvasive methods for assessing gas exchange. Airway management, oxygen therapy, and mechanical ventilation, important therapies in the critical care unit, are also discussed.

REVIEW OF RESPIRATORY ANATOMY AND PHYSIOLOGY

The primary function of the respiratory system is gas exchange. Oxygen and carbon dioxide are exchanged via the respiratory system to provide adequate oxygen to the cells and to remove carbon dioxide, the by-product of metabolism, from the cells. The respiratory system is divided into (1) the upper airway, (2) the lower airway, and (3) the lungs.[49] The upper airway conducts gas to and from the lower airway, and the lower airway provides gas exchange at the alveolar-capillary membrane. The anatomical structure of the respiratory system is shown in Figure 9-1.

Upper Airway

The upper airway consists of the nasal cavity and the pharynx. The nasal cavity conducts air, filters large foreign particles, and warms and humidifies air. When an artificial airway is placed, these natural functions of the airway are bypassed. The nasal cavity also is responsible for voice resonance, smell, and sneeze reflexes. The throat, or pharynx, transports both air and food.

Lower Airway

The lower airway consists of the larynx, trachea, right and left mainstem bronchi, bronchioles, and alveoli. The larynx is the narrowest part of the conducting airways in adults and contains the vocal cords. The larynx is partly covered by the epiglottis, which prevents aspiration of food, liquid, or saliva into the lungs during swallowing. The passage through the vocal cords is the glottis (Figure 9-2).

The trachea warms, humidifies, and filters air. Cilia in the trachea propel mucus and foreign material upward through the airway. At about the level of the fifth thoracic vertebra (sternal angle, or angle of Louis), the trachea branches into the right and left mainstem bronchi, which conduct air to the respective lungs. This bifurcation is referred to as the *carina*. The right mainstem bronchus is shorter, wider, and straighter than the left. The bronchi further branch into the bronchioles and finally the terminal bronchioles, which supply air to the alveoli. Mucosal cells in the bronchi secrete mucus that lubricates the airway and traps foreign materials, which are moved by the cilia upward to be expectorated or swallowed.

The alveoli are the distal airway structures and are responsible for gas exchange at the capillary level. The alveoli consist of a single layer of epithelial cells and fibers that permit expansion and contraction. The type II cells inside the alveolus secrete surfactant, which coats the inner surface and prevents it from collapsing. A network of pulmonary capillaries covers

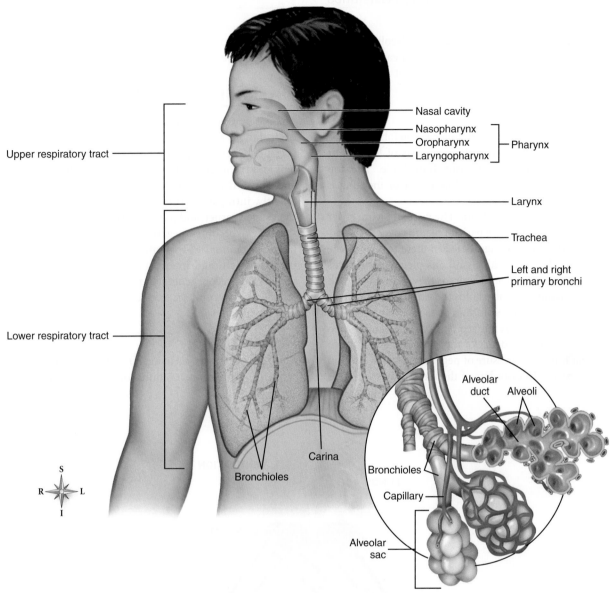

FIGURE 9-1 Anatomy of the upper and lower respiratory tracts. The inset shows the grapelike clusters of alveoli and their rich blood supply, which supports the exchange of oxygen and carbon dioxide. (From Patton KT and Thibodeau GA. *Anatomy and Physiology.* 7th ed. St. Louis: Mosby; 2010.)

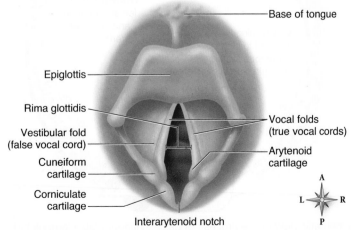

FIGURE 9-2 The vocal cords and glottis. (From Patton KT, Thibodeau GS. *Anatomy and Physiology.* 7th ed. St. Louis: Mosby; 2010.)

the alveoli. Gas exchange occurs between the alveoli and these capillaries.[49,61] The large combined surface area and single cell layer of the alveoli promote very efficient diffusion of gases.

Lungs

The lungs consist of lobes; the left lung has two lobes, and the right lung has three lobes. Each lobe consists of lobules, or segments, that are supplied by one bronchiole. The top of each lung is the apex, and the lower part of the lung is the base.

The lungs are covered by pleura. The visceral pleura cover the lung surfaces, whereas the parietal pleura cover the internal surface of the thoracic cage. Between these two layers the pleural space is formed, which contains pleural fluid. This thin fluid lubricates the pleural layers as they slide across each other during breathing. It also holds the two pleurae together because it creates surface tension, an attractive force between liquid molecules. It is this surface tension between the two pleurae, opposing the tendency of the elastic lung to want to collapse, that leads to a pressure of negative 5 cm H_2O within the pleural space.[27] In disorders of the pleural space, such as pneumothorax, this negative pressure is disrupted, leading to collapse of the lung and the need for a chest tube.

PHYSIOLOGY OF BREATHING

The basic principle behind the movement of gas in and out of the lung is that gas travels from an area of higher to lower pressure. During inspiration, the diaphragm lowers and flattens and the intercostal muscles contract, lifting the chest up and outward to increase the size of the chest cavity. Subsequently, intrapleural pressure becomes even more negative than stated earlier, and intraalveolar pressure (the pressure in the lungs) becomes negative, causing air to flow into the lungs *(inspiration)*.[27] Expiration is a passive process in which the diaphragm and intercostal muscles relax and the lungs recoil. This recoil generates positive intraalveolar pressure relative to atmospheric pressure, and air flows out of the lungs *(expiration)*.[69]

Gas Exchange

The process of gas exchange (Figure 9-3) consists of four steps: (1) ventilation, (2) diffusion at pulmonary capillaries,

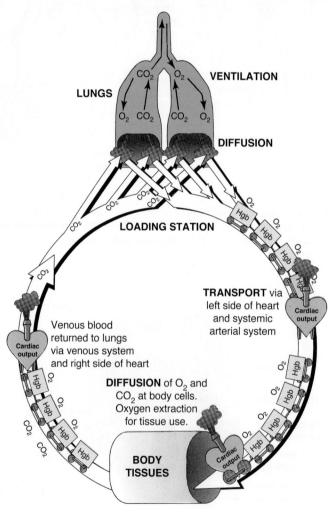

FIGURE 9-3 Schematic view of the process of gas exchange. *Hgb,* Hemoglobin. (Modified from Alspach J. *AACN Instructor's Resource Manual for AACN Core Curriculum for Critical Care Nursing.* 4th ed. Philadelphia: Saunders; 1992.)

(3) perfusion (transportation), and (4) diffusion to the cells.[27,69,70]

1. Ventilation is the movement of gases (oxygen and carbon dioxide) in and out of the alveoli.
2. Diffusion of oxygen and carbon dioxide occurs at the alveolar-capillary membrane (Figure 9-4). The driving force to move the gas from the alveoli to the capillary and vice versa is the pressure of the gases across the alveolar-capillary membrane. Diffusion is the movement of gas molecules from an area of higher to lower pressure. Oxygen pressure is higher in the alveoli than in the capillaries, thus promoting oxygen diffusion from the alveoli into the blood. Carbon dioxide pressure is higher in the capillaries, thus promoting the diffusion of carbon dioxide into the alveoli for elimination during exhalation.
3. The oxygenated blood in the pulmonary capillary is transported via the pulmonary vein to the left side of the heart. The oxygenated blood is perfused and transported to the tissues.
4. Diffusion of oxygen and carbon dioxide occurs at the cellular level based on pressure gradients. Oxygen diffuses from blood into the cells, and carbon dioxide leaves the cells and diffuses into the blood in a process called internal

respiration. Carbon dioxide is transported via the vena cava to the right side of the heart and into the pulmonary capillaries where it diffuses into the alveoli and is eliminated through exhalation.

Regulation of Breathing

The rate, depth, and rhythm of ventilation are controlled by respiratory centers in the medulla and pons. When the carbon dioxide level is high or the oxygen level is low, chemoreceptors in the respiratory center, carotid arteries, and aorta send messages to the medulla to regulate respiration. In persons with normal lung function, high levels of carbon dioxide stimulate respiration. However, patients with chronic obstructive pulmonary disease (COPD) maintain higher levels of carbon dioxide as a baseline, and their ventilatory drive in response to increased carbon dioxide levels is blunted. In these patients, the stimulus to breathe is hypoxemia, a low level of oxygen in the blood.[27]

Respiratory Mechanics
Work of Breathing

The work of breathing (WOB) is the amount of effort required for the maintenance of a given level of ventilation. When the lungs are not diseased, the respiratory muscles manage the WOB using unlabored respirations. The respiratory pattern changes automatically to manage an increased WOB when lung disease is present, and the patient may use accessory muscles. As the WOB increases, more energy must be expended to obtain adequate ventilation, which requires proportionately more oxygen and glucose. If the WOB becomes too high, respiratory failure ensues and mechanical ventilatory support is warranted.[51,53]

Compliance

Compliance is a measure of the distensibility, or stretchability, of the lung and chest wall. The lungs are primarily made up of elastin and collagen fibers that in disease states become less elastic, leading to so-called stiff lungs. *Distensibility* refers to how easily the lung is stretched when the respiratory muscles work and expand the thoracic cavity. Compliance, a clinical measurement of the lung's distensibility, is defined as the change in lung volume per unit of pressure change.[51,69]

Various pathological conditions such as pulmonary fibrosis, acute respiratory distress syndrome (ARDS), and pulmonary edema lead to low pulmonary compliance. In these situations, the patient must generate more work to breathe to create negative pressure to inflate the stiff lungs. Compliance is also decreased in obesity secondary to the increased mass of the chest wall.

In emphysema, destruction of lung tissue and enlarged air spaces cause the lungs to lose their elasticity, which increases compliance. The lungs are more distensible in this situation, require lower pressures for ventilation, and may collapse during expiration, causing air to become trapped in the distal airways.

Monitoring changes in compliance provides an objective clinical indicator of changes in the patient's lung condition

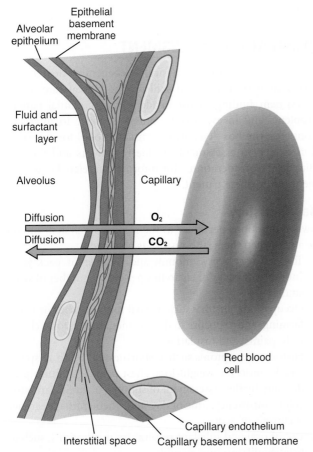

FIGURE 9-4 Diffusion of oxygen and carbon dioxide at the alveolar-capillary membrane. (From Hall JE, Guyton AC. *Guyton and Hall Textbook of Medical Physiology.* 12th ed. Philadelphia: Saunders; 2011.)

and ability to ventilate, especially the mechanically ventilated patient with decreased lung compliance. Compliance of the lung tissue is best measured under static conditions (no airflow), and is achieved by instituting a 2-second inspiratory hold maneuver with the mechanical ventilator.[51,53] Static compliance in patients with normal lungs usually ranges from 50 to 170 mL/cm H_2O.[69] This means that for every 1-cm H_2O change of pressure in the lungs, the volume of gas increases by 50 to 170 mL. A single measurement of compliance is not useful in monitoring patient progress; it is important to trend compliance over time.

Dynamic compliance is measured while gases are flowing during breathing; it measures not only lung compliance but also airway resistance to gas flow. The normal value for dynamic compliance is 50 to 80 mL/cm H_2O.[69] Dynamic compliance is easier to measure because it does not require breath holding or an inspiratory hold; however, it is not a pure measurement of lung compliance. A decrease in dynamic compliance may signify a decrease in compliance or an increase in resistance to gas flow.

The respiratory therapist (RT) or nurse measures compliance in the mechanically ventilated patient to identify trends in the patient's condition. Compliance can easily be obtained on most modern ventilators when the operator requests it using the menu options. Poor compliance requires higher ventilatory pressures to achieve adequate lung volume. Higher ventilatory pressures place the patient at increased risk for complications, such as volutrauma.

Resistance

Resistance refers to the opposition to the flow of gases in the airways. Factors that affect airway resistance are airway length, airway diameter, and the flow rate of gases. Airway resistance is increased when the airway is lengthened or narrowed, as with an artificial airway, or when the natural airway is narrowed by spasms (bronchoconstriction), the presence of mucus, or edema. Finally, resistance increases when gas flow is increased, as with increased breathing effort or when a patient requires mechanical ventilation. When resistance increases, more effort is required by the patient to maintain gas flow. If the patient is unable to generate the increased WOB, the amount of gas flow the patient produces decreases. Thus increasing airway resistance may result in reduced lung volume and inadequate ventilation.[27,69]

LUNG VOLUMES AND CAPACITIES

Air volume within the lung is measured with an instrument called a *spirometer*. Lung volumes and capacities (two or more lung volumes added together) are important for determining adequate pulmonary function, and are shown graphically in Figure 9-5. Descriptions of the lung volumes and capacities are provided in Table 9-1. Measurements of lung volumes and capacities allow the practitioner to assess baseline pulmonary function and to monitor the improvement or progression of pulmonary diseases and patient response to therapy. For example, when the patient performs incentive

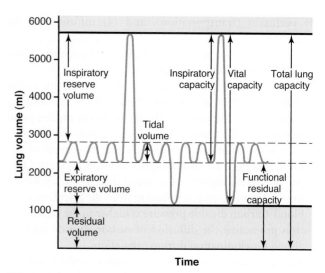

FIGURE 9-5 Lung volumes and capacities. (From Hall JE, Guyton AC. *Guyton and Hall Textbook of Medical Physiology* 12th ed. Philadelphia: Saunders; 2011.)

spirometry, the nurse and RT assess the patient's inspiratory capacity and trend its improvement or decline over time and with interventions. Lung capacities decline gradually with aging.

RESPIRATORY ASSESSMENT

The ability to perform a physical assessment of the respiratory system is an essential skill for the critical care nurse. Assessment findings assist in identifying potential patient problems and in evaluating patient response to interventions. See the box "Geriatric Considerations" for information related to assessment of elderly patients and the box "Bariatric Considerations" for information related to assessment of the obese patient.

Health History

Several questions pertinent to the respiratory system should be asked when the health history is obtained:

1. Tobacco use: type, amount, and number of pack-years (number of packs of cigarettes per day × number of years smoking)
2. Occupational history such as coal mining, asbestos work, farming, and exposure to dust, fumes, smoke, toxic chemicals, paints, and insulation
3. History of symptoms such as shortness of breath, dyspnea, cough, anorexia, weight loss, chest pain, or sputum production; further assessment of sputum, including amount, color, consistency, time of day, and whether its appearance is chronic or acute
4. Use of oral and inhalant respiratory medications, such as bronchodilators and steroids
5. Use of over-the-counter or street inhalant drugs
6. Allergies: medication, food, or environmental
7. Dates of last chest radiograph and tuberculosis screening

TABLE 9-1   LUNG VOLUMES AND CAPACITIES

NAME	DEFINITION	AVERAGE	FORMULA
Volumes*			
Tidal volume (V_T)	Volume of a normal breath	500 mL	
Inspiratory reserve volume (IRV)	Maximum amount of gas that can be inspired at the end of a normal breath (over and above the V_T)	3000 mL	
Expiratory reserve volume (ERV)	Maximum amount of gas that can be forcefully expired at the end of a normal breath	1200 mL	
Residual volume (RV)	Amount of air remaining in the lungs after maximum expiration	1300 mL	
Capacities			
Inspiratory capacity (IC)	Maximum volume of gas that can be inspired at normal resting expiration; the IC distends the lungs to their maximum amount	3500 mL	$IC = V_T + IRV$
Functional residual capacity (FRC)	Volume of gas remaining in the lungs at normal resting expiration	2500 mL	$FRC = ERV + RV$
Vital capacity (VC)	Maximum volume of gas that can be forcefully expired after maximum inspiration	4700 mL	$VC = V_T + IRV + ERV$
Total lung capacity (TLC)	Volume of gas in the lungs at end of maximum inspiration	6000 mL	$TLC = V_T + ERV + RV$

*Volumes are average in a 70-kg young adult. There is a range of normal values that varies by age, height, body size, and gender. Volumes are less in women than men when height and age are equal.

GERIATRIC CONSIDERATIONS

Physiological Changes with Aging
- ↓ Chest wall distensibility (costal cartilage calcifies)
- ↓ Alveolar surface area (enlarged alveoli)
- ↓ Alveolar elasticity
- ↓ Lung volume
- ↓ Diffusing capacity
- ↓ Physiological compensatory mechanisms in response to hypercapnea or hypoxia
- Weaker respiratory muscles
- Decreased cough and gag

Assessment Changes
Normal Findings Because of Aging Process
- Kyphosis
- Barrel chest
- ↓ Chest expansion
- Lower PaO_2 levels on ABG

Increased Risk for
- Secretion retention and pneumonia
- Poor gas exchange
- Mental status changes as an early sign of gas exchange problems
- Aspiration
- Respiratory distress
- Respiratory failure

ABG, Arterial blood gas; *PaO2*, partial pressure of oxygen in arterial blood.
Data from Miller CA. (2012). Respiratory function. In CA Miller (Ed.) *Nursing for Wellness in Older Adults*, 6th ed. Philadelphia: Lippincott, Williams & Wilkins; West JB. (2011). *Respiratory Physiology: The Essentials* (9th ed.). Baltimore, MD: Lippincott Williams & Wilkins.

BARIATRIC CONSIDERATIONS

Physiological Changes with Obesity
- Diaphragm is cephaloid-displaced, especially in the supine position, resulting in ↓ lung volumes
- Collapse of small airways and alveoli
- Decreased lung compliance and increased airway resistance
- Fatty infiltration of respiratory muscles
- Increased oxygen consumption to perform the work of breathing due to increased mass of thorax
- Increased fat distribution within the soft tissue of the airway
- Increased fat distribution in the neck, causing redundant skin folds

Assessment Changes Related to Obesity
- Increased respiratory rate
- Decreased breath sounds
- ↓ Chest expansion
- Snoring
- Dyspnea at rest or with talking
- Lower PaO_2 levels on ABG
- Decreased quality of portable CXR

Increased Risk for
- Atelectasis
- Poor gas exchange
- Respiratory distress
- Respiratory failure
- Obesity hypoventilation syndrome (OHS), also known as obstructive sleep apnea
- Difficult intubation
- Difficult ventilation with a bag-valve-mask device
- Complications related to tracheostomy

ABG, Arterial blood gas; *CXR,* chest x-ray; *PaO₂,* partial pressure of oxygen in arterial blood.
From Siela D, (2009). Pulmonary aspects of obesity in critical care. *Critical Care Nursing Clinics of North America,* 21(3), 301-310.

Physical Examination
Inspection

Inspection provides an initial clue for potential acute and chronic respiratory problems. The head, neck, fingers, and chest are inspected for abnormalities.

The chest is observed for shape, breathing pattern, and chest excursion. During inspiration, chest wall excursion should be symmetrical. Asymmetrical excursion is usually associated with unilateral ventilation problems. The trachea is normally in a midline position; a tracheal shift may occur with a tension pneumothorax. Signs of acute respiratory distress include labored respirations, irregular breathing pattern, use of accessory muscles, asymmetrical chest movements, chest-abdominal asynchrony, open-mouthed breathing, or gasping breaths. Cyanosis is a late sign of hypoxemia and should not be relied on as an early warning of distress. Other indications

Cheyne-Stokes Respirations gradually increase in depth, then become more shallow; followed by a period of apnea

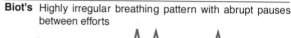

Biot's Highly irregular breathing pattern with abrupt pauses between efforts

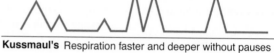

Kussmaul's Respiration faster and deeper without pauses

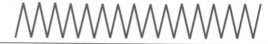

Apneustic Respirations prolonged, gasping, followed by extremely short, inefficient expiration

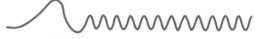

FIGURE 9-6 Breathing patterns.

of respiratory abnormalities include pallor or rubor, pursed-lip breathing, jugular venous distention, prolonged expiratory phase of breaths, poor capillary refill, clubbing of fingers, and a barrel-shaped chest.[68]

The respiratory rate (RR) should be counted for a full minute in critically ill patients. The normal RR is 12 to 20 breaths per minute, and expiration is usually twice as long as inspiration (inspiration-to-expiration ratio is 1:2). The normal breathing pattern is regular and even with an occasional sigh, and is called *eupnea. Tachypnea,* a RR of greater than 20 breaths per minute, may occur with anxiety, fever, pain, anemia, low PaO_2, and elevated $PaCO_2$. *Bradypnea,* a RR of less than 10 breaths per minute may occur in central nervous system disorders including administration or ingestion of central nervous system depressant medications or alcohol, severe metabolic alkalosis, and fatigue. The depth of respirations is as important as the rate and provides information about the adequacy of ventilation. Alterations from normal rate and depth should be documented and reported.

Several abnormal breathing patterns (Figure 9-6) are possible and should be reported.[68] *Cheyne-Stokes respirations* have a cyclical respiratory pattern. Deep, increasingly shallow respirations are followed by a period of apnea that lasts approximately 20 seconds, but the period may vary and progressively lengthen. Therefore, the duration of the apneic period is timed for trending. The cycle repeats after each apneic period. Cheyne-Stokes respirations may occur in central nervous system disorders and congestive heart failure. *Biot's respirations,* or cluster breathing, are cycles of breaths that vary in depth and have varying periods of apnea. Biot's respirations are seen with brainstem injury. *Kussmaul's respirations* are deep, regular, and rapid (usually more than 20 breaths per minute), and are commonly observed in diabetic ketoacidosis and other disorders that cause metabolic acidosis. *Apneustic respirations* are gasping inspirations followed by short, ineffective expirations. They are often associated with lesions to the pons.

Palpation

Palpation is frequently performed simultaneously with inspection. Palpation is used to evaluate chest wall excursion, tracheal deviation, chest wall tenderness, subcutaneous crepitus, and tactile fremitus. The chest wall should not be tender to palpation; tenderness is usually associated with inflammation or trauma, including rib fractures. *Subcutaneous crepitus* or *subcutaneous emphysema* is the presence of air beneath the skin surface that has escaped from the airways or lungs. It is palpated with the fingertips and may feel like crunching Rice Krispies under the skin. The temptation to further palpate should be resisted, because palpation promotes air dissection in the skin layers. Subcutaneous air may result from chest trauma, such as rib fractures, and from barotrauma. It indicates that the lungs or airways are not intact.

Percussion

The chest may be percussed to identify respiratory disorders such as hemothorax, pneumothorax, and consolidation. In percussion, the middle finger of one hand is tapped twice by the middle finger of the opposite hand placed against the patient's chest. The vibrations produced by tapping create different sounds, depending on the density of the underlying tissue being percussed. Five sounds may be audible on percussion: resonance (normal), dullness (tissue more dense than normal as in consolidation), flatness (absence of air as in lung collapse), hyperresonance (increased amount of air as in emphysema), and tympany (large amount of air as in pneumothorax).[68]

Auscultation

Lung sounds are routinely assessed every 4 hours in critically ill patients using the diaphragm of the stethoscope pressed firmly against the chest wall. The stethoscope should be placed directly on the patient's chest; sounds are difficult to distinguish if they are auscultated through the patient's gown or clothing. The friction of chest hair on the stethoscope may mimic the sound of crackles; wetting the chest hair may reduce this sound. In addition, the stethoscope tubing should not rest against skin or objects such as sheets, bed rails, or ventilator circuitry during auscultation.[51]

A systematic sequence should be used during auscultation, with sounds from one side of the chest wall compared with those from the other (Figure 9-7). Auscultation is best performed with the patient sitting in an upright position and breathing deeply in and out through the mouth. It may not be feasible for a critically ill patient to assume a sitting position for auscultation. In this circumstance, auscultation of the anterior and lateral chest is often performed. However, every opportunity should be taken to turn the patient and auscultate the chest posteriorly. When the patient has an artificial airway, the trachea should be auscultated for the presence of an air leak.

Breath Sounds

The nurse listens carefully for both normal and abnormal, or *adventitious,* breath sounds. Types of normal breath sounds include bronchial (larynx, trachea), bronchovesicular (large central airways), and vesicular (smaller airways). Adventitious sounds the nurse must be familiar with and able to report include crackles, rhonchi, wheezes, pleural friction rub, and stridor (Table 9-2). Breath sounds may be decreased because of the presence of fluid, air, or increased tissue density. Shallow respirations can also mimic decreased breath

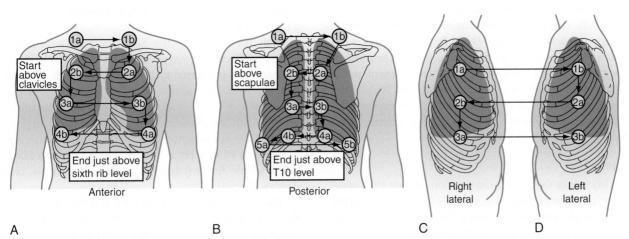

FIGURE 9-7 Systematic method for palpation, percussion, and auscultation of the lungs in anterior **(A)**, posterior **(B)**, and lateral regions **(C** and **D)**. The techniques should be performed systematically to compare right and left lung fields.

TABLE 9-2   ADVENTITIOUS BREATH SOUNDS

SOUND/DESCRIPTION	CAUSE	CLINICAL SIGNIFICANCE	ADDITIONAL DESCRIPTORS/ COMMENTS
Crackles—discontinuous, explosive, bubbling sounds of short duration	Air bubbling through fluid or mucus, or alveoli popping open on inspiration	Atelectasis, fluid retention in small airways (pulmonary edema), retention of mucus (bronchitis, pneumonia), interstitial fibrosis	Fine: soft, short duration Coarse: loud, longer duration Wet or dry May disappear after coughing, suctioning, or deep inspiration if alveoli remain inflated
Rhonchi—coarse, continuous, low-pitched, sonorous, or rattling sound	Air movement through excess mucus, fluid, or inflamed airways	Diseases resulting in airway inflammation and excess mucus (e.g., pneumonia, bronchitis, or excess fluid, as in pulmonary edema)	Inspiratory and/or expiratory; may clear or diminish with coughing if caused by airway secretions
Wheezes—high- or low-pitched whistling, musical sound heard during inspiration and/or expiration	Air movement through narrowed airway, which causes airway wall to oscillate or flutter	Bronchospasm, as in asthma, partial airway obstruction by tumor, foreign body or secretions, inflammation, or stenosis	High or low pitched; inspiratory and/or expiratory
Stridor—high-pitched, continuous sound heard over upper airway; a crowing sound	Air flowing through constricted larynx or trachea	Partial obstruction of upper airway, as in laryngeal edema, obstruction by foreign body, epiglottitis	Potentially life-threatening
Pleural friction rub—coarse, grating, squeaking, or scratching sound, as when two pieces of leather rub together	Inflamed pleura rubbing against each other	Pleural inflammation, as in pleuritis, pneumonia, tuberculosis, chest tube insertion, pulmonary infarction	Occurs during breathing cycle and is eliminated by breath holding Need to discern from pericardial friction rub, which continues despite breath holding

sounds; therefore the patient must take deep breaths during auscultation. The breath sounds should be carefully documented and abnormalities reported.

Arterial Blood Gas Interpretation

The ability to interpret ABG results rapidly is an essential critical care skill. ABG results reflect oxygenation, adequacy of gas exchange, and acid-base status. Blood for ABG analysis is obtained from either a direct arterial puncture (radial, brachial, or femoral artery) or an arterial line. ABGs aid in patient assessment and must be interpreted in conjunction with the patient's physical assessment findings, clinical history, and previous ABG values (Table 9-3). Noninvasive measures of gas exchange have reduced the frequency of ABG measurements.

Oxygenation

The ABG values that reflect oxygenation include the partial pressure of oxygen dissolved in arterial blood (PaO_2) and the arterial oxygen saturation of hemoglobin (SaO_2). Approximately 3% of the available oxygen is dissolved in plasma. The remaining 97% of the oxygen attaches to hemoglobin in red blood cells, forming oxyhemoglobin.[69]

Partial pressure of arterial oxygen. The normal PaO_2 is 80 to 100 mm Hg at sea level. The PaO_2 decreases in the elderly; the value for persons 60 to 80 years of age usually ranges from 60 to 80 mm Hg.

Arterial oxygen saturation of hemoglobin. The SaO_2 is the percentage of hemoglobin saturated with oxygen and is normally 92% to 99%. The SaO_2 is very important because it represents the primary way oxygen is transported to the tissues. The SaO_2 is measured directly from an arterial blood sample or continuously monitored indirectly with the use of a pulse oximeter (SpO_2).

Both the PaO_2 and the SaO_2 are used to assess oxygenation. Decreased oxygenation of arterial blood (PaO_2 <60 mm Hg) is referred to as *hypoxemia*, which may present with numerous symptoms described in Box 9-1. A patient with a PaO_2 of less than 60 mm Hg requires immediate intervention with supplemental oxygen to treat the hypoxemia while further assessment is done to identify the cause. A PaO_2 of less than 40 mm Hg is life-threatening because oxygen is not available for metabolism. Without treatment, cellular death will occur.[27,70]

The relationship between the PaO_2 and the SaO_2 is shown in the S-shaped *oxyhemoglobin dissociation curve* (Figure 9-8). The upper portion of the curve (PaO_2 >60 mm Hg) is flat. In this area of the curve, large changes in the PaO_2 result in only small changes in SaO_2. For example, the normal PaO_2 of 80 to 100 mm Hg is associated with an SaO_2 of 92% to 100%. If the PaO_2 decreases from 80 to 60 mm Hg, the SaO_2 decreases from 92% to 90%. Although this example reflects a drop in PaO_2, the patient is not immediately compromised,

TABLE 9-3   BLOOD GAS INTERPRETATION

STATUS	pH	PCO₂	HCO₃⁻	BASE EXCESS
Respiratory Acidosis				
Uncompensated	↓ 7.35	↑ 45	Normal	Normal
Partially compensated	↓ 7.35	↑ 45	↑ 26	↑ +2
Compensated	7.35-7.45	↑ 45	↑ 26	↑ +2
Respiratory Alkalosis				
Uncompensated	↑ 7.45	↓ 35	Normal	Normal
Partially compensated	↑ 7.45	↓ 35	↓ 22	↓ −2
Compensated	7.40-7.45	↓ 35	↓ 22	↓ −2
Metabolic Acidosis				
Uncompensated	↓ 7.35	Normal	↓ 22	↓ −2
Partially compensated	↓ 7.35	↓ 35	↓ 22	↓ −2
Compensated	7.35-7.45	↓ 35	↓ 22	↓ −2
Metabolic Alkalosis				
Uncompensated	↑ 7.45	Normal	↑ 26	↑ +2
Partially compensated*	↑ 7.45	↑ 45	↑ 26	↑ +2
Compensated*	7.40-7.45	↑ 45	↑ 26	↑ +2
Combined Respiratory and Metabolic Acidosis	↓ 7.35	↑ 45	↓ 22	↓ −2
Combined Respiratory and Metabolic Alkalosis	↑ 7.45	↓ 35	↑ 26	↑ +2

*Partially compensated or compensated metabolic alkalosis generally is rarely seen clinically because of the body's mechanism to prevent hypoventilation.

Modified from Kacmarek RM, Dimas S, & Mack CW. (2005). Acid-base balance and blood gas interpretation. In RM Kacmarek, S Dimas, & CW Mack (Eds.), *The Essentials of Respiratory Care*. St. Louis: Mosby.

BOX 9-1   SIGNS AND SYMPTOMS OF HYPOXEMIA

Integumentary System
- Pallor
- Cool, dry
- Cyanosis (late)
- Diaphoresis (late)

Respiratory System
- Dyspnea
- Tachypnea
- Use of accessory muscles

Cardiovascular System
- Tachycardia
- Dysrhythmias
- Chest pain
- Hypertension early, followed by hypotension
- Increased heart rate early, followed by decreased heart rate

Central Nervous System
- Anxiety
- Restlessness
- Confusion
- Fatigue
- Combativeness/agitation
- Coma

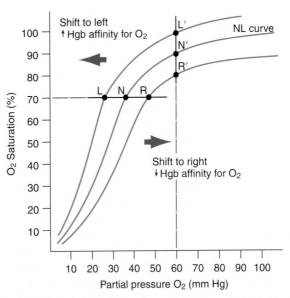

FIGURE 9-8 Oxyhemoglobin dissociation curve. A PaO₂ of 60 mm Hg correlates with an oxygen saturation of 90%. When the PaO₂ falls below 60 mm Hg, small changes in PaO₂ are reflected in large changes in oxygen saturation. Shifts in the oxyhemoglobin curve are shown. *L*, Left shift; *N*, normal; *R*, right shift. (From Alspach J. *AACN Instructor's Resource Manual for AACN Core Curriculum for Critical Care Nursing.* 5th ed. Philadelphia: Saunders; 2001.)

because the hemoglobin responsible for carrying oxygen to all the tissues is still well saturated with oxygen.

The critical zone of the oxyhemoglobin dissociation curve occurs when the PaO_2 decreases to less than 60 mm Hg. At this point, the curve slopes sharply, and small changes in PaO_2 are reflected in large changes in the oxygen saturation. These changes in SaO_2 may cause a significant decrease in oxygen delivered to the tissues.[69,70]

As shown in Figure 9-8, the oxyhemoglobin dissociation curve may shift under certain conditions. When the curve shifts to the right, a decreased hemoglobin affinity for oxygen exists; therefore oxygen is more readily released to the tissues. Conditions that cause a right shift include acidemia, increased temperature, and increased levels of the glucose metabolite 2,3-diphosphoglycerate (2,3-DPG), which occurs in anemia, chronic hypoxemia, and low cardiac output states. When conditions exist where the curve has shifted to the right, the PaO_2 is higher than expected at the normal curve.[69]

When the curve shifts to the left, hemoglobin affinity for oxygen increases and hemoglobin clings to oxygen. Conditions that cause a left shift include alkalemia, decreased temperature, high altitude, carbon monoxide poisoning, and a decreased 2,3-DPG level. Common causes of decreased 2,3-DPG include administration of stored bank blood, septic shock, and hypophosphatemia.[27,70] With a left shift, the PaO_2 is lower than expected at the normal curve. Therefore, if the patient's SpO_2 is 92%, an ABG should be drawn to assess whether hypoxemia is present.

Ventilation and Acid-Base Status

Blood gas values that reflect ventilation and acid-base or metabolic status include the partial pressure of carbon dioxide ($PaCO_2$), pH, and bicarbonate (HCO_3^-).[27,69,70]

pH. The concentration of hydrogen ions (H^+) in the blood is referred to as the *pH*. The normal pH range is 7.35 to 7.45 (exact value, 7.40). If the H^+ level increases, the pH decreases (becomes <7.35) and the patient is said to have *acidemia*. Conversely, a decrease in H^+ level results in an increase in the pH (>7.45), and the patient is said to have *alkalemia*.

Partial pressure of arterial carbon dioxide. $PaCO_2$ is the partial pressure of carbon dioxide (CO_2) dissolved in arterial plasma. The $PaCO_2$ is regulated by the lungs and has a normal range of 35 to 45 mm Hg. A $PaCO_2$ of less than 35 mm Hg indicates respiratory alkalosis; a $PaCO_2$ greater than 45 mm Hg indicates respiratory acidosis. The respiratory system controls the $PaCO_2$ by regulating ventilation (the patient's rate and depth of breathing). If the patient hypoventilates, carbon dioxide is retained, leading to respiratory acidosis ($PaCO_2$ >45 mm Hg). Conversely, if a patient hyperventilates, excess carbon dioxide is excreted by the lungs, resulting in respiratory alkalosis ($PaCO_2$ <35 mm Hg).[69] Conditions that cause respiratory acidosis and alkalosis are noted in Box 9-2.

Sodium bicarbonate. Whereas H^+ ions are an acid in the body, HCO_3^- is a base, a substance that neutralizes or buffers acids. HCO_3^- is regulated by the kidneys. Its normal range is 22 to 26 mEq/L. An HCO_3^- level greater than 26 mEq/L

BOX 9-2 CAUSES OF COMMON ACID-BASE ABNORMALITIES

Respiratory Acidosis: Retention of CO_2
- Hypoventilation
- CNS depression (anesthesia, narcotics, sedatives, drug overdose)
- Respiratory neuromuscular disorders
- Trauma: spine, brain, chest wall
- Restrictive lung diseases
- Chronic obstructive pulmonary disease
- Acute airway obstruction (late phases)

Respiratory Alkalosis: Hyperventilation
- Hypoxemia
- Anxiety, fear
- Pain
- Fever
- Stimulants
- CNS irritation (e.g., central hyperventilation)
- Excessive ventilatory support (bag-valve-mask, mechanical ventilation)

Metabolic Acidosis
Increased Acids
- Diabetic ketoacidosis
- Renal failure
- Lactic acidosis
- Drug overdose (salicylates, methanol, ethylene glycol)

Loss of Base
- Diarrhea
- Pancreatic or small bowel fluid loss

Metabolic Alkalosis
Gain of Base
- Excess ingestion of antacids
- Excess administration of sodium bicarbonate
- Citrate in blood transfusions

Loss of Metabolic Acids
- Vomiting
- Nasogastric suctioning
- Low potassium and/or chloride
- Diuretics (loss of chloride and/or potassium)

CNS, Central nervous system; *CO₂*, carbon dioxide.

---

indicates metabolic alkalosis, whereas an HCO_3^- level less than 22 mEq/L indicates metabolic acidosis. Conditions that cause metabolic acidosis and alkalosis are noted in Box 9-2.

Buffer systems. The body regulates acid-base balance through buffer systems, which are substances that minimize the changes in pH when either acids or bases are added. For example, acids are neutralized through combination with a base, and vice versa. The most important buffering system, the bicarbonate buffer system, accounts for more than half of the total buffering and is activated as the H^+ concentration increases. HCO_3^- combines with H^+ to form carbonic acid (H_2CO_3), which breaks down into carbon dioxide (which is excreted through the lungs) and water (H_2O). The equation for this mechanism is as follows:

$$H^+ + HCO_3^- \longrightarrow H_2CO_3 \longrightarrow H_2O + CO_2$$

The bicarbonate buffering system operates by using the lungs to regulate CO_2 and the kidneys to regulate HCO_3^-.[35,69,70]

Base excess or base deficit. The base excess or base deficit is reported on most ABG results. This lab value reflects the sum of all of the buffer bases in the body, the total buffer base. The normal range for base excess/base deficit is -2 to $+2$ mEq/L. In metabolic acidosis, the body's buffers are used up in an attempt to neutralize the acids, and a base deficit occurs. In metabolic alkalosis, the total buffer base increases and the patient will have a base excess. All metabolic acid-base disturbances are accompanied by a change in the base excess/base deficit, making it a very reliable indicator of metabolic acid-base disorders.[35] In pure respiratory acid-base disturbances, the base excess/base deficit is normal; however, once compensation occurs, the base excess/base deficit changes.

Compensation. Compensation involves mechanisms that normalize the pH when an acid-base imbalance occurs. The kidneys attempt to compensate for respiratory abnormalities, whereas the lungs attempt to compensate for metabolic problems. The lungs quickly respond to compensate for a primary metabolic acid-base abnormality For example, in metabolic acidosis, the depth and rate of ventilation is increased in an effort to blow off more CO_2 (acid). Conversely in metabolic alkalosis, the rate and depth of ventilation may be decreased in an effort to retain acid.[27]

The kidneys compensate for primary respiratory acid-base abnormalities by excreting excess H^+ and retaining HCO_3^-. The renal system activates more slowly taking up to 2 days to regulate acid-base balance. The kidneys excrete HCO_3^- when respiratory alkalosis is present, and retain HCO_3^- when respiratory acidosis is present.[27,35] The renal and respiratory systems exist in harmony to maintain acid-base balance (Figure 9-9).

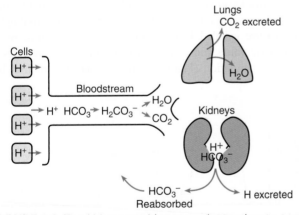

FIGURE 9-9 The kidneys and lungs work together to compensate for acid-base imbalances in the respiratory or metabolic systems. *HCO₃⁻,* Bicarbonate; *H₂CO₃,* carbonic acid. (Modified from Harvey MA. *Study Guide to the Core Curriculum for Critical Care Nursing.* 3ʳᵈ ed. Philadelphia: Saunders; 2000.)

Steps In Arterial Blood Gas Interpretation

Systematic analysis of ABG values involves five steps.[51] Table 9-3 lists lab values associated with acid-base abnormalities. Critical ABG values are noted in the box, "Laboratory Alert."

> ### ⚠ LABORATORY ALERT
> #### *Arterial Blood Gas Critical Values**
>
> | |
> |---|
> | PaO_2 <60 mm Hg |
> | $PaCO_2$ >50 mm Hg |
> | pH <7.25 or >7.60 |
>
> *These are critical values only if they differ from baseline values (i.e., an acute change). Some patients with pulmonary disease tolerate highly "abnormal" arterial blood gas values.
> *PaCO₂,* Partial pressure of carbon dioxide in arterial blood; *PaO₂,* partial pressure of oxygen in arterial blood.

Step 1: Look at each number individually and label it. Decide whether the value is high, low, or normal and label the finding. For example, a pH of 7.50 is high and labeled as alkalemia.

Step 2: Evaluate oxygenation. Oxygenation is analyzed by evaluating the PaO_2 and the SaO_2. Hypoxemia is present and considered a significant problem when the PaO_2 falls to less than 60 mm Hg or the SaO_2 falls to less than 90%. A complete assessment must take into account the level of supplemental oxygen a patient is receiving when the ABG is drawn.

Step 3: Determine acid-base status. Assess the pH to determine the acid-base status. A pH of 7.40 is the absolute normal. If the pH is less than 7.4, the primary disorder is acidosis. If the pH is greater than 7.4, the primary disorder is alkalosis. Therefore, even if the pH is within the normal range, noting whether it is on the acid or alkaline side of 7.40 is important.

Step 4: Determine whether primary acid-base disorder is respiratory or metabolic. Assess the $PaCO_2$, which reflects the respiratory system, and the HCO_3^- level, which reflects the metabolic system, to determine which one is altered in the same manner as the pH. The ABG results may reflect only one disorder (respiratory or metabolic). However, two primary acid-base disorders may occur simultaneously (mixed acid-base imbalance). For example, during cardiac arrest, both respiratory acidosis and metabolic acidosis commonly occur because of hypoventilation and lactic acidosis. Use the base excess to confirm your interpretation of the primary acid-base disturbance, especially if the disorder is mixed.

Step 5: Determine whether any form of compensatory response has taken place. Compensation refers to a return to a normal blood pH by means of respiratory or renal mechanisms. The system opposite the primary disorder attempts the compensation. For example, if a patient has respiratory acidosis, such as occurs in COPD (low pH, high $PaCO_2$), the kidneys respond by retaining more HCO_3^- and excreting H^+. Conversely, if a patient has metabolic acidosis, such as occurs in diabetic ketoacidosis (low pH, low HCO_3^-), the lungs respond by hyperventilation and excretion of carbon dioxide (respiratory alkalosis).[27,69] So if the $PaCO_2$ and the HCO_3^-

BOX 9-3 EXAMPLES OF ARTERIAL BLOOD GASES AND COMPENSATION

Example 1

PaO_2	80 mm Hg (normal)
pH	7.30 (low; acidosis)
$PaCO_2$	50 mm Hg (high; respiratory acidosis)
HCO_3^-	22 mEq/L (normal)
SaO_2	95% (normal)

Interpretation: Normal oxygenation, respiratory acidosis; no compensation.

Example 2

PaO_2	80 mm Hg (normal)
pH	7.32 (low; acidosis)
$PaCO_2$	50 mm Hg (high; respiratory acidosis)
HCO_3^-	28 mEq/L (high; metabolic alkalosis)
SaO_2	95% (normal)

Interpretation: Normal oxygenation, partly compensated respiratory acidosis. The arterial blood gases are only partly compensated because the pH is not yet within normal limits.

Example 3

PaO_2	80 mm Hg (normal)
pH	7.36 (acid side of normal)
$PaCO_2$	50 mm Hg (high; respiratory acidosis)
HCO_3^-	29 mEq/L (high; metabolic alkalosis)
SaO_2	95% (normal)

Interpretation: Normal oxygenation, completely (fully) compensated respiratory acidosis. The pH is now within normal limits; therefore complete compensation has occurred.

HCO_3^-, Bicarbonate; $PaCO_2$, partial pressure of carbon dioxide in arterial blood; PaO_2, partial pressure of oxygen in arterial blood; SaO_2, saturation of hemoglobin with oxygen in arterial blood.

are abnormal in the same direction, then compensation is occurring.

Compensation may be absent, partial, or complete. Compensation is absent if the system opposite the primary disorder is within normal range. If compensation has occurred but the pH is still abnormal, compensation is referred to as partial. Compensation is complete if compensatory mechanisms are present and the pH is within normal range. The body does not overcompensate.[69,70] Examples of ABG compensation are shown in Box 9-3.

Noninvasive Assessment of Gas Exchange

Intermittent ABG results have been the gold standard for the monitoring of gas exchange and acid-base status. Improvements in technology for noninvasive assessment of gas exchange by pulse oximetry and capnography have reduced the number of ABG samples obtained in critically ill patients.

Assessment of Oxygenation

Pulse oximetry. Pulse oximetry measures the saturation of oxygen in pulsatile blood (SpO_2) which reflects the SaO_2.

The oxyhemoglobin dissociation curve (see Figure 9-8) shows the relationship between SaO_2 and PaO_2 and provides the basis for pulse oximetry. The sensor that measures SpO_2 is placed on the patient's finger, toe, ear, or forehead where blood flow is not diminished. Light emitted from the sensor is absorbed by hemoglobin with oxygen, or hemoglobin without oxygen providing the necessary information for the device to calculate the percent hemoglobin saturated with oxygen in the pulsatile (arterial) blood. Critically ill patients have continuous pulse oximetry. SpO_2 values are sometimes "spot checked" in patients who are less acutely ill. Pulse oximetry values are used to monitor a patient's response to treatment (e.g., ventilator changes, suctioning, inhalation therapy, body position changes) by following trends in oxygen saturation. However, SpO_2 only measures fluctuation in oxygenation and cannot be used to assess carbon dioxide levels.[51,57]

To ensure accurate SpO_2 readings, the nurse must ensure that the sensor is placed correctly on a warm, well-perfused area and an adequate pulsatile signal is detected. Several factors affect the accuracy of SpO_2 values. Artifact from patient motion or edema at the sensor site may prevent an accurate measurement. The SpO_2 measurements may be lower than the actual SaO_2 if the perfusion to the sensor site is reduced (e.g., limb ischemia, or inflated blood pressure cuff), or in the presence of sunlight, fluorescent light, nail polish or artificial nails, and intravenous dyes. The SpO_2 measurements may be higher than the actual SaO_2 reported by ABG analysis if the patient has an abnormal hemoglobin, such as methemoglobin or carboxyhemoglobin.[28,35]

Assessment of Ventilation

End-tidal carbon dioxide monitoring. End-tidal carbon dioxide monitoring ($ETCO_2$) is the noninvasive measurement of alveolar CO_2 at the end of exhalation when CO_2 concentration is at its peak.[35,65] It reflects alveolar CO_2 level, which in turn reflects the arterial CO_2 ($PaCO_2$) and therefore is used to monitor and assess trends in the patient's ventilatory status. Expired gases are sampled from the patient's airway and are analyzed by a CO_2 sensor that uses infrared light to measure exhaled CO_2 at the end of inspiration. Both a numeric value and a waveform are provided for assessment of ventilation (Figure 9-10).[22,35,65] The sensor may be

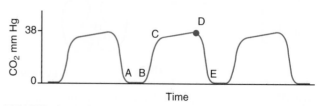

FIGURE 9-10 Capnogram or graphic display of exhaled carbon dioxide (CO_2). Rise in the waveform from *A* to *D* represents CO_2 leaving the lung. Point *D* is where end-tidal CO_2 is measured and represents the highest concentration of exhaled alveolar CO_2.

attached to an adaptor on the endotracheal tube (ETT) or the tracheostomy tube. A nasal cannula with a sidestream capnometer can be used in patients without an artificial airway.[51] The sampling port should be placed as close as possible to the patient's airway.

Normally, $ETCO_2$ values average 2 to 5 mm Hg less than the $PaCO_2$ in individuals with normal lung and cardiac function.[35] To determine the baseline correlation between $ETCO_2$ and $PaCO_2$, the $ETCO_2$ is measured at the same time an ABG is obtained. $ETCO_2$ is subtracted from the $PaCO_2$, providing an index known as the $PaCO_2$-$ETCO_2$ gradient. For example, if a blood gas shows that the $PaCO_2$ is 40 mm Hg and simultaneously the $ETCO_2$ is noted to be 36 mm Hg, the $PaCO_2$-$ETCO_2$ gradient is +4. Knowing the gradient allows for noninvasive assessment of the patient's ventilation by trend monitoring the $ETCO_2$ and inferring the $PaCO_2$ by use of the gradient.[51]

$ETCO_2$ monitoring is used to evaluate ventilation for trending data when precision is not essential. Clinical applications of $ETCO_2$ monitoring include assessment of the patient's response to ventilator changes and respiratory treatments, determining the proper position of the ETT, trending CO_2 in patients with traumatic brain injury or subarachnoid hemorrhage, or detecting disconnection from the ventilator.[22,65] The most common pitfall of $ETCO_2$ monitoring is believing that the value reflects only the patient's ventilatory status. Changes in exhaled CO_2 may occur because of changes not only in ventilation, but also in CO_2 production (metabolism), transport of CO_2 to the lung, and accuracy of the equipment. For example, a decreased $ETCO_2$ value could indicate decreased alveolar ventilation, a reduction in lung perfusion as in hypotension or pulmonary embolus, a reduction in metabolic production of CO_2 as in hypothermia or return to normothermia after fever, or obstruction of the CO_2 sampling tube.[22,65]

Colorimetric carbon dioxide detector. Disposable colorimetric $ETCO_2$ detectors are routinely used after intubation to differentiate tracheal from esophageal intubation (Figure 9-11).[35] When CO_2 is detected, the color of the indicator changes, verifying correct tube placement.

OXYGEN ADMINISTRATION

Oxygen is administered to treat or prevent hypoxemia. Oxygen may be supplied by various sources such as piped into wall devices, oxygen tanks, or oxygen concentrators. The amount of oxygen being administered to the patient is described as the fraction of inspired oxygen (FiO_2). Oxygen concentrations are reported in percentages, whereas the FiO_2 is reported as a decimal. Devices can deliver low (<35%), moderate (35% to 60%), or high (>60%) oxygen concentrations.[30,35]

Oxygen delivery devices are classified into two general categories: low-flow systems (nasal cannula, simple face mask, partial-rebreather mask, and non-rebreather mask), and high-flow systems (air-entrainment or Venturi mask and high-flow nasal cannula).[30,51] Low-flow systems deliver

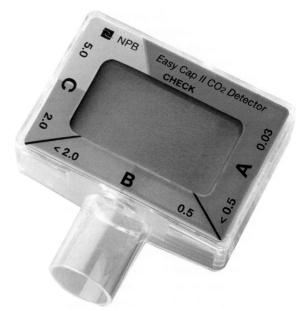

FIGURE 9-11 Disposable colorimetric carbon dioxide (CO_2) detector for confirming endotracheal tube placement. Detection of CO_2 confirms tube placement in the lungs because the only source of CO_2 is the alveoli. (Image used by permission from Nellcor Puritan Bennett LLC, Boulder, Colorado, doing business as Covidien.)

oxygen at flow rates that are less than the patient's inspiratory demand for gas; total patient demand is not met. Low-flow system devices require that the patient entrain, or draw in, room air along with the delivered O_2 enriched gas. FiO_2 cannot be precisely controlled or predicted, because it is determined not only by the amount of oxygen delivered but also the patient's ventilatory pattern and thus the amount of air the patient entrains. For example, if the patient's ventilation increases, the delivered FiO_2 decreases because the patient entrains a larger percentage of room air. Conversely, if the patient's ventilation decreases, the oxygen delivered is less diluted and the FiO_2 rises.[30,51] In high-flow systems, the flow of oxygen enriched gas is sufficient for the patient's total inspiratory demand. The FiO_2 remains fairly constant. In general, for delivery of a consistent FiO_2 to a patient with a variable (deep, irregular, shallow) ventilatory pattern, a high-flow system should be used.

The successful administration of oxygen therapy is important in treating hypoxemia. When administering oxygen, it is important to consider not only the adequacy of the flow delivered by a device, but also fit and function. To ensure proper fit and function, the nurse or RT inspects the patient's face to assess how well the oxygen delivery device is positioned and whether the airway is patent. The oxygen-connecting tubing is traced back to the gas source origin to ensure that it is connected. Finally, it is important to ensure that the gas source is oxygen and that it is turned on and set properly.

Humidification

Humidification of oxygen is recommended when O_2 flow is greater than 4 L/min to prevent the mucous membranes from drying. At lower flow rates, the patient's natural humidification system provides adequate humidity.[21,49,69] The nurse monitors the quantity and quality (consistency) of the patient's secretions to determine the adequacy of humidification. If the secretions are thick despite adequate humidification of the delivered gases, the patient needs systemic hydration.

Humidification is also an important element of ventilator management. It is essential to maintain the inspired gas reaching the patient's airway at as close to 37° C and 100% relative humidity as possible.[30,69] Two approaches are used to provide humidification. One method functions by actively passing the dry inspired gas through a water-based humidification system before it reaches the patient's airway. The second method is to attach a heat-moisture exchanger (HME) to the ventilator circuit. The HME functions as an artificial "nose" to warm and humidify the patient's inspired breath with his or her own expired moisture and body heat.

During mechanical ventilation, frequent inspection of the humidification unit is needed. If a water-based humidification is used, routine checks include maintaining the water reservoir level and removing condensate from loops in the ventilator circuit. During manipulation of the circuit tubing, it is important to prevent emptying the condensate into the patient's airway. This can lead to contamination of the patient's airway as well as breathing difficulty.[33] If an HME is used, it must be inspected regularly for accumulation of patient secretions in the device, which could result in partial or complete obstruction, increased airway resistance, and increased WOB.[21]

Oxygen Delivery Devices
Nasal Cannula

The nasal cannula is relatively comfortable to wear and easy to secure on the patient. In adult patients, nasal cannulas provide oxygen concentrations between 24% and 44% oxygen at flow rates up to 6 L/min.[30,35] An increase in oxygen flow rate by 1 L/min generally increases oxygen delivery by 4% (e.g., 2 L/min nasal cannula delivers 28% of oxygen, whereas 3 L/min provides 32%). Flow rates higher than 6 L/min are not effective in increasing oxygenation because the capacity of the patient's anatomical reservoir in the nasopharynx is surpassed. An important nursing intervention for patients receiving oxygen via nasal cannula is to assess the skin above the ears for skin breakdown. It may be necessary to pad the tubing over the ear with gauze.

High Flow Nasal Cannula

Oxygen delivered at rates ranging from 15 to 40 L/min is known as high-flow therapy and has historically has been delivered with face masks. However, the delivery of high-flow therapy, which provides high concentrations of oxygen ranging from 60% to 90% and greater is possible through a nasal cannula when it is properly humidified with a special high-flow system. Compliance with therapy is usually better with a nasal cannula because the patient is more comfortable and can eat, drink, and talk. The high-flow system fills the patient's nasopharynx so that it becomes a reservoir of oxygen, thereby improving the oxygen delivered to the alveoli with each breath. It is important to collaborate with the RT to ensure the water in the system remains sufficient to humidify the high flow of gas.

Simple Face Mask

Placing a mask over the patient's face creates an additional oxygen reservoir beyond the patient's natural anatomical reservoir. The mask should fit tight and the flow rate set to at least 5 L/min to prevent rebreathing carbon dioxide. Oxygen is delivered at flow rates of 5 to 12 L/min, which provides concentrations of 30% to 60%.[35] The patient should be instructed about the importance of wearing the mask as applied. The inside of the mask should be cleaned as needed, and the skin should be assessed for areas of pressure.[30]

Face Masks with Reservoirs

Both the partial rebreathing and non-rebreathing masks are similar to the design of a simple face mask, but with the addition of an oxygen reservoir bag. The reservoir increases the amount of oxygen available to the patient during inspiration and allows for the delivery of concentrations of 35% to 60% (partial rebreather) or 60% to 80% (non-rebreather) dependent on the flowmeter setting, the fit of the mask, and the patient's respiratory pattern. The main difference between these two devices is that the non-rebreather mask has one-way valves between the mask and reservoir bag and over one of the exhalation ports. These valves ensure the patient breathes a high concentration of oxygen-enriched gas from the reservoir with each breath (Figure 9-12). The flow rate on the meter should be set to prevent the reservoir bag from deflating no more than one half during inspiration for the partial rebreather, and to prevent the bag from deflating for the non-rebreather.[30] Either mask may be used in the critically ill patient with severe hypoxemia in an effort to prevent the need for endotracheal intubation and mechanical ventilation.

Venturi or Air-Entrainment Mask

The Venturi or air-entrainment mask appears much like a simple face mask; however, it has a jet adapter placed between the mask and the tubing to the oxygen source. The jet adapters come in various sizes and are often color coded to the FiO_2 they deliver. The appropriate oxygen flow rate is often inscribed on the adapter (Figure 9-13). The Venturi mask delivers a fixed FiO_2. Because the level of oxygen can be closely regulated, the Venturi mask is commonly used in the hypoxemic patient with chronic pulmonary disease for whom the delivery of excessive oxygen could depress the respiratory drive.[30,35]

Aerosol and Humidity Delivery Systems

The goal of adding humidity to the inspired gases is to prevent dehydration of the airways and secretions secondary to breathing dry medical gases. The high-humidity face mask or face tent is an option for patients who do not have artificial airways (Figure 9-14). High-flow devices used for administering

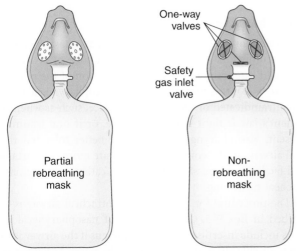

FIGURE 9-12 Partial rebreathing and non-rebreathing oxygen masks. (From Kacmarek RM, Dimas S, Mack CW. *The Essentials of Respiratory Care.* 4th ed. St. Louis: Mosby; 2005.)

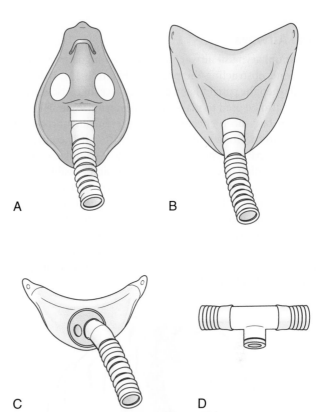

FIGURE 9-14 Devices used to apply high-flow, high-humidity oxygen therapy. **A,** Aerosol mask. **B,** Face tent. **C,** Tracheostomy collar. **D,** Briggs T-piece. (From Kacmarek RM, Dimas S, Mack CW. *The Essentials of Respiratory Care.* 4th ed. St. Louis: Mosby; 2005.)

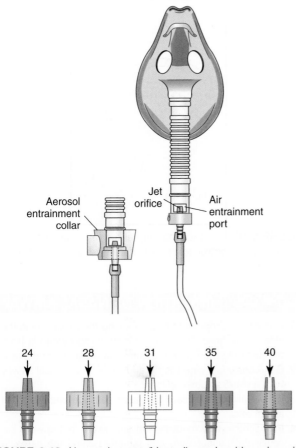

FIGURE 9-13 Air-entrainment (Venturi) mask with various jet orifices. Each orifice provides a specific delivered FiO_2. (Modified from Kacmarek RM, Dimas S, Mack CW. *The Essentials of Respiratory Care.* 4th ed. St. Louis: Mosby; 2005.)

humidified oxygen to patients with an artificial airway are the T-piece and the tracheostomy mask/collar. Humidity is added through a nebulizer that delivers a fixed FiO_2. The initial flow rate is set at 10 L/min and is adjusted so that a constant mist is seen coming from the exhalation port[30,35,51]

Manual Resuscitation Bag (Variable Performance)

A manual resuscitation bag, or bag-valve device, is used to ventilate and oxygenate a patient manually (see Chapter 10). The device is attached to a face mask or connected directly to an ETT or tracheostomy tube to ventilate the patient. When used on an emergency basis, the bag-valve device should have a reservoir attached to increase the FiO_2. The oxygen flowmeter attached to the bag is set at 15 L/min.[51]

AIRWAY MANAGEMENT

Positioning

A patent airway is essential to adequate ventilation and is a priority of nursing care. When the airway is partially or totally obstructed the first method for reinstating a patent airway is proper head position with the head-tilt/chin-lift or jaw thrust. An airway adjunct such as the oral or nasopharyngeal airway may be needed to help maintain the airway.

Oral Airways

The oropharyngeal airway prevents the tongue from falling back and obstructing the pharynx (Figure 9-15). It is indicated when the patient has a depressed level of consciousness. It may also be used to make ventilation with a manual resuscitation bag more effective, or to prevent an unconscious patient from biting and occluding an ETT. It is contraindicated in a patient who is awake because it stimulates the gag reflex, resulting in discomfort, agitation, and possibly emesis. It is important to choose the proper size oral airway: too short an airway forces the patient's tongue back into the pharynx and too long stimulates the gag reflex.[58,60] Nursing care includes assessing the lips and tongue for signs of pressure ulceration and suctioning the oropharynx of accumulated secretions.[51] The technique for inserting an oral airway is described in Box 9-4.

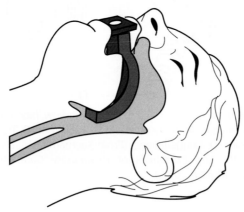

FIGURE 9-15 Maintaining a patent airway with an oral airway. (Modified from Shilling A, Durbin CG. Airway management. In: Cairo JM, ed. *Mosby's Respiratory Care Equipment*. 8th ed. St. Louis: Mosby; 2010.)

BOX 9-4   INSERTION OF ORAL AIRWAY

1. Choose the proper size by measuring the airway on the patient. Airway should extend from the edge of the patient's mouth to the ear lobe.
2. Suction mucus from the mouth using a tonsil (Yankauer) tip catheter.
3. Turn the airway upside down with its tip against the hard palate and slide airway into mouth until the soft palate is reached; then rotate the airway to match the curvature of the tongue into the proper position.
4. An alternative method to step 3 is to use a tongue blade to depress the patient's tongue while inserting the airway, matching its curvature to that of the tongue.
5. Advance tip to back of mouth. Ensure end of airway rests between the teeth but does not compress the lips against the teeth, which would cause injury.
6. Assess airway patency, breath sounds, and chest movement. Noises indicating upper airway obstruction should be absent.
7. Maintain the patient's proper head alignment after airway insertion.

Nasopharyngeal Airways

The nasopharyngeal airway, also known as a nasal airway or nasal trumpet, is a soft rubber or latex tube placed in the nose and extending to the posterior portion of the pharynx (Figure 9-16). It is indicated when an oropharyngeal airway is contraindicated or too difficult to place, such as when the patient's jaw is tight during a seizure, or if oral trauma is present. Nasopharyngeal airways are better tolerated than oral airways in the conscious patient, are more comfortable, and facilitate the passage of a suction catheter during nasotracheal suctioning.

The procedure for inserting a nasotracheal airway is described in Box 9-5. Complications of nasopharyngeal airways include insertion into the esophagus if the airway is too long, nosebleeds, and ulceration of the nares. Extended use of nasopharyngeal airways is not recommended because of an increased risk for sinusitis or otitis.

Endotracheal Intubation

Intubation refers to the insertion of an ETT into the trachea through either the mouth or the nose. Advantages of oral versus nasal endotracheal intubation are listed in Box 9-6. The ETT (Figure 9-17, *A*) is typically made of a polyvinyl

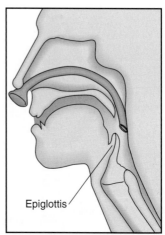

Epiglottis

FIGURE 9-16 The nasopharyngeal airway is used to relieve upper airway obstruction and to facilitate passage of a suction catheter.

BOX 9-5   INSERTION OF NASAL AIRWAY

1. Choose the proper size by positioning the airway along the side of the head. The proper length airway extends from the nostril to the earlobe, or just past the angle of the jaw.
2. Generously lubricate the tip and sides of the nasal airway with a water-soluble lubricant.
3. If time allows, lubricate the nasal passage with a topical anesthetic.
4. Insert the airway medially and downward, not upward because the nasopharynx lies directly behind the nares. It may be necessary to rotate the airway slightly.
5. After insertion, assess airway patency, breath sounds, and chest movement.

BOX 9-6   ORAL VERSUS NASOTRACHEAL INTUBATION

Oral Intubation

Advantages

- Quickly performed, emergency airway
- Larger tube facilitates secretion removal and bronchoscopy; creates less airway resistance
- Less kinking of tube
- Preferred method; less sinusitis and otitis media

Disadvantages

- Discomfort
- Mouth care more difficult to perform
- Impairs ability to swallow
- May increase oral secretion production
- May cause irritation and ulceration of the mouth
- Greater risk of self-extubation
- More difficult to communicate by mouthing words
- Patient may bite on airway, reducing gas flow

Nasotracheal Intubation

Advantages

- Greater patient comfort and tolerance
- Better mouth care possible
- Fewer oral complications
- Less risk of accidental extubation
- Facilitates swallowing of oral secretions
- Communication by mouthing words enhanced

Disadvantages

- More difficult to place
- Possible epistaxis during insertion
- Increases risk for sinusitis and otitis media
- May be more difficult to perform
- Secretion removal more difficult because of smaller tube diameter
- Increases work of breathing associated with smaller diameter tube

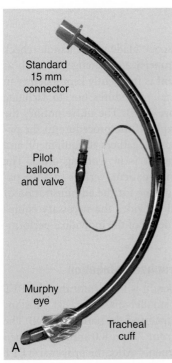

Standard 15 mm connector

Pilot balloon and valve

Murphy eye

Tracheal cuff

A

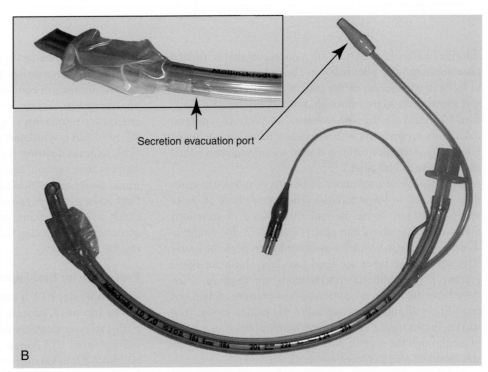

Secretion evacuation port

B

FIGURE 9-17 A, Endotracheal tube. **B,** Hi-Lo Evac endotracheal tube. Note suction port above the cuff for removal of pooled secretions. (From Shilling A, Durbin CG. Airway management. In: Cairo JM, ed. *Mosby's Respiratory Care Equipment.* 8th ed. St. Louis: Mosby; 2010.)

Outcomes of Endotracheal Tubes with Subglottic Secretion Drainage

Problem

Specialized endotracheal tubes (ETT) have been developed with the target of reducing ventilator-associated pneumonia (VAP). One such tube has an additional port for subglottic secretion drainage (SSD-ETT). Outcomes of such devices need to be evaluated.

Clinical Question

What is the impact of the SSD-ETT on preventing VAP?

Evidence

A meta-analysis of 13 randomized clinical trials was conducted. VAP was reduced in 12 of the trials. The overall risk for VAP was reduced by 50%. Use of the SSD-ETT also resulted in a reduction in the critical care length of stay and duration of mechanical ventilation. In subjects who developed VAP, the onset was delayed in those with the SSD-ETT.

Implications for Nursing

Despite strong evidence as to the outcomes associated with the SSD-ETT, the tubes have not been widely adopted. Primary reasons for nonuse are the higher costs associated with the devices, and ensuring that patients who may benefit from the tube get intubated with the specialized devices. Nurses can assist in developing protocols for implementing the SSD-ETT in clinical practice, such as availability of the tube on crash carts and in the emergency department. When a patient has an SSD-ETT, the nurse must collaborate with the respiratory therapist to ensure that the suction port is connected to the suction regulator at the correct pressure and that it is draining appropriately. Periodic flushing of the suction port with air is needed.

Level of Evidence

A—Meta-analysis

Reference

Muscedere J, Rewa O, Mckechnie K, Jiang X, Laporta D, & Heyland DK. Subglottic secretion drainage for the prevention of ventilator-associated pneumonia: a systematic review and meta-analysis. *Critical Care Medicine* 2011;39, 1985-1991.

---

chloride or silicone material with a distal cuff that is inflated via a one-way valve pilot balloon. The purpose of the cuff is to facilitate ventilation of the patient by sealing the trachea and allowing air to pass through, not around the ETT. Standard ETT cuffs are the high-volume, low-pressure type, and most cuffs are inflated with air (some tubes have a foam-filled cuff). The pilot balloon is used to monitor and adjust cuff pressure as indicated.[58]

ETTs capable of continuous suctioning of subglottic secretions are used in some facilities. These tubes have an extra suction port just above the cuff for removal of secretions that accumulate above the cuff (Figure 9-17, *B*). Evidence shows a decrease in ventilator-associated pneumonia by nearly 50% when these tubes are used (see box, "Evidence-Based Practice").[14,15] Additional interventions are required when these tubes are in place. Continuous low-pressure suction not exceeding −20 mm Hg is applied to the suction lumen. The suction lumen must remain patent. Administration of a bolus of air through the suction port is often needed to relieve obstruction and maintain continuous suction.

Intubation is performed to establish an airway, assist in secretion removal, protect the airway from aspiration in patients with a depressed cough and gag, and provide mechanical ventilation. Personnel who are trained and skilled in intubation perform the procedure: anesthesiologists, nurse anesthetists, acute care nurse practitioners, emergency department physicians, intensivists, RTs, and some paramedics.[51] Intubation may be performed emergently on a patient in cardiac or respiratory arrest, or electively in a patient with impending respiratory failure.

The nurse must be familiar with and be able to gather intubation equipment quickly. The nurse also needs to know how to connect the laryngoscope blade to the handle, check to see that it illuminates properly, and change the bulb as needed. Intubation equipment is frequently kept together in an emergency cart or special procedures box to facilitate emergency intubation (Figure 9-18). The nurse notifies the RT to obtain a ventilator, explains the procedure to the patient, removes dentures if present, gathers all equipment, and ensures that suction equipment is in working order. The nurse assists in positioning the patient, verifies that the patient has a patent intravenous line for the administration of fluids and medications, and provides the necessary equipment while anticipating the needs of the individual performing the intubation.

Procedure for Oral Endotracheal Intubation

The proper size ETT is chosen; it is important that the ETT not be too small, because a smaller-diameter ETT substantially increases airway resistance and the patient's WOB. The average-sized ETT ranges from 7.5 to 8.0 mm for women and from 8.0 to 9.0 mm for men.[58] After the proper size ETT is selected, the cuff is inflated to check for symmetry and any leaks. A plastic-coated malleable stylet may be used to stiffen the ETT to facilitate insertion, but it should be carefully placed inside the ETT to avoid its protrusion beyond the end of the ETT. The ETT is lubricated with a water-soluble lubricant to facilitate passage through the structures of the oropharynx.

The laryngoscope is attached to the appropriate size and type of blade (straight or curved) based on the patient's anatomy and the preference of the clinician performing the intubation. Blade sizes range from 0 to 4. The average-sized adult is intubated with a size-3 blade.[60] Optional equipment

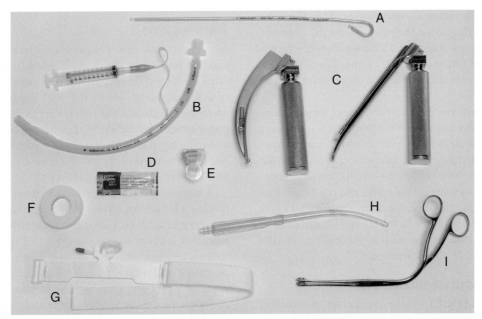

FIGURE 9-18 Equipment used for endotracheal intubation: **A,** stylet (disposable); **B,** endotracheal tube with 10-mL syringe for cuff inflation; **C,** laryngoscope handle with attached curved blade *(left)* and straight blade *(right)*; **D,** water-soluble lubricant; **E,** colorimetric CO_2 detector to check tube placement; **F,** tape or **G,** commercial device to secure tube; **H,** Yankauer disposable pharyngeal suction device; **I,** Magill forceps (optional). Additional equipment, not shown, includes suction source and stethoscope.

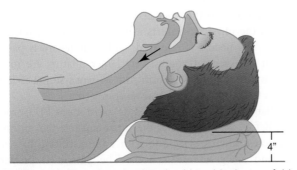

FIGURE 9-19 Elevating the head with a blanket or folded towels places the patient in the "sniffing position" to facilitate endotracheal intubation.

includes a fiberoptic laryngoscope or equipment for video-assisted intubation.

The patient is placed in a "sniffing" position to facilitate visualization of the glottis, or vocal cords. Placing a folded towel or bath blanket under the head may help to achieve this position (Figure 9-19). Time permitting, the patient is premedicated with a sedative and possibly a paralytic agent to allow for easier manipulation of the mandible and visualization of the glottis. The patient is then hyperoxygenated with 100% oxygen by using a bag-valve device connected to a face mask. The intubation procedure should be performed within 30 seconds. If the intubation is difficult and additional attempts are required

to secure the airway, the patient must be manually ventilated between each intubation attempt.

The person doing the intubation, while taking care not to damage the patient's teeth or other structures, inserts the laryngoscope blade into the patient's mouth to visualize the vocal cords. If secretions and vomitus are present, the oral cavity is suctioned. A rigid tonsil tip suction (e.g., Yankauer) is very efficient in removing thick secretions and is often used. When the tube is properly inserted about 5 to 6 cm beyond the vocal cords into the trachea, the laryngoscope and stylet are removed and the ETT cuff is inflated.[58,60]

Procedure for Nasotracheal Intubation

Two approaches to nasal intubation are possible: blind and direct visualization.[60] The equipment for nasotracheal intubation is the same as for oral intubation with the addition of Magill forceps. The naris selected for the ETT passage is prepared with a topical vasoconstricting agent to reduce bleeding, and an anesthetic agent. One option is to lubricate the ETT with a water-soluble gel containing 2% lidocaine. The patient is positioned as indicated by the preference of the person performing the intubation: semi-Fowler, high Fowler, or supine.

After the patient's naris and the ETT have been prepared, the ETT is inserted "blindly"; that is, no laryngoscope is used to visualize the cords. The ETT is advanced toward the glottis as the intubator listens to the intensity of the patient's breathing. Blind intubation can be performed only in the patient who is capable of spontaneous respirations. The closer the intubator comes to the glottis, the more intense the sound of air movement becomes until the ETT passes through the vocal cords and moves into the trachea. The passage of the ETT beyond the vocal cords usually elicits a cough from the patient and vocal silence.

Because some patients have atypical upper airway anatomy, nasal intubation can also be performed through direct visualization. In this method, the practitioner uses a laryngoscope and Magill forceps, or fiberoptic bronchoscopy, for the procedure. When the tube reaches the oropharynx, the laryngoscope is inserted to visualize the cords, and the Magill forceps are used to grasp the tube just above the ETT cuff and direct it between the vocal cords. With nasal intubation, the correct placement level of the ETT at the naris is usually 28 cm for males and 26 cm for females.[58]

Verification of Endotracheal Tube Placement

Correct placement of the ETT in the trachea (versus incorrect placement in the esophagus) is verified by clinical assessment and confirmation devices. Clinical assessment includes auscultation of the epigastrium and lung fields, and observing for bilateral chest expansion.[66] Failure to hear breath sounds while hearing air over the epigastrium represents esophageal rather than tracheal intubation. Breath sounds are equal bilaterally when the tube is placed correctly. Intubation of the right mainstem bronchus is common because the right mainstem is straighter than the left, and the ETT is occasionally placed deeper in the trachea than necessary. Right mainstem bronchus intubation is suspected when unilateral expansion of the right chest is observed during ventilation and the breath sounds are louder on the right than left.

Another method of assessment is done with a confirmation device. Monitoring devices to confirm ETT placement include either a disposable $ETCO_2$ detector, or a bulb aspiration device (esophageal detector device). The disposable $ETCO_2$ detector is attached to the end of the ETT. This device changes color when carbon dioxide is detected and is a highly reliable method of confirming tracheal (versus esophageal) intubation.[58,60] Another option is to attach an aspiration device that is similar to a bulb syringe. The device is compressed and deflated and is attached to the ETT. If the tube is in the trachea, the bulb inflates rapidly. If the tube is in the esophagus, filling is delayed. Pulse oximetry also assists in assessment of tube placement. SpO_2 will fall if the esophagus has been inadvertently intubated, and it may be decreased in right mainstem intubation. Finally, a portable chest radiograph is ordered to confirm tube placement.[51]

The tip of the ETT should be approximately 3 to 4 cm above the carina.[60] Once the placement is confirmed, the centimeter depth marking at the lip or naris should be noted in the medical record. An indelible marker can be used to mark the ETT at the lip or naris. These nursing measures assist with ongoing monitoring of proper tube position. The nurse and RT collaborate to ensure the ETT is properly secured with tape or a commercial device to prevent dislodging. Figure 9-20 shows two methods for securing the ETT.

Tracheostomy

A tracheostomy tube provides an airway directly into the anterior portion of the neck. Tracheostomy tubes are indicated for long-term mechanical ventilation, long-term secretion management, protecting the airway from aspiration when the cough and gag reflexes are impaired, bypassing an upper airway obstruction that prevents placement of an ETT, and reducing the WOB associated with an ETT. The tracheostomy tube reduces the WOB because it is shorter than an ETT and airflow resistance is less.[18,66]

A tracheostomy is the preferred airway for the patient requiring a long-term airway who is able to transfer to a progressive care unit, because it is associated with several advantages.[66] It is better tolerated than an ETT; therefore patients may require less sedation or restraint use. A patient may be permitted oral intake if swallowing studies demonstrate absence of aspiration. Oral hygiene is more easily performed, and some tube designs allow for talking and therefore facilitate patient communication.

There is no clearly defined time for when a tracheostomy should be performed. If mechanical ventilation and an artificial airway are projected to be needed for a prolonged period, the decision to perform a tracheostomy should be made early.[17]

The tracheostomy has traditionally been a surgical technique performed in the operating room. However, a percutaneous dilatational tracheostomy (PDT) procedure may be performed safely at the bedside by a trained physician.[17] The PDT is performed by making a small incision into the anterior neck down to the trachea. Once this location has been reached, the physician inserts a needle and sheath into the trachea. The needle is removed, and a guidewire is passed through the sheath. Progressively larger dilators are introduced over the guidewire until the patient's stoma is large enough to accommodate a tracheostomy tube.[17,18]

Collaboratively, the nurse and RT assist in the PDT procedure. Before the procedure, the nurse ensures that intravenous access lines are accessible for administration of sedatives and analgesic medications. The patient is properly positioned, and the height of the bed is adjusted relative to the individual performing the procedure. Sterile supplies are gathered, and sterility is maintained throughout the procedure. Physiological parameters are monitored continuously and documented at least every 15 minutes throughout the PDT, and for a least an hour after the procedure.[51]

The most significant postprocedure complication of PDT is accidental decannulation. When a patient undergoes a surgical tracheostomy, the trachea is surgically attached to the skin. This promotes prompt identification of the tract and reinsertion of the tracheal tube should it become dislodged. With a PDT, the trachea is not secured in this way, and a mature tract takes approximately 2 weeks to form. Accidental decannulation and attempted reinsertion of the airway during this time may result in difficulty securing the airway, bleeding, tracheal injury, and death. Oral intubation may be required if the airway becomes dislodged or needs to be replaced.[51]

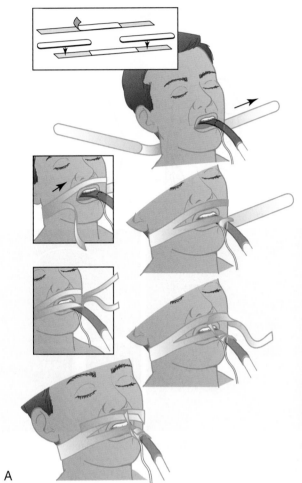

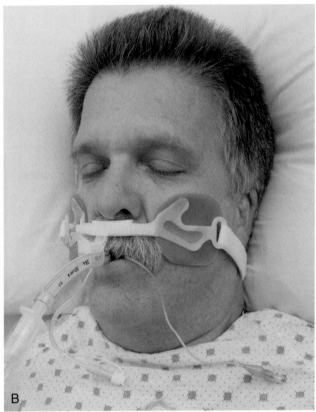

FIGURE 9-20 Two methods for securing the endotracheal tube: tape **(A)** and harness device **(B).** Harness device shown is the SecureEasy Endotracheal Tube Holder. Nonelastic headgear reduces the risk of self-extubation. A soft bite block prevents tube occlusion. (**B** Reprinted with permission, Cleveland Clinic Center for Medical Art & Photography © 2011-2012. All rights reserved.)

Tracheostomy Tube Designs

Tracheostomy tubes come in a variety of sizes and styles, and are primarily made of plastic. Design features are shown in Figure 9-21. The flange lies against the patient's neck and has an opening on both ends for the placement of tracheostomy ties for securing the airway. Similar to the ETT, some tracheostomy tubes have a distal cuff and pilot balloon. An important part of the tracheostomy system is the obturator, which is inserted into the trachea tube during insertion. The rounded end of the obturator extends just beyond the end of the tracheostomy tube and creates a smooth tip, allowing for easy entry into the stoma. The obturator is removed after tube insertion to allow for air passage through the trachea. It must be kept in a visible location in the patient's room should emergency reinsertion of a misplaced tube be necessary. In this situation the obturator is inserted into the tracheostomy to create a rounded, smooth end promoting reentry into the stoma without tissue injury.[51]

Cuffed versus uncuffed tracheostomy tubes. Critically ill patients who need mechanical ventilation require cuffed tubes to ensure delivery of ventilation and prevent aspiration. The cuff may be a conventional low-pressure, high-volume type, or it may be constructed of foam. The foam-cuff tube may prevent trauma to the airway because of the low pressure exerted to the airway, and it is sometimes used for patients who have difficulty maintaining a good seal with conventional cuffed tracheostomy tubes. Many other types of tracheostomy tubes are available.[58,60,66] An uncuffed tracheostomy tube is used for long-term airway management in a patient who does not require mechanical ventilation and is at low risk of aspiration. For example, a patient with a neurological injury may require a tracheostomy for airway management and secretion removal. Metal tracheostomy tubes are uncuffed.[63]

Single- versus double-cannula tracheostomy tubes. Tracheostomy tubes may have one or two cannulas. A single-cannula

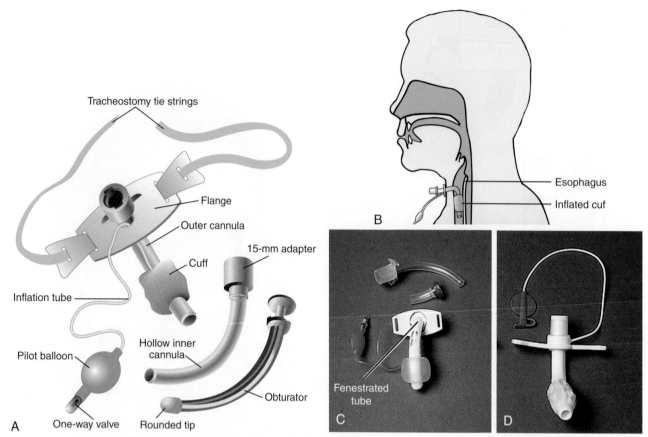

FIGURE 9-21 A, General design features of the tracheostomy tube. **B,** Trach tube in place. **C,** Fenestrated tracheostomy tube (see text for description). **D,** Fome cuff tracheostomy tube. (From Lewis SL, Dirkson SR, Heitkemper MM, et al. *Medical-Surgical Nursing.* 8th ed. St. Louis: Mosby; 2011.)

tube does not have an inner cannula, whereas a double-cannula tube has both an inner and outer cannula. The inner cannula is removable to facilitate cleaning of the inner lumen and to prevent tube occlusion from accumulated secretions. Inner cannulas can be reusable or disposable. Cuffed tracheostomy tubes with disposable inner cannulas are commonplace in the critical care unit.

Fenestrated tracheostomy tube. The fenestrated tracheostomy tube has a hole in the outer cannula that allows air to flow above the larynx. The tube functions as a standard tracheostomy tube when the inner cannula is in place. When the inner cannula is removed, the fenestrated tracheostomy tube assists in weaning a patient from the tracheostomy by gradually allowing the patient to breathe through the natural upper airway. The fenestrated tube also allows the patient to emit vocal sounds, thereby facilitating communication.[60,66] To use a cuffed fenestrated tracheostomy tube for speaking or to promote breathing through the natural airway, the inner cannula is carefully removed and the cuff is deflated. The inner cannula must be reinserted and the cuff reinflated for eating, suctioning, mechanical ventilation, or use of a bag-valve device.[51]

Speaking tracheostomy valves. One-way speaking valves are available to allow patients with a tracheostomy an opportunity to speak. Although these valves can be used in both ventilated and nonventilated patients, they can be used only in patients capable of initiating and maintaining spontaneous ventilation.[60] Examples of these adjunctive devices include the Passy-Muir Valve (Passy-Muir, Inc., Irvine, CA) and the Shiley Phonate Speaking Valve (Covidien, Boulder, CO). For the speaking valve to work correctly, the valve is connected to the tracheostomy tube, the cuff on the tracheostomy tube is deflated, and the patient is allowed to breathe and exhale through the natural airway. The valve itself is a one-way device allowing gas to enter through it into the tracheostomy tube and to the patient. Because this is a one-way valve, exhaled gas exits the trachea via the natural airway, past the deflated cuff of the tracheostomy tube and through the vocal cords.[58]

If a speaking valve is used in conjunction with mechanical ventilation, it must be used with a tracheostomy tube, not an ETT. The delivered tidal volume (V_T) must be increased to ensure an adequate volume to ventilate the patient because a portion of the delivered V_T is lost via the deflated tracheostomy cuff.[51] While the valve is in place, the patient is carefully assessed for respiratory stability and tolerance. Monitoring includes measurements of the patient's SpO$_2$, heart rate, RR, and blood pressure; observations about the patient's anxiety level and perception of the experience; and assessment of the patient's WOB. Management of secretions is another important nursing intervention.[5]

Endotracheal Suctioning

Patients with an artificial airway need to be suctioned to ensure airway patency because the normal protective ability to cough and expel secretions is impaired. Suctioning is performed according to a standard procedure to prevent complications such as hypoxemia, airway trauma, infection, and increased intracranial pressure in patients with head injury. Suctioning also stimulates the cough reflex and promotes the mobilization and removal of secretions.

Because suctioning is associated with complications, it is performed only as indicated by physical assessment and not according to a predetermined schedule. Indications for endotracheal suctioning include visible secretions in the tube, frequent coughing, presence of rhonchi, oxygen desaturation, a change in vital signs (e.g., increased or decreased heart rate or RR), dyspnea, restlessness, increased peak inspiratory pressure (PIP), or high-pressure ventilator alarms.[12,51] The number of suction passes is usually one to three; however, suctioning should be continued until secretions are removed. Suction duration is limited to 10 to 15 seconds and rest periods are provided between suction passes.

Key points related to endotracheal suctioning are discussed in Box 9-7. Hyperoxygenation with 100% oxygen should be performed for 30 seconds before suctioning, during the procedure, and immediately after suctioning.[12] Most ventilators have a built-in suction mode that delivers 100% oxygen for a short period (e.g., 2 minutes). Hyperoxygenation can also be administered with a bag-valve device. If the patient does not tolerate suctioning with hyperoxygenation alone, hyperinflation may be used. Hyperinflation involves the delivery of breaths 1.0 to 1.5 times the V$_T$ and is performed by giving the patient three to five breaths before and between suctioning attempts using either the ventilator or bag-valve device.[12]

The closed tracheal, or in-line, suction catheter is an alternative to the single use suction catheter. The closed tracheal suction system consists of a suction catheter enclosed in a plastic sheath that is attached to the patient's ventilator circuit and airway (Figure 9-22). The device assists in maintaining oxygenation during suctioning, reduces symptoms associated with hypoxemia, maintains positive end-expiratory pressure (PEEP), and protects staff from the patient's secretions; the data are inconsistent regarding its cost-effectiveness.[19,34] Depending on the institution, closed suctioning may be used on all ventilated patients; or it may be used for specific indications, such as for clinically unstable patients receiving high levels of PEEP, and for those requiring frequent suctioning.[45,63]

Saline instillation into the trachea during suctioning should not be routinely performed.[52] Although use of saline

---

BOX 9-7 KEY POINTS FOR ENDOTRACHEAL SUCTIONING

- Suction only as indicated by patient assessment.
- Choose the proper-size device. The diameter of the suction catheter should be no more than half the diameter of the artificial airway.
- Assemble equipment: suction kit with two gloves or closed suction system (CSS), sterile water or saline for rinsing the catheter. The CSS is attached to the ventilator circuit, usually by a respiratory therapist.
- Set the suction regulator at 80 to 120 mm Hg.
- Use sterile technique for suctioning.
- Hyperoxygenate the patient via the ventilator circuit before, between, and after suctioning.
- Gently insert suction catheter until resistance is met, then pull back 1 cm.
- Suction the patient no longer than 10 to 15 seconds while applying intermittent or constant suction.
- Repeat endotracheal suctioning until the airway is clear.
- Rinse the catheter with sterile saline after endotracheal suctioning is performed.
- Suction the mouth and oropharynx with the single-use suction catheter, suction swabs, or a tonsil suction device.
- Auscultate the lungs to assess effectiveness of suctioning, and document findings.
- Document the amount, color, and consistency of secretions.

- *Steps specific to closed suctioning* (in addition to those just noted):
  - Using the dominant hand, insert the suction catheter into the airway until resistance is met. Simultaneously, use the nondominant hand to stabilize the artificial airway.
  - Withdraw the suction catheter while depressing the suction valve; be careful to not angle the wrist of the hand while withdrawing the catheter, because kinking of the catheter and loss of suction may occur.
  - Ensure that CSS catheter is completely withdrawn from the airway. A marking is visible on the suction catheter when it is properly withdrawn.
  - Rinse the catheter after the procedure. Connect a small vial or syringe of normal saline for tracheal instillation (without preservatives) to the irrigation port, and simultaneously instill the saline into the port while depressing the suction control.
  - Keep the CSS suction catheter out of the patient's reach to avoid accidental self-extubation.

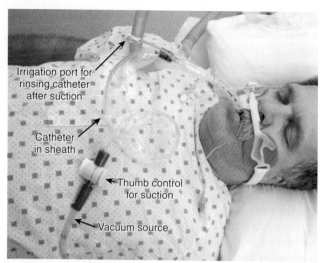

FIGURE 9-22 Closed tracheal suction device. (Reprinted with permission, Cleveland Clinic Center for Medical Art & Photography © 2011-2012. All rights reserved.)

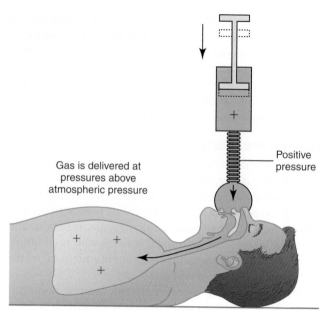

FIGURE 9-23 Concept of positive-pressure ventilation.

was a common practice for many years, saline instillation is associated with problems such as oxygen desaturation, washing organisms in the ETT into the lower airway, and patient discomfort.[1,10,46,55] Purported benefits of liquefying secretions and increasing volume of secretions removed are not proven. Adequate patient hydration and airway humidification, rather than saline instillation, facilitate secretion removal.

MECHANICAL VENTILATION

The purpose of mechanical ventilation is to support the respiratory system until the underlying cause of respiratory failure can be corrected. Most ventilatory support requires an artificial airway; however, it may be applied without an artificial airway and is called noninvasive ventilation.

Indications

Mechanical ventilation is warranted for patients with acute respiratory failure who are unable to maintain adequate gas exchange as reflected in the ABGs. A clinical definition of respiratory failure is as follows:

- $PaO_2 \leq 60$ mm Hg on a FiO_2 greater than 0.5 (oxygenation)
- $PaCO_2 \geq 50$ mm Hg, with a pH of 7.25 or less (ventilation)[35,53]

The patient may also demonstrate progressive physiological deterioration such as rapid, shallow breathing and an increase in the WOB as evidenced by increased use of the accessory muscles of ventilation, abnormal breathing patterns, and complaints of dyspnea. As lifesaving therapy, the purpose of mechanical ventilation is to support the respiratory system while a treatment plan is instituted to correct the underlying abnormality.[35,51,52]

Positive-Pressure Ventilation

In the critical care setting, most patients are treated with positive-pressure ventilation. This method uses positive pressure to force air into the lungs via an artificial airway, as illustrated in Figure 9-23. Movement of gases into the lungs through the use of *positive pressure* is the opposite of spontaneous breathing. Spontaneous ventilation begins when energy is expended to contract the muscles of respiration. This enlarges the thoracic cavity, increases *negative pressure* within the chest and lungs, and results in the flow of air, at atmospheric pressure, into the lungs. If mechanical ventilators could mimic the intrathoracic pressures present during spontaneous ventilation, it would be ideal. Negative-pressure ventilators, which originated with the iron lung, perform in this manner; however, these ventilators are for management of chronic conditions. Many of the complications of mechanical ventilation are related to air being forced into the lungs under positive pressure.

Ventilator Settings

In most institutions in the United States and Canada, ventilators are set up and managed by RTs. However, the nurse must be familiar with selected values on the control panel or graphic interface unit to assess ventilator settings, patient response to ventilation, and alarms. Representative control panels and screens of ventilators are shown in Figure 9-24. Although the control panel of a microprocessor type of ventilator can appear overwhelming, it is important for the nurse to learn to identify the common screen views that provide the settings and patient data that are integral to patient assessment. The nurse must know the basic ventilator settings of mode of ventilation, FiO_2, V_T, set RR rate, PEEP, and pressure support. Additional settings of inspiratory-to-expiratory (I:E) ratio, sensitivity, and sigh are also discussed to provide a basis for the nurse to knowledgeably communicate with the RT and provider.[51]

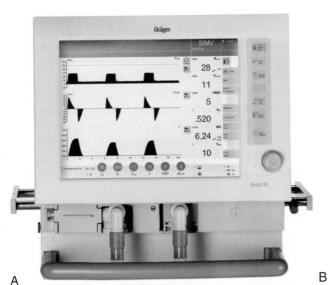
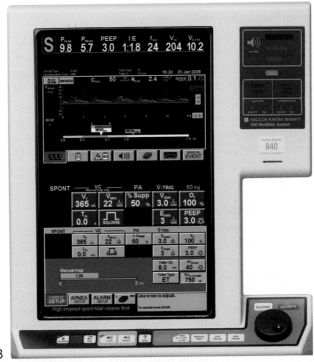

FIGURE 9-24 Examples of mechanical ventilators and their control panels and graphic interface unit (GIU). **A,** Dräger Evita XL. **B,** Puritan Bennett 840 Ventilator GIU. (**A** Copyright Drägerwerk AG & Co. KGa, Lubeck. All rights reserved. **B** Image used by permission from Nellcor Puritan Bennett LLC, Boulder, Colorado, doing business as Covidien.)

Fraction of Inspired Oxygen

The FiO$_2$ is set from 0.21 (21% or room air) to 1.00 (100% oxygen). The initial FiO$_2$ setting is based on the patient's immediate physiological needs and should be set to whatever is necessary to maintain a PaO$_2$ between 60 and 100 mm Hg and/or a SpO$_2$ of *at least* 90%. After the patient is stabilized, the setting is adjusted based on ABG or pulse oximetry values.

Tidal Volume

The amount of air delivered with each preset breath is the V$_T$. The V$_T$ is dictated by body weight and by the patient's lung characteristics (compliance and resistance), and it is set to ensure that excessive stretch and pressure on the lung tissue is avoided. A starting point for the V$_T$ setting is 6 to 8 mL/kg of ideal body weight with the lowest value recommended in patients with obstructive airway disease or ARDS.[7,31,35] The parameters monitored to avoid excessive pressure are the PIP and plateau airway pressure (Pplat). These pressures should remain below 40 cm H$_2$O and 30 cm H$_2$O, respectively.[7] The V$_T$ setting can be reduced if the resulting airway pressures are nearing the maximum. Conversely, if the airway pressures are acceptable and a larger V$_T$ is needed to remove CO$_2$, it can be increased. When choosing and adjusting the V$_T$ setting, the goal is to achieve the lowest Pplat while maintaining gas exchange and patient comfort.

Respiratory Rate

The RR is the frequency of breaths (f) set to be delivered by the ventilator. The RR is set as near to physiological rates (14 to 20 breaths per minute) as possible. Frequent changes in the RR are often required based on observation of the patient's WOB and comfort, and assessment of the PaCO$_2$ and pH. During initiation of mechanical ventilation, many patients require full ventilatory support. The RR at this time is selected on the basis of the V$_T$, to achieve a minute ventilation (VE) that maintains an acceptable acid-base status (VE = RR × V$_T$). As the patient becomes capable of participating in the ventilatory work, the ventilator RR is decreased, or the mode of ventilation is changed, to encourage more spontaneous breathing.

Inspiratory-to-Expiratory Ratio

The I:E ratio is the duration of inspiration in comparison with expiration. In spontaneous ventilation, inspiration is shorter than expiration. When a patient undergoes mechanical ventilation, the I:E ratio is usually set at 1:2 to mimic this pattern of spontaneous ventilation; that is, 33% of the respiratory cycle is spent in inspiration and 66% in the expiratory phase. Longer expiratory times, I:E ratio of 1:3 or 1:4, may be needed in patients with COPD to promote more complete exhalation and reduce air trapping.[35,51,53]

Inverse Inspiratory-to-Expiratory Ratio

Inspiratory-to-expiratory (I:E) ratios such as 1:1, 2:1, and 3:1 are called inverse I:E ratios. An inverse I:E ratio is used to improve oxygenation in patients with noncompliant lungs, such as in ARDS. During the traditional I:E ratio of 1:2, alveoli in noncompliant lungs may not have sufficient time to reopen during the shorter inspiratory phase, and may collapse during the longer expiratory phase. An inverse I:E ratio allows unstable alveoli time to fill and prevents them from collapsing, because the next inspiration begins before the alveoli reach a volume where they can collapse.[35,51]

Positive End-Expiratory Pressure

PEEP is the addition of positive pressure into the airways during expiration. PEEP is measured in cm H_2O. Typical settings for PEEP are 5 to 20 cm H_2O, although higher levels may be used to treat refractory hypoxemia. Because positive pressure is applied at end expiration, the airways and alveoli are held open, and oxygenation improves. PEEP increases oxygenation by preventing collapse of small airways and maximizing the number of alveoli available for gas exchange (Figure 9-25). By recruiting more alveoli for gas exchange and by holding them open during expiration, the functional residual capacity improves, resulting in better oxygenation.

Many mechanically ventilated patients routinely receive 3 to 5 cm H_2O of PEEP, a value often referred to as *physiological PEEP*. This small amount of PEEP is thought to mimic the normal "back pressure" created in the lungs by the epiglottis in the spontaneously breathing patient that is removed by the displacement of the epiglottis by the artificial airway.

PEEP is often added to decrease a high FiO_2 that may be required to achieve adequate oxygenation. For example, a patient may require a FiO_2 of 0.80 to maintain a PaO_2 of 85 mm Hg. By adding PEEP, it may be possible to decrease the FiO_2 to a level where oxygen toxicity in the lung is not a concern (<0.5) while maintaining an adequate PaO_2.[53] The nurse monitors the PEEP level by observing the pressure level displayed on the ventilator's analog and graphic displays. When no PEEP is set, the pressure reading on the graphic display should be zero at end expiration. When PEEP is applied, the pressure reading does not return to zero at the end of the breath, and the display shows the amount of PEEP.

Although PEEP is often essential for treatment, it is associated with adverse effects. Problems related to PEEP occur as a result of the increase in intrathoracic pressure. These problems include a decrease in cardiac output secondary to decreased venous return, volutrauma or barotrauma, and increased intracranial pressure resulting from impedance of venous return from the head, Whenever the level of PEEP is increased, the nurse should evaluate the patient's hemodynamic response through physical assessment and by available hemodynamic parameters. Management of decreased cardiac output secondary to PEEP includes ensuring the patient has adequate intravascular volume (preload) and administering fluids as needed. If the cardiac output remains inadequate, an inotropic agent such as dobutamine should be considered. Optimal PEEP is defined as the amount of PEEP that affords the best oxygenation without resulting in adverse hemodynamic effects or pulmonary injury.[35,51]

Auto-PEEP. Auto-PEEP is the spontaneous development of PEEP caused by gas trapping in the lung resulting from insufficient expiratory time and incomplete exhalation. These trapped gases create positive pressure in the lung. Both set PEEP and auto-PEEP have the same physiological effects; therefore it is important to know when auto-PEEP is present so it can be managed properly.[35,51,53]

Causes of auto-PEEP formation include rapid RR, high VE demand, airflow obstruction, and inverse I:E ratio ventilation. Auto-PEEP cannot be detected by the ventilator pressure manometer until a special maneuver is performed. This maneuver involves instituting a 2-second end-expiratory pause, which allows the ventilator to read the pressure deep in the lung. The airway pressure manometer reading therefore reflects total PEEP, which is the set PEEP and auto-PEEP added together. To determine auto-PEEP, the following calculation is performed:

$$\text{Auto-PEEP} = \text{Total PEEP} - \text{Set PEEP}$$

Sensitivity

Sensitivity determines the amount of patient effort needed to initiate gas flow through the circuitry on a patient-initiated breath. The sensitivity is set so that the ventilator is "sensitive" to the patient's effort to inspire. If the sensitivity is set too low, the patient must generate more work to trigger gas flow. If it is set too high, auto-cycling of the ventilator may occur, resulting in patient-ventilator dyssynchrony, because the ventilator cycles into the inspiratory phase when the patient is not ready for a breath.[51,53]

Patient Data

The nurse and RT ensure that the ventilator settings are consistent with the physician's orders. The ventilator control panel or graphic interface unit also provides valuable information regarding the patient's response to mechanical ventilation. These patient data include exhaled tidal volume (EV_T), PIP, and total RR.

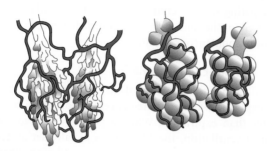

FIGURE 9-25 Effect of application of positive end-expiratory pressure (PEEP) on the alveoli. (Modified from Pierce LNB. *Management of the Mechanically Ventilated Patient.* Philadelphia: Saunders; 2007.)

Exhaled Tidal Volume

The EV_T is the amount of gas that comes out of the patient's lungs on exhalation. The EV_T is not a ventilator setting. It is considered patient data that indicates the patient's response to mechanical ventilation. This is the most accurate measure of the volume received by the patient and therefore is monitored at least every 4 hours and more often as indicated. Although the prescribed V_T is set on the ventilator control panel, it is not guaranteed to be delivered to the patient. Volume may be lost because of leaks in the ventilator circuit, around the cuff of the airway, or via a chest tube if there is a pleural air leak.[50] The volume actually received by the patient, regardless of mode of ventilation, must be confirmed by monitoring the EV_T on the display panel of the ventilator. If the EV_T deviates from the set V_T by 50 mL or more, the nurse and RT must troubleshoot the system to identify the source of gas loss.[50]

Peak Inspiratory Pressure

The PIP is the maximum pressure that occurs during inspiration. The amount of pressure necessary to ventilate the patient increases with increased airway resistance (e.g., secretions in the airway, bronchospasm, biting the ETT) and decreased lung compliance (e.g., pulmonary edema, worsening infiltrate or ARDS, pleural space disease). The PIP should never be allowed to rise above 40 cm H_2O, because higher pressures can result in ventilator-induced lung injury.[7,62]

The nurse should monitor and record the PIP at least every 4 hours and with any change in patient condition that could increase airway resistance or decrease compliance.[50] Increasing PIP or values greater than 40 cm H_2O should be immediately reported so that interventions can be ordered to improve lung function, ventilator settings can be adjusted to reduce the inspiratory pressure, or both.

Total Respiratory Rate

The total RR equals the number of breaths delivered by the ventilator (set rate) plus the number of breaths initiated by the patient. Assessing the total RR provides data regarding the patient's contribution to the WOB, or whether the ventilator is performing all of the work. It also provides an assessment of the ability of the set RR and V_T to meet VE demands. The total RR is a very sensitive indicator of overall respiratory stability.[50] For example, if the patient is on assist/control ventilation at a set RR of 10 breaths per minute, and the total RR for 1 minute is 16, the patient is initiating 6 breaths above the set rate of 10. If the patient is on synchronized intermittent mandatory ventilation at a set RR of 8 breaths per minute, and the total RR is 12 breaths per minute with good spontaneous V_T for body weight, the patient is tolerating the mode of ventilation. If the patient's total RR increases to 26 breaths per minute, this finding indicates that something has changed and the patient needs to be reassessed for causes of the increased rate, such as fatigue, pain, or anxiety. Treatment is based on the identified cause.

Modes of Mechanical Ventilation

Modes of mechanical ventilation describe how breaths are delivered to the patient. Modes of ventilation are classified as volume, pressure, or dual modes. This classification is based on the variable that the ventilator maintains at a preset value during inspiration.[50] In a volume mode of ventilation, the set V_T is maintained during inspiration. In a pressure mode of ventilation, pressure is set and does not vary throughout inspiration. An understanding of the basic volume and pressure modes of ventilation provides a solid foundation for the nurse to learn the dual modes.

Volume Ventilation

In volume ventilation, V_T is constant for every breath delivered by the ventilator. The ventilator is set to allow airflow into the lungs until a preset volume has been reached. A major advantage of this mode is that the V_T is delivered, regardless of changes in lung compliance or resistance. However, the PIP varies in this mode, depending on compliance and resistance. Assist/control (A/C; Figure 9-26, *A*) and synchronized intermittent mandatory ventilation (SIMV; Figure 9-26, *B*) are modes of volume ventilation.

Assist/control ventilation. The volume A/C (V–A/C) mode of ventilation delivers a preset number of breaths of a preset V_T. The patient may trigger additional spontaneous breaths between the ventilator-initiated breaths. When the patient initiates a breath by exerting a negative inspiratory effort, the ventilator delivers an assisted breath of the preset V_T. The V_T of the assisted breaths is constant for both ventilator-initiated and patient-triggered breaths. The V–A/C mode ensures that the patient receives adequate ventilation, regardless of spontaneous efforts. The V–A/C mode is indicated when it is desirable for the ventilator to perform the bulk of the WOB. The only work the patient must perform is the negative inspiratory effort required to trigger the ventilator on the patient-initiated breaths. The A/C mode is useful in a patient with a normal respiratory drive but whose respiratory muscles are too weak or unable to perform the WOB (e.g., patient emerging from general anesthesia or with pulmonary disease such as pneumonia).[53] A disadvantage of V–A/C ventilation is that respiratory alkalosis may develop if the patient hyperventilates because of anxiety, pain, or neurological factors. Respiratory alkalosis is treated or prevented by providing sedation or analgesia as needed, or changing to SIMV.[35] Another disadvantage is that the patient may rely on the ventilator and not attempt to initiate spontaneous breathing if ventilatory demands are met.

During V–A/C ventilation, the nurse monitors several parameters. These include the total RR, to determine whether the patient is initiating spontaneous breaths; the EV_T, to ensure that the set V_T is delivered; the PIP, to determine whether it is increasing (indicating a change in compliance or resistance, which needs to be further evaluated); the patient's sense of comfort and synchronization with the ventilator; and the acid-base status.[50]

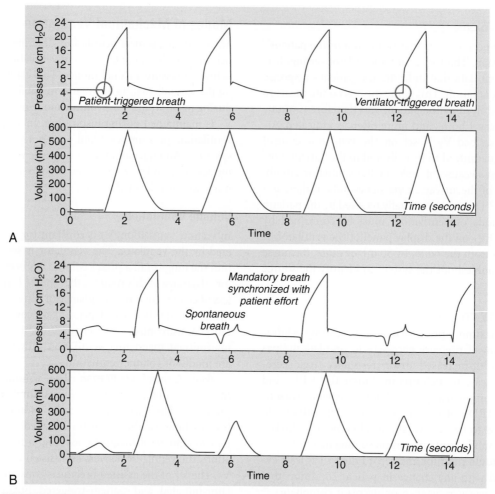

FIGURE 9-26 Waveforms of volume-controlled ventilator modes. **A,** Volume assist/control (V–A/C) ventilation. The patient may trigger additional breaths above the set rate. The ventilator delivers the same volume for ventilator-triggered and patient-triggered (assisted) breaths. **B,** Synchronized intermittent mandatory ventilation (SIMV). Both spontaneous and mandatory breaths are graphed. Mandatory breaths receive the set tidal volume (V_T). V_T of spontaneous breaths depends on work patient is capable of generating, lung compliance, and airway resistance.

Synchronized intermittent mandatory ventilation. The volume SIMV mode of ventilation delivers a set number of breaths of a set V_T, and between these mandatory breaths the patient may initiate spontaneous breaths. If the patient initiates a breath near the time a mandatory breath is due, the delivery of the mandatory breath is synchronized with the patient's spontaneous effort to prevent patient-ventilator dyssynchrony. The volume of the spontaneous breaths depends on the patient's respiratory effort. The main difference between the SIMV and V–A/C modes is the volume of the patient-initiated breaths. Patient-initiated breaths in A/C ventilation result in the patient receiving a set V_T. In SIMV, the V_T of spontaneous breaths is variable because it depends on patient effort and lung characteristics.[50,51]

The SIMV mode helps to prevent respiratory muscle weakness associated with mechanical ventilation because the patient contributes to the WOB. SIMV is indicated when it is desirable to allow patients to breathe at their own RR and assist in maintaining a normal $PaCO_2$, or when hyperventilation has occurred in the V–A/C mode. SIMV is also indicated for weaning patients from mechanical ventilation. As the SIMV rate is lowered, the patient initiates more spontaneous breaths, assuming a greater portion of the ventilatory work. As the patient demonstrates the ability to take on even more WOB, the mandatory breath rate is decreased accordingly. However, compared with other weaning modalities, SIMV is associated with the longest weaning and lowest success rate.[5,20]

During SIMV, the nurse monitors the total RR to determine whether the patient is initiating spontaneous breaths, and the patient's ability to manage the WOB. If the total RR increases, the V_T of the spontaneous breaths is assessed for adequacy. An adequate spontaneous V_T is 5 to 7 mL/kg of ideal body weight. A rising total RR may indicate that the patient is beginning to fatigue, resulting in a more shallow and rapid respiratory pattern. This pattern may lead to

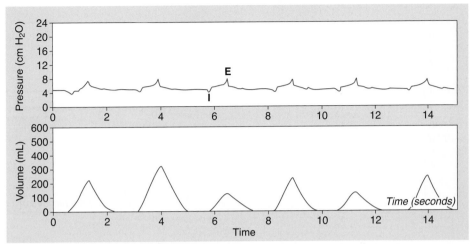

FIGURE 9-27 Continuous positive airway pressure (CPAP) is a spontaneous breathing mode. Positive pressure at end expiration splints alveoli and supports oxygenation. Note that the pressure does not fall to zero, indicating the level of CPAP. *E,* Expiration; *I,* inspiration.

atelectasis, a further increase in the WOB, and the need for greater ventilatory support.[50,51] The nurse monitors the EV_T of both the mandatory and spontaneous breaths to ensure that the set V_T is being delivered with the mandatory breaths, and that the spontaneous V_T is adequate. As in A/C ventilation, the nurse assesses the PIP, the patient's sense of comfort and synchronization with the ventilator, and the acid-base status.

Pressure Ventilation

In pressure ventilation the ventilator is set to allow air to flow into the lungs until a preset inspiratory pressure has been reached. The V_T the patient receives is variable and depends on lung compliance and airway and circuit resistance. Patients with normal lung compliance and low resistance will have better delivery of V_T for the amount of inspiratory pressure set.[35,50,51,53] An advantage of pressure-controlled modes is that the PIP can be reliably controlled for each breath the ventilator delivers. A disadvantage is that hypoventilation and respiratory acidosis may occur since delivered V_T varies; therefore, the nurse must closely monitor EV_T.[51] Pressure modes include continuous positive airway pressure, pressure support, pressure control, pressure-controlled inverse-ratio ventilation, and airway pressure–release ventilation.

Continuous positive airway pressure. Continuous positive airway pressure (CPAP) is positive pressure applied throughout the respiratory cycle to the spontaneously breathing patient (Figure 9-27). The patient must have a reliable respiratory drive and adequate V_T because no mandatory breaths or other ventilatory assistance is given. The patient performs all the WOB. CPAP provides pressure at end expiration, which prevents alveolar collapse and improves the functional residual capacity and oxygenation.[35,50] CPAP is identical to PEEP in its physiological effects. CPAP is the correct term when the end-expiratory pressure is applied in the spontaneously breathing patient. PEEP is the term used for

the same setting applied to the patient is receiving an additional form of respiratory support (e.g., A/C, SIMV, pressure support). CPAP is indicated as a mode of weaning, when the patient has adequate ventilation but requires end-expiratory pressure to stabilize the alveoli and maintain oxygenation. Because the ventilator is used to deliver CPAP during weaning, the nurse can monitor the adequacy of the patient's EV_T, alarms can be set to detect low EV_T and apnea, and mechanical breaths can be delivered in the event of apnea.[51]

CPAP can also be administered via a nasal or face mask. Typically, a nasal CPAP system is used to keep the airway open in patients with obstructive sleep apnea.

Pressure support. Pressure support (PS) is a mode of ventilation in which the patient's spontaneous respiratory activity is augmented by the delivery of a preset amount of inspiratory positive pressure. PS may be used as a stand-alone mode (Figure 9-28) or in combination with other modes, such as SIMV, to augment the V_T of the spontaneous breaths (Figure 9-29). The positive pressure is applied throughout inspiration, thereby promoting the flow of gas into the lungs, augmenting the patient's spontaneous V_T, and decreasing the WOB associated with breathing through an artificial airway and the ventilatory circuit.[35,50,53] Typical levels of PS ordered for the patient are 6 to 12 cm H_2O. The V_T is variable, determined by patient effort, the amount of PS applied, and the compliance and resistance of the patient and ventilator system. EV_T must be closely monitored during PS; if it is inadequate, the level of PS is increased. PS may increase patient comfort because the patient has greater control over the initiation and duration of each breath. PS promotes conditioning of the respiratory muscles since the patient works throughout the breath; this may facilitate weaning from the ventilator.

Pressure assist/control. Pressure assist/control (P–A/C) is a mode of ventilation in which there is a set RR, and every breath is augmented by a set amount of inspiratory pressure.

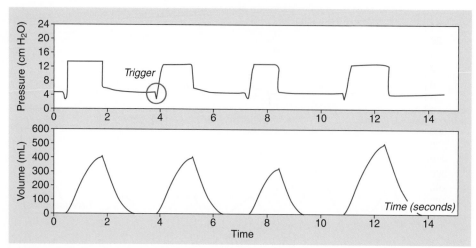

FIGURE 9-28 Pressure support ventilation requires the patient to trigger each breath, which is then supported by pressure on inspiration. Patient may vary amount of time in inspiration, respiratory rate, and tidal volume (V_T).

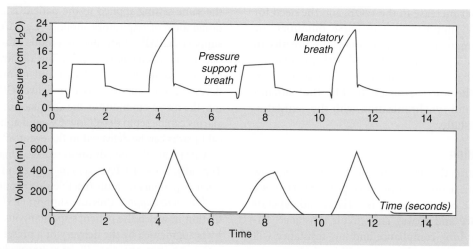

FIGURE 9-29 Synchronized intermittent mandatory ventilation (SIMV) with pressure support (PS). SIMV breaths receive set tidal volume (V_T). Pressure support is applied to the spontaneous, patient-triggered breaths.

If the patient triggers additional breaths beyond the mandatory breaths, those breaths are augmented by the set amount of inspiratory pressure (Figure 9-30). Just as with PS, there is no set V_T. The V_T the patient receives is variable and determined by the set inspiratory pressure, the patient's lung compliance, and circuit and airway resistance. The typical pressure in P–A/C ranges from 15 to 25 cm H_2O, which is higher than a PS level because P–A/C is indicated for patients with ARDS, or those with a high PIP during traditional volume ventilation. Because the lungs are noncompliant in these conditions, higher inspiratory pressure levels are needed to achieve an adequate V_T. P–A/C reduces the risk of barotrauma while maintaining adequate oxygenation and ventilation. During P–A/C, the nurse must be familiar with all the ventilator settings: the level of pressure, the set RR, the FiO_2,

and the level of PEEP. The nurse monitors the total RR to evaluate whether the patient is initiating spontaneous breaths, and EV_T for adequacy of volume.[50]

Pressure-controlled inverse-ratio ventilation. With pressure-controlled inverse-ratio ventilation (PC-IRV), the patient receives P–A/C ventilation as described, and the ventilator is set to provide longer inspiratory times. The I:E ratio is inversed to increase the mean airway pressure, open and stabilize the alveoli, and improve oxygenation. PC-IRV is indicated for patients with noncompliant lungs such as in ARDS, when adequate oxygenation is not achieved despite high FiO_2, PEEP, or positioning. Because the reverse I:E ratio ventilation is uncomfortable, the patient must be sedated and possibly paralyzed to prevent ventilator dyssynchrony and oxygen desaturation.[50,53]

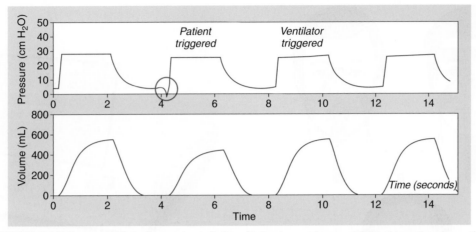

FIGURE 9-30 Pressure assist/control ventilation. Patient can trigger additional breaths above the set rate. Patient- and ventilator-triggered breaths receive the same inspiratory pressure.

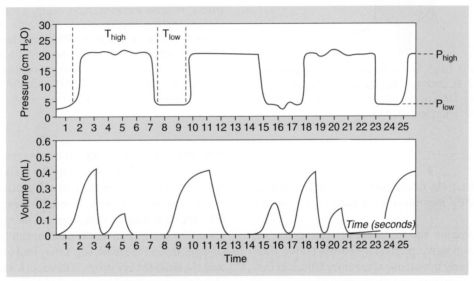

FIGURE 9-31 Airway pressure–release ventilation.

Airway pressure–release ventilation. Airway pressure–release ventilation (APRV) is a mode of ventilation that provides two levels of CPAP, one during inspiration and the other during expiration, while allowing unrestricted spontaneous breathing at any point during the respiratory cycle (Figure 9-31). APRV starts at an elevated pressure, the CPAP level or pressure high (P_{HIGH}), followed by a release pressure, pressure low (P_{LOW}). After the airway pressure release, the P_{HIGH} level is restored.[23] The time spent at P_{HIGH} is known as time high (T_{HIGH}) and is generally prolonged, 4 to 6 seconds. The shorter release period (P_{LOW}) is known as time low (T_{LOW}) and is generally 0.5 to 1.1 seconds. When observing the pressure waveform, APRV is similar to PC-IRV; however, unlike PC-IRV, the patient has unrestricted spontaneous breathing. The patient is more comfortable on APRV, and

neither deep sedation nor paralysis is needed. APRV assists in providing adequate oxygenation while lowering PIP. It is indicated as an alternative to V–A/C or P–A/C for patients with significantly decreased lung compliance, such as those with ARDS.[26,35,50]

Noninvasive Positive-Pressure Ventilation

Noninvasive positive-pressure ventilation (NPPV) is the delivery of mechanical ventilation without an ETT or tracheostomy tube. NPPV provides ventilation via (1) a face mask that covers the nose, mouth, or both; (2) a nasal mask or pillow; or (3) a full face mask (Figure 9-32). Complications associated with an artificial airway are reduced, such as vocal cord injury and ventilator-associated pneumonia, and sedation needs are less. During NPPV, the patient can eat and

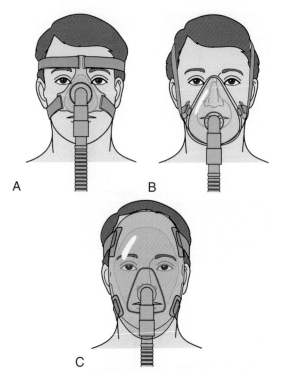

FIGURE 9-32 Masks used for noninvasive positive-pressure ventilation. **A,** Nasal. **B,** Oronasal. **C,** Total face mask. (Redrawn from Mims BC, Toto KH, Luecke LE, et al. *Critical Care Skills.* 2nd ed. Philadelphia: Saunders; 2003.)

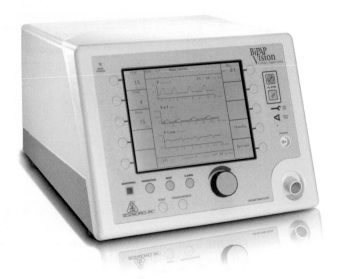

FIGURE 9-33 Noninvasive positive-pressure ventilation (NPPV) may be administered through a mask with the BiPAP Vision ventilator. This ventilator is capable of operating in four modes: pressure support (PS); spontaneous/timed (S/T) mode, which is pressure support with backup pressure control; timed (T), which is pressure control; and continuous positive airway pressure (CPAP). (Courtesy Phillips Healthcare, Andover, Massachusetts.)

speak, and is free from the discomfort of an artificial airway. Treatment with NPPV may prevent the need for intubation in many patients.

NPPV is indicated for the treatment of acute exacerbations of COPD, cardiogenic pulmonary edema (along with other treatments), early hypoxemic respiratory failure in immunocompromised patients, and obstructive sleep apnea. It may also be used to prevent reintubation in a patient who has been extubated but is having respiratory distress, and to provide ventilatory support while an acute problem is treated in patients for whom intubation is undesirable, such as those with "do not intubate" orders.[50] Contraindications to NPPV include apnea, cardiovascular instability (hypotension, uncontrolled dysrhythmias, and myocardial ischemia), claustrophobia, somnolence, high aspiration risk, viscous or copious secretions, inability to clear secretions, recent facial or gastroesophageal surgery, craniofacial trauma, and burns.[35,50]

NPPV can be delivered with critical care ventilators or a ventilator specifically designed to provide NPPV (Figure 9-33). Modes delivered can be pressure or volume; however, pressure modes are better tolerated. The most common modes of ventilation delivered via NPPV are pressure support or pressure control with PEEP and CPAP.

During NPPV, it is important for the nurse to work with the RT to ensure the right size and type of mask is chosen, and that it fits snugly enough to prevent air leaks. The nurse monitors the mask and the skin under the mask edges for signs of breakdown. If signs of excess pressure are noted, interventions include repositioning the mask, placing a layer of wound care dressing on the skin as a protective shield, or trying another type of mask. If mouth breathing is a problem with the nasal mask, a chin strap can be applied, or the mask should be changed to an oronasal or full face mask. Leakage of gases around the mask edges may lead to drying of the eyes and the need for eye drops. The mouth and airway passages should be monitored for excessive drying, and a humidification system applied as indicated. The nurse also monitors the total RR, the EV_T to ensure it is adequate, and the PIP.[50,51]

High Frequency Oscillatory Ventilation

High frequency oscillatory ventilation (HFOV) delivers subphysiological tidal volumes at extremely fast rates (300 to 420 breaths per minute). It is indicated in patients with noncompliant lungs and hypoxemia where conventional ventilation results in high airway pressures. This strategy stabilizes the alveoli and improves gas mixing, thereby improving oxygenation. The small tidal volumes limit peak pressure, preventing overdistention and protecting the lung from further injury. At the same time, collapse of the alveoli at end-expiration is limited through the use of higher end-expiratory pressure. HFOV is delivered with a specialized ventilator that uses a diaphragm, much like a stereo speaker, driven by a piston creating a constant flow of gases in and out of the lung (Figure 9-34). Ventilator settings control the amount, timing, and speed of piston movement. The nurse must learn new monitoring parameters when caring for a patient on HFOV.

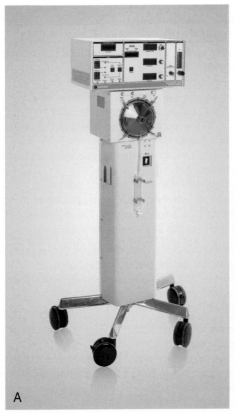
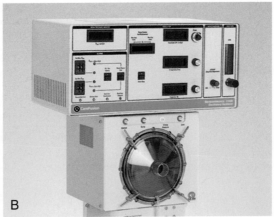

FIGURE 9-34 A, SensorMedics 3100B High Frequency Oscillatory Ventilator. **B,** Enlarged view. (Courtesy CareFusion, San Diego, California.)

Advanced Methods and Modes of Mechanical Ventilation

Microprocessor ventilators offer a wide range of options for mechanical ventilation. However, other forms of ventilatory support are available. These advanced techniques are usually ordered to treat patients with respiratory failure that is refractory to conventional treatment. These techniques include, but are not limited to, high-frequency jet ventilation, extracorporeal membrane oxygenation, and inhaled nitric oxide. Specialized equipment and training are essential for these advanced treatments.

Respiratory Monitoring During Mechanical Ventilation

Nurses and RTs routinely monitor many parameters while a patient receives mechanical ventilation. Monitoring done to assess the patient's response to treatment and to anticipate and plan for the ventilator weaning process includes physical assessment of the patient and assessment of the ventilator system: airway, circuitry, accuracy of ventilator settings, and patient data. Physical assessment includes vital signs and hemodynamic parameters, patient comfort and WOB, synchrony of patient's respiratory efforts with the ventilator, breath sounds, amount and quality of respiratory secretions, and assessment of the chest drain system if present. ABG results, pulse oximetry, and

$ETCO_2$ values are evaluated to assess oxygenation and ventilation.[20,51,57,65] Patient data evaluated from the ventilator include EV_T (mandatory, spontaneous, and assisted breaths), total RR, and PIP. Further assessment of the PIP may require direct measurements of airway resistance and static lung compliance. The ventilator system should be checked by the nurse at least every 4 hours. The RT performs a more detailed assessment of the ventilator's functioning, including alarms and the appropriateness of alarm settings.

Alarm Systems

Alarms are an integral part of mechanical ventilation because this equipment provides vital life support functions. Alarms warn of technical or patient events that require attention or action; therefore knowledge about alarms and how to troubleshoot them is essential. Two important rules must be followed to ensure patient safety:

1. Never shut off alarms. It is acceptable to silence alarms for a preset delay while working with a patient, such as during suctioning. However, alarms are never shut off.
2. Manually ventilate the patient with a bag-valve device if unable to troubleshoot alarms quickly or if equipment failure is suspected. A bag-valve device must be readily available at the bedside of every patient who is mechanically ventilated.

TABLE 9-4	MANAGEMENT OF COMMON VENTILATOR ALARMS	
ALARM	**DESCRIPTION**	**INTERVENTION**
High peak pressure	Set 10 cm H_2O above average PIP Triggered when pressure increases anywhere in circuit Ventilator responds by terminating inspiratory phase to avoid pressure injury (barotrauma)	Assess for kinks in endotracheal tube or ventilator circuit and correct Assess for anxiety and level of sedation patient biting or gagging on tube; administer medications if warranted, use airway securing device with bite block Observe for coughing, auscultate lung sounds for need for suctioning or bronchodilator Use communication assistive devices for patient who is attempting to talk Empty water from water traps if indicated Assess for worsening pulmonary pathology resulting in reduction in lung compliance (i.e., pulmonary edema) Notify RT and/or physician if alarm persists
Low pressure Low PEEP/CPAP	Set 10 cm H_2O below average PIP Set 3-5 cm H_2O below set PEEP/CPAP Triggered when pressure decreases in circuit	Assess for leaks in ventilator circuit or disconnection of ventilator circuit from airway; reconnect If malfunction is noted, manually ventilate patient with bag-mask device Notify RT to troubleshoot alarm
Low exhaled tidal volume Low minute ventilation (VE)	Set 10% below the set VT and the patients average VE Ensures adequate alveolar ventilation	Assess for disconnection of ventilator circuit from airway; reconnect Assess for disconnection in any part of the ventilator circuit; reconnect Assess for leak in cuff of artificial airway by listening for audible sounds around the airway and using device to measure cuff pressure; inflate as needed Assess for new or increasing air leak in a chest drain system; connect if system-related, notify provider if patient-related Assess for changes in lung compliance, increase in airway resistance, or patient fatigue in patient on a pressure mode of ventilation
High exhaled tidal volume High minute ventilation (VE)	Set 10% above the set VT and the patients average VE	Assess cause for increased RR or VT such as anxiety, pain, hypoxemia, metabolic acidosis; treat Assess for excess water in tubing; drain appropriately
Apnea alarm	Set for <20 seconds Warns when no exhalation detected Ventilator will default to a backup controlled mode if one is set	Assess for cause of lack of spontaneous respiratory effort (sedation, respiratory arrest, neurological condition); physically stimulate patient, encourage patient to take a deep breath, reverse sedatives or narcotics Manually ventilate patient while RT and/or provider are notified to modify ventilator settings to provide more support

CPAP, Continuous positive airway pressure; *PEEP,* positive end-expiratory pressure; *PIP,* peak inspiratory pressure; *RT,* respiratory therapist; *VE,* minute ventilation; *VT,* tidal volume.

When an alarm sounds, the first thing to do is to look at the patient. If the patient is disconnected from the ventilator circuit, quickly reconnect the patient to the machine. If the circuit is connected to the airway, quickly assess whether the patient is in distress, and whether he or she is adequately ventilated and oxygenated. The nurse quickly assesses the patient's level of consciousness, airway, RR, oxygen saturation level, heart rate, color, WOB, chest wall movement, and lung sounds. The ventilator display is observed to identify the status message related to the alarm, and the alarm is silenced while the cause of the alarm is determined. Immediate action is required if the patient is in acute distress with labored respirations, an abnormal breathing pattern, pallor and diaphoresis, deterioration in breath sounds, or decreasing SpO_2.[53] The nurse quickly disconnects the patient from the ventilator and manually ventilates with a bag-valve device while a second caregiver, often the RT, further assesses the problem. If the patient is not in respiratory distress, the nurse uses the assessment data gathered to proceed with problem solving. Table 9-4 provides an overview of management of common ventilator alarms.

Complications of Mechanical Ventilation

Numerous complications are associated with intubation and mechanical ventilation. Many complications can be prevented or treated rapidly through vigilant nursing care.[51] Best

Implementation of the Ventilator Bundle

The ventilator bundle of care should be implemented in all patients who receive mechanical ventilation.[32] This bundle is a group of evidence-based recommendations that has been demonstrated to improve outcomes. It is expected that all interventions in the bundle be implemented unless contraindicated:

- Maintain head of bed elevation at 30 to 45 degrees
- Interrupt sedation each day to assess readiness to wean from ventilator
- Provide prophylaxis for deep vein thrombosis
- Administer medications for peptic ulcer disease prophylaxis
- Daily oral care with chlorhexidine[4,32] (NOTE: The Institute of Healthcare Improvement [IHI] added this element to the ventilator bundle. Recommended chlorhexidine solution strength is 0.12%. Other bundles recommend oral care with antiseptics and do not specify a particular solution.)

practice includes implementation of the "ventilator bundle" for all mechanically ventilated patients to prevent complications and improve outcomes (see box, "Clinical Alert").

Airway Problems

Endotracheal tube out of position. The ETT can become dislodged if it is not secured properly during procedures such as oral care or changing the ETT securing device, during transport, or if the patient is anxious or agitated and attempts to pull out the tube. The ETT may be displaced upward, resulting in the cuff being positioned between or above the vocal cords. Conversely, the tube may advance too far into the airway and press on the carina or move into the right mainstem bronchus. Symptoms include absent or diminished breath sounds in the left lung and unequal chest excursion. The nurse should notify the provider of these findings so the cuff can be let down, the tube gently retracted as needed, and the cuff properly reinflated.

Whenever the ETT is manipulated, the nurse must assess for bilateral chest excursion, auscultate the chest for bilateral breath sounds after the procedure, and reassess tube position at the lip. A quick check of the centimeter markings can determine whether the tube has advanced or pulled out of proper position. When a serious airway problem cannot be quickly resolved, the nurse attempts to manually ventilate the patient to assess airway patency. If the patient cannot be ventilated and the tube is not obviously displaced or the patient is not biting the airway, the nurse should attempt to pass a suction catheter through the airway to determine whether it is obstructed. If the catheter cannot be passed and the patient has spontaneous respirations, the cuff is deflated to allow air to pass around the tube. If the patient still cannot be adequately ventilated, the airway must be removed and the patient is ventilated with a bag-valve device while preparing for emergent reintubation.[35,53]

Unplanned extubation. The patient may intentionally or inadvertently remove the airway. The two most frequent methods by which self-extubation occurs are (1) by using the tongue, and (2) by leaning forward or scooting downward so the patient uses his or her hands to remove the tube.[4,54] Unplanned extubation can also occur as a result of patient care. For example, the tube can be dislodged if the ventilator circuit or closed suction catheter pulls on the ETT during procedures such as turning. Despite vigilant nursing care, unplanned extubation may result. Strategies for preventing an unplanned extubation are described in Box 9-8.

Laryngeal and tracheal injury. Damage to the larynx and trachea can occur because of tube movement and excess pressure exerted by the distal cuff. The nurse should prevent the patient from excessive head movement, especially flexion and extension, which result in the tube moving up and down in the airway, causing abrasive injury. An intervention for preventing tracheal damage from the cuff is routine cuff pressure monitoring (Figure 9-35). Pressures should not exceed 25 to 30 cm H_2O (18 to 22 mm Hg).[58,61,64,66] Various commercial devices are available to measure cuff pressures quickly and easily. The nurse works with the RT to ensure an appropriate cuff volume and pressure.

Damage to the oral or nasal mucosa. Tape or commercial devices that secure the ETT can cause breakdown of the lip and oral mucosa. Nasal intubation may result in skin breakdown on the nares and also a higher risk of sinusitis. Ongoing assessment and skin care assist in preventing damage to the mouth and nose. The ETT should be repositioned daily to prevent pressure necrosis.

BOX 9-8   STRATEGIES FOR UNPLANNED OR SELF-EXTUBATION

- Provide patient education regarding the purpose of the artificial airway and reassurance that it will be removed as soon as the patient can breathe independently.
- Provide adequate analgesia and sedation.
- Monitor all intubated patients vigilantly; assess for risks for self-extubation (distress, disorientation).
- Apply protective devices (e.g., soft wrist restraints, arm immobilizers, mitts) according to hospital standards of practice.
- Adequately secure the endotracheal tube around the patient's head, not just to the face.
- Cut the end of the endotracheal tube to 2 inches beyond the fixation point.
- Provide support for the ventilator tubing and closed suction systems; keep these items out of the patient's reach.
- Use two staff members when repositioning an endotracheal tube.
- Educate the family to assist in monitoring the patient.
- Extubate the patient in a timely manner when the patient meets established criteria.

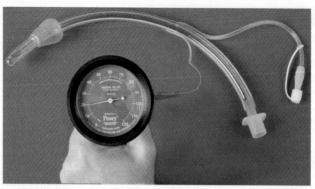

FIGURE 9-35 Monitoring endotracheal tube cuff pressures. (Reprinted with permission, Cleveland Clinic Center for Medical Art & Photography © 2011-2012. All rights reserved.)

PULMONARY SYSTEM

Trauma. *Barotrauma*, which means pressure trauma, is the injury to the lungs associated with mechanical ventilation. In barotrauma, alveolar injury or rupture occurs as a result of excessive pressure, excessive peak inflating volume (volutrauma), or both.[7,35] Barotrauma may occur when the alveoli are overdistended, such as with positive-pressure ventilation, PEEP, and high V_T. The alveoli rupture or tear so that air escapes into various parts of the thoracic cavity, causing subcutaneous emphysema (air in the tissue space), pneumothorax or tension pneumothorax, pneumomediastinum, pneumopericardium, or pneumoperitoneum. Signs and symptoms of barotrauma include high PIP and mean airway pressures, decreased breath sounds, tracheal shift, subcutaneous crepitus, new air leak or increase in air leak in a chest drainage system, and symptoms associated with hypoxemia.

A life-threatening complication is a tension pneumothorax. When tension pneumothorax occurs, pressurized air enters the pleural space. Air is unable to exit the pleural space and continues to accumulate. Air in the pleural space causes an increase in intrathoracic pressure, increasing amounts of lung collapse, shifting of the heart and great vessels to the opposite thorax (mediastinal shift), tachycardia, and hypotension. Treatment consists of immediate insertion of a chest tube or a needle thoracostomy. Whenever a pneumothorax is suspected in a patient receiving mechanical ventilation, the patient should be removed from the ventilator and ventilated with a bag-valve device until a needle thoracostomy is performed or a chest tube is inserted.

Lung tissue injury induced by local or regional overdistending volume is called *volutrauma*. The damage that occurs to the lung is similar to the pathological findings of early ARDS and is probably the result of local stress and strain on the alveolar-capillary membrane. Volutrauma results in increased permeability of the alveolar-capillary membrane, pulmonary edema, accumulation of white blood cells and protein in the alveolar spaces, and reduced surfactant production. Because it is difficult to determine the exact distribution of volume in a patient's lung, pressure is used as a surrogate for volume. The PIP is kept below 40 cm H_2O and/or the Pplat is kept at less than 30 cm H_2O as lung protective strategies to prevent both volutrauma and barotrauma.[35]

Oxygen toxicity. The exposure of the pulmonary tissues to high levels of oxygen can lead to pathological changes. The degree of injury is related to the duration of exposure and to the FiO_2, not to the PaO_2. The first sign of oxygen toxicity, tracheobronchitis, is caused by irritant effects of oxygen. Prolonged exposure to high FiO_2 may lead to changes in the lung that mimic ARDS. As a general rule, an FiO_2 up to 1.0 may be tolerated for up to 24 hours. However, the goal is to lower the FiO_2 to less than 0.60.[30] Absorption atelectasis is another problem associated with high FiO_2. Nitrogen is needed to prevent collapse of the alveoli. When the FiO_2 is 1.0, alveolar collapse and atelectasis result from a lack of nitrogen in the distal air spaces.

Respiratory acidosis or alkalosis. Acid-base disturbances may occur secondary to V_T and RR settings on the ventilator. For example, if a patient is receiving A/C ventilation set at 10 breaths per minute but the patient's RR is 28 breaths per minute because of pain or anxiety, respiratory alkalosis may occur. If the ventilator is set at a low RR (e.g., 2 to 6 breaths per minute) and the patient does not have an adequate drive to initiate additional breaths, respiratory acidosis may occur. Ideally the V_T and RR are set to achieve a VE that ensures a normal $PaCO_2$ level.

Infection. Patients with artificial airways who are receiving mechanical ventilation are at an increased risk of ventilator-associated pneumonia (VAP) because normal upper airway defense mechanisms are bypassed. About 10% to 20% of ventilated patients develop VAP.[56] The incidence is highest in the first 5 days of mechanical ventilation.[2] The principal mechanism for the development of VAP is aspiration of colonized gastric and oropharyngeal secretions. Factors that contribute to VAP include poor oral hygiene, aspiration, contaminated respiratory therapy equipment, poor hand washing by caregivers, breach of aseptic technique when suctioning, inadequate humidification or systemic hydration, and decreased ability to produce an effective cough because of the artificial airway.[44] Specific strategies to reduce VAP include the following:

- Elevate head of the bed 30 to 45 degrees if not medically contraindicated to prevent reflux and aspiration of gastric contents. Elevation of the head of the bed is associated with a 26% risk reduction in pneumonia.[16]
- Prevent drainage of ventilator circuit condensate into the patient's airway. Always discard condensate and never drain it back into the humidifier.[11]
- Practice proper hand hygiene and wear gloves when handling respiratory secretions.
- Use an ETT with a lumen for aspirating subglottic secretions that pool above the airway cuff.[11]
- Ensure secretions are aspirated from above the cuff before cuff deflation or tube removal.[11]
- Provide comprehensive oral hygiene that includes a mechanism for dental plaque removal and reduction of bacterial burden in the oral cavity.[11]
- Use noninvasive mechanical ventilation when possible.

Determination of VAP has low sensitivity and specificity. The Centers for Disease Control along with a team of experts has recommended surveillance for ventilator-associated conditions, including infectious and non-infectious causes. See box, "Clinical Alert, Ventilator-Associated Conditions".

! CLINICAL ALERT

Ventilator-Associated Conditions

The Centers for Disease Control has proposed surveillance for ventilator-associated conditions (VAC), including infectious and non-infectious types. Following a baseline period of stability or improvement for 2 or more days on mechanical ventilation, VAC will be determined by indicators of worsening oxygenation: 1) Need to increase FiO_2 by .20 or higher for two or more days; or 2) Need to increase PEEP by 3 cm H_2O for two or more days.

From http://www.cdc.gov/nhsn/PDFs/vae/CDC_VAE_CommunicationsSummary-for-compliance_20120313.pdf. Accessed May 20, 2012.

Dysphagia and aspiration. Artificial airways increase the risk of upper airway injury which in turn affects upper airway mechanics and protective reflexes and can have negative effects on swallowing physiology.[3] Patients intubated 48 hours or longer are at risk for disordered swallowing which can lead to aspiration and pneumonia. Reports of dysphagia following intubation vary widely, ranging from 3% to 83%, and are mostly due to a wide assortment of assessment methods and instruments.[62] Although many factors contribute to dysphagia, the artificial airway interferes with the ability to execute an efficient and safe swallow. After extubation or tracheostomy, the transition to oral feedings may be appropriate; however, before oral feedings are initiated a speech therapy evaluation for swallowing is recommended, because many patients have difficulty with swallowing and are prone to aspiration after prolonged intubation.[3] Simple bedside tests for dysphagia before and after extubation are emerging as methods to identify this potentially serious complication.[13]

CARDIOVASCULAR SYSTEM

Hypotension and decreased cardiac output may occur with mechanical ventilation and PEEP, secondary to increased intrathoracic pressure, which can result in decreased venous return. The hemodynamic effects of mechanical ventilation are more pronounced in patients with hypovolemia or poor cardiac reserve. Patients with a high PIP who receive PEEP of greater than 10 cm H_2O may need a hemodynamic monitor to assess volume status and cardiac output. Management of hypotension and decreased cardiac output involves the administration of volume to ensure an adequate preload, followed by administration of inotropic agents as necessary.

Gastrointestinal System

Stress ulcers and gastrointestinal bleeding may occur in patients who undergo mechanical ventilation. All patients undergoing mechanical ventilation should receive medications for stress ulcer prophylaxis.[32] Enteral feeding is initiated as soon as possible, and the patient is monitored for gross and occult blood in the gastric aspirate and stools. Other interventions include identification and reduction of stressors, communication and reassurance, and administration of anxiolytic or sedative agents, as necessary based on standardized assessment tools (see Chapter 5).

Nutritional support is required for all patients who require mechanical ventilation (see Chapter 6). Inadequate nutrition may occur if the patient is not started on early nutritional support or receives inadequate supplemental nutrition.[47] The type of formula may need to be modified for ventilated patients. Excess CO_2 production may occur with high-carbohydrate feedings and place a burden on the respiratory system to excrete the CO_2, increasing the WOB.[47] Formulas developed for the patient with pulmonary disorders may be indicated.[42]

An essential nursing intervention for the intubated patient who receives enteral nutrition is to reduce the risk of aspiration. The nurse must keep the head of the bed elevated at least 30 degrees during enteral feeding.[16]

Psychosocial Complications

Several psychosocial hazards may occur because of mechanical ventilation. Patients may experience stress and anxiety because they require a machine for breathing. If the ventilator is not set properly or if the patient resists breaths, patient-ventilator dyssynchrony may occur. The noise of the ventilator and the need for frequent procedures, such as suctioning, may alter sleep and wake patterns. In addition, the patient can become psychologically dependent on the ventilator.[23]

NURSING CARE

Nursing care of the patient who requires mechanical ventilation is complex. The nurse must provide care to the patient by using a holistic approach, including competent delivery of a highly sophisticated technology. A detailed plan of care is described in the box, "Nursing Care Plan for the Mechanically Ventilated Patient."

Text continued on p. 212

for the Mechanically Ventilated Patient

NURSING DIAGNOSIS

Impaired Spontaneous Ventilation related to respiratory muscle fatigue, acute respiratory failure, metabolic factors

PATIENT OUTCOMES

- Spontaneous ventilation with normal ABGs; free of dyspnea or restlessness
- No complications associated with mechanical ventilation

NURSING INTERVENTIONS	RATIONALES
• Have bag-valve device and suctioning equipment readily available	• Be prepared in the event of airway incompetency; maintain airway patency
• Maintain artificial airway; secure ETT or tracheostomy with tape or commercial devices; prevent unplanned extubation (see Box 9-8)	• Ensure maintenance of an adequate airway to facilitate mechanical ventilation; prevent unintended removal of artificial airway

• Assess position of artificial airway:
  • Auscultate for bilateral breath sounds
  • Evaluate placement on chest x-ray
  • Once proper position is confirmed, mark the position (cm marking) of the ETT with an indelible pen and note position of the tube at the lip line as part of routine assessment
	• Maintain an adequate airway by ensuring that artificial airway in the proper position

• Monitor oxygenation and ventilation at all times, and respond to changes:
  • Vital signs
  • Total respiratory rate
  • Exhaled tidal volume of ventilator-assisted and patient-initiated breaths
  • Oxygen saturation
  • End-tidal CO_2
  • Mental status and level of consciousness
  • Signs and symptoms of hypoxemia (see Box 9-1)
  • ABGs
	• Ensure adequate oxygenation, ventilation and acid-base balance; identify when ventilator setting changes are indicated

• Assess respiratory status at least every 4 hours and respond to changes:
  • Breath sounds anteriorly and posteriorly
  • Respiratory pattern
  • Chest excursion
  • Patient's ability to initiate a spontaneous breath
	• Ensure patient is breathing comfortably and is not expending excessive energy on the work of breathing; identify reportable changes

• Reposition ETT from side to side every 24 hours; assess and document skin condition[66]
  • Note placement of tube at lip line
  • Use two staff members for procedure
  • Suction secretions above the ETT cuff before repositioning tube
  • After the procedure, assess position of tube at lip and auscultate for bilateral breath sounds
	• Prevent skin breakdown from the tube, tape, or airway securing device; prevent aspiration of oral secretions and ventilator-associated pneumonia; and ensure that tube remains in proper position after manipulation

• Monitor cuff pressure of ETT or tracheostomy and maintain within therapeutic range[61]	• Prevent complications associated with overinflation or underinflation of ETT cuff
• Maintain integrity of mechanical ventilator circuit; monitor ventilator settings; respond to ventilator alarms; keep tubing free of moisture by draining away from the patient and using devices such as water traps to facilitate drainage of moisture	• Ensure safe administration of mechanical ventilation; maximize ventilation and prevent aspiration of contaminated condensate
• Monitor serial chest radiographs	• Assess for correct position of ETT and improvement or worsening of pulmonary conditions

• Implement a multiprofessional plan of care to address underlying pulmonary condition
  • Coordinate with RT, MD, and multiprofessional team
  • Evaluate response to lung expansion bronchial hygiene and pulmonary medication therapies
  • Mobilize patient as much as possible (i.e., turning, progressive upright mobility, lateral rotation therapy)
  • Consider pronation therapy in refractive hypoxemia
  • Ensure adequate hydration, nutrition, and electrolyte balance
	• Mechanical ventilation only supports the respiratory system until the underlying condition is treated or resolved; well-coordinated team effort is essential to avoid fragmentation of care

NURSING INTERVENTIONS	RATIONALES
• Implement a multiprofessional plan of care to maintain patient comfort, mobility, nutrition, and skin integrity; support patient and family	• Prevent complications associated with mechanical ventilation and bed rest; foster patient and family well-being

NURSING DIAGNOSIS

Ineffective Airway Clearance related to ETT, inability to cough, thick secretions, fatigue

PATIENT OUTCOMES
• Airway free of secretions
• Clear lung sounds

NURSING INTERVENTIONS	RATIONALES
• Assess need for suctioning (rising PIP, high pressure or low exhaled V_T alarm on ventilator, audible/visible secretions, rhonchi on auscultation)	• Indicate possibility of airway obstruction with secretions and need for suctioning
• Suction as needed according to standard of practice (see Box 9-7)	• Remove secretions; maintain patent airway; improve gas exchange
• Assess breath sounds, PIP and exhaled V_T after suctioning	• Assess effectiveness of suctioning; breath sounds should improve, PIP should decrease in volume mode, EVT should increase
• If tracheal secretions are thick, assess hydration of patient and humidification of ventilator; avoid instillation of normal saline	• Assist in thinning secretions for easier removal; saline has not shown to be effective and is associated with hypoxemia and increased risk of infection
• Reposition the patient frequently	• Mobilize secretions, improve gas exchange

NURSING DIAGNOSIS

Risk for Infection related to endotracheal intubation and Risk for Aspiration of oropharyngeal secretions

PATIENT OUTCOMES
• Absence of ventilator-associated pneumonia

NURSING INTERVENTIONS	RATIONALES
• Maintain head of bed at 30 degrees or greater	• Decrease risk for aspiration of oropharyngeal and gastric secretions
• Monitor temperature every 4 hours; assess amount, color, consistency, and odor of secretions; notify physician if secretions change	• Identify signs of infection
• Use good hand-washing techniques; wear gloves for procedures, including closed suctioning; use aseptic technique for suctioning	• Prevent transmission of bacteria to the patient
• Implement a comprehensive oral care protocol that includes oral suction at least every 4 hours and brushing teeth at least every 12 hours	• Remove dental plaque and bacteria from the oropharynx, and prevent aspiration of contaminated oral secretions
• Maintain integrity of ETT cuff; keep cuff pressure between 20 and 30 cm H_2O	• Prevent aspiration of oropharyngeal secretions

NURSING DIAGNOSIS

Risk for Ineffective Protection related to ventilator dependence, PEEP, decreased pulmonary compliance, and issues related to mechanical ventilator (settings, alarms, disconnection)

PATIENT OUTCOME
• Free of ventilator-induced lung injury

NURSING INTERVENTIONS	RATIONALES
• Assess prescribed ventilator settings every 2 hours (mode, set rate, VT, FiO_2, PEEP); ensure that alarms are on	• Ensure that patient is receiving therapy as ordered; promote patient safety
• Assess PIP at least every 4 hours	• Identify elevations in PIP, which may indicate worsening lung function, need to adjust pulmonary therapies or ventilator settings to ensure PIP does not exceed 40 cm H_2O

Continued

◎ **NURSING CARE PLAN—cont'd**

for the Mechanically Ventilated Patient

NURSING INTERVENTIONS	RATIONALES

• Assess tolerance to ventilatory assistance and monitor for patient-ventilator asynchrony; notify RT and licensed provider of potential need to adjust ventilator settings
  • Patient's respiratory cycle out of phase with ventilator
  • High pressure, low EVT alarms
  • Subjective report of breathlessness
  • Labored respirations, especially increased effort on inspiration
  • Tachypnea
  • Anxiety, agitation
	• Provide cues of condition improving or worsening; may indicate need for suctioning or need to adjust ventilator settings that are insufficient to meet patients ventilatory needs

• Assess for signs of pneumothorax every 4 hours or with changes; if symptomatic, determine need for manual ventilation and prepare for chest tube insertion:
  • Subcutaneous crepitus
  • Unequal chest excursion
  • Unilateral decrease in breath sounds
  • Restlessness
  • Increasing PIP
  • Tracheal shift
  • Decreasing SpO_2
	• Early detection of impaired ventilation so emergency chest tube insertion can be efficiently performed

• Respond to all ventilator alarms	• Provide immediate intervention in response to specific alarm; promote patient safety

NURSING DIAGNOSIS

Anxiety and related to need for mechanical ventilation, impaired verbal communication, change in environment, unmet needs, fear of death

PATIENT OUTCOMES

• Calm and cooperative

NURSING INTERVENTIONS	RATIONALES
• Assess patient every 4 hours for signs of anxiety; administer sedation as indicated and assess response using standardized sedation assessment tools	• Identify presence or absence (or relief) of anxiety; standardized tools facilitate communication among team members and assessment of trends
• Collaborate with physician to develop a sedation plan if anxiety or agitation that is not due to pain or delirium impairs ventilation	• Promote effectiveness of mechanical ventilation and patient ventilator synchrony; pain is managed with analgesics, delirium will be worsened by sedation
• Assess respiratory pattern for synchrony with ventilator	• Respiratory efforts that are asynchronous with the ventilator result in discomfort, anxiety, dyspnea, and abnormal ABGs

• Talk to patient frequently; establish method for communication that is appropriate for the patient's native language and abilities; speak slowly and do not shout; expect frustration
  • Yes/no questions
  • Clipboard with paper and pencil
  • Picture communication boards
  • Computerized systems
  • Lip reading
  • Devices that allow the patient to speak
	• Promote communication with the patient and help to identify needs, assess responses to treatment, and reduce anxiety; strategies must be culturally appropriate to facilitate patient understanding

• Implement interventions to reduce anxiety:
  • Calm and reassuring presence
  • Simple explanations before and during procedures
  • Call light within reach
  • Family visitation
  • Diversionary activities, such as music or television at appropriate intervals
  • Promote regular sleep/wake cycle and daytime activity
	• Assist in preventing and/or relieving fear and anxiety
	• Promote rest, healing and recovery

◎ NURSING CARE PLAN—cont'd

for the Mechanically Ventilated Patient

NURSING INTERVENTIONS	RATIONALES
• Collaborate with the healthcare team to develop strategies to reduce anxiety and maximize effectiveness of mechanical ventilation: changes in settings, sedation, analgesia, complementary and alternative therapies	• Medications are frequently needed as an adjunct during mechanical ventilation; complementary therapies such as touch, massage, reflexology, music therapy, and meditation may also be effective

NURSING DIAGNOSIS

Risk for Decreased Cardiac Output related to effects of positive pressure ventilation, PEEP, volume depletion or overload

PATIENT OUTCOME
• Adequate cardiac output

NURSING INTERVENTIONS	RATIONALES
• Assess for hypotension, tachycardia, dysrhythmias, decreased level of consciousness, cool skin, mottling	• Indicate decreased cardiac output
• Measure hemodynamic profile at least every 4 hours if hemodynamic monitoring device is in place; reassess after any ventilator setting changes that affect V_T, PEEP, or PIP	• Assess filling pressure and cardiac output, and identify trends
• Alert the physician to changes in cardiac output and hemodynamic profile	• Ventilator settings, especially PEEP, may need to be adjusted; therapies to improve oxygenation may need to be added (lung expansion, bronchial hygiene, rotation, placing prone, etc.) so PEEP can be reduced and oxygenation maintained
• Maintain optimum fluid balance	• Additional volume may be needed, especially if patient is receiving PEEP; fluid retention may also occur
• Administer other medications as ordered (e.g., inotropic agents or diuretics)	• Medications may be needed to optimize cardiac output and/or relieve fluid retention

NURSING DIAGNOSIS

Dysfunctional Ventilatory Weaning Response related to ineffective airway clearance, sleep-pattern disturbances, inadequate nutrition, pain, anemia, abdominal distention, debilitated condition, and psychological factors

PATIENT OUTCOME
• Liberation from mechanical ventilation
• Adequate ABG values
• Respiratory pattern and rate WNL
• Effective secretion clearance

NURSING INTERVENTIONS	RATIONALE
• Assess patient's readiness to wean (see Box 9-10)	• Identify readiness to begin the weaning process using validated parameters
• Provide weaning method based on protocols and research evidence (see Box 9-9)	• Protocol-driven weaning is an effective strategy for systematic ventilator liberation that reduces ventilator days and ICU and hospital length of stay
• Collaborate with the healthcare team to provide mechanical ventilation modes, patient coaching, and progressive mobility that supports respiratory muscle training	• Promote respiratory conditioning that facilitates patient's ability to resume the work of breathing
• Promote rest and comfort throughout the weaning process, especially between weaning trials; identify strategies that result in relaxation and comfort; ensure that environment is safe and comfortable	• Facilitate weaning from mechanical ventilation
• Support patients in setting goals for weaning	• Promote rehabilitation and give patients some control in the process
• Collaborate with the healthcare team to determine the most effective strategies for weaning those with severe dysfunctional breathing patterns	• Various strategies may be needed to wean the patient; ongoing assessment is essential to determine the most effective strategy

Continued

◎ **NURSING CARE PLAN—cont'd**

for the Mechanically Ventilated Patient

NURSING INTERVENTIONS	RATIONALES

• Implement strategies that maximize tolerance of weaning:
  • Titrate sedation and analgesia to a level at which patient is calm and cooperative with absence of respiratory depression
  • Schedule when patient is rested
  • Avoid other procedures during weaning
  • Position patient upright to allow for full expansion with abdominal compression on diaphragm
  • Promote normal sleep-wake cycle
  • Limit visitors to supportive persons
  • Coach through periods of anxiety
	• Strategies assist in ensuring that patient is rested, with an adequate level of consciousness and decreased anxiety and in an optimal position for lung expansion; weaning efforts will be maximized

• Terminate weaning if patient is unable to tolerate the process (see Box 9-11)	• Maintain adequate ventilation and gas exchange; prevent fatigue of respiratory muscles
• Consider referring patients with prolonged ventilator dependence to an alternative setting	• Alternative settings specialize in weaning patients who are "difficult to wean"

ABG, Arterial blood gas; *CO,* cardiac output; *CO₂,* carbon dioxide; *ETT,* endotracheal tube; *FiO₂,* fraction of inspired oxygen; *ICU,* intensive care unit; *PEEP,* positive end-expiratory pressure; *PIP,* peak inspiratory pressure; *PS,* pressure support; *RR,* respiratory rate; *SpO₂,* oxygen saturation as measured by pulse oximetry; *V_T,* tidal volume; *WNL,* within normal limits.
Based on data from Gulanick M, & Myers JL. (2011). *Nursing Care Plans: Diagnoses, Interventions, and Outcomes* (7th ed.). St. Louis: Mosby.

Communication

Communication difficulties are common because of the artificial airway. The lack of vocal expression has been identified by patients as a major stressor that elicits feelings of panic, isolation, anger, helplessness, and sleeplessness.[24] Patients express a need to know and to make themselves understood. They need constant reorientation, reassuring words emphasizing a caregiver's presence, and point-of-care information that painful procedures done to them are indeed necessary and helpful. In addition, touch, eye contact, and positive facial expressions are beneficial in relieving anxiety.[44] Caregivers who attempt to individualize communication with intubated patients by using a variety of methods provide patients a greater sense of control, encourage participation in their own care, and minimize cognitive disturbances.[24]

Head nods, mouthing words, gestures, and writing are identified as the most frequently used method of nonverbal communication among intubated ICU patients, but they are often inhibited by wrist restraints.[29] Communication with gestures and lip reading can convey some basic needs; however, augmentative devices may facilitate even better communication. Although writing is sometimes used, critically ill patients are often too weak or poorly positioned to write, or they lack the concentration to spell. A picture board with icons representing basic needs and the alphabet that can be easily cleaned between patients should be available in every ICU. A board with pictures improved communication for patients after cardiothoracic surgery and was preferred by a small group of critical care survivors who were interviewed about augmentative communication methods.[48] Family members can serve as a communication link between the patient and the care providers. It is important to reassure the patient that the loss of their voice is temporary and that speech will be possible after the tube is removed.

Maintaining Comfort and Reducing Distress

Intubation, mechanical ventilation, advanced methods for ventilation (e.g., inverse-ratio ventilation), and suctioning contribute to patient discomfort and distress. Patients often need both pharmacological and nonpharmacological methods to manage discomfort and to treat anxiety.[67] Strategies to promote patient comfort are discussed in-depth in Chapter 5.

Medications

Commonly used medications include analgesics, sedatives, and neuromuscular blocking agents; many patients need a combination of these drugs.[36,38] Medications are chosen based on the hemodynamic stability of the patient, the diagnosis, and the desired patient goals and outcomes. It is very important that the nurse, RT, and physician all use the same objective sedation and analgesia scoring systems to promote unambiguous assessment and communication. In some institutions, nurses use decision trees or algorithms to guide initiation and titration of medications to targeted sedation and analgesia goals.[6] Medications are tapered or discontinued when the patient is ready to be weaned from mechanical ventilation.

Analgesics, such as morphine and fentanyl, are administered to provide pain relief. Sedatives, such as dexmedetomidine, benzodiazepines, and propofol, are given to sedate the patient, reduce anxiety, and promote synchronous breathing with the ventilator. Benzodiazepines promote amnesia but are also associated with an increase in delirium.[33] Patients who have acute lung injury or increased intracranial pressure, or who require nontraditional modes of mechanical ventilation may require deep sedation or therapeutic paralysis with neuromuscular blocking agents. Chemical paralysis must be discontinued before attempting to wean the patient from mechanical ventilation.[33]

When sedation of the mechanically ventilated patient is indicated it must be titrated to a specific goal agreed upon by the multiprofessional team. Insufficient sedation may precipitate ventilator dyssynchrony and physiological alterations in thoracic pressures and gas exchange. Inadequate sedation is also associated with unplanned extubation. Oversedation and prolonged sedation are associated with a longer duration of mechanical ventilation and lengths of stay in the critical care unit and hospital.[36] Prolonged duration of mechanical ventilation predisposes the patient to an increased risk of VAP, lung injury, and other complications. Depth of sedation also contributes to delayed weaning from mechanical ventilation. Since sedation, duration of mechanical ventilation, and ventilator weaning are tightly interrelated, the nurse must ensure that the patient is maintained on the lowest dose and lightest level of sedation as possible. "Daily interruption," "sedation vacation," or a "spontaneous awakening trial" to evaluate the patient's cognitive status, to reduce the overall dose of sedation, and to determine what dose, if any, sedation is needed to achieve a calm, cooperative patient is an important nursing intervention.[33,37] Optimal sedation of the mechanically ventilated patient is present when the patient resides at a state in which patient-ventilator harmony exists and the patient remains capable of taking spontaneous breaths in readiness for weaning, when appropriate.[37,38] Some patients may achieve this state without sedative agents. Administering sedatives intermittently and as needed rather than continuously is another strategy the nurse should consider.

Nonpharmacological Interventions

Nonpharmacological, complementary, and alternative medicine strategies can be used to reduce distress, promote patient-ventilator synchrony, and maintain a normal cognitive state.[67] The nurse creates a healing environment by involving the patient and family in the plan of care, reducing excess noise and light stimulation, providing a reassuring presence, and minimizing unnecessary patient stimulation to promoting a normal sleep-wake cycle. Adequate rest and frequent reorientation are also important for the prevention of delirium. A progressive mobility plan reduces deconditioning and promotes endurance of the respiratory muscles to facilitate ventilator liberation. Daytime exercise may also promote a more restful nighttime sleep.

Complementary and alternative strategies may also be helpful in reducing distress and promoting rest. Examples of these strategies include meditation, guided imagery and relaxation, prayer, music therapy, massage, accupressure, therapeutic touch, herbal products and dietary supplements, and presence.[67] Nurses should ask the family and patient if they are already using complementary strategies and, if so, incorporate them as possible. The goal of learning to incorporate these therapies into practice is to reduce patient distress, promote sleep, and create a healing environment conducive to reducing ventilator days.

WEANING PATIENTS FROM MECHANICAL VENTILATION

Mechanical ventilation is a therapy designed to support the respiratory system until the underlying disease or indication for mechanical ventilation is resolved. The team caring for a ventilated patient should always be planning for how the patient will be weaned or "liberated" from the ventilator. Another term for liberation is discontinuation of ventilator support. In general, patients who require short-term ventilatory support, defined as 3 days or less of mechanical ventilation, are weaned quickly.[9,40] Conversely, weaning patients who require long-term ventilatory support, is usually a slower process and may be characterized by periods of success as well as setbacks. Reduction of ventilator support can be done as the patient demonstrates the ability to resume part of or all of the WOB.

Approach to Weaning Using Best Evidence

A systematic approach to weaning is indicated for patients. Based on a comprehensive review of the research, evidenced-based guidelines for ventilator weaning were developed.[39-41] Box 9-9 summarizes these guidelines. Weaning protocols managed by nurses and RTs, as compared with traditional weaning directed by physicians, result in a reduction of ventilator days and shorter stays in the ICU and hospital.[37] The protocol should clearly define the method or screening tool to determine the patient's readiness to wean, the method and duration of the weaning trial, and when to terminate a weaning trial versus proceed with requesting an order for extubation. The weaning plan should include methods to facilitate respiratory muscle work along with adequate rest.[40,51] See the box, "QSEN Exemplar," for an example of teamwork and collaboration during the weaning process.

Assessment for Readiness to Wean (Wean Screen)

Before initiating the weaning trial, the patient is screened for readiness using parameters that have been associated with ventilator discontinuation success (Box 9-10). Weaning assessment tools are useful in assessing a patient's strengths and factors that may interfere with successful weaning. Patients are usually able to wean when the underlying disease process is resolving, they are hemodynamically stable, and they are able to initiate an inspiratory effort.[40] Therefore assessment of the neurological, cardiovascular, and respiratory systems provides a sufficient screen in most patients requiring a ventilator for only a short period.

Patients who require long-term mechanical ventilation (>72 hours) may have more physiological factors that affect weaning, such as inadequate nutrition and respiratory muscle deconditioning. A tool that provides a more comprehensive or multidimensional assessment of weaning readiness, as well as a baseline score from which to measure patient progress once

BOX 9-9   EVIDENCE-BASED GUIDELINES FOR WEANING FROM MECHANICAL VENTILATION

1. Identify causes for ventilator dependence if the patient requires ventilation for longer than 24 hours.
2. Conduct a formal assessment to determine a high potential for successful weaning:
   - Evidence of reversal of underlying cause of respiratory failure
   - Adequate oxygenation (PaO_2/FiO_2 >150-200; positive end-expiratory pressure <5-8 cm H_2O; FiO_2 <0.4-0.5) and pH (>7.25)
   - Hemodynamic stability
   - Able to initiate an inspiratory effort
3. Conduct a spontaneous breathing trial (SBT). During the SBT, evaluate respiratory pattern, adequacy of gas exchange, hemodynamic stability, and comfort. A patient who tolerates a SBT for 30 to 120 minutes should be considered for permanent ventilator discontinuation.
4. If a patient fails an SBT, determine the cause for the failed trial. Provide a method of ventilatory support that is nonfatiguing and comfortable. Correct reversible causes, and attempt a SBT every 24 hours if the patient meets weaning criteria.
5. Assess airway patency and the ability of the patient to protect the airway to determine whether to remove the artificial airway from a patient who has been successfully weaned.
6. In postsurgical patients, provide anesthesia/sedation strategies and ventilator management aimed at early extubation.
7. Develop weaning protocols that the nurse and respiratory therapist can implement.
8. Consider a tracheostomy when it becomes apparent that the patient will require prolonged ventilator assistance. Patients with the following conditions may benefit most from early tracheostomy:
   - High levels of sedation
   - Marginal respiratory mechanics (e.g., tachypnea) associated with work of breathing
   - Psychological benefit from ability to eat and speak
   - Enhanced mobility to promote physical therapy efforts and psychological support
9. Conduct slow-paced weaning in a patient who requires prolonged mechanical ventilation. Wean a patient to 50% of maximum ventilator support before daily SBT. Then initiate SBTs with gradual increase in duration of the SBT.
10. Unless evidence of irreversible disease exists (e.g., high cervical spine injury), do not consider a patient to be ventilator dependent until 3 months of weaning attempts have failed.
11. Transfer a patient who has failed weaning attempts but is medically stable to a facility that specialize in management of ventilator-dependent patients.

FiO₂, Fraction of inspired oxygen; *PaO₂*, partial pressure of oxygen in arterial blood; *SBT*, spontaneous breathing trial.
Based on data from MacIntyre N. (2009). Discontinuing mechanical ventilatory support. In NR Macintyre and RD Branson (Eds.) *Mechanical Ventilation* 2nd ed., St. Louis: Saunders Elsevier, pp. 317-324; MacIntyre N, Cook D, & Ely E. (2001). Evidence-based guidelines for weaning and discontinuing mechanical ventilatory support: A collective task force facilitated by the American College of Chest Physicians; the American Association for Respiratory Care; and the American College of Critical Care Medicine. *Chest, 120,* 375S-395S; MacIntyre NR. (2004). Evidence-based ventilator weaning and discontinuation. *Respiratory Care, 49,* 830-836.

QSEN EXEMPLAR

Teamwork and Collaboration

Successful weaning of patients from mechanical ventilation requires a team approach. Led by a clinical nurse specialist (CNS), a hospital established a multiprofessional ventilator team composed of a pulmonologist, critical care nurses, stepdown unit nurses, respiratory therapist, speech therapist, physical therapist, clinical pharmacist, case manager, social worker, chaplain, and home care personnel. Every patient in the facility who was mechanically ventilated for more than 3 days received a comprehensive evaluation by the CNS. The CNS met with the patient, family, physician, and unit staff to identify potential issues that could impact the weaning process. Patients meeting criteria were then presented at the weekly "Vent Team" meeting. Individualized weaning plans were developed for each patient. Additional concerns related to mechanical ventilation including nutrition, communication, mobility and function, pain and anxiety, infection risk, patient and family coping, end-of-life concerns, spirituality, and discharge preparation were addressed, and plans of care were modified as required. Patient outcomes included improved transitions between nursing units, reduction in ventilator days, reduction in ventilator-acquired pneumonia, and reduced length of stay. Team members proactively worked with patients and families to address end-of-life issues and to plan terminal weaning as appropriate. A team approach was used to transition patients who required ongoing mechanical ventilation for conditions such as amytrophic lateral sclerosis and spinal cord injury to the care of the family provider in the home setting.

BOX 9-10 ASSESSMENT PARAMETERS INDICATING READINESS TO WEAN

Underlying Cause for Mechanical Ventilation Resolved
- Improved chest x-ray findings
- Minimal secretions
- Normal breath sounds

Hemodynamic Stability; Adequate Cardiac Output
- Absence of hypotension
- Minimal vasopressor therapy

Adequate Respiratory Muscle Strength
- Respiratory rate <25-30 breaths/min
- Negative inspiratory pressure or force that exceeds −20 cm H_2O
- Spontaneous tidal volume 5 mL/kg
- Vital capacity 10-15 mL/kg
- Minute ventilation 5-10 L/min
- Rapid shallow breathing index <105

Adequate Oxygenation Without a High FiO_2 and/or a High PEEP
- PaO_2 >60 mm Hg with FiO_2 0.4-0.5
- PaO_2/FiO_2 >150-200
- PEEP <5-8 cm H_2O

Absence of Factors that Impair Weaning
- Infection
- Anemia
- Fever
- Sleep deprivation
- Pain
- Abdominal distention; bowel abnormalities (diarrhea or constipation)
- Mental readiness to wean: calm, minimal anxiety, motivated
- Minimal need for sedatives and other medications that may cause respiratory depression

FiO_2, Fraction of inspired oxygen; *PaO_2,* partial pressure of oxygen in arterial blood; *PEEP,* positive end-expiratory pressure.

weaning is begun, is the Burns Wean Assessment Program (BWAP). The BWAP has been scientifically tested in critically ill patients.[9] The BWAP evaluates nonpulmonary factors that impact weaning success, such as hematocrit; fluids, electrolytes, and nutrition; anxiety, pain, and rest; bowel function; and physical conditioning and mobility. Pulmonary factors assessed with the BWAP include RR and pattern; secretions; neuromuscular disease and deformities; airway size and clearance; and ABGs.

The nurse must collaborate with RT and physician, using data and weaning assessment tools to identify readiness for weaning and factors that may impede successful weaning.[37,52] When a patient continues to not be ready to wean or is not successful at a weaning trial, these factors should be assessed and optimized to promote patient success in future weaning endeavors.

Weaning Process (Weaning Trial)

Table 9-5 describes weaning methods. Patients are assessed and monitored throughout the weaning process; therefore the nurse must organize work to remain vigilant throughout the trial. Four methods of reducing ventilatory support are used: SIMV, PS, T-piece, or CPAP. Studies do not demonstrate one method to be superior to the others; however, they do show that weaning takes longer with SIMV.[5,20,40] Current evidenced-based practice guidelines recommend the use of a spontaneous breathing trial (SBT) for weaning. PS, T-piece, and CPAP qualify as spontaneous breathing modes, whereas SIMV, because of the provision of mandatory breaths, does not. The SBT for up to 2 hours (90 to 120 minutes) provides a direct assessment of spontaneous breathing capabilities and

has been shown to be the most effective way to shorten the ventilator discontinuation process.[40]

The weaning procedure is explained to the patient and family in a manner that promotes reassurance and minimizes anxiety. The patient should be adequately rested and positioned optimally for diaphragm function and lung expansion, such as sitting. Baseline parameters are obtained: vital signs, heart rhythm, ABGs or pulse oximetry/ETCO2 values, and neurological status. The patient is monitored during the weaning process for tolerance or intolerance to the procedure. Although the patient is required to increase participation in the WOB, caregivers must ensure that the patient does not become fatigued by the weaning effort and become compromised.[8,35] Box 9-11 provides a list of physiological parameters that are monitored to identify that the patient is not tolerating the weaning process. If these signs of intolerance develop, the weaning trial is stopped and mechanical ventilation is resumed at ventilator settings that provide full ventilatory support.[52]

Many respiratory and nonrespiratory factors can impact weaning success. Increased oxygen demands occur with infection, fever, anemia, pain, or asking the patient to perform another activity such as physical therapy during the trial, and can impair weaning. Other factors to assess for are decreased respiratory performance from malnutrition, overuse of sedatives or hypnotics, sleep deprivation, and abdominal distention. Factors involving equipment or technique, such as time of day or method for weaning, should also be examined. Psychological factors to evaluate include apprehension and fear, helplessness, and depression.[28,67] Each factor should be systematically assessed and optimized to promote weaning success.

TABLE 9-5   WEANING METHODS

| MODE | WEANING TECHNIQUE | |
	DESCRIPTION	STRATEGIES
Spontaneous Breathing Trial Gradual reconditioning through trials of spontaneous breathing effort	Every breath is spontaneous and patient performs all the work of breathing Attempt daily if patient passes wean screen Successful when patient remains stable for 90-120 minutes	Alternating periods of resting on full ventilator support with advancing periods of gradually reduced support Ratio of rest periods to time on trial based on patient's response Amount of time to liberate patient varies; may be days to weeks Indicated for significantly deconditioned patients
Pressure Support Provides inspiratory support to overcome resistance to gas flow through ventilator circuit and artificial airway	PS of 5 cm H_2O + 5 cm H_2O PEEP	Begin at level of PS that ensures normal RR and V_T Gradual reduction in PS in 2-5 cm H_2O increments Gradually lengthen intervals at reduced levels of support Discontinue when patient stable for 2 hours or longer at 5 cm H_2O PS
T-Piece Patient performs all the WOB No ventilator alarms for apnea, decreased VT, etc.	Remove patient from ventilator and provide humidified oxygen via a T-piece adaptor attached to the ETT or tracheostomy tube	May start with trial as short as 5 minutes Increase time on T-piece as tolerated with adequate rest periods (6-8 hours) on full ventilatory support Discontinue when patient stable on T-piece for at least 2 hours, often longer
CPAP Useful when patient requires PEEP to maintain oxygenation Patient performs all the WOB Ventilator will provide alarms for apnea, high RR, or low EVT	CPAP of 5 cm H_2O	CPAP of 5 cm H_2O May start with trial as short as 5 minutes Increase time on CPAP as tolerated with adequate rest periods (6-8 hours) on full ventilatory support Discontinue when patient stable on CPAP for at least 2 hours, often longer
SIMV	Not applicable, not a spontaneous breathing mode	Decrease the number of mandatory (machine) breaths in increments of 2 as tolerated Discontinue when patient stable on SIMV of 2-4 for 2 hours, often longer

cm H_2O, Centimeters of water; *CPAP*, continuous positive airway pressure; *ETT*, endotracheal tube; *EV_T*, exhaled tidal volume; *PEEP*, positive end-expiratory pressure; *PS*, pressure support; *RR*, respiratory rate; *SIMV*, synchronous intermittent mandatory ventilation; *V_T*, tidal volume; *WOB*, work of breathing.

BOX 9-11   CRITERIA FOR DISCONTINUING WEANING

Respiratory
- Respiratory rate >35 breaths/min or <8 breaths/min
- Spontaneous V_T <5 mL/kg ideal body weight
- Labored respirations
- Use of accessory muscles
- Abnormal breathing pattern: chest/abdominal asynchrony
- Oxygen saturation <90%

Cardiovascular
- Heart rate changes more than 20% from baseline
- Dysrhythmias (e.g., premature ventricular contractions or bradycardia)
- Ischemia: ST-segment elevation
- Blood pressure changes more than 20% from baseline
- Diaphoresis

Neurological
- Agitation, anxiety
- Decreased level of consciousness
- Subjective discomfort

V_T, Tidal volume.

Extubation

If the patient demonstrates tolerance to the weaning procedure and can sustain spontaneous breathing for 90 to 120 minutes, then the second step to ventilator discontinuation, the decision to extubate (remove the ETT), may be made. Consideration must be given to the need for the airway for secretion clearance; therefore the patient must have a good cough and require suctioning no more than every 2 hours. If the patient has a tracheostomy, the patient may be liberated from the ventilator but the tracheostomy is maintained to facilitated airway clearance. If the decision is made to extubate, the ETT should be suctioned thoroughly before removal. Secretions that may have pooled above the cuff should be aspirated, the balloon of the ETT is deflated, and the ETT is removed during inspiration.[11,50,66] Once extubated, the patient is assessed for stridor, hoarseness, changes in vital signs, or low SpO_2, which may indicate complications.[63] Noninvasive ventilation may be used to avert reintubation in some patients.[41]

CASE STUDY

Mr. P., age 65 years, was transferred to the critical care unit from the emergency department after successful resuscitation from a cardiac arrest sustained out of the hospital. Initial diagnosis based on laboratory results and electrocardiography is acute anterior myocardial infarction. It is suspected that Mr. P. aspirated gastric contents during the cardiac arrest. He opens his eyes to painful stimuli. He is orally intubated and receiving mechanical ventilation. He is on assist-control ventilation, respiratory rate set at 12 breaths/min, FiO_2 of 0.40, PEEP 5 cm H_2O, V_T 700 mL. An arterial blood gas is drawn upon arrival to the critical care unit and shows the following values: pH, 7.33; $PaCO_2$, 40 mm Hg; HCO_3^-, 20 mEq/L; PaO_2, 88 mm Hg; and SaO_2, 99%. A decision is made to maintain the initial ventilator settings. The following day, Mr. P.'s chest radiograph shows progressive infiltrates. His oxygen saturation is dropping below 90% and he is demonstrating signs of hypoxemia: increased heart rate and premature ventricular contractions. Arterial blood gas analysis at this time shows pH, 7.35; $PaCO_2$, 43 mm Hg; HCO_3^-, 26 mEq/L; PaO_2, 58 mm Hg; and SaO_2, 88%. The physician orders the FiO_2 increased to 0.50, and PEEP increased to 10 cm H_2O.

Questions

1. What were the results of Mr. P.'s first arterial blood gas analysis? What factors are contributing to these results?
2. What factor is contributing to Mr. P.'s worsening condition the day after hospital admission?
3. Interpret the arterial blood gases done the day after the cardiac arrest.
4. Why did the physician change the ventilator settings after the second set of arterial blood gases?
5. What must the nurse assess after the addition of the PEEP? Why is this especially important for Mr. P.?

SUMMARY

Skills in establishing and maintaining a patent airway, providing oxygen therapy, initiating mechanical ventilation, and ongoing patient assessment are essential for critical care nurses. Care of the patient requiring mechanical ventilation is common practice in the critical care unit; therefore it is essential that the nurse apply knowledge and skills to effectively care for these vulnerable patients.

CRITICAL THINKING EXERCISES

1. Based on your knowledge of clinical disorders, identify different clinical conditions that could cause problems with the following steps in gas exchange:
   a. Ventilation
   b. Diffusion
   c. Perfusion (transportation)
2. Your patient has the following arterial blood gas results: pH, 7.28; PaO_2, 52 mm Hg; SaO_2, 84%; $PaCO_2$, 55 mm Hg; HCO_3^-, 24 mEq/L.
   a. What is your interpretation of this arterial blood gas?
   b. What clinical condition or conditions could cause the patient to have these arterial blood gas results?
3. Your patient requires mechanical ventilation for treatment. The pressure alarm keeps going off for a few seconds at a time, even though you have just suctioned the patient. What nursing assessments and potential actions are warranted at this time?
4. You are caring for a patient who has been mechanically ventilated for 2 weeks. Physically, the patient meets all the criteria to begin weaning from mechanical ventilation. What parameters should the nurse monitor to assess tolerance of weaning?
5. Your patient is being ventilated with noninvasive positive-pressure ventilation with a nasal mask. The patient is mouth breathing and the ventilator is alarming low exhaled tidal volume. What interventions should the nurse take to ensure the patient receives adequate ventilation?

REFERENCES

1. Ackerman MH, Mick DJ. Instillation of normal saline before suctioning in patients with pulmonary infections: a prospective randomized controlled trial. *American Journal of Critical Care*. 1998;7:261-266.

2. American Thoracic Society. Guidelines for the management of adults with hospital-acquired, ventilator-associated, and healthcare-associated pneumonia. *American Journal of Respiratory and Critical Care Medicine*. 2005;171:388-416.

3. Baumgartner CA, Bewyer E, Bruner D. Management of communication and swallowing in intensive care. *AACN Advance Critical Care*. 2008;19:433-443.

4. Bouza C, Garcia E, Diaz M, et al. Unplanned extubation in orally intubated medical patients in the intensive care unit: a prospective cohort study. *Heart and Lung*. 2007;36:270-276.

5. Brochard L, Rauss A, Benito S, et al. Comparison of three methods of gradual withdrawal from ventilatory support during weaning from mechanical ventilation. *American Journal of Respiratory and Critical Care Medicine*. 1994;150:896-903.

6. Brook AD, Ahrens TS, Schaiff R, et al. Effect of a nursing-implemented sedation protocol on the duration of mechanical ventilation. *Critical Care Medicine*. 1999;27:2609-2615.

7. Brower R, Matthay M, Morris A, et al. Ventilation with lower tidal volumes as compared with traditional tidal volumes for acute lung injury and the acute respiratory distress syndrome: the acute respiratory distress syndrome network. *New England Journal of Medicine*. 2000;342:1301-1308.

8. Burns SM. AACN protocols for practice: weaning from mechanical ventilation. In: Burns SM, ed. *AACN Protocols for Practice: Care of the Mechanically Ventilated Patient*. 2nd ed., pp. 97-160. Boston: Jones & Bartlett; 2007.

9. Burns SM, Fisher C, Tribble SS, et al. Multifactor clinical score and outcome of mechanical ventilation weaning trials: Burns wean assessment program. *American Journal of Critical Care*. 2010;(19)5:431-440.

10. Celik SA, Kanan NA. A current conflict: use of isotonic sodium chloride solution on endotracheal suctioning in critically ill patients. *Dimensions of Critical Care Nursing*. 2006;25(1):11-14.

11. Centers for Disease Control and Prevention. Guidelines for preventing health-care associated pneumonia. *MMWR. Morbidity and Mortality Weekly Report*. 2004;53:(RR-3).

12. Chulay M, Seckel MA. Suctioning: endotracheal or tracheostomy tube. In: Lynn-McHale Weigand DJ, ed. *AACN Procedure Manual for Critical Care*. 6th ed., 80-104. St. Louis: Elsevier Saunders; 2011.

13. Colonel P, Houze MH, Vert H, et al. Swallowing disorders as a predictor of unsuccessful extubation: a clinical evaluation. *American Journal of Critical Care*. 2008;17:504-510.

14. DePew CL. Subglottic secretion drainage: a literature review. *AACN Advanced Critical Care*. 2007;18:366-379.

15. Dezfulian C, Shojania K, Collard HR, et al. Subglottic secretion drainage for preventing ventilator-associated pneumonia: a meta-analysis. *American Journal of Medicine*. 2005;118:11-18.

16. Drakulovic MB, Torres A, Bauer TT, et al. Supine body position as a risk factor for nosocomial pneumonia in mechanically ventilated patients: a randomised trial. *Lancet*. 1999;354:1851-1858.

17. Durbin CG Jr. Indications for and timing of tracheostomy. *Respiratory Care*. 2005;50:483-487.

18. Durbin CG, Jr. Techniques for performing tracheostomy. *Respiratory Care*. 2005;50:488-496.

19. El Masry A, Williams PF, Chipman DW, et al. The impact of closed endotracheal suctioning systems on mechanical ventilator performance. *Respiratory Care*. 2005;50:345-353.

20. Esteban A, Frutos F, Tobin MJ, et al. A comparison of four methods of weaning patients from mechanical ventilation. Spanish Lung Failure Collaborative Group. *New England Journal of Medicine*. 1995;332:345-353.

21. Fink J. Humidity and aerosol therapy. In: Cairo JM, Pilbeam SP, eds. *Mosby's Respiratory Care Equipment*. 8th ed. St. Louis: Mosby; 2010.

22. Good VS, Luehrs P. Continuous end-tidal carbon dioxide monitoring. In: Lynn DJ, Lynn-McHale Weigand DJ, ed. *AACN Procedure Manual for Critical Care*. 6th ed., pp. 106-127. St. Louis: Elsevier Saunders; 2011.

23. Grossbach I, Chlan L, Tracy MF. Overview of mechanical ventilatory support and management of patient- and ventilator-related responses. *Critical Care Nurse*. 2011;31:30-45.

24. Grossbach I, Stranberg S, Chlan L. Promoting effective communication for patients receiving mechanical ventilation. *Critical Care Nurse*. 2011;31(3):46-61

25. Gulanick M, Myers JL. *Nursing Care Plans: Nursing Diagnosis and Intervention*. 7th ed. St. Louis: Mosby; 2011.

26. Habashi NM. Other approaches to open-lung ventilation: airway pressure release ventilation. *Critical Care Medicine*. 2005;33:S228-S240.

27. Hall JE, Guyton AC. *Textbook of Medical Physiology*. 12th ed. Philadelphia: Saunders Elsevier; 2011.

28. Happ MB, Swigart VA, Tate JA, et al. Family presence and surveillance during weaning from prolonged mechanical ventilation. *Heart and Lung*. 2007;36:47-57.

29. Happ MB, Tuite P, Dobbin K, et al. Communicating ability, method, and content among nonspeaking nonsurviving patients treated with mechanical ventilation in the intensive care unit. *American Journal of Critical Care*. 2004;13(3):210-220.

30. Heuer AJ, Scanlan CL. Medical gas therapy. In: Wilkins RL, Stoller JK, Kacmarek RM, eds. *Egan's Fundamentals of Respiratory Care*. 8th ed., pp. 868-920. St. Louis: Mosby Elsevier; 2009.

31. Hickling KG. Lung-protective ventilation in acute respiratory distress syndrome: protection by reduced lung stress or by therapeutic hypercapnia? *American Journal of Respiratory and Critical Care Medicine*. 2000;162:2021-2022.

32. Institute for Healthcare Improvement. Getting started kit: prevent ventilator associated pneumonia. *How to Guide*. Available at www.ihi.org; 2007

33. Jacobi J, Fraser GL, Coursin DB, et al. Clinical practice guidelines for the sustained use of sedatives and analgesics in the critically ill adult. *Critical Care Medicine*. 2002;30:119-141.

34. Jongerden IP, Rovers MM, Grypdonck MH, et al. Open and closed endotracheal suction systems in mechanically ventilated intensive care patients: a meta-analysis. *Critical Care Medicine*. 2007;35:260-270.

35. Kacmarek RM, Dimas S, Mack CW. *The Essentials of Respiratory Care*. St. Louis: Mosby; 2005.

36. Kollef MH, Levy NT, Ahrens TS, et al. The use of continuous I.V. sedation is associated with prolongation of mechanical ventilation. *Chest*. 1998;114:541-548.

37. Kollef MH, Shapiro SD, Silver P, et al. A randomized, controlled trial of protocol-directed versus physician-directed weaning from mechanical ventilation. *Critical Care Medicine*. 1997;25:567-574.

38. Luer J. Sedation and neuromuscular blockade in the mechanically ventilated patient. In: Burns SM, ed. *AACN Protocols for Practice: Care of the Mechanically Ventilated Patient.* 2nd ed., pp. 253-284. Boston: Jones & Bartlett; 2007.

39. MacIntyre N. Discontinuing mechanical ventilatory support. In: MacIntyre NR, Branson RD, eds. *Mechanical Ventilation.* 2nd ed., St. Louis: Saunders Elsevier; 2009.

40. MacIntyre N, Cook D, Ely E. Evidence-based guidelines for weaning and discontinuing mechanical ventilatory support: a collective task force facilitated by the American College of Chest Physicians; the American Association for Respiratory Care; and the American College of Critical Care Medicine. *Chest.* 2001;120:375S-395S.

41. MacIntyre NR. Evidence-based ventilator weaning and discontinuation. *Respiratory Care.* 2004;49:830-836.

42. Malone AM. The use of specialized enteral formulas in pulmonary disease. *Nutrition in Clinical Practice.* 2004;19:557.

43. Miller CA. Respiratory function. In: Miller CA, ed. *Nursing for Wellness in Older Adults.* 6th ed. Philadelphia: Lippincott, Williams & Wilkins; 2012.

44. Muscedere IP. Comprehensive evidence-based clinical practice guidelines for ventilator associated pneumonia prevention. *Journal Critical Care.* 2007;23:126-137.

45. Niel-Weise BS, Snoeren RL, van den Broek PJ. Policies for endotracheal suctioning of patients receiving mechanical ventilation: a systematic review of randomized controlled trials. *Infection Control and Hospital Epidemiology.* 2007;28:531.

46. O'Neal PV, Grap MJ, Thompson C, et al. Level of dyspnoea experienced in mechanically ventilated adults with and without saline instillation prior to endotracheal suctioning. *Intensive and Critical Care Nursing.* 2001;17:356-363.

47. Parrish CR, Krenitsky J, Willcutts K. Nutritional support for mechanically ventilated patients. In: Burns SM, ed. *AACN Protocols for Practice: Care of the Mechanically Ventilated Patient.* 2nd ed., pp. 191-244. Boston: Jones & Bartlett; 2007.

48. Patak L, Gawlinski A, Fung NI, et al. Communication boards in critical care: patients' views. *Applied Nursing Research.* 2006;19:182-190.

49. Patton KT, Thibodeau GA. Anatomy of the respiratory system. In: Thibodeau GA, Patton KT, eds. *Anatomy and Physiology,* 7th ed., pp. 777-817. St. Louis: Mosby Elsevier; 2010.

50. Pierce LNB. Invasive and noninvasive modes and methods of mechanical ventilation. In: Burns SM, ed. AACN *Protocols for Practice: Care of the Mechanically Ventilated Patient.* 2nd ed., pp. 59-89. Boston: Jones & Bartlett; 2007.

51. Pierce LNB. *Management of the Mechanically Ventilated Patient.* 2nd ed. Philadelphia: Saunders; 2007.

52. Pilbeam SP. Discontinuation of and weaning from mechanical ventilation. In: Pilbeam SP, Cairo JM, eds. *Mechanical Ventilation: Physiological and Clinical Applications.* 4th ed., pp. 443-471. St. Louis: Mosby; 2006.

53. Pilbeam SP, Cairo JM. *Mechanical Ventilation: Physiological and Clinical Applications.* 4th ed. St. Louis: Mosby; 2006.

54. Richmond AL, Jarog DL, Hanson VM. Unplanned extubation in adult critical care. Quality improvement and education payoff. *Critical Care Nurse.* 2004;24:32-37.

55. Ridling DA, Martin LD, Bratton SL. Endotracheal suctioning with or without instillation of isotonic sodium chloride solution in critically ill children. *American Journal of Critical Care.* 2003;12:212-219.

56. Safdar N, Dezfulian C, Collard HR, et al. Clinical and economic consequences of ventilator-associated pneumonia: A systematic review. *Critical Care Medicine.* 2005;33:2184-2193.

57. Schutz SL. Oxygen saturation monitoring with pulse oximetry. In: Lynn-McHale Weigand DJ, ed. *AACN Procedure Manual for Critical Care.* 6th ed., 121-137. St. Louis: Elsevier Saunders; 2011.

58. Shilling A, Durbin CG. Airway management. In: Cairo J, ed. *Mosby's Respiratory Care Equipment.* 8th ed. St. Louis: Mosby Elsevier; 2010.

59. Siela D. Pulmonary aspects of obesity in critical care. *Critical Care Nursing Clinics of North America.* 2009;21(3):301-310.

60. Simmons KF, Scanlan CL. Airway management. In: Wilkins RL, Stoller JK, Scanlan CL, Kacmarek RM, eds. *Egan's Fundamentals of Respiratory Care.* 9th ed., pp. 694-765. St. Louis: Mosby Elsevier; 2009.

61. Skillings K, Curtis B. Tracheal tube cuff care. In: Lynn-McHale Weigand DJ, ed. *AACN Procedure Manual for Critical Care.* Philadelphia: Saunders; 2010.

62. Skoretz SA, Flowers HL, Martino R. The incidence of dysphagia following endotracheal intubation. *Chest.* 2010;137: 665-673.

63. Sole ML, Byers JF, Ludy JE, et al. A multisite survey of suctioning techniques and airway management practices. *American Journal of Critical Care.* 2003;12:220-230.

64. Sole ML, Xiaogang S, Talber S, et al. Evaluation of an intervention to maintain endotracheal tube cuff pressure within therapeutic range. *American Journal of Critical Care.* 2011;20:109-118.

65. St. John RE. End-tidal CO_2 monitoring. In: Burns SM, ed. *AACN Protocols for Practice: Noninvasive Monitoring.* 2nd ed. Boston: Jones & Bartlett; 2006.

66. St. John RE, Seckel MA. Airway management. In: Burns SM, ed. *AACN Protocols for Practice: Care of the Mechanically Ventilated Patient.* 2nd ed. Boston: Jones & Bartlett; 2007.

67. Tracy MF, Chlan L. Nonpharmacologic interventions to manage common symptoms in patients receiving mechanical ventilation. *Critical Care Nurse.* 2011;31:19-29.

68. Weber J, Kelly JH. Thorax and lungs. *Health Assessment in Nursing.* 4th ed., Philadelphia: Lippincott, Williams & Wilkins; 2010.

69. West JB. *Respiratory Physiology: the Essentials.* 9th ed. Baltimore, MD: Lippincott Williams & Wilkins; 2011.

70. Wilkins RL. Gas exchange and transport. In: Wilkins RL, Stoller JK, Kacmarek RM, eds. *Egan's Fundamentals of Respiratory Care.* 9th ed., pp. 238-268. St. Louis: Mosby Elsevier; 2009.

10

Rapid Response Teams and Code Management

Deborah G. Klein, MSN , RN, APRN-BC, CCRN, FAHA

⊖volve WEBSITE

Many additional resources, including self-assessment exercises, are located on the Evolve companion website at http://evolve.elsevier.com/Sole.

- Review Questions
- Mosby's Nursing Skills Procedures

- Animations
- Video Clips

INTRODUCTION

Code, code blue, code 99, and *Dr. Heart* are terms frequently used in hospital settings to refer to emergency situations that require lifesaving resuscitation and interventions. Codes are called when patients have a cardiac and/or respiratory arrest or a life-threatening cardiac dysrhythmia that causes a loss of consciousness. (The generic term *arrest* is used in this chapter to refer to these conditions.) Regardless of cause, patient survival and positive outcomes depend on prompt recognition of the situation and immediate institution of basic and advanced life support measures. *Code management* refers to the initiation of a code and the lifesaving interventions performed when a patient arrests.

Rapid response teams (RRTs) have recently been implemented to address changes in a patient's clinical condition *before* a cardiac and/or respiratory arrest occurs. The intent of a RRT is to prevent the cardiac and/or respiratory arrest from ever occurring. The Institute for Healthcare Improvement and The Joint Commission National Patient Safety Goals require hospitals to implement systems that enable healthcare workers to request additional assistance from a specially trained individual(s) when the patient's condition appears to be worsening.[13,25]

This chapter discusses the role of RRTs in preventing cardiopulmonary arrest, the roles of the personnel involved in a code, and equipment that must be readily available to support interventions of the RRT or during a code. Basic and advanced life support measures are presented, including medications commonly used during a code. For the most up-to-date information, the reader should contact the American Heart Association (AHA) for current recommendations for basic and advanced cardiac life support or access materials on the AHA website. Care of the patient after a code is discussed, including the use of therapeutic hypothermia.

In the absence of a written order from a physician to withhold resuscitative measures, cardiopulmonary resuscitation (CPR) and a code must be initiated when a patient has a cardiopulmonary arrest. Ideally, the physician, family, and patient (if possible) make the decision whether CPR is to be performed before resuscitative measures are needed. However, it is the physician who makes the decision to terminate resuscitation efforts in progress. Decisions about resuscitation status often create ethical dilemmas for the nurse, patient, and family (see Chapter 3).

All personnel involved in hospital patient care should have basic life support (BLS) training, including how to operate an automated external defibrillator (AED). This training is also recommended for the lay public through the Heartsaver courses offered through the AHA. Advanced cardiac life support (ACLS) provider training is available through the AHA and is strongly recommended for anyone working in critical care.

RAPID RESPONSE TEAMS

The goal of the RRT is to ensure that interventions are available quickly when patient conditions become unstable before an actual cardiopulmonary arrest. Failure to recognize changes in a patient's condition until major complications, including death, have occurred is referred to as "failure to rescue."[8] Conditions associated with failure to rescue include respiratory failure, acute cardiac failure, acute changes in level of consciousness, hypotension, dysrhythmias, pulmonary edema, and sepsis.[15] Up to 80% of patients having an in-hospital cardiac arrest have signs of physiological instability as evidenced by changes in heart rate, blood pressure, and/or respiratory status in the 24 hours before cardiac arrest.[11,16] The RRT concept is based on identification of patients at risk, early notification of a specific team of responders, rapid intervention by the response team, and ongoing evaluation of the team's performance.[14]

A RRT provides a resource team that can be called to the bedside 24 hours a day, 7 days a week, to assess patients outside the critical care unit and intervene as needed; they also support and educate the nursing staff.[26] Composition of the RRT varies—some are composed of a critical care nurse, a respiratory therapist, and a physician. Other members may include an acute care nurse practitioner, a clinical nurse specialist, or a physician's assistant. The RRT may be called upon any time a staff member is concerned about changes in a patient's condition, including heart rate, systolic blood pressure, respiratory rate, pulse oximetry saturation, mental status, urinary output, or laboratory values. Some institutions empower family members to activate the RRT if they identify a change in the patient's condition.

The development of criteria to facilitate early identification of physiological deterioration helps nurses to determine whether the RRT should be called for a bedside consultation. Once the RRT is activated, both personnel and equipment are brought to the patient's bedside within minutes. The equipment that the RRT carries ranges from a stethoscope to more complex monitoring equipment, including portable electrocardiogram (ECG) monitor, pulse oximetry monitor, oxygen delivery system, intravenous (IV) supplies, and medications. Point-of-care testing equipment to perform finger-stick blood glucose, arterial blood gas analysis, hemoglobin and hematocrit, and basic metabolic panel may be available. ACLS algorithms, standing medical orders, and evidence-based protocols guide RRT interventions. Data on RRT calls and patient outcomes are reviewed to develop strategies to prevent clinical deterioration and optimize outcomes for patients who are assessed by the RRT. Early research on the activation of RRTs demonstrated a reduction in cardiac arrests, critical care unit length of stay, and the incidence of acute illness, such as respiratory failure, stroke, severe sepsis, and acute kidney injury.[27] However, a recent systematic literature review and meta-analysis of 1.3 million patients found that implementation of a RRT was not associated with lower hospital mortality rates in hospitalized adults.[7]

ROLES OF CAREGIVERS IN CODE MANAGEMENT

Prompt recognition of a patient's arrest and rapid initiation of BLS and ACLS measures are essential for improved patient outcomes. The first person to recognize that a patient has had an arrest should call for help, instruct someone to "call a code," call for a defibrillator/AED, and begin CPR. One-person CPR is continued until additional help arrives.

Code Team

Key personnel are notified to assist with code management. An overhead paging system or individual pagers may be used to contact personnel, depending on hospital policies. Most hospitals have code teams that are designated to respond to codes (Table 10-1). The code team usually consists of a physician, critical care or emergency department nurses, a nursing supervisor, a nurse anesthetist or anesthesiologist, a respiratory therapist, a pharmacist or pharmacy technician, an ECG technician, and a chaplain. The code team responds to the code and works in conjunction with the patient's nurse and primary physician, if present. If a code team does not exist,

TABLE 10-1	ROLES AND RESPONSIBILITIES OF CODE TEAM MEMBERS
TEAM MEMBER	**PRIMARY ROLE**
Leader of the code (usually a physician)	Directs code. Makes diagnoses and treatment decisions
Primary nurse	Provides information to code leader. Measures vital signs. Assists with procedures. Administers medications
Second nurse	Coordinates use of the crash cart. Prepares medications. Assembles equipment (intubation, suction)
Nursing supervisor	Controls the crowd. Contacts the attending physician. Assists with medications and procedures. Ensures that a bed is available in critical care unit. Assists with transfer of patient to critical care unit
Nurse or assistant	Records events on designated form
Anesthesiologist or nurse anesthetist	Intubates patient. Manages airway and oxygenation
Respiratory therapist	Assists with ventilation and intubation. Obtains blood sample for ABG analysis. Sets up respiratory equipment/mechanical ventilator
Pharmacist or pharmacy technician	Assists with medication preparation. Prepares intravenous infusions
ECG technician	Obtains 12-lead ECG
Chaplain	Supports family

ABG, Arterial blood gas; *ECG,* electrocardiogram.

any available trained personnel usually respond. Teamwork during a code is essential (see box, "QSEN Exemplar").

Leader of the Code

The person who directs, or "runs," the code is responsible for making diagnoses and treatment decisions. The leader is usually a physician who is preferably experienced in code management, such as an intensivist or emergency department physician. However, the leader may be the patient's primary physician or another physician who is available and qualified for the task. If several physicians are present, one assumes responsibility for being the code team leader and should be the only person giving orders for interventions, to avoid confusion and conflict. In some small hospitals, codes may be directed by a nurse trained in ACLS. In this situation, standing physician orders are needed to guide and support the nurse's decision making.

The leader of the code needs as much information about the patient as possible to make treatment decisions. Necessary information includes the reason for the patient's hospitalization, the patient's current treatments and medications, the patient's code status, and the events that occurred immediately before the code. If possible, the code leader should not perform CPR or other tasks. The leader should give full attention to assessment, diagnosis, and treatment decisions to direct resuscitative efforts.

Code Nurses

Primary nurse. The patient's primary nurse should be free to relate information to the person directing the code. The primary nurse may also start IV lines, measure vital signs, administer emergency medications, assist with procedures, or defibrillate the patient as directed by the code leader (if the primary nurse is qualified).

Second nurse. The major task of the second nurse present is to coordinate the use of the crash cart. This nurse must be thoroughly familiar with the layout of the cart and the location of items. This nurse locates, prepares, and labels medications and IV fluids, and also assembles equipment for intubation, suctioning, and other procedures, such as central line insertion. An additional nurse or assistant records the code events on a designated form (code record).

Nursing supervisor. The nursing supervisor responds to the code to assist in whatever manner is needed. Frequently, more people respond to a code than are needed. One job of the supervisor is to limit the number of people in the code to only those necessary and those there for learning purposes. This approach decreases crowding and confusion. Other responsibilities may include contacting the patient's primary physician, relaying information to the staff and family, and ensuring that all the necessary equipment is present and functioning. If the patient must be transferred to the critical care unit, the supervisor may also ensure that a critical care bed is available and coordinate the transfer.

Anesthesiologist or Nurse Anesthetist

The anesthesiologist or nurse anesthetist assumes control of the patient's ventilation and oxygenation. This team member intubates the patient to ensure an adequate airway and to facilitate ventilation. The primary or second nurse assists with the setup and checking of intubation equipment.

Respiratory Therapist

The respiratory therapist usually assists with manual ventilation of the patient before and after intubation. The therapist may also obtain a blood sample for arterial blood gas analysis, set up oxygen and ventilation equipment, and suction the patient. In some institutions, the respiratory therapist performs intubation.

Pharmacist or Pharmacy Technician

In some hospitals, a pharmacist or pharmacy technician responds to codes. This person may prepare medications and mix IV infusions for administration during the code. The pharmacist may also calculate appropriate medication doses based on the patient's weight. Frequently, pharmacy staff members are also responsible for bringing additional medications. At the termination of the code, pharmacy staff may replenish the crash cart medications and ensure pharmacy charges to the patient's account.

Electrocardiogram Technician

In some hospitals, an ECG technician responds to codes. This person is available to obtain 12-lead ECGs that may be ordered to assist with diagnosis and treatment.

Chaplain

As a code team member, the hospital chaplain can be very helpful in comforting and waiting with the patient's family. The chaplain or other support person usually takes the family to a quiet, private area for waiting and remains with them

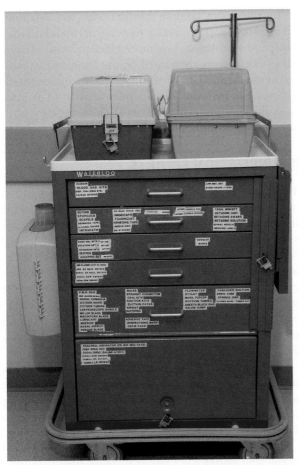

FIGURE 10-1 A typical crash cart.

during the code. This person may also be able to check on the patient periodically to provide the family a progress report.

Other Personnel

Other personnel should be available to run errands, such as taking blood samples to the laboratory or obtaining additional supplies. Meanwhile, other patients need monitoring and care. Only staff members necessary for the code should remain; others should attend to the other patients.

EQUIPMENT USED IN CODES

While the first person to recognize a code calls for help and begins life support measures, another team member immediately brings the crash cart and defibrillator to the patient's bedside (Figure 10-1). Crash carts vary in organization and layout, but they all contain the same basic emergency equipment and medications. Many hospitals have standardized crash carts, so anyone responding to a code is familiar with the location of the items on the cart. In other hospitals, the makeup and organization of the crash cart are unique to each unit. Whether carts are standardized or unique to an individual unit, nurses responding to codes must be familiar with them.

Most carts have equipment stored on top and in several drawers. Table 10-2 lists equipment on a typical crash cart. Equipment such as back boards and portable suction machines may be attached to the cart. Larger equipment is stored on the top of the cart or in a large drawer; smaller items, such as medications and IV equipment, are in the smaller drawers.

TABLE 10-2	**TYPICAL CONTENTS OF A CRASH CART**
MAIN ITEMS	**SPECIFIC SUPPLIES**
Back Cardiac board	
Side Portable suction machine, bag-valve device, and oxygen tubing	Suction device with canister and tubing, face mask, and oxygen tank Container for disposing of needles, syringes, and other sharp items
Top Monitor-defibrillator with recorder, clipboard with code record and drug calculation reference sheets	ECG leads, electrodes, conductive gel or adhesive electrode pads; possible transcutaneous pacemaker or combination unit
Airway equipment drawer or box	Oral and nasal airways, ETTs, stylet, laryngoscope handle and curved and straight blades, lubricating jelly, 10-mL syringes, and tape, exhaled CO_2 detector
IV equipment drawer	IV catheters of various sizes, tape, syringes, needles and needleless adaptors, IV fluids (NS, Ringer's lactate solution, and D_5W); and IV tubing
Medication drawer or box	All IV push emergency medications in prefilled syringes if available, sterile water and NS for injection, and IV infusion emergency medications (see Table 10-4)
Miscellaneous supply drawer	Sterile and nonsterile gloves, suction catheters, nasogastric tubes, chest tubes, blood pressure cuff, blood collection tubes, sutures, pacemaker magnet, extra ECG recording paper, gauze pads, face masks
Procedure kits	Arterial blood gas, tracheotomy, intraosseous insertion kit, central line insertion kit, chest tube tray

CO_2, Carbon dioxide; D_5W, 5% dextrose in water; *ECG*, electrocardiogram; *ETTs*, endotracheal tubes; *IV*, intravenous; *NS*, normal saline.

A back or "cardiac" board is usually located on the back or side of the cart. It is placed under the patient as soon as possible to provide a hard, level surface for the performance of chest compressions. Alternatively, some hospital bed headboards are removable for use as a cardiac board. The patient is either lifted up or logrolled to one side for placement of the board. Care should be taken to protect the patient's cervical spine if injury is suspected.

A monitor-defibrillator is located on top of the cart or on a separate cart. The patient's cardiac rhythm is monitored via the leads and electrodes or through adhesive electrode pads on this machine. A "quick look" at the patient's cardiac rhythm can also be obtained by placing the defibrillation paddles on the chest. In the hospital setting, continuous monitoring via the electrodes is preferable to intermittent use of the defibrillation paddles for a quick look at the rhythm. The monitor must have a strip-chart recorder for documenting the patient's ECG rhythm for the code record. Newer monitor/defibrillator units include capabilities for transcutaneous pacing and an AED. Some patient care units may use an AED for initial code management.

A bag with an attached face mask (bag-mask device) and oxygen tubing is usually kept on the crash cart. The tubing is connected either to a wall oxygen inlet or to a portable oxygen tank on the crash cart. Supplemental oxygen is always used with the bag-mask device. Airway management supplies are located in one of the drawers. Some institutions have a separate box containing airway management supplies.

Another drawer contains IV supplies and solutions. Normal saline (NS) and Ringer lactate solution are the IV fluids most often used. A 5% dextrose in water solution (D_5W) in 250- and 500-mL bags is used to prepare vasoactive infusions.

Emergency medications fill another drawer or may be located in a separate box. These include IV push medications and medications that must be added to IV fluids for continuous infusions. Most IV push medications are available in prefilled syringes. Several drugs that are given via a continuous infusion (e.g., lidocaine, dopamine) are also available as premixed bags. Medications are discussed in depth later in the Pharmacological Intervention during a Code section of this chapter.

Other important items on the cart include a suction device with a canister and tubing and suction catheters, nasogastric tubes, and a blood pressure cuff. Various kits used for tracheotomy, central line insertion, and intraosseous insertion are also frequently kept on the crash cart.

The crash cart and defibrillator are usually checked by nursing staff at designated time intervals (every shift or every 24 hours) to ensure that all equipment and medications are present and functional. Once the cart is fully stocked, it should be kept locked, to prevent borrowing of supplies and equipment.

The nurse can become familiar with the location of items on the cart by being responsible for checking it. Management of the code is more efficient when the nurse knows where items are located on the crash cart, as well as how to use them. Many institutions require nursing staff to participate in periodic "mock" codes to assist in maintaining skills. Multiprofessional team simulations also provide excellent opportunities for skill development.

RESUSCITATION EFFORTS

The flow of events during a code requires a concentrated team effort. BLS is provided until the code team arrives. Once help arrives, CPR is continued by use of the two-person technique. Priorities during cardiac arrest are high-quality CPR and early defibrillation. Other tasks such as connecting the patient to an ECG monitor, starting IV lines, attaching an oxygen source to the bag-mask device, and setting up suction are performed by available personnel as soon as possible. The activities that occur during the code are summarized in Table 10-3. Often, several activities are performed simultaneously.

The code team should be alerted to the patient's code status. Individuals may have advance directives documenting their wishes. This document provides instructions to family members, physicians, and other healthcare providers (see Chapter 3).

Many states have implemented "no CPR" options. The patient, who usually has a terminal illness, signs a document requesting "no CPR" if there is a loss of pulse or if breathing stops. In some states, this document directs the patient to wear a "no CPR" identification bracelet. In the event of a code, the bracelet alerts the responders that CPR efforts are prohibited. The responders should respect the person's wishes.

Basic Life Support

The goal of BLS is to support or restore effective circulation, oxygenation, and ventilation with return of spontaneous circulation. Early CPR and early defibrillation with an AED are stressed.[2] CPR must be initiated immediately in the event of an arrest to improve the patient's chance of survival.

The 2010 AHA Guidelines for CPR recommend a change in the BLS sequence from A-B-C (airway, breathing, circulation) to C-A-B (chest compressions, airway, breathing) and determining whether defibrillation is needed. BLS providers must be trained in the use of an AED (discussed in detail in the Electrical Therapy section of this chapter). Assessment is a part of each step, and the steps are performed in order (Box 10-1). The following summary is adapted from the AHA standards.[3]

TABLE 10-3	FLOW OF EVENTS DURING A CODE	
PRIORITIES	**EQUIPMENT FROM CART**	**INTERVENTION**
Recognition of arrest		Assess code status, call for help, assess for absence of breathing, initiate CPR
Arrival of code team, crash cart, cardiac monitor-defibrillator, AED	Cardiac board Bag-mask device with oxygen tubing Oral airway Oxygen and regulator if not already at bedside	Place patient on cardiac board Ventilate with 100% oxygen with oral airway and bag-mask device Continue chest compressions
Identification of team leader		Assess patient Direct and supervise team members Solve problems Obtain patient history and determine events leading up to the code
Rhythm diagnosis	Cardiac monitor defibrillator AED 12-Lead ECG machine	Attach limb leads or adhesive electrode pads, but do not interrupt CPR
Prompt defibrillation if indicated	Defibrillator/AED	Use correct algorithm
Intubation (if ventilation inadequate and trained personnel available)	Suction equipment Laryngoscope Endotracheal tube and other intubation equipment Stethoscope Exhaled CO_2 detector or waveform capnography	Connect suction equipment Intubate patient (interrupt CPR no more than 10 seconds) Confirm tube position: listen over bilateral lung fields; observe chest movement; confirm with secondary measure (exhaled CO_2 detector or waveform capnography) Secure tube Oxygenate
Venous access	Peripheral or central IV equipment IO insertion kit IV tubing, infusion fluid (NS)	Insert peripheral IV into antecubital sites Insert IO needle Central line may be inserted by physician
Drug administration	Drugs as ordered (and in anticipation, based on algorithms)	Use correct algorithm

Ongoing assessment of the patient's response to therapy during resuscitation		Assess frequently:
		  Pulse generated with CPR
		  Adequacy of artificial ventilation
		  Arterial blood gases or other laboratory studies
		  Spontaneous pulse after any intervention or rhythm change
		  Spontaneous breathing with return of pulse
		  Blood pressure, if pulse is present
		  Decision to stop, if no response to therapy

Drawing arterial and venous blood specimens	Arterial puncture and venipuncture equipment	Draw specimens Treat as needed, based on results
Documentation	Code record	Accurately record events while resuscitation is in progress Record rhythm strips during the code
Controlling or limiting crowd		Dismiss those not required for bedside tasks
Family notification		Keep family informed of patient's condition Notify outcome with sensitivity Explore options for family presence during code
Transfer of patient to critical care unit		Ensure bed assigned for patient Transfer with adequate personnel and emergency equipment
Critique		Evaluate events of code and express feelings

AED, Automated external defibrillator; *CO₂*, carbon dioxide; *CPR*, cardiopulmonary resuscitation; *ECG*, electrocardiogram; *IO*, intraosseous; *IV*, intravenous; *NS*, normal saline.
Based on data from Neumar RW, Otto CW, Link MS, Kronick SL, Shuster M, Callaway CW, et al. (2010). *Part 8: adult advanced cardiovascular life support: 2010 American Heart Association Guidelines for Cardiopulmonary Resuscitation and Emergency Cardiovascular Care. Circulation. 122* (18 Suppl 3):S729-S767; American Heart Association. (2011). *ACLS Provider Manual.* Dallas, TX: Author.

Responsiveness

The first intervention is to assess unresponsiveness by tapping or shaking a patient and shouting, "Are you OK?" The patient is positioned on his or her back, and assessed for absent or abnormal breathing by looking at the chest. If the patient is unresponsive, the nurse calls for help by shouting to fellow caregivers or by using the nurse-call system. If the patient must be turned to the supine position, the head and body are turned as a unit to prevent possible injury.

Circulation and Chest Compressions

The second step of CPR is to ensure adequate circulation. The presence or absence of a carotid pulse is assessed for 5 to 10 seconds to detect bradycardia. The pulse is assessed even if the patient is attached to a cardiac monitor because artifact or a loose lead may mimic a cardiac dysrhythmia. The nurse checks the patient's carotid pulse on the side nearest the nurse.

If a pulse is present, rescue breathing is initiated at a rate of 10 to 12 breaths per minute, or 1 breath every 5 to 6 seconds. The pulse is assessed every 2 minutes for no longer than 10 seconds. If the pulse is absent, the nurse begins cardiac compressions. The patient is placed supine on a firm surface (cardiac board). Proper hand position is essential for performing compressions. The location for compressions is the lower half of the sternum in the center of the chest between the nipples. The heel of one hand is placed on the lower half of the sternum. The heel of the second hand is placed on top of the first hand so the hands are overlapped and parallel. Using both hands, the nurse begins compressions by depressing the sternum 2.0 inches for the average adult and then

letting the chest return to its normal position. Compressions are performed at a rate of at least 100 per minute ("hard and fast"). The compression-ventilation ratio is 30 compressions to 2 breaths.

Every effort is made to minimize interruptions in chest compressions. CPR is continued until the monitor-defibrillator/AED arrives, electrode pads are placed, and the AED is ready to analyze the rhythm. Shocks are provided as indicated. After each shock, immediately resume CPR beginning with compressions for 2 minutes.

Airway

There are two methods for opening the airway to provide breaths: head-tilt/chin-lift (Figure 10-2) and jaw thrust. The head-tilt/chin-lift is performed by placing one hand on the victim's forehead and tilting the head back. The fingers of the other hand are placed under the bony part of the lower jaw near the chin. The jaw is then lifted to bring the chin forward. Two people are usually needed to perform the jaw thrust and provide breaths with a bag-mask device. A jaw thrust is used when a head or neck injury is suspected.

The first person who arrives to help should activate the code team. Some units and emergency departments have an emergency call system that can be activated from the patient's room by the pressing of a button. If the nurse is alone and an emergency call system is not available, the nurse presses the nurse-call system and begins CPR. When the call is answered the nurse states, "Call a code!"

Breathing

Barrier devices must be available in the workplace for individuals who are expected to perform CPR. In the hospital setting, these include a pocket mask at every patient's bedside; critical care units often have a bag-mask device available for each patient.

Ventilation of the patient with a bag-mask device requires that an open airway be maintained. Frequently, an oral airway is used to keep the airway patent and to facilitate ventilation. The bag-mask device is connected to an oxygen source set at 15 L/min. The face mask is positioned and sealed over the patient's mouth and nose after opening the airway. The patient is manually ventilated with the bag-mask device (Figure 10-3). Personnel should be properly trained to use the bag-mask device effectively.

Advanced Cardiac Life Support

For cardiac or respiratory emergencies, many institutions follow the AHA standards for ACLS. The tools of management are the BLS survey followed by the ACLS survey.[2]

The BLS survey focuses on early CPR and early defibrillation. The ABCDs of ACLS are the same as for BLS: airway, breathing, and compressions or circulation. "D" refers to differential diagnosis or searching, finding, and treating reversible causes.

Airway

Airway management involves reassessment of original techniques established in BLS. Endotracheal intubation provides

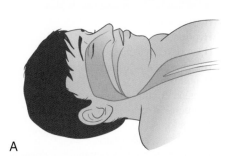
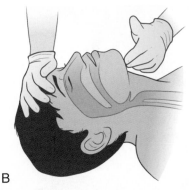

FIGURE 10-2 Head-tilt/chin-lift technique for opening the airway. **A,** Obstruction by the tongue. **B,** Head-tilt/chin-lift maneuver lifts tongue relieving airway obstruction.

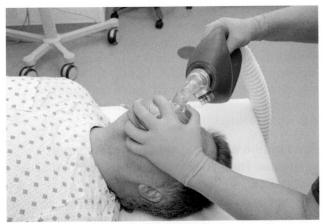

FIGURE 10-3 Rescue breathing with bag-mask device. (Reprinted with permission, Cleveland Clinic Center for Medical Art & Photography © 2011-2012. All rights reserved.)

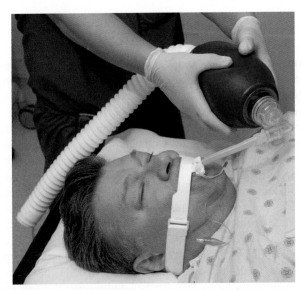

FIGURE 10-4 Ventilation with a bag-valve device connected to endotracheal tube.

definitive airway management and should be performed if needed by properly trained personnel during the resuscitation effort.[2] The benefit of endotracheal intubation is weighed against the effects of interrupting chest compressions. If bag-mask ventilation is adequate, endotracheal intubation may be deferred until the patient fails to respond to initial CPR and defibrillation or until spontaneous circulation returns.

Techniques of endotracheal intubation are discussed in Chapter 9. Once intubated, the patient is manually ventilated with a bag-valve device attached to the endotracheal tube (ETT; Figure 10-4). The bag-valve device should have a reservoir and be connected to an oxygen source to deliver 100% oxygen while providing a tidal volume of 6 to 7 mL/kg. Chest compressions are not stopped for ventilations. Chest compressions are delivered continuously at a rate of 100 per minute. Ventilations are delivered one breath every 6 to 8 seconds or approximately 8 to 10 breaths per minute.

Breathing

Breathing assessment determines whether the ventilatory efforts are causing the chest to rise. If the patient is intubated,

ETT placement is confirmed by bilateral breath sounds and observation of chest movement with ventilation. Continuous waveform capnography (discussed in more detail later) is recommended for monitoring and confirming correct placement of the ETT. A secondary method of assessing ETT placement may be done with an exhaled carbon dioxide (CO_2) detector or esophageal detector device (Figure 10-5).[2] If no chest expansion is present with bag-valve ventilation, the ETT has mistakenly been placed in the esophagus and is removed immediately. A chest radiograph confirms placement after the code.

Circulation

Circulation initially focuses on chest compressions, attachment of electrodes and leads to the monitor-defibrillator, rhythm identification, IV and/or intraosseous (IO) access, and medication administration. If ventricular fibrillation or

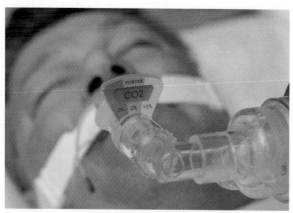

FIGURE 10-5 End-tidal carbon dioxide detector connected to an endotracheal tube. Exhaled carbon dioxide reacts with the device to create a color change indicating correct endotracheal tube placement.

BOX 10-2	**REVERSIBLE CAUSES OF CARDIAC ARREST**

Hypovolemia
Hypoxia
Hydrogen ion (acidosis)
Hypokalemia or hyperkalemia
Hypothermia
Tension pneumothorax
Tamponade, cardiac
Toxins (drug overdose)
Thrombosis, pulmonary
Thrombosis, coronary (massive myocardial infarction)

pulseless ventricular tachycardia is identified, high energy unsynchronized shocks are delivered followed by two minutes of chest compressions with ventilation. IV access for medication administration is then obtained. A patent IV is necessary during an arrest for the administration of fluids, medications, or both. IO cannulation may be performed when IV access is not available, and it is recommended by the AHA as the primary alternative to IV access.[2] IO cannulation provides access to the bone marrow and is a rapid, safe, and reliable route for administering medications, blood, and IV fluid during resuscitation. Commercially available kits facilitate IO access in adults. Endotracheal administration of medications may be considered; however, tracheal absorption of medications is poor, and optimal dosing is not known. Medications that can be administered through the ETT until IV access is established are epinephrine, lidocaine, and vasopressin.[2]

Most critically ill patients have an IV access. If the patient does not have IV access or needs additional IV access, a large-bore IV should be inserted. The antecubital vein is the first target for IV access. Other areas for IV insertion include the dorsum of the hands and the wrist. If a peripheral IV cannot be started, the physician inserts a central line for IV access. The IO route is an option if IV access is difficult.

NS is the preferred IV fluid because it expands intravascular volume better than dextrose. When any medication is administered by the peripheral IV route, it is best followed with a 20-mL bolus of IV fluid and elevation of the extremity for about 10 to 20 seconds to enhance delivery to the central circulation.

Differential Diagnosis

Differential diagnosis involves searching for, finding, and treating reversible causes of the cardiopulmonary arrest. Cardiac dysrhythmias that result in cardiac arrests have many possible causes (Box 10-2). The lethal dysrhythmias include ventricular fibrillation/pulseless ventricular tachycardia (VF/VT), asystole, and pulseless electrical activity (PEA). Other dysrhythmias that may lead to a cardiopulmonary arrest include symptomatic bradycardias and symptomatic tachycardias. Algorithms for treating these rhythm disorders have been established by the AHA.[2] Because these algorithms periodically change, critical actions in the management of these dysrhythmias are summarized rather than publishing the algorithms.

Recognition and Treatment of Dysrhythmias
Ventricular Fibrillation and Pulseless Ventricular Tachycardia

The most common initial rhythms in witnessed sudden cardiac arrest are VF or pulseless VT. When VF is present, the heart quivers and does not pump blood. The treatment for VF and pulseless VT is the same.

Critical actions.
- Initiate the BLS survey. Begin CPR until a defibrillator is available. Defibrillate as soon as possible because early CPR and defibrillation increase the chance of survival and a good neurological outcome.
- Give one shock and resume CPR beginning with chest compressions. If a biphasic defibrillator is available, use the dose at which that defibrillator has been shown to be effective for terminating VF (typically 120 joules [J] to 200 J). If the dose is not known, use the maximum dose available. If a monophasic defibrillator is available, use an initial shock of 360 J and use 360 J for subsequent shocks. Resume CPR immediately beginning with chest compressions for 5 cycles or about 2 minutes. One cycle consists of 30 compressions followed by 2 ventilations. After 5 cycles of CPR, check rhythm. (Monophasic versus biphasic defibrillation is discussed in the Electrical Therapy section of this chapter.)
- If VF/VT persists, continue CPR, charge the defibrillator, and obtain IV/IO access. Give one shock (biphasic defibrillator, use same joules as first shock or higher; monophasic defibrillator, use 360 J). Resume CPR immediately, beginning with chest compressions for 5 cycles or about 2 minutes.

- When IV or IO access is available, administer epinephrine, 1 mg IV/IO every 3 to 5 minutes, if VF persists. One dose of vasopressin, 40 units IV/IO, may substitute the first or second dose of epinephrine. Check rhythm after 2 minutes or 5 cycles of CPR. If VF/VT persists, resume CPR immediately beginning with chest compressions for 5 cycles or 2 minutes, and charge the defibrillator.
- Give one shock (biphasic defibrillator, use same joules as first shock or higher; monophasic defibrillator, use 360 J). Resume CPR immediately for 5 cycles or about 2 minutes.
- Consider giving an antidysrhythmic medications either before or after the shock; however, there is no evidence that an antidysrhythmic medication given during a cardiac arrest increases survival to discharge.[2] If administered, amiodarone is the first choice, followed by lidocaine and magnesium sulfate. Dosages and administration are discussed in the Pharmacological Intervention during a Code section of this chapter.
- Reassess the patient frequently. Search for and treat the underlying cause of the cardiac arrest. Check for return of pulse, spontaneous respirations, and blood pressure. Resume CPR if appropriate.

Pulseless Electrical Activity and Asystole

The goal in treating any rhythm without a pulse is to determine and treat the probable underlying cause of this condition. PEA, an organized rhythm without a pulse, is often associated with clinical conditions that can be reversed if they are identified early and treated appropriately.[2] Asystole is the absence of electrical activity on the ECG and has a poor prognosis. It is essential to search for and treat reversible causes of asystole for resuscitation efforts to be successful.

Critical actions

- Initiate the BLS survey. Initiate CPR for 5 cycles or 2 minutes. IV/IO access is obtained. Endotracheal intubation is only performed if ventilations with a bag-mask device are ineffective.
- Consider possible causes and treat (see Box 10-2).
- Confirm asystole by ensuring lead and cable connections are correct, ensuring that the power is on, and verifying asystole in another lead. An additional lead confirms or rules out the possibility of a fine VF.
- Check rhythm for no longer than 10 seconds. If no rhythm is present (e.g., asystole), resume CPR for 5 cycles or 2 minutes. If organized electrical activity is present, palpate a pulse for at least 5 seconds but no longer than 10 seconds. If no pulse is present (e.g., PEA), resume CPR starting with chest compressions for 5 cycles or 2 minutes.
- When IV or IO access is available, administer epinephrine, 1 mg IV/IO every 3 to 5 minutes, or vasopressin, 40 units IV/IO, to replace the first or second dose of epinephrine. CPR is not stopped for drug administration. Consider endotracheal intubation.
- Resume CPR for 5 cycles or 2 minutes, and then check the rhythm and pulse.
- Continue the ACLS survey while identifying underlying causes and initiating related interventions.

> ### BOX 10-3 SIGNS AND SYMPTOMS OF POOR PERFUSION ASSOCIATED WITH BRADYCARDIA
>
> **Signs**
> - Hypotension
> - Orthostatic hypotension
> - Diaphoresis
> - Pulmonary congestion
> - Pulmonary edema
>
> **Symptoms**
> - Chest pain
> - Shortness of breath
> - Decreased level of consciousness
> - Weakness
> - Fatigue
> - Dizziness
> - Syncope

- Consider termination of resuscitative efforts if a reversible cause is not rapidly identified and treated, and the patient fails to respond to the BLS and ACLS surveys. The decision to terminate resuscitative efforts in the hospital is the responsibility of the treating physician and is based on consideration of many factors, including time from collapse to CPR, time from collapse to first defibrillation attempt (if shockable rhythm present), comorbid disease, prearrest state, initial rhythm at time of arrest, and response to resuscitative measures.

Symptomatic Bradycardia

This category encompasses two types: *bradycardia,* a heart rate less than 60 beats per minute (e.g., third degree heart block), or *symptomatic bradycardia,* any heart rhythm that is slow enough to cause hemodynamic compromise (Box 10-3). When bradycardia is the cause of the symptoms, the heart rate is generally less than 50 beats per minute. The cause of the bradycardia must be considered. For example, hypotension associated with bradycardia may be caused by dysfunction of the myocardium or hypovolemia, rather than by a conduction system or autonomic nervous system disturbance.

Critical actions

- Perform ACLS survey. Maintain a patent airway and assist breathing as necessary. Provide oxygen if patient hypoxic as determined by pulse oximetry. Monitor blood pressure, heart rate, and pulse oximetry. Obtain a 12-lead ECG. Establish IV access. Search for and treat possible contributing factors.
- Determine if signs and symptoms of poor perfusion are present and if they are related to the bradycardia (see Box 10-3). If adequate perfusion is present, observe and monitor.

- If poor perfusion is present, administer atropine, 0.5 mg IV every 3 to 5 minutes to a total dose of 3 mg. Atropine is not indicated in second-degree atrioventricular (AV) block type II or third-degree AV block.
- If atropine is ineffective, prepare for transcutaneous pacing. If used, analgesics or sedatives may need to be given because patients often find the pacing stimulus that is delivered with this therapy uncomfortable.
- Consider epinephrine or dopamine infusion if pacing is not effective. Both dopamine and epinephrine infusions may be used with symptomatic bradycardia if low blood pressure is associated with the bradycardia.

Unstable Tachycardia

Tachycardia is defined as a heart rate greater than 100 beats per minute. *Unstable tachycardia* occurs when the heart beats too fast for the patient's clinical condition. The treatment of this group of dysrhythmias involves the rapid recognition that the patient is symptomatic and that the signs and symptoms are caused by the tachycardia. Generally, if the heart rate is less than 150 beats per minute, it is unlikely that the symptoms of instability are caused by the tachycardia. Synchronized cardioversion and antidysrhythmic therapy may be needed.[2]

Critical actions

- Perform the BLS and ACLS survey. Assess the patient and recognize the signs of cardiovascular instability, including increased work of breathing (tachypnea, intercostal retractions, paradoxical abdominal breathing) and hypoxia as determined by pulse oximetry. Provide supplemental oxygen, assess blood pressure, and establish IV access. Determine cardiac rhythm.
- Assess the degree of instability. If the patient has hypotension, altered mental status, signs of shock, chest discomfort, or acute heart failure, prepare for synchronized cardioversion. If the ECG complex is regular and narrow, consider administration of adenosine.
- If cardioversion is indicated, premedicate with sedation if patient is conscious. Cardioversion is an uncomfortable procedure.
- Perform synchronized cardioversion at the appropriate energy level. Supraventricular tachycardia and atrial flutter often respond to energy levels as low as 50 J. If the initial 50 J fails, the energy dose is increased stepwise for subsequent attempts. In unstable atrial fibrillation, start at 200 J monophasic or 120 to 200 J biphasic, and increase the energy dose stepwise for subsequent cardioversion attempts. Cardioversion for monomorphic ventricular tachycardia with a pulse should be initiated at 100 J monophasic or biphasic and increased stepwise for subsequent attempts.[2]
- Reassess the patient and rhythm and consider further monitoring and antidysrhythmic therapy including adenosine, procainamide, or amiodarone.

Electrical Therapy

The therapeutic use of electrical current has expanded over the past several years with the addition and increased use of the AED. This section addresses the use of electricity in code management for the purposes of defibrillation, cardioversion, and transcutaneous (external) pacing.

Defibrillation

The only effective treatment for VF and pulseless VT is defibrillation. VF deteriorates into asystole if not treated. VF may occur as a result of coronary artery disease, myocardial infarction, electrical shock, drug overdose, near drowning, and acid-base imbalance.

Definition. Defibrillation is the delivery of an electrical current to the heart through the use of a defibrillator (Figure 10-6). The current can be delivered through the chest wall by use of external paddles or adhesive electrode pads ("hands off" defibrillation) connected to cables. Smaller internal paddles may be used to deliver current directly to the heart during cardiac surgery when the chest is open and the heart is visualized. Defibrillation works by completely depolarizing the heart and disrupting the impulses that are causing the dysrhythmia. Because the heart is completely depolarized, the sinoatrial node or other pacemaker can resume control of the heart's rhythm.

Defibrillation delivers energy or current in waveforms. *Monophasic* waveforms deliver current in one direction. More recently, defibrillators have been developed that deliver biphasic current. *Biphasic* waveforms deliver current that

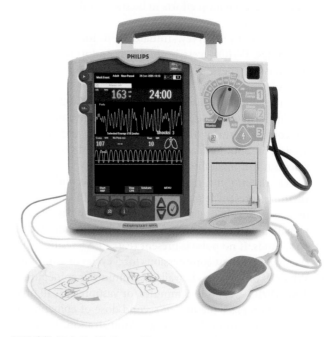

FIGURE 10-6 Defibrillator. (Courtesy Philips Healthcare, Andover, Massachusetts.)

flows in a positive direction for a specified duration and then reverses and flows in a negative direction. As a result, less joules are needed for defibrillation. Biphasic defibrillation is at least as effective as monophasic defibrillation, and in some reports is more effective in converting VF with fewer shocks.[2]

Procedure. Using conductive materials during defibrillation reduces transthoracic impedence and enhances the flow of electrical current through the chest structures. Conductive materials include paddles with electrode paste, gel pads, or adhesive electrode pads.

Two methods exist for paddle or pad placement for external defibrillation. The standard or anterior paddle placement is used most often. In the anterior method, one paddle or adhesive electrode pad is placed at the second intercostal space to the right of the sternum, and the other paddle or adhesive electrode pad is placed at the fifth intercostal space, midaxillary line, to the left of the sternum (Figure 10-7). The alternative method is

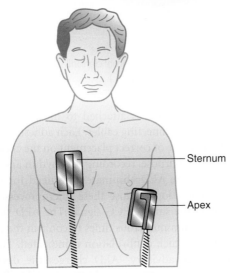

FIGURE 10-7 Paddle placement for defibrillation.

anteroposterior placement. Adhesive electrode pads are used because of the difficulty in correctly placing the paddles. The anterior electrode pad is placed at the left anterior precordial area, and the posterior electrode pad is placed at the left posterior-infrascapular area or at the posterior-infrascapular area (Figure 10-8). Refer to the manufacturer's instructions for exact placement of the electrode pads.

The amount of energy delivered is referred to as joules, or watt-seconds (w-s). For monophasic defibrillation, 360 J is used for all shocks. For biphasic defibrillation, refer to the manufacturer's instructions for the amount of joules to be delivered to the patient. If the recommended dose is unknown, use the maximum dose available.[2]

For the shock to be effective, some type of conductive medium is placed between the paddles and the skin. In the past, gel has been used to conduct the electricity. If gel is used, it is important to cover the paddles completely with the gel. Commercially prepared defibrillator gel pads are available that facilitate defibrillation and also prevent burns on the patient's skin that may occur when paddles are used. Adhesive electrode pads used in "hands-off" defibrillation also have conductive gel. No data suggest that one is better than the other; however, adhesive electrode pads reduce the risk of current arcing, facilitate monitoring of the patient's underlying rhythm, and allow the rapid delivery of a shock when needed. Therefore adhesive electrode pads are recommended instead of paddles to enhance the delivery of the electrical current.[2]

The defibrillator is charged to the desired setting. The paddles are placed firmly on the patient's chest. Firm pressure is needed to facilitate skin contact and to reduce the impedance to the flow of current. Safety is essential during the procedure to prevent injury to the patient and the personnel assisting with the procedure. The person performing the defibrillation ensures that all personnel are standing clear of the bed and visually checks to see that no one is in contact with the patient or bed. It is important that this step not be

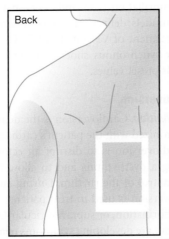
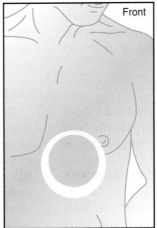
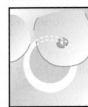

FIGURE 10-8 Anteroposterior placement of adhesive electrode pads for defibrillation or transcutaneous pacing.

BOX 10-4 PROCEDURE FOR EXTERNAL DEFIBRILLATION

- Apply adhesive electrode pads or gel pads to the patient's chest (or apply conductive gel to paddles).
- Turn on the defibrillator.
- Select the energy level.
- If using paddles, position the paddles on the patient's chest.
- If using adhesive electrode pads, connect the electrode cable to the defibrillator.
- Ensure that all personnel (including yourself) are clear of the patient, the bed, and any equipment that is connected to the patient.
- Charge the defibrillator to the desired setting.
- Shout "Clear. I am going to shock on three," and look to verify that all personnel are clear.
- If using paddles, apply firm pressure on both paddles.
- Shout "One, two, three. Shocking."
- Deliver shock by depressing buttons on each paddle simultaneously. If using adhesive electrode pads, press the "shock" button on the defibrillator.
- Resume cardiopulmonary resuscitation.

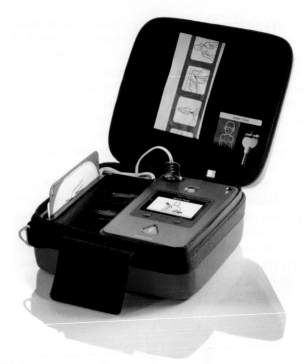

FIGURE 10-9 Automated external defibrillator. (Courtesy Philips Healthcare, Bothell, Washington.)

---

omitted when hands-off defibrillation is used. The announcement, "Clear. I am going to shock on three," provides an audible check that no one is touching the patient. "One, two, three, shocking," is announced as the shock is delivered. CPR is resumed immediately, beginning with chest compressions for 5 cycles or 2 minutes. Then the patient's rhythm and pulse are checked. Rhythm strips are recorded during the procedure to document response. The procedure for defibrillation is summarized in Box 10-4.

Complications of defibrillation include burns on the skin and damage to the heart muscle. Arcing of electricity or a spark can occur if the paddles are not firmly placed on the skin, excessive conductive gel is used, or the skin is wet. Arcing has also been noted when patients have medication patches with aluminized backing (e.g., nitroglycerin, nicotine, pain medication); therefore these patches should be removed and the area cleansed before defibrillation. Body jewelry such as nipple rings should also be removed before defibrillation to reduce the risk for arcing of electricity during the procedure.

Automated External Defibrillation

The AED extends the range of personnel trained in the use of a defibrillator and shortens the time between code onset and defibrillation. The AED is considered an integral part of emergency cardiac care.

Definition. The AED is an external defibrillator with rhythm analysis capabilities (Figure 10-9). It is used to achieve early defibrillation. Because of the ease of use, AEDs may be placed on medical-surgical patient units, emergency response vehicles, and in public places.

Indications. The AED should be used only when a patient is in cardiac arrest (unresponsive, absent or abnormal breathing, and no pulse). Confirmation that the patient is in cardiac arrest must be obtained before attaching the AED.[3]

Procedure. The AED is attached to the patient by two adhesive pads and connecting cables. Each adhesive electrode pad depicts an image of correct placement on the chest. These pads serve a dual purpose: recording the rhythm and delivering the shock. The AED eliminates the need for training in rhythm recognition because these microprocessor-based devices analyze the surface ECG signal. The AED "looks" at the patient's rhythm numerous times to confirm the presence of a rhythm for which defibrillation is indicated. The semi-automatic "shock advisory" AED charges the device and "advises" the operator to press a button to defibrillate. The fully automated AED requires only that the operator attach the defibrillation pads and turn on the device (Box 10-5). Both models deliver AHA-recommended energy levels for the treatment of VF/pulseless VT. They are not designed to deliver synchronous shocks and will shock VT if the rate exceeds preset values.

Cardioversion

Definition. Cardioversion is the delivery of a shock that is synchronized with the patient's cardiac rhythm. The purpose of cardioversion is to disrupt an ectopic pacemaker that is causing a dysrhythmia and to allow the sinoatrial node to take control of the rhythm. During an emergency situation, cardioversion is used to treat patients with VT, atrial flutter, atrial fibrillation, or supraventricular tachycardia who have a pulse but are developing symptoms related to poor perfusion, such as hypotension and a decreased level of consciousness. Elective cardioversion is used to treat stable atrial flutter and atrial fibrillation.

Cardioversion is similar to defibrillation, except the delivery of energy is synchronized to occur during ventricular

BOX 10-5   PROCEDURE FOR AUTOMATED EXTERNAL DEFIBRILLATOR (AED) OPERATION

- Turn the power on.
- Attach the AED connecting cables to the AED "box."
- Attach the adhesive electrode pads to the patient:

  Place one electrode pad on the upper right sternal border directly below the clavicle.

  Place the other electrode pad lateral to the left nipple, with the top margin of the pad a few inches below the axilla.

  The correct position of the electrode pads is often displayed on the electrode pads.

- Attach the AED connecting cables to the adhesive electrode pads.
- Clear personnel from the patient (no one should be touching the patient), and press the "analyze" button to start rhythm analysis.
- Listen or read the message "shock indicated" or "no shock indicated."
- Clear personnel from the patient, and press the "shock" button if shock is indicated.

BOX 10-6   PROCEDURE FOR SYNCHRONIZED CARDIOVERSION

- Ensure that emergency equipment is readily available.
- Explain the procedure to the patient.
- Sedate the conscious patient unless unstable or rapidly deteriorating.
- Attach monitor leads to the patient. Ensure that the monitor displays the patient's rhythm clearly without artifact.
- Apply the adhesive electrode pads (recommended) or defibrillator gel pads to the patient's chest (or apply conductive gel to the paddles).
- Turn on the defibrillator to "synchronous" mode.
- Observe the rhythm on the monitor to determine that the R wave is properly sensed and marked (usually with a spike) (see Figure 10-11).
- Select the appropriate energy level.
- If using paddles, position the paddles on the patient's chest and apply firm pressure.
- Announce "Charging defibrillator. Stand clear." Ensure that all personnel (including yourself) are clear of the patient, the bed, and any equipment that is connected to the patient.
- Press the "Charge" button on the defibrillator.
- Shout "Clear. I am going to shock on three," and look to verify that all personnel are clear.
- Shout "One, two, three. Shocking."
- Deliver synchronized shock by depressing the buttons on each paddle simultaneously or press the shock button on the defibrillator if using adhesive electrode pads. Keep the buttons depressed until the shock has been delivered.
- After the cardioversion, observe the patient's heart rhythm to determine effectiveness.

depolarization (peak of the QRS complex). Delivering the shock during the QRS complex prevents the shock from being delivered during repolarization (T wave), often termed the vulnerable period. If a shock is delivered during this vulnerable period (Figure 10-10), VF may occur. Because the purpose of cardioversion is to disrupt the rhythm rather than completely depolarize the heart, less energy is usually required. Cardioversion can be performed with energy levels as low as 50 J. The amount of energy is gradually increased until the rhythm is converted.

Procedure. The procedure for cardioversion (Box 10-6) is similar to that for defibrillation. However, the defibrillator is set in the "synchronous" mode for the cardioversion. The R waves are sensed by the machine and are noted by "spikes" or other markings on the monitor of the defibrillator (Figure 10-11). It is important to assess that all R waves are properly sensed. When it is time to deliver the shock, the buttons on the paddles must remain depressed until the shock is delivered because energy is discharged only during the QRS complex. When a patient is undergoing cardioversion on a nonemergency basis,

sedation is given before the procedure. Rhythm strips are recorded during cardioversion to document response.

Special Situations

Patients at risk for sudden cardiac death may have an implanted ICD/permanent pacemaker that delivers shocks

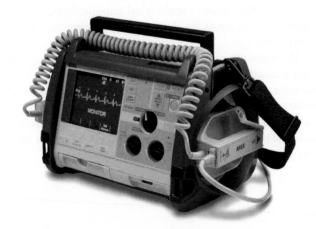

FIGURE 10-11 Monitor/defibrillator demonstrating marked R waves for cardioversion. (Courtesy Zoll Medical, Burlington, Massachusetts.)

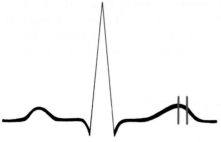

FIGURE 10-10 Approximate location of the vulnerable period. (From Conover MB. *Understanding Electrocardiography.* 8th ed. St. Louis: Mosby; 2003.)

directly to the heart muscle if a life-threatening dysrhythmia is detected. These devices are easily identified because they create a hard lump beneath the skin of the upper chest or abdomen. When a patient with a permanent pacemaker or ICD requires defibrillation, placing the paddle near the generator is avoided. Although damage to the device rarely occurs, the device can absorb much of the current of defibrillation from the adhesive electrode pads or paddles, block the shock delivery, and reduce the chance of success. The adhesive electrode pad or paddle should be placed to either side and not directly on top of the implanted device.[2]

A patient may have an ICD with dual-chamber pacing capabilities. Nurses should become familiar, whenever possible, with the type of therapy the patient's device has been programmed to deliver. By the time VF/VT is recognized on the monitor, the rhythm should also have been recognized by the ICD. If a successful shock by the ICD has not occurred when the rhythm is noted on the monitor, standard code management is initiated. If external defibrillation is unsuccessful, the location of the adhesive electrode pads or paddles on the chest should be changed. Anterior-posterior placement may be more effective than anterior-apex placement. External defibrillation of a patient while the ICD is firing does not harm the patient or the ICD. ICDs and permanent pacemakers are insulated from damage caused by conventional external defibrillation. There is no danger to personnel if the ICD discharges while staff members are touching the patient. However, the shock may be felt and has been compared to the sensation of contact with an electrical outlet. The pacing and sensing thresholds of the pacemaker or ICD are assessed after external defibrillation.

Transcutaneous Cardiac Pacing

Definition. Transcutaneous (external noninvasive) cardiac pacing is used during emergency situations to treat symptomatic bradycardia (hypotension, acutely altered mental status, ischemic chest pain, signs of shock, heart failure) that has not responded to atropine. Transcutaneous pacing is not recommended for asystole. In this method of pacing, the heart is stimulated with externally applied, adhesive electrode pads that deliver the electrical impulse. Impulse conduction occurs across the chest wall to stimulate the cardiac contraction.

The transcutaneous pacemaker may be a freestanding unit with a monitor and a pacemaker. Most models incorporate a monitor, a defibrillator, and an external pacemaker into one system (Figure 10-12). The advantages of transcutaneous pacemakers include easy operation in an emergent situation, minimal training, and none of the risks associated with invasive pacemakers.

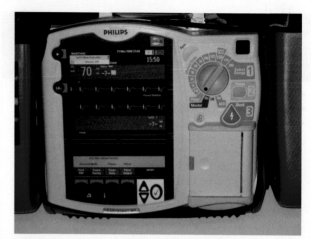

FIGURE 10-12 Transcutaneous pacemaker-defibrillator. (Courtesy Philips Healthcare, Andover, Massachusetts.)

Procedure. The procedure for transcutaneous pacing (Box 10-7) involves the placement of adhesive electrode pads anteriorly and posteriorly on the patient (see Figure 10-8). The electrodes are connected to the external pacemaker allowing for hands-off pacing. The pacemaker is set in either asynchronous or demand modes. Some devices permit only demand pacing. In the asynchronous mode, the pacemaker generates a rhythm without regard to the patient's own rhythm. In the demand mode, the pacemaker fires only if the patient's heart rate falls below a preset limit determined by the operator (e.g., 60 beats per minute). The milliamperes (mA) output is adjusted to stimulate a paced beat, usually 2 mA above the dose at which consistent capture is observed.

The electrical and mechanical effectiveness of pacing is assessed. The electrical activity is noted by a pacemaker "spike" that indicates that the pacemaker is initiating electrical activity. The spike is followed by a broad QRS complex (Figure 10-13). Mechanical activity is noted by palpating a pulse during electrical activity. In addition, the patient has signs of improved cardiac output, including increased blood pressure and improved skin color and skin temperature. If the external pacemaker is effective, the patient may need to have a temporary transvenous pacemaker inserted, depending on the cause of the bradycardia.

The alert patient who requires transcutaneous pacing may experience some discomfort. Because the skeletal muscles are stimulated as well as the heart muscle, the patient may experience a tingling, twitching, or thumping feeling that ranges from mildly uncomfortable to intolerable. Sedation, analgesia, or both may be indicated.

BOX 10-7	PROCEDURE FOR TRANSCUTANEOUS PACEMAKER

- If the patient is alert, explain the procedure.
- Clip excess hair from the patient's chest. Do not shave hair.
- Apply the anterior electrode to the chest. The electrode is centered at the fourth intercostal space to the left of the sternum.
- Apply the posterior electrode on the patient's back to the left of the thoracic spine.
- Connect the electrode cable to the pacemaker generator.
- Turn the unit on. Choose pacing mode (asynchronous or demand).
- Set the pacemaker parameters for heart rate (60 beats per minute) and output (2 mA above the dose at which consistent capture is observed) according to the manufacturer's instructions.
- Adjust the heart rate based on the patient's clinical response.
- Assess the adequacy of pacing:
  - Pacemaker spike and QRS complex (capture)
  - Heart rate and rhythm
  - Blood pressure
  - Level of consciousness
- Observe for patient discomfort. The patient may need sedation and/or analgesia.
- Anticipate follow-up treatment (e.g., insertion of a temporary transvenous pacemaker).

PHARMACOLOGICAL INTERVENTION DURING A CODE

Medications that are administered during a code depend on several factors: the cause of the arrest, the patient's cardiac rhythm, the physician's preference, and the patient's response. The goals of treatment are to reestablish and maintain optimal cardiac function, to correct hypoxemia and acidosis, and to suppress dangerous cardiac ectopic activity. In addition, medications are used to achieve a balance between myocardial oxygen supply and demand, to maintain adequate blood pressure, and to relieve heart failure. Because of the rapid and profound effects these drugs can have on cardiac activity and hemodynamic function, continuous ECG monitoring is essential, and hemodynamic monitoring should be instituted as soon as possible after the code. IV push medications given peripherally are followed by flushing with at least 20 mL of IV fluid to ensure central circulation. In addition, because of the precise dosages and careful administration required with these medications, infusion pumps are used when continuous infusions are given. IV infusion rates are tapered slowly, with frequent monitoring of clinical effectiveness.

The following drugs are included in ACLS guidelines and represent those medications most frequently used in code management.[2] Actions and uses, and dosages for each medication, as well as side effects and nursing implications, are discussed in this section and are summarized in Table 10-4.

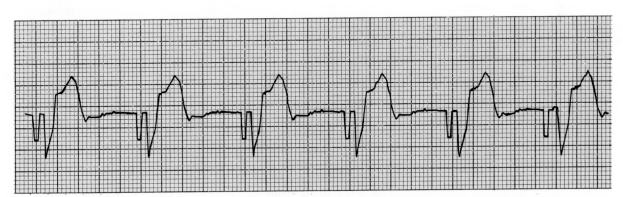

FIGURE 10-13 Electrical capture of transcutaneous pacemaker. Note the pacemaker spikes followed by a wide QRS complex and a tall T wave.

TABLE 10-4   PHARMACOLOGY

Medications Frequently Used in Code Management

MEDICATION	ACTION/USE	DOSE/ROUTE	SIDE EFFECTS	NURSING IMPLICATIONS
Adenosine (Adenocard)	Slows conduction in AV node and interrupts AV nodal reentry circuits *Use:* Initial drug of choice for supraventricular dysrhythmias	6 mg rapid IV bolus over 1-3 seconds, followed by 20 mL rapid NS flush; if no response in 1-2 minutes, give 12 mg repeat dose and flush; may repeat 12 mg dose if necessary	Headache, facial flushing dyspnea, bronchospasm, and chest pain; may cause asystole up to 15 seconds	Half-life 10 seconds; higher dose needed with theophyline, lower dose with dipyridamole or after cardiac transplantation
Amiodarone (Cordarone)	↓Membrane excitability, prolongs action potential to terminate VT or VF *Use:* Treatment and prophylaxis of recurrent VF and hemodynamically unstable VT; rapid atrial dysrhythmias	*Cardiac arrest:* 300 mg IV/IO push followed by dose of 150 mg *Recurrent VF/VT:* 150 mg IV over 10 minutes (15 mg per minute); may repeat 150 mg IV every 10 minutes as needed; followed by 360 mg infusion for 6 hours (1 mg/min) then 540 mg for next 18 hours (0.5 mg/min) for a maximum dose of 2.2 g over 24 hours	Bradycardia, hypotension; use with caution on preexisting conduction system abnormalities	Monitor for symptomatic sinus bradycardia, PR, QRS, and QT prolongation. Central venous catheter infusion site preferred with in-line filter
Atropine	↑SA node automaticity and AV node conduction activity *Use:* Symptomatic bradycardia	*Bradycardia:* 0.5 mg IV every 3-5 minutes to maximum dose of 3 mg 2-3 mg in 10 mL NS or sterile water may be given via ETT	Tachycardia, increased myocardial oxygen consumption and ischemia	Consider transcutaneous pacing, dopamine infusion, or epinephrine infusion if atropine is ineffective
Dopamine (Intropin)	*Moderate doses:* stimulates beta receptors to ↑contractility *High doses:* stimulates alpha receptors *Use:* Hypotension not related to hypovolemia	*Moderate doses* (2-10 mcg/kg/min): ↑Contractility and cardiac output *High doses* (10-20 mcg/kg/min): vasoconstriction and ↑systemic vascular resistance *IV infusion:* 400-800 mg in 250 mL D₅W = 1600-3200 mcg/mL; infuse at 2-5 mcg/kg/min and titrate as needed to maximum 50 mcg/kg/min	Tachycardia, increased dysrhythmias	Extravasation may cause necrosis and sloughing Administer through a central line if possible
Epinephrine (Adrenalin)	↑Contractility, automaticity, systemic vascular resistance, and arterial blood pressure; improves coronary and cerebral perfusion *Use:* VF, pulseless VT, PEA, asystole; consider after atropine as an alternative infusion to dopamine in symptomatic bradycardia	1 mg IV/IO, or 2-2.5 mg in 10 mL sterile water or NS via ETT; may repeat every 3-5 minutes *IV infusion:* 1 mg in 250 mL NS; infuse at 1-10 mcg/min and titrate as needed	Tachycardia, hypertension	In a cardiac arrest may be used as a continuous infusion for hypotension

TABLE 10-4   PHARMACOLOGY
Medications Frequently Used in Code Management—cont'd

MEDICATION	ACTION/USE	DOSE/ROUTE	SIDE EFFECTS	NURSING IMPLICATIONS
Lidocaine (Xylocaine)	Suppresses ventricular dysrhythmias, raises fibrillation threshold. *Use:* Alternative to amiodarone in cardiac arrest from VF and VT	*VF/VT:* 1-1.5 mg/kg IV/IO, followed by 0.5-0.75 mg/kg every 5-10 minutes to maximum of 3 doses of 3 mg/kg; may be given by ETT at dose of 2-4 mg/kg in 10 mL sterile water or NS; follow with continuous IV infusion at 1-4 mg/min. *IV infusion:* 1 g in 250 mL or 2 g in 500 mL = 4 mg/mL	Neurological toxicity if drug level excessive	Lower dose if impaired hepatic blood flow
Magnesium	Essential for enzyme reactions and sodium-potassium pump, ↓ postinfarction dysrhythmias. *Use:* Torsades de pointes, hypomagnesemia	*Cardiac arrest:* 1-2 g in 10 mL of D₅W IV/IO over 5-20 min. *Nonarrest:* 1-2 g in 50-100 mL of D₅W IV, over 5-60 min followed by infusion of 0.5 to 1 g/hr	Flushing, bradycardia, hypotension, respiratory depression	Monitor serum magnesium levels
Norepinephrine (Levophed)	Stimulates alpha receptors to cause arterial and venous vasoconstriction; Stimulates beta receptors to increase contractility. *Use:* Hypotension uncorrected by other medications	Continuous IV infusion at 0.1-0.5 mcg/kg/min (0.5-1 mcg/min), titrated upward as needed to maximum of 30 mcg/min. *IV infusion:* 4 mg in 250 mL D₅W	Myocardial ischemia	Administer through central line, if possible; extravasation may cause necrosis and sloughing
Oxygen	↑ Arterial oxygen content and tissue oxygenation. *Use:* Cardiopulmonary arrest, chest pain, hypoxemia	100% in a code via bag-valve device with mask		Monitor pulse oximetry values
Sodium bicarbonate	Preexisting metabolic acidosis, hyperkalemia or tricyclic antidepressant overdose. Counteracts metabolic acidosis by binding with hydrogen ions to produce water and carbon dioxide	1 mEq/kg IV push initially; subsequent doses based on bicarbonate levels		Ensure adequate CPR, oxygenation, and ventilation
Vasopressin	Nonadrenergic, peripheral vasoconstriction. *Use:* Alternative vasopressor to epinephrine in VF, pulseless VT, asystole or PEA	40 units IV/IO push (one dose only). May be given via ETT; dilute in 10 mL sterile water or NS	Myocardial ischemia	May be useful in place of epinephrine in VF, pulseless VT, asystole or PEA

AV, Atrioventricular; *CPR,* cardiopulmonary resuscitation; *D₅W,* 5% dextrose in water; *ETT,* endotracheal tube; *IO,* intraosseous; *IV,* intravenous; *NS,* normal saline; *PEA,* pulseless electrical activity; *SA,* sinoatrial; *VF,* ventricular fibrillation; *VT,* ventricular tachycardia.
Based on data from Neumar RW, Otto CW, Link MS, Kronick SL, Shuster M, Callaway CW, et al. (2010). Part 8: adult advanced cardiovascular life support: 2010 American Heart Association Guidelines for Cardiopulmonary Resuscitation and Emergency Cardiovascular Care. *Circulation.* 122(18 Suppl 3):S729-S767; American Heart Association. (2011). *Advanced cardiac life support provider manual.* Dallas, TX; Gahart BL. & Nazareno AR. (2011). *2011 Intravenous medications.* St. Louis: Mosby.

Oxygen

Oxygen is essential to resuscitation and has several pharmacological considerations. Oxygen is used to treat hypoxemia, which exists in any arrest situation as a result of lack of adequate gas exchange, inadequate cardiac output, or both. Artificial ventilation without supplemental oxygen does not correct hypoxemia. In addition, the success of other medications and interventions, such as defibrillation, depends on adequate oxygenation and normal acid-base status.

Oxygen can be delivered via bag-mask device, bag-valve device to an ETT, or other airway adjuncts. During an arrest, 100% oxygen is administered.

Epinephrine (Adrenalin)

Epinephrine is a potent vasoconstrictor. Because of its alpha-adrenergic and beta-adrenergic effects (Box 10-8), epinephrine increases systemic vascular resistance and arterial blood pressure, as well as heart rate, contractility, and automaticity of cardiac pacemaker cells. Because of peripheral vasoconstriction, blood is shunted to the heart and brain. Epinephrine also increases myocardial oxygen requirements.

Epinephrine is indicated for the restoration of cardiac electrical activity in an arrest. In addition, epinephrine increases automaticity and the force of contraction, an effect that makes the heart more susceptible to successful defibrillation. Epinephrine is used to treat VF or pulseless VT that is unresponsive to initial defibrillation, asystole, and PEA.

During a code, epinephrine may be given by the IV or IO route or through an ETT. The IV dosage is 1.0 mg (10 mL of a 1:10,000 solution) and is repeated every 3 to 5 minutes as needed. When given through the ETT, 2 to 2.5 mg is diluted in 10 mL of NS or sterile water.

Epinephrine may be administered by continuous infusion to increase the heart rate or blood pressure. Dilution is 1 mg in 250 or 500 mL of D_5W or NS. The infusion is started at 1 mcg/min and is titrated according to the patient's response in a range of 2 to 10 mcg/min. In a situation other than cardiac arrest, because epinephrine increases myocardial oxygen requirements, the nurse must monitor the patient closely for signs of myocardial ischemia.

BOX 10-8	**EFFECTS OF ADRENERGIC RECEPTOR STIMULATION**

Alpha
- Vasoconstriction
- Increased contractility

Beta$_1$
- Increased heart rate
- Increased contractility

Beta$_2$
- Vasodilation
- Relaxation of bronchial, uterine, and gastrointestinal smooth muscle

---

Vasopressin

Vasopressin is recommended as an alternative to epinephrine administration in VF unresponsive to shock.[2] At high doses, vasopressin is a potent vasoconstrictor. A single dose of 40 units IV/IO is recommended. Repeat doses are not necessary because the drug has a 10- to 20-minute half-life. Administration of the drug is not recommended for conscious patients with coronary artery disease because severe angina can result from the vasoconstriction. If necessary, vasopressin may be given via an ETT after it is diluted in 10 mL of NS or sterile water.

Atropine

Atropine is used to increase the heart rate by decreasing the vagal tone. It is indicated for patients with symptomatic bradycardia. Routine use of atropine during PEA or asystole is no longer recommended because it is unlikely to be of benefit.[3] For symptomatic bradycardia, atropine 0.5 mg IV is given and repeated every 3 to 5 minutes as needed (for a total of 3 mg) to maintain a heart rate greater than 60 beats per minute or until adequate tissue perfusion is achieved as indicated by blood pressure and level of consciousness. If atropine is ineffective in maintaining the heart rate and adequate tissue perfusion, consider transcutaneous pacing, dopamine infusion (2 to 10 mcg/kg/min) or an epinephrine infusion (2 to 10 mcg/min). If necessary, atropine may be given via an ETT. The dose for ETT administration is 2 to 3 mg diluted in 10 mL of NS or sterile water. Atropine is used cautiously in acute coronary ischemia or myocardial infarction because the increased heart rate may worsen ischemia or increase infarction size.[2]

Amiodarone (Cordarone)

Amiodarone is a unique antidysrhythmic possessing some characteristics of all groups of antidysrhythmic drugs. It reduces membrane excitability, and by prolonging the action potential and retarding the refractory period, it facilitates the termination of VT and VF. It also has alpha-adrenergic and beta-adrenergic blocking properties. Many antidysrhythmic agents, despite their effectiveness in suppression of dysrhythmias, also have a propensity to exacerbate dysrhythmias. This property is known as *proarrhythmia* or *prodysrhythmia*. Administration of amiodarone is rarely associated with prodysrhythmias. It is less likely to produce hypotension and myocardial depression than is procainamide. Amiodarone has the added benefit of dilating coronary arteries and increasing coronary blood supply. Amiodarone also decreases systemic vascular resistance, and in patients with impaired left ventricular function it can improve cardiac pump function.

IV amiodarone is indicated for treatment and prophylaxis of recurring VF and unstable VT refractory to other treatment. In cardiac arrest, it is administered when VF and pulseless VT is not responsive to CPR, defibrillation and vasopressors. It is also given in supraventricular tachycardia for rate control or conversion of atrial fibrillation or flutter, especially in patients with heart failure. During cardiac arrest it is administered as a 300 mg IV/IO loading bolus. If VF/pulseless VT persists, a second loading dose of 150 mg IV/IO may be given in 3 to 5 minutes. For recurrent VF/pulseless VT, a bolus dose of 150 mg IV may be administered over 10 minutes (15 mg per minute) that may be repeated every 10 minutes as needed. This may be followed by an infusion of 360 mg over the next 6 hours (1 mg/min), and then a maintenance infusion of 540 mg over the next 18 hours (0.5 mg/min) for a maximum cumulative dose of 2.2 gm over 24 hours. Adverse reactions include hypotension and bradycardia, which can be prevented by slowing the infusion rate or treating the patient with fluids, vasopressors, chronotropic medications, or temporary pacing.

Lidocaine (Xylocaine)

Lidocaine is an antidysrhythmic drug that suppresses ventricular ectopic activity. It depresses the ventricular conduction system and reduces automaticity. Lidocaine is used when amiodarone is not available in cardiac arrest from VT and VF. It is also used in the suppression of ventricular ectopy (premature ventricular contractions).

During a code, a bolus dose of 1 to 1.5 mg/kg of lidocaine is administered by IV/IO push. Additional boluses of 0.5 to 0.75 mg/kg may be administered every 5 to 10 minutes, as needed, until a maximum of 3 doses or a total of 3 mg/kg has been given. If IV or IO access is not available, 2 to 4 mg/kg of lidocaine diluted in 10 mL of NS or sterile water may be given through the ETT.

If lidocaine is successful in treating the cardiac dysrhythmia, a continuous infusion should be started at 1 to 4 mg/min. Dilution is 1 g mixed in 250 mL of D_5W, or 2 g can be mixed in 500 mL. Both solutions deliver 4 mg/mL, the standard dilution.

Dosages of lidocaine should be decreased in patients with impaired hepatic blood flow (as occurs in heart failure, left ventricular dysfunction), and in elderly patients. Blood levels are monitored, and the patient is assessed for central nervous system disturbances that may indicate lidocaine toxicity. Common side effects of lidocaine include lethargy, confusion, tinnitus, muscle twitching, seizures, bradycardia, and paresthesias.

Adenosine (Adenocard)

Adenosine is the initial drug of choice for the diagnosis and treatment of supraventricular dysrhythmias. Adenosine slows conduction through the AV node and interrupts AV node reentrant electrical conduction, which is the cause of most supraventricular dysrhythmias. It is effective in restoring normal sinus rhythm in patients with paroxysmal supraventricular tachycardia, including that caused by Wolff-Parkinson-White syndrome. Adenosine does not convert supraventricular rhythms that do not involve the sinoatrial or AV node, such as atrial fibrillation, atrial flutter, atrial tachycardia, and VT. However, adenosine may produce a brief AV node block, thereby assisting with the diagnosis of these rhythms.

Adenosine has an onset of action of 10 to 40 seconds and duration of 1 to 2 minutes; therefore, it is administered rapidly. The initial dose is a 6 mg IV push over 1 to 3 seconds, followed by a 20-mL rapid saline flush. A period of asystole lasting as long as 15 seconds may occur after adenosine administration from suppression of AV node conduction. A second and third dose of 12 mg may be given 1 to 2 minutes later if the first dose is ineffective in converting the rhythm. Common side effects include transient facial flushing (from mild dilation of blood vessels in the skin), dyspnea, coughing (from mild bronchoconstriction), and chest pain.

Magnesium

Magnesium is essential for many enzyme reactions and for the function of the sodium-potassium pump. It also acts as a calcium channel blocker and slows neuromuscular transmission. Hypomagnesemia is associated with a high frequency of cardiac dysrhythmias, including refractory VF. Magnesium administered IV may terminate or prevent recurrent torsades de pointes in patients who have a prolonged QT interval. Torsades de pointes is a form of VT characterized by QRS complexes that change amplitude and appearance (polymorphic) and appear to twist around the isoelectric line (Figure 10-14). The QRS complexes may deflect downward for a few beats and then upward for a

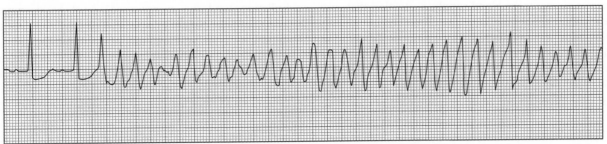

FIGURE 10-14 Torsades de pointes. The QRS complex seems to spiral around the isoelectric line. (From Urden LD, Stacy KM, Lough ME. *Critical Care Nursing: Diagnosis and Management.* 6th ed. St. Louis: Mosby; 2010.)

few beats. When VF/pulseless VT cardiac arrest is associated with torsades de pointes, 1 to 2 g of magnesium sulfate diluted in 10 mL of D_5W is given IV/IO over 5 to 20 minutes. In nonarrest situations, a loading dose of 1 to 2 g mixed in 50 to 100 mL of D_5W is given over 5 to 60 minutes. Slower rates are recommended in a stable patient. The side effects of rapid magnesium administration include hypotension, bradycardia, flushing, and respiratory depression. Serum magnesium levels are monitored to avoid hypermagnesemia.

Sodium Bicarbonate

A patient who has experienced an arrest quickly becomes acidotic. The acidosis results from two sources: (1) no blood flow during the arrest, and (2) low blood flow during CPR. Effective ventilation with supplemental oxygen and rapid restoration of tissue perfusion by CPR and spontaneous circulation are the best mechanisms to correct these causes of acidosis.

Limited data support the administration of sodium bicarbonate during cardiac arrest.[17] Sodium bicarbonate buffers the increased numbers of hydrogen ions present in metabolic acidosis. It is beneficial in treating preexisting metabolic acidosis, hyperkalemia, or tricyclic antidepressant overdose.

The initial dosage of sodium bicarbonate is 1 mEq/kg by IV push. When possible, bicarbonate therapy should be guided by the bicarbonate concentration or calculated base deficit from arterial blood gas analysis or laboratory measurement. Sodium bicarbonate should not be mixed or infused with any other medication because it may precipitate or cause deactivation of other medications.

Dopamine (Intropin)

The indication for dopamine is symptomatic hypotension in the absence of hypovolemia. It is the second-line medication for symptomatic bradycardia (after atropine). Its effects are dose related. At rates of 2 to 10 mcg/kg/min, myocardial contractility increases from alpha- and beta-adrenergic stimulation, causing enhanced cardiac contractility, increased cardiac output, increased heart rate, and increased blood pressure. At rates greater than 10 mcg/kg/min, systemic vascular resistance markedly increases as a result of generalized vasoconstriction produced from alpha-adrenergic stimulation. At doses greater than 20 mcg/kg/min, marked vasoconstriction occurs. Myocardial workload is increased without an increase in coronary blood supply, a situation that may cause myocardial ischemia.

Dopamine is administered by continuous IV infusion starting at 2 to 5 mcg/kg/min, and the dose is titrated upward to patient response. A dilution of 400 to 800 mg of dopamine in 250 to 500 mL of D_5W delivers 1600 to 3200 mcg/mL. The lowest dose necessary for blood pressure control should be used to minimize side effects and to ensure adequate perfusion of vital organs.

In addition to causing myocardial ischemia, dopamine may also cause cardiac dysrhythmias, such as tachycardia and premature ventricular contractions. Necrosis and sloughing

---

GERIATRIC CONSIDERATIONS

- Many elderly patients in the hospital would not want their stated resuscitation preferences followed if they were to lose their decision-making capacity. They would prefer that their family and physician make resuscitation decisions for them.[22]
- Elderly patients have an increased incidence of complications from chest compressions, including rib fractures, sternal fractures, pneumothorax, and hemothorax.
- Declines in hepatic and renal functioning occur in the elderly that may result in higher-than-desired serum drug concentrations and adverse drug reactions with standard therapeutic dosing regimens.
- Beta-adrenergic receptors on the myocardium in the elderly are less responsive to changes in heart rate and cardiac contractility. Heart rate responses to beta-blocker (propranolol, metoprolol) and parasympathetic (atropine) medications are less.
- A decline in heart rate and slowing of conduction through the atrioventricular node result in a narrow therapeutic range for cardiovascular medications.
- Cardiopulmonary resuscitation is less likely to be effective in patients older than 70 years with comorbidities, unwitnessed arrest, terminal arrhythmias (asystole, pulseless electrical activity), cardiopulmonary resuscitation duration greater than 15 minutes, metastatic cancer, sepsis, pneumonia, renal failure, trauma, and acute and sustained hypotension.[23]

---

of tissue may occur if the drug infiltrates; therefore, it should be infused into a central line if possible. Phentolamine, 5 to 10 mg in 10 to 15 mL of NS, can be injected into the infiltrated area to prevent necrosis.

DOCUMENTATION OF CODE EVENTS

A detailed chronological record of all interventions must be maintained during a code.[12] One of the first actions of the nurse team leader or nursing supervisor is to ensure that someone is assigned to record information throughout the code. Documentation includes the time the code is called, the time CPR is started, any actions that are taken, and the patient's response (e.g., presence or absence of a pulse, heart rate, blood pressure, cardiac rhythm). Intubation and defibrillation (and the energy used) must be documented, along with the patient's response. The time and sites of IV initiations, types and amounts of fluids administered, and medications given to the patient are all accurately recorded. Rhythm strips are recorded to document events and response to treatment. Many hospitals have standardized code records (Figure 10-15) that list actions and medications, and include spaces for the time of interventions and any comments. It is best if information can be recorded directly on the code record during the code to ensure that all information is obtained. The code record is signed by the code team and becomes part of the patient's permanent record.

Cleveland Clinic
EMERGENCY RESPONSE FORM
Page 1 of 2

For scanning accuracy, affix patient label within this outlined box.
Patient Name: ______
Clinic Number: ______

DATE: ____/____/____
LOCATION OF EVENT ______
WITNESSED EVENT ☐ NO ☐ YES
CHECK IF PRESENT AT ONSET OXYGEN DEVICE (L/minute or FiO2:) ______
☐ ETT ☐ VENT ☐ IV ACCESS
MONITOR: ☐ ECG ☐ RR ☐ pOx
CONSCIOUS AT ONSET: ☐ YES ☐ NO
PULSE AT ONSET: ☐ YES ☐ NO
RESPIRATION AT ONSET: ☐ YES ☐ NO
RHYTHM AT ONSET: ☐ NSR ☐ A FIB ☐ BRADY ☐ ASYS ☐ PEA
☐ VFIB ☐ VTACH ☐ SVT ☐ PACED ☐ OTHER ______

CCF102713

PRECIPITATING EVENTS: ______

WEIGHT: ______

Cleveland Clinic
EMERGENCY RESPONSE FORM
Page 2 of 2

For scanning accuracy, affix patient label within this outlined box.
Patient Name: ______
Clinic Number: ______

DATE: ____/____/____
MEDICATIONS ADMINISTERED FOR INTUBATION:
☐ Etomidate ___mg ☐ Succinylcholine ___mg ☐ Rocuronium ___mg
☐ Vecuronium ___mg ☐ Mikazolam ___mg ☐ Other: ______
PATIENT INTUBATED AT: ______
SIZE OF ETT: ______
LOCATION: ___ CM @ LIPLINE
CONFIRMATION: ☐ $^{+}ETCO_2$ ☐ OTHER:
(√) CHECK AT LEAST ONE ADDITIONAL
☐ DIRECT VISUALIZATION ☐ BIL. BREATH SOUNDS ☐ ABSENCE OF GASTRIC INFLATION
IMPEDENCE THRESHOLD DEVICE: ☐ YES ☐ NO
ANESTHESIA: ______ PRINT NAME

OUTCOME:
PATIENT EXPIRED AT: ______
PATIENT TRANSFERRED AT: ______
PATIENT TRANSFERRED TO: ______
PATIENT REMAINED AT: ______
FAMILY NOTIFIED AT: ______

DNR ☐ YES ☐ NO	TIME	RHYTHM	HEART RATE	DEFIB/CARDIO-JOULES ☐ AED ☐ BI ☐ MONO	CHEST COMPRESSIONS (√)	PULSE c̄ COMPRESSIONS (√)	B.P. ☐ ART ☐ NIBP ☐ MANUAL	O_2 SATURATION	RESPIRATORY RATE	BVM (√)	CONFIRMATION OF AIRWAY (√)	INTRAVENOUS PUSH INJECTIONS: AMIODARONE	ATROPINE	Ca CHLORIDE	EPINEPHRINE	LIDOCAINE	MAGNESIUM SULFATE	PHENYLEPHRINE	SODIUM BICARBONATE	VASOPRESSIN			I.V. FLUIDS	CONTINUOUS I.V. INFUSIONS: AMIODARONE	DOPAMINE	EPINEPHRINE	NOREPINEPHRINE			SIGNIFICANT EVENTS (example: ABG results, CT insertion, code status change, other medications, etc.)
				within 3 minutes of VT/VF: shocks at least 2 minutes apart	begin less than 1 minute if no pulse						Confirmation every 10 minutes				within 5 minutes of pulseless rhythm					40 units may use once - 1st or 2nd dose of epi				Adult 450mg/250ml D5W	Adult 800mg/250ml D5W	Adult 4mg/250ml D5W	Adult 4mg or 16mg/250ml D5W			

Medication Nurse (Preparation): ______ SIGNATURE   DRUG BOX #: ______
Medication Nurse (Administration): ______ SIGNATURE   CRASH CART #: ______
Recording Nurse: ______ SIGNATURE   Respiratory Therapist: ______ SIGNATURE
1027 13 REV. 2/11   WHITE - CHART COPY

L.I.P. IN CHARGE OF RESUSCITATION: ______ (SIGNATURE VERIFIES SHEET REVIEWED AND AGREEMENT) PRINT NAME ______ SIGNATURE
STAFF MD/FELLOW PRESENT AT RESUSCITATION ______ SIGNATURE
Post Resuscitation Care: ☐ Vital Signs ☐ Echo ☐ Labs ☐ Chest X ray ☐ 12 ECG ☐ ABG
YELLOW - Mail to HS2-03   1027 13 REV. 2/11

FIGURE 10-15 Sample of a code record used for documenting activities during a code. (Courtesy Cleveland Clinic, Cleveland, Ohio.)

CARE OF THE PATIENT AFTER RESUSCITATION

Systematic post–cardiac arrest care after return of spontaneous circulation (ROSC) can improve patient survival with good quality of life.[2,5,19] Postresuscitation goals include optimizing cardiopulmonary function and tissue perfusion, transporting the patient to an appropriate critical car unit capable of providing post–cardiac arrest care, and identifying and treating the precipitating causes of the arrest to help prevent another arrest. This is achieved by advanced airway placement, maintenance of blood pressure and oxygenation, control of dysrhythmias, advanced neurological monitoring, and the use of therapeutic hypothermia.

After ROSC an adequate airway and support of breathing must be initiated. The unconscious patient will require an advanced airway or endotracheal intubation. When securing the endotracheal tube, ties that pass circumferentially around the patient's neck are avoided because venous return to the brain could become obstructed. The head of the bed should be elevated 30 degrees if tolerated to reduce the incidence of cerebral edema, aspiration, and ventilatory associated pneumonia.

Waveform capnography is recommended to confirm and continuously monitor the position of the ETT, especially during patient transport.[19] Waveform capnography measures the partial pressure of CO_2 at the end of expiration ($ETCO_2$). It can be continuously measured as a numeric value with a graphic display of the exhaled waveform over time (Figure 10-16). A heated sensor is placed in the airway circuit between the ETT and the ventilator tubing. The exhaled gas flows directly over the sensor, providing a measurement of $ETCO_2$. When the ETT is correctly placed, a normal waveform is seen with $ETCO_2$ rising on expiration, sustaining a plateau, and returning to baseline on inspiration (see Figure 10-16). A sudden loss of $ETCO_2$ with a waveform at baseline indicates incorrect ETT placement or cardiac arrest. The patient's airway should be assessed immediately. The normal range of $ETCO_2$ is 35 to 45 mm Hg. Waveform capnography should be used in addition to breath sound auscultation and direct visualization of the larynx. If not available, an end-tidal carbon dioxide detector placed on the ETT (see Figure 10-5) or esophageal detector device may be used.

Although 100% oxygen may have been used during the initial resuscitation, the lowest inspired oxygen concentration to maintain SpO_2 94% (via pulse oximetry) and PaO_2 at approximately 100 mm Hg (via arterial blood gas) should be used. Excessive ventilation (too fast or too much) is avoided because it may increase intrathoracic pressure and decrease cardiac output. The decrease in $PaCO_2$ seen with hyperventilation can also decrease cerebral blood flow. Manual ventilations with a bag-valve device are performed at 10 to 12 breaths per minute and titrated to achieve a $ETCO_2$ of 35 to 45 mm Hg or a $PaCO_2$ of 40 to 45 mm Hg.

The major determinant of CO_2 delivery to the lungs is cardiac output. If ventilation is relatively constant, $ETCO_2$ will correlate with cardiac output during CPR. Therefore waveform capnography could be used to evaluate the effectiveness of CPR compressions.[29] A chest x-ray is performed soon after arrival in the critical care unit to verify ETT placement.

Continuous ECG monitoring continues after ROSC, during transport to the critical care unit, and throughout critical care unit care stay until no longer deemed necessary. IV access is obtained if not already established and position and function of any IV catheter is verified. An IO catheter emergently placed during the code should be replaced by IV access. If the patient is hypotensive (systolic blood pressure less than 90 mm Hg) fluid boluses of 1 to 2 liters normal saline or lactated Ringer solution are considered. Cold fluid may be used if therapeutic hypothermia will be initiated. Vasoactive medications including dopamine (5 to 10 mcg/kg/min), norepinephrine (0.1 to 0.5 mcg/kg/min) or epinephrine (1 to 10 mcg/min) may be initiated

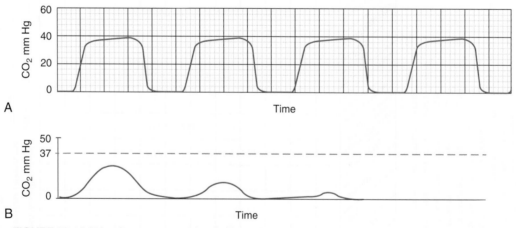

FIGURE 10-16 Waveform capnography. **A,** Normal waveform indicating adequate ventilation pattern ($ETCO_2$ 35 to 40 mm Hg). **B,** Abnormal waveform indicating airway obstruction or obstruction in breathing circuit ($ETCO_2$ decreasing).

and titrated to achieve a systolic blood pressure of 90 mm Hg or a mean arterial blood pressure of 65 mm Hg. Metabolic acidosis may be seen after cardiac arrest and is often corrected as adequate perfusion is restored. Blood pressure and heart rate are recorded at least every 30 minutes during continuous infusions of vasoactive medications. If antidysrhythmic medications were used successfully during the code, additional doses may be repeated to achieve adequate blood levels, or continuous infusions may be administered. Other medications may be given to improve cardiac output and myocardial oxygen supply.

One of the most common causes of cardiac arrest is cardiovascular disease and coronary ischemia.[2] Therefore a 12-lead ECG should be obtained as soon as possible to determine the presence of ST elevation or new bundle branch block. If there is a high suspicion of acute myocardial infarction (AMI), protocols for treatment and coronary reperfusion are implemented. An arterial line and pulmonary artery catheter are frequently inserted after a code to facilitate hemodynamic assessment and patient treatment. An indwelling urinary catheter is inserted to monitor urinary output hourly. A nasogastric tube is inserted if bowel sounds are absent and in patients with a decreased level of consciousness who are mechanically ventilated.

Neurological prognosis is difficult to determine during the first 72 hours post–cardiac arrest. This time frame is usually extended in patients who are being cooled.[6] Therefore serial neurological exams are performed, including response to verbal commands or physical stimulation, pupillary response to light, presence of corneal reflex, spontaneous eye movement, gag, cough, and spontaneous breaths. Patients with post–cardiac arrest cognitive dysfunction may display agitation. In addition, the presence of an ETT may result in pain, discomfort, and anxiety. Intermittent or continuous IV sedation, analgesia, or both can be used to achieve specific goals (see Chapter 5). Seizure activity is common following cardiac arrest. Serial head computed tomography (CT) scans and electroencephalography (EEG) monitoring may be performed if the patient is comatose and/or has seizures. Management of patient care continues to focus on the differential diagnosis to identify reversible causes of the arrest and the underlying pathophysiology including electrolyte abnormalities. Hyperglycemia may occur post–cardiac arrest. The optimum blood glucose concentration and strategies are not known for patients post–cardiac arrest.[19] However, a target range of 144 to 180 mg/dL has been shown to decrease the risk of hyperglycemia after cardiac arrest.[19] See the box, "Laboratory Alert," which summarizes critical electrolyte values.

Emotional support is an important aspect of care after an arrest. Fear of death or of a recurrence of the arrest is common. Survivors often feel the need to discuss their experience in depth, and nurses should listen objectively and provide psychological support. In addition to the patient, many other people are affected when a code occurs. Family members, roommates and other patients, and staff members are all affected by the emergency.

Research supports the benefits of family presence during a code. Families who have been present during a code describe the benefits as knowing that everything possible was being done for their loved one, feeling supportive and helpful to the patient and staff, sustaining patient-family relationships, providing a

---

! LABORATORY ALERT

Electrolyte Values

LABORATORY TEST	CRITICAL VALUE	SIGNIFICANCE
Sodium (Na)	<136 or >145 mEq/L	Implications for polarization of heart muscle via K^+/Na^+ pump
Potassium (K)	<3.5 or >5.3 mEq/L	Affects cardiac conduction and contraction Maintains cardiac cell homeostasis ECG: *Hypokalemia:* depressed ST segments, flat or inverted T wave, presence of U wave *Hyperkalemia:* tall, peaked T waves, disappearance of P waves, widening of QRS; can progress to asystole
Calcium (Ca)	<8.8 or >10.2 mg/dL	Affects cardiac cell action potential and contraction ECG: *Hypocalcemia:* prolonged QT interval *Hypercalcemia:* shortened QT interval
Magnesium (Mg)	<1.3 or >2.5 mEq/L	Affects contraction of cardiac muscle and promotes vasodilation that may reduce preload, alter cardiac output, and reduce systemic blood pressure ECG: *Hypomagnesemia:* flat or inverted T waves, ST segment depression, prolonged QT interval *Hypermagnesemia:* peaked T waves, bradycardia, signs of depressed contractility

ECG, Electrocardiogram.

sense of closure on a life shared together, and facilitating the grief process.[9,17] Family members should be given the option of being present at the bedside (see Chapter 2).[1]

Therapeutic Hypothermia After Cardiac Arrest

Studies have indicated that fever resulting from brain injury or ischemia exacerbates the degree of permanent neurological damage after cardiac arrest and contributes to an increased length of stay. The higher the body temperature is after a cardiac arrest, the poorer is the neurological recovery. Lower body temperature after cardiac arrest is associated with better neurological recovery (see box, "Evidence-Based Practice, Therapeutic Hypothermia").[28] Induced hypothermia to a core body temperature of 32° C to 34° C for 12 to 24 hours may be beneficial in reducing neurological impairment after out-of-hospital VF arrest when initiated within minutes of ROSC.[5,24] In addition, these patients are more likely to survive to hospital discharge.[4] Hypothermia decreases the metabolic rate by 6% to 7% for every decrease of 1° C in temperature. Because cerebral metabolic rate for oxygen is the main determinant of cerebral blood flow, inducing hypothermia may improve oxygen supply and reduce oxygen consumption in the ischemic brain. The AHA recommends that comatose adult patients (who lack meaningful response to verbal commands) with ROSC after out-of-hospital VF cardiac arrest be cooled to 32° C to 34° C for 12 to 24 hours.[17] Induced hypothermia should be considered for comatose adult patients with ROSC after in-hospital cardiac arrest of any initial rhythm, or after out-of-hospital cardiac arrest with an initial rhythm of PEA or asystole.[17]

Although data support cooling to 32° C to 34° C, the optimal temperature has not been determined. In addition, the optimal method, time of onset and duration, and rewarming rate are not known. Multiple methods for inducing hypothermia include ice packs, cooling blankets, specialized cooling pads that adhere to the skin, ice-cold isotonic IV fluids, or an endovascular device using a central catheter and an external heat exchange system. Several commercially available cooling systems are available to initiate and maintain therapeutic hypothermia. In one system, iced solution is circulated through specialized external pads that adhere to the skin (Figure 10-17). Another system uses an endovascular catheter that circulates iced solution through a closed system of balloons (Figure 10-18). Both systems have closed feedback allowing continuous adjustment in the temperature of the iced solution to maintain a core preset temperature. Ice-cold isotonic IV fluid (30 mL/kg of saline 0.9% or Ringer lactate solution) can be infused to initiate cooling, but it must be combined with another method to maintain hypothermia.[17] Hypothermia should be initiated as soon as possible after resuscitation, however, the optimal duration of hypothermia has not been defined. The patient's core body temperature should be continuously monitored using an esophageal thermometer, bladder catheter with a temperature probe, or pulmonary artery catheter if one is placed. Axillary, oral, and tympanic temperature probes do not measure core body temperature changes and should not be used during therapeutic hypothermia. A secondary source of temperature measurement should be considered

---

EVIDENCE-BASED PRACTICE

Therapeutic Hypothermia after Resuscitation from Nonshockable Initial Rhythms

Problem
Therapeutic hypothermia has been increasingly used in clinical practice to improve outcomes after cardiac arrest.

Question
Does induced hypothermia benefit adult patients who present with nonshockable initial rhythms?

Evidence
Kim and colleagues reviewed the results of two randomized and 12 nonrandomized studies. Therapeutic hypothermia in management of patients with nonshockable rhythms was associated with reduced mortality, but little effect on neurological outcomes. The authors note that most studies had a high risk for bias and that the overall quality of evidence for review was low. They emphasize that randomized clinical trials are needed to assess the outcomes of therapeutic hypothermia in this patient population.

Implications for Nursing
Patients presenting with nonshockable initial rhythms have a high mortality rate and risk of negative neurological outcomes. Most hospitals have identified protocols for implementation of therapeutic hypothermia after cardiac arrest and do not consider if the

arrest was secondary to a shockable rhythm associated with better outcomes versus a nonshockable rhythm, such as asystole, which is associated with poor outcomes. It is important for nurses to implement therapeutic hypothermia protocols for survivors of cardiac arrest who meet eligibility criteria. Until further trials indicate which patients benefit most from this therapy, nurses must be knowledgeable of the preferred methods for cooling in their institution, cool the patient to the desired level of hypothermia, provide medications to support patient comfort during hypothermia, monitor for potential complications of hypothermia, and rewarm the patient gradually according to established protocols. Skills in neurological assessment before, during, and after the procedure are also essential.

Level of Evidence
C—Meta-analysis of studies with low quality of evidence

References
Kim YM, Yim HW, Jeong SH, Klem ML, & Callaway CW. Does therapeutic hypothermia benefit adult cardiac arrest patients presenting with non-shockable initial rhythms? A systematic review and meta-analysis of randomized and non-randomized studies. *Resuscitation.* 2011;83(12)188-196.

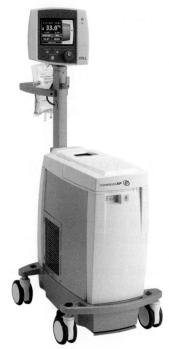

FIGURE 10-18 Thermagard XP. (Courtesy Zoll, Chelmsford, Massachusetts.)

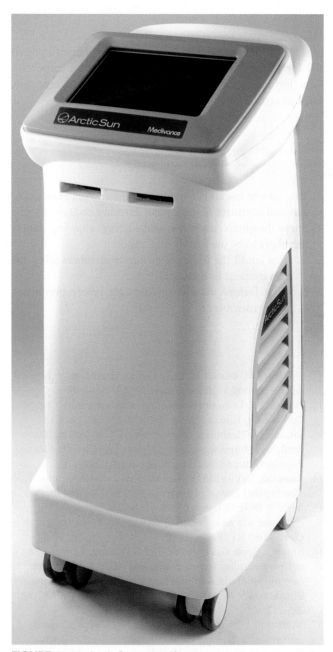

FIGURE 10-17 Arctic Sun 5000. (Courtesy Medivance, Louisville, Colorado.)

especially if a closed feedback cooling system is used for temperature management.

Shivering is anticipated during cooling and rewarming as part of the normal physiological process to a change in body temperature. Shivering increases oxygen consumption especially during the induction of hypothermia where it actually generates heat, making it more difficult to cool. Shivering is controlled with IV sedatives, analgesics, and neuromuscular blockade medications, however, these medications can also mask seizure activity. Therefore continuous EEG monitoring is recommended to identify any seizure activity that occurs during therapeutic hypothermia.[21]

There are potential complications associated with hypothermia including bleeding, infection, and metabolic and electrolyte disturbances.[18] Coagulopathy occurs with hypothermia, and any bleeding should be controlled before inducing hypothermia. Bleeding may be seen following invasive procedures (coronary angiography with antiplatelet therapy or anticoagulation, intraaortic balloon pump placement) but is not associated with increased mortality.[18] Hypothermia suppresses ischemia-induced inflammatory reactions that occur after cardiac arrest, resulting in an increased risk of infection. Pneumonia is common in unconscious patients and may not be related to hypothermia. Bloodstream infections have occurred more frequently with the use of endovascular catheters as compared to noninvasive cooling methods, but these infections have not been associated with increased mortality.[20] Nurses must insure infection prevention strategies are followed, including correct central line maintenance, VAP prevention, and good hand-washing technique.

Hyperglycemia occurs with hypothermia because of increased stress and the release of endogenous and exogenous catecholamines. Hyperglycemia should be managed with an IV insulin infusion to achieve appropriate glycemic control. During cooling, potassium, magnesium, phosphate, and calcium levels may decrease and are corrected as needed. During the rewarming process these electrolyte levels may rise. Some hypothermia protocols require that potassium replacement stop 8 hours before initiating slow, controlled rewarming to prevent increased potassium levels.

After 24 hours of cooling, rewarming proceeds slowly (0.25° C to 0.5° C per hour) to prevent sudden vasodilation, hypotension, and shock.[13]

SUMMARY

Positive patient outcomes depend on the healthcare team members' ability to recognize problems rapidly and to intervene effectively. When a patient has a cardiac or respiratory arrest, or both, in the hospital, BLS and ACLS measures must be initiated immediately. How the code team functions and how interventions are carried out affect the patient's potential for recovery. Thus code management is an important topic for anyone involved in the care of patients, especially those in critical care areas.

CRITICAL THINKING EXERCISES

1. A surgical patient on a general nursing unit has just been successfully defibrillated with the use of an AED by the nursing staff. He is being manually ventilated with a bag-mask device. Identify the current nursing priorities and their rationales.
2. You are the second nurse to respond to a code. The first nurse is administering CPR. Describe your first actions and their rationales.
3. Your patient has an ICD/permanent pacemaker. How would care and treatment of this patient differ in a code situation?
4. Some hospitals are now considering allowing family members to be present during a code.
   a. How could the presence of family members affect the management of the code?
   b. What factors should you consider before permitting family members to be present?

REFERENCES

1. AACN. AACN practice alert: Family presence during resuscitation and invasive procedures. Available at http://www.aacn.org/WD/Practice/Docs/PracticeAlerts/Family%20Presence%2004-2010%20final.pdf; 2010. Accessed September 4, 2011.
2. American Heart Association. *Advanced Cardiac Life Support Provider Manual*. Dallas, TX: Author; 2011.
3. American Heart Association. *BLS for Healthcare Providers*. Dallas, TX: Author; 2011.
4. Arrich J, Holzer M, Herkner H. Cochrane corner: hypothermia for neuroprotection in adults after cardiopulmonary resuscitation. *Anesthesia Analgesia*. 2010;110(4):1339.
5. Bernard SA, Gray TW, Buist MD, et al. Treatment of comatose survivors of out-of-hospital cardiac arrest with induced hypothermia. *New England Journal of Medicine*. 2002;346(8):557-563.
6. Booth CM, Boone PH, Tomlinson G. Is this patient dead, vegetative, or severely neurologically impaired? Assessing outcome for comatose survivors of cardiac arrest. *Journal of the American Medical Association*. 2004;291(7):870-879.
7. Chan PS, Jain R, Nallmothu BK. Rapid response teams: a systematic review and meta-analysis. *Archives of Internal Medicine*. 2010;170(1):18-26.
8. DeVita MA, Bellomo R, Hillman K, et al. Findings of the first consensus conference on medical emergency teams. *Critical Care Medicine*. 2006;34(12):2463-2478.
9. Egging D, Crowley M, Arruda T, et al. Emergency Nurses Resources. Family presence during invasive procedures and resuscitation in the emergency department. *Journal of Emergency Nursing*. 2011;37(5):469-473.
10. Geocadin RG, Koenig MA, Stevens RD, et al. Intensive care for brain injury after cardiac arrest: Theraputic hypothermia and related neuroprotective strategies. *Critical Care Clinics*. 2007;22:619-636.
11. Hillman KM, Bristow PJ, Chey T, et al. Antecedents to hospital deaths. *Internal Medicine Journal*. 2001;31:343-348.
12. Howard PK. Documentation of resuscitation events. *Critical Care Nursing Clinics of North America*. 2005;17(1):39-43.
13. Institute for Healthcare Improvement. *Rapid Response Teams*. Available at http://www.ihi.org/explore/RapidResponseTeams/Pages/default.aspx; Accessed September 4, 2011.
14. Jones DA, DeVita MA, Bellomo R. Rapid response teams. *New England Journal of Medicine*. 2011;365(2):139-146.
15. Jones D, Duke G, Green J, et al. Medical emergency team syndrome and an approach to their management. *Critical Care*. 2006;10(1):R30.
16. Krause J, Smith G, Prytherch D, et al. A comparison of antecedents to cardiac arrests, deaths, and emergency intensive care admissions in Australia, New Zealand, and the United Kingdom. The ACA-DEMIA study. *Resuscitation*. 2004;62(3):275-282.
17. Neumar RW, Otto CW, Link MS, et al. Part 8: adult advanced cardiovascular life support: 2010. American Heart Association Guidelines for Cardiopulmonary Resuscitation and Emergency Cardiovascular Care. *Circulation*. 2010;22(18 suppl 3):S729-S767.
18. Nielsen N, Sunde K, Hovdenes J, et al. Adverse events and their relation to mortality in out-of-hospital cardiac arrest patients treated with therapeutic hypothermia. *Critical Care Medicine*. 2011;39(1):57-64.
19. Peberdy MA, Callaway CW, Neuman RW, et al. Part 9: post-cardiac arrest care: 2010. American Heart Association Guidelines for Cardiopulmonary Resuscitation and Emergency Cardiovascular Care. *Circulation*. 2010;122(18 suppl 3):S768-S786.
20. Pichon N, Amiel JB, Francois B, et al. Efficacy of and tolerance to mild induced hypothermia after out-of-hospital cardiac arrest using an endovascular cooling system. *Critical Care*. 2007;11(3):R71.

21. Polderman KH, Ingelbord H. Therapeutic hypothermia and controlled nomothermia in the intensive care unit: practical considerations, side effects, and cooling methods. *Critical Care Medicine.* 2009;37(3):1101-1120.

22. Puchalski CM, Zhong Z, Jacobs MM, et al. Patients who want their family and physician to make resuscitation decisions for them: observations from SUPPORT and HELP. *Journal of the American Geriatrics Society.* 2000;48(suppl 5):S84-S90.

23. Robinson EM. Ethical analysis of cardiopulmonary resuscitation for elders in acute care. *AACN Clinical Issues.* 2002;13(1):132-144.

24. The Hypothermia after Cardiac Arrest Study Group. Mild therapeutic hypothermia to improve the neurologic outcome after cardiac arrest. *New England Journal of Medicine.* 2002;346(8):549-556.

25. The Joint Commission. 2009 *National Patient Safety Goals.* Available at http://www.jointcommission.org/patientsafety/nationalpatientsafetygoals/; Accessed September 4, 2011.

26. Thomas K, Force MV, Rasmussen D, et al. Rapid response teams: challenges, solutions, and benefits. *Critical Care Nurse.* 2007;27(1):20-27.

27. Winters BD, Pham JC, Hunt EA, et al. Rapid response systems: A systematic review. *Critical Care Medicine.* 2007;35(5):1238-1243.

28. Zeiner A, Holzer M, Sterz F, et al. Hyperthermia after cardiac arrest is associated with an unfavorable neurologic outcome. *Archives of Internal Medicine.* 2001;161(16):2007-2012.

29. Zwerneman K. End-tidal carbon dioxide monitoring: a vital sign worth watching. *Critical Care Nursing Clinics of North America.* 2006;18(2):217-225.

PART 3

Nursing Care During Critical Illness

CHAPTER

11

Shock, Sepsis, and Multiple Organ Dysfunction Syndrome

Kathleen Hill, MSN, RN, CCNS-CSC

℮volve WEBSITE

Many additional resources, including self-assessment exercises, are located on the Evolve companion website at http://evolve.elsevier.com/Sole.
- Review Questions
- Mosby's Nursing Skills Procedures
- Animations
- Video Clips

INTRODUCTION

Shock is a clinical syndrome characterized by inadequate tissue perfusion that results in cellular, metabolic, and hemodynamic derangements. Impaired tissue perfusion occurs when there is an imbalance between cellular oxygen supply and cellular oxygen demand. Shock can result from ineffective cardiac function, inadequate blood volume, or inadequate vascular tone. The effects of shock are not isolated to one organ system; instead, all body systems may be affected. Shock can progress to organ failure and death unless compensatory mechanisms reverse the process, or clinical interventions are successfully implemented. Shock frequently results in systemic inflammatory response syndrome (SIRS) and multiple organ dysfunction syndrome (MODS). Shock is associated with many causes and a variety of clinical manifestations. Patient responses to shock and treatment strategies vary, thus presenting a challenge to the healthcare team in assessment and management.

This chapter discusses the various clinical conditions that create the shock state including hypovolemia, cardiogenic shock, distributive shock (anaphylactic, neurogenic, and septic shock), and obstructive shock. The progression of shock to SIRS and MODS is also described. The pathophysiology, clinical presentation, and definitive and supportive management of each type of shock state are reviewed.

REVIEW OF ANATOMY AND PHYSIOLOGY

The cardiovascular system is a closed, interdependent system composed of the heart, blood, and vascular bed. Arteries, arterioles, capillaries, venules, and veins make up the vascular

bed. The microcirculation, the portion of the vascular bed between the arterioles and the venules, is the most significant portion of the circulatory system for cell survival. Its functions are the delivery of oxygen and nutrients to cells, the removal of waste products of cellular metabolism, and the regulation of blood volume. In addition, the vessels of the microcirculation constrict or dilate selectively to regulate blood flow to cells in need of oxygen and nutrients.

The structure of the microcirculation differs according to the function of the tissues and organs it supplies; however, all of the vascular beds have common structural characteristics (Figure 11-1). As oxygenated blood leaves the left side of the heart and enters the aorta, it flows through progressively smaller arteries until it flows into an arteriole. Arterioles are lined with smooth muscle, which allows these small vessels to change diameter and, as a result, to direct and adjust blood flow to the capillaries. From the arteriole, blood enters a metarteriole, a smaller vessel that branches from the arteriole at right angles. Metarterioles are partially lined with smooth muscle, which also allows them to adjust diameter size and to regulate blood flow into capillaries.

Blood next enters the capillary network by passing through a muscular precapillary sphincter. Capillaries are narrow, thin-walled vascular networks that branch off the metarterioles. This network configuration increases the surface area to allow for greater fluid and nutrient exchange. It also decreases the velocity of the blood flow to prolong transport time through the capillaries. Capillaries have no contractile ability and are not responsive to vasoactive chemicals, electrical or mechanical stimulation, or pressure across their walls. The precapillary sphincter is the only means of regulating blood flow into a capillary. When the

250

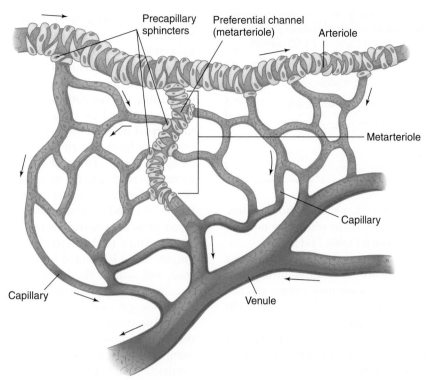

FIGURE 11-1 Microcirculation. (From McCance KL, Huether SE. *Pathophysiology. The Biologic Basis for Disease in Adults and Children.* 6th ed. St. Louis: Mosby; 2010.)

precapillary sphincter constricts, blood flow is diverted away from a capillary bed and directed to one that supplies tissues in need of oxygen and nutrients. The capillary bed lies close to the cells of the body, a position that facilitates the delivery of oxygen and nutrients to the cells.

Once nutrients are exchanged for cellular waste products in the capillaries, blood enters a venule. These small muscular vessels are able to dilate and constrict, offering postcapillary resistance for the regulation of blood flow through capillaries. Blood then flows from the venule and enters the larger veins of the venous system. Another component of the microcirculation consists of the arteriovenous anastomoses that connect arterioles directly to venules. These muscular vessels are able to shunt blood away from the capillary circulation and send it directly to tissues in need of oxygen and nutrients.

Blood pressure is determined by cardiac output and systemic vascular resistance (SVR). Blood pressure is decreased whenever there is a decrease in cardiac output (hypovolemic, cardiogenic, or obstructive shock) or SVR (neurogenic, anaphylactic, or septic shock). Changing pressures within the vessels as blood moves from an area of high pressure within the arteries and passes to the venous system, which has lower pressures, facilitate the flow of blood. The force of resistance opposes blood flow; thus as resistance increases, blood flow decreases. Resistance is determined by three factors: (1) vessel length, (2) blood viscosity, and (3) vessel diameter. Increased resistance occurs with increased vessel length, increased blood viscosity, and decreased blood vessel diameter. Vessel diameter is the most important determinant of resistance.

As the pressure of blood within the vessel decreases, the diameter of the vessel decreases, resulting in decreased blood flow. The critical closing pressure and the resultant cessation of blood flow occur when blood pressure decreases to a point at which it is no longer able to keep the vessel open.

The delivery of oxygen to tissues and cells is required for the production of cellular energy (adenosine triphosphate [ATP]). The delivery of oxygen (DO_2) requires an adequate hemoglobin level to carry oxygen, adequate functioning of the lungs to oxygenate the blood and saturate the hemoglobin (SaO_2), and adequate cardiac functioning (cardiac output) to transport the oxygenated blood to the tissues and cells. Any impairment in the DO_2, or any increase in the consumption of oxygen by the tissues (VO_2), causes a decrease in oxygen reserve (as indicated by the mixed venous oxygen saturation [SvO_2]), which may result in tissue hypoxia, depletion of the supply of ATP, lactic acidosis, organ dysfunction, and potentially death.

Pathophysiology

Diverse events can initiate the shock syndrome. Shock begins when the cardiovascular system fails to function properly because of an alteration in at least one of the four essential circulatory components: blood volume, myocardial contractility, blood flow, or vascular resistance. Under healthy circumstances, these components function together to maintain circulatory homeostasis. When one of these components fails, the others compensate. However, as compensatory mechanisms fail, or if more than one of the

TABLE 11-1	CLASSIFICATION OF SHOCK
TYPE OF SHOCK	PHYSIOLOGICAL ALTERATION
Hypovolemic	Inadequate intravascular volume
Cardiogenic	Inadequate myocardial contractility
Obstructive	Obstruction of blood flow
Distributive Anaphylactic Neurogenic Septic	Inadequate vascular tone

circulatory components is affected, a state of shock ensues. Shock states are classified according to which one of these components is adversely affected (Table 11-1).

Shock is not a single clinical entity but a life-threatening response to alterations in circulation resulting in impaired tissue perfusion. As the delivery of adequate oxygen and nutrients decreases, impaired cellular metabolism occurs. Cells convert from aerobic to anaerobic metabolism. Less energy in the form of ATP is produced. Lactic acid, a by-product of anaerobic metabolism, causes tissue acidosis. Cells in all organ systems require energy to function, and this resultant tissue acidosis impairs cellular metabolism. Shock is not selective in its effects—all cells, tissues, and organ systems suffer as a result of the physiological response to the stress of shock and decreased tissue perfusion. The end result is organ dysfunction because of decreased blood flow through the capillaries that supply the cells with oxygen and nutrients (Figure 11-2).

Stages of Shock

Although the response to shock is highly individualized, a pattern of stages progresses at unpredictable rates. If each stage of shock is not recognized and treated promptly, progression to the next stage occurs. The pathophysiological events and associated clinical findings for each stage are summarized in Table 11-2.

Stage I: Initiation

The process of shock is initiated by subclinical hypoperfusion that is caused by inadequate DO_2, inadequate extraction of oxygen, or both. No obvious clinical indications of hypoperfusion are noted in this stage although hemodynamic alterations, such as a decrease in cardiac output, are noted if invasive hemodynamic monitoring is used for patient assessment.

Stage II: Compensatory Stage

The sustained reduction in tissue perfusion initiates a set of neural, endocrine, and chemical compensatory mechanisms in an attempt to maintain blood flow to vital organs and to restore homeostasis. During this stage, symptoms become apparent, but shock may still be reversed with minimal morbidity if appropriate interventions are initiated.

Neural compensation. Baroreceptors (which are sensitive to pressure changes) and chemoreceptors (which are sensitive to chemical changes) located in the carotid sinus and aortic arch detect the reduction in arterial blood pressure. Impulses are relayed to the vasomotor center in the medulla oblongata, stimulating the sympathetic branch of the autonomic nervous system to release epinephrine and norepinephrine from the adrenal medulla. In response to this catecholamine release, both heart rate and contractility increase to improve cardiac output. Dilation of the coronary arteries occurs to increase perfusion to the myocardium to meet the increased demands for oxygen. Systemic vasoconstriction and redistribution of blood occurs. Arterial vasoconstriction improves blood pressure, whereas venous vasoconstriction augments venous return to the heart, increasing preload and cardiac output. Blood is shunted from the kidneys, gastrointestinal tract, and skin to the heart and brain. Bronchial smooth muscles relax, and respiratory rate and depth are increased, improving gas exchange and oxygenation. Additional catecholamine effects include increased blood glucose levels as the liver is stimulated to convert glycogen to glucose for energy production; dilation of pupils; and peripheral vasoconstriction and increased sweat gland activity resulting in cool, moist skin.

Endocrine compensation. In response to the reduction in blood pressure, messages are also relayed to the hypothalamus, which stimulates the anterior and posterior pituitary gland. The anterior pituitary gland releases adrenocorticotropic hormone (ACTH), which acts on the adrenal cortex to release glucocorticoids and mineralocorticoids (e.g., aldosterone). Glucocorticoids increase the blood glucose level by increasing the conversion of glycogen to glucose (glycogenolysis) and causing the conversion of fat and protein to glucose (gluconeogenesis). Mineralocorticoids act on the renal tubules causing the reabsorption of sodium and water, resulting in increased intravascular volume and blood pressure. The renin-angiotensin-aldosterone system (Figure 11-3) is stimulated by a reduction of pressure in the renal arterioles of the kidneys and/or by a decrease in sodium levels as sensed by the kidney's juxtaglomerular apparatus. In response to decreased renal perfusion, the juxtaglomerular apparatus releases renin. Renin circulates in the blood and reacts with angiotensinogen to produce angiotensin I. Angiotensin I circulates through the lungs, where it forms angiotensin II, a potent arterial and venous vasoconstrictor that increases blood pressure and improves venous return to the heart. Angiotensin II also activates the adrenal cortex to release aldosterone.

Antidiuretic hormone (ADH) is released by the posterior pituitary gland in response to the increased osmolality of the blood that occurs in shock. The overall effects of endocrine compensation result in an attempt to combat shock by providing the body with glucose for energy and by increasing the intravascular blood volume.

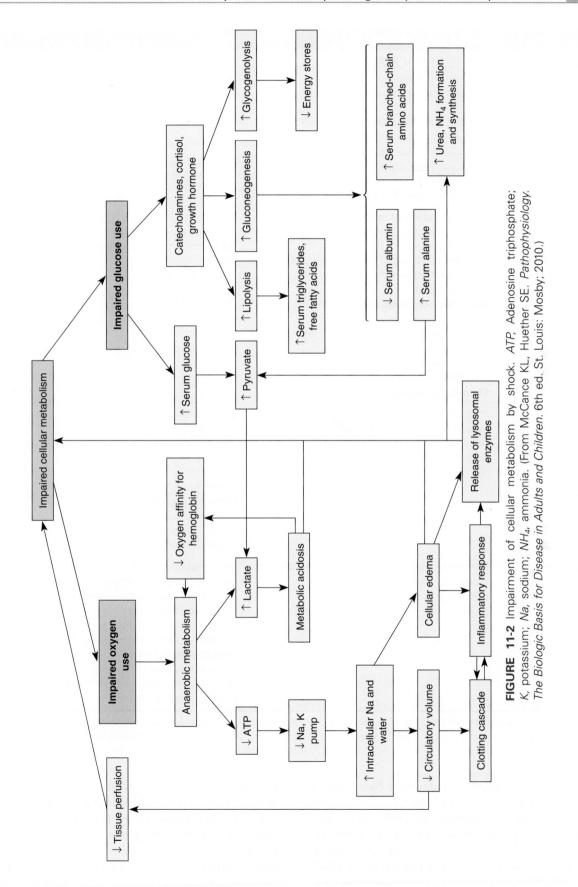

FIGURE 11-2 Impairment of cellular metabolism by shock. *ATP,* Adenosine triphosphate; *K,* potassium; *Na,* sodium; *NH4,* ammonia. (From McCance KL, Huether SE. *Pathophysiology. The Biologic Basis for Disease in Adults and Children.* 6th ed. St. Louis: Mosby; 2010.)

TABLE 11-2	STAGES OF SHOCK	
STAGE OF SHOCK	**PHYSIOLOGICAL EVENTS**	**CLINICAL PRESENTATION**
I: Initiation	↓ Tissue oxygenation caused by: ↓ Intravascular volume (hypovolemic) ↓ Myocardial contractility (cardiogenic) Obstruction of blood flow (obstructive) ↓ Vascular tone (distributive) Septic (mediator release) Anaphylactic (histamine release) Neurogenic (suppression of SNS)	No observable clinical indications ↓ CO may be noted with invasive hemodynamic monitoring
II: Compensatory	**Neural compensation by SNS** ↑ Heart rate and contractility Vasoconstriction Redistribution of blood flow from nonessential to essential organs Bronchodilation **Endocrine compensation** (RAAS, ADH, glucocorticoids release) Renal reabsorption of sodium, chloride, and water Vasoconstriction Glycogenolysis and gluconeogenesis **Chemical compensation**	↑ Heart rate (except neurogenic) Narrowed pulse pressure Rapid, deep respirations causing respiratory alkalosis Thirst Cool, moist skin Oliguria Diminished bowel sounds Restlessness progressing to confusion Hyperglycemia ↑ Urine specific gravity and ↓ creatinine clearance
III: Progressive	Progressive tissue hypoperfusion Anaerobic metabolism with lactic acidosis Failure of sodium-potassium pump Cellular edema	Dysrhythmias ↓ BP with narrowed pulse pressure Tachypnea Cold, clammy skin Anuria Absent bowel sounds Lethargy progressing to coma Hyperglycemia ↑ BUN, creatinine, and potassium Respiratory and metabolic acidosis
IV: Refractory	Severe tissue hypoxia with ischemia and necrosis Worsening acidosis SIRS MODS	Life-threatening dysrhythmias Severe hypotension despite vasopressors Respiratory and metabolic acidosis Acute respiratory failure Acute respiratory distress syndrome Disseminated intravascular coagulation Hepatic dysfunction/failure Acute kidney injury Myocardial ischemia/infarction/failure Cerebral ischemia/infarction

ADH, Antidiuretic hormone; *BP,* blood pressure; *BUN,* blood urea nitrogen; *CO,* cardiac output; *MODS,* multiple organ dysfunction syndrome; *RAAS,* renin-angiotensin-aldosterone system; *SIRS,* systemic inflammatory response syndrome; *SNS,* sympathetic nervous system.

Chemical compensation. As pulmonary blood flow is reduced, ventilation-perfusion imbalances occur. Initially, alveolar ventilation is adequate, but the perfusion of blood through the alveolar capillary bed is decreased. Chemoreceptors located in the aorta and carotid arteries are stimulated in response to this low oxygen tension in the blood. Consequently, the rate and depth of respirations increase. As the patient hyperventilates, carbon dioxide is excreted and respiratory alkalosis occurs. A reduction in carbon dioxide levels and the alkalotic state cause vasoconstriction of cerebral blood vessels. This vasoconstriction, coupled with the reduced oxygen tension, may lead to cerebral hypoxia and ischemia. The overall effects of chemical compensation result in an attempt to combat shock by increasing oxygen supply; however, cerebral perfusion may decrease.

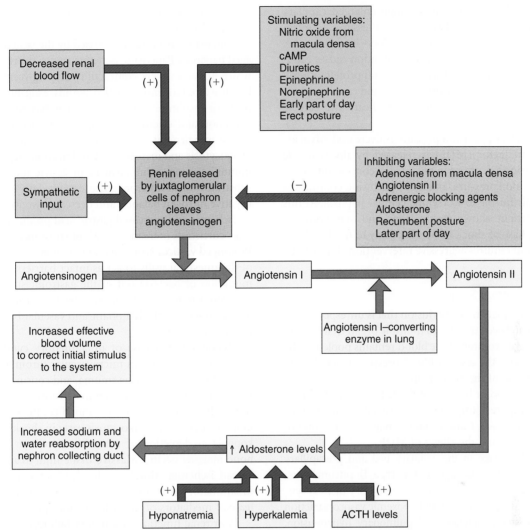

FIGURE 11-3 The feedback mechanisms regulating aldosterone secretion. *ACTH,* Adrenocorticotropic hormone; *cAMP,* cyclic adenosine monophosphate. (From McCance KL, Huether SE. *Pathophysiology. The Biologic Basis for Disease in Adults and Children.* 6th ed. St. Louis: Mosby; 2010.)

Stage III: Progressive Stage

If the cause of hypoperfusion is not corrected or if the compensatory mechanisms continue without reversing the shock, profound hypoperfusion results with further patient deterioration. Vasoconstriction continues in the systemic circulation. Although this effect shunts blood to vital organs, the decrease in blood flow leads to ischemia in the extremities, weak or absent pulses, and altered body defenses. Prolonged vasoconstriction results in decreased capillary blood flow and cellular hypoxia. The cells convert to anaerobic metabolism, producing lactic acid, which leads to metabolic acidosis. Anaerobic metabolism produces less ATP than aerobic metabolism, which reduces the energy available for cellular metabolism. The lack of ATP also causes failure of the sodium-potassium pump. Sodium and water accumulate

within the cell, resulting in cellular swelling and a further reduction in cellular function.

The microcirculation exerts the opposite effect and dilates to increase the blood supply to meet local tissue needs. Whereas the arterioles remain constricted in an attempt to keep vital organs perfused, the precapillary sphincters relax, allowing blood to flow into the capillary bed. Meanwhile, postcapillary sphincters remain constricted. As a result, blood flows freely into the capillary bed but accumulates in the capillaries as blood flow exiting the capillary bed is impeded. Capillary hydrostatic pressure increases, and fluid is pushed from the capillaries into the interstitial space, causing interstitial edema. This intravascular to interstitial fluid shift is further aggravated by the release of histamine and other inflammatory mediators that increase capillary permeability, along with the loss of proteins through enlarged capillary pores, which decreases capillary oncotic pressure. As intravascular blood volume decreases, the blood becomes more viscous and blood flow is slowed. This situation causes capillary sludging as red blood cells, platelets, and proteins clump together. The loss of intravascular volume and capillary pooling further reduce venous return to the heart and cardiac output.

Coronary artery perfusion pressure is decreased. Myocardial depressant factor (MDF) is released by the ischemic pancreas, causing a decrease in myocardial contractility. Cardiac output, blood pressure, and tissue perfusion continue to decrease, contributing to worsening cellular hypoxia. At this point, the patient shows classic signs and symptoms of shock. This phase of shock responds poorly to fluid replacement alone and requires aggressive interventions if it is to be reversed.

Stage IV: Refractory Stage

Prolonged inadequate tissue perfusion that is unresponsive to therapy ultimately contributes to multiple organ dysfunction and death. A large volume of the blood remains pooled in the capillary bed, and the arterial blood pressure is too low to support perfusion of the vital organs.

Dysrhythmias occur because of the failure of the sodium-potassium pump, resulting from decreased ATP, hypoxemia, ischemia, and acidosis. Cardiac failure may occur because of ischemia, acidosis, and the effects of MDF.

Endothelial damage in the capillary bed and precapillary arterioles, along with damage to the type II pneumocytes, which make surfactant, leads to acute respiratory distress syndrome (ARDS). Hypoxemia causes hypoxemic vasoconstriction of the pulmonary circulation and pulmonary hypertension. Ventilation-perfusion mismatch occurs because of disturbances in both ventilation and perfusion. Pulmonary edema may result from disruption of the alveolar-capillary membrane, ARDS, heart failure, or overaggressive fluid resuscitation.

When cerebral perfusion pressure is significantly impaired, loss of autoregulation occurs, resulting in brain ischemia. Cerebral infarction may occur. Sympathetic nervous system dysfunction results in massive vasodilation, depression of cardiac and respiratory centers results in bradycardia and bradypnea, and impaired thermoregulation results in poikilothermism.

Renal vasoconstriction and hypoperfusion of the kidney decreases the glomerular filtration rate. Prolonged ischemia causes acute kidney injury with acute tubular necrosis. Metabolic acids accumulate in the blood, worsening the metabolic acidosis caused by lactic acid production during anaerobic metabolism.

Hypoperfusion damages the reticuloendothelial cells, which recirculate bacteria and cellular debris, thereby predisposing the patient to bacteremia and sepsis. Damage to hepatocytes causes the liver to be unable to detoxify drugs, toxins, and hormones, conjugate bilirubin, or synthesize clotting factors. Hepatic dysfunction causes a decreased ability to mobilize carbohydrate, protein, and fat stores, which results in hypoglycemia.

Pancreatic enzymes are released by the ischemic and damaged pancreas. Pancreatic ischemia causes the release of MDF, which impairs cardiac contractility. Hyperglycemia may occur because of endogenous corticosteroids, exogenous corticosteroids, or insulin resistance. This hyperglycemia results in dehydration and electrolyte imbalances related to osmotic diuresis; impairment of leukocyte function causing decreased phagocytosis and increased risk of infection; depression of the immune response; impairment in gastric motility; shifts in substrate availability from glucose to free fatty acids or lactate; negative nitrogen balance; and decreased wound healing.

Ischemia and increased gastric acid production caused by glucocorticoids increase the risk of stress ulcer development. Prolonged vasoconstriction and ischemia lead to the inability of the intestinal walls to act as intact barriers to prevent the migration of bacteria out of the gastrointestinal tract. This may result in the translocation of bacteria from the gastrointestinal tract into the lymphatic and vascular beds, increasing the risk for sepsis.

Hypoxia and release of inflammatory cytokines impair blood flow and result in microvascular thrombosis. Sluggish blood flow, massive tissue trauma, and consumption of clotting factors may cause disseminated intravascular coagulation (DIC). The bone marrow mobilizes the release of white blood cells, causing leukocytosis early in shock and then leukopenia as depletion of white blood cells in blood and in bone marrow occurs. Massive tissue injury caused by widespread ischemia stimulates the development of a systemic inflammatory response syndrome (SIRS) with a massive release of mediators of the inflammatory process.

Poor renal function, respiratory failure, and impaired cellular function aggravate the existing state of acidosis, which contributes to further fluid shifts, loss of vasomotor tone, and relative hypovolemia. Alterations in the cardiovascular system and continued acidosis cause a reduction in heart rate, impaired myocardial contractility, and a further decrease in cardiac output and tissue perfusion. Cerebral ischemia occurs because of the reduction in cerebral blood flow. Consequently, the sympathetic nervous system is stimulated, an effect that aggravates the existing vasoconstriction, increasing afterload and decreasing cardiac output. Prolonged cerebral ischemia eventually causes the loss of sympathetic nervous system response, and vasodilation and bradycardia result. The patient's decreasing blood pressure and heart rate cause a lethal decrease in tissue perfusion, multisystem organ failure that is unresponsive to therapy, and ultimately brain death and cardiopulmonary arrest.

Systemic Inflammatory Response Syndrome

SIRS is widespread inflammation that can occur in patients with diverse disorders such as infection, trauma, shock, pancreatitis, or ischemia.[8] It may result from or lead to MODS. SIRS is most frequently associated with sepsis. Sepsis is defined as infection associated with SIRS.[8]

The inflammatory cascade maintains homeostasis through a balance between proinflammatory and antiinflammatory processes. Inflammation is normally a localized process; SIRS is a systemic response associated with the release of mediators. These mediators cause an increase in the permeability of the endothelial wall, shifting fluid from the intravascular space into extravascular spaces, including the interstitial space. Intravascular volume is reduced, resulting in a condition of relative hypovolemia. Other mediators cause microvascular clotting, impaired fibrinolysis, and widespread vasodilation.

Effects of Aging

The effects of aging diminish the body's ability to tolerate shock states. As the body ages, the left ventricular wall thickens, ventricular compliance decreases, and calcification and fibrosis of the heart valves occur. Stroke volume and, resultantly, cardiac output are reduced. There is a decreased sensitivity of the baroreceptors and a diminished heart rate response to sympathetic nervous system stimulation in the early stage of shock. Older adults are more likely to be prescribed beta-blockers, which also decrease the heart rate response. Arterial walls lose elasticity causing an increase in SVR, which increases the myocardial oxygen demand and decreases the responsiveness of the arterial system to the effects of catecholamines.

Aging causes decreased lung elasticity, decreased alveolar perfusion, decreased alveolar surface area, and thickening of the alveolar-capillary membrane. These changes limit the body's ability to increase blood oxygen levels during shock states. The ability of the kidney to concentrate urine decreases with age, which limits the body's ability to conserve water when required.

The immune system loses effectiveness with age, referred to as immunosenescence. This increases the risk of infection and sepsis, especially with illness, injury, or surgery. Older adults are also at greater risk for anaphylaxis since they have been exposed to more antigens and therefore have antibodies to more antigens.

ASSESSMENT

An understanding of the pathophysiology of shock and identification of patients at risk are essential for the prevention of shock. Assessment focuses on three areas: history, clinical presentation, and laboratory studies. The logical approach is to review the history of the patient and then assess the systems most sensitive to a lack of oxygen and nutrients. The patient's history may include an identifiable predisposing factor or cause of the shock state.

Clinical Presentation

Multiple body systems are affected by the shock syndrome. The clinical presentation specific to each classification of shock is discussed later (also see boxes, "Clinical Alert," and "Geriatric Considerations").

! CLINICAL ALERT
Shock

ASSESSMENT	SIGNIFICANCE
Change in vital signs, hemodynamic parameters, sensorium	Secondary to decreased tissue perfusion and initiation of compensatory mechanisms
Decreased urine output, rising BUN and creatinine levels	Secondary to initiation of compensatory mechanisms and decreased renal perfusion
Tachypnea, hypoxemia, worsening chest x-ray	Related to development of acute respiratory distress syndrome secondary to hypoperfusion
Petechiae, ecchymosis, bleeding from puncture sites, overt or occult blood in urine, stool, gastric aspirate, tracheal aspirate	Related to development of disseminated intravascular coagulation secondary to shock, SIRS
Hypoglycemia, increase in liver enzymes	Related to hepatic dysfunction secondary to hypoperfusion

BUN, Blood urea nitrogen; *SIRS*, systemic inflammatory response syndrome.

GERIATRIC CONSIDERATIONS

- Decreased skin turgor makes assessment of fluid status more difficult
- Dehydration is common, and may increase the risk for hypovolemia
- Infection is common in the elderly and is one of the top causes of death; several factors contribute to infection:
  - Changes in skin and mucous membranes
  - Increased risk for influenza, pneumonia, cancer, and autoimmune diseases
  - Nutritional deficits associated with poor nutrition, weight loss, low albumin levels, poor oral hygiene, and altered mental status
  - Medications that affect the immune system

Central Nervous System

The central nervous system is the most sensitive to changes in the supply of oxygen and nutrients. It is the first system affected by changes in cellular perfusion. Initial responses of the central nervous system to shock include restlessness, agitation, and anxiety. As the shock state progresses, the patient becomes confused and lethargic because of the decreased perfusion to the brain. As shock progresses, the patient becomes unresponsive.

Cardiovascular System

A major focus of assessment is blood pressure. It is important for the nurse to know the patient's baseline blood pressure.

During the compensatory stage, innervation of the sympathetic nervous system results in an increase in myocardial contractility and vasoconstriction, which results in a normal or slightly elevated systolic pressure, an increased diastolic pressure, and a narrowed pulse pressure. As the shock state progresses, the systolic blood pressure decreases, but the diastolic pressure remains normal, resulting in a narrowed pulse pressure. This narrowed pulse pressure may precede changes in heart rate.[10]

Definitions vary, but a decrease in systolic blood pressure to less than 90 mm Hg is considered hypotensive. If the patient is hypertensive, a decrease in systolic pressure of 40 mm Hg from the usual systolic pressure is considered severely hypotensive. Auscultated blood pressure in shock may be significantly inaccurate because of peripheral vasoconstriction. If blood pressure is not audible, the approximate systolic pressure can be assessed by palpation or ultrasound (Doppler) devices. If the brachial pulse is readily palpable, the approximate systolic pressure is 80 mm Hg. Corresponding blood pressure for palpation of the femoral and carotid pulses is 70 and 60 mm Hg, respectively. Intra-arterial pressure monitoring may be indicated to directly measure blood pressure to obtain accurate readings and guide therapy.

The rate, quality, and character of major pulses (i.e., carotid, radial, femoral, dorsalis pedis, and posterior tibial) are evaluated. In shock states, the pulse is often weak and thready. The pulse rate is increased, usually greater than 100 beats per minute, through stimulation of the sympathetic nervous system as a compensatory response to the decreased cardiac output and increased demand of the cells for oxygen. In later stages of shock, the pulse slows, possibly from release of MDF.

Normal compensatory responses to shock may be altered if the patient is taking certain medications. Negative inotropic agents, such as propranolol and metoprolol, are widely used in the treatment of angina, hypertension, and dysrhythmias. These agents work primarily by blocking the effects of the beta branch of the sympathetic nervous system, and cause a decrease in heart rate and cardiac output. A patient who is taking these medications has an altered ability to respond to the stress of shock and may not exhibit the typical signs and symptoms such as tachycardia and anxiety.

Assessment of the jugular veins provides information regarding the volume and pressure in the right side of the heart. It is an indirect method of evaluating the central venous pressure. Neck veins are distended in patients with obstructive or cardiogenic shock and are flat in hypovolemic shock.

Capillary refill assesses the ability of the cardiovascular system to maintain perfusion to the periphery. The normal response to pressure on the nail beds is blanching; the color returns to a normal pink hue 1 to 2 seconds after the pressure is released. A delay in the return of color indicates peripheral vasoconstriction. Capillary refill provides a quick assessment of the patient's overall cardiovascular status, but this assessment is not reliable in a patient who is hypothermic or has peripheral circulatory problems.

A central venous catheter may be inserted to aid in the differential diagnosis of shock, to administer and monitor therapies, and to evaluate the preload of the heart. Normally, the central venous pressure (or right atrial pressure [RAP]) is 2 to 6 mm Hg. When blood volume decreases (hypovolemic shock), or the vascular capacitance increases (distributive shock), the central venous pressure decreases. In cardiogenic shock, the central venous pressure is increased because of poor myocardial contractility and high filling pressure in the ventricles. In obstructive shock secondary to cardiac tamponade or tension pneumothorax, the central venous pressure is high.

A pulmonary artery (PA) catheter is a useful tool for diagnosing and treating the patient in shock. The risks associated with catheter insertion and central line-associated bloodstream infection must be weighed against the clinical information obtained from this invasive diagnostic device (see box, "QSEN Exemplar"). The PA catheter can give information regarding cardiac dynamics, fluid balance, and effects of vasoactive agents. Preload, which is measured by RAP for the right ventricle and by the pulmonary artery occlusion pressure (PAOP) for the left ventricle, is used to assess fluid balance. Cardiac output and index, afterload, and stroke work indices can also be assessed with a PA catheter (refer to Chapter 8). Table 11-3 describes hemodynamic values and alterations in each classification of shock. Critical care management involves optimizing cardiac

QSEN EXEMPLAR

Quality Improvement

Central line–associated bloodstream infections (CLABSI) and ventilator-associated pneumonia (VAP) are common causes of morbidity and mortality in critically ill patients. The Rhode Island Collaborative is a partnership of 11 hospitals including 23 critical care units that sought to study outcomes of bundled infection prevention interventions. Best practice protocols were selected based upon a Michigan-based quality improvement project. Interventions associated with CLABSI prevention included: hand washing, full barrier precautions during central line insertion, chlorhexidine skin cleansing, avoidance of femoral insertion sites, and timely removal of unnecessary central line catheters. Head-of-the-bed elevation, deep vein thrombosis prophylaxis, gastric ulcer prophylaxis, daily assessment for weaning appropriateness, and appropriate management of sedation comprised VAP preventative strategies. Additionally, a comprehensive safety program was implemented in each participating unit. In an effort to promote a culture of safety, practitioners were empowered to stop procedures where safety was potentially compromised. The bundled intervention protocols were associated with significant, sustained statewide declines in CLABSI and VAP rates, thus reducing the risk for sepsis.

Reference

DePalo VA, McNicoll L, Cornell M, Rocha JM, Adams L, & Pronovost PJ. The Rhode Island collaborative: a model for reducing central line-associated bloodstream infection and ventilator-assisted pneumonia statewide. *Quality and Safety in Healthcare*, 2010;19, 555-561.

TABLE 11-3   HEMODYNAMIC ALTERATIONS IN SHOCK STATES

HEMODYNAMIC PARAMETER, NORMAL VALUE	HYPOVOLEMIC	CARDIOGENIC	OBSTRUCTIVE	DISTRIBUTIVE SEPTIC	ANAPHYLACTIC	NEUROGENIC
Heart rate 60-100 beats/min	High	High	High	High	High	Normal or low
Blood pressure	Normal → Low	Normal → Low	Normal → Low	Normal → Low	Normal → Low	Normal → Low
Cardiac output 4-8 L/min	Low	Low	Low	High then low	Normal → Low	Normal → Low
Cardiac index 2.5-4.0 L/min/m²	Low	Low	Low	High then low	Normal → Low	Normal → Low
RAP 2-6 mm Hg	Low	High	High	Low to variable	Low	Low
PAOP 8-12 mm Hg or PADP 8-15 mm Hg	Low	High	High if impaired diastolic filling or high LV afterload; Low if high RV afterload	Low to variable	Low	Low
SVR 770-1500 dynes/sec/cm⁻⁵	High	High	SVR Low PVR High	Low to variable	Low	Low
SvO₂ 60%-75%	Low	Low	Low	High then low	Low	Low

LV, Left ventricular; *PADP,* pulmonary artery diastolic pressure; *PAOP,* pulmonary artery occlusion pressure; *PVR,* pulmonary vascular resistance; *RAP,* right atrial pressure; *RV,* right ventricular; *SvO₂,* mixed venous oxygen saturation; *SVR,* systemic vascular resistance.

output, and minimizing myocardial oxygen consumption. If an oximetric PA catheter is inserted, mixed venous oxygen saturation (SvO₂) is measured. The SvO₂ reflects the amount of oxygen bound to hemoglobin in the venous circulation and reflects the balance between oxygen delivery (DO₂) and consumption (VO₂). If the SvO₂ is less than 60%, either the DO₂ is inadequate or the VO₂ is excessive. The SvO₂ is decreased in all forms of shock except in early septic shock, where the poor oxygen extraction causes SvO₂ to be high. The SvO₂ is useful in identifying the type of shock and in evaluating the effectiveness of treatment. Continuous measurement of central venous oxygenation (ScvO₂) can also be obtained using a fiberoptic central venous catheter rather than an oximetric PA catheter. ScvO₂ correlates to SvO₂ and is easier to obtain in emergent situations.[30]

Respiratory System

In the early stage of shock, respirations are rapid and deep. The respiratory center responds to shock and metabolic acidosis with an increase in respiratory rate to eliminate carbon dioxide. Direct stimulation of the medulla by chemoreceptors alters the respiratory pattern. As the shock state progresses, metabolic wastes accumulate and cause generalized muscle weakness, resulting in shallow breathing with poor gas exchange.

Although pulse oximetry is commonly used to measure arterial oxygen saturation (SpO₂), it must be used with caution in patients in shock because decreased peripheral circulation may result in inaccurate readings. Arterial blood gas analysis provides a more accurate assessment of oxygenation.

Renal System

Renal hypoperfusion and decreased glomerular filtration rate cause oliguria (urine output <0.5 mL/kg/hr). The renin-angiotensin-aldosterone system is activated, which promotes the retention of sodium and the reabsorption of water in the kidneys, further decreasing urinary output. This prerenal cause of acute kidney injury is manifested by concentrated urine and an increased blood urea nitrogen level, while the serum creatinine level remains normal. If the decreased perfusion is prolonged, acute tubular necrosis, a form of intrarenal failure, occurs and creatinine levels increase.

Gastrointestinal System

Hypoperfusion of the gastrointestinal system results in a slowing of intestinal activity with decreased bowel sounds, distention, nausea, and constipation. Paralytic ileus and ulceration with bleeding may occur with prolonged hypoperfusion. Damage to the microvilli allows translocation of bacteria from the gastrointestinal tract to the lymphatic and systemic circulation, increasing the risk of infection and sepsis in the already compromised critically ill patient.

Hypoperfusion of the liver leads to decreased function and alterations in liver enzyme levels such as lactate dehydrogenase (LDH) and aspartate aminotransferase (AST). If decreased perfusion persists, the liver is not able to produce coagulation factors, detoxify drugs, or neutralize invading microorganisms. Clotting disorders, drug toxicity concerns, and increased susceptibility for infection occur.

Hematological System

The interaction between inflammation and coagulation enhances clotting and inhibits fibrinolysis, leading to clotting in the microcirculatory system and bleeding. An increased consumption of platelets and clotting factors occurs, causing a consumptive coagulopathy. The inability of the liver to manufacture clotting factors also contributes to the coagulopathy. A decreased platelet count, decreased clotting factors, and prolonged clotting times are seen with coagulopathy. Petechiae and ecchymosis may occur, along with blood in the urine, stool, gastric aspirate, and/or tracheal secretions. The clotting in the microcirculation causes peripheral ischemia manifested by acrocyanosis and necrosis of digits and extremities. Leukocytosis frequently occurs, especially in early septic shock. Leukopenia occurs later because of consumption of white blood cells.

Integumentary System

Skin color, temperature, texture, turgor, and moisture level are evaluated. Cyanosis may be present; however, it is a late and unreliable sign. The patient may exhibit central cyanosis, seen in the mucous membranes of the mouth and nose; or peripheral cyanosis, evident in the nails and earlobes. While turgor is frequently used to determine the presence of interstitial dehydration, elderly adults have decreased skin elasticity, making this evaluation misleading.

Laboratory Studies

Laboratory studies assist in the differential diagnosis of the patient in shock (see box, "Laboratory Alert"). However, by the time many of the laboratory values are altered, the patient is in the later stages of shock. The clinical picture is often more useful for early diagnosis and immediate treatment.

! LABORATORY ALERT

Shock

DIAGNOSTIC STUDY	CRITICAL VALUE	SIGNIFICANCE
Chemistry Studies		
Glucose	<70 or >100 mg/dL	Frequently ↑ early shock, ↓ late shock ↑ Impairs immune response
Blood urea nitrogen	>20 mg/dL	↑ Hypoperfusion (prerenal failure) ↑ Gastrointestinal bleeding and catabolism
Creatinine	>1.2 mg/dL	↑ Acute kidney injury
Sodium	<136 or >145 mEq/L	↓ Hemodilution from replacement of excessive hypotonic fluid ↑ Hemoconcentration from fluid loss
Chloride	>108 mEq/L	↑ Excess infusion of normal saline; may cause hyperchloremic acidosis
Potassium	<3.5 or >5.3 mEq/L	↓ Excessive loss of potassium ↑ Impaired elimination from acute kidney injury Observe for cardiac dysrhythmias
Lactate	>2.2 mEq/L	↑ Hypoxia leading to anaerobic metabolism and production of lactic acid
AST	>20 units/L	↑ Hepatic impairment
LDH	>102 units/L	↑ Hepatic impairment, renal impairment, intestinal ischemia, or myocardial infarction
Hematology Studies		
WBCs	<4500 or >11,000/microliter	↑ Stress response; significant increase indicates infection ↓ Late shock due to consumption of WBCs
Hemoglobin	<12 g/dL	↓ Blood loss
Hematocrit	<35%	↓ Blood loss ↑ Dehydration and hemoconcentration
Arterial Blood Gases		
pH	<7.35 or >7.45	↑ Early shock—respiratory alkalosis due to hyperventilation ↓ Late shock—metabolic acidosis due to lactic acidosis
PaCO₂	<35 or >45 mm Hg	↓ Early shock—respiratory alkalosis due to hyperventilation
PaO₂	<80 mm Hg	↓ Hypoxemia; may indicate pulmonary edema or ARDS
HCO₃⁻	<22 mEq/L	↓ Late shock—metabolic acidosis caused by hypoxia, anaerobic metabolism, and lactic acidosis

ARDS, Acute respiratory distress syndrome; *AST,* aspartate aminotransferase; *HCO₃⁻,* bicarbonate; *LDH,* lactate dehydrogenase; *PaCO₂,* partial pressure of arterial carbon dioxide; *PaO₂,* partial pressure of arterial oxygen; *WBCs,* white blood cells.

Serum lactate level is a measure of the overall state of shock, regardless of the cause. The lactate level is an indicator of decreased oxygen delivery to the cells and of the adequacy of treatment. Elevated lactate levels produce an acidic environment and decreased arterial pH. The serum lactate level correlates with the degree of hypoperfusion.

MANAGEMENT

Management of the patient in shock consists of identifying and treating the cause of the shock as rapidly as possible. Care is directed toward correcting or reversing the altered circulatory component (e.g., blood volume, myocardial contractility, obstruction, or vascular resistance) and reversing tissue hypoxia. A combination of fluid, pharmacological, and mechanical therapies are implemented to maintain tissue perfusion and improve oxygen delivery. These interventions include increasing the cardiac output and cardiac index,

increasing the hemoglobin level, and increasing the arterial oxygen saturation. Efforts are also aimed toward minimizing oxygen consumption. Specific management for each classification of shock is discussed later. Nursing interventions are summarized in the box, "Evidence-Based Practice."

Maintenance of Circulating Blood Volume and Adequate Hemoglobin Level

Regardless of the cause, shock produces profound alterations in fluid balance. Therefore patients experiencing absolute hypovolemia (hypovolemic shock) or relative hypovolemia (distributive shock) require the administration of intravenous (IV) fluids to restore intravascular volume, maintain oxygen-carrying capacity, and establish the hemodynamic stability necessary for optimal tissue perfusion. The choice of fluid and the volume and rate of infusion depend on the type of fluid lost, the patient's hemodynamic status, and coexisting conditions.

EVIDENCE-BASED PRACTICE

Nursing Interventions for Shock

Problem
Severe sepsis and septic shock result in mortality rates greater than 20%.[1] Evidence-based practice guidelines have been published by the Surviving Sepsis Campaign (SSC) to facilitate medical management.[2,3] Patients also require expert nursing knowledge and skill to recognize the possible development of sepsis and the delivery of competent care of the patient with sepsis to improve their survival and quality of life after hospitalization.[1]

Clinical Question
What nursing interventions are recommended in caring for patients with severe sepsis or septic shock?

Evidence
1. Early enteral nutrition started in the first 24 to 48 hours after admission to a critical care unit **(Level of Evidence: A).**
   Patients require nutrition that not only meets higher caloric requirements, but also supports the immune system and promotes cellular repair.[6] Early enteral nutrition assists the intestinal mucosa in maintaining its barrier function and can reduce the risk for infection by as much as 30% to 40%.[7]
2. A plan for pressure ulcer prevention and management **(Level of Evidence: D).**
   The hemodynamic alterations associated with shock and sepsis, and use of vasoactive medications, combined with comorbid conditions, limited mobility, and altered sensation place the patient at higher risk for the development of pressure ulcers.[4] Frequent turning, reduction of friction and shear, pressure redistribution through the use of special mattress surfaces are all within the control of the bedside nurse.[5]

Implications for Nursing
These two basic nursing interventions should be a regular feature of nursing care in the ICU patient with sepsis or multiple organ dysfunction. The interventions may require the

nurse to initiate a multiprofessional collaboration with other team members—dieticians, wound care specialists, pharmacists, physicians—to fully implement them; but it is the nurse who provides the attentiveness in initiating and maintaining these interventions.

References
1. Aitken L, Williams G, Harvey M, Blot S, Kleinpell R, Labeau S, et al. Nursing considerations to complement the Surviving Sepsis Campaign guidelines. *Critical Care Medicine.* 2011; 39(7),1800-1818.
2. Dellinger RP, Carlet JM, Masur H, et al. Surviving Sepsis Campaign guidelines for management of severe sepsis and septic shock. *Critical Care Medicine.* 2004;32, 858-873.
3. Dellinger RP, Levy MM, Carlet JM, et al. Surviving Sepsis Campaign: International guidelines for management of severe sepsis and septic shock: 2008. *Critical Care Medicine.* 2008;36, 296-327.
4. Elliott R, McKinley S, Fox V. Quality improvement program to reduce the prevalence of pressure ulcers in an intensive care unit. *American Journal of Critical Care.* 2008;17, 328–334.
5. European Pressure Ulcer Advisory Panel (EPUAP) and National Pressure Ulcer Advisory Panel. (2009). *Prevention and Treatment of Pressure Ulcers: Quick Reference Guide.* Washington DC: National Pressure Ulcer Advisory Panel available at: http://www.npuap.org/Final_Quick_Prevention_for_web_2010.pdf. Accessed July 26, 2011.
6. Martindale RG, McClave SA, Vanek VW, et al. Guidelines for the provision and assessment of nutrition support therapy in the adult critically ill patient: Society of Critical Care Medicine and American Society for Parenteral and Enteral Nutrition: Executive Summary. *Critical Care Medicine.* 2009;37, 1757–1761.
7. Simpson F. & Doig GS. Parenteral vs. enteral nutrition in the critically ill patient: A meta-analysis of trials using the intention to treat principle. *Intensive Care Medicine.* 2005;31,12–23.

Benefits of IV fluid administration include increased intravascular volume, increased venous return to the right side of the heart, optimal stretching of the ventricle, improved myocardial contractility, and increased cardiac output. However, these effects may be dangerous to the patient in cardiogenic shock because large volumes of fluid overwork an already failing heart. Instead, cardiogenic shock is managed primarily with medications that reduce both preload and afterload.

Fluid administration is adjusted based on changes in blood pressure, urine output, hemodynamic values, diagnostic test results, and the clinical picture of the patient's response to treatment. Values obtained from hemodynamic monitoring also assist in monitoring effects of treatment. Generally, volume replacement continues until an adequate mean arterial pressure (65 to 70 mm Hg) is achieved and evidence of end-organ tissue perfusion is reestablished, as evidenced by improvement in the level of consciousness, urinary output, and peripheral perfusion.

Patients in severe shock may require immediate, rapid volume replacement. The IV infusion rate can be increased by using a blood pump to administer fluids under pressure, by using large-bore infusion tubing, or by using a rapid-infusion device. Infusion pumps are used to rapidly and accurately administer large volumes of fluids. Administration of large volumes of room-temperature fluids can rapidly drop core body temperature and cause hypothermia. Fluid-related hypothermia causes alterations in cardiac contractility and coagulation. For this reason, large volumes of fluids should be infused through warming devices (Figure 11-4).

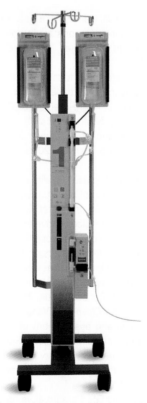

FIGURE 11-4 Level 1 rapid infuser. (Courtesy Level 1, Inc., Rockland, Massachusetts.)

Intravenous Access

IV access is needed to administer fluids and medications. The patient in shock requires a minimum of two IV catheters, one in a peripheral vein and one in a central vein. Peripheral access via a large-gauge catheter (14- or 16-gauge) in a large vein in the antecubital fossa provides a route for rapid administration of fluids and medications. Establishing IV routes in a patient in shock is challenging because peripheral vasoconstriction and venous collapse make access difficult.

A central venous catheter is inserted for large-volume replacement and is also used to monitor central venous pressures. Central venous catheters are commonly inserted into the subclavian, internal jugular, or femoral veins. An upper extremity insertion site is preferred over the femoral vein.[25] Multilumen catheters, which provide multiple access ports, allow the concurrent administration of fluid, medication, and blood products. A PA catheter may be inserted to monitor hemodynamic pressures and guide fluid replacement.

Fluid Challenge

Once IV access is established, a fluid challenge may be performed to assess the patient's hemodynamic response to fluid administration. Various methods for administering a fluid challenge exist. Typically, a rapid infusion of 250 mL (up to 2 L) of a crystalloid solution is initiated first. Nursing responsibilities include obtaining the baseline hemodynamic measurements, administering the fluid challenge, and assessing the patient's response. A fluid challenge algorithm is helpful in guiding fluid resuscitation (Figure 11-5).

Types of Fluids

The choice of fluids depends on the cause of the volume deficit, the patient's clinical status, and the physician's preference. Although the nurse is not responsible for selecting the infusion or transfusion, an understanding of the rationale for the prescribed fluid and the expected effects is needed to assess patient outcomes. The nurse carefully monitors the patient's response to fluid therapy.

Blood, blood products, crystalloids, and colloids are used alone, or in combination, to restore intravascular volume. Crystalloids are infused until diagnostic testing and blood typing and crossmatching are completed. Colloids are avoided in situations where there is an increase in capillary permeability, as in sepsis and septic shock, anaphylactic shock, and early burn injury. A systematic review of 30 randomized controlled trials found no benefit in giving colloids over crystalloids, and recommended against the administration of colloids in most patient populations. In critically ill patients with hypovolemia, administration of albumin was associated with a higher risk of death.[9] A Cochrane Review demonstrated no difference in mortality between the use of crystalloid solution or colloids in the resuscitation of critically ill patients.[26]

Crystalloids are inexpensive and readily available. Crystalloids are classified by tonicity. Isotonic solutions have approximately the same tonicity as plasma (osmolality, 250 to 350 mOsm/L). Lactated Ringer's (LR) solution and 0.9% normal

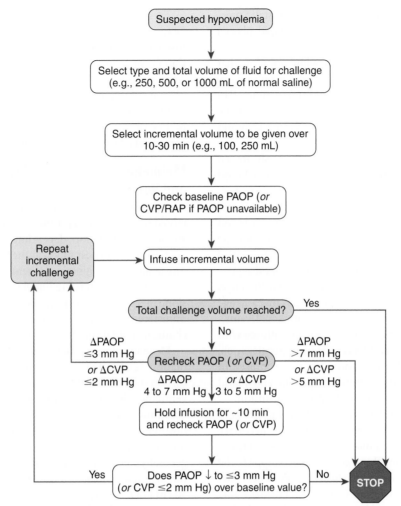

FIGURE 11-5 Fluid challenge algorithm. *CVP,* Central venous pressure; *PAOP,* pulmonary artery occlusion pressure. (Adapted from Kruse JA, Fink MP, Carlson RW. *Saunders Manual of Critical Care.* Philadelphia: Saunders; 2003.)

saline are isotonic solutions that are commonly infused. These solutions move freely from the intravascular space into the tissues. Traditionally, 3 mL of crystalloid solution is administered to replace each 1 mL of blood loss. LR solution closely resembles plasma and may be the only fluid replacement required if blood loss is less than 1500 mL. LR solution contains lactate, which is a salt that the liver converts to bicarbonate, so it counteracts metabolic acidosis if the liver function is normal. LR should not be infused in patients with impaired liver function or severe lactic acidosis. Although 0.9% normal saline is an isotonic solution, its side effects include hypernatremia, hypokalemia, and hyperchloremic metabolic acidosis. Solutions of 5% dextrose in water and 0.45% normal saline are hypotonic and are not used for fluid resuscitation. Hypotonic solutions rapidly leave the intravascular space, causing interstitial and intracellular edema.

When large volumes of crystalloids are infused, the patient is at risk of developing hemodilution of red blood cells and plasma proteins. Hemodilution of red blood cells impairs

oxygen delivery if the hematocrit value is decreased and the cardiac output cannot increase enough to compensate. Hemodilution of plasma proteins decreases colloid osmotic pressure and places the patient at risk of developing pulmonary edema. Elderly patients are at increased risk of developing pulmonary edema and may require invasive hemodynamic monitoring to guide fluid resuscitation.

Colloids contain proteins that increase osmotic pressure. Osmotic pressure holds and attracts fluid into blood vessels, thereby expanding plasma volume. Because colloids remain in the intravascular space longer than crystalloids, smaller volumes of colloids are given in shock states. Albumin and plasma protein fraction (Plasmanate) are naturally occurring colloid solutions that are infused when the volume loss is caused by a loss of plasma rather than blood, such as in burn injury (see Chapter 20), peritonitis, and bowel obstruction. Typing and crossmatching of albumin and plasma protein fraction are not required. Pulmonary edema is a potential complication of colloid administration, resulting from increased pulmonary capillary permeability or increased capillary hydrostatic pressure in the pulmonary vasculature created by rapid plasma expansion.

Hetastarch (Hespan) is a synthetic colloid solution that acts as a plasma expander but carries less risk for pulmonary edema. Side effects include altered prothrombin time (PT) and activated partial thromboplastin time (aPTT) and the potential for circulatory overload. No more than 1 L should be administered in a 24-hour period.[10]

Blood products, packed red blood cells, fresh frozen plasma, and platelets are administered to treat major blood loss. Typing and crossmatching of these products are performed to identify the patient's blood type (A, B, AB, O) and Rh factor, and to ensure compatibility with the donor blood to prevent transfusion reactions. In extreme emergencies, the patient may be transfused with type-specific or O-negative blood, which is considered the universal donor blood type.

Transfusions require an IV access with at least a 20-gauge, preferably an 18-gauge or larger, catheter (a 22- or 23-gauge needle or catheter may be used in adults with small veins). Solutions other than 0.9% normal saline are not infused with blood because they cause red blood cells to aggregate, swell, and burst. In addition, IV medications are never infused in the same port with blood. Appropriate patient and blood identification is necessary before starting any transfusion.

Transfusions are administered with a blood filter to trap debris and clots. Frequent patient assessment is necessary during a blood transfusion to monitor for adverse reactions. In the event of a reaction, the transfusion is stopped, the transfusion tubing is disconnected from the IV access site, and the vein is kept open with an IV of 0.9% normal saline solution. The patient is assessed, and the physician and laboratory are notified. All transfusion equipment (bag, tubing, and remaining solutions) and any blood or urine specimens obtained are sent to the laboratory according to hospital policy. The events of the reaction, interventions used, and patient response to treatment are documented.

The transfusion administration time varies with the particular blood product used and the individual patient circumstances. Documentation of the transfusion includes the blood product administered, baseline vital signs, start and completion time of the transfusion, volume of blood and fluid, assessment of the patient during the transfusion, and any nursing actions taken.

Packed red blood cells increase the blood volume and therefore provide more oxygen-carrying capability to the tissues. One unit of packed red blood cells increases the hematocrit value by about 3% and the hemoglobin value by 1 g/dL. Typing and crossmatching of packed red blood cells are required. Red blood cells tend to aggregate because of the fibrinogen coating; therefore, washed red blood cells may be given. Acidosis, hyperkalemia, and coagulation problems are associated with transfusions of banked blood older than 24 hours. Massive transfusion (approximately 10 units) is associated with decreased 2,3-diphosphoglycerate (2,3-DPG), causing a shift of the oxyhemoglobin dissociation curve to the left, which impairs the delivery of oxygen to the tissues.

Fresh frozen plasma is administered to replace all clotting factors except platelets. When massive transfusions are infused, fresh frozen plasma is given rapidly to restore coagulation factors. One unit of fresh frozen plasma is given for every 4 to 5 units of packed red blood cells transfused. Typing and crossmatching of fresh frozen plasma are required.

Platelets are given rapidly to help control bleeding caused by low platelet counts (usually <50,000/microliter). Typing of platelets, but not crossmatching, is required.

Maintenance of Arterial Oxygen Saturation and Ventilation

Airway maintenance is the top priority. The airway is maintained by proper head position, use of oral or nasopharyngeal airways, or intubation, depending on the patient's condition. Suctioning and chest physical therapy facilitate secretion removal and help maintain a patent airway.

Oxygen is administered to elevate the arterial oxygen tension, thereby improving tissue oxygenation. Oxygen is administered by methods ranging from nasal cannula to mechanical ventilation, depending on the patient's condition.

Mechanical ventilation is used to maintain adequate ventilation as reflected by a normal partial pressure of arterial carbon dioxide ($PaCO_2$) level. Another benefit of mechanical ventilation in a patient with shock is to reduce the work of breathing and the associated increase in oxygen consumption. Tidal volumes and inspiratory pressures are kept low to prevent ventilator-induced lung injury. Tidal volumes are generally between 6 and 8 mL/kg of ideal body weight, and the inspiratory plateau pressures are maintained at less than 30 cm H_2O.[35] Positive end-expiratory pressure (PEEP) is used to maintain alveolar recruitment and may protect against ventilator-induced lung injury by preventing the repetitive opening and collapsing of the alveoli.[29] Newer ventilator modes, such as the pressure-regulated volume-controlled mode, aid in keeping inspiratory pressures low.

Sedation or neuromuscular blockade is considered to reduce oxygen consumption. Arterial blood gases, pulse oximetry, and hemodynamic monitoring aid in the evaluation of oxygen consumption and delivery.

Pharmacological Support

Pharmacological management of shock is based on the manipulation of the determinants of cardiac output: heart rate, preload, afterload, and contractility. Figure 11-6 describes therapies used to manipulate these parameters. These drugs are preferably administered through a central venous catheter. Hemodynamic monitoring is often used to assess the effectiveness of medications. Older adults are particular sensitive to the physiological impact of medications and the deleterious effects of polypharmacy. Table 11-4 describes medications that are commonly administered in shock.

Cardiac Output

Low or high heart rates and dysrhythmias decrease cardiac output. Chronotropic drugs and antidysrhythmic agents are given as indicated. In neurogenic shock, sinus bradycardia

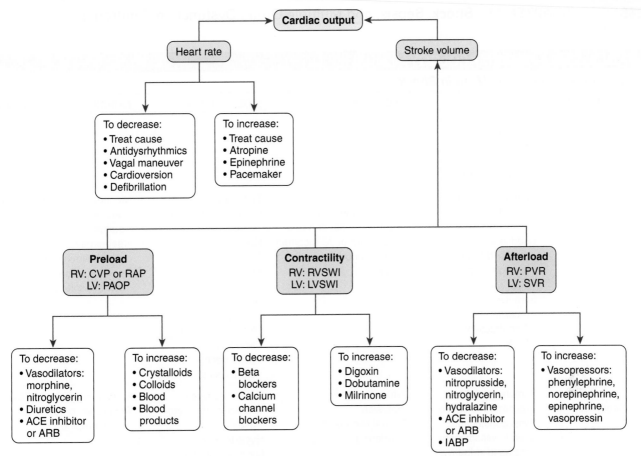

FIGURE 11-6 Therapeutic manipulation of cardiac output and myocardial oxygen consumption. *ACE,* Angiotensin-converting enzyme; *ARB,* angiotensin receptor blocker; *CVP,* central venous pressure; *IABP,* intra-aortic balloon pump; *LV,* left ventricle; *LVSWI,* left ventricular stroke work index; *PAOP,* pulmonary artery occlusion pressure; *PVR,* pulmonary vascular resistance; *RAP,* right atrial pressure; *RV,* right ventricle; *RVSWI,* right ventricular stroke work index; *SVR,* systemic vascular resistance. (Adapted from Dennison RD. *Pass CCRN!* 3rd ed. St. Louis: Mosby; 2007.)

TABLE 11-4 PHARMACOLOGY

Medications Commonly Used in Shock

MEDICATION	ACTION/USE	DOSE/ROUTE	SIDE EFFECTS	NURSING IMPLICATIONS
Dobutamine (Dobutrex)	Stimulates primarily beta₁ receptors to ↑ contractility and ↑ heart rate and cause vasodilation in low CO states	2-20 mcg/kg/min IV infusion Central venous catheter preferred	Tachycardia Dysrhythmias Hypotension Nausea, vomiting Dyspnea Headache Anxiety Paresthesia Palpitations Chest pain	Monitor BP, HR, ECG, PAP, PAOP, SVR, CO, and CI Use cautiously in patients with hypertension, myocardial ischemia, or ventricular dysrhythmias Replace volume before initiation of infusion Do not administer with alkaline solutions
Dopamine (Intropin)	Used in low CO states or vasodilatory states (distributive shock) to restore vascular tone Dose-dependent effect At 2-10 mcg/kg/min stimulates beta₁ receptors to ↑ contractility and ↑ HR	2-20 mcg/kg/min IV infusion and titrated upward as necessary to (maximum of 50 mcg/kg/min) Central venous catheter preferred	Tachycardia Dysrhythmias Nausea, vomiting Dyspnea Headache Palpitations Chest pain in patients with coronary artery disease Tissue necrosis if extravasation occurs	Monitor HR, BP, ECG, PAP, PAOP, SVR, CO, CI, and urine output Treat cause of ↓ BP before initiating (e.g., hypovolemia treated with fluid resuscitation) Wean slowly Treat extravasation with phentolamine (Regitine) Do not administer with alkaline solutions

Continued

TABLE 11-4   PHARMACOLOGY—cont'd

Medications Commonly Used in Shock

MEDICATION	ACTION/USE	DOSE/ROUTE	SIDE EFFECTS	NURSING IMPLICATIONS
Dopamine (Intropin)—cont'd	At 10-20 mcg/kg/min stimulates alpha receptors to cause vasoconstriction and increased SVR			
Norepinephrine (Levophed)	Stimulates alpha receptors to cause vasoconstriction Used in vasodilatory states (distributive shock) to restore vascular tone Stimulation of beta receptors to ↑ contractility and ↑ HR	2-12 mcg/min IV infusion and titrated upward as needed to a maximum of 30 mcg/min Central venous catheter preferred	Tachycardia Ventricular dysrhythmias Hypertension Anxiety Headache Tremor Dizziness Chest pain Metabolic (lactic) acidosis Tissue necrosis if extravasation occurs	Monitor BP, HR, ECG, urine output, and neurological status Treat extravasation with phentolamine (Regitine) Do not administer with alkaline solutions
Phenylephrine (Neosynephrine)	Stimulates alpha receptors to cause vasoconstriction Used in vasodilatory states (distributive shock) to restore vascular tone	2-10 mcg/kg/min IV infusion Central venous catheter preferred	Reflex bradycardia Ventricular dysrhythmias Hypertension Nausea, vomiting Paresthesia Palpitations Anxiety Restlessness Headache Tremor Chest pain	Monitor HR, BP, and ECG Treat reflex bradycardia with atropine
Vasopressin	Vasoconstriction via smooth muscle contraction of all parts of capillaries, arterioles, and venules Used in vasodilatory states (distributive shock) to restore vascular tone	0.01 to 0.03 unit/min IV infusion Central venous catheter preferred	↓ HR ↑ BP Fever Hyponatremia Abdominal cramps Tremor Headache Seizures Coma Chest pain and myocardial ischemia	
Nitroglycerin	Vasodilation by direct smooth muscle relaxation, predominantly venous Used in preload and/or afterload reduction (cardiogenic shock) Dose-dependent effect Arterial dilation only if infusion >1 mcg/kg/min	Initial dose 5-10 mcg/min IV infusion; increase by 5-10 mcg/min every 5 minutes until desired results are achieved (control of chest pain and decreased preload)	↑ or ↓ HR ↑ or ↓ BP Palpitations Weakness Apprehension Flushing Dizziness Syncope Headache	Monitor HR, BP, and urine output Monitor RAP, PAP, PAOP, SVR, CO, and CI if pulmonary artery catheter present Use cautiously in hypotension Administer in glass bottle via non–polyvinyl chloride tubing

TABLE 11-4 PHARMACOLOGY—cont'd

Medications Commonly Used in Shock

MEDICATION	ACTION/USE	DOSE/ROUTE	SIDE EFFECTS	NURSING IMPLICATIONS
Nitroprusside (Nipride)	Vasodilation by direct smooth muscle relaxation, predominantly arterial. Used in preload and/or afterload reduction (cardiogenic shock)	0.5-10 mcg/kg/min IV infusion	Nausea, vomiting, abdominal pain, Headache, Tinnitus, Dizziness, Diaphoresis, Apprehension, Hypotension, Tachycardia, Palpitations, Hypoxemia (nitroprusside-induced intrapulmonary thiocyanate toxicity)	Monitor HR, BP, urine output, and neurological status. Monitor for patient thiocyanate toxicity (metabolic acidosis, confusion, hyperreflexia, and seizures). Serum thiocyanate levels drawn daily if drug is used longer than 72 hours. Treatment includes amyl nitrate, sodium nitrate, and/or sodium thiosulfate. Protect from light by wrapping with opaque material (e.g., aluminum foil)

All medications should be administered via volumetric infusion pump.
BP, Blood pressure; *CI,* cardiac index; *CO,* cardiac output; *D₅W,* 5% dextrose in water; *ECG,* electrocardiogram; *HR,* heart rate; *IV,* intravenous; *NS,* normal (0.9%) saline; *PAOP,* pulmonary artery occlusion pressure; *PAP,* pulmonary artery pressure; *RAP,* right atrial pressure; *SVR,* systemic vascular resistance.

secondary to cervical spinal cord injury does not usually require therapy. However, if the bradycardia is significant and results in decreased perfusion, atropine or a temporary pacemaker may be required.

Preload

In hypovolemic and distributive shock, fluid administration is the primary treatment to increase preload. In cardiogenic shock, the myofibrils are overstretched and the preload needs to be reduced. Venous vasodilators or diuretics are administered to reduce preload.

Afterload

Afterload is low in distributive shock. In this situation, agents that cause vasoconstriction are administered to increase vascular tone and tissue perfusion pressure. Examples of vasoconstrictive drugs include phenylephrine, norepinephrine, epinephrine, or vasopressin. These drugs increase blood pressure and SVR. A negative effect of drugs that increase afterload is an increase in the myocardial oxygen demand. Accurate measurement/calculation of SVR and PVR via a pulmonary artery catheter assists in assessment.

Vasopressors should not be administered in hypovolemic shock because these patients require volume replacement. Administration of vasopressors in hypovolemia causes vasoconstriction and further diminishes tissue perfusion.

In cardiogenic shock, the afterload needs to be reduced. The use of arterial vasodilators to reduce afterload may be limited by the patient's blood pressure. In situations where hypotension prevents the use of arterial vasodilators, an intraaortic balloon pump is used to decrease afterload.

Contractility

Drugs that increase contractility, such as dobutamine, may be administered in cardiogenic shock. Although drugs that decrease contractility (e.g., beta-blockers) may be used to decrease myocardial oxygen consumption in patients with coronary artery disease, they are contraindicated in a patient in shock.

Other Medications

Other drugs used to manage shock include sedatives, analgesics, insulin, corticosteroids, and antibiotics. Although respiratory acidosis is treated by improving ventilation, metabolic acidosis caused by lactic acidosis is best treated by improving the aspects of DO₂: SaO₂, hemoglobin level, and cardiac output. Arterial blood gas analysis and serum lactate levels are used to guide treatment.

Hyperglycemia is common in patients in shock, especially patients with septic shock. Data suggest that intensive insulin therapy to maintain serum glucose levels less than 150 mg/dL reduces morbidity and mortality in critically ill patients.[37]

Low–molecular weight heparin is frequently prescribed for deep vein thrombosis prophylaxis. An H₂-receptor antagonist (ranitidine [Zantac] or proton pump inhibitor (pantoprazole [Protonix]) is frequently prescribed for peptic ulcer prophylaxis.

Maintenance of Body Temperature

The patient's temperature is monitored frequently. Care is directed toward maintaining normal body temperature. Hypothermia depresses cardiac contractility and impairs cardiac output and oxygen delivery. Hypothermia also impairs the coagulation pathway, which can result in a significant coagulopathy. Hypothermia is anticipated when fluids are infused rapidly, and use of a fluid warmer should be considered. Patients should be kept warm and comfortable, but not overly warmed. Excessive warmth increases the oxygen demand on an already stressed cardiovascular system.

Nutritional Support

Nutritional support is essential for patient survival. The goals of nutritional support are to initiate enteral intake as soon as possible and to maintain sufficient caloric intake to assist in the healing process. Early enteral feeding decreases hypermetabolism, minimizes bacterial translocation, decreases diarrhea, and decreases length of stay. Nutritional requirements of the patient in shock are highly variable depending on the degree of hemodynamic stability, the cause of shock, and the patient's age, gender, and preexisting diseases. Enteral feeding is the preferred method, and immune-boosting formulas may be prescribed. Administration of enteral nutrition may be limited by paralytic ileus, gastric dilation, or both, which are common in shock. Total parenteral nutrition is given if patients are unable to tolerate enteral feeding (see Chapter 6).[3]

Maintenance of Skin Integrity

The decreased perfusion seen in shock can precipitate injury to the skin. Meticulous skin care is required to promote skin integrity. The patient is turned at frequent intervals, and lotion is applied. Pressure-relieving devices, such as therapeutic beds or mattresses, may be indicated. Therapeutic beds with automatic rotation features do not substitute for the pressure relief afforded by manual turning and positioning. Lotion moisturizes the skin to reduce the effects of shear and friction generated when the patient is repositioned in the bed. The heels should be elevated off the surface of the bed with pillows or with pressure-relief boots.

Psychological Support

Nursing interventions also focus on identifying the impact of the illness on the patient and the family. Nursing interventions include providing information, which is essential for the psychological well-being of the patient and the family, and may help to give them a sense of understanding and control of the situation. Since shock has a high mortality, a discussion should be initiated regarding life-sustaining therapies (see Chapters 2 and 3).

NURSING DIAGNOSIS

The primary nursing diagnosis for all patients in shock is altered tissue perfusion. This diagnosis may be related to decreased tissue perfusion, myocardial contractility, vascular resistance, obstruction, or a combination of these. The nurse provides care to support tissue perfusion of the patient in shock until definitive care is underway. Supportive care is aimed at maintenance of organ function (see box, "Nursing Care Plan for the Patient in Shock").

◎ NURSING CARE PLAN

for the Patient in Shock

NURSING DIAGNOSIS
Altered tissue perfusion related to decreased blood volume (hypovolemic shock); decreased myocardial contractility (cardiogenic shock); impaired circulatory blood flow (obstructive shock); and widespread vasodilatation (septic, anaphylactic, or neurogenic shock)

PATIENT OUTCOMES
Adequate Tissue Perfusion
- Alert and responsive
- Skin warm and dry with good turgor
- Vital signs and hemodynamic parameters within normal limits (see Table 11-3)
- Systolic and diastolic blood pressure within 20 mm Hg of baseline
- Heart rate 60 to 100 beats per minute
- Oxygen saturation 90% or greater
- Normal body temperature
- Strong peripheral pulses
- Balanced intake and output
- Stable body weight
- Urine output at least 0.5 mL/kg/hr
- Normal serum and urine laboratory values and ABG results
- Adequate pain management
- Absence of complications (ARDS, DIC, acute kidney injury, hepatic failure, MODS)

⊚ NURSING CARE PLAN—cont'd

for the Patient in Shock

NURSING INTERVENTIONS	RATIONALES
• Monitor for early symptoms of shock (see Table 11-2)	• Initiate early support to improve outcomes and reduce risk of complications, organ failure, and death
• Establish or maintain patent airway	• Provide adequate gas exchange
• Monitor oxygenation: pulse oximetry, ABGs, SvO₂; administer oxygen to maintain SpO₂ at least 90%	• Assess for need for supplemental oxygen; ensure adequate oxygen delivery to the tissues
• Prepare for intubation and mechanical ventilation as needed	• Mechanical ventilation is frequently required to ensure adequate ventilation and reduce the work of breathing
• Establish intravenous access; use large-bore catheters (14 or 16 gauge); obtain central venous access, if possible	• Provide rapid fluid administration; central IV access allows for fluid and drug administration without the concerns of peripheral infiltration and irritation
• Control bleeding through the application of pressure or surgical intervention	• Prevent blood loss
• Administer fluids as ordered (crystalloids, colloids, blood products)	• Maintain tissue perfusion
• Consider warming fluids before infusing	• Reduce hypothermia and its complications
• Replace blood components as indicated; obtain laboratory specimen for type and crossmatch	• Replace volume loss associated with blood loss; prevent transfusion reaction
• Evaluate patient's response to fluid challenges and blood product administration: improved vital signs, level of consciousness, urinary output, hemodynamic values, and serum and urine laboratory values	• Monitor response to treatment
• Monitor for clinical indications of fluid overload (↑ HR, ↑ RR, dyspnea, crackles) when fluids are administered rapidly	• Assess for signs of volume overload in response to treatment
• Monitor cardiopulmonary status: HR, RR, BP, MAP, skin color, temperature, and moisture, capillary refill, hemodynamic values, cardiac rhythm, neck veins, lung sounds	• Monitor response to treatment
• Monitor level of consciousness	• Assess perfusion of the central nervous system
• Monitor gastrointestinal status: abdominal distention, bowel sounds, gastric pH, vomiting, large enteral feeding residual	• Assess perfusion of the gastrointestinal system and prevent potential complications
• Monitor fluid balance: I&O, daily weights, amount and type of drainage (chest tube, nasogastric, wounds)	• Evaluate need for continued fluid volume support
• Monitor serial serum values: Hct, Hgb, WBC, PT, aPTT, D-dimer, platelets, ABGs, chemistry profile, lactate, cultures	• Evaluate response to treatment
• Assess and treat pain and discomfort: monitor pain level; administer analgesics; implement comfort and relaxation measures (turning, repositioning, skin care, music); maintain appropriate room temperature; evaluate patient's response	• Promote patient comfort and evaluate response to pain management
• Administer medications as prescribed and specific for the classification of shock (see Table 11-4)	• Improve outcomes and reduce complications
• Provide wound care as indicated and evaluate healing	• Promote wound healing and prevent infection
• Provide adequate nutritional support; collaborate with dietitian about patient's nutritional needs; promote early enteral feed (if tolerated)	• Promote optimum cell function and healing; reduce complications
• Provide psychological support for patient, family, and others	• Reduce the stress response and physiological demand; promote family functioning
• Evaluate patient response to interventions and adjust treatments accordingly; monitor for complications	• Monitor patient response to determine need for modification of treatment and/or nursing care

ABG, Arterial blood gas; *aPTT*, activated partial thromboplastin time; *ARDS*, acute respiratory distress syndrome; *BP*, blood pressure; *DIC*, disseminated intravascular coagulation; *Hct*, hematocrit; *Hgb*, hemoglobin; *HR*, heart rate; *I&O*, intake and output; *IV*, intravenous; *MAP*, mean arterial pressure; *MODS*, multiple organ dysfunction syndrome; *PT*, prothrombin time; *RR*, respiratory rate; *SpO₂*, oxygen saturation by pulse oximetry; *SvO₂*, mixed venous oxygen saturation; *WBC*, white blood cell.

Based on data from Gulanick M and Myers JL. *Nursing Care Plans: Diagnoses, Interventions, and Outcomes*, 7th edition, St. Louis: Mosby; 2011.

SPECIFIC CLASSIFICATIONS OF SHOCK

Table 11-5 provides a summary of the classifications of shock.

Hypovolemic Shock

Hypovolemic shock occurs when the circulating blood volume is inadequate to fill the vascular network. Intravascular volume deficits may be caused by external or internal losses of either blood or fluid. In these situations, the intravascular blood volume is depleted and unavailable to transport oxygen and nutrients to tissues. The severity of hypovolemic shock is dependent upon the volume deficit, the acuity of volume loss, the type of fluid lost, and the age and preinjury health status of the patient.

External volume deficits include loss of blood, plasma, or body fluids. The most common cause of hypovolemic shock is hemorrhage. External loss of blood may occur after traumatic injury, surgery, or obstetrical delivery or with coagulation alterations (hemophilia, thrombocytopenia, DIC, and anticoagulant medications). External plasma losses may be seen in patients with burn injuries who have significant fluid shifts from the intravascular space to the interstitial space (see Chapter 20. Excessive external loss of fluid may occur through the gastrointestinal tract via suctioning, upper gastrointestinal bleeding, vomiting, diarrhea, reduction in oral fluid intake, or fistulas; through the genitourinary tract as a result of excessive diuresis, diabetes mellitus with polyuria, diabetes insipidus, or Addison disease; or through the skin secondary to diaphoresis without fluid and electrolyte replacement.

Blood or body fluids may be sequestered within the body outside the vascular bed. Internal sequestration of blood may be seen in patients with a ruptured spleen or liver, hemothorax, hemorrhagic pancreatitis, fractures of the femur or pelvis, and dissecting aneurysm. Internal sequestration of body fluids includes ascites, peritonitis, and peripheral edema. Fluid sequestration is also seen in patients with intestinal obstruction, which causes fluid to leak from the intestinal capillaries into the lumen of the intestine.

Fluid losses may be obvious or subtle. Assessment includes weighing dressings; measuring drainage from chest or nasogastric tubes; monitoring potential sites for bleeding, such as surgical wounds, or IV or intraarterial catheter sites after removal; and considering insensible losses, such as perspiration. Abdominal girth is measured periodically in patients in whom occult bleeding may be suspected or in those with ascites. Daily weights are obtained by using the same scale with the patient wearing the same clothing at approximately the same time each day. Evaluation of the hematocrit is useful in determining whether blood or fluid was lost. In a patient with blood loss, the hematocrit will be decreased, whereas in a patient with fluid loss, the hematocrit will be increased.

TABLE 11-5	SUMMARY OF CLASSIFICATIONS OF SHOCK		
CLASSIFICATION	**POSSIBLE CAUSES**	**CLINICAL PRESENTATION**	**MANAGEMENT**
Hypovolemic shock	*External loss of blood:* GI hemorrhage Surgery Trauma *External loss of fluid:* Diarrhea Diuresis Burns *Internal sequestration of blood fluid:* Hemoperitoneum Retroperitoneal hemorrhage Hemothorax Hemomediastinum Dissecting aortic aneurysm Femur or pelvic fracture Ascites Pleural effusion	↑ HR ↓ BP Tachypnea Oliguria Cool, pale skin Decreased mental status Flat neck veins ↓ CO, CI, RAP, PAP, PAOP ↑ SVR ↓ SvO_2 ↑ *Hematocrit:* if from dehydration ↓ *Hematocrit:* if from blood loss	Eliminate and treat the cause Replace lost volume with appropriate fluid
Cardiogenic shock	Myocardial infarction Myocardial contusion Cardiomyopathy Myocarditis Severe heart failure Dysrhythmias Valvular dysfunction	↑ HR Dysrhythmias ↓ BP Chest pain Tachypnea Oliguria Cool, pale skin ↓ Mentation	Improve contractility with inotropic agents Mechanical support Emergency revascularization Reduce preload Reduce afterload Prevent/treat dysrhythmias

TABLE 11-5	SUMMARY OF CLASSIFICATIONS OF SHOCK—cont'd		
CLASSIFICATION	POSSIBLE CAUSES	CLINICAL PRESENTATION	MANAGEMENT
Cardiogenic shock—cont'd	Ventricular septal rupture	Left ventricular failure Right ventricular failure ↓ CO, CI ↑ RAP, PAP, PAOP, SVR ↓ SvO$_2$	

Obstructive shock	*Impaired diastolic filling:*
	  Cardiac tamponade
	  Tension pneumothorax
	  Constrictive pericarditis
	  Compression of great veins
	Increased right ventricular afterload:
	  Pulmonary embolism (PE)
	  Severe pulmonary hypertension
	  Increased intrathoracic pressure
	Increased left ventricular afterload:
	  Aortic dissection
	  Systemic embolization
	  Aortic stenosis
	  Abdominal hypertension
		↑ HR
		Dysrhythmias
		↓ BP
		Chest pain
		Dyspnea
		Oliguria
		Cool, pale skin
		Decreased mental status
		Jugular venous distention
		Cardiac tamponade: muffled heart sounds, pulsus paradoxus
		Tension pneumothorax: diminished breath sounds on affected side, tracheal shift away from affected side
		Pulmonary embolism: right ventricular failure
		Aortic dissection: ripping chest pain, pulse differences between left and right side, widened mediastinum
		↓ CO, CI
		↑ or normal RAP, PAP, PAOP
		↑ PVR, ↓ SVR
		↓ SvO$_2$
			Eliminate source of obstruction or compression
			Pericardiocentesis for cardiac tamponade
			Fibrinolytics, anticoagulants for PE
			Emergency decompression for tension pneumothorax

Anaphylactic shock	*Foods:* fish, shellfish, eggs, milk, wheat, strawberries, peanuts, tree nuts (pecans, walnuts), food additives *Drugs:* antibiotics, ACE inhibitors, aspirin, local anesthetics, narcotics, barbiturates, contrast media, blood and blood products, allergic extracts *Bites or stings:* venomous snakes, wasps, hornets, spiders, jellyfish, stingrays, deer flies, fire ants *Chemicals:* latex, lotions, soap, perfumes, iodine-containing solutions	↑ HR; dysrhythmias ↓ BP Chest pain Tachypnea Flushed, warm to hot skin Oliguria Restlessness, change in LOC, seizures Nausea, vomiting, abdominal cramping, diarrhea Dyspnea, cough, stridor, wheezing, dysphagia Urticaria, angioedema, hives ↓ CO, CI ↓ RAP, PAP, PAOP, SVR ↓ SvO$_2$ ↑ IgE	Remove offending agent or slow absorption: remove stinger; apply ice to sting or bite; discontinue drug, dye, blood; lavage stomach if antigen ingested; flush skin with water Maintain airway, oxygenation, and ventilation; intubation may be necessary Modify or block the effects of mediators: epinephrine, antihistamines, steroids Maintain MAP
Neurogenic shock	General or spinal anesthesia Epidural block Cervical spinal cord injury *Drugs:* barbiturates, phenothiazines, sympathetic blocking agents	↓ HR ↓ BP Hypothermia Warm, dry, flushed skin Oliguria Neurological deficit ↓ CO, CI ↓ RAP, PAP, PAOP, SVR ↓ SvO$_2$	Eliminate and treat the cause Maintain MAP Maintain adequate heart rate VTE prophylaxis

Continued

TABLE 11-5	SUMMARY OF CLASSIFICATIONS OF SHOCK—cont'd		
CLASSIFICATION	**POSSIBLE CAUSES**	**CLINICAL PRESENTATION**	**MANAGEMENT**
Septic shock	*Immunosuppression:* Extremes of age Malnutrition Alcoholism or drug abuse Malignancy History of splenectomy Chronic health problems Immunosuppressive therapies *Significant bacteremia:* Invasive procedures and devices Traumatic wounds or burns GI infection or untreated disease Peritonitis Food poisoning Prolonged hospitalization Translocation of GI bacteria (associated with NPO status)	*Early, hyperdynamic, warm:* ↑ HR Normal or ↓ BP ↑ Pulse pressure Skin warm, flushed Confusion Oliguria ↑ CO, CI ↓ RAP, PAP, PAOP, SVR ↑ SvO₂ *Late, hypodynamic, cold:* ↑ HR ↓ BP ↓ Pulse pressure Skin cool, pale ↓ LOC Anuria Hypothermia ↓ CO, CI Variable RAP, PAP, PAOP, SVR ↓ SvO₂ Positive culture	Good hand-washing techniques Avoid invasive procedures Identify source of infection Meticulous oral and airway care Meticulous catheter and wound care Avoid NPO status: initiate and maintain enteral nutrition Antibiotics as indicated by culture results Control hyperthermia Maintain MAP

ACE, Angiotensin-converting enzyme; *BP,* blood pressure; *CI,* cardiac index; *CO,* cardiac output; *GI,* gastrointestinal; *HR,* heart rate; *IgE,* immunoglobulin; *LOC,* level of consciousness; *MAP,* mean arterial pressure; *NPO,* nothing by mouth; *PAOP,* pulmonary artery occlusion pressure; *PAP,* pulmonary artery pressure; *PE,* pulmonary embolism; *PVR,* pulmonary vascular resistance; *RAP,* right atrial pressure; *SvO₂,* mixed venous oxygen saturation; *SVR,* systemic vascular resistance; *VTE,* venous thromboembolism.

Hypovolemic shock results in a reduction of intravascular volume and a decrease in venous return to the right side of the heart. Ventricular filling pressures (preload) are reduced, resulting in a decrease in stroke volume and cardiac output. As the cardiac output decreases, blood pressure decreases and tissue perfusion decreases. Figure 11-7 summarizes the pathophysiology of hypovolemic shock.

Patients with hypovolemic shock present with signs and symptoms as a result of poor organ perfusion, including altered mentation ranging from lethargy to unresponsiveness; rapid, deep respirations; cool, clammy skin with weak, thready pulses; tachycardia; and oliguria. Hypovolemic shock resulting from hemorrhage is classified according to the volume of blood lost and the resultant effects on the level of consciousness, vital signs, and urine output (Table 11-6).

An increase in abdominal girth may be an indicator of abdominal bleeding or fluid loss into the abdomen. Ultrasonography is performed to determine the presence of abdominal bleeding or fluid loss. If bleeding or fluid loss is found, computed tomography may be obtained to pinpoint sources of bleeding, (hypovolemic shock) or locate possible abscesses, which can cause sepsis.

Management of hypovolemic shock focuses on identifying, treating, and eliminating the cause of the hypovolemia and replacing lost fluid. Examples of treating the cause include surgery, antidiarrheal medication for diarrhea, and insulin for hyperglycemia. The type of fluid lost is considered when determining fluid replacement. Isotonic crystalloids such as normal saline are generally used first, although blood and blood products may be administered if the patient is bleeding. The 3-for-1 rule is used which recommends the replacement of 300 mL of isotonic solution for every 100 mL of blood lost. Hemodynamic monitoring provides objective data to guide fluid replacement. Patients receiving blood replacement are likely to require less than 3 times the lost volume.[2] Hypertonic saline (3%) expands the intravascular volume by creating an osmotic effect that displaces water from the intracellular space. Administration of hypertonic saline is an alternative in trauma patients because less volume is required.[2]

Cardiogenic Shock

Cardiogenic shock can occur when the heart fails to act as an effective pump. A decrease in myocardial contractility results in decreased cardiac output and impaired tissue perfusion. Cardiogenic shock is one of the most difficult types of shock to treat and carries a hospital mortality of 67%.[13]

The most common cause of cardiogenic shock is an extensive left ventricular myocardial infarction. A correlation exists between the amount of myocardial damage and the likelihood of cardiogenic shock. If 40% or more of the left ventricle is damaged, the likelihood of cardiogenic shock increases. Other causes of cardiogenic shock include

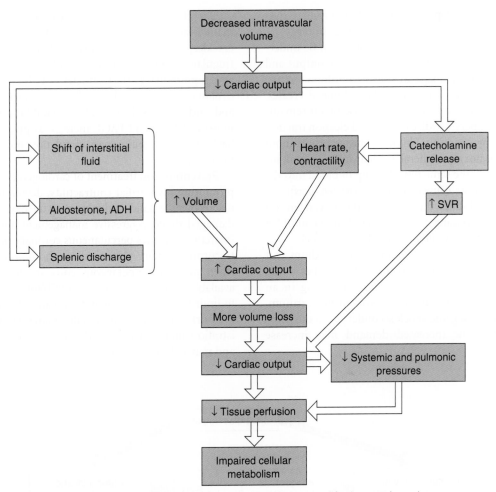

FIGURE 11-7 Hypovolemic shock. This type of shock becomes life threatening when compensatory mechanisms *(orange boxes)* are overwhelmed by continuous loss of intravascular volume. *ADH,* Antidiuretic hormone; *SVR,* systemic vascular resistance. (From McCance KL, Huether SE. *Pathophysiology. The Biologic Basis for Disease in Adults and Children.* 6th ed. St. Louis: Mosby; 2010.)

TABLE 11-6	SEVERITY OF HEMORRHAGIC SHOCK			
	CLASS			
INDICATORS	I	II	III	IV
Blood loss (% blood volume)	<15%	15%-30%	30%-40%	>40%
Blood loss (mL)	<750	750-1500	1500-2000	>2000
Heart rate per minute	<100	100-120	120-140	>140
Blood pressure	Normal	Normal	Decreased	Decreased
Pulse pressure	Normal or increased	Decreased	Decreased	Decreased
Respiratory rate per minute	14-20	20-30	30-40	>35
Urine output (mL/hr)	>30	20-30	<20	Negligible
CNS/mental status	Slightly anxious	Mildly anxious	Anxious, confused	Confused, lethargy
Fluid replacement	Crystalloid	Crystalloid	Crystalloid and blood	Crystalloid and blood

CNS, Central nervous system.
Adapted from American College of Surgeons' Committee on Trauma. (2008). *Advanced trauma life support (ATLS) program for doctors student manual* (8th ed.). Chicago: American College of Surgeons.

dysrhythmias, cardiomyopathy, myocarditis, valvular dysfunction, severe heart failure, and structural disorders.[13]

The pathophysiology of cardiogenic shock can be understood by reviewing cardiac dynamics of cardiac output and stroke volume. When damage to the myocardium occurs, contractile force is reduced and stroke volume decreases. Ventricular filling pressures increase because blood remains in the cardiac chambers. Cardiac output and ejection fraction decrease causing hypotension. This hypotension brings about a reflex compensatory peripheral vasoconstriction and increased afterload. At the same time, backup of blood into the pulmonary circulation causes decreased oxygen perfusion across alveolar membranes, thus reducing the oxygen tension in the blood and decreasing cellular metabolism. Figure 11-8 summarizes the pathophysiology of cardiogenic shock.

An increased demand is placed on the myocardium as it attempts to increase perfusion to the cells. The heart rate increases as a compensatory mechanism, resulting in an increased oxygen demand on an overworked myocardium. In patients with cardiogenic shock secondary to acute myocardial infarction, the increased demand may increase infarction size.

The clinical presentation of cardiogenic shock includes manifestations of left ventricular failure (S_3 heart sound, crackles, dyspnea, hypoxemia) and right ventricular failure (jugular venous distention, peripheral edema, hepatomegaly). A pulmonary artery catheter is useful in trending hemodynamic parameters. In cardiogenic shock, cardiac output and cardiac index decrease; however, RAP, pulmonary artery pressure (PAP), and PAOP increase as pressure and volume back up into the pulmonary circulation and the right side of the heart.

Prevention and treatment of cardiogenic shock is aimed at promoting myocardial contractility, decreasing the myocardial oxygen demand, and increasing the oxygen supply to the damaged tissue. Aggressive management after a myocardial infarction includes percutaneous coronary interventions, intracoronary stent placement, or both, fibrinolytic agents when primary percutaneous coronary intervention is not available, glycoprotein IIb/IIIa inhibitors, and beta-blockers to limit the size of the infarction. Pain relief and rest reduce the workload of the heart and the infarct size. Oxygen administration increases oxygen delivery to the ischemic muscle and may help save myocardial tissue.[18]

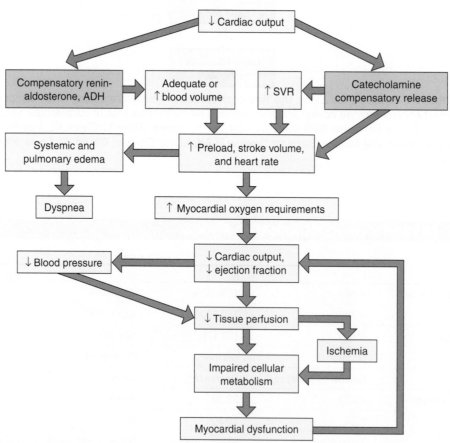

FIGURE 11-8 Cardiogenic shock. *ADH,* Antidiuretic hormone; *SVR,* systemic vascular resistance. Shock becomes life threatening when compensatory mechanisms *(orange boxes)* cause increased myocardial oxygen requirements. (From McCance KL, Huether SE. *Pathophysiology. The Biologic Basis for Disease in Adults and Children.* 6th ed. St. Louis: Mosby; 2010.)

Pharmacological agents are administered to decrease preload (RAP, PAOP), decrease afterload (SVR), increase stroke volume, increase cardiac index, and increase contractility (see Table 11-4). Diuretics (e.g., furosemide) and venous vasodilators (e.g., morphine, nitroglycerin, nitroprusside) reduce preload and venous return to the heart. Nitroglycerin at low doses (<1 mcg/kg/min) causes venous vasodilation to decrease preload. At higher doses (>1 mcg/kg/min) arterial vasodilation decreases afterload. These drugs must be used cautiously because they may cause hypotension, thereby contributing to further cellular hypoperfusion.

Positive inotropic agents (e.g., dobutamine) are given to increase the contractile force of the heart. As contractility increases, ventricular emptying improves, filling pressures decrease (RAP, PAOP), and stroke volume improves. The improved stroke volume increases cardiac output and improves tissue perfusion. However, positive inotropic agents also increase myocardial oxygen demand and must be used cautiously in patients with myocardial ischemia.

Afterload reduction may be achieved by the cautious administration of arterial vasodilators (e.g., nitroprusside) to decrease SVR, increase stroke volume, and increase cardiac index. Blood pressure must be carefully monitored to keep the mean arterial pressure above 65 mm Hg to ensure organ perfusion. Significant hypotension may limit the use of arterial vasodilators, as coronary artery perfusion pressure may be reduced and worsen myocardial ischemia. In this situation, afterload reduction is achieved through the insertion of an intraaortic balloon pump (IABP).

The *IABP* is a cardiac assist device that provides *counterpulsation therapy* concurrently with pharmacological support. IABP therapy is initiated by inserting a dual-chambered balloon into the descending thoracic aorta via the femoral artery. The balloon is inserted percutaneously at the patient's bedside or under fluoroscopy. The tip of the balloon is positioned just distal to the left subclavian artery (Figure 11-9). Correct placement is verified by chest x-ray.

The IABP improves coronary artery perfusion, reduces afterload, and improves perfusion to vital organs. The balloon is inflated mechanically with helium. Inflation and deflation are automatically timed with the cardiac cycle. The IABP inflates during diastole when the aortic valve is closed. The inflation cycle displaces blood backward and forward simultaneously. The backward flow increases perfusion to the coronary arteries, and the forward flow increases perfusion to vital organs. Balloon deflation occurs just before systole and left ventricular ejection. This sudden deflation, along with the displacement of blood that occurred during diastole, reduces the pressure in the aorta and decreases afterload and myocardial oxygen demand. Desired outcomes for a patient in cardiogenic shock with an IABP include decreased SVR, diminished symptoms of myocardial ischemia (chest pain, ST-segment elevation), and increased stroke volume and cardiac output.

Counterpulsation therapy with an IABP requires a high degree of nursing skill because of the complexity of the

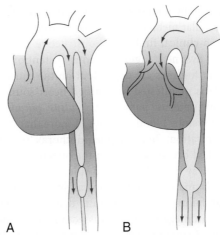

FIGURE 11-9 Intraaortic balloon pump. The balloon is deflated during systole **(A)** and inflated during diastole **(B)**.

equipment and the need for frequent monitoring. Many institutions require nurses to be credentialed in managing the patient with an IABP. Limb ischemia and embolic phenomena are potential complications that must be assessed. Other complications include dissection of the aorta, infection, ineffective pumping, and technical problems. Use of the IABP is contraindicated in patients with aortic valve insufficiency or aortic aneurysm.

Ventricular assist devices (VADs) may be used temporarily to support a failing ventricle that has not responded to IABP therapy and pharmacological therapy. VADs are used to treat cardiogenic shock by allowing the ventricle to recover or to support the patient awaiting cardiac transplant as a bridge to transplant. They can be used to support the left ventricle, the right ventricle, or both ventricles. VADs vary in design and technology. In general, they consist of an external pump, which diverts blood from the failing ventricle or ventricles and pumps it back into the aorta (left VAD [LVAD]), the pulmonary artery (right VAD [RVAD]), or both great vessels (Bi-VAD). The use of VADs requires extensive training and advanced nursing care. These devices are not typically available in community hospitals.

Obstructive Shock

Obstructive shock (also known as extracardiac obstructive shock) occurs when there is a physical impairment to adequate circulatory blood flow. Causes of obstructive shock include impaired diastolic filling (cardiac tamponade, tension pneumothorax, constrictive pericarditis, compression of the great veins), increased right ventricular afterload (pulmonary embolism, severe pulmonary hypertension, increased intrathoracic pressures), and increased left ventricular afterload (aortic dissection, systemic embolization, aortic stenosis). Obstruction of the heart or great vessels either impedes venous return to the right side of the heart or prevents effective pumping action of the heart. This results in decreased cardiac output, hypotension, decreased tissue perfusion, and impaired cellular metabolism (Figure 11-10).

Common clinical findings in obstructive shock include chest pain, dyspnea, jugular venous distention, and hypoxia. Other findings are dependent on the cause. Cardiac tamponade is manifested by muffled heart sounds, hypotension, and pulsus paradoxus. *Pulsus paradoxus* is a decrease in systolic blood pressure of more than 10 mm Hg during inspiration. Tension pneumothorax is manifested by diminished breath sounds on the affected side and tracheal shift away from the affected side. Massive pulmonary embolism is manifested by clinical indications of right ventricular failure (jugular venous distention, peripheral edema, hepatomegaly). Aortic dissection is manifested by complaints of ripping chest pain that radiates to the back, pulse differences between the left and right side, and a widened mediastinum on chest x-ray, echocardiogram, or computed tomography scan.

Obstructive shock may be prevented or treated, or both, by aggressive interventions to relieve the source of the compression or obstruction. Cardiac tamponade may be relieved by a *pericardiocentesis,* or the removal of fluid from the pericardial sac. A tension pneumothorax from blunt or penetrating chest injuries may be relieved by a needle *thoracentesis* to remove the accumulated intrathoracic pressure. The risk of pulmonary embolism may be reduced by early surgical reduction of long bone fractures, devices to enhance circulation in immobile patients (e.g., sequential compression devices), range-of-motion exercises, and prophylactic anticoagulant therapy.

Distributive Shock

Distributive shock, also known as vasogenic shock, describes several different types of shock that present with widespread vasodilation and decreased SVR. Neurogenic, anaphylactic, and septic shock are forms of distributive shock. Vasodilation increases the vascular capacity; however, the blood volume is unchanged, resulting in a relative hypovolemia. This causes a decrease in venous return to the right side of the heart and a reduction in ventricular filling pressures. Anaphylactic shock and septic shock are also complicated by an increase in capillary permeability, which decreases intravascular volume, further compromising venous return. Eventually, in all forms of distributive shock, stroke volume, cardiac output, and blood pressure decrease, resulting in decreased tissue perfusion and impaired cellular metabolism.

Neurogenic Shock

Neurogenic shock occurs when a disturbance in the nervous system affects the vasomotor center in the medulla. In healthy persons, the vasomotor center initiates sympathetic stimulation of nerve fibers that travel down the spinal cord and out to the periphery. There, they innervate the smooth muscles of the blood vessels to cause vasoconstriction. In neurogenic shock, there is an interruption of impulse transmission or a blockage of sympathetic outflow resulting in vasodilation, inhibition of baroreceptor response, and impaired thermoregulation. Consequently, these reactions create vasodilation with decreased SVR, venous return, preload, and cardiac output and a relative hypovolemia. Figure 11-11 summarizes the pathophysiology of neurogenic shock.

Causes of neurogenic shock include injury or disease of the upper spinal cord, spinal anesthesia, nervous system damage, administration of ganglionic and adrenergic blocking agents, and vasomotor depression. Patients who have a cervical spinal cord injury may experience a permanent or temporary interruption in sympathetic nerve stimulation. Spinal anesthesia may extend up the spinal cord and may block sympathetic nerve impulses from the vasomotor center. Vasomotor depression may be seen with deep general anesthesia, injury to the medulla, administration of drugs, severe pain, and hypoglycemia.

The most profound features of neurogenic shock are bradycardia with hypotension from the decreased sympathetic activity. The skin is frequently warm, dry, and flushed. Hypothermia develops from uncontrolled heat loss. Venous pooling in the lower extremities promotes the formation of deep vein thrombosis, which can result in pulmonary embolism. A neurological deficit may be evident.

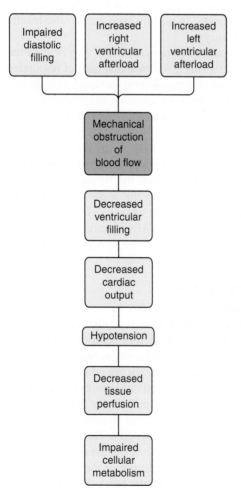

FIGURE 11-10 Obstructive shock.

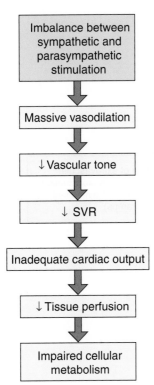

```
┌─────────────────────┐
│   Imbalance between  │
│    sympathetic and  │
│    parasympathetic  │
│      stimulation    │
└─────────────────────┘
          │
          ▼
┌─────────────────────┐
│  Massive vasodilation│
└─────────────────────┘
          │
          ▼
┌─────────────────────┐
│   ↓ Vascular tone   │
└─────────────────────┘
          │
          ▼
┌─────────────────────┐
│        ↓ SVR        │
└─────────────────────┘
          │
          ▼
┌─────────────────────┐
│ Inadequate cardiac output│
└─────────────────────┘
          │
          ▼
┌─────────────────────┐
│  ↓ Tissue perfusion │
└─────────────────────┘
          │
          ▼
┌─────────────────────┐
│   Impaired cellular │
│      metabolism     │
└─────────────────────┘
```

FIGURE 11-11 Neurogenic shock. *SVR,* Systemic vascular resistance. (From McCance KL, Huether SE. *Pathophysiology. The Biologic Basis for Disease in Adults and Children.* 6th ed. St. Louis: Mosby; 2010.)

Management focuses on treating the cause, including reversal of offending drugs or glucose administration for hypoglycemia. Immobilization of spinal injuries with traction devices (halo brace to maintain alignment) or surgical intervention to stabilize the injury assists in preventing severe neurogenic shock. For patients receiving spinal anesthesia, elevating the head of the bed may prevent the progression of the spinal blockade up the cord. IV fluids are infused to treat hypotension; however, they must be given cautiously to prevent fluid overload and cerebral or spinal cord edema.[6] Vasopressors are frequently required to maintain perfusion. Alpha- and beta-adrenergic agents, such as dopamine or norepinephrine, are preferred because pure alpha-adrenergic agents, such as phenylephrine, are associated with persistent bradycardia.[17] Hypothermia is common so the patient is rewarmed slowly, because rapid rewarming may cause vasodilation and worsen the patient's hemodynamic status. Atropine is used for symptomatic bradycardia; however, a temporary or permanent pacemaker may be required.

Anaphylactic Shock

A severe allergic reaction can precipitate a second form of distributive shock known as anaphylactic shock. Antigens, which are foreign substances to which someone is sensitive, initiate an antigen-antibody response. Table 11-5 lists some common antigens causing anaphylaxis.

Once an antigen enters the body, antibodies (immunoglobulin E [IgE]) are produced that attach to mast cells and basophils. The greatest concentrations of mast cells are found in the lungs, around blood vessels, in connective tissue, and in the uterus. Mast cells are also found to a lesser extent in the kidneys, heart, skin, liver, and spleen and in the omentum of the gastrointestinal tract. Basophils circulate in the blood. Both mast cells and basophils contain histamine and histamine-like substances, which are potent vasodilators.

The initial exposure (primary immune response) to the antigen does not usually cause any harmful effects; however, subsequent exposures to the antigen may cause an anaphylactic reaction (secondary immune response). The antigen-antibody reaction causes cellular breakdown and the release of powerful vasoactive mediators from the mast cells and basophils. These mediators cause bronchoconstriction, excessive mucus secretion, vasodilation, increased capillary permeability, inflammation, gastrointestinal cramps, and cutaneous reactions that stimulate nerve endings, causing itching and pain. Figure 11-12 summarizes the pathophysiology of anaphylactic shock. The combined effects result in decreased blood pressure, relative hypovolemia caused by the vasodilation and fluid shifts, and symptoms of anaphylaxis that primarily affect the skin, respiratory, and gastrointestinal systems.

Obtaining a thorough history of allergies and drug reactions, especially reactions to drugs with similar structures, is an important strategy to prevent anaphylactic shock. For example, if patients are allergic to penicillin, they are likely to have a reaction to ampicillin (Principen), carbenicillin (Geopen), or nafcillin sodium. The response to IV administration of medications, particularly antibiotics, is monitored. Injecting small amounts of a drug before the entire dose is given is recommended to assist in detecting a possible reaction. Care is taken during the transfusion of blood or blood products, which can result in allergic reactions. The patient receiving any of these products is observed closely for any signs of an allergic reaction.

The clinical presentation of anaphylactic shock includes flushing, pruritus, urticaria, and angioedema (swelling of eyes, lips, tongue, hands, feet, genitalia). Cough, runny nose, nasal congestion, hoarseness, dysphonia, and dyspnea are common because of upper airway obstruction from edema of the larynx, epiglottis, or vocal cords. Stridor may occur as a result of laryngeal edema. Lower airway obstruction may result from diffuse bronchoconstriction and cause wheezing and chest tightness. Tachycardia and hypotension occur, and the patient may show signs of pulmonary edema. Gastrointestinal symptoms of nausea, vomiting, cramping, abdominal pain, and diarrhea may also occur. Neurological symptoms include lethargy and decreased consciousness. Elevated levels of IgE are seen on laboratory analysis.

Goals of therapy are to remove the antigen, reverse the effects of the mediators, and promote adequate tissue perfusion. If the anaphylactic reaction results from medications, contrast dye, or blood or blood products, the infusion is immediately stopped. Airway, ventilation, and circulation are

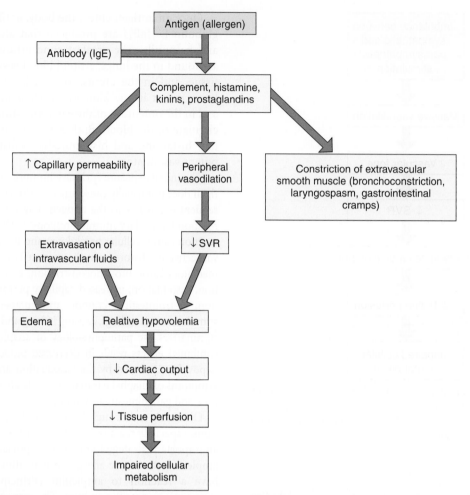

FIGURE 11-12 Anaphylactic shock. *IgE,* Immunoglobulin E; *SVR,* systemic vascular resistance. (From McCance KL, Huether SE. *Pathophysiology. The Biologic Basis for Disease in Adults and Children.* 6th ed. St. Louis: Mosby; 2010.)

supported. Laryngeal edema may be severe enough to require intubation or cricothyrotomy if swelling is so severe that an endotracheal tube cannot be placed. Oxygen is administered to keep the SpO_2 greater than 90%. Removal of the offending agent is achieved by removing the stinger, administering antivenom, stopping the drug, performing gastric lavage, or flushing the skin.[31]

Epinephrine is the drug of choice for treating anaphylactic shock. Epinephrine is an adrenergic agent that promotes bronchodilation and vasoconstriction. For mild reactions, epinephrine 0.1 to 0.25 mg (1.0 to 2.5 mL of a 1:10,000 solution) is administered intramuscularly or subcutaneously. The dose may be repeated at 20- to 30-minute intervals until anaphylaxis is resolved. To block histamine release, diphenhydramine (Benadryl), an H_1-receptor blocker, or ranitidine, an H_2-receptor blocker, may decrease some of the cutaneous symptoms of anaphylaxis, but both are considered second-line treatment.[31] Corticosteroids such as methylprednisolone (Solu-Medrol) are used to reduce inflammation. Fluid replacement, positive inotropic agents, and vasopressors may be required.

Septic Shock

Septic shock is one component of a continuum of progressive clinical insults including SIRS, sepsis, and MODS. In the past, there has been confusion about what these various syndromes represented. Because of this confusion and the complexity of these syndromes, consensus definitions were identified in 1992[8] and were reviewed in 2001.[21] The 2001 consensus group took the definitions a step further by identifying diagnostic criteria for sepsis. The intent of the criteria is to provide a tool to recognize and diagnose sepsis quickly, prompt the search for an infectious source, and to initiate the appropriate therapy. None of the diagnostic criteria are specific for sepsis because these parameters can be altered by other conditions. The definitions and diagnostic criteria are presented in Table 11-7. Invasion of the host by a microorganism or an infection begins the process that may progress to sepsis, followed by severe sepsis and septic shock, which progresses to MODS.

Once a microorganism has invaded a host, an inflammatory response is initiated to restore homeostasis. SIRS occurs, leading to release of inflammatory mediators or cytokines,

TABLE 11-7   CLINICAL CONDITION, DIAGNOSTIC CRITERIA, AND MANAGEMENT IN THE CONTINUUM OF SEPSIS

CLINICAL CONDITION AND DEFINITION	DIAGNOSTIC CRITERIA	MANAGEMENT
Infection: Inflammatory response to microorganisms	Fever	Administer antibiotics Surgical excision or drainage of source of infection
SIRS: Systemic inflammatory response to a clinical insult including infection, pancreatitis, ischemia, trauma, or hemorrhagic shock	Tachycardia (HR ≥90 beats/min) Respiratory rate >20 breaths/min or $PaCO_2$ <32 mm Hg Temperature >38° C (hyperthermia) or <36° C (hypothermia)	Administer antibiotics Remove source of infection Maintain adequate ventilation and oxygenation Replace fluid
Sepsis: Systemic response to infection manifested by two or more of the symptoms noted with SIRS	Leukocytosis (WBC count >12,000 cells/microliter) or leukopenia (WBC count <4000 cells/microliter) or >10% immature bands	Antipyretics
Severe sepsis: Sepsis associated with organ dysfunction.	As above with evidence of impaired systemic perfusion and organ function, possibly including lactic acidosis, oliguria, or acute change in mental status	Administer antibiotics Remove source of infection Maintain adequate ventilation and oxygenation Maximize oxygen delivery; minimize oxygen demand Replace fluid Administer vasoactive medications Correct acid-base abnormalities Monitor and support organ function Consider hydrocortisone if poor response to fluids and vasoactive medication[12]
Septic shock: Sepsis with hypotension despite adequate fluid resuscitation, along with perfusion abnormalities	Hypotension Lactic acidosis, oliguria, acute change in mental status Patients receiving inotropic agents or vasopressors may not exhibit hypotension	Administer antibiotics Maintain adequate ventilation and oxygenation Maximize oxygen delivery; minimize oxygen demand Replace fluid Administer vasoactive medications Correct acid-base abnormalities Monitor and support organ function Consider hydrocortisone if poor response to fluids and vasoactive medication[12]
MODS: Altered organ function in acutely ill patients	See Table 11-9	Maintain adequate ventilation and oxygenation Maximize oxygen delivery; minimize oxygen demand Perform dialysis Monitor and support organ function Monitor clotting studies and bleeding

HR, Heart rate; *MODS,* multiple organ dysfunction syndrome; *PaCO2,* partial pressure of arterial carbon dioxide; *SIRS,* systemic inflammatory response syndrome; *WBC,* white blood cell.
Definitions modified from Dellinger RP, Levy MM, Carlet JM, Bion J, Parker M, Jaeschke R, et al. Surviving Sepsis Campaign: International guidelines for management of severe sepsis and septic shock: 2008. *Critical Care Medicine,* 2008;36(1), 298-327.

which are produced by the white blood cells. SIRS can also occur as a result of trauma, shock, pancreatitis, or ischemia.[12] For reasons not completely understood, SIRS may progress to septic shock and MODS (Figure 11-13). Cytokines are proinflammatory or antiinflammatory. Proinflammatory cytokines including tumor necrosis factor, interleukin-1α, and

interleukin-β produce pyrogenic responses and initiate the hepatic response to infection. Antiinflammatory cytokines including nitric oxide, lipopolysaccharide, and interleukin-1–receptor antagonist are compensatory, ensuring that the effect of the proinflammatory mediators does not become destructive. In sepsis, continued activation of proinflammatory

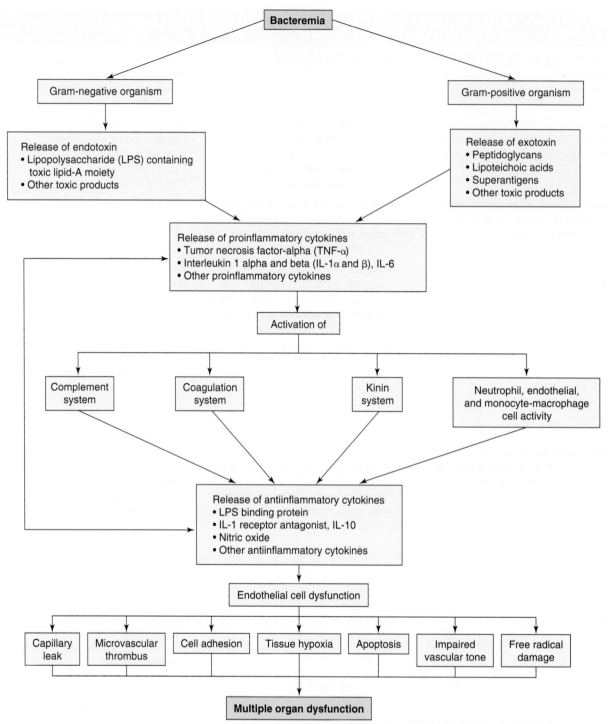

FIGURE 11-13 Sepsis and septic shock pathophysiology. (Modified from McCance KL, Huether SE. *Pathophysiology. The Biologic Basis for Disease in Adults and Children.* 6th ed. St. Louis: Mosby; 2010.)

cytokines overwhelms the antiinflammatory cytokines and excessive systemic inflammation results.

A state of enhanced coagulation occurs through stimulation of the coagulation cascade, with a reduction in the levels of activated protein C and antithrombin III. This results in the generation of thrombin and the formation of microemboli that impair blood flow and organ perfusion.

Fibrinolysis is activated in response to the activation of the coagulation cascade to promote clot breakdown. However, activation is followed by inhibition, further promoting coagulopathy. This imbalance among inflammation, coagulation, and fibrinolysis results in systemic inflammation, widespread coagulopathy, and microvascular thrombi that impair tissue perfusion, leading to MODS.

TABLE 11-8 **STAGES OF SEPTIC SHOCK**	
EARLY (HYPERDYNAMIC; LOOKS LIKE INFECTION)	**LATE (HYPODYNAMIC; LOOKS LIKE SHOCK)**
Clinical Presentation	
Tachycardia	Tachycardia
Pulses bounding	Pulses weak and thready
Blood pressure: normal or low	Hypotension
Wide pulse pressure	Narrow pulse pressure
Skin warm, flushed	Skin cool, pale
Hyperpnea	Bradypnea or tachypnea
Change in mental status (irritability and confusion)	↓ Level of consciousness (lethargy or coma)
Oliguria	Anuria
Hyperthermia	Hypothermia
Hemodynamic Parameters	
↑ CO/CI	↓ CO/CI
↓ RAP/PAP/PAOP	RAP/PAP/PAOP variable
↓ SVR	SVR variable
↑ SvO₂	↓ SvO₂
Diagnostic Findings	
ABGs: respiratory alkalosis with hypoxemia	ABGs: metabolic acidosis with hypoxemia
↑ PT and aPTT	↑ PT and aPTT
↓ Platelets	↓ Platelets
↑ WBC count	↓ WBC count
↑ Glucose	↓ Glucose
	↑ BUN, creatinine
	↑ Serum arterial lactate
	↑ Amylase, lipase
	↑ AST, ALT, LDH

ABGs, Arterial blood gases; *ALT,* alanine aminotransferase; *aPTT,* activated partial thromboplastin time; *AST,* aspartate aminotransferase; *BUN,* blood urea nitrogen; *CI,* cardiac index; *CO,* cardiac output; *LDH,* lactic dehydrogenase; *PAOP,* pulmonary artery occlusion pressure; *PAP,* pulmonary artery pressure; *PT,* prothrombin time; *RAP,* right atrial pressure; *SvO₂,* oxygen saturation of venous blood; *SVR,* systemic vascular resistance; *WBC,* white blood cell.

These inflammatory mediators also damage the endothelial cells that line blood vessels, producing profound vasodilation and increased capillary permeability. Initially, this results in tachycardia, hypotension, and low SVR. Although norepinephrine and the renin-angiotensin-aldosterone system are activated in response to this clinical state, they are unable to enter the cells, and hypotension and vasodilation persist. In contrast, the plasma levels of the antidiuretic hormone (ADH or vasopressin) are low despite the presence of hypotension. The exact mechanism that creates this low concentration is not known; however, administering a continuous vasopressin infusion significantly increases blood pressure in septic shock.[20]

Once sepsis is present, it can progress to septic shock. Septic shock is sepsis with hypotension that is unresponsive to fluid resuscitation along with signs of inadequate organ perfusion such as metabolic acidosis, acute encephalopathy, oliguria, hypoxemia, or coagulation disorders. The clinical course of septic shock is frequently differentiated between the early (warm, hyperdynamic) phase and the late (cold, hypodynamic) phase (Table 11-8).

Factors that increase the risk of developing sepsis are categorized as either situations that cause immunosuppression or situations that cause significant bacteremia (see Table 11-5). Sepsis is infection with SIRS and is the systemic response to infection. SIRS is present if two or more of the clinical manifestations of SIRS are identified (see Table 11-7). Sepsis can advance to severe sepsis with hypotension, chills, decreased urine output, decreased skin perfusion, poor capillary refill, skin mottling, decreased platelets, petechiae, hyperglycemia, and unexplained changes in mental status.[14]

Prevention of sepsis is promoted by preventing infections, including proper hand washing, use of aseptic technique, and awareness of the patient at risk. The critically ill patient is debilitated and has many potential portals of entry for bacterial invasion. Meticulous technique is required during procedures such as suctioning, dressing changes, and wound care and when handling catheters or tubes. Frequent assessment of temperature, wounds, and laboratory results including white blood cell count, differential counts, and cultures is important for the identification of infection.

Gram-negative bacteria such as *Escherichia coli,* *Klebsiella* species, or *Pseudomonas* species are a common cause of infections in adults. Common sites of infection include the pulmonary system, urinary tract, gastrointestinal system, and wounds. Urinary tract infection is an often overlooked cause of secondary bloodstream infections. Minimizing the use of indwelling catheters by assessing daily their need and promptly removing unnecessary catheters is recommended.[25,28]

Gram-positive bacteria such as *Staphylococcus aureus* can also lead to sepsis and septic shock. These bacteria release a potent toxin that exerts its effects within hours. Gram-positive infection has been associated with the use of tampons in menstruating women (known as toxic shock syndrome); however, it is also seen after vaginal and cesarean delivery and in patients with surgical wounds, abscesses, infected burns, abrasions, insect bites, herpes zoster, cellulitis, septic abortion, and osteomyelitis. In addition, the bacteria may be transmitted from mother to newborn. Management includes antimicrobial therapy, removal of the source of infection if one is found, fluid resuscitation, and vasoactive medication to improve cardiac performance.

Pneumonia is a common trigger for sepsis. Ventilator-associated pneumonia (VAP) is a significant risk factor for the development of sepsis. Several strategies have been identified that reduce the risk of ventilator-associated pneumonia and are easily implemented. These include providing regular oral care with chlorhexidine-based antiseptic to intubated patients, and reducing the number of ventilator circuit changes.[1,3,12] VAP prevention measures also include venous thromboembolism (VTE) prophylaxis, stress ulcer prophylaxis, and ventilator weaning trials. This capacity is assessed with a "sedation vacation," a planned holding of sedation to evaluate the patient's ability to wean from the ventilator. Another strategy is the use of an endotracheal tube with a dorsal lumen to allow continuous suction of secretions from the subglottic area.[15]

Timely identification of the causative organism and the initiation of appropriate antibiotics improve survival of patients with sepsis or septic shock.[16] Any catheter suspected to be a source of infection should be removed. Surgery may be required to locate the source of infection, drain an abscess, and/or debride any necrosis.

Before antibiotic therapy is initiated, culture and sensitivity tests of blood, urine, sputum, wound, tip of a catheter, and any suspicious site are obtained. This helps to identify the source of the infection, the type of organisms, and which antibiotics should be used.[27] However, the need for early administration of antibiotics, preferably within 1 hour, requires the initial antibiotic selection be directed toward the most likely organism, and frequently, empirical and broad-spectrum antibiotics are initiated.[12] Antibiotics may be changed after Gram stain results (approximately 4 hours) or culture and sensitivity results (approximately 72 hours) are available. Antibiotics are discontinued if the cause of the sepsis is not bacterial. Unfortunately, antibiotics do not act on the immune response to infection and do not directly improve tissue perfusion.

Early goal-directed therapy has been shown to decrease mortality in patients with severe sepsis and septic shock and

is advocated for the first 6 hours of sepsis resuscitation.[29,36] Early goal-directed therapy includes administration of IV fluids to keep the central venous pressure at 8 mm Hg or greater (but not >15 mm Hg) and the heart rate at less than 110 beats per minute, administration of vasopressors to keep the mean arterial pressure at 65 mm Hg or greater, and administration of dobutamine, packed red blood cells, or both to keep the central venous oxygen saturation (ScvO$_2$) at 70% or greater.[12,36,40]

Isotonic crystalloid solutions are infused for fluid resuscitation. Colloids are likely to leak out of the vascular bed into the interstitium because of increased capillary permeability. Vasopressors, frequently norepinephrine or dopamine, are used to increase SVR and mean arterial pressure. Vasopressin may be added to norepinephrine, especially when high doses of norepinephrine are required.[23] Advantages of vasopressin include decreasing exogenous catecholamines and increasing the release of cortisol and ACTH.[20] In addition, vasopressin causes vasoconstriction without the adverse effects of tachycardia and ventricular ectopy seen with catecholamines such as dopamine or norepinephrine. Dobutamine may be used to increase the myocardial contractility and improve the cardiac index and DO$_2$ in patients with a decreased ScvO$_2$. If the patient's hematocrit is less than 30%, the administration of packed red blood cells is advocated to increase DO$_2$.[32]

Elevated cardiac troponin levels and elevated brain natriuretic peptide (BNP) indicate left ventricular dysfunction and a poor prognosis in patients with sepsis and septic shock.[22,38] ACTH-stimulated cortisol levels may be measured because poor ACTH-cortisol responses are associated with a high mortality.[11] Corticosteroids have been shown to reduce mortality for those patients with sepsis or septic shock who have an inadequate response to the ACTH stimulation test.[5] Routine use of corticosteroids, however, is not recommended because of the effects on glucose homeostasis, the risk for infection, and the potential for myopathy.[34]

In severe sepsis, the patient has excessive coagulation, inflammation, and impaired fibrinolysis. Recombinant human activated protein C (drotrecogin alfa [Xigris]) is an antiinflammatory, antithrombotic, and profibrinolytic agent that reduces the inflammatory, clotting, and bleeding responses to sepsis. It has been shown to reduce mortality in patients with severe sepsis with dysfunction of two organ systems.[7] Continued evaluation has failed to show a survival benefit for patients with severe sepsis and septic shock. The manufacturer announced a voluntary recall from the market in October 2011 (www.fda.gov/Drugs/DrugSafety/ucm277114.htm).

Hyperglycemia and insulin resistance are common in the patient with sepsis. The effect is even more significant in patients with MODS caused by sepsis.[37] Guidelines published in 2008[12] recommend frequent glucose testing and intensive IV insulin protocols to maintain blood glucose levels at less than 150 mg/dL. Data from the NICE-SUGAR trial[24] suggest that the target be less than 180 mg/dL. On the basis of those results, normal blood glucose levels may not be the clinical goal.

Although pyrogens (polypeptides that produce fever) aid in activation of the immune response, temperature reduction is considered for core body temperatures of 41° C or higher because of the significant increase in oxygen consumption. Treatment of fever includes physiological cooling (ice packs, tepid baths, cooling blanket, or misting) along with administration of antipyretics (acetaminophen, ibuprofen, or aspirin). Care must be taken to avoid overcooling because hypothermia adversely affects oxygen delivery and may result in shivering, which increases oxygen consumption.

Many experimental therapies have been advocated for sepsis and septic shock. Plasmapheresis may remove endotoxin and other harmful substances produced by either the infective organism or the inflammatory process.[19] Immunoglobulins may also be prescribed, especially in patients who are immunocompromised.[19]

MULTIPLE ORGAN DYSFUNCTION SYNDROME

MODS is the progressive dysfunction of two or more organ systems as a result of an uncontrolled inflammatory response to severe illness or injury. Organ dysfunction can progress to organ failure and death. The most common causes of MODS are sepsis and septic shock; however, MODS can occur after any severe injury or disease process that activates a massive systemic inflammatory response including any classification of shock. The immune system and the body's response to stress can cause maldistribution of circulating volume, global tissue hypoxia, and metabolic alterations that result in damage to organs. Failure of two or more organs is associated with an estimated 45% to 55% mortality, 80% mortality when three or more organ systems fail, and 100% mortality if three or more organ systems fail for longer than 4 days.[4]

Damage to organs may be primary or secondary. In *primary MODS* there is direct injury to an organ from shock, trauma, burn injury, or infection with impaired perfusion that results in dysfunction. Decreased perfusion may be localized or systemic. As a result of this insult, the stress response and inflammatory response are activated with the release of catecholamines and activation of mediators that affect cellular activity (Figure 11-14).

Secondary MODS is a consequence of widespread systemic inflammation that results in dysfunction of organs not involved with the initial insult. It occurs in response to altered regulation of the acute immune and inflammatory responses. Failure to control the inflammatory response leads to excessive production of inflammatory cells and biochemical mediators that cause widespread damage to vascular endothelium and organ damage. The interaction of injured organs then leads to self-perpetuating inflammation with maldistribution of blood flow and hypermetabolism.

Maldistribution of blood flow refers to the uneven distribution of flow to various organs and between the large vessels

and capillary beds. It is caused by vasodilation, increased capillary permeability, selective vasoconstriction, and impaired microvascular circulation. This impaired blood flow leads to impaired tissue perfusion and a decreased oxygen supply to the cells. The organs most severely affected are the lungs, splanchnic bed, liver, and kidneys.

Hypermetabolism with altered carbohydrate, fat, and lipid metabolism is initially compensatory to meet the body's increased demands for energy. Eventually, hypermetabolism becomes detrimental, placing tremendous demands on the heart as cardiac output increases up to twice the normal value. Hyperglycemia occurs as gluconeogenesis by the liver increases and glucose use by the cells decreases.

The decreased oxygen delivery to the cells (from maldistribution of blood flow) and increased oxygen needs of the cells (from hypermetabolism) create an imbalance in oxygen supply and demand. In MODS, the amount of oxygen consumed becomes dependent on the amount of oxygen that can be delivered to the cells. Hypoxemia, cellular acidosis, and impaired cellular function result with the development of multiple organ failure.

The clinical presentation of MODS is caused by inflammatory mediator damage, tissue hypoxia, and hypermetabolism. Damage to the organs is usually sequential rather than simultaneous. The first system frequently affected is the pulmonary system, with acute ARDS developing within 12 to 24 hours after the initial insult. Coagulopathy frequently develops, followed by renal, hepatic, and intestinal impairment.[33] Failure of the cardiovascular system, neurological system, or both, are frequently fatal events. MODS progresses from minor dysfunction of one or multiple organs to multiple organs requiring support.

Criteria used in the diagnoses of organ dysfunction are described in Table 11-9. Pulmonary dysfunction is manifested by tachypnea, hypoxemia despite high levels of supplemental oxygen, and chest x-ray changes. Hematological dysfunction is manifested by petechiae, bleeding, thrombocytopenia, prolonged PT and aPTT, increased fibrin split products, and a positive D-dimer. The earliest sign of hepatic dysfunction is hypoglycemia, which is followed by jaundice, increased liver enzymes and bilirubin, prolonged PT, and decreased albumin. The first indication of intestinal dysfunction is frequently intolerance of enteral feedings with abdominal distention and increased retention volumes. Renal dysfunction is evidenced by oliguria to anuria, increased blood urea nitrogen and creatinine, and fluid and electrolyte imbalance. Tachycardia (frequently with dysrhythmias), hypotension, and hemodynamic alterations indicate cardiovascular dysfunction. Finally, cerebral dysfunction is manifested by a change in level of consciousness, confusion, and focal neurological signs such as hemiparesis. The final response to MODS is hypotension that is unresponsive to fluids and vasopressors, and cardiac arrest.

Management of MODS focuses on prevention and support. The initial source of inflammation must be eliminated or controlled. A secondary insult must be avoided. Potential

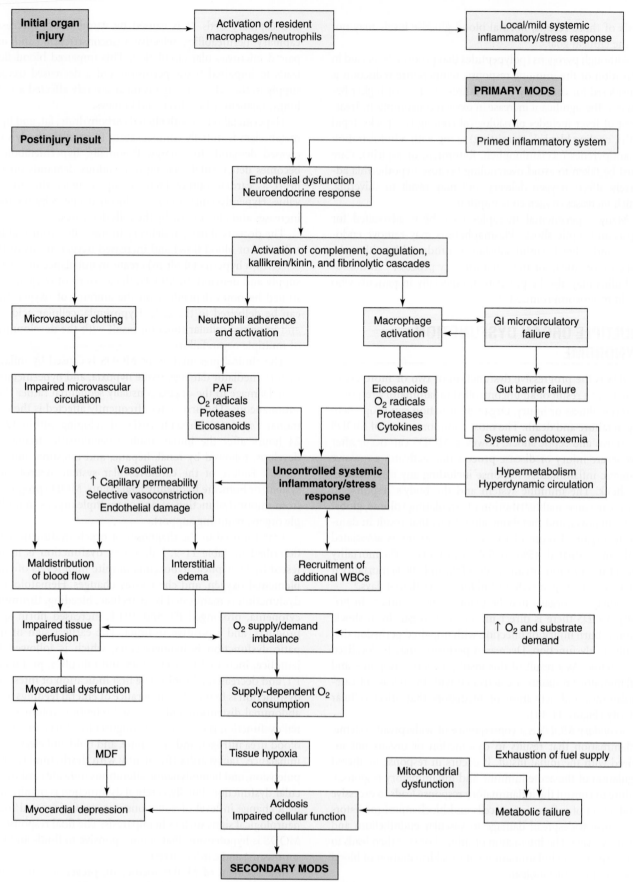

FIGURE 11-14 Pathogenesis of multiple organ dysfunction syndrome. *GI,* Gastrointestinal; *MDF,* myocardial depressant factor; *MODS,* multiple organ dysfunction syndrome; *PAF,* platelet activating factor; *WBCs,* white blood cells. (Modified from McCance KL, Huether SE. *Pathophysiology. The Biologic Basis for Disease in Adults and Children.* 6th ed. St. Louis: Mosby; 2010.)

TABLE 11-9	MULTIPLE ORGAN DYSFUNCTION SYNDROME	
SYSTEM	**DYSFUNCTION**	**CLINICAL PRESENTATION**
Pulmonary	Acute respiratory distress syndrome	Predisposing factor such as shock or sepsis Unexplained hypoxemia ($\downarrow$ PaO_2, $\downarrow$ SaO_2) Dyspnea Tachypnea PaO_2/FiO_2 ratio <300 for acute lung injury and <200 for ARDS Bilateral pulmonary infiltrates on chest x-ray PAOP <18 mm Hg
Cardiovascular	Hyperdynamic or hypodynamic	See Table 11-8
Hematological	Disseminated intravascular coagulation	Fibrin split products >1:40 or D-dimer >2 mg/L Thrombocytopenia Prolonged PT and aPTT INR >1.5 Bleeding Petechiae
Renal	Acute tubular necrosis	Oliguria $\uparrow$ Serum creatinine, $\uparrow$ BUN Urinary sodium >20 mEq/L
Liver	Hepatic dysfunction/failure	$\uparrow$ Serum bilirubin $\uparrow$ AST, ALT, LDH Jaundice Hepatomegaly $\uparrow$ Serum ammonia $\downarrow$ Serum albumin
Central nervous system	Cerebral ischemia/infarction	Lethargy Altered level of consciousness Fever
Metabolic	Lactic acidosis	$\uparrow$ Serum lactate level

ALT, Alanine transaminase; *aPTT*, activated partial thromboplastin time; *AST*, aspartate transaminase; *BUN*, blood urea nitrogen; *FiO₂*, fraction of inspired oxygen; *INR*, international normalized ratio; *LDH*, lactic dehydrogenase; *PaO₂*, partial pressure of arterial oxygen; *PAOP*, pulmonary artery occlusion pressure; *PT*, prothrombin time; *SaO₂*, arterial oxygen saturation.

sites of infection are removed, including debriding necrotic tissue, draining abscesses, reducing the number of invasive procedures performed, and removing hematomas. Goals are to control infection, provide adequate tissue oxygenation, restore intravascular volume, and support organ function. Antibiotics are administered. SpO_2 is maintained between 88% and 92%, hemoglobin levels should be above 7 to 9 g/dL, and an SvO_2 greater than 70% is desired. Aggressive fluid therapy with isotonic crystalloid solutions is initiated early during systemic vasodilation to promote oxygen delivery to the tissues.

Support for each organ must be provided. Respiratory failure is managed with mechanical ventilation with low tidal volumes, high oxygen concentrations, and positive end-expiratory pressures (see Chapter 14). Adequate nutrition and metabolic support is provided with enteral feedings

(see Chapter 6). Acute kidney injury is managed with continuous renal replacement therapies or hemodialysis (see Chapter 15). Inotropic drugs (low-dose dopamine or dobutamine) or vasopressors (norepinephrine or vasopressin) may be needed to maximize cardiac contractility and maintain cardiac output.

PATIENT OUTCOMES

The expected outcome for the patient in shock is that the patient will have improved tissue perfusion. Specific patient outcomes include alertness and orientation; normotension; warm, dry skin; adequate urine output; hemodynamic and laboratory values within normal limits; absence of infection; and intact skin. The patient should be resting quietly.

CASE STUDY

Mr. R., a 33-year-old man, was involved in a motor vehicle crash in which he sustained chest injuries. Mr. R., the driver, was not wearing his seat belt, and the steering wheel was bent. At the scene, Mr. R. was unresponsive. After placing a cervical collar to stabilize his neck, the paramedics performed endotracheal intubation and provided ventilation with 100% oxygen via a bag-valve device. Vital signs included a palpable systolic blood pressure (BP) of 60 mm Hg and a heart rate of 136 beats per minute. Mr. R.'s skin was pale, cold, and clammy with a delay in capillary refill. Peripheral pulses were weak and thready. Two 14-gauge peripheral intravenous catheters were inserted, and lactated Ringer's solution was infused at a wide open rate. He was transported to the emergency department on a backboard. The initial assessment in the emergency department noted that his palpable BP had increased to 90 mm Hg, and heart rate was 125 beats per minute. He was restless in response to pain, with no other purposeful responses. Pupils were equal and reactive to light. Chest expansion was unequal, and breath sounds were markedly diminished on the right side. A chest x-ray documented a 70% hemopneumothorax on the right side, and a 36-French chest tube was inserted at the eighth intercostal space at the right midaxillary line. Immediately, 2000 mL of blood was drained from the chest, and an additional 500 mL of drainage was recorded in the next 30 minutes. Initial laboratory results were:

Hemoglobin: 9 g/dL
Prothrombin time: 15 seconds
Hematocrit: 31%
Partial thromboplastin time: 47 seconds
Platelets: 274,000/microliter
Red blood cells: 2.9 million/microliter
White blood cells: 5300/microliter

An indwelling urinary catheter was inserted, and 80 mL of clear, yellow urine immediately drained. Fluid resuscitation was continued to maintain a systolic BP at 90 to 100 mm Hg. Mr. R. was taken immediately to the operating room, where a right thoracotomy was performed, with repair of the right axillary artery. In the operating room, his vital signs remained stable with continued fluid resuscitation of crystalloids, blood, and fresh frozen plasma.

After surgery, he was admitted to the critical care unit, where his BP was 116/70 mm Hg, heart rate was 90 beats per minute, and respiration rate was 24 breaths per minute on the ventilator (assist/control mode with a rate of 20 breaths per minute). He was responsive to commands and denied pain. He was medicated with morphine, 4 mg intravenous push every hour for pain. Laboratory results were:

Hemoglobin: 11 g/dL
Prothrombin time: 18.7 seconds
Hematocrit: 34%
Partial thromboplastin time: 71.7 seconds
Platelets: 180,000/microliter
Fibrinogen: 76 mg/dL
Red blood cells: 4.8 million/microliter
White blood cells: 5300/microliter

Arterial blood gases (on assisted ventilation with FiO_2 0.60):
pH: 7.30
$PaCO_2$: 40 mm Hg
PaO_2: 90 mm Hg
SaO_2: 92%
HCO_3^-: 17 mEq/L

Questions

1. What type of shock did Mr. R. demonstrate at the scene, and what components of his assessment supported this diagnosis?
2. Mr. R.'s initial assessment indicates that he is in which stage of shock?
3. In the emergency department, Mr. R. received lactated Ringer's solution for fluid resuscitation. Is this the appropriate solution at this time?
4. Explain Mr. R.'s arterial blood gas results. What treatment is indicated?
5. Describe the nursing care Mr. R. will receive in the first 24 hours after his surgery.
6. Describe the risk factors Mr. R. has for developing sepsis.

▌ S U M M A R Y

The risk of shock is a common threat for all patients. Its causes are many, and treatment for shock is varied and complex. Complications of shock are related to the metabolic and tissue changes that result. If the normal compensatory mechanisms are not supported by effective therapeutic interventions, the pathological consequences perpetuate a vicious cycle of shock. The cycle is initiated by ischemia to the cells. Ischemia results in anaerobic metabolism, which leads to an accumulation of lactic acid and metabolic acidosis. This acidosis potentially leads to irreversible changes in the cells, organ failure, multiorgan failure, and death.

Prevention is the primary goal; it is accomplished through the identification of high-risk patient conditions and early interventions. Successful management relies on accurate nursing assessments, data analysis, implementation of definitive interventions, and evaluation of patient response to treatment. Shock is a crisis for the patient, family, nurse, and healthcare team. A multiprofessional approach of clinical expertise combined with caring assists the patient in reaching a positive outcome.

CRITICAL THINKING EXERCISES

1. Several people are admitted to the critical care unit, including (1) a 79-year-old man with a small anterior myocardial infarction and no prior cardiac history, (2) a 47-year-old man being given contrast media during a diagnostic procedure, (3) a 17-year-old adolescent with a cervical spine injury after a diving accident, and (4) a 72-year-old woman who was admitted with a bowel perforation caused by intestinal malignancy. Discuss what additional assessment information is needed to determine which of these patients has the potential to develop shock and the rationale for your decision.

2. A patient was admitted from the emergency department after a motorcycle crash in which he sustained blunt abdominal trauma. IV access was established in the internal jugular and left antecubital veins, and lactated Ringer's solution was infused. The results of initial computed tomography scan of the abdomen were negative. On admission to the critical care unit, you review the results of the hematological profile. Explain the rationale for the alterations in these values.
   a. Hemoglobin: 9.1 g/dL
   b. Hematocrit: 31.1%
   c. Platelets: 274,000/microliter
   d. Red blood cells: 2.9 million/microliter
   e. White blood cells: 9800/microliter
   f. Prothrombin time: 15 seconds
   g. Activated partial thromboplastin time: 38 seconds

3. Describe factors in the critically ill patient that increase susceptibility to the development of severe sepsis and septic shock. Describe how these can be prevented.

4. Differentiate between the early, hyperdynamic phase and the late, hypodynamic phase of septic shock.

5. Which type of shock is associated with the following hemodynamic changes?
   a. Bradycardia, decreased SVR, decreased SvO_2
   b. Increased RAP, PAP, PAOP, increased SVR, increased SvO_2
   c. Tachycardia, decreased SVR, increased SvO_2
   d. Decreased RAP, PAP, PAOP, increased SVR, decreased SvO_2
   e. Tachycardia, decreased SVR, decreased SvO_2

REFERENCES

1. Ahrens T, Vollman K. Severe sepsis management: are we doing enough? *Critical Care Nurse*. 2003;23(suppl 5):2-15.
2. Aitken L, Williams G, Harvey M, et al (2011). Nursing considerations to complement the Surviving Sepsis Campaign guidelines. *Critical Care Medicine*. 2011;39(7):1800-1818.
3. American College of Surgeons' Committee on Trauma. *Advanced Trauma Life Support (ATLS) for Doctors Student Manual*. 8th ed. Chicago: American College of Surgeons; 2008.
4. Angus DC, Linde-Zwirble WT, Lidicker J, et al. (2001). Epidemiology of severe sepsis in the United States: analysis of incidence, outcome, and associated costs of care. *Critical Care Medicine*. 2001;29(7):1303-1310.
5. Annane D, Sebille V, Charpentier C, et al. Effect of treatment with low doses of hydrocortisone and fludrocortisone on mortality in patients with septic shock. *Journal of the American Medical Association*. 2002;288(7):862-871.
6. Barker E. *Neuroscience Nursing. A Spectrum of Care*. 3rd ed. St. Louis: Mosby; 2007.
7. Bernard GR, Vincent J-L, Laterre P-F, et al. Efficacy and safety of recombinant human activated protein C for severe sepsis. *New England Journal of Medicine*. 2001;344(10):699-709.
8. Bone R, Sprung C, Sibbald W. Definitions for sepsis and organ failure. *Critical Care Medicine*. 1992;20(6):724.
9. Cochrane Injuries Group Albumin Reviewers. Human albumin administration in critically ill patients: systematic review of randomized controlled trials. *British Medical Journal*. 1998;317:235-240.
10. Cottingham C. Resuscitation of traumatic shock. *AACN Advanced Critical Care*. 2006;17(3):317-326.
11. deJong MFC, Beishuizen A, Spijkstra J-J, et al. Relative adrenal insufficiency as a predictor of disease severity, mortality, and beneficial effects of corticosteroid therapy in septic shock. *Critical Care Medicine*. 2007;35(8):1-8.
12. Dellinger RP, Levy MM, Carlet JM, et al. Surviving Sepsis Campaign: international guidelines for management of severe sepsis and septic shock: 2008. *Critical Care Medicine*. 2008;36(1):298-327.
13. Goldberg RJ, Spencer FA, Gore JM, et al. Thirty-year trends (1975 to 2005) in the magnitude of, management of, and hospital death rates associated with cardiogenic shock in patients with acute myocardial infarction: a population-based perspective. *Circulation*. 2009;119(9):1211.
14. Kleinpell RM. The role of the critical care nurse in the assessment and management of the patient with severe sepsis. *Critical Care Nursing Clinics of North America*. 2003;15(1):27-34.
15. Kollef MH. Prevention of hospital-associated pneumonia and ventilator-associated pneumonia. *Critical Care Medicine*. 2004;32(6):1396-1405.
16. Kortgen A, Niederprum P, Bauer M. Implementation of an evidence-based "standard operating procedure" and outcome in septic shock. *Critical Care Medicine*. 2006;34(3):943-949.
17. Kruse JA, Fink MP, Carlson RW. *Saunders Manual of Critical Care*. Philadelphia: Saunders; 2003.
18. Kushner FG, Hand M, Smith SC, et al. 2009 focused updates: ACC/AHA guidelines for the management of patients with ST-elevation myocardial infarction (updating the 2004 guideline and 2007 focused update) and ACC/AHA/SCAI guidelines on percutaneous coronary intervention (updating the 2005 guideline and 2007 focused update) a report of the American College of Cardiology Foundation/American Heart Association Task Force on Practice Guidelines). *Journal of the American College of Cardiology*, 2009;54(23):2205-2241.

19. Kyles DM, Baltimore J. Adjunctive use of plasmapheresis and intravenous immunoglobulin therapy in sepsis: a case report. *American Journal of Critical Care.* 2005;14(2):109-112.

20. Lee CS. Role of exogenous arginine vasopressin in the management of catecholamine-refractory septic shock. *Critical Care Nurse.* 2006;26(6):17-23.

21. Levy MM, Fink MP, Marshall JC, et al. 2001 SCCM/ESICM/ACCP/ATS/SIS International Sepsis Definitions Conference. *Critical Care Medicine.* 2003;31(4):1250-1256.

22. Maeder M, Fehr T, Rickli H, et al. Sepsis-associated myocardial dysfunction: diagnostic and prognostic impact of cardiac troponins and natriuretic peptides. *Chest.* 2006;129(5):1349-1366.

23. Moore FA, McKinley BA, Moore EE. The next generation in shock resuscitation. *Lancet.* 2004;363:1988-1996.

24. NICE-SUGAR Study Investigators. Finfer S, Chittock DR, Su SY, et al. *New England Journal of Medicine.* 2009;360(13):1283-1297.

25. O'Grady N, Alexander M, Burns L, et al. Guidelines for the Prevention of Intravascular Catheter-Related Infections. *Clinical Infectious Diseases.* 2011;52(9):1087-1099.

26. Perel P, Roberts I. Colloids versus crystalloids for fluid resuscitation in critically ill patients. *Cochrane Database Systematic Review.* 2007;(3):CD000567.

27. Picard KM, O'Donoghue SC, Young-Kershaw DA, et al. Development and implementation of a multidisciplinary sepsis protocol. *Critical Care Nurse.* 2006;26(3):43-54.

28. Rebmann T, Greene LR. Preventing catheter-associated urinary tract infections: an executive summary of the Association for Professionals in Infection Control and Epidemiology, Inc., Elimination Guide. *American Journal of Infection Control.* 2010;38(8):644-646.

29. Rivers E, Nguyen B, Havstad S, et al. Early goal-directed therapy in the treatment of severe sepsis and septic shock. *New England Journal of Medicine.* 2001;345(19):1368-1377.

30. Rivers EP, Ander DS, Powell D. Central venous oxygen saturation monitoring in the critically ill patient. *Current Opinion in Critical Care.* 2001;7(3):204-211.

31. Sampson H. Second symposium on the definition and management of anaphylaxis: summary report. *Journal of Allergy and Clinical Immunology.* 2006;117(2)

32. Shapiro NI, Howell MD, Talmor D, et al. Implementation and outcomes of the Multiple Urgent Sepsis Therapies (MUST) protocol. *Critical Care Medicine.* 2006;34(4):1025-1032.

33. Sharma S, Kumar A. Septic shock, multiple organ failure, and acute respiratory distress syndrome. *Current Opinion in Pulmonary Medicine.* 2003;(3):199-209.

34. Shorr A. *Clinical Challenges in Critical Care Medicine. Managing Severe Sepsis.* CME activity adapted from American Thoracic Society (ATS) 103rd International Conference May 18-23, 2007, San Francisco, CA. Available at www.medscape.com/viewprogram/7302_pnt; 2007 Accessed November 25, 2007.

35. The Acute Respiratory Distress Syndrome Network. Ventilation with lower tidal volumes as compared with traditional tidal volumes for acute lung injury and the acute respiratory distress syndrome. *New England Journal of Medicine.* 2000;342:1301-1308.

36. Trzeciak S, Dellinger RP, Abate NL, et al. Translating research to clinical practice: a 1-year experience with implementing early goal-directed therapy for septic shock in the emergency department. *Chest.* 2006;129(2):225-232.

37. van den Berghe G, Wouters P, Weekers F, et al. Intensive insulin therapy in critically ill patients. *New England Journal of Medicine.* 2001;345(19):1359-1367.

38. Varpula M, Pulkki K, Karlsson S, et al. Predictive value of N-terminal pro-brain natriuretic peptide in severe sepsis and septic shock. *Critical Care Medicine.* 2007;35(5):1277-1283.

39. Vincent JL, Bernard GR, Beale R, et al. Drotrecogin alfa (activated) treatment in severe sepsis from the global open-label trial ENHANCE: Further evidence for survival and safety and implications for early treatment. *Critical Care Medicine.* 2005;33(10):2266-2277.

40. Vincent JL, Gerlach H. Fluid resuscitation in severe sepsis and septic shock: an evidence-based review. *Critical Care Medicine.* 2004;32(suppl):S451-S454.

Cardiovascular Alterations

Colleen Walsh-Irwin, MS, RN, CCRN, ANP

⊖volve WEBSITE

Many additional resources, including self-assessment exercises, are located on the Evolve companion website at http://evolve.elsevier.com/Sole.

- Review Questions
- Mosby's Nursing Skills Procedures

- Animations
- Video Clips

INTRODUCTION

Care of the patient with alterations in cardiac status present unique challenges due to potential serious hemodynamic changes that can affect the prognosis of the critically ill patient. The critical care nurse needs both theoretical knowledge and practice-related understanding of the common cardiac diseases to have the sound clinical judgment necessary for making rapid and accurate decisions. The purpose of this chapter is to identify and explore common cardiac alterations that are likely to be encountered by the critical care nurse caring for adult patients with compromised cardiac status, and to describe the nursing care to optimize patient outcomes.

NORMAL STRUCTURE AND FUNCTION OF THE HEART

The heart muscle is approximately the size of a person's closed fist and lies within the mediastinal space of the thoracic cavity between the lungs, directly under the lower half of the sternum, and above the diaphragm (Figure 12-1). It is covered by the pericardium, which has an inner visceral layer and an outer parietal layer. Certain diseases can cause this covering to become inflamed and can subsequently diminish the effectiveness of the heart as a pump. Several cubic milliliters of lubricating fluid are present between these layers. Some pathological conditions can increase the amount and the consistency of this fluid, affecting the pumping ability of the heart. The heart muscle itself is composed of three layers. The outer layer, or epicardium, covers the surface of the heart and extends to the great vessels; the

middle, muscular layer, or myocardium, is responsible for the heart's pumping action; and the inner endothelial layer, or endocardium, covers the heart valves and the small muscles associated with the opening and closing of those valves. These layers are damaged or destroyed when a patient has a myocardial infarction (MI).

Functionally, the heart is divided into right-sided and left-sided pumps that are separated by a septum. The right side is considered to be a low-pressure system, whereas the left side is a high-pressure system. Each side has an atrium that receives the blood, and a ventricle that pumps it out. The right atrium receives deoxygenated blood from the body through the superior vena cava and inferior vena cava. Blood travels from the atrium to the ventricles by means of a pressure gradient between the chambers. The right ventricle pumps the deoxygenated blood to the lungs through the pulmonary artery for oxygen and carbon dioxide exchange. The left atrium receives the newly oxygenated blood by way of the pulmonary veins from the lungs, and the left ventricle pumps the oxygenated blood through the aorta to the systemic circulation (Figure 12-2).

The four cardiac valves maintain the unidirectional blood flow through the chambers of the heart. The valves also assist in producing the pressure gradient needed between the chambers for the blood to flow through the heart. There are two types of valves: the atrioventricular (AV) valves, which separate the atria from the ventricles; and the semilunar (SL) valves, which separate the pulmonary artery from the right ventricle and the aorta from the left ventricle (Figure 12-3). The AV valves are the tricuspid valve, which

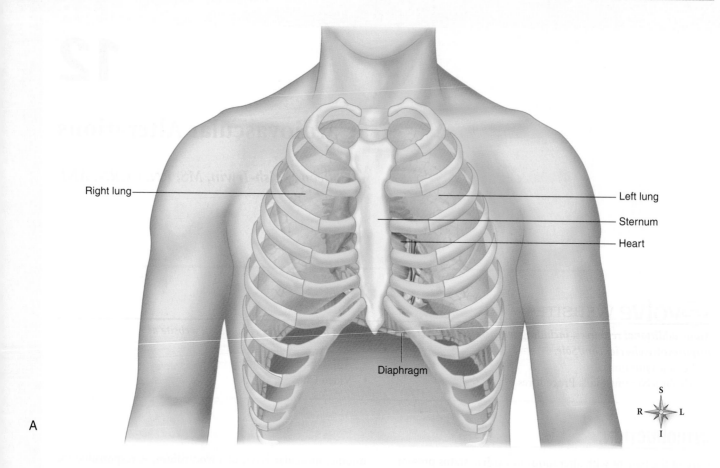

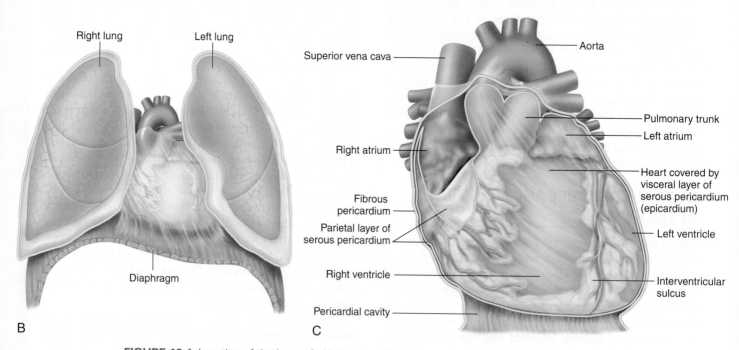

FIGURE 12-1 Location of the heart. **A,** Heart in mediastinum showing relationship to lungs and other anterior thoracic structures. **B,** Anterior view of isolated heart and lungs. Portions of the parietal pleura and pericardium have been removed. **C,** Detail of heart resting on diaphragm with pericardial sac opened.

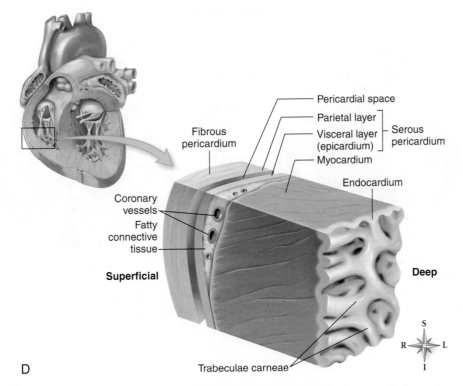

D

FIGURE 12-1, cont'd D, Wall of the heart. The cutout section of the heart wall shows the outer fibrous pericardium and the parietal and visceral layers of the serous pericardium (with the pericardial space between them). Note that a layer of fatty connective tissue is located between the visceral layer of the serous pericardium (epicardium) and the myocardium. Note also that the endocardium covers beamlike projections of myocardial muscle tissue, called *trabeculae carneae.* (From Patton KT, Thibodeau GA. *Anatomy and Physiology.* 8th ed. St. Louis: Mosby; 2013.)

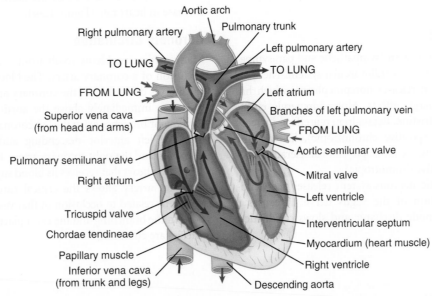

FIGURE 12-2 Structures that direct blood flow through the heart. (From McCance KL, Huether SE. *Pathophysiology. The Biologic Basis for Disease in Adults and Children.* 6th ed. St. Louis: Mosby; 2010.)

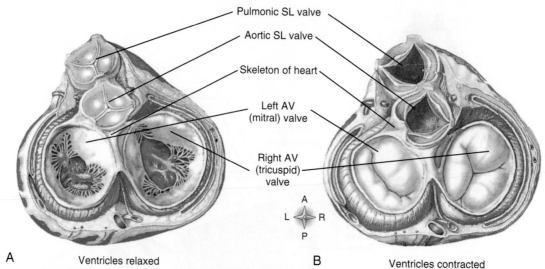

FIGURE 12-3 A, The atrioventricular (AV) valves in the open position and the semilunar (SL) valves in the closed position. **B,** The AV valves in the closed position and the SL valves in the open position. (From Patton KT, Thibodeau GA. *Anatomy and Physiology.* 7th ed. St. Louis: Mosby; 2010.)

lies between the right atrium and the right ventricle, and the mitral valve, located between the left atrium and the left ventricle. Each AV valve is anchored by chordae tendineae to the papillary muscles on its ventricular floor. The semilunar valves are the pulmonic valve, which lies between the right ventricle and the pulmonary artery, and the aortic valve, located between the left ventricle and the aorta. These semilunar valves are not anchored by chordae tendineae. Instead, their closing is passive and is caused by differences in pressure between the chamber and the respective great vessel.

Autonomic Control

The autonomic nervous system (sympathetic and parasympathetic) exerts control over the cardiovascular system. The sympathetic nervous system releases norepinephrine, which has alpha- and beta-adrenergic effects. Alpha-adrenergic effects cause arterial vasoconstriction. Beta-adrenergic effects increase sinus node discharge (positive chronotropic), increase the force of contraction (positive inotropic), and accelerate the AV conduction time (positive dromotropic).

The parasympathetic nervous system releases acetylcholine through stimulation of the vagus nerve. It causes a decrease in the sinus node discharge and slows conduction through the AV node.

In addition to this innervation, receptors help to control cardiovascular function. The first receptors are the *chemoreceptors,* which are sensitive to changes in the partial pressure of arterial oxygen (PaO_2), the partial pressure of arterial carbon dioxide ($PaCO_2$), and pH blood levels. Chemoreceptors stimulate the vasomotor center in the medulla; this center controls vasoconstriction and vasodilation. Second are *baroreceptors,* which are sensitive to stretch and pressure. If blood pressure increases, the baroreceptors cause the heart rate to decrease. If the blood pressure decreases, the baroreceptors stimulate an increase in heart rate (Figure 12-4).

Coronary Circulation

Many cardiac problems result from a complete or a partial occlusion of a coronary artery. The blood supply to the myocardium is derived from the coronary arteries that branch off the aorta immediately above the aortic valve (Figure 12-5). Two major branches exist: the left coronary artery, which splits into the left anterior descending and the left circumflex branches; and the right coronary artery. Knowledge of the portion of the heart that receives its blood supply from a particular coronary artery allows the critical care nurse to anticipate problems related to occlusion of that vessel (Box 12-1). Variations in the branching and the exact placement of the coronary arteries are common.

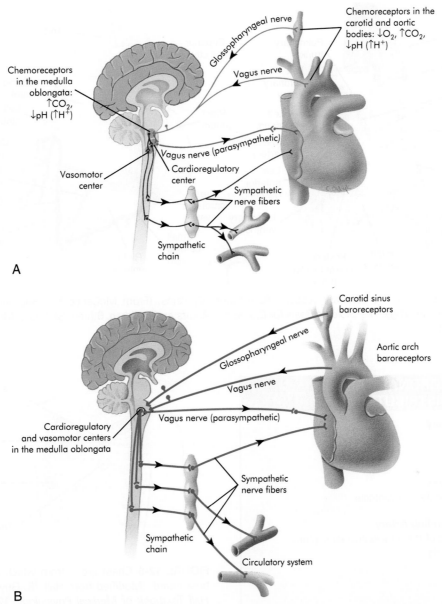

FIGURE 12-4 A, Chemoreceptor and **B,** baroreceptor reflex control of blood pressure. (From Seeley RR, Stephens TD, Tate P: *Anatomy and Physiology.* 3rd ed. St. Louis: Mosby; 1995.)

Blood flow to the coronary arteries occurs during ventricular diastole, when the aortic valve is closed and the sinuses of Valsalva are filled with blood. Myocardial fibers are relaxed at this time, thus promoting blood flow through the coronary vessels. The coronary veins return blood from the coronary circulation back into the heart through the coronary sinuses to the right and left atria.

Other Cardiac Functions

Knowledge of properties of cardiac muscle and the normal conduction system of the heart is essential since many patients have cardiac dysrhythmias (see Chapter 7). Hemodynamic concepts of the cardiovascular system are also important in understanding pathological disorders such as heart failure (HF). (Refer to Chapter 8 for hemodynamic content.)

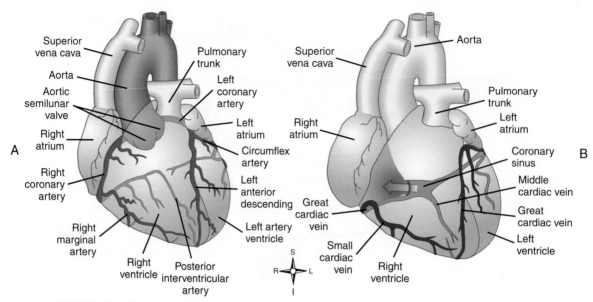

FIGURE 12-5 The coronary vessels. **A,** Arteries. **B,** Veins. (From McCance KL, Huether SE. *Pathophysiology. The Biologic Basis for Disease in Adults and Children.* 6th ed. St. Louis: Mosby; 2010.)

BOX 12-1	CORONARY ARTERY DISTRIBUTION

Right Coronary Artery
- Right atrium
- Right ventricle
- Sinoatrial node
- Atrioventricular bundle
- Posterior portion of the left ventricle

Left Anterior Descending Artery
- Anterior two thirds of the intraventricular septum
- Anterior left ventricle

Circumflex Artery
- Left atrium
- Posterior left ventricle

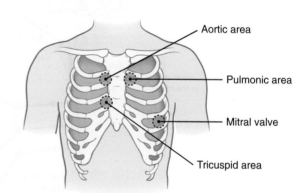

FIGURE 12-6 Chest areas from which each valve sound is best heard. (Modified from Hall JE, Guyton AC. *Guyton and Hall Textbook of Medical Physiology.* 12th ed. Philadelphia: Saunders; 2011.)

Heart Sounds

The vibrations produced by vascular walls, flowing blood, heart muscle, and heart valves create sound waves known as heart sounds. Auscultation of these sounds with a stethoscope over the heart provides valuable information about valve and cardiac function (Figure 12-6). Ventricular systole occurs when the pulmonic and aortic valves open to allow blood to be pumped to the lungs (right ventricle-pulmonic valve) and systemic circulation (left ventricle-aortic valve). Ventricular diastole occurs when the tricuspid and mitral valves open to allow the ventricles to fill with blood.

The first heart sound is known as S_1. This sound has been described as "lub." It is caused by closure of the tricuspid and mitral valves. It is best heard at the apex of the heart (fifth intercostal space, left midclavicular line) and represents the beginning of ventricular systole.

The second heart sound is known as S_2. It has been described as "dub" and is caused by closure of the pulmonic and aortic valves. It is best heard at the second intercostal space at the left or right sternal border and represents the beginning of ventricular diastole. The first and second heart sounds are best heard with the diaphragm of the stethoscope.

A third heart sound, S₃ or ventricular or protodiastolic gallop, is a normal variant in young adults, but usually represents a pathological process in the older adult. The sound is caused by rapid left ventricular filling and may be produced at the time when the heart is already overfilled or poorly compliant. The S₃ sound is low pitched and can best be heard with the bell of the stethoscope at the fifth intercostal space, at the left midclavicular line. It occurs immediately after S₂. Together with S₁ and S₂, S₃ produces a "lub-dubba" or "ken-**tuk**'e" sound. S₃ is often heard in patients with HF or fluid overload.

A fourth heart sound, S₄ or presystolic or atrial gallop, is produced from atrial contraction that is more forceful than normal. Together with S₁ and S₂, S₄ produces a "te-lubb-dubb" or "**ten**'-ne-see" sound. S₄ can be normal in elderly patients, but it is often heard after an acute myocardial infarction (AMI), when the atria contract more forcefully against ventricles distended with blood.

In the severely failing heart, all four sounds (S₄, S₁, S₂, and S₃) may be heard, producing a "gallop" rhythm (quadruple gallop), so named because it sounds like the hoof beats of a galloping horse. It can best be heard with the bell of the stethoscope at the fifth intercostal space, at the left midclavicular line. In addition, it is often documented S₄, S₁, S₂, S₃ because of the order in which the sounds are heard. Summation gallop is when the third and fourth heart sounds are superimposed and is usually an indication of heart disease.

Heart Murmur

A heart murmur is a sound caused by turbulence of blood flow through the valves of the heart. A murmur is usually a rumbling, blowing, harsh, or musical sound. It is important to distinguish the sound, anatomical location, loudness, and intensity of a murmur and determine whether extra heart sounds are heard. Table 12-1 gives a grading of heart murmurs.

TABLE 12-1	GRADING OF HEART MURMURS
Intensity of Murmur Graded from I to VI Based on Increasing Loudness	
Grade I	Lowest intensity, usually not audible by inexperienced providers
Grade II	Low intensity, usually audible by inexperienced providers
Grade III	Medium intensity without a thrill
Grade IV	Medium intensity with a thrill
Grade V	Loudest murmur audible when stethoscope is placed on the chest; associated with a thrill
Grade VI	Loudest intensity, audible when stethoscope is removed from chest; associated with a thrill

Murmurs are audible when a septal defect is present; when a valve (usually aortic or mitral) is stenosed, or when the valve leaflets fail to approximate (valve insufficiency). The presence of a new murmur warrants special attention, particularly in a patient with AMI. A papillary muscle may have ruptured, causing the mitral valve to not close correctly, which can be indicative of severe damage and impending complications (HF and pulmonary edema). Auscultation of heart sounds is a skill developed from practice in listening to many different patients' hearts and in correlating the sounds heard with the patients' pathological conditions.

CORONARY ARTERY DISEASE

Coronary artery disease (CAD) is a broad term used to refer to the narrowing or occlusion of the coronary arteries. Other terms used to describe CAD include coronary heart disease and atherosclerotic heart disease.

Pathophysiology

CAD is the progressive narrowing of one or more coronary arteries by atherosclerosis. CAD results in ischemia when the internal diameter of the coronary vessel is reduced by 70% (Figure 12-7).[27]

Atherosclerosis is an inflammatory disease progressing from endothelial injury to fatty streak, plaque, and complex lesion. The process begins with injury to the endothelium due to cardiac risk factors such as smoking, hypertension, diabetes, and hyperlipidemia (Box 12-2). Once injury occurs, endothelial cells become inflamed causing release of cytokines. Macrophages adhere to the injured endothelium and release enzymes and toxic oxygen radicals that create oxidative stress, oxidize low-density lipoproteins (LDLs) and further injure the vessel. Inflammation with oxidative stress and activation of macrophages occurs. Oxidized LDL penetrate the arterial wall and are engulfed by macrophages, creating foam cells (Figure 12-8). Accumulation of foam cells lead to fatty streak formation.[31] By the age of 20 years, most individuals have fatty streaks, an accumulation of serum lipoproteins in the intima of the vessel wall, in their coronary arteries.[19] The dysfunctional formation of a fatty streak leads to the presence of fibrotic plaque. Growth factors are also released, including angiotensin II, fibroblast growth factor, and platelet-derived growth factor, which stimulate smooth muscle proliferation in the affected vessel. Over time, a collagen cap is formed from connective tissue (fibroblasts and macrophages) and LDL (Figure 12-7, C).

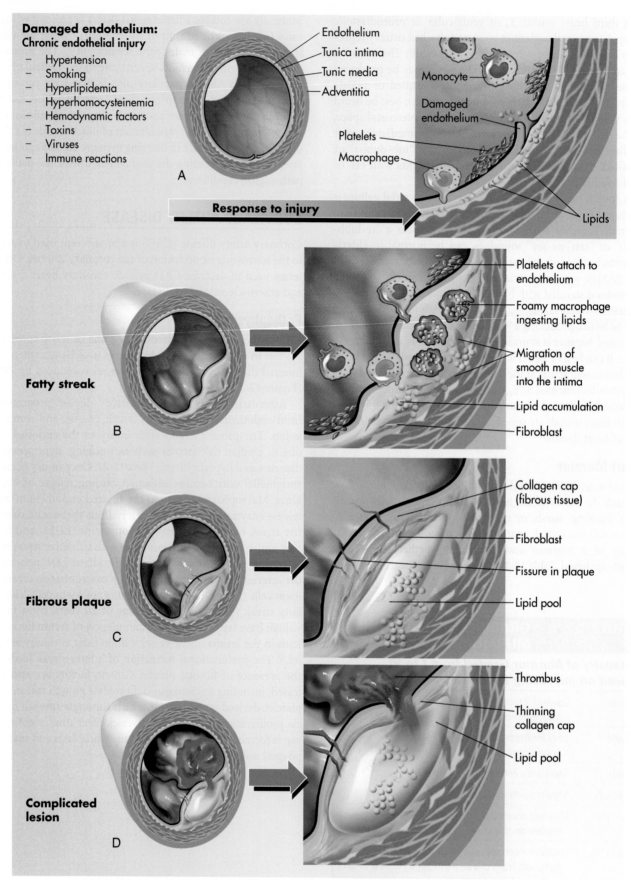

Damaged endothelium:
Chronic endothelial injury

- Hypertension
- Smoking
- Hyperlipidemia
- Hyperhomocysteinemia
- Hemodynamic factors
- Toxins
- Viruses
- Immune reactions

A

Endothelium
Tunica intima
Tunic media
Adventitia

Monocyte
Damaged endothelium
Platelets
Macrophage

Response to injury

Lipids

Fatty streak

B

Platelets attach to endothelium
Foamy macrophage ingesting lipids
Migration of smooth muscle into the intima
Lipid accumulation
Fibroblast

Fibrous plaque

C

Collagen cap (fibrous tissue)
Fibroblast
Fissure in plaque
Lipid pool

Complicated lesion

D

Thrombus
Thinning collagen cap
Lipid pool

FIGURE 12-7 Progression of atherosclerosis. **A,** Damaged endothelium. **B,** Fatty streak. **C,** Fibrous plaque. **D,** Complicated lesion. (From McCance KL, Huether SE. *Pathophysiology. The Biologic Basis for Disease in Adults and Children.* 6th ed. St. Louis: Mosby; 2010.)

BOX 12-2   RISK FACTORS FOR CORONARY ARTERY DISEASE

Several risk factors predispose persons to coronary artery disease (CAD). Some risk factors cannot be changed (e.g., gender, heredity, and age). Other risk factors are modifiable: smoking, high blood cholesterol, high blood pressure, physical inactivity, overweight or obesity, and diabetes.

Gender
Men have a greater risk of heart attacks than women and have heart attacks earlier in life.

Heredity
Family history of early heart disease is an unmodifiable risk for CAD. A positive history is defined as having a first degree relative (parent, sister, brother, or child) with CAD having been diagnosed before age 55 years in male relatives and before age 65 years in female relatives.[33]

Age
Men in their mid 40s, and women once they reach menopause, are considered at higher risk for CAD.

Smoking
Smokers have a higher risk of CAD. Smoking increases low-density lipoprotein (LDL) levels and damages the endothelium of coronary vessels. These are predisposing factors for the development of atherosclerosis. Smoking also causes vasoconstriction of coronary vessels, thus decreasing blood supply.

Blood Cholesterol
Serum cholesterol or lipid levels play a key role in the development of atherosclerosis. Elevated total cholesterol (>200 mg/dL) is considered a risk factor for CAD. Cholesterol is insoluble in plasma and must be transported by lipoproteins that are soluble. High-density lipoproteins (HDLs) are considered the good cholesterol. HDLs assist in transporting cholesterol to the liver for removal. A high HDL level (>40 mg/dL for men and >50 mg/dL

for women) may reduce the incidence of CAD, whereas a low HDL level (<40 mg/dL) is considered a risk factor for developing CAD.

LDLs are considered the bad cholesterol. LDLs transport and deposit cholesterol to the arterial vessels, thus facilitating the process of atherosclerosis. An LDL level <100 mg/dL is optimal. Other non-HDL lipoproteins also contribute to the development of CAD. Very-low-density lipoproteins are largely composed of triglycerides and contribute to an increased risk of CAD.

High Blood Pressure
A blood pressure (BP) greater than 120/80 mm Hg is considered prehypertension. A BP greater than 140/89 mm Hg or taking antihypertensive medication is a risk factor for CAD. Hypertension causes direct injury to the vasculature, leading to the development of CAD. Oxygen demands are also increased. The heart muscle enlarges and weakens over time, thereby increasing the workload of the heart.

Physical Inactivity
Lack of physical activity is a risk factor for CAD. Regular aerobic exercise reduces the incidence of CAD. Exercise also helps to control other risk factors such as high blood pressure, diabetes, and obesity.

Overweight and Obesity (See Bariatric Considerations)
Obesity increases the atherogenic process and predisposes persons to CAD. In addition, obesity is related to hypertension and diabetes, two other major risk factors. The waist-to-hip ratio and body mass index (BMI) are important assessments.

Diabetes
Diabetes is associated with increased levels of LDL and triglycerides. Glycation associated with diabetes decreases the uptake of LDL by the liver and increases the hepatic synthesis of LDL.

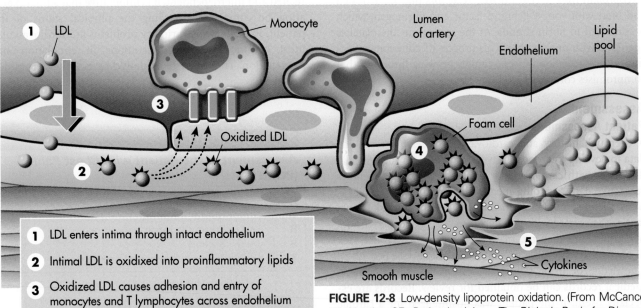

1   LDL enters intima through intact endothelium

2   Intimal LDL is oxidixed into proinflammatory lipids

3   Oxidized LDL causes adhesion and entry of monocytes and T lymphocytes across endothelium

4   Monocytes differentiate into macrophages and then consume large amounts of LDL, transforming into foam cells

5   Foam cells release growth factors (cytokines) that encourage atherosclerosis

FIGURE 12-8 Low-density lipoprotein oxidation. (From McCance KL, Huether SE. *Pathophysiology. The Biologic Basis for Disease in Adults and Children.* 6th ed. St. Louis: Mosby; 2010; Modified from Crawford MH, Dim Arco JP, eds: *Cardiology.* London: Mosby-Wolfe; 2001.)

BARIATRIC CONSIDERATIONS

Obesity is a risk factor of coronary artery disease (CAD). Persons with a greater proportion of fat through the abdomen ("apple-shaped") have been shown to have a higher incidence of CAD than those with greater fat distribution over the hips ("pear-shaped"). The waist-to-hip ratio is used to help identify this risk. Body mass index is another way to determine the degree of overweight.

Bariatric surgery may result in improved cardiac function and may assist in preventing heart failure. Weight loss in patients with morbid obesity has been associated with changes in left ventricular structure and improved right ventricular function.

Reference

Garza CA, Pellikka PA, Somers VK, Sarr MG, Collazo-Clavell ML, Korenfeld Y, Lopez-Jimenez F. Structural and functional changes in left and right ventricles after major weight loss following bariatric surgery for morbid obesity. *American Journal of Cardiology*. 2010;105:550-556.

BOX 12-3 QUESTIONING OF ACTIVITIES FOR STRESS REDUCTION

- What, if any, is the critically ill patient's exercise routine, including the type, amount, and regularity of the activity?
- What is the critically ill patient's daily food pattern and intake?
- What is the critically ill patient's sleep pattern?
- What are the critically ill patient's habitual social patterns in using tobacco, alcohol, drugs, coffee, tea, and caffeinated sodas?

Plaques may rupture, with the contents interacting with blood, producing a thrombus. The thrombus can occlude a coronary artery, with resulting injury and infarction. Rupture of the plaque starts the coagulation cascade with the initiation of thrombin production, the conversion of fibrinogen to fibrin, and platelet aggregation at the site. After injury to the endothelium, platelets are exposed to proteins that bind to receptors, causing adhesion of platelets at the site of injury. Next, the platelets are activated and change shape. They release thromboxane A_2 and serotonin. Each platelet has thousands of glycoprotein IIb/IIIa (Gp IIb/IIIa) receptors that are activated and bind with von Willebrand factor and fibrinogen, which is converted to fibrin strands. At the same time, the platelets aggregate with one another. This process of adhesion, activation, and aggregation causes a rapidly growing thrombus that compromises coronary blood flow.[31]

Assessment

Patient Assessment

A thorough history and cardiovascular assessment provide data to develop a comprehensive plan of care for the critically ill patient with cardiovascular disease. The history includes subjective data regarding medical history, prior hospitalizations, allergies, and family medical history. Several risk factors that are associated with CAD are also assessed: hypertension, hyperlipidemia, diabetes, male gender, age, tobacco use, lack of physical activity, obesity, and family history (see Box 12-2). Knowledge of prior hospitalizations is also important so medical records can be obtained for review. Records are especially useful if the patient was hospitalized for a cardiac event or underwent cardiac diagnostic testing. Information regarding the patient's current medications, both prescription and over-the-counter, includes assessment of the patient's understanding and use of these medications. For example,

when considering nitroglycerin (NTG) administration, it is necessary to know the history of the patient's use of phosphodiesterase type 5 (PDE5) inhibitors taken for erectile dysfunction, such as sildenafil (Viagra). These medications potentiate the hypotensive effects of nitrates such as NTG; thus concurrent use is contraindicated. It is also important to determine whether the patient has any food or drug allergies.

A psychosocial or personal history is important for the planning of the critically ill patient's care. This history includes major stress events and everyday stressors (Box 12-3).

Before beginning the physical examination, the nurse determines recent and recurrent symptoms that may be related to the patient's current problems. Such information gathering includes the presence or absence of fatigue, fluid retention, dyspnea, irregular heartbeat (palpitations), and chest pain (see box, "Clinical Alert: Assessment of the Patient with Chest Pain [PQRST]"). The physical examination itself encompasses all the body systems and is not limited to the cardiovascular system. Because all the body systems are interrelated and interdependent, it is imperative that a total evaluation be completed regarding the physical status of the patient. Patients whose primary problems are cardiovascular most commonly exhibit alterations in circulation and oxygenation. Thus all systems should be examined from this perspective.

⚠ CLINICAL ALERT

Assessment of the Patient with Chest Pain (PQRST)

P	Provocation
Q	Quality
R	Region/Radiation
S	Severity
T	Timing (when began) and Treatment

The examination is performed in an orderly, organized manner and involves the techniques of inspection, palpation, percussion, and auscultation. A baseline assessment is provided in Table 12-2.

TABLE 12-2	MAJOR SYSTEMS ASSESSMENT FOR CARDIOVASCULAR DISEASE
SYSTEM	**ASSESSMENT**
Neurological	Level of consciousness, orientation to person, place, time, events; presence of hallucinations, depression, withdrawal, restlessness, apprehensiveness, irritability, cooperativeness, response to tactile stimuli; type, location of pain; how pain is relieved; trembling; pupils (size, equality, response); paresthesias; eye movements; hand grips (strength and equality); leg movement
Skin	Color (mottling, cyanosis, pallor), temperature, dryness, turgor, presence of rashes, broken areas, pressure areas, urticaria, incision site, wounds
Cardiovascular	BP (bilaterally); apical heart rate and radial pulses; pulse deficit; monitor leads on patient in correct anatomical placement; regularity of rhythm, presence of ectopy; PR interval, QRS, and QT intervals; heart sounds; presence of abnormalities (rubs, gallops, clicks); neck vein distention with head of bed at what angle; edema (sacral and dependent); calf pain; varicosities; presence of pulses: bilateral carotid, radial, femoral, posterior tibial, dorsalis pedis; capillary refill in extremities; hemodynamic measurements; temporary pacemaker settings; medications to maintain BP or rhythm
Respiratory	Rate, depth, and quality of respirations; oxygen needs; accessory muscle use; cough, sputum: type, color, suctioning frequency; symmetry of chest expansion and breath sounds, breath sounds (crackles, wheezing); interpretation of ABGs; chest tube with description of drainage, fluctuation in water seal, bubbling, suction applied; tracheostomy or endotracheal tube; ventilator used; ventilator settings; ventilator rate versus patient's own breaths
Gastrointestinal	Abdominal size and softness, bowel sounds, nausea and vomiting, bowel movement, dressing and/or drainage, NG tube with description of drainage, feeding tube: type and frequency of feedings, drains
Genitourinary	Voiding or indwelling urinary catheter, urine color, quality and quantity; vaginal or urethral drainage
Intravenous	Volume of fluid, type of solution, rate; intravenous site condition
Wounds	Dry or drainage, type, color, amount, odor; hematoma, inflamed, drains, hemovac, dressing changes, cultures

ABG, Arterial blood gas; *BP*, blood pressure; *NG*, nasogastric.

Diagnostic Studies

Many diagnostic studies are fundamental for the care and treatment of critically ill patients with CAD. The following sections contain brief descriptions of common diagnostic studies the cardiac patient may encounter.

12-Lead electrocardiography (ECG; also commonly referred to as EKG). This noninvasive test is usually preliminary to most other tests performed. It is useful in identification of rhythm disturbances, pericarditis, pulmonary diseases, left ventricular hypertrophy, and myocardial ischemia, injury, and infarction. The importance of this basic test should not be underestimated.

Chest x-ray. The chest x-ray is usually performed in the anteroposterior view. The chest x-ray study is used for detecting cardiomegaly, cardiac positioning, degree of fluid infiltrating the pulmonary space or pericardial space, and other structural changes that may affect the physical ability of the heart to function in a normal manner.

Holter monitor. This test is used to detect suspected dysrhythmias. The patient is connected to a small portable recorder (about the size of a large cellular phone) by three to five electrodes; the recorder is worn for 24 to 48 hours. The patient engages in normal daily activities, and keeps a log of all activities and symptoms during the monitoring period. The recording is analyzed for abnormalities and correlated with the documented activities and symptoms.

Exercise tolerance test (ETT) or stress test. This is a noninvasive test in which the patient is connected to an ECG machine while exercising. Physical stress causes an increase in myocardial oxygen consumption. If oxygen demand exceeds supply, ischemia may result. The stress test is used to document exercise-induced ischemia, and it can identify those individuals prone to cardiac ischemia during activity when resting ECGs are normal. The exercise usually involves pedaling a stationary bike or walking on a treadmill. The patient is constantly monitored, the pulse and blood pressure are checked at intervals, and the ECG printout is analyzed at the end of the testing period. Changes in the ST segments of the ECG can indicate ischemia. Beta-blockers are often held the morning of an ETT so that an adequate heart rate can be attained during the test. Patients return to their room or go home after the heart rate returns to baseline.

Pharmacological stress testing. If a patient is physically unable to perform the exercise, a pharmacological stress test can be done. This is done in conjunction with radionuclide scintigraphy or echocardiography. Medications such as regadenoson, dipyridamole, or adenosine are used because they cause vasodilation of normal coronary arteries. If an area of the blood vessel is stenosed, it does not dilate and shows up as hypoperfusion with radionuclide scanning, or as hypokinesis with echocardiography. Alternatively, dobutamine can be used, which increases heart rate and contractility. Areas that are not perfused well because of blockages are evident when scanned.

Nuclear stress testing. This test can be done with exercise to increase the sensitivity of the test and/or be used for patients who have an ECG that precludes an accurate interpretation of ST-segment changes. It is also used in conjunction with medications for patients who cannot walk on a treadmill. Technetium-99m and thallium-201 are radionuclides given intravenously to image the heart at rest and at stress (induced either by exercise or use of a pharmacological agent). The stress images are compared to the rest images. Perfusion defects seen on rest and stress images are evidence of infarct, whereas defects noted on stress that are normal during the rest study indicate ischemia.

Echocardiography. This is a noninvasive, acoustic imaging procedure that uses ultrasound to visualize the cardiac structures and the motion and function of cardiac valves and chambers. A transducer placed on the chest wall sends ultrasound waves at short intervals. The reflected sound waves, termed echoes, are displayed on a graph for interpretation. Echocardiography is used to assess valvular function, evaluate congenital defects, measure size of cardiac chambers, evaluate cardiac disease progression, evaluate ventricular function, diagnose myocardial tumors and effusions, and, to a lesser degree, measure cardiac output. Ventricular function is evaluated by obtaining an ejection fraction. The ejection fraction is the percentage of blood ejected from the left ventricle during systole, normally 55% to 60%.

Transesophageal echocardiography. This test provides ultrasonic imaging of the heart from a view behind the heart. In transesophageal echocardiography (TEE), an ultrasound probe is fitted on the end of a flexible gastroscope, which is inserted into the posterior pharynx and advanced into the esophagus. TEE shows a clear picture because the esophagus is against the back of the heart and parallel to the aorta. TEE is indicated to visualize prosthetic heart valves, mitral valve function, aortic dissection, vegetative endocarditis, congenital heart defects in adults, cardiac masses and tumors, and embolic phenomena. It is also used intraoperatively to assess left ventricular function. Patients should fast (except for medications) for 6 to 8 hours before the examination. During the procedure, vital signs, cardiac rhythm, and oxygen saturation are monitored. After the procedure, the patient is unable to eat until the gag reflex returns. A rare complication of TEE is esophageal perforation, with signs of sore throat, dysphagia, stiff neck, and epigastric or substernal pain that worsens with breathing and movement, or pain in the back, abdomen, or shoulder.

Multigated blood pool study. The multigated blood pool study (MUGA) scan is used to assess left ventricular function. An isotope is injected and images of the heart are taken during systole and diastole to assess the ejection fraction of the heart. An ejection fraction of 55% to 60% and symmetrical contraction of the left ventricle are considered normal test results.

Cardiac magnetic resonance imaging. Magnetic resonance imaging (MRI) is a noninvasive test used to evaluate tissues, structures, and blood flow. MRI is a technique that uses magnetic resonance to create images of hydrogen. These images are created as the ions are emitted, picked up, and fed into a computer that reconstructs the image that can differentiate between healthy and ischemic tissue. MRI is used to diagnose or evaluate coronary artery disease, aortic aneurysm, congenital heart disease, left ventricular function, cardiac tumors, thrombus, valvular disease, and pericardial disorders. One of the advantages of MRI is that it does not involve exposure to ionizing radiation. Contrast can be used with MRI to enhance results.

MRI cannot be performed on patients with pacemakers, defibrillators, cochlear implants, or some types of brain clips (used for aneurysms). The test can be very stressful for patients who are claustrophobic, and in these situations, open MRI may be indicated. ECG monitoring is difficult to use during MRI; therefore critically ill patients may not be good candidates for this procedure. Specialized monitors have been developed specifically for use in MRI to facilitate cardiac monitoring when indicated.

Cardiac catheterization and angiography. This is an invasive procedure that can be divided into two stages (right-sided and left-sided catheterization). Cardiac catheterization is used to measure pressures in the chambers of the heart, cardiac output, and blood gas content; confirm and evaluate the severity of lesions within the coronary arteries; and to assess left ventricular function.

Right-sided catheterization is performed by placing a pulmonary artery catheter in the femoral or brachial vein and then carefully advancing it into the right atrium, right ventricle, and pulmonary artery. The healthcare provider measures pressures in the right atrium, right ventricle, and pulmonary artery, and the pulmonary artery occlusion pressure. Oxygen saturations can be measured if indicated (i.e., valve disease or septal defect).

Left-sided catheterization is performed to visualize coronary arteries, to note the area and extent of lesions within the native vessel walls and bypass grafts, to evaluate angina-related spasms, to locate areas of infarct, and to perform interventions such as percutaneous angioplasty or stent placement.

Left-sided catheterization is performed by cannulation of a femoral, brachial, or radial artery. The procedure entails positioning a catheter into the aorta at the proximal end of the coronary arteries. Dye is injected into the arteries, and a radiographic picture is recorded as the dye progresses or fails to progress through the coronary circulation. In addition, dye is injected into the left ventricle, and the amount of dye ejected with the next systole is measured to determine the ejection fraction.

After the procedure the catheters are removed. To prevent bleeding from the arterial site, a vascular sealing device made of collagen (e.g., AngioSeal), a clip-mediated device (e.g., StarClose), or a stitch device (e.g., Perclose) may be used to close the puncture site in the artery. A hemostatic bandage (e.g., QuickClot) can also be used. If a sealing or stitch device is not used, firm pressure is applied for 15 to 30 minutes. Commercial devices (e.g., FemoStop; Figure 12-9) are available to assist in applying pressure to the site. Depending on the diagnostic study results and the patient's status, patients are usually discharged within 6 to 8 hours of completion of the test.

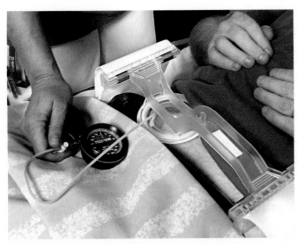

FIGURE 12-9 FemoStop in correct position. (Courtesy RADI Medical Systems, Inc. Sweden.)

BOX 12-4	NURSING CARE AFTER CARDIAC CATHETERIZATION AND ANGIOGRAPHY

- Maintain the patient on bed rest (time varies depending on the size of the catheter used and the method for preventing arterial bleeding).
- Keep the extremity used for catheter insertion immobile.
- Observe the insertion site for bleeding or hematoma, especially if the patient is receiving postprocedure anticoagulant therapy.
- Mark the hematoma with a marker around outer perimeter, to aid in assessing for an increase in bleeding.
- Assess for bruits.
- Maintain head-of-bed elevation no higher than 30 degrees.
- Monitor peripheral pulses, color, and sensation of the extremity distal to insertion site (every 15 minutes × 4; every 30 minutes × 4; every 1 hour × 2). In addition, monitor the opposite extremity pulse to assess for presence of equal pulses and color, and sensation bilaterally.
- Observe cardiac rhythm.
- Encourage fluid intake if not contraindicated.
- Monitor intake and output.
- Observe for an adverse reaction to dye (angiography).
- Assess for chest pain, back pain, and shortness of breath and notify health care provider.

Nursing care for a patient undergoing cardiac catheterization involves the preprocedure instruction (the procedure will be performed using local anesthesia, and the patient may feel a warm or hot flush sensation or flutter of the catheter as it moves about) and the postprocedure instruction. The postprocedure routine is noted in Box 12-4.

Electrophysiology study. An electrophysiology study is an invasive procedure that involves the introduction of an electrode catheter percutaneously from a peripheral vein or artery into the cardiac chamber or sinuses and the performance of programmed electrical stimulation of the heart. Electrophysiology studies aid in recording intracardiac ECGs, diagnosing cardiac conduction defects, evaluating the effectiveness of antidysrhythmic medications, determining the proper choice of pacemaker programming, and mapping the cardiac conduction system before ablation.

Laboratory Diagnostics

Other diagnostic measures include the evaluation of serum electrolyte studies and cardiac enzymes. Because many books are available regarding the reading and interpretation of laboratory values, this section presents a brief overview of the more important blood studies that should or may need to be assessed in the patient with a cardiovascular alteration.[10]

Serum electrolytes. Electrolytes are important in maintaining the function of the cardiac conduction system. Imbalances in sodium, potassium, calcium, and magnesium can result in cardiac dysrhythmias. Therefore analysis of serum electrolytes is a routine part of the assessment and treatment of the cardiac patient. Table 12-3 reviews ECG changes that may alert the nurse to possible electrolyte abnormalities.

Serum enzymes. Enzymes are proteins that are produced by all living cells and released into the bloodstream. When cells are injured or diseased, more enzymes are released. Assessments of enzyme levels released from cardiac muscle are useful in the diagnosis of AMI.[9]

- *Creatine kinase (CK)* enzymes increase within 2 to 6 hours after the onset of myocardial muscle damage. Peak levels occur within 18 to 36 hours, and levels return to baseline in 3 to 6 days. Total CK can be elevated from a variety of diseases and conditions, such as muscle injury and acute renal failure and therefore is nonspecific.

TABLE 12-3	ECG CHANGES ASSOCIATED WITH ELECTROLYTE IMBALANCES	
ELECTROLYTE IMBALANCE	**PANIC VALUE**	**MANIFESTATIONS**
Hypokalemia	<2.5 mEq/L	U wave, increased ventricular ectopy
Hyperkalemia	>6.6 mEq/L	Tall, peaked T waves, conduction blocks, ventricular fibrillation
Hypocalcemia	<7.0 mg/dL	Prolonged ST segment and QT interval
Hypercalcemia	>12.0 mg/dL	Shortened ST segment and QT interval
Hypomagnesemia	<0.5 mEq/L	Prolonged PR and QT intervals, broad, flat T waves, PVCs, ventricular tachycardia or fibrillation
Hypermagnesemia	>3.0 mEq/L	Prolonged PR and QT intervals, widened QRS

PVCs, Premature ventricular contractions.
Modified from Chernecky CC, & Berger BJ. (2008). *Laboratory tests and diagnostic procedures* (5th ed.). Philadelphia: Saunders.

- CK_2-MB (heart) is a fraction of the total CK that is specific for cardiac muscle. Normal values of CK_2-MB are 0% to 6% of the total CK, or 0.3 to 4.9 ng/mL. Values are elevated after AMI, cardiac surgery, and blunt cardiac trauma. The initial rise in CK_2-MB levels after an AMI occurs within 4 to 8 hours after the onset of damage. Peak levels occur in 18 to 24 hours, and levels return to baseline within 3 days. Total CK and CK_2-MB are usually ordered at the initial assessment and serially at 8, 16, and 24 hours after the onset of chest pain to assist in the diagnosis of AMI.
- Troponin I and troponin T. Serum troponin levels are useful in the early diagnosis of AMI. Levels are normally undetectable in healthy people and elevate as early as 1 hour after myocardial cell injury. Testing for troponin can be done quickly in the field or the emergency department and aids in the early diagnosis of AMI. The normal value of troponin I is less than 0.5 mcg/L, and that of troponin T is less than 0.1 mcg/L.
- Myoglobin. Serum myoglobin is released within 30 to 60 minutes after AMI. Normal values are less than 72 ng/mL in men, and less than 58 ng/mL in women. Myoglobin levels rise before CK and CK_2-MB and are useful in the early diagnosis of AMI. Myoglobin alone is not specific for AMI, but when used in combination with other tests, it can aid in the diagnosis. Some institutions order myoglobin levels every 2 hours. A doubling of levels from one sample to the next sample is indicative of AMI.

Nursing Diagnoses

CAD is a broad diagnostic area, and thus several nursing diagnostic categories apply. With the complications of CAD, such as angina, MI, and HF, the diagnostic categories are more specific. Nursing diagnoses of patients with CAD include the following:

- Pain related to decreased coronary artery tissue perfusion
- Anxiety/fear related to treatments and invasive procedures used for diagnostic testing
- Knowledge deficit related to understanding of anatomy and pathophysiology of the heart and its functions, complexity of treatment, new condition, emotional state
- Health-seeking behaviors related to desire for information regarding altered health status or a disease process or condition

Interventions
Nursing Interventions

Nursing interventions are patient centric and encompass health assessment and patient education. Assessment of the patient's psychosocial status and family support, as well as the patient's history and physical examination findings, are used to guide interventions. The nurse instructs the patient about risk factor modification and signs and symptoms of progression of CAD that warrant medical treatment.

Medical Management

The goals of medical management are to reduce the risk factors for progression of CAD. This includes achieving target levels of LDL. The National Cholesterol Education Project of the National Heart, Lung, and Blood Institute recommends that an optimal LDL level is less than 100 mg/dL, but the target level should be adjusted in relation to the patient's number of major risk factors for CAD.[4] These include family history, age, smoking, hypertension, and diabetes. The key to lessening the burden of coronary heart disease in the United States is primary prevention, and one way this can be accomplished is through thorough management of cholesterol levels (see box, "Laboratory Alert," for LDL, high-density lipoproteins [HDL], and triglyceride levels).

Strategies for risk factor modification include a low-fat, low-cholesterol diet, exercise, weight loss, smoking cessation, and control of other risks such as diabetes and hypertension. If LDL levels are not at target values after 6 months of risk factor modification, patients are started on lipid-lowering medications.

Medications to reduce serum lipid levels. Lipid-lowering drugs include statins, bile acid resins, ezetimibe, and nicotinic acid (Table 12-4). The statins are officially classified as 3-hydroxy-3-methylglutaryl-coenzyme A (HMG-CoA) reductase inhibitors. The statins lower LDL more than other types of lipid-lowering drugs. They work by slowing the production of cholesterol and increasing the liver's ability to remove LDL from the body. Some commonly used drugs are lovastatin, atorvastatin, pravastatin, simvastatin, and rosuvastatin. The drugs are well tolerated by most patients. It is recommended that statins be given as a single dose in the evening because the body makes more cholesterol at night.

! LABORATORY ALERT

Target Lipid Levels

RISKS	TARGET LOW-DENSITY LIPOPROTEIN LEVEL	TARGET HIGH-DENSITY LIPOPROTEIN LEVEL	TARGET TRIGLYCERIDE LEVEL
No CAD; 0-1 risk factors	<160 mg/dL	>60 mg/dL	<190 mg/dL
No CAD; 2 or more risk factors	<130 mg/dL	>60 mg/dL	<160 mg/dL
CAD or CAD risk equivalent (other atherosclerotic disease, diabetes, multiple risks)	<100 mg/dL	>60 mg/dL	<130 mg/dL

CAD, Coronary artery disease.

TABLE 12-4 PHARMACOLOGY

Medications for Lowering Cholesterol and Triglycerides

Antilipemic Agents (HMG-CoA Reductase Inhibitors)

Indications: used to lower total and LDL cholesterol and to help reduce the risk of acute myocardial infarction and stroke

Mechanism of action: competitively inhibit HMG-CoA reductase, the enzyme that catalyzes the rate-limiting step in cholesterol biosynthesis, resulting in lower total and LDL cholesterol levels with increased HDL cholesterol

MEDICATION	DOSE/ROUTE	SIDE EFFECTS AND NURSING CONSIDERATIONS
Lovastatin (Altocor, Mevacor)	10-80 mg PO once daily (in the evening) or in two divided doses	Headache, dizziness, constipation, weakness, and increased creatine phosphokinase (CPK) levels Instruct patient to take with evening meal. Report severe muscle pain, or weakness, which can be a sign of rhabdomyolysis, a serious side effect. Obtain baseline liver function and lipid profile tests before starting therapy, every 2 months for first year, then at 6 and 12 months, or when dose increased. Do not give in pregnancy. Instruct patient about a low-cholesterol diet.
Atorvastatin (Lipitor)	10-80 mg PO daily	Same
Fluvastatin (Lescol)	20-80 mg daily PO at bedtime	Same
Pravastatin (Pravachol)	10-80 mg daily PO at bedtime	Same
Rosuvastatin (Crestor)	5-40 mg daily PO at bedtime	Same
Simvastatin (Apo-Simvastatin, Zocor)	5-80 mg daily PO at bedtime	Same as above. The FDA has mandated no more new prescriptions of 80 mg. Patients that have been stable for over a year may continue to take 80 mg. Also, no more than 20 mg for patients taking amlodipine or ranolazine, and no more than 10 mg for patients on amiodarone, verapamil, or diltiazem. Contraindicated in patients on gemfibrozil; antifungal medications including itraconazole, ketoconazole, posaconazole; antibiotics such as erythromycin, clarithromycin, telithromycin; and HIV protease inhibitors such as nefazodone, cyclosporine, and danazol.

Antilipemic Agents (Bile Acid Sequestrants)

Indications: used to manage hypercholesterolemia

Mechanism of action: form a nonabsorbable complex with bile acids in the intestine, inhibiting enterohepatic reuptake of intestinal bile salts, which increases the fecal loss of bile salt–bound LDL cholesterol

MEDICATION	DOSE/ROUTE	SIDE EFFECTS AND NURSING CONSIDERATIONS
Cholestyramine (Novo-Cholamine, Prevalite, Questran, Questran-Light)	*Powder:* 4-24 g 1-2 times a day *Tablet:* 4-16 g 1-2 times a day	Constipation, heartburn, nausea, flatulence, vomiting, abdominal pain, and headache Instruct patient to mix powder with fluid or applesauce. Do not take dry, avoid inhaling product. Patient should take other medications at least 1 hour before taking this medication. Patient should report any stomach cramping, pain, blood in stool, and unresolved nausea or vomiting. Monitor cholesterol and triglyceride levels before and during therapy. Use during pregnancy must be cautious, weighing benefits of use against the possible risks involved.
Colesevelam (Welchol)	625 mg, 3 tablets BID with meals	Same
Colestipol (Colestid)	*Powder:* 5-30 g mixed with liquid in divided doses *Tablet:* 2 g daily-BID, max 16 g/day	Same
Ezetimibe (Zetia)	*Tablet:* One tablet once a day by mouth with or without food	Headache, dizziness, diarrhea, sore throat, runny nose, sneezing, and joint pain. Monitor for signs of liver failure. Follow low-cholesterol, low-fat diet. Keep a written list of all prescription and nonprescription medicines as well as vitamins, minerals, or other dietary supplements.

Continued

TABLE 12-4 PHARMACOLOGY

Medications for Lowering Cholesterol and Triglycerides—cont'd

Antilipemic Agent (Miscellaneous, Niacin)

Indications: adjunctive treatment of hyperlipidemia
Mechanism of action: inhibits VLDL synthesis

MEDICATION	DOSE/ROUTE	SIDE EFFECTS AND NURSING CONSIDERATIONS
Nicotinic acid (Niacin)	1.5-2 g daily in 3 divided doses *Sustained release*: 500 mg at bedtime, max 2000 mg/day	Headache, flushing, bloating, flatulence, and nausea Instruct patient to take it as directed and not to exceed recommended dosage. Should be taken after meals. Patient should report persistent gastrointestinal disturbances or changes in color of urine or stool. Take with aspirin to reduce flushing.

Antilipemic Agent (Fibric Acid)

Indications: treatment of hypertriglyceridemia in patients who have not responded to dietary intervention
Mechanism of action: inhibits biosynthesis of VLDL, increases HDL, and decreases triglycerides

Gemfibrozil (Lopid)	600 mg BID PO	Stomach upset, fatigue, headache, diarrhea, and nausea. Instruct patient to take before breakfast and dinner. May take with milk or meals if gastrointestinal upset occurs. Patient should report severe abdominal pain, nausea, or vomiting. Use during pregnancy must be weighed against the possible risks.
Fenofibrate (Tricor)	67-200 mg PO	Nausea, abdominal pain, increased liver enzymes, rash, headaches

BID, Twice daily; *HDL,* high-density lipoprotein; *HMG-CoA,* 3-hydroxy-3-methylglutaryl-coenzyme A; *LDL,* low-density lipoprotein; *PO,* orally; *VLDL,* very-low-density lipoprotein.
From Skidmore-Roth L. (2011). *Mosby's 2011 Nursing Drug Reference.* St. Louis: Mosby.

LDL levels are reassessed in 4 to 6 weeks, and dosages are adjusted as needed.[28] A disadvantage of the medications is that they can cause liver damage; therefore it is important to ensure that the patient has liver enzymes drawn periodically to assess liver function. The medications can also cause myopathies, although rare, and patients are instructed to contact their healthcare provider if they develop any muscle aches.

The bile acid resins combine with cholesterol-containing bile acids in the intestines to form an insoluble complex that is eliminated through feces. These drugs lower LDL levels by 10% to 20%. Bile acid resins include cholestyramine and colestipol. The drugs are mixed in liquid and are taken twice daily. They are associated with side effects such as nausea and flatulence and are contraindicated in biliary obstruction. The drugs interfere with absorption of many medications. It is recommended that other medications be given 1 hour before or 4 hours after administration of the resins to promote absorption.[11]

Ezetimibe (Zetia) works in the digestive tract by blocking the absorption of cholesterol from food. It is often used in conjunction with other cholesterol reducing medications. Ezetimibe can cause liver disease; therefore liver function tests need to be monitored and the drug is contraindicated in severe hepatic disease. Although the drug lowers lipid levels, it has not been proven to reduce heart disease. The medication is also being tested in combination with statins to achieve LDL goals.

Nicotinic acid, or niacin, reduces total cholesterol, LDL, and triglyceride levels, and it increases HDL. The drug is available over-the-counter; however, its use in lowering cholesterol must be under the supervision of a healthcare provider. A long-acting, once-daily dose, is available by prescription. The drug dosage is gradually increased to the maximum effective daily dose. Common side effects include a metallic taste in mouth, flushing, and increased feelings of warmth. Major side effects include hepatic dysfunction, gout, and hyperglycemia. Because nicotinic acid affects the absorption of other drugs, it must be given separately from other medications. Administering niacin with food and aspirin can reduce some of the side effects.[28]

If triglyceride levels are elevated, patients may be prescribed agents that specifically lower triglyceride levels. One agent is gemfibrozil, a fibric acid derivative that lowers triglycerides and increases HDL levels. This drug is associated with many gastrointestinal side effects.

If a patient does not respond adequately to single-drug therapy, combined-drug therapy is considered to lower LDL levels further. For example, statins may be combined with bile acid resins. Patients must be carefully monitored when two or more lipid-lowering agents are given simultaneously.

Medications to prevent platelet adhesion and aggregation. Drugs are often prescribed for the patient with CAD to reduce platelet adhesion and aggregation. A single dose of 81 to 325 mg of an enteric-coated aspirin per day is commonly prescribed. To prevent platelet aggregation, other agents that may be prescribed with aspirin such as clopidogrel (Plavix) or prasugrel (Effient). In addition, Brilinta (ticagrelor) has just been approved.

Patient Outcomes

Several outcomes are expected after treatment. These include relief of pain; less anxiety related to the disease; adherence to health behavior modification to reduce cardiovascular risks; and the ability to describe the disease process, causes, factors contributing to the symptoms, and the procedures for disease or symptom control.

ANGINA

Angina is chest pain or discomfort caused by myocardial ischemia that occurs from an imbalance between myocardial oxygen supply and demand. CAD and coronary artery spasms are common causes of angina.

Pathophysiology

Angina (from the Latin word meaning *squeezing*) is the chest pain associated with myocardial ischemia; it is transient and does not cause cell death; but it may be a precursor to cell death from MI. The neural pain receptors are stimulated by accelerated metabolism, chemical changes and imbalances, and/or local mechanical stress resulting from abnormal myocardial contractions. The oxygen circulating via the vascular system to the myocardial cells decreases, causing ischemia to the tissue, resulting in pain.

Angina occurs when oxygen demand is higher than oxygen supply. Box 12-5 shows factors influencing oxygen supply and demand that may result in angina.

Types of Angina

Different types of angina exist: stable, unstable, and variant. *Stable angina* occurs with exertion and is relieved by rest. It is sometimes called chronic exertional angina. *Unstable angina* pain is often more severe, may occur at rest, and requires more frequent nitrate therapy. It is sometimes described as crescendo (increasing) in nature. During an unstable episode, the ECG may show ST-segment depression, T-wave inversions, or no changes at all. The patient has an increased risk of MI within 18 months of onset of unstable angina; therefore medical or surgical interventions, or both, are warranted. Patients are often hospitalized for diagnostic workup and treatment. The treatment of unstable angina is discussed more completely in the section, "Acute Coronary Syndrome."

Variant, or *Prinzmetal, angina* is caused by coronary artery spasms. It often occurs at rest and without other precipitating factors. The ECG shows a marked ST elevation (usually seen only in AMI) during the episode. The ST segment returns to normal after the spasm subsides. AMI can occur with prolonged coronary artery spasm, even in the absence of CAD.

Assessment

Assessment of the patient with actual or suspected angina involves continual observation of the patient and monitoring of signs, symptoms, and diagnostic findings. The patient must be monitored for the type and degree of pain (see box, "Clinical Alert: Symptoms of Angina").

> **! CLINICAL ALERT**
> ### *Symptoms of Angina*
>
> - Pain is frequently retrosternal, left pectoral, or epigastric. It may radiate to the jaw, left shoulder, or left arm.
> - Pain may be associated with dyspnea, light-headedness, or diaphoresis.
> - Pain can be described as chest pressure, burning, squeezing, heavy, or smothering.
> - Pain usually lasts 1 to 5 minutes.
> - Classic placing of clenched fist against the chest (sternum) may be seen, or may be absent if the sensation is confused with indigestion.
> - Pain usually begins with exertion and subsides with rest.

The precipitating factors that can be identified as bringing on an episode of anginal pain include physical or emotional stress, exposure to temperature extremes, and ingestion of a heavy meal. It is important to know what factors alleviate the anginal pain, including stopping activity or exercise and taking nitroglycerin sublingual tablets or spray.

Diagnostic Studies

Diagnostic studies for angina include the following: history and physical examination, including assessment of pain and precipitating factors; laboratory data, including blood studies for anemia (hemoglobin and hematocrit values), cardiac enzymes (CK_2-MB, cardiac troponin I, cardiac troponin T levels), and cholesterol and triglyceride levels; ECGs during resting periods; stress testing; and coronary angiography. Complications of untreated or unstable angina include MI,

> **BOX 12-5 FACTORS THAT INFLUENCE OXYGEN DEMAND AND SUPPLY**
>
> **Increased Oxygen Demand**
> - **Increased heart rate:** exercise, tachydysrhythmias, fever, anxiety, pain, thyrotoxicosis, medications, ingestion of heavy meals, adapting to extremes in temperature
> - **Increased preload:** volume overload
> - **Increased afterload:** hypertension, aortic stenosis, vasopressors
> - **Increased contractility:** exercise, medications, anxiety
>
> **Reduced Oxygen Supply**
> - Coronary artery disease
> - Coronary artery spasms
> - Anemia
> - Hypoxemia

HF, dysrhythmias, psychological depression, and sudden death.

Nursing Diagnoses

Several nursing diagnoses and interventions are identified for patients with angina. These include the following[11]:

- Acute chest pain related to myocardial ischemia
- Knowledge deficit related to unfamiliarity with disease process and treatment
- Activity intolerance related to chest pain, side effects of prescribed medications, imbalance between oxygen supply and demand

Interventions

Nursing Interventions

Nursing interventions for the patient with angina are aimed at assessing the patient's description of pain, noting exacerbating factors and measures used to relieve the pain; evaluating whether this is a chronic problem (stable angina) or a new presentation; assessing for appropriateness of performing an ECG to evaluate ST-segment and T-wave changes; monitoring vital signs during chest pain and after nitrate administration; and monitoring the effectiveness of interventions.

The patient is instructed to relax and rest at the first sign of pain or discomfort, and to notify the nurse at the onset of any type of chest pain so that nitrates and oxygen can be administered. The nurse also offers assurance and emotional support by explaining all treatments and procedures and by encouraging questions. The nurse begins to assess the patient's knowledge level regarding the causes of angina, diagnostic procedures, the treatment plan, and risk factors for CAD. For those patients that smoke, readiness to quit should be assessed. Smoking cessation is encouraged. Patients who wish to stop smoking can be referred to the American Heart Association, American Lung Association, or American Cancer Society for support groups and interventions.

Medical Interventions

Unstable angina can be treated by conservative management, early intervention with percutaneous intervention, or surgical revascularization. Conservative intervention for the patient experiencing angina includes the administration of nitrates, beta-adrenergic blocking agents, calcium channel blocking agents, and ranolazine (Table 12-5). Angioplasty, stenting, and bypass surgery are approaches to revascularization.

TABLE 12-5 PHARMACOLOGY

Drugs for Acute Coronary Syndromes

Nitrates

Indications: angina

Mechanism of action: directly relaxes smooth muscle, which causes vasodilation of the systemic vascular bed; decrease myocardial oxygen demands; secondary effect is vasodilation of responsive coronary arteries

MEDICATION	DOSE/ROUTE	SIDE EFFECTS AND NURSING CONSIDERATIONS
Nitroglycerin (Tridil, Nitro-Bid, Nitro-Dur, Nitrostat)	*SL:* 0.4 mg SL every 5 minutes for up to 3 doses *Topical:* 0.5-2 inches every 6 hours *Transdermal:* One patch each day *IV:* continuous infusion started at 5 mcg/min and titrated up to 200 mcg/min maximum	Headache, flushing, tachycardia, dizziness, and orthostatic hypotension Instruct patient to call 911 if chest pain does not subside after the third SL dose. For topical dosing, patient should have a nitrate-free interval (10-12 hours/day) to avoid development of tolerance. Instruct patient not to combine nitrate use with medications used for treatment of erectile dysfunction (e.g., vardenafil, tadalafil, sildenafil).
Isosorbide dinitrate (Isordil)	*PO:* 5-40 mg BID-TID	Same
Isosorbide mononitrate (Imdur)	*PO:* 30-60 mg every day; maximum daily dose 240 mg	Same Do not crush or dissolve.

Beta-Blockers

Indications: used to treat angina, acute myocardial infarction, dysrhythmias and heart failure

Mechanism of action: block beta-adrenergic receptors, which results in decreased sympathetic nervous system response such as decreased heart rate, blood pressure, and cardiac contractility

MEDICATION	DOSE/ROUTE	SIDE EFFECTS AND NURSING CONSIDERATIONS
Metoprolol (Lopressor, Toprol XL)	*PO:* 50-100 mg BID *PO Toprol XL:* 12.5-200 mg daily *IV:* 5 mg	Bradycardia, hypotension, atrioventricular blocks, asthma attacks, fatigue, impotence, may mask hypoglycemic episodes.

TABLE 12-5   **PHARMACOLOGY**

Drugs for Acute Coronary Syndromes—cont'd

MEDICATION	DOSE/ROUTE	SIDE EFFECTS AND NURSING CONSIDERATIONS
		Teach patient to take pulse and blood pressure on regular basis and not to abruptly stop taking beta-blockers. Close glucose monitoring is needed if diabetic. Patient should have ECG monitoring during IV administration. Monitor for worsening signs of heart failure.
Propranolol (Inderal)	*PO:* 80-320 mg in divided doses 2-4 times a day *IV:* 0.5-3.0 mg IVP at rate of 1 mg/minute	Same
Labetalol (Trandate, Normodyne)	*PO:* 200-400 mg BID *IV:* 2 mg over 2 minutes at 10-minute intervals; slow IVP	Same Acts on both alpha, beta$_1$, and beta$_2$ receptors During IV administration, monitor blood pressure continuously; maximum effect occurs within 5 minutes.
Carvedilol (Coreg)	*PO:* 3.125-50 mg BID	Same; take with meals. Dose is doubled every 2 weeks until desired effect.

Calcium Channel Blockers

Indications: used to treat hypertension, tachydysrhythmias, vasospasms, and angina

Mechanism of action: inhibit the flow of calcium ions across cellular membranes, with resulting increased coronary blood flow and myocardial perfusion and decreased myocardial oxygen requirements

MEDICATION	DOSE/ROUTE	SIDE EFFECTS AND NURSING CONSIDERATIONS
Verapamil (Calan, Isoptin)	*PO:* 80-120 mg TID	Dizziness, flushing, headaches, bradycardia, atrioventricular blocks, and hypotension. Teach patient to monitor pulse and blood pressure, especially if taking nitrates and/or beta-blockers. Tablets cannot be crushed or chewed. Instruct patient to make position changes slowly.
Nifedipine (Procardia)	*PO:* 10 mg TID *PO sustained release:* 30-60 mg daily	Same Important that short-acting formulation (capsule) is swallowed whole and not punctured or chewed.
Diltiazem (Cardizem, Cardizem CD)	*PO:* 30 mg QID *PO sustained release:* 120-360 mg daily	Same

Antiplatelet Agents

Indications: unstable angina, acute myocardial infarction, and coronary interventions

Mechanism of action: inhibit clotting mechanisms within the clotting cascade or prevent platelet aggregation

MEDICATION	DOSE/ROUTE	SIDE EFFECTS AND NURSING CONSIDERATIONS
Aspirin	*PO:* 81-325 mg daily	Bleeding, epigastric discomfort, bruising, and gastric ulceration Instruct patient to take medication with food. Do not crush or chew the enteric-coated forms. Instruct patient to be aware of additive effects with OTC drugs containing aspirin or salicylate or other NSAIDs.
Clopidogrel (Plavix)	*PO:* 300-mg loading dose, then 75 mg daily (in combination with aspirin)	Same
Prasugrel (Effient)	*PO:* 60-mg loading dose, then 10 mg daily	Anemia, edema, headaches, dizziness. Not recommended for patients >75 years of age, weighing <60 kg, or with history of TIA.
Ticagrelor (Brilinta)	*PO:* 180-mg (two 90-mg tablets) loading dose (in combination with 325 mg aspirin), then 90 mg daily (with 81 mg aspirin)	Contraindicated in patients with history of intracranial hemorrhage, active pathological bleeding, or severe hepatic impairment. Higher incidence of bradydysrhythmias noted in clinical studies. Comparison of ticagrelor vs. clopidogrel reported a higher incidence of bleeding (11.6% vs 11.2%) and dyspnea (14% vs 8%).

Continued

TABLE 12-5 PHARMACOLOGY

Drugs for Acute Coronary Syndromes—cont'd

Glycoprotein IIb/IIIa Inhibitors

Indications: acute coronary syndromes and coronary intervention patients

Mechanism of action: antiplatelet agent and glycoprotein IIb/IIIa inhibitor; act by binding to the glycoprotein IIb/IIIa receptor site on the surface of the platelet

MEDICATION	DOSE/ROUTE	SIDE EFFECTS AND NURSING CONSIDERATIONS
Abciximab (ReoPro)	*IV:* 0.25 mg/kg IV bolus followed by a continuous infusion at 0.125 mg/kg/min for 12 hours	Bleeding, bruising, hemorrhage, thrombocytopenia, and hypotension. Avoid IM injections and venipunctures. Observe and teach patient bleeding precautions and activities to avoid that may cause injury. Assess infusion insertion site for bleeding or hematoma formation. Assess puncture site used for coronary intervention frequently. Abciximab is not reversible because of its binding to platelets. For hemorrhage, give fresh frozen plasma and platelets. Monitor CBC and aPTT daily.
Tirofiban (Aggrastat)	*IV:* 0.4 mcg/kg/min for 30 minutes, then continued at 0.1 mcg/kg/min for 12-24 hours. Reduce loading and maintenance infusion by 50% in patients with impaired renal function (creatinine clearance <30 mL/min)	Same. Tirofiban stops working when the infusion is discontinued. Platelet function is restored 4 hours after stopping the infusion.
Eptifibatide (Integrilin)	*IV:* 180 mcg/kg loading dose over 2 minutes, followed by continuous infusion of 2 mcg/kg/min for 18-24 hours or until hospital discharge. Reduce maintenance dose by 50% (to 1 mcg/kg/minute) in patients with creatinine clearance <50 mL/min; contraindicated if creatinine clearance <20 mL/min. Concurrent aspirin, thienopyridine, and heparin therapy is recommended	Same. Eptifibatide stops working when the infusion is discontinued. Platelet function is restored 4 hours after stopping the infusion.

Antithrombin Agents

Indications: prevention of or delay in thrombus formation

Mechanism of action: enhances inhibitory effects of antithrombin III, preventing conversion of fibrinogen to fibrin and prothrombin to thrombin

MEDICATION	DOSE/ROUTE	SIDE EFFECTS AND NURSING CONSIDERATIONS
Heparin	*IV:* 5000-7000 units bolus, followed by infusion of 1000 units/hr, titrated to aPTT	Bleeding, bruising, thrombocytopenia. Monitor aPTT. Monitor for signs of bleeding and hematoma formation. Avoid IM injections. Do not rub the site after giving the injection. Increased bleeding risk when dosing unfractioned heparin in patients with renal insufficiency. The aPTT should be monitored aggressively and the patient should be evaluated closely for signs and symptoms of bleeding.
Enoxaparin (Lovenox)	*Subcutaneous:* 1 mg/kg every 12 hours, in conjunction with aspirin. For patients with creatinine clearances <30 mL/minute, dosage is 1 mg/kg every 24 hours.	Bleeding, bruising, local site hematomas, and hemorrhage. Instruct patient to report persistent chest pain, unusual bleeding or bruising. Do not rub the site after giving the injection.

TABLE 12-5 PHARMACOLOGY
Drugs for Acute Coronary Syndromes—cont'd

Analgesic
Indications: pain relief and anxiety reduction during acute myocardial infarction
Mechanism of action: binds to opioid receptors in the central nervous system and causes inhibition of ascending pain pathways, altering perception and response to pain

MEDICATION	DOSE/ROUTE	SIDE EFFECTS AND NURSING CONSIDERATIONS
Morphine	*IV:* 2-4 mg IVP every 5-10 minutes	Hypotension, respiratory depression, apnea, bradycardia, nausea, and restlessness. Titrated for chest pain. Monitor level of consciousness, blood pressure, respiratory rate, and oxygen saturation during therapy. Effects are reversed with naloxone (Narcan).

Angiotensin-Converting Enzyme Inhibitors
Indications: used to treat hypertension, heart failure, and patients after myocardial infarction
Mechanism of action: prevent the conversion of angiotensin I to angiotensin II resulting in lower levels of angiotensin II, which causes an increase in plasma renin activity and a reduction of aldosterone secretion; also inhibit the remodeling process after myocardial injury

MEDICATION	DOSE/ROUTE	SIDE EFFECTS AND NURSING CONSIDERATIONS
Enalapril (Vasotec)	*PO:* 2.5-40 mg BID	Hypotension, bradycardia, renal impairment, cough, and orthostatic hypotension. Monitor urine output. Monitor potassium levels. Avoid use of NSAIDs. Instruct patient to avoid rapid change in position such as from lying to standing. Contraindicated in pregnancy.
Fosinopril (Monopril)	*PO:* 20-40 mg daily or BID	Same
Captopril (Capoten)	*PO:* 6.25 mg TID increasing gradually to 100 mg TID	Same

aPTT, Activated partial thromboplastin time; *BID,* twice daily; *CBC,* complete blood count; *ECG,* electrocardiogram; *IVP,* intravenous push; *NSAIDs,* nonsteroidal antiinflammatory drugs; *OTC,* over-the-counter; *PO,* orally; *QID,* four times daily; *SL,* sublingual; *TID,* three times daily. From Skidmore-Roth L. (2011). *Mosby's 2011 Nursing Drug Reference.* St. Louis: Mosby.

Nitrates are the most common medications for angina. They are direct-acting smooth muscle relaxants that cause vasodilation of the peripheral or systemic vascular bed.[28] Nitrate therapy is beneficial because it decreases myocardial oxygen demand. The vasodilating effect causes relief of pain and lowering of blood pressure. Nitroglycerin is available in quick-acting forms such as sublingual tablets or spray, or intravenous infusion. Long-acting forms are delivered orally or by ointments and skin patches (transdermal). Oral isosorbide (Isordil, Ismo, Imdur) is another vasodilator. Side effects of these vasodilators include headache, flushing, tachycardia, dizziness, and orthostatic hypotension. Instructions for NTG therapy are detailed in Box 12-6.

Beta-adrenergic blocking agents may also be used to treat angina. They block adrenergic receptors, thereby decreasing heart rate, blood pressure, and cardiac contractility.[28] Examples include atenolol, metoprolol, propranolol, labetalol, carvedilol, nadolol, timolol, and pindolol. The side effects of these agents include bradycardia, AV block, asthma attacks, depression, erectile dysfunction, hypotension, memory loss, and masking of hypoglycemic episodes. The patient is taught to take these agents as prescribed, not to stop taking them abruptly, and to monitor heart rate and blood pressure at regular intervals.

Calcium channel blockers inhibit the flow of calcium ions across cellular membranes, an effect that causes direct increases in coronary blood flow and myocardial perfusion.[28] These drugs are used for treating tachydysrhythmias, vasospasms, and hypertension, as well as for treating angina. Calcium channel blockers are divided into two categories: dihydropyridines and non-dihydropyridines. Dihydropyridines are primarily used to treat hypertension. These drugs typically end in "pine," such as amlodipine,

BOX 12-6 INSTRUCTIONS REGARDING NITROGLYCERIN

If the client is discharged on sublingual or buccal nitroglycerin, instruct client to:

- Have tablets readily available.
- Take a tablet before strenuous activity and in stressful situations.
- Take one tablet when chest pain occurs and another every 5 minutes up to a total of three times if necessary; obtain emergency medical assistance if pain persists.
- Place the tablet under the tongue or in the buccal pouch and allow it to dissolve thoroughly.
- Store tablets in a tightly capped, original container away from heat and moisture.
- Replace tablets every 6 months or sooner if they do not relieve discomfort.
- Avoid rising to a standing position quickly after taking nitroglycerin.
- Recognize that dizziness, flushing, and mild headache are common side effects.
- Report fainting, persistent or severe headache, blurred vision, or dry mouth.
- Avoid drinking alcoholic beverages.
- Caution use of drugs for erectile dysfunction (e.g., Viagra, Levitra) when taking nitrates because hypotensive effects are exaggerated.

If nitroglycerin skin patches are prescribed:

- Provide instructions about correct application, skin care, the need to rotate sites and to remove the old patch, and frequency of change.
- The patch should only be worn 12 to 14 hours per day to prevent development of nitrate tolerance.

From Skidmore-Roth, L. (2011). *Mosby's 2011 Nursing Drug Reference*. St. Louis: Mosby.

felodipine, nifedipine, and isradipine. Non-dihydropyridines such as verapamil (Calan, Isoptin) and diltiazem (Cardizem) are more effective for treating angina and dysrhythmias. The side effects of calcium channel blockers include dizziness, flushing, headaches, decreased heart rate, and hypotension. Ankle edema is a major side effect with the dihydropyridine-type calcium channel blocker. When prescribed a calcium channel blocker, the patient is taught to monitor blood pressure for hypotension and heart rate for bradycardia, especially if the agents are taken in combination with nitrates and beta-blockers.

Outcomes

The outcomes for patients with angina are that they will verbalize relief of chest discomfort, appear relaxed and comfortable, verbalize an understanding of angina pectoris and its management, describe their own cardiac risk factors and strategies to reduce them, and perform activities within limits of their ischemic disease, as evidenced by absence of chest pain or discomfort and no ECG changes reflecting ischemia.[11]

ACUTE CORONARY SYNDROME

Acute coronary syndrome (ACS) includes the diagnoses of unstable angina (UA) (previously defined) as well as acute myocardial infarction (AMI). AMI is defined as non–ST segment elevation myocardial infarction (NSTEMI) or ST segment elevation myocardial infarction (STEMI) by ECG characteristics. Prompt recognition and treatment results in improved outcomes for all ACSs.[24]

Pathophysiology

AMI is caused by an imbalance between myocardial oxygen supply and demand. This imbalance is the result of decreased coronary artery perfusion. Most cases of AMI are secondary to atherosclerosis. Other causes (<5%) include coronary artery spasm, coronary embolism, and blunt trauma. Reduced blood flow to an area of the myocardium causes significant and sustained oxygen deprivation to myocardial cells. Normal functioning is disrupted as ischemia and injury lead to eventual cellular death. Myocardial dysfunction occurs as more cells become involved.

Prolonged ischemia from cessation of blood flow to the cardiac muscle results in infarction and evolves over time. Cardiac cells can withstand ischemic conditions for 20 minutes; after that period, irreversible myocardial cell damage and cellular death begins. The amount of cell death increases, extending from the endocardium to the epicardium, as the duration of the occlusion increases. The extent of cell death determines the size of the MI. Contractility in the infarcted area becomes impaired. A nonfunctional zone and a zone of mild ischemia with potentially viable tissue surround the infarct. The ultimate size of the infarct depends on the fate of this ischemic zone. Early interventions, such as the administration of thrombolytics, can restore perfusion to the ischemic zone and can reduce the area of myocardial damage.

Based on the ECG, AMI is classified as a STEMI or NSTEMI. STEMI usually occurs because of plaque rupture leading to complete occlusion of the artery. NSTEMI usually results from a partially occluded coronary vessel. Most infarcts occur in the left ventricle; however, right ventricular infarction commonly occurs in patients with inferior wall infarction.[4] The treatment for a RV infarct is usually fluid therapy. Patients with right ventricular infarctions require cardiac pacing more frequently than left ventricular infarcts secondary to conduction defects, which are common.

The severity of the MI is determined by the success or lack of success of the treatment and by the degree of collateral circulation present at that particular part of the heart muscle. The *collateral circulation* consists of the alternative routes, or channels, that can develop in the myocardium in response to chronic ischemia or regional hypoperfusion. Through this small network of extra vessels, blood flow can be improved to the threatened myocardium.

TABLE 12-6	MYOCARDIAL INFARCTION BY SITE, ELECTROCARDIOGRAPHIC CHANGES, AND COMPLICATIONS		
LOCATION OF MI	**PRIMARY SITE OF OCCLUSION**	**PRIMARY ECG CHANGES**	**COMPLICATIONS**
Inferior MI	RCA (80%-90%) LCX (10%-20%)	II, III, aV_F	First- and second-degree heart block, right ventricular infarction
Inferolateral MI	LCX	II, III, aV_F, V_5, V_6	Third-degree heart block, left HF, cardiomyopathy, left ventricular rupture
Posterior MI	RCA or LCX	No lead truly looks at posterior surface Look for reciprocal changes in V_1 and V_2—tall, broad R waves; ST depression and tall T waves Posterior leads V_7, V_8, and V_9 may be recorded and evaluated	First-, second-, and third-degree heart blocks, HF, bradydys-rhythmias
Anterior MI	LAD	V_2-V_4	Third-degree heart block, HF, left bundle branch block
Anterior-septal MI	LAD	V_1-V_3	Second- and third-degree heart block
Lateral MI	LAD or LCX	V_5, V_6, I, aVL	HF
Right ventricular	RCA	V_4R Right precordial leads V_1R-V_6R may be recorded and evaluated	Increased RAP, decreased cardiac output, bradydysrhyth-mias, heart blocks, hypoten-sion, cardiogenic shock

AV, Atrioventricular; *ECG,* electrocardiographic; *HF,* heart failure; *LAD,* left anterior descending; *LCX,* left circumflex artery; *MI,* myocardial infarction; *RAP,* right atrial pressure; *RCA,* right coronary artery.

Assessment

Patient Assessment

Patient assessment includes close observation to identify the classic signs and symptoms of AMI. Chest pain is the paramount symptom. It may be severe, crushing, tight, squeezing, or simply a feeling of pressure. It can be precordial, substernal, or in the back, radiating to the arms, neck, or jaw. The skin may be cool, clammy, pale, and diaphoretic; the patient's color may be dusky or ashen; and slight hyperthermia may be present. The patient may be dyspneic and tachypneic, and may feel faint or have intermittent loss of sensorium. Nausea and vomiting commonly occur. Hypotension may be present and is often associated with dysrhythmias, particularly ventricular ectopy, bradycardia, tachycardia, or heart block. The type of dysrhythmia present depends on the area of the MI. The patient may be anxious or restless, or may exhibit certain behavioral responses including denial, depression, and a sense of impending doom. *Women are more likely to have atypical signs and symptoms* such as fatigue, diaphoresis, indigestion, arm or shoulder pain, nausea, and vomiting.[23]

Some individuals have ischemic episodes without knowing it, thereby having a *silent* infarction. These occur with no presenting signs or symptoms. This is more common in diabetic patients secondary to neuropathy. Assessment of a patient experiencing an AMI takes all the foregoing signs and

symptoms into account during the history and physical examination. Risk factors for an AMI are also considered.

Diagnosis

Diagnosis of AMI is based on symptoms, analysis of a 12-lead ECG, and cardiac enzyme values. The ECG is inspected for ST-segment elevation (>1 mm) in two or more contiguous leads. ST-segment depression ($\geq$0.5 mm) and new onset left bundle branch block also suggest an AMI. The type of AMI can be determined by the particular coronary artery involved and the blood supply to that area (Table 12-6).

Elevated serum cardiac enzymes are used to confirm the diagnosis of AMI: total CK, CK_2-MB, troponins I and T, and myoglobin. These tests are ordered immediately when a diagnosis of AMI is suspected and periodically (usually every 6-8 hours) during the first 24 hours to assess for increasing levels. Emergency cardiac catheterization may be performed in institutions with interventional cardiology services. Criteria for the diagnosis of ACS are summarized in Table 12-7.

Nursing Diagnoses

Nursing diagnoses and collaborative problems for the patient with AMI are described in the "Nursing Care Plan for the Patient with Acute Myocardial Infarction."

TABLE 12-7   CRITERIA FOR DIAGNOSIS OF ACUTE CORONARY SYNDROME

MAJOR CRITERIA	MINOR CRITERIA	
A diagnosis of an ACS can be made if one or more of the following major criteria are present:	In the absence of a major criterion, a diagnosis of ACS requires the presence of at least one item from both columns I and II	
	I	**II**
• ST-elevation or left bundle branch block (LBBB) in the setting of recent (<24 hours) or ongoing angina • New, or presumably new, ST-segment depression (≥0.05 mV) or T-wave inversion (≥0.2 mV) with rest symptoms • Elevated serum markers of myocardial damage (i.e., troponin I, troponin T, and CK$_2$-MB)	• Prolonged (i.e., >20 minutes) chest, arm/shoulder, neck, or epigastric discomfort • New onset chest, arm/shoulder, neck, or epigastric discomfort at rest, minimal exertion or ordinary activity • Previously documented chest, arm/shoulder, neck, or epigastric discomfort which has become distinctly more frequent or longer in duration	• Typical or atypical angina • Male age >40 years or female age >60 years • Known CAD • Heart failure, hypotension, or transient mitral regurgitation by examination • Diabetes • Documented extracardiac vascular disease • Pathological Q-waves on ECG • Abnormal ST-segment or T-wave abnormalities not known to be new

ACS, Acute coronary syndrome; *CAD,* coronary artery disease; *CK$_2$-MB,* creatine kinase MB band; *ECG,* electrocardiogram.
From Veterans Health Administration, Department of Defense. (2003). *VA/DoD clinical practice guideline for management of ischemic heart disease.* Washington, D.C.: Veterans Health Administration, Department of Defense.

◎ NURSING CARE PLAN

for the Patient with Acute Myocardial Infarction

NURSING DIAGNOSIS
Acute Chest Pain related to myocardial infarction, ischemia, or reduced coronary artery blood flow

PATIENT OUTCOMES
Chest pain relieved
• Verbalizes relief of pain
• Appears comfortable

NURSING INTERVENTIONS	RATIONALES

• Assess for characteristics of AMI pain:
  • Occurs suddenly
  • More intense
  • Quality varies
  • Not relieved with rest or nitrates
  • Atypical symptoms in older patients, women, and patients with diabetes and heart failure
	• Assist in identification of AMI to provide early treatment

• Note time since onset of first episode of chest pain; if less than 6 hours, patient may be a candidate for thrombolytic therapy	• Provide timely intervention
• Assess prior treatments for pain; patient may have taken sublingual nitroglycerin and a single dose of aspirin before arriving to hospital	• Assess response to prior treatment; assess need for aspirin as part of treatment protocol
• Monitor heart rate and blood pressure during pain episodes and during medication administration	• Assess nonverbal indicators of pain and response to treatment
• Assess baseline ECG for signs of MI: T and ST changes and development of Q waves and compare to previous ECGs if available	• Identify ischemia, injury, evolving AMI
• Monitor serial cardiac enzymes	• Assist in diagnosis and confirmation of AMI
• Continually reassess chest pain and response to medication; ongoing pain signifies prolonged myocardial ischemia and warrants immediate intervention	• Assess response to treatment; ensure that pain is controlled
• Assess for contraindications to thrombolytic agents; absolute contraindications include active internal bleeding, bleeding diathesis, or history of hemorrhagic stroke or intracranial hemorrhage	• Ensure that medication is administered safely when warranted; prevent complications associated with the medication

⊚ NURSING CARE PLAN

for the Patient with Acute Myocardial Infarction—cont'd

NURSING INTERVENTIONS	RATIONALES
• Assess for relative contraindications or warning conditions	• Risks of thrombolytic agents are weighed against benefits
• Maintain bed rest during periods of pain	• Reduce oxygen demand of the heart
• Administer oxygen therapy at 4-6 L/min; maintain oxygen saturation above 90%	• Ensure adequate oxygenation to the myocardium to prevent further damage
• Initiate IV nitrates according to protocol	• Nitrates are both coronary dilators and peripheral vasodilators causing hypotension
• Administer morphine sulfate according to unit protocol	• Reduce the workload on the heart through venodilation
• Administer IV beta-blockers according to protocol	• Reduce mortality in acute-phase MI
• Administer oral aspirin	• Decrease platelet aggregation to improve mortality
• Administer angiotensin-converting enzyme inhibitors	• Reduce progression to heart failure and death in patients with large MIs with LV dysfunction and in diabetic patients having an MI
• Administer thrombolytic agents according to unit protocol	• Restore perfusion
• Monitor for signs of bleeding: puncture sites, gingival bleeding, and prior cuts; observe for presence of occult or frank blood in urine, stool emesis, and sputum	• Assess for complications of thrombolytic therapy so that treatment can be initiated as needed
• Assess for intracranial bleeding by frequent monitoring of neurological status; changes in mental status, visual disturbances, and headaches are frequent signs of intracranial bleeding	• Assess for complication of intracranial bleeding associated with thrombolytic therapy
• Administer IV heparin according to unit protocol adjusting aPTT dose to 1.5 to 2 times normal	• Maintain coronary artery vessel patency after thrombolysis
• Prepare for possible cardiac catheterization, percutaneous transluminal coronary angioplasty or stent or coronary artery bypass graft surgery if signs of reperfusion are not evident and infarction evolves or if primary angioplasty is indicated	• Facilitate rapid intervention to restore coronary artery perfusion

NURSING DIAGNOSIS

Decreased Cardiac Output related to dysrhythmias, sympathetic nervous system stimulation, or electrolyte imbalances

PATIENT OUTCOMES

Normal cardiac rhythm with adequate cardiac output

• Strong peripheral pulses	• Good capillary refill
• Normal blood pressure	• Adequate urine outputs
• Clear breath sounds	• Clear mentation

NURSING INTERVENTIONS	RATIONALES
• Monitor heart rate and rhythm continuously; anticipate common dysrhythmias—PVCs, ventricular tachycardia, atrial flutter, and atrial fibrillation	• Detect and treat dysrhythmias
• Assess for signs of decreased cardiac output	• Identify complications to ensure timely treatment
• Monitor PR, QRS, and QT intervals	• Detect abnormal conduction of impulses early
• Monitor continuous ECG in appropriate leads	• See Chapter 7 for best practice for monitoring
• Institute treatment according to advanced cardiac life support (ACLS) guidelines or unit protocol	• Surveillance may prevent lethal dysrhythmias
• Assess peripheral and central pulses	• Detect reduced stroke volume and cardiac output
• Assess for mental status changes—restlessness and anxiety	• Detect early signs of hypoxemia
• Assess respiratory rate, rhythm, and breath sounds; rapid, shallow respirations and presence of crackles, wheezes or Cheyne-Stokes respirations	• Assess respiratory symptoms associated with low cardiac output
• Assess urine output via indwelling urinary catheter	• Assess adequacy of renal perfusion
• Auscultate for presence of S_3, S_4, or systolic murmur	• S_3 denotes LV dysfunction; S_4 indicates a noncompliant ventricle; a systolic murmur may be caused by papillary muscle rupture

Continued

for the Patient with Acute Myocardial Infarction—cont'd

NURSING INTERVENTIONS	RATIONALES
• Assess pulse oximetry and arterial blood gas results; maintain oxygen saturation of at least 90%	• Ensure adequate oxygenation
• If inferior wall MI, evaluate right-sided 12-lead ECG; assess for signs of a right ventricular MI and right ventricular failure (see Box 12-12)	• Identify right ventricular MI and potential complication of right-sided heart failure
• Anticipate insertion of hemodynamic monitoring catheter	• Guide management of fluids and medications
• Administer IV fluids	• Maintain fluid balance
• Monitor for signs of left and right ventricular failure (Box 12-12)	• For left-sided failure anticipate diuretics, vasodilators, inotropics, and oxygen as indicated
	• For right-sided failure anticipate fluid resuscitation and possible inotropic and peripheral vasodilator therapy
• Carefully administer nitrates and morphine sulfate for pain	• Reduced preload and filling pressures associated with these medication may compromise cardiac output

NURSING DIAGNOSIS

Fear related to change in health status, threat of death, threat to self-concept, critical care environment

PATIENT OUTCOMES

Fear is decreased or resolved
• Verbalizes reduced fear
• Demonstrates positive coping mechanisms

NURSING INTERVENTIONS	RATIONALES
• Assess level of fear noting nonverbal communication	• Identify fear and anxiety
• Assess coping factors	• Coping patterns are highly individualized
• Acknowledge awareness of patient's fears	• Validate feelings and communicate acceptance of those feelings
• Allow patient to verbalize fears of dying	• May reduce anxiety
• Offer realistic assurances of recovery	• Reduce anxiety by providing accurate information
• Maintain confident, assured manner	• Staff anxiety may be perceived by the patient
• Explain care provided and rationale so it is understandable	• Allay anxiety; lack of understanding can add to fear
• Assure the patient that monitoring will ensure prompt intervention	• Provide a measure of safety
• Reduce unnecessary external stimuli	• Anxiety may escalate with excessive noise
• Provide diversional materials	• Decrease anxiety and prevent feelings of isolation
• Establish rest periods	• Ensure dedicate periods to facilitate physical and mental rest
• Refer to other support persons as appropriate	• Additional specialty expertise may be required
• Administer mild sedative as prescribed	• Medication may be required to reduce anxiety

NURSING DIAGNOSIS

Risk for Activity Intolerance related to weakness or imbalance between oxygen supply and demand

PATIENT OUTCOMES

Tolerates progressive activity
• Heart rate and blood pressure within expected range and no complaints of dyspnea or fatigue
• Verbalizes realistic expectations for progressive activity

NURSING INTERVENTIONS	RATIONALES
• Assess respiratory and cardiac status before initiating activity	• Physical deconditioning may occur with prolonged bed rest
• Observe and document response to activity	• Assess response to activity progression
• Encourage adequate rest	• Provide time for energy conservation and recovery
• Provide small, frequent meals	• Facilitate digestion and reduce energy needs
• Instruct patient not to hold breath while exercising or moving about in bed and not to strain for bowel movements	• Valsalva maneuver affects endocardial repolarization
• Maintain progression of activity per cardiac rehabilitation protocol	• Provide gradual increase in activity as tolerated
• Provide emotional support when increasing activity	• Reduce anxiety about overexertion

AMI, Acute myocardial infarction; *aPTT,* activated partial thromboplastin time; *ECG,* electrocardiogram; *IV,* intravenous; *LV,* left ventricular; *PVCs,* premature ventricular contractions; *RAP,* right atrial pressure.
Based on data from Gulanick M and Myers JL. *Nursing Care Plans: Diagnoses, Interventions, and Outcomes,* 7th ed. St. Louis, Mosby, 2011.

Complications

Complications of AMI include cardiac dysrhythmias, heart failure, thromboembolism, rupture of a portion of the heart (e.g., ventricular wall, interventricular septum, or papillary muscle), pericarditis, infarct extension or recurrence, and cardiogenic shock (see Chapter 11). Dysrhythmias, heart failure, and pericarditis are discussed later in this chapter.

Medical Interventions

Treatment goals for AMI are to establish reperfusion, reduce infarct size, prevent and treat complications, and provide emotional support and education.[11] Medical treatment of AMI is aimed at relieving pain, providing adequate oxygenation to the myocardium, preventing platelet aggregation, and restoring blood flow to the myocardium through thrombolytic therapy or acute interventional therapy, such as angioplasty. Hemodynamic monitoring is also used to assess cardiac function and to monitor fluid balance in some patients.

Pain Relief

The initial pain of AMI is treated with morphine sulfate administered by the IV route. The dose is 2 to 4 mg IV push over 5 minutes. Patients must be observed for hypotension and respiratory depression (see Table 12-5).

Nitrates. Nitroglycerin (NTG) may be given to reduce the ischemic pain of AMI. NTG increases coronary perfusion because of its vasodilatory effects. It is usually started at doses of 5 to 10 mcg/min IV and titrated to a total dose of 50 to 200 mcg/min until chest pain is absent, pulmonary artery occlusion pressure decreases, and/or systolic blood pressure decreases. Caution should be used in administering NTG to patients with inferior or right ventricular infarctions because it can lead to profound hypotension.

Oxygen

Oxygen administration is important for assisting the myocardial tissue to continue its pumping activity and for repairing the damaged tissue around the site of the infarct. Treatment with oxygen via nasal cannula at 4 to 6 L/min assists in maintaining oxygenation. Rest also helps to improve oxygenation. The goal is to maintain oxygen saturation above 90%. However, recent guidelines suggest that routine use of supplemental oxygen may not be necessary in patients with uncomplicated ACS without signs of heart failure or hypoxemia.[24]

Antidysrhythmics

Dysrhythmias are common after AMI. Drugs to treat cardiac dysrhythmias are administered when the heart's natural pacemaker develops an abnormal rate or rhythm (see Chapter 7).

Prevention of Platelet Aggregation

Alterations in platelet function contribute to occlusion of the coronary arteries. Aspirin (325 mg) is given immediately to all patients with suspected AMI. Aspirin blocks synthesis of thromboxane A_2, thus inhibiting aggregation of platelets. In addition, a thienopyridine, such as clopidogrel (Plavix), prasugel (Effient), or ticagrelor (Brilinta); or a Gp IIb/IIIa inhibitor may added.[33] Heparin is used with other antiplatelet agents.

Thrombolytic Therapy

One common treatment for STEMI is thrombolytic therapy. Research has shown that occlusion of the coronary vessel does not cause immediate myocardial cell death. Ischemia begins within minutes of the vessel occlusion, and prolonged injury results in AMI.[26] The goals are to dissolve the lesion that is occluding the coronary artery and to increase blood flow to the myocardium. For treatment to be considered, the patient must be symptomatic for less than 6 hours, have pain for 20 minutes that was unrelieved by NTG, and have a 12-lead ECG with an ST-segment elevation of 1 mm or greater in two or more contiguous ECG leads or an ST-segment depression of 0.5 mm or greater. Table 12-8 lists some of the common thrombolytics currently available.

A summary of the use of thrombolytics includes the following:
- Fibrinolysis reduces mortality and salvages myocardium in STEMI.
- Fibrinolysis is not effective in the treatment of unstable angina or NSTEMI.
- Thrombolysis should be instituted within 30 to 60 minutes of arrival. The sooner treatment is initiated, the better the outcome.
- Patients treated within the first 70 minutes of onset of symptoms have 75% reduction in mortality rates and greater than 50% reduction in infarct size.
- The worst possible complication of fibrinolysis is intracranial hemorrhage. Bleeding from puncture sites commonly occurs.

Nursing care of the patient includes rapid identification of whether the patient is a suitable candidate for IV thrombolytics, thus ensuring as little delay as possible before the therapy; and screening for contraindications. Next, the nurse secures three vascular access lines and obtains necessary laboratory data. Initial ECG monitoring is documented before starting the infusion, at various times throughout the infusion, and at the end of the infusion. Finally, the patient is monitored for complications, including reperfusion dysrhythmias (premature ventricular contractions, sinus bradycardia, accelerated idioventricular rhythm, or ventricular tachycardia), oozing at venipuncture sites, gingival bleeding, reocclusion or reinfarction, and symptoms of hemorrhagic stroke.

TABLE 12-8   PHARMACOLOGY

Thrombolytics

MEDICATION	DOSE/ROUTE	HALF-LIFE
Alteplase (tissue plasminogen activator; t-PA)	*3-hour infusion:* For adults weighing >65 kg, 100-mg dose; administer 60 mg over the first hour (6-10 mg as IV bolus over 1-2 minutes followed by infusion of remaining dose), 20 mg over second hour, and 20 over third hour For adults weighing <65 kg, 1.25 mg/kg dose; administer 60% first hour (6%-10% as a IV bolus followed by infusion of remaining dose), 20% over second hour, and 20% over third *Accelerated 90-minute infusion:* For adults weighing >67 kg, 100-mg dose; administer 15-mg bolus IV over 1-2 minutes, followed by infusion of 50 mg over the first 30 minutes, and 35 mg over next 60 minutes For adults weighing ≤67 kg, administer 15-mg bolus IV over 1-2 minutes, followed by infusion of 0.75 mg/kg over the first 30 minutes (not to exceed 50 mg), and 0.50 mg/kg over next 60 minutes (not to exceed 35 mg)	4-5 minutes
Reteplase (r-PA)	10 units IV bolus; repeat 10-unit dose in 30 minutes; administer over 2 minutes. Give through a dedicated IV line Do not give repeat bolus if serious bleeding occurs after first IV bolus	13-16 minutes
Tenecteplase (TNK)	Total dose 30 to 50 mg, based on weight (see package insert) given IV over 5 seconds	20-24 minutes
Streptokinase (SK)	1.5 million units IV infusion over 60 minutes	23 minutes

IV, Intravenous.
From Skidmore-Roth L. (2011). *Mosby's 2011 Nursing Drug Reference.* St. Louis: Mosby.

Percutaneous Coronary Intervention

Primary percutaneous coronary intervention (PCI) is performed in the management of AMI with improved outcomes over thrombolytic therapy. PCI should be performed within 90 minutes of arrival to the emergency department, with a target of less than 60 minutes (termed *door to balloon time*).[16] Primary PCI has been demonstrated to be more effective than thrombolysis in opening acutely occluded arteries in settings where it can be rapidly performed by experienced interventional cardiologists.[16] If patients present to a facility without PCI capabilities, they should be transferred to a PCI-capable facility to receive a PCI within 90 minutes of being assessed, or triaged to receive fibrinolytic therapy at the receiving facility.

Facilitated Percutaneous Coronary Intervention

Facilitated PCI is the use of additional agents, fibrinolysis, Gp IIb/IIIa inhibitors, or both to pretreat the patient awaiting primary PCI. It was thought that facilitated PCI would improve outcomes; however, administration of these agents before PCI is associated with higher rates of death, reinfarction, and bleeding complications. Therefore facilitated PCI is not recommended; PCI is the preferred treatment.

Additional research is needed to test if fibrinolytic therapy is preferable to delayed PCI in facilities without an interventional cardiology service. American College of Cardiology guidelines recommend treating the affected vessel when feasible and deferring surgical or PCI-based revascularization of other vessels until the patient's condition has stabilized and the most appropriate treatment strategy has been determined.[16]

Medications

Several medications may be ordered for the patient with AMI. Patients whose chest pain symptoms are suggestive of serious illness need immediate assessment in a monitored unit and early therapy to include an IV line, oxygen, aspirin, NTG, and morphine. Early therapy consists of aspirin, heparin or low–molecular weight heparin, nitrates, beta-blockers, clopidogrel, bivalirudin, and fondaparinux.

Nitrates. Nitrates are vasodilators that reduce pain, increase venous capacitance, and reduce platelet adhesion and aggregation. Sublingual NTG is often given in the emergency department. IV NTG is effective for relieving ischemia (see Table 12-5).

Beta-blockers. Beta-blockers are used to decrease heart rate, blood pressure, and myocardial oxygen consumption. Morbidity and mortality after AMI have been reduced by the use of beta-blockers. Commonly used drugs include metoprolol, atenolol, and carvedilol. The patient is carefully assessed for hypotension and bradycardia. Beta-blockers should be started within 24 hours of AMI unless otherwise contraindicated.

Angiotensin-converting enzyme inhibitors. After an AMI, the area of ventricular damage changes shape or *remodels*. The ventricle becomes thinner and balloons out, thus reducing contractility. Cardiac tissue surrounding the area of infarction undergoes changes that can be categorized as (1) myocardial stunning (a temporary loss of contractile function that persists for hours to days after perfusion has been restored); (2) hibernating myocardium (tissue that is persistently ischemic and undergoes metabolic adaptation to prolong myocyte survival until perfusion can be restored); and (3) myocardial remodelling (a process mediated by angiotensin II, aldosterone, catecholamines, adenosine, and inflammatory cytokines that causes myocyte hypertrophy and loss of contractile function in the areas of the heart distant from the site of infarctions). Angiotensin-converting enzyme inhibitors (ACEI) should be started within 24 hours to reduce the incidence of ventricular remodelling. The drugs can be discontinued if the patient exhibits no signs of ventricular dysfunction (see Table 12-5). ACEIs should be prescribed for patients with UA, NSTEMI, STEMI with a left ventricular ejection fraction (LVEF) of 40% or less, and patients with a history of hypertension, diabetes or chronic kidney disease unless contraindicated.[4] The most common side effect with ACEI is cough, which is chronic and nonproductive. If side effects occur with ACEI, angiotensin receptor blockers (ARBs) should be initiated.[2]

Novel Stem Cell Treatment

Autologous bone marrow stem cell therapy is being used to prevent ventricular remodeling and improve cardiac function. The stem cells are implanted either within the heart or the heart muscle (see box, "Evidence-Based Practice").

Outcomes

Patient outcomes are generalized to encompass the wide spectrum of patients who have experienced an AMI, uncomplicated or complicated, that require medical or surgical intervention. Outcomes include verbalization of relief of pain and fear, adequate cardiac output, ability to tolerate progressive activity, and demonstration of positive coping mechanisms.

INTERVENTIONAL CARDIOLOGY

Several interventions are done to treat ACS. Primary PCI is recommended for treatment of acute STEMI. The goal is to treat the patient to prevent AMI. Intervention is also used after AMI to prevent further damage of the myocardium. PCIs consist of percutaneous transluminal coronary angioplasty (PTCA or angioplasty), percutaneous transluminal coronary rotational atherectomy, directional coronary atherectomy, laser atherectomy, and intracoronary stenting. An early, invasive PCI procedure is indicated for patients with UA/NSTEMI who are hemodynamically unstable or continue to have angina, or have an elevated risk for clinical events.[33] For the purposes of this book, only PTCA and stenting are

EVIDENCE-BASED PRACTICE

Stem Cell Therapy to Improve Cardiac Function

Problem
Novel treatments are needed to prevent ventricular remodeling and improve cardiac function. Remodeling occurs after acute myocardial infarction and can lead to heart failure. Bone marrow stem cell therapy has been studied for about a decade.

Clinical Question
Does bone marrow stem cell therapy prevent ventricular remodelling and improve cardiac function?

Evidence
Strauer and Steinhoff provide an excellent discussion of the role of bone marrow stem cell therapy in the treatment of acute myocardial infarction. They summarize the research and also depict graphically the process of getting stem cells to the cardiac muscle. Tuty Kuswardhani and Soetjitno conducted a systematic review and meta-analysis of 10 randomized controlled trials to assess effect of therapy on cardiac function and secondary outcomes. In comparison to placebo, the analysis found stem cell therapy superior in improving left ventricular function. Therapy was not associated with a reduction in mortality, but it protected patients from recurrent myocardial infarction and rehospitalizations for heart failure. They concluded that stem cell therapy was effective and safe.

Implications for Nursing
Rehospitalization for heart failure secondary to ventricular remodeling after an infarction is a common occurrence. Novel treatment is needed to prevent these physiological changes from occurring. Nurses need to be aware of novel and cutting-edge therapies to improve patient outcomes. Knowledge of stem cell therapy is therefore important to understand. Since the stem cell therapy is autologous, the procedure is safe, clinically justified, and should not be associated with ethical issues related to the practice. Related nursing care is similar to that of post–cardiac catheterization.

Level of Evidence
A—Meta-analysis

References
Strauer B-E, & Steinhoff G. 10 Years of intracoronary and intramyocardial bone marrow stem cell therapy of the heart. *Journal of the American College of Cardiology,* 2011;58:1095-1104.
Tuty Kuswardhani RA, & Soejitno A. Bone marrow-derived stem cells as an adjunctive treatment for acute myocardial infarction: A systematic review and meta-analysis. *Acta Medica Indonesiana,* 2011;43(3):168-177.

discussed. The postprocedure care for all patients who undergo PCI consists of the same interventions.

Percutaneous Transluminal Coronary Angioplasty

The purpose of PTCA is to compress intracoronary plaque to increase blood flow to the myocardium. It is usually the treatment of choice for patients with uncompromised collateral flow, noncalcified lesions, and lesions not present at bifurcations of vessels. PTCA is performed in the cardiac catheterization laboratory. A balloon catheter is inserted in the manner of coronary angiography, but it is threaded into the occluded coronary artery and is advanced with the use of a guidewire across the lesion. The balloon is inflated under pressure one or several times to compress the lesion (Figure 12-10).

The optimal goal after PTCA is open coronary arteries (Figure 12-11). This procedure best treats fixed, noncalcified lesions that are accessible for dilation. Single-vessel disease remains the classic indication for PTCA. PTCA is not recommended for a lesion of the left main coronary artery.[15]

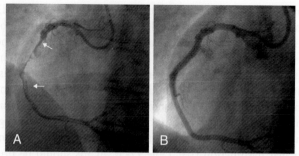

FIGURE 12-11 A, A thrombotic occlusion of the right coronary artery is noted *(arrows)*. **B,** Right coronary artery is opened and blood flow restored following angioplasty and placement of a 4-mm stent. (From Lewis SL. *Medical-Surgical Nursing: Assessment and Management of Clinical Problems.* St. Louis: Mosby; 2011.)

Complications

Complications of PTCA are commonly due to the angiography and include hematoma at the catheter insertion site, AMI, stroke or transient ischemic attack, pseudoaneurysm,

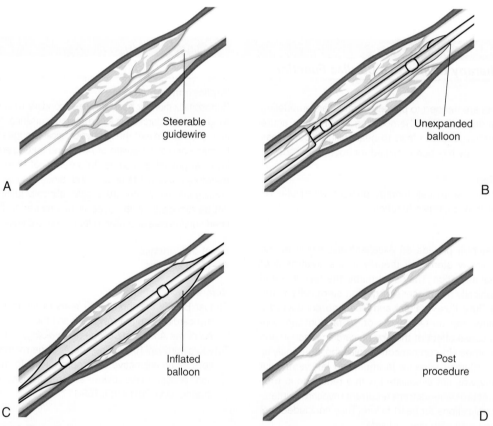

FIGURE 12-10 Coronary angioplasty procedure. **A-D,** Order of procedure. (From Moser DK, Riegel B. *Cardiac Nursing.* St. Louis: Mosby; 2008.)

dysrhythmias, infection, acute kidney injury, and coronary artery dissection. Mortality rates for PTCA are less than 1%, with the risk of AMI less than 1.5%.[33]

Intracoronary Stent

Intracoronary stents are tubes that are implanted at the site of stenosis to widen the arterial lumen by squeezing atherosclerotic plaque against the artery's walls (as does PTCA). However, the stent also keeps the lumen open by providing structural support. Stent designs differ, but most designs have springs, slots, or mesh tubes about 15 mm in length, with some resembling the spiral bindings used in notebooks. These are tightly wrapped around a balloon catheter, which is inflated to implant the stent.

The procedure for placing a stent is similar to the procedure in PTCA, in which the patient first undergoes cardiac angiography for identification of occlusions in coronary arteries. The balloon catheter bearing the stent is inserted into the coronary artery, and the stent is positioned at the desired site. The balloon is inflated, thereby expanding the stent, which squeezes the atherosclerotic plaque and intimal flaps against the vessel wall. After the balloon is deflated and removed, the stent remains, holding the plaque and other matter in place and providing structural support to keep the artery from collapsing (Figure 12-12).[27]

Aggressive anticoagulation therapy before, during, and after the procedure is necessary for the prevention of coagulation. Before sheath removal, peripheral perfusion is monitored because the sheath may cause occlusion of the femoral artery. Peripheral pulses, skin color, and temperature are monitored. The insertion site is inspected for any oozing or bleeding. After sheath removal, hemostasis is maintained with manual pressure, a femoral compression device, or an arterial puncture sealing device. Pain management and proper hydration aid in recovery. Retroperitoneal bleeding or impaired perfusion may occur after sheath removal. Restenosis can occur as a result of neointimal growth because of the body's natural defense when the inner intimal lining is injured, even slightly, as happens with stent placement. Restenosis occurs in 30% to 40% of patients who undergo this procedure. The Gp IIb/IIIa inhibitors are used after stent placement to prevent acute reocclusion through prevention of platelet aggregation.

After a stent procedure, a patient must take antiplatelet agents such as aspirin and clopidogrel,[27] prasugrel, or ticagrelor. Aspirin is used indefinitely at dose ranges of 81 to 162 mg. Oral clopidogrel, 75 mg/day, should be added to aspirin for 3 to 12 months; it may be used as short as 30 days or given indefinitely. Antibiotics are no longer indicated post stent for prophylaxis protection of endocarditis.[33]

Therapies in intracoronary stenting have advanced using both bare metal stents and drug-eluting stents. Normal reaction from the body to vascular injury is neointimal (new intimal cell) growth. When a stent is placed, minor damage to the inner lining of the artery occurs; thus the body's natural defense is to grow new intimal cells to repair the damage, leading to in-stent restenosis.

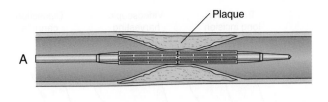
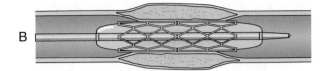
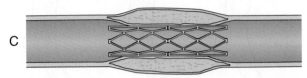

FIGURE 12-12 Placement of coronary artery stent. **A,** The stent is positioned at the site of the lesion. **B,** The balloon is inflated, expanding the stent. The balloon is then deflated and removed. **C,** The implanted stent is left in place. (From Lewis SL. *Medical-Surgical Nursing: Assessment and Management of Clinical Problems.* St. Louis: Mosby; 2011.)

Drug-eluting stents have the benefit of having an antiproliferative medication coating that reduces in-stent thrombosis. Medication is released slowly over 2 to 4 weeks from the stent to reduce the risk of neointimal growth.[27]

Surgical Revascularization

Surgical approaches used for revascularization include coronary revascularization by coronary artery bypass graft (CABG), minimally invasive CABG, and transmyocardial revascularization (TMR).

Coronary Artery Bypass Graft

CABG is a surgical procedure in which the ischemic area or areas of the myocardium are revascularized by implantation of the internal mammary artery or bypassing of the coronary occlusion with a saphenous vein graft or radial artery graft. The indications for CABG are chronic stable angina that is refractory to other therapies, significant left main coronary occlusion (>50%), triple-vessel CAD, unstable angina pectoris, left ventricular failure, lesions not amenable to PTCA, and PTCA failure.[27]

CABG is performed in the operating room while the patient receives general anesthesia and is intubated. One approach is to make a midsternal, longitudinal incision into the chest cavity. Surgery is done either with cardiopulmonary bypass or without (*off-pump*). During cardiopulmonary bypass, blood is pumped through an oxygenator, or heart-lung machine, to receive oxygen. Cardioplegia solution is used to stop the heart so surgery can be performed.

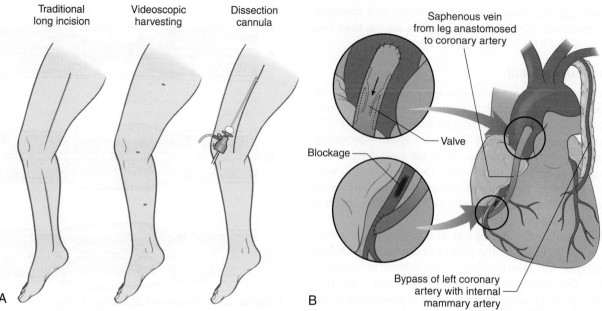

FIGURE 12-13 Coronary artery bypass graft surgery. **A,** Saphenous vein is harvested from the leg using either a traditional long incision or less invasive videoscopic harvesting. **B,** The vein is then anastomosed to the coronary artery.

The coronary arteries are visualized, and a segment of the saphenous vein is grafted or anastomosed to the distal end of the vessel, with the proximal end of the graft vessel anastomosed to the aorta (Figure 12-13). The internal mammary artery is often used for creating an artery-to-artery graft. Internal mammary revascularization has better long-term patency than saphenous vein grafts. It is the preferred graft for lesions of the left anterior descending coronary artery.

Once grafting is done, the cardiopulmonary bypass (if used) is progressively discontinued, chest and mediastinal tubes are inserted, and the chest is closed. Box 12-7 gives information related to chest and mediastinal tubes.[31]

Minimally Invasive Coronary Artery Surgery

Minimally invasive coronary artery surgery is also called limited-access coronary artery surgery.[2] It has been evaluated as an alternative to the standard methods for CABG. Two commonly used approaches include port-access coronary artery bypass (PACAB or PortCAB) and minimally invasive coronary artery bypass (MIDCAB).

In PACAB, the heart is stopped, and the patient undergoes cardiopulmonary bypass. Small incisions (ports) are made in the patient's chest. The surgical team passes instruments through the ports to perform the bypasses using the internal mammary artery, saphenous vein, or radial artery. Procedures to replace damaged valves through limited-access ports are also being done.

The goal of MIDCAB is to avoid using cardiopulmonary bypass. It is performed while the patient's heart is still beating and is intended for use when only one or two arteries will be bypassed. MIDCAB uses a combination of small holes or ports in the chest and a small incision made directly over the coronary artery to be bypassed. The internal mammary artery is commonly used for the graft. The surgeon views and performs the attachment directly, so the artery to be bypassed must be right under the incision.

The American Heart Association's Council on Cardiothoracic and Vascular Surgery has been carefully monitoring these two procedures. MIDCAB appears to be easier on the patient and less expensive than CABG. However, complications may require an open-chest procedure.[2] As these surgical procedures are refined so that they are no more invasive than angioplasty, they will become more common.

Robotically-assisted heart surgery is another type of minimally invasive heart surgery. The cardiac surgeons use a computer console to control surgical instruments on thin robotic arms. Like the other two minimally invasive surgeries just discussed, smaller incisions and quicker recovery times are the primary benefits.

Management after Cardiac Surgery

Patients are usually admitted directly to the critical care unit after cardiac surgery. The patient often has a pulmonary artery catheter, arterial catheter, peripheral IV lines, pleural chest tubes, mediastinal tubes, and an indwelling urinary catheter. The patient is usually mechanically ventilated in the immediate postoperative period. The nurse assesses the patient often and provides rapid interventions to help the patient recover from anesthesia and to prevent complications. The nurse-to-patient ratio is often 1:1 during the first few hours after surgery or until the patient is extubated. Nursing care for these patients is summarized in Box 12-8.

BOX 12-7   KEY POINTS FOR MAINTAINING PLEURAL CHEST AND MEDIASTINAL TUBES

Definitions
- **Pleural chest tube:** The tube is inserted into the pleural space to maintain the normal negative pressure and to facilitate respiration. It is inserted after cardiac surgery if the pleural space is opened. It is also inserted as treatment for pneumothorax or hemothorax.
- **Mediastinal tube:** The tube is inserted into the mediastinal space to provide drainage after cardiac surgery.
- **Drainage system:** A water-seal system assists in maintaining negative pressures (chest tube). Some devices are designed to function without water (dry). Suction (up to 20 cm H_2O) is often applied to facilitate drainage.
- **Autotransfusion:** Reinfusion of autologous drainage from the system back to the patient.

Baseline Assessment
- Make sure that all connections are tight: insertion site to the chest drainage system, suction control chamber to the suction unit.
- Assess that the dressing over insertion site is dry and intact.
- Palpate for subcutaneous crepitus around the insertion site and chest wall.
- Auscultate breath sounds bilaterally.
- Observe the color and consistency of fluid in the collecting tubing (more accurate assessment than fluid in the drainage system); mark the fluid level on the drainage system.
- Assess the drainage system for proper functioning (read instructions for the device being used).
- Check the water in the water-seal level; the water level should fluctuate with respirations in chest tubes (not in mediastinal tubes).
- Check suction control and be sure that suction is on, if ordered.
- Check for intermittent bubbling in the water-seal chamber; it indicates an air leak from the pleural space (pleural tube).

Maintaining the Chest Drainage System
- Keep the tubing coiled on the bed near the patient.
- Record drainage in the medical record per protocol; notify the provider of excessive drainage (volume to report determined by unit parameters or written order; volume varies depending on purpose of the tube and time since insertion).
- Change the dressing according to unit protocol.
- Splint the insertion site to facilitate coughing and deep breathing.
- Ensure that drainage flows into the drainage system by facilitating gravity drainage; *milking* and *stripping* the tubes are not recommended because these procedures generate high negative pressures in the system.
- If the patient is transported (or ambulated) disconnect the drainage system from suction and keep it upright below the level of the chest. Do not clamp the tube.
- Chest x-ray studies are done immediately after insertion and usually daily thereafter.

Assisting with Removal
- Chest and mediastinal tubes are usually removed by the provider.
- Ensure adequate pain medication before removal.
- Apply an occlusive dressing to the site after removal.
- A chest x-ray study is usually done after removal.

Autotransfusion
- An autotransfusion collection system is attached to the chest drainage device.
- Anticoagulants may be ordered to be added to the autotransfusion system (citrate-phosphate-dextrose, acid-phosphate-dextrose, or heparin); these are not usually necessary with mediastinal drainage.
- Reinfuse drainage within the time frame specified by unit policy. It is recommended that reinfusion begin within 6 hours of initiating the collection, and reinfused to the patient within a 4-hour period.
- Evacuate air from the autotransfusion bag; air embolism may occur unless all air is removed.
- Attach a microaggregate filter and infuse via gravity or a pressure bag

BOX 12-8   NURSING INTERVENTIONS AFTER CARDIAC SURGERY

- Monitor for hypotension; administer fluids and vasopressors as ordered or based on protocol.
- Assess for hypovolemia; monitor and trend output from the pleural chest and mediastinal tubes and urine output.
- Monitor hemodynamic pressures, SvO_2, stroke index, cardiac index, PAOP, and RAP; treat the patient per protocol.
- Rewarm the patient gradually (if applicable).
- Monitor and treat fluid and electrolytes, hemoglobin, hematocrit, renal function, and coagulation studies.
- Provide pain relief.

- Monitor for complications: intraoperative AMI, dysrhythmias, heart failure, cardiac tamponade, thromboembolism, impaired renal function, pneumonia, pneumothorax, pleural effusion, cerebral ischemia, or stroke.
- Wean from mechanical ventilation per protocol; extubate; promote pulmonary hygiene every 1 to 2 hours while the patient is awake.
- Assess wounds and provide incisional care per hospital protocol.
- Gradually increase the patient's activity.
- Provide emotional support to the patient and family.

PAOP, Pulmonary artery occlusion pressure; *RAP,* right atrial pressure; *SvO_2,* mixed venous oxygen saturation.

Complications of Cardiac Surgery

Patients who have had cardiac surgery should be closely monitored for complications such as dysrhythmias (atrial fibrillation, atrial flutter, ventricular tachycardia, ventricular fibrillation), MI, shock, pericarditis, pericardial effusion, and cardiac tamponade. The critical care nurse taking care of a patient who has just undergone CABG must have quick critical thinking skills and the ability to assess the whole picture, while prioritizing interventions that need to be performed.

MECHANICAL THERAPIES

Transmyocardial Revascularization

In transmyocardial revascularization (TMR), a high-energy laser creates channels from the epicardial surface into the left ventricular chamber. This procedure is also called *laser revascularization*. The purpose of TMR is to increase perfusion directly to the heart muscle. It is performed on patients who are poor candidates for CABG and whose symptoms are refractory to medical treatment. To do this procedure, a surgeon makes an incision on the left side of the chest and inserts a laser into the chest cavity. With the laser, the surgeon makes channels (1 mm) through the heart's left ventricle in between heartbeats. The laser is fired when the chamber is full of blood so the blood can protect the inside of the heart. Twenty to 40 channels are created.[3] Then the surgeon applies pressure on the outside of the heart. This seals the outer openings but lets the inner channels stay open, to allow oxygen-rich blood to flow through the heart muscle.

TMR has received Food and Drug Administration approval for use in patients with severe angina who have no other treatment options. It has produced early promising results in that the angina of 80% to 90% of patients who have had this procedure has significantly improved (at least 50%) through 1 year after surgery. There are still limited follow-up data as to how long the benefits of this procedure might last.[3] Improvement in symptoms usually occurs over time, not immediately. TMR will not replace CABG or angioplasty as a common method of treating CAD. TMR may be used for patients who are high-risk candidates for a second bypass or angioplasty, for example, patients whose blockages are too diffuse to be treated with bypass alone, or some patients with heart transplants who develop atherosclerosis.

Enhanced External Counterpulsation

Enhanced external counterpulsation (EECP) is a treatment used for angina when the patient is not a candidate for bypass surgery or percutaneous coronary intervention. EECP uses cuffs wrapped around the patients legs to increase arterial blood pressure and retrograde aortic blood flow during diastole. Sequential pressure, using compressed air, is applied from the lower legs to the upper thighs. These treatments take place over the course of a few hours per day for several weeks. There are no definite data that EECP reduces ischemia; however, there is evidence to support a reduction in angina.[21]

CARDIAC DYSRHYTHMIAS

Cardiac dysrhythmias have many causes such as CAD, AMI, electrolyte imbalances, and HF. The various dysrhythmias and patient assessment are discussed in Chapter 7. Emergency treatments of dysrhythmias include medications, transcutaneous pacemakers, and cardioversion and defibrillation (see Chapter 10). Other drugs that may be used to manage dysrhythmias are shown in Table 12-9. Additional surgical and electrical treatments are discussed in the following sections.

Radiofrequency Catheter Ablation

Radiofrequency catheter ablation is a method used to treat dysrhythmias when medications, cardioversion, or both, are not effective or not indicated. The objective of catheter ablation is to permanently interrupt electrical conduction or activity in a region of dysrhythmogenic cardiac tissue. Indications for radiofrequency catheter ablation include the presence of dysrhythmias such as ventricular tachycardia, atrial fibrillation, atrial flutter, and AV nodal reentry tachycardia. The most predominant group are those patients with symptomatic paroxysmal atrial fibrillation.[30]

Radiofrequency ablation is performed percutaneously. The procedure begins with a diagnostic electrophysiology (EP) study to map the areas to be ablated. A catheter with an electrode is positioned at the accessory (abnormal) pathway, and mild, painless radiofrequency energy (similar to microwave heat) is transmitted to the pathway, causing coagulation and necrosis in the conduction fibers without destroying the surrounding tissue. This stops the area from conducting the extra impulses that cause the tachycardia. After each ablation attempt, the patient is retested until there is no recurrence of the tachycardiac rhythm.

A radiofrequency ablation technique called circumferential radiofrequency ablation is used to treat atrial fibrillation. The lines of electrical conduction that may contribute to atrial fibrillation are located where the pulmonary veins connect to the left atrium. Radiofrequency ablation is done in a circular pattern around each pulmonary vein opening. In addition, pulmonary vein isolation may be used to determine sites for ablation.[30]

Pacemakers

Temporary pacemakers are used to treat patients urgently who are waiting for a permanent pacemaker placement or to treat transient bradydysrhythmias. Temporary pacemakers types are external (transcutaneous) or transvenous. External pacing requires large electrodes that are attached to the chest (see Chapter 10). This type of pacing is quite uncomfortable for the patients because of the current of electricity that is required to pace the heart; therefore it is only used on an emergency basis. Transvenous pacing uses a wire passed through the venous system into the heart and connected to an external pulse generator. This type is more comfortable, but is only used for a short period of time due to the risk of infection and venous thrombosis.[13]

TABLE 12-9 PHARMACOLOGY
Medications Used to Treat Dysrhythmias

MEDICATION	INDICATIONS	MECHANISM OF ACTION	DOSE/ROUTE	SIDE EFFECTS	NURSING IMPLICATIONS
Diltiazem (Cardizem)	Atrial fibrillation/flutter SVT	Inhibits calcium ion influx into vascular smooth muscle and myocardium	*IV*: 0.25 mg/kg actual body weight over 2 minutes May repeat in 15 minutes at dose of 0.35 mg/kg actual body weight *Infusion*: 5-15 mg/hour × 24 hours	Hypotension, edema, dizziness, bradycardia	Often used in conjunction with digoxin for rate control Not used in heart failure Observe for dysrhythmias
Amiodarone (Cordarone)	Atrial fibrillation/flutter SVT Ventricular dysrhythmias	Prolongs action potential phase 3	*IV*: 150 mg IV in 100 mL 5% dextrose/water over 10 minutes (15 mg/min). Follow with infusion of 360 mg over next 6 hours at 1 mg/min rate (mix 900 mg in 500 ml solution; 1.8 mg/mL). Follow with maintenance infusion of 540 mg over remaining 18 hours (0.5 mg/min). Maintenance infusion can be continued at 0.5 mg/min for 2 to 3 weeks *PO*: For life-threatening dysrhythmias, loading dose of 800-1600 mg/day for 1-3 weeks; decrease dose to 600-800 mg/day for 1 month decrease to lowest therapeutic dose, usually 400 mg/day	Bradycardia, complete atrioventricular block, hypotension Multiple side effects (thyroid, pulmonary, hepatic, neurological, dermatological)	Long half-life Monitor cardiac rhythm Obtain baseline pulmonary and liver function tests
Flecainide (Tambocor)	Ventricular dysrhythmias	Decreases conduction in all parts of the heart; stabilizes cardiac membrane	*PO*: 50-100 mg every 12 hours; increase as needed, not to exceed 400 mg/day	Hypotension, bradycardia, heart block, blurred vision, respiratory depression	Interacts with many other drugs; check drug guide Monitor cardiac rhythm Monitor intake and output Assess electrolytes Assess for central nervous system symptoms
Sotalol (Betapace)	Ventricular dysrhythmias	Nonselective beta-blocker	*PO*: 80 mg BID Increase to 240-320 mg/day	Hematological disorders, bronchospasm	Monitor blood pressure and pulse rate Check baseline liver and renal function before beginning therapy Monitor hydration Watch for QT prolongation Teach patient not to decrease drug abruptly
Ibutilide (Corvert)	Atrial fibrillation/flutter	Prolongs duration of action potential and refractory period	*IV*: 1 mg IV push over 10 minutes; may repeat after 10 minutes	Hypotension, bradycardia, sinus arrest	Monitor cardiac rhythm Assess for central nervous system symptoms Use usually restricted to electrophysiology personnel
Propafenone (Rythmol)	Ventricular dysrhythmias	Stabilizes cardiac membranes; depresses action potential phase 0	*PO*: 150 mg every 8 hours; 450-900 mg/day	Ventricular dysrhythmias, heart failure, dizziness, nausea/vomiting, altered taste	Monitor cardiac rhythm Use in patients without structural heart disease

BID, Twice daily; *ECG,* electrocardiogram; *IV,* intravenous; *PO,* orally; *SVT,* supraventricular tachycardia.
From Skidmore-Roth L. (2011). *Mosby's 2011 Nursing Drug Reference.* St. Louis: Mosby.

TABLE 12-10 THE NASPE/BPEG GENERIC (NBG) PACEMAKER CODE (REVISED 2000)

POSITION	I	II	III	IV	V
Category:	**Chamber(s) paced**	**Chamber(s) sensed**	**Response to sensing**	**Rate modulation**	**Multisite pacing**
	O = None	**O** = None	**O** = None	**O** = None	**O** = None
	A = Atrium	**A** = Atrium	**T** = Triggered	**R** = Rate modulation	**A** = Atrium
	V = Ventricle	**V** = Ventricle	**I** = Inhibited		**V** = Ventricle
	D = Dual (A + V)	**D** = Dual (A + V)	**D** = Dual (T + I)		**D** = Dual (A + V)
Manufactures' designation:	**S** = Single (A or V)	**S** = Single (A or V)			

From Bernstein AD, Daubert J-C, Fletcher RD, Hayes DL, Lüderitz B, Reynolds DW, Schoenfeld MH, Sutton R. The Revised NASPE/BPEG Generic Code for antibradycardia, adaptive-rate, and multisite pacing. *Journal of Pacing and Clinical Electrophysiology* 2002;25:260-264.

Permanent pacemakers are used to treat conduction disturbances of the heart. Guidelines for implantation of pacemakers were most recently updated in 2008. They include sinus node dysfunction, atrioventricular block, neurocardiogenic syncope, and some tachycardias.[10] Biventricular pacemakers are used to treat heart failure and will be discussed along with implantable cardioverter-defibrillators. Pacemakers are inserted in the operating room, cardiac catheterization lab, or electrophysiology lab depending on the facility. Depending on the indication, the patient may require atrial and/or ventricular pacing. Leads are inserted through the venous system and into the right atrium and/or right ventricle. A pulse generator is attached to the leads and implanted under the skin, usually on the left side of the chest. Pacemakers are powered by lithium batteries that last approximately 7 to 10 years, at which point a new pulse generator is implanted and attached to the existing functioning leads.

Pacemakers are referred to by a lettered code used to describe their basic function. This code has been modified by the North American Society of Pacing and Electrophysiology and the British Pacing and Electrophysiology Group, currently known as Heart Rhythm Society. The code uses three or four letters to define the chamber paced, chamber sensed, response to pacing, and rate responsiveness, if rate response is being used (Table 12-10).[7]

Cardiac resynchronization therapy (CRT) is permanent pacing with an additional lead placed in the left ventricle. It is indicated to provide therapy for patients with heart failure, with a widened QRS complex and left ventricular ejection fraction of 35% or less, who are on maximum medical therapy and remain symptomatic.[10] Cardiac resynchronization therapy involves biventricular pacing to synchronize contractions of both ventricles. This improves symptoms of heart failure, decreases mortality, and decreases hospital readmissions. It can be implanted as pacemaker device or, as is more common, in combination with a defibrillator.

Defibrillators

Implantable cardioverter-defibrillators (ICDs) are placed in patients for primary or secondary prevention of potentially lethal dysrhythmias. In primary prevention, they are indicated

BOX 12-9 INDICATIONS FOR AN IMPLANTABLE CARDIOVERTER-DEFIBRILLATOR

- Cardiac arrest resulting from ventricular fibrillation (VF) or ventricular tachycardia (VT) not produced by a transient or reversible cause or in the event of AMI when revascularization cannot be done
- Spontaneous sustained VT in association with structural heart disease
- Syncope of undetermined origin with clinically relevant, hemodynamically significant sustained VT or VF induced during electrophysiological study
- Nonsustained VT in patients with coronary artery disease, prior myocardial infarction, left ventricular dysfunction, and inducible VF or sustained VT during electrophysiological study
- Patients with left ventricular ejection fraction of 30% or less, at least 40 days after myocardial infarction and 3 months after coronary revascularization
- Patients with left ventricular ejection fracture less than 35%, NYHA Class II-III in nonischemic heart disease or ischemic heart disease with no coronary revascularization on optimal medical therapy

From Gami A S, Hayes D L, & Friedman P A. (2008). Indications for Pacemakers, ICDs and CRT. In D L Hayes & P A Friedman (Eds.), *Cardiac Pacing, Defibrillation and Resynchronization* (2nd ed.). West Sussex: Wiley-Blackwell.

for patients who are at risk of sudden cardiac death (SCD) such as patients with heart failure, patients who have genetic mutations that put them at risk for ventricular dysrhythmias, and certain congenital and structural heart diseases.[10] In secondary prevention, they are implanted in patients who have survived cardiac arrest or sustained ventricular tachycardia (VT). Current indications for ICD therapy are listed in Box 12-9. ICDs are also able to detect fast heart rates, and when necessary deliver a shock to the heart to stop the abnormal heart rhythm.

ICDs are implanted in the same manner as pacemakers by electrophysiologists (cardiologists who specialize in cardiac

BOX 12-10   PATIENT AND FAMILY TEACHING FOR AN IMPLANTABLE CARDIOVERTER-DEFIBRILLATOR

Preprocedural Teaching
- Device and how it works
- Lead and generator placement
- Implantation procedure
- Educational materials from the manufacturer

Postprocedural Teaching
- Site care and symptoms of complications
- Hematoma at the site is most common when patient takes anticoagulant or antiplatelet medications
- Restricting activity of the arm on the side of the implant
- Identification (Medic Alert jewelry and ICD card)
- Diary of an event if the device fires
- Response if the device fires (varies from falling, tingling, or discomfort to no awareness of the shock); family members need to help in assessment
- Safety measures:
  - Avoid strong magnetic fields (no magnetic resonance imaging)
  - Avoid sources of high-power electricity
  - Keep cellular phones at least 6 inches from the ICD
- Inform airline security personnel about the device; avoid the metal detector; the security wand may be used but should not be left over the device
- The defibrillator therapy must be turned off for surgical procedures using electrocautery
- Everyday activities:
  - Hairdryers, microwaves, and razors are safe
  - Sexual activity can be resumed; tachycardia associated with sexual activity may cause the device to fire; rate adjustments may be needed; If shock occurs during sexual activity, it will not harm the partner
  - Avoid driving for 6 months if the patient has a history of sudden cardiac arrest
- Testing of the device requiring additional electrophysiological studies
- Replacement of the device
- Instruction of family members in cardiopulmonary resuscitation and in how to contact emergency personnel
- Support groups in the local community

ICD, Implantable cardioverter-defibrillator.

rhythms). All ICDs are developed with pacemaker capabilities in the rare instance when the patient needs backup pacing after receiving an ICD shock. ICDs are also capable of providing CRT for patients that require it.

Pacemaker and ICD functions are periodically checked in the office and at home using telemonitoring. These checks help to ensure proper functioning of the devices, and determine when the battery needs to be replaced. The patient is instructed to carry a wallet identification card at all times (see additional patient and family teaching in Box 12-10). Although newer devices are being designed for MRI compatibility, patients who currently have these devices are restricted from undergoing an MRI.

HEART FAILURE

Heart failure (HF) is a complex clinical syndrome that results from the heart's inability to pump blood sufficiently to meet the metabolic demands of the body.[8] HF can result from any structural or functional cardiac disorder that impairs the ability of the ventricle to fill or eject blood. CAD is the primary underlying cause of HF; however, several nonischemic causes have been identified: hypertension, valvular disease, exposure to myocardial toxins, myocarditis, untreated tachycardia, alcohol abuse, and sometimes unidentifiable causes (which result in idiopathic dilated cardiomyopathy).

The cardinal manifestations of HF are dyspnea, fatigue, exercise intolerance, and fluid retention, which may lead to pulmonary and peripheral edema. Signs and symptoms of HF consist of progressive exertional dyspnea, paroxysmal nocturnal dyspnea, orthopnea, fatigability, loss of appetite, abdominal bloating, nausea or vomiting, and eventual organ system dysfunction, particularly the renal system as the failure advances.

The American Heart Association and American College of Cardiology developed a classification system for HF. A patient is classified from stage A to D, based on results of physical examination, diagnostic tests, and clinical symptoms. This terminology helps in understanding that HF is often a progressive condition and worsens over time. HF can be asymptomatic (stages A and B, pre-HF) or symptomatic (stages C and D).[12] HF also has a classification system based on symptoms. The New York Heart Association (NYHA) Heart Failure Symptom Classification System is used to determine functional limitations, and it is also an indicator of prognosis. Class I refers to no symptoms with activity, up to Class IV which indicates dyspnea with little or no exertion.[12] The two classification systems can be used with each other (Table 12-11).

Pathophysiology

HF is impaired cardiac function of one or both ventricles. HF is also classified as systolic or diastolic. Systolic HF results from impaired pumping of the ventricles. Diastolic HF results from impaired filling or relaxation of the ventricles. The most common type of HF is left-sided systolic dysfunction. Right-sided dysfunction is usually a consequence of left-sided HF; however, it can be a primary cause of HF after a right ventricular MI, or it may be secondary to pulmonary pathology. Selected causes of HF are noted in Box 12-11.[12]

TABLE 12-11   ACC/AHA 2001 STAGING COMPARED TO NYHA FUNCTIONAL CLASSIFICATION

ACC/AHA		NYHA	
A	At high risk of developing HF, but without structural heart disease or symptoms of HF	None	
B	Structural heart disease or symptoms of HF	I	Asymptomatic
C	Structural heart disease with prior or current symptoms of HF	II	Symptomatic with moderate exertion
		III	Symptomatic with minimal exertion
		IV	Symptomatic with rest
D	Refractory HF requiring specialized interventions	IV	Symptomatic with rest

ACC, American College of Cardiology; *AHA,* American Heart Association; *HF,* heart failure; *NYHA,* New York Heart Association.
From Institute for Clinical Systems Improvement (ICSI): Health Care Guideline: Heart failure in adults (August 2011). http://www.icsi.org/heart_failure_2/heart_failure_in_adults_.html

BOX 12-11   CAUSES OF HEART FAILURE

Left Heart Systolic Failure
- Myocardial infarction
- Coronary artery disease
- Cardiomyopathy
- Hypertension
- Valvular heart disease
- Tachydysrhythmias
- Toxins: cocaine, ethanol, chemotherapy agents
- Myocarditis
- Pregnancy postpartum cardiomyopathy

Left Heart Diastolic Failure
- Myocardial infarction
- Coronary artery disease
- Hypertrophic heart disease
- Pericarditis
- Infiltrative disease: amyloid sarcoid
- Radiation therapy to the chest
- Age
- Hypertension

Right Heart Systolic Failure
- Right ventricular infarction
- Left-sided heart failure
- Pulmonary embolus
- Pulmonary hypertension
- Chronic obstructive pulmonary disease
- Septal defects

Right Heart Diastolic Failure
- Right ventricular hypertrophy
- Infiltrative disease: amyloid, sarcoid
- Radiation therapy to the chest

In left-sided HF, the left ventricle cannot pump efficiently. The ineffective pumping action causes a decrease in cardiac output, leading to poor perfusion. The volume of blood remaining in the left ventricle increases after each beat. As this volume increases, it backs up into the left atrium and pulmonary veins and into the lungs, causing congestion. Eventually, fluid accumulates in the lungs and pleural spaces, causing increased pressure in the lungs. Gas exchange (oxygen and carbon dioxide) in the pulmonary system is impaired. The backflow can continue into the right ventricle and right atrium and into the systemic circulation (right-sided HF).

When gas exchange is impaired and carbon dioxide increases, the respiratory rate increases to help eliminate the excess carbon dioxide. This phenomenon causes the heart rate to increase, pumping more blood to the lungs for gas exchange. The increased heart rate results in the pumping of more blood from the systemic circulation into the cardiopulmonary circulation, which is already dangerously overloaded, thus a vicious cycle ensues.

As the heart begins to fail to meet the body's metabolic demands, several compensatory mechanisms are activated to improve cardiac output and tissue perfusion. The most noteworthy of these neurohormonal systems are the renin-angiotensin-aldosterone system and the adrenergic nervous system. These interrelated systems act in concert to redistribute blood to critical organs in the body by increasing peripheral vascular tone, heart rate, and contractility. The activation of these diverse systems may account for many of the symptoms of HF and may contribute to the progression of the syndrome. Although these responses may be initially viewed as compensatory, many of them are or become counterregulatory and lead to adverse effects.[8]

The *renin-angiotensin-aldosterone system* plays a major role in the pathogenesis and progression of HF. Angiotensin II is a potent vasoconstrictor and promotes salt and water retention by stimulation of aldosterone release. Sodium

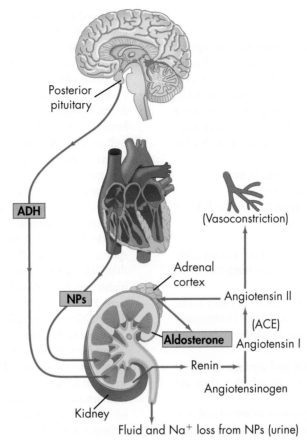

Posterior pituitary

ADH

NPs

(Vasoconstriction)

Adrenal cortex

Angiotensin II

(ACE)

Aldosterone

Angiotensin I

Renin

Angiotensinogen

Kidney

Fluid and Na⁺ loss from NPs (urine)

FIGURE 12-14 Three mechanisms that influence total plasma volume. *ACE*, Angiotensin converting enzyme; *ADH*, antidiuretic hormone; *Na⁺*, sodium; *NPs*, natriuretic peptides. (From McCance KL, Huether SE. *Pathophysiology. The Biologic Basis for Disease in Adults and Children.* 6th ed. St. Louis: Mosby; 2010; Modified from Thibodeau GA, Patton KT: *Anatomy and Physiology.* 5th ed. St. Louis: Mosby; 2003.)

reabsorption increases, and this, in turn, increases blood volume. In patients with impaired function, the heart is unable to handle the extra volume effectively, resulting in edema (peripheral, visceral, and hepatic) (Figure 12-14).

The *adrenergic nervous system* is activated. Although this is initially beneficial in preserving cardiac output and systemic blood pressure, chronic activation is deleterious. Activation (1) produces tachycardia, thereby decreasing preload and contributing to a further decrease in stroke index; (2) causes vasoconstriction, which increases afterload, further decreasing stroke index; and (3) increases contractility, which increases myocardial oxygen demand, thereby decreasing contractility and possibly decreasing stroke index. These changes are progressive. In time, the ventricle dilates, hypertrophies, and becomes more spherical. This process of cardiac remodeling generally precedes symptoms by months or even years.[8]

Assessment

Patient assessment includes the identification of the cause of both right-sided and left-sided HF, the signs and symptoms, and precipitating factors as well as diagnostic studies. Signs and symptoms of HF are presented in Box 12-12.[8]

BOX 12-12 SIGNS AND SYMPTOMS OF HEART FAILURE

Left-Sided Heart Failure: Poor Pump
- Dyspnea/orthopnea
- Cheyne-Stokes
- Paroxysmal nocturnal dyspnea
- Cough (orthopnea equivalent)
- Fatigue or activity intolerance
- Diaphoresis
- Pulmonary crackles
- Elevated pulmonary capillary occlusion pressure
- S_3 and S_4 gallop
- Tachycardia
- Tachypnea
- Hepatojugular reflux

Right Sided Heart Failure: Excess Volume
- Jugular venous distention
- Liver engorgement (hepatomegaly) with ascites in severe cases
- Edema
- Loss of appetite, nausea, vomiting
- Elevated central venous or right atrial pressure

Diagnosis

In diagnosing HF, it is important to identify the etiology or precipitating factors. It is also important to determine whether ventricular dysfunction is systolic or diastolic because therapies are different. Ischemia is responsible for most cases of HF. Identifying ischemia as a cause of HF is important because a majority of these patients may benefit from revascularization.

Diagnosis of the patient with suspected HF includes the following:

- *A complete history including precipitating factors*
- *Physical examination, including assessment of:*
  - Intravascular volume, with examination of neck veins and presence of hepatojugular reflux
  - Presence or absence of edema
  - Perfusion status, which includes blood pressure, quality of peripheral pulses, capillary refill, and temperature of extremities
  - Lung sounds, which may not be helpful. In many cases, the lung fields are clear when the patient is obviously congested, a reflection of chronicity of the disease and adaptation.
- *Chest x-ray study* to view heart size and configuration and to check the lung fields to determine whether they are clear or opaque (fluid filled)
- *Hemodynamic monitoring with pulmonary artery catheter.* Mixed venous oxygen saturation, stroke index, cardiac index, and pulmonary artery pressures are important parameters to assess in the most critically ill patients, especially those who do not respond to conventional therapy. Noninvasive methods of determining hemodynamic parameters also helpful (see Chapter 8).
- *Noninvasive imaging of cardiac structures.* The single most useful test in evaluating patients with HF is the echocardiogram, which can evaluate ventricular enlargement, wall motion abnormalities, valvular structures. It will also determine the left ventricular ejection fraction (LVEF).
- *Arterial blood gases to assess oxygenation and acid-base status*
- *Serum electrolytes.* Many electrolyte imbalances are seen in patients with HF. A low serum sodium level is a sign of advanced or end-stage disease; a low potassium level is associated with diuresis; a high potassium level is seen in renal impairment; blood urea nitrogen and creatinine levels are elevated in low perfusion states, renal impairment, or with overdiuresis.
- *Complete blood count to assess for anemia*
- *B (brain)-type natriuretic peptide (BNP).* BNP is a cardiac hormone secreted by ventricular myocytes in response to wall stretch. BNP and ProBNP assays are useful in the diagnosis of patients with dyspnea of unknown etiology.[11] BNP is a good marker for differentiating between pulmonary and cardiac causes of dyspnea.[9] Plasma concentrations of BNP reflect the severity of HF. In decompensated HF, the BNP concentration increases as a response to wall stress or stretch. As the HF is treated, BNP is used to assess the response to therapies. The normal BNP concentration is less than 100 pg/mL. A BNP level greater than 500 pg/mL is highly specific and indicates increased mortality risk short-term. Patients are at increased risk of readmission and death if the BNP concentration remains persistently elevated at the time of discharge.[11] BNP is not a good indicator of heart failure for patients with chronic renal insufficiency.
- *Liver function studies.* The liver often becomes enlarged with tenderness because of hepatic congestion. Serum transaminase and bilirubin levels are elevated with diminished liver function. Function usually returns once the patient is treated and euvolemic.
- *ECG.* Intraventricular conduction delays are common. Left bundle branch blocks are often associated with structural abnormalities. Patients frequently have premature ventricular contractions, premature atrial contractions, and atrial dysrhythmias. Sinus tachycardia at rest implies substantive cardiac decompensation, and detection of this occurrence is essential.

Nursing Diagnoses

Many nursing diagnoses are associated with HF, such as decreased cardiac output, fluid volume excess, and activity intolerance. See the "Nursing Care Plan for the Patient with Heart Failure" for nursing diagnoses, outcomes, interventions, and rationale.

◎ NURSING CARE PLAN

for the Patient with Heart Failure

NURSING DIAGNOSIS

Decreased Cardiac Output related to increased preload or afterload, decreased cardiac contractility, dysrhythmias, impaired diastolic function

PATIENT OUTCOMES

Adequate cardiac output

- Clear lung sounds
- No shortness of breath
- Absence of or reduced edema

NURSING INTERVENTIONS	RATIONALES
• Assess rate and quality of apical and peripheral pulses	• Assess for compensatory tachycardia
• Assess BP for orthostatic changes	• Low CO as well as vasodilating medications may alter adequate perfusion
• Assess for presence of S_3 and S_4 heart sounds	• Assess left ventricular ejection or reduced compliance
• Assess lung sounds	• Crackles reflect fluid accumulation
• Assess for complaints of fatigue or altered activity tolerance	• Common in low CO states
• Assess urine output	• Assess renal perfusion
• Determine mental status changes, restlessness, irritability	• Assess for alteration in cerebral perfusion
• Assess oxygen saturation; administer supplemental oxygen to maintain saturation above 90%	• Ensure adequate oxygenation
• Monitor serum electrolytes	• Assess risk factors for dysrhythmias
• Assess BNP	• Elevated with increased left ventricular filling pressures
• Monitor for signs/symptoms of digitalis toxicity	• Therapeutic and toxic margin is narrow
• Weigh and evaluate trends	• Assess for fluid volume status
• Administer medications	• Many medications needed to improve CO; assess response
• Optimize preload	• Promote adequate CO
• Increased preload—restrict fluids and sodium	
• Decreased preload—increase fluids	
• Consider invasive hemodynamic monitoring	• Provide data to guide treatment

NURSING DIAGNOSIS

Excess Fluid Volume related to impaired cardiac contractility and decreased cardiac output

PATIENT OUTCOMES

Optimal fluid balance

- Stable weight
- Absence of or reduction in edema
- Clear lung sounds

NURSING INTERVENTIONS	RATIONALES
• Monitor and trend daily weight	• Weight gain of 2-3 lb in a day or 5 lb in 1 week indicates excess fluid volume
• Assess for presence of edema over ankles, feet, sacrum, and dependent areas	• Symmetrical dependent edema is characteristic in HF
• Auscultate for adventitous lung sounds and assess for labored breathing	• Elevation of pulmonary pressure shifts fluid to interstitial and alveolar spaces
• Assess for JVD, ascites, nausea, and vomiting	• Right-sided HF increases venous pressure and fluid congestion
• Assess electrolyte imbalances—low potassium, low sodium, low magnesium, and elevated creatinine levels	• Monitor for side effects of diuretics
• Consider hemofiltration or ultrafiltration for excess fluid volume	• Remove excess fluid volume
• Position patient comfortably with head of bed elevated	• Decrease orthopnea

Continued

◎ NURSING CARE PLAN

for the Patient with Heart Failure—cont'd

NURSING DIAGNOSIS

Risk for Electrolyte Imbalance related to changes in volume status, decreased renal perfusion, diuretics, low-sodium diet

PATIENT OUTCOMES

Electrolytes within normal range

NURSING INTERVENTIONS	RATIONALES
• Monitor serum electrolyte levels	
• Hyponatremia	• Hyponatremia may be dilutional
• Hypokalemia	• Require higher safety range for normal potassium
• Hypomagnesemia	• Dysrhythmias increase risk of sudden death
• Hypernatremia	• Hypernatremia is caused by large loss of water
• Hyperkalemia	• Coadministration of ACE inhibitors, ARBs, or aldosterone blockers can cause potassium retention, especially if decreased renal function worsens as well
• Place on cardiac monitor	• Assess for dysrhythmias associated with electrolyte imbalances
• Administer diuretics	• Restore water and sodium balance
• Administer electrolyte supplements by mouth or intravenously: provide appropriate diet with foods that contain supplements	• Prevent electrolyte imbalances via medication and/or diet

NURSING DIAGNOSIS

Activity Intolerance related to decreased cardiac output, deconditioning, sedentary lifestyle, imbalance between oxygen supply and demand, insufficient sleep and rest, lack of motivation, depressions

PATIENT OUTCOMES

Improved activity tolerance
• Able to perform required activities of daily living
• Verbalizes and uses energy conservation techniques

NURSING INTERVENTIONS	RATIONALES
• Assess patient's current level of activity	• Assess baseline activity
• Observe and document response to activity	• HR increases >20 beats/min; BP drop of >20 mm Hg, dyspnea, light-headedness, and fatigue signify abnormal responses to activity
• Monitor sleep pattern and amount of sleep during night and day	• Provide adequate rest to facilitate progression of activity
• Evaluate need for oxygen with activity	• Compensate for increased oxygen demand
• Teach energy conservation techniques	• Reduce oxygen consumption
• Sit for tasks	
• Push rather than pull	
• Slide rather than lift	
• Store frequently used items within reach	
• Organize a work-rest-work schedule	
• Provide emotional support and encouragement	• Promote positive reinforcement to guide activity progression

◎ NURSING CARE PLAN

for the Patient with Heart Failure—cont'd

NURSING DIAGNOSIS

Disturbed Sleep Pattern related to anxiety or fear, physical discomfort, shortness of breath, medication schedule and effects or side effects

PATIENT OUTCOMES

Adequate sleep and rest
- Verbalizes improvement in hours and quality of sleep
- Appears rested and more alert
- Need for daytime napping decreases

NURSING INTERVENTIONS	RATIONALES
• Assess sleep patterns	• Provide baseline assessment
• Assess for nocturia, dyspnea, orthopnea, PND, and fear of PND	• Assess for common issues associated with sleep disturbances
• Plan medication schedules to allow uninterrupted period and avoid waking up to use the bathroom	• Promote periods of uninterrupted sleep
• Avoid caffeine, smoking, and eating 2 hours before sleep	• Promote relaxation and sleep
• Encourage patient to elevate HOB	• Reduce pulmonary congestion and nighttime dyspnea
• Review how to summon for help during the night	• Reduce anxiety and fear that may disrupt sleep patterns

NURSING DIAGNOSIS

Deficient Knowledge related to unfamiliarity with pathology, treatment, and medications; lack of information literacy, ineffective teaching-learning in past hospitalizations, cognitive limitations, depression

PATIENT OUTCOME

Adequate knowledge of disease and treatment
- Patient or significant others and verbalize causes, treatment, and care related to HF

NURSING INTERVENTIONS	RATIONALE
• Assess knowledge of causes, treatment, and care related to HF as well as best learning style (i.e., reading, listening, demonstration, etc.)	• Provide a base for educational planning
• Identify misconceptions regarding care	• Identify baseline knowledge and misperceptions that need to be corrected
• Educate about normal heart and circulation, HF disease process, symptoms, dietary modifications, activity guidelines, medications, psychological aspects of illness, goals of therapy, and community resources	• Reduce symptoms and readmission for exacerbation
• Use teach-back methods and encourage questions	• Verify understanding of information

ACE, Angiotensin converting enzyme; *ARB*, angiotensin II receptor blocker; *BP*, blood pressure; *CO*, cardiac output; *HF*, heart failure; *HOB*, head of bed; *HR*, heart rate; *JVD*, jugular venous distention; *PND*, paroxysmal nocturnal dyspnea.
Based on data from Gulanick M and Myers JL. *Nursing Care Plans: Diagnoses, Interventions, and Outcomes*, 7th ed. St. Louis, Mosby; 2011.

Interventions

Medical and nursing interventions for the patient with HF consist of a threefold approach: (1) treatment of the existing symptoms, (2) prevention of complications, and (3) treatment of the underlying cause. For example, some patients with HF can be treated by controlling hypertension or by repairing or replacing abnormal heart valves.

Treatment of existing symptoms includes the following:

1. *Improve pump function, fluid removal, and enhanced tissue perfusion* (Tables 12-12 and 12-13)[11]

   a. First-line medications include ACE inhibitors, angiotensin receptor blockers, and diuretics. Once symptoms and volume status are stable, a beta-blocker (metoprolol, carvedilol, bisoprolol) should be added. An ACE inhibitor and beta-blocker form the cornerstone of the treatment for HF.[11] Angiotensin receptor blockers (candesartan and valsartan) are also indicated even before trying an ACE inhibitor.

   b. Additional drug therapies include digoxin, spironolactone, eplerenone, hydralazine, and nitrates.

   c. Inotropes—dobutamine, dopamine, and milrinone—have failed to demonstrate improved mortality in the treatment of severe decompensated HF although they may improve symptoms at end of life.[11]

   d. Nesiritide (Natrecor) is administered IV to patients with acutely decompensated HF who have dyspnea at rest or with minimal activity. The best candidates for therapy are those who have clinical evidence of fluid overload, increased central venous pressure, or both.[12]

2. *Reduce cardiac workload and oxygen consumption*

   a. The intraaortic balloon pump is an invasive strategy to preserve coronary flow in the presence of severe, acute decompensated HF. It is used to stabilize patients with marked hemodynamic instability to allow time for insertion of a left ventricular assist device (LVAD).[27]

   b. LVADs are capable of partial to complete circulatory support for short- to long-term use. They assist the failing heart and maintain adequate circulatory pressure. LVADs attach to the patient's own heart and leave the patient's heart intact, and they have the potential for removal. At present, the LVAD is therapy for patients with terminal HF and has been used in patients who are not eligible for heart transplant.[12]

   c. Biventricular pacing. Patients with chronic HF may exhibit dyssynchronous contraction of the left ventricle, resulting from abnormal electrical conduction pathways. The abnormality leads to increased symptoms of heart failure. Cardiac resynchronization therapy through biventricular pacing involves placing a ventricular lead in the right ventricle and another lead down the coronary sinus to the left ventricle. Both ventricles are stimulated simultaneously, resulting in a synchronized contraction that improves cardiac performance and exercise tolerance as well as decreasing hospitalizations and mortality.[8]

   d. Nursing measures that reduce cardiac workload and oxygen consumption are to schedule rest periods and to encourage patients to modify their activities of daily living. Activity is advanced as tolerated. Patients with HF derive tremendous benefit from formal cardiac rehabilitation to improve activity tolerance and endurance.

3. *Optimize gas exchange through supplemental oxygen and diuresis*

   a. Evaluate the airway, the degree of respiratory distress, and the need for supplemental oxygenation by pulse oximetry, arterial blood gas measurement, or both. Patients are more comfortable in semi-Fowler position. Adjust oxygen delivery. Consider noninvasive ventilatory support such as continuous positive airway pressure (CPAP) or bilevel positive airway pressure (BiPAP). CPAP and BiPAP have demonstrated effectiveness in the management of HF and often reduce the need for intubation.[11]

   b. Diurese aggressively. Administer IV diuretics; furosemide and bumetanide are the preferred diuretics. Ethacrynic acid is useful if the patient has a serious sulfa allergy. Torsemide is also used. These agents are characterized by quick onset; diuresis is expected 15 to 30 minutes after administration. Intravenous loop diuretic administration is preferred over intravenous thiazide diuretic administration. The goal is to achieve euvolemia, which may take days. When the patient is euvolemic, oral medications are restarted.

   c. Patients with severe HF are often considered at high risk for thromboembolic events due to stasis of blood in the atria and ventricles as well as venous stasis due to poor circulation. Anticoagulation is often used in these patients for those reasons, however, the research is lacking in support of this[11,17]

   d. Control of sodium and fluid retention involves fluid restriction of 2 L/day and sodium restriction of 2 g/day. Sodium restriction alone may provide substantial benefits for patients with HF.[11] Dietary counseling includes a discussion about fluid balance management and the importance of avoiding excess sodium or water intake, or both. Referral to a dietician should be considered for all patients.

   e. Daily weights are a priority in these patients.

Nurses make a tremendous impact by teaching and enforcing these concepts throughout the hospital stay. Patients may find it easier to continue these habits at discharge if their importance is stressed throughout hospitalization (see box, "QSEN Exemplar").

TABLE 12-12 · MEDICATION SUBSETS FOR HEART FAILURE

MEDICATION	MANAGEMENT OF HEART FAILURE
ACE inhibitors	Slow disease progression, improve exercise capacity, and decrease hospitalization and mortality
Angiotensin II receptor antagonists	Reduce afterload and improve cardiac output. Can be used for patients with ACE-inhibitor cough
Hydralazine/Isosorbide dinitrate	Vasodilator effect; useful in patients intolerant to ACE inhibitors
Diuretics	Manage fluid overload
Aldosterone antagonists	Manage HF associated with LV systolic dysfunction (<35%) while receiving standard therapy, including diuretics
Digoxin	Improve symptoms, exercise tolerance, and quality of life; no effect on mortality
Beta-blockers	Manage HF associated with LV systolic dysfunction (<40%); well tolerated in most patients, including those with comorbidities such as diabetes mellitus, chronic obstructive lung disease, and peripheral vascular disease

ACE, Angiotensin-converting enzyme; *HF,* heart failure; *LV,* left ventricular.

TABLE 12-13 · PHARMACOLOGY

Specific Medications for Heart Failure

Angiotensin-Converting Enzyme Inhibitors (ACE-Is)

Indications: used to treat hypertension, heart failure, and patients after myocardial infarction

Mechanism of action: prevent the conversion of angiotensin I to angiotensin II resulting in lower levels of angiotensin II, thus causing an increase in plasma renin activity and a reduction of aldosterone secretion; also inhibit the remodeling process after myocardial injury

MEDICATION	DOSE/ROUTE	SIDE EFFECTS AND NURSING CONSIDERATIONS
Enalapril (Vasotec)	*PO:* 2.5-20 mg BID	Hypotension, bradycardia, renal impairment, cough, and orthostatic hypotension. Do not give IV enalapril to patients with unstable heart failure or acute myocardial infarction. Monitor urine output and potassium levels. Avoid use of NSAIDs. Instruct patient to avoid rapid change in position such as from lying to standing. Contraindicated in pregnancy.
Fosinopril (Monopril)	*PO:* 10-40 mg daily	Same
Captopril (Capoten)	*PO:* 6.25-100 mg TID	Same

Diuretics

Indication: for the management of edema or fluid volume overload associated with heart failure and hepatic or renal disease

Mechanism of action: inhibit reabsorption of sodium and chloride in the ascending loop of Henle and distal renal tubule, interfering with the chloride-binding cotransport system, causing increased excretion of water, sodium, chloride, magnesium, and calcium

MEDICATION	DOSE/ROUTE	SIDE EFFECTS AND NURSING CONSIDERATIONS
Furosemide (Lasix)	*PO/IV:* 20-600 mg BID	Orthostatic hypotension, vertigo, dizziness, gout, hypokalemia, cramping, diarrhea or constipation, hearing impairment, tinnitus (rapid IV administration). Monitor laboratory results, especially potassium levels. Monitor cardiovascular and hydration status regularly. In decompensated patients, use IV route until euvolemic status is reached. Administer first dose early in the day and second dose late in afternoon, to prevent sleep disturbance.
Bumetanide (Bumex)	*PO/IV/IM:* 0.5-10 mg daily	Same
Torsemide (Demadex)	*PO/IV:* 10-200 mg daily Maximum 200 mg daily	Same
Metolazone (Zaroxolyn)	*PO:* 5-20 mg daily	Increased diuretic effect occurs when it is given with furosemide and other loop diuretics. Administer 30 minutes before IV loop diuretic.
Ethacrynic acid (Edecrin)	*PO:* 50-200 mg daily	Same Used when patient has a sulfa allergy.

Continued

TABLE 12-13	**PHARMACOLOGY**

Specific Medications for Heart Failure—cont'd

Beta-Blockers

Indications: used to treat angina, AMI, and heart failure

Mechanism of action: block beta-adrenergic receptors, with resulting decreased sympathetic nervous system responses such as decreases in heart rate, blood pressure, and cardiac contractility in heart failure may improve systolic function over time

MEDICATION	DOSE/ROUTE	SIDE EFFECTS AND NURSING CONSIDERATIONS
Metoprolol (Lopressor)	*PO:* 50-450 mg daily *IV:* 5 mg IVP *PO Toprol XL:* 25-200 mg daily	Bradycardia, hypotension, atrioventricular blocks, asthma attacks, fatigue, impotence, may mask hypoglycemic episodes. Teach patient to take pulse and blood pressure on regular basis. Patient should not abruptly stop taking these drugs. Close glucose monitoring if the patient is diabetic. Patients should be started on the lowest dose and slowly titrated to the maximum dose over 4-6 weeks to relieve symptoms.
Carvedilol (Coreg)	*PO:* 12.5-50 mg daily	Same Better tolerated on a full stomach.
Bisoprolol (Concor)	*PO:* 2.5-20 mg daily	Same

Aldosterone Receptor Antagonist

Indication: management of edema associated with excessive aldosterone secretion

Mechanism of action: competes with aldosterone for receptor sites in distal renal tubules, increasing sodium chloride and water excretion while conserving potassium and hydrogen ions; may block the effect of aldosterone on arterial smooth muscle

MEDICATION	DOSE/ROUTE	SIDE EFFECTS AND NURSING CONSIDERATIONS
Spironolactone (Aldactone)	*PO:* 25-200 mg daily	Monitor serum potassium and renal function; drug is potassium sparing.
Eplerenone (Inspra)	*PO:* 50 mg daily; increase to 50 mg BID if inadequate response after 4 weeks	Monitor blood pressure closely, especially at 2 weeks. Monitor potassium and sodium levels.

Inotropes

Indication: treatment of cardiac decompensation from heart failure, shock, or renal failure

Mechanism of action: augment cardiac output by increasing contractility and enhancing tissue perfusion; agents listed use different mechanisms

MEDICATION	DOSE/ROUTE	SIDE EFFECTS AND NURSING CONSIDERATIONS
Digoxin (Lanoxin)	*PO/IV:* 0.125-0.5 mg daily	Heart block, asystole, visual disturbances (blurred or yellow vision), confusion/mental disturbances, nausea, vomiting, diarrhea. Monitor serum concentrations; digoxin possesses a narrow therapeutic range and toxicity can be life-threatening. Maintain serum potassium levels; hypokalemia increases risk of digoxin toxicity. Monitor heart rate and notify provider if rate is <50 beats/min. Treatment of digoxin toxicity is digoxin immune fab (DigiFab).
Dopamine (Intropin)	*IV infusion:* 1-50 mcg/kg/min titrated to desired response Always administer into large vein via infusion device	Frequent ventricular ectopy, tachycardia, anginal pain, vasoconstriction, headache, nausea, or vomiting. Extravasation into surrounding tissue can cause tissue necrosis and sloughing. Monitor heart rate/rhythm and blood pressure closely. Dopamine is frequently used to treat hypotension because of its peripheral vasoconstrictor action. It is often used with dobutamine. Thus blood pressure is maintained by increased cardiac output (dobutamine) and vasoconstriction (dopamine). Monitor the IV site frequently.
Dobutamine (Dobutrex)	*IV infusion:* 2.5-40 mcg/kg/min titrated to desired response Always administer into large vein via infusion device	Increased heart rate, ventricular ectopy, hypotension, angina, headache, nausea, and local inflammatory changes. Drug has been used in outpatient settings (continuous at home or intermittent infusions in office) in patients with end-stage heart failure to stabilize symptoms. Monitor heart rate/rhythm and blood pressure closely.

TABLE 12-13 PHARMACOLOGY

Specific Medications for Heart Failure—cont'd

MEDICATION	DOSE/ROUTE	SIDE EFFECTS AND NURSING CONSIDERATIONS
Milrinone (Primacor)	*IV:* Loading dose of 50 mcg/kg over 10 minutes, followed by continuous infusion 0.375-0.75 mcg/kg/min Always administer into large vein via infusion device	Same as dobutamine
Inamrinone (Inocor)	*IV:* Loading dose of 0.75 mg/kg over 2 to 3 minutes, followed by continuous infusion of 5 to 10 mcg/kg/min May give additional bolus of 0.75 mcg/kg/min 30 minutes after starting therapy Do not exceed total daily dose of 10 mg/kg	Same as dobutamine Do not administer furosemide and inamrinone through the same IV line because precipitation occurs

Brain Natriuretic Peptide

Indication: decompensated congestive heart failure

Mechanism of action: exogenous form of hormone produced by myocardial myocytes as a result of myocardial stress and stretching; vasodilates both veins and arteries and has a positive neurohormonal effect by decreasing aldosterone, and positive renal effects by increasing diuresis and natriuresis

MEDICATION	DOSE/ROUTE	SIDE EFFECTS AND NURSING CONSIDERATIONS
Nesiritide (Natrecor)	*IV:* Loading dose of 2mcg/kg followed by infusion of 0.01 mcg/kg/min	Hypotension, enhanced diuresis, electrolyte imbalances (hypokalemia) Patients will usually respond quickly to therapy. Infusions generally run for 24 hours but can continue for days in the severely decompensated patient

Nitrates

Indications: to reduce afterload, elevated systemic vascular resistance

Mechanism of action: directly relax smooth muscle, which causes vasodilation of the peripheral vascular bed; decrease myocardial oxygen demands

MEDICATION	DOSE/ROUTE	SIDE EFFECTS AND NURSING CONSIDERATIONS
Nitroglycerin (Tridil)	*IV infusion:* 5 mcg/min, titrated to a maximum of 200 mcg/min	Headache, dizziness, flushing, orthostatic hypotension Monitor blood pressure closely. Titrate to effect

Angiotensin Receptor Blockers

Indications: hypertension, heart failure; used in patients who cannot tolerate use of ACE-Is

Mechanism of action: selective and competitive angiotensin II receptor antagonists; block the vasoconstrictor and aldosterone-secreting effects of angiotensin II

MEDICATION	DOSE/ROUTE	SIDE EFFECTS AND NURSING CONSIDERATIONS
Valsartan (Diovan)	*PO:* 40 mg daily BID up to 320 mg total daily dose	Hypotension, diarrhea, dyspepsia, upper respiratory infection Avoid use of NSAIDs, such as indomethacin or naproxen, which may cause renal impairment.
Candesartan (Atacand)	*PO:* 4-32 mg daily or BID	Same

BID, Twice daily; *IM,* intramuscular; *IV,* intravenous; *IVP,* intravenous push; *NSAIDs,* nonsteroidal antiinflammatory drugs; *PO,* orally; *TID,* three times daily.

Cardiac transplantation is a therapeutic option of last resort for patients with end-stage HF. Patients who have severe cardiac disability refractory to expert management and who have a poor prognosis for 6-month survival are optimal candidates. For many patients with symptomatic HF and ominous objective findings (ejection fraction <20%, stroke volume <40 mL, severe ventricular dysrhythmias), timing of the surgery is difficult. A further consideration may be the quality of life, which is a judgment made between the patient and physicians.

Once the crisis stage has passed and the patient is stabilized, the precipitating factors for the complications must be addressed and treated. Treatment consists of surgical or catheter-based interventions as addressed for a patient with a MI, such as CABG, PTCA or stent, and pharmacological therapy (ACE inhibitors, beta-blocker); valve replacement or repair for valvular heart disease; restoration of sinus rhythm if atrial fibrillation or flutter and tachydysrhythmias are present; and management of risk factors such as hypertension, hyperlipidemia, diabetes, and obesity. Compliance with medications and sodium restriction is continually and vigilantly readdressed.

Complications

Complications of HF can be devastating. Interventions must be provided to avoid extending the existing conditions or allowing the development of new, life-threatening complications. Two specific complications for which the patients are monitored are pulmonary edema and cardiogenic shock.

Pulmonary Edema

The failing heart is sensitive to increases in afterload. In some patients with HF, when systolic blood pressure is 150 mm Hg or higher, pulmonary edema will ensue. The pulmonary vascular system becomes full and engorged. The results are increasing volume and pressure of blood in pulmonary vessels, increasing pressure in pulmonary capillaries, and leaking of fluid into the interstitial spaces of lung tissue.

Pulmonary edema greatly reduces the amount of lung tissue space available for gas exchange and results in clinical symptoms of extreme dyspnea, cyanosis, severe anxiety, diaphoresis, pallor, and blood-tinged, frothy sputum. Arterial blood gas results indicate severe respiratory acidosis and hypoxemia.

Patients with persistent volume overload may be candidates for continuous IV diuretics, ultrafiltration, or hemodialysis.[11] Loop diuretics given as an IV bolus are considered along with an IV infusion. Furosemide is the most commonly used loop diuretic, with the dose adjusted upward if the patient is currently on oral doses. The diuretic effect occurs in 30 minutes, with the peak effect in 1 to 2 hours.[28] IV torsemide or bumetanide are alternative loop diuretics.

The pharmacological characteristics of loop diuretics are similar. Continuous infusion of loop diuretics is considered if the patient does not respond to intermittent dosing. In addition, combinations of diuretics with different mechanisms of action are considered. Thiazide diuretics such as metolazone are often added. Monitoring hourly urinary output assists in determining the effectiveness of the diuretic therapy.

Although diuretic therapy is important, it is also critical to lower the blood pressure and cardiac filling pressures. Intravenous NTG is administered and titrated until the blood pressure is controlled, resulting in a reduction in both preload and afterload.[11] Patients who do not demonstrate improvement in symptoms require more aggressive treatment. A NTG infusion is initiated at 10 to 20 mcg/min, and initial titration is in increments of 10 mcg/min at intervals of 3 to 5 minutes, guided by patient response. The maximum dose is 200 mcg/min. Other care requirements for the administration of NTG include the use of non–polyvinyl chloride tubing. If this tubing is not available and traditional polyvinyl chloride tubing must be used, then the initial dose for NTG starts at 25 mcg/min IV. Patients who do not respond to aggressive diuretics and nitroglycerin may be a candidate for nesitiride (Natrecor), a natriuretic peptide.[11]

Cardiogenic Shock

Cardiogenic shock is the most acute and ominous form of pump failure. Cardiogenic shock can be seen after a severe MI, with dysrhythmias, decompensated HF, pulmonary embolus, cardiac tamponade, and ruptured abdominal aortic aneurysm. Often, the outcome of cardiogenic shock is death. Cardiogenic shock and its treatment are discussed in depth in Chapter 11. Outcomes for the patient with HF are included in the nursing care plan.

PERICARDITIS

Pericarditis is acute or chronic inflammation of the pericardium. It may occur as a consequence of AMI or secondary to kidney injury (uremic pericarditis), infection, radiation therapy, connective tissue diseases, or cancer.[25] The pericardium has an inner and outer layer with a small amount of lubricating fluid between the layers. When the pericardium becomes inflamed, the amount of fluid between the two layers increases (pericardial effusion). This squeezes the heart and restricts its action and may result in cardiac tamponade. Chronic inflammation can result in constrictive pericarditis, which leads to scarring. The epicardium may thicken and calcify (see Figure 12-1).

The patient with pericarditis usually has precordial pain; this pain frequently radiates to the shoulder, neck, back, and arm and is intensified during deep inspiration, movement, coughing, and even swallowing. Other signs and symptoms may include a pericardial friction rub, dyspnea, weakness, fatigue, a persistent temperature elevation, an increased white blood cell count and sedimentation rate, and an increased anxiety level.[25] Pulsus paradoxus may be noted while auscultating the blood pressure. Pain due to pericarditis is usually positional and pleuritic (worse with inspiration and cough).

Detection of a pericardial friction rub is the most common method of diagnosing pericarditis. The friction rub is usually heard best on inspiration with the diaphragm of the stethoscope placed over the second, third, or fourth intercostal spaces at the sternal border. It is best heard when the patient is leaning forward. Friction rubs have been described as grating, scraping, squeaking, or scratching sounds. This rubbing sound results from an increase in fibrous exudate between the two irritated pericardial layers.

The ECG is useful in confirming the diagnosis of pericarditis because it is abnormal in 90% of patients with acute pericarditis. There are diffuse concave ST-segment elevation and PR-segment deviations opposite to P-wave polarity. T waves progressively flatten and invert, with generalized T-wave inversions present in most or all leads.[25] In echocardiogram is also useful in diagnosis to visualize the effusion.

The treatment of patients with pericarditis involves relief of pain (analgesic agents or antiinflammatory agents, such as colchicine and ibuprofen), antibiotics if the causative agent is bacterial, and treatment of other systemic symptoms.[25]

Approximately 15 to 50 mL of fluid is in the pericardial space. Excess fluid compresses the heart chambers, limits the filling capacity of the heart, and may result in tamponade. Treatment of cardiac tamponade includes inserting a needle into the pericardial space to remove the fluid (pericardiocentesis). In extreme cases, surgery may be required to remove part of the pericardium (pericardial window).

ENDOCARDITIS

Infective endocarditis occurs when microorganisms circulating in the bloodstream attach onto an endocardial surface. It is caused by various microbes, and frequently involves the heart valves. Endocarditis is classified as one of three types: native valve endocarditis (NVE), acute and subacute; prosthetic valve endocarditis (PVE), early and late; and intravenous drug abuse (IVDA) endocarditis.[7] *Staphylococcus aureus* is the most common causative pathogen in endocarditis. *Streptococcus* and *Enterococcus* organisms are often seen in subacute NVE.[7] Certain preexisting heart conditions increase the risk of developing endocarditis: implantation of an artificial (prosthetic) heart valve, a history of previous endocarditis, and heart valves damaged by conditions such as rheumatic fever, congenital heart defects, or valve defects.[6]

Infectious lesions, referred to as *vegetation,* form on the heart valves. These lesions have irregular edges, creating a cauliflower-like appearance. The mitral valve is the most common valve to be affected.[6] The vegetative process can grow to involve the chordae tendineae, papillary muscles, and conduction system. Therefore the patient may have dysrhythmias or acute HF. Patients with IVDA endocarditis usually do not have underlying structural disease.

The clinical presentation of patients with acute infectious endocarditis includes high fever and shaking chills. Other clinical manifestations of endocarditis include night sweats, cough, weight loss, general malaise, weakness, fatigue, headache, musculoskeletal complaints, new murmurs, and symptoms of HF. Skin abnormalities associated with septic emboli may also be seen: Janeway lesions (lesions that are often hemorrhagic and present on the palms and soles), Osler nodes (red-purple lesions on fingers or toes), splinter hemorrhages, and Roth spots (retinal hemorrhages). Skin lesions are referred to as the peripheral stigmata of endocarditis.[20]

Treatment of endocarditis involves diagnosing the infective agent and treating with the appropriate intravenous antibiotics for 4 to 6 weeks. Valve replacement surgery may be indicated in severe cases.[20] Prevention is important, and antibiotic prophylaxis is recommended for high-risk patients prior to procedures.

VASCULAR ALTERATIONS

The aorta is the largest blood vessel in the body both in length and diameter. Shaped like a walking cane, the aorta is an artery that carries blood from the heart. It extends from the aortic valve to the abdomen.[6] Its many branches supply blood to all other areas of the body. The aorta is divided into the thoracic and abdominal aorta (Figure 12-15).

The thoracic aorta is divided into the ascending aorta, the aortic arch, and the descending aorta. The thoracic aorta begins at the aortic root, which supports the bases of the three aortic valve leaflets.[5] The round segment, or cane handle, is

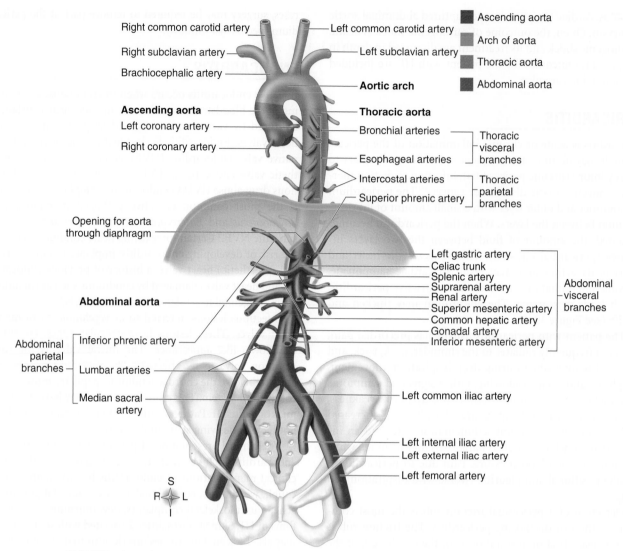

FIGURE 12-15 Anatomy of the aorta and its major branches. (From Patton KT, Thibodeau GA. *Anatomy and Physiology*. 8th ed. St. Louis: Mosby; 2013.)

the ascending aorta and the aortic arch. Branches of the ascending aorta include the right and left coronary arteries, which feed the myocardium. The arch vessels include the innominate artery, which branches into the right subclavian artery and right common carotid artery, and the left common carotid and left subclavian arteries. These branches send blood to the head and the upper extremities. The descending thoracic aorta, the long segment of the cane, is to the left of the midline of the chest. Branches of the descending aorta are the intercostal arteries. These arteries are the major blood supply to the distal spinal cord.

The abdominal aorta begins at the level of the diaphragm. At the umbilicus, it bifurcates into the iliac arteries. Abdominal branches include the celiac artery, the superior and inferior mesenteric arteries, and the renal arteries.

Aortic Aneurysms

The word *aneurysm* comes from the Greek *aneurysma*, which means "widening." An aneurysm is a diseased area of an artery causing dilatation and thinning of the wall. An aneurysm may be further classified as a false (pseudoaneurysm) or true aneurysm (Figure 12-16). A false aneurysm results from a complete tear in the arterial wall. Blood leaks from the artery to form a clot. Connective tissue is then laid down around this cavity. One example of a false aneurysm is an arterial wall tear resulting from an arterial puncture in the groin area. Anastomotic aneurysms are false aneurysms found at any graft-host artery anastomosis. True aneurysms include fusiform, saccular, and dissecting aneurysms. Fusiform or spindle-shaped aneurysms are generally found in the abdominal aorta and are the most common. A saccular aneurysm is a bulbous pouching of the artery usually found in the thoracic aorta.

Abdominal aortic aneurysms (AAA) are divided into thoracic aortic, thoracoabdominal aortic, and abdominal aortic types.

Atherosclerosis and degeneration of elastin and collagen are the underlying causes in most cases. They are also associated with certain connective tissue disorders such as Marfan syn-

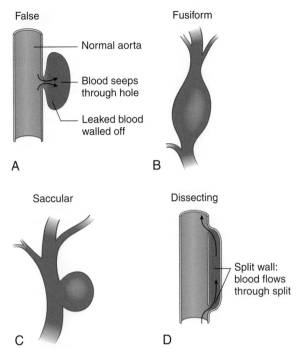

False
Fusiform

— Normal aorta

— Blood seeps through hole

— Leaked blood walled off

A   B

Saccular
Dissecting

Split wall: blood flows through split

C   D

FIGURE 12-16 The four types of aneurysms. **A,** False. **B,** Fusiform. **C,** Saccular. **D,** Dissecting.

drome (see box, "Genetics: Marfan Syndrome"). Aneurysms are frequently hereditary, with a predominance in males. Risk factors of atherosclerosis such as age, smoking, hyperlipidemia, hypertension, and diabetes are also risk factors for aortic aneurysms.[18]

Most aneurysms are asymptomatic and are found on routine physical examination, or when testing for another disease entity. Back or abdominal pain may be noted with AAA. The goal of treatment is avoidance of rupture, which is dramatic and often fatal. Risk of rupture is related to the size of the aneurysm, with aneurysms larger than 6 cm carrying the greatest risk. Patients should be followed closely for changes in size of the aneurysm.

Treatment of an aneurysm is based on the symptoms of the patient and the size of the aneurysm. Thoracic aortic or thoracoabdominal aortic aneurysms larger than 5.5 to 6.0 cm, and abdominal aortic aneurysms 5.0 cm or larger are usually surgically repaired. Patients with smaller aneurysms are followed up diagnostically for any change in size. For

GENETICS

Marfan Syndrome

Advances in genetic disorders have resulted in new insights into the pathogenesis of disease, particularly in understanding the expression of proteins whose alteration or deficiency causes disease. One cardiovascular disease that illustrates this type of advance in the biologic basis of disease is Marfan syndrome (MFS). This single gene disorder demonstrates an autosomal dominant pattern of inheritance, which means that each child of an affected parent has a 50% chance of receiving a disease-causing gene variant. Further, it is highly penetrant, meaning that nearly all carriers develop the disease.[5] However, there is marked variation in phenotypes, even within families. New understanding of the molecular mechanisms underlying the pathogenesis of MFS helps explain the variety of abnormalities manifested.[2]

Most cases of MFS are caused by a mutation in the *FBN1* gene, located on chromosome 15. This gene codes for fibrillin-1, a glycoprotein that is found in both elastic and nonelastic tissues.[2] Fibrillin-1 helps form the complexes that anchor elastic fibers and regulates messengers associated with growth of long bones and cardiovascular tissue remodelling. Generally, it is missense mutations in the *FBN1* gene that alter a single amino acid out of the 2871 proteins that build fibrillin-1. The altered genetic code results in a changed structure, delayed secretion, or enhanced destruction of fibrillin-1. The reduction in effective fibrillin-1 results in connective-tissue weakness and explains the structural defects in the lens of the eyes, blood vessels, heart valves and skin. Altered regulation of growth factors explains bone overgrowth and skin and muscle hypoplasia in MFS.[4]

About 75% of MFS is inherited, but another 25% of individuals develop the disease from de novo mutations, meaning that the mutation occurred in the egg or sperm or in the early embryo.[2] Whether inherited or a new alteration, variation exists in

the number and severity of symptoms, despite inheriting a similarly altered gene. Thus, despite high penetrance, the presence of a *FBN1* MFS variant gene does not predict the onset or severity of disease. The diagnosis of MFS is based on the presence of a positive family history and the number of organ systems with MFS-related defects. Genetic testing is available from a wide variety of laboratories[6] and mutations of the *FBN1* gene can be detected in more than 90% of patients with MFS.[7] While genetic testing is sensitive to MFS, it is not specific, in that *FBN1* variations are associated with other hereditary connective tissue disorders such as bicuspid aortic valve or Ehlers-Danlos syndrome.[2]

The phenotypes—clinical manifestations—that are most commonly associated with MFS are aortic aneurysm (especially thoracic); dilation of the root of the aorta where it is connected to the left ventricle; tall stature with especially long arms, legs, fingers, and toes; a protruding or indented sternum; enlargement of the dural membrane surrounding the lower spine or brainstem (i.e., dural ectasia); and discoloration of the lens of the eye. Individuals can also present with blebs or emphysema-like changes in the lung with possible spontaneous pneumothorax, inguinal or incisional hernias, skin stretch marks (i.e., striae), joint hypermobility, and visual disorders such as myopia or early cataracts.[1,5] Aortic aneurysm and dissection in MFS is associated with high morbidity and mortality.

Management of MFS is tailored to each individual's manifestation of the disease. For individuals who have cardiovascular manifestations of MFS, interventions typically include beta-blockers and angiotensin converting enzyme inhibitors or selective angiotensin-2 receptor blockers to control blood pressure and slow the progression of widening in the aorta.[3,4] Clinicians also advise individuals to restrict contact sports and weight lifting. Definitive treatment is surgical intervention on the aortic

Continued

GENETICS

Marfan Syndrome—cont'd

root and ascending aorta to prevent dissection. Patients with MFS and their family members may be referred by clinicians for genetic testing and genetic counseling, including psychosocial support and risk assessment.

References

1. Braverman AC, Thompson RW, Sanchez LA. Disease of the Aorta. In RO Bonow, DL Mann, DP Zipes, P Libby, (Eds.), _Braunwald's Heart Disease: A Textbook of Cardiovascular Medicine_ (9th ed). Philadelphia: Saunders, 2012.
2. Canadas V, Vilacosta I, Bruna I, Fuster V. Marfan syndrome. Part 1: pathophysiology and diagnosis. _Nature Reviews Cardiology._ 2010;7(5), 256-265.
3. Canadas V, Vilacosta I, Bruna I, Fuster V. Marfan syndrome. Part 2: treatment and management of patients. _Nature Reviews Cardiology._ 2010;7(5), 266-276.
4. Dietz HC. New therapeutic approaches to mendelian disorders. _New England Journal of Medicine._ 2010;363(9), 852-863.
5. Lashley FR. _Clinical genetics in nursing practice._ 3rd ed. New York: Springer, 2006.
6. National Center for Biotechnology Information. GeneTests. Seattle, WA: National Center for Biotechnology Information, National Institutes of Health; 1993-2011 [cited 2011 May 15. Available from: http://www.ncbi.nlm.nih.gov/sites/GeneTests/.
7. National Marfan Foundation. Molecular Testing Port Washington, New York: National Marfan Association; 2011 [updated 2011; cited 2011 May 20]; Available from: http://www.marfan.org/marfan/2550/Molecular-Testing.

patients with small aortic abdominal aneurysms, smoking cessation is emphasized because there is evidence that smoking leads to faster expansion and rupture of an aneurysm.[5,14]

Aortic Dissection

Aortic dissection is a life-threatening emergency that requires immediate medical attention. Dissection is a tear in the intimal layer of the vessel creating a "false" lumen, causing blood flow diversion into the false lumen. Sudden, severe chest pain is the most common presenting symptom of aortic dissection. Dissections are divided into two categories: Stanford type A (proximal) and type B (distal). Type A is more concerning because it involves the ascending aorta and therefore dissection can extend into the coronary and arch vessels. It usually presents as severe anterior chest pain. Type B is confined to the descending thoracic and abdominal aorta and is often associated with pain between the scapulae. Ascending dissections are more common in younger patients, especially those with Marfan syndrome. Immediate treatment is directed at controlling blood pressure to 100 to 120 mm Hg, and decreasing the force of contraction of the heart. Therefore beta-blockers are the initial pharmacological treatment of choice. Emergency surgery is warranted to prevent death. Once rupture occurs, the overall 30-day survival rate is only 11%.[14,18]

Nursing Assessment

Knowledge of anatomy is the key factor in the treatment and care of patients with aortic aneurysms. Presentation of symptoms, intraoperative risk, and postoperative care are often location dependent. Blood flow to aortic branches may be hindered by the aneurysm itself, or embolization of thrombus may cause signs and symptoms such as chest pain, transient ischemic attacks, arm paresthesia with arch location, transient paralysis with descending aorta involvement, or abdominal or flank pain with AAA. In addition, systolic blood pressure may be different in each arm if the dissection occludes one of the subclavian arteries. A murmur may be auscultated if the dissection results in aortic regurgitation.[18]

Diagnostic Studies

1. _Physical examination._ Disparity in blood pressure measurements may be noted between the right and left arms or between the arms and legs, or a diminished pulse may be found in one of the limbs. Palpation reveals decreased or absent peripheral pulses. The patient may have a history of paresthesia, transient ischemic attacks, lower extremity or buttock claudication, and/or back or abdominal pain.
2. _Imaging studies._ Abdominal ultrasound, Computed tomography, angiography, TEE, and MRI are accurate diagnostic tools for abdominal aneurysms.

Treatment

Open surgical or endovascular repair is the treatment for large aortic aneurysms.[14] The open or conventional repair of aortic aneurysm is the endoaneurysmal repair (Figure 12-17). This surgery requires a midline, transverse anterior, or a retroperitoneal approach.

Endovascular aneurysm repair (EVAR) or thoracic endovascular aneurysm repair (TEVAR) is less invasive and refers to percutaneous stent placement in the descending thoracic or thoracoabdominal aorta. Both method and approach depend on the surgeon's preference and the patient's anatomy.[1] Through a small opening in the exposed femoral artery, an intraluminal sheathed stent is introduced, placed, and deployed with fluoroscopic guidance. The repair is usually successful, with less than 2% of patients who have to be converted to open repair.[1] Care of the vascular surgery patient is detailed in Box 12-13.

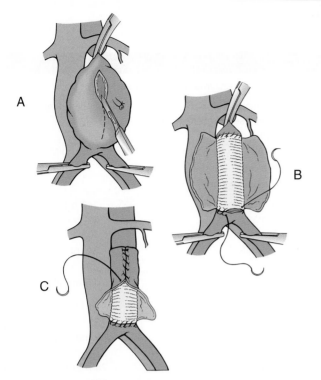

FIGURE 12-17 Surgical repair of an abdominal aortic aneurysm. **A,** The aneurysmal sac is incised. **B,** The synthetic graft is inserted. **C,** The native aortic wall is sutured over the synthetic graft (From Wipke-Tevis DD, Rich K, *Nursing Management Vascular Disorders.* In Lewis SL, et al. *Medical-Surgical Nursing: Assessment and Management of Clinical Problems.* 8th ed. St. Louis: Mosby; 2011.)

BOX 12-13   NURSING INTERVENTIONS AFTER AORTIC SURGERY

- Monitor vital signs every 1 hour (postrecovery stage): pulse; assess for tachycardia and irregular rhythms.
- Blood pressure: keep the patient normotensive; hypertension causes bleeding; give vasodilators per protocol. Hypotension causes organ ischemia; give fluids and vasoconstrictors.
- Monitor hemodynamic pressures: SvO$_2$, stroke index, cardiac index; PAOP and RAP; and treat per protocols.
- Assess for hypovolemia: monitor output from chest tubes, drains, and urine output every 1 hour.
- Assess for hypothermia: rewarm the patient per protocol.
- Monitor fluid and electrolytes, hemoglobin, hematocrit, renal function, and coagulation studies.
- Monitor the radial, dorsalis pedis, and posterior tibial pulses every 1 hour; use Doppler studies as needed. Assess the ankle-brachial index every 2 hours or as ordered.
- Monitor for complications: intraoperative AMI, dysrhythmias, heart failure, cardiac tamponade, thromboembolism, impaired renal function, pneumonia, pneumothorax, pleural effusion, cerebral ischemia, or stroke.
- Implement ventilator bundle of care (see Chapter 9), wean from mechanical ventilation and extubate as soon as possible; promote pulmonary hygiene.
- Assess wounds and provide incisional care per protocol.
- Organize nursing care; control environmental stimuli.
- Gradually increase the patient's activity.
- Provide emotional support to the patient and family; assess the family's level of understanding; discuss the postoperative course.
- For abdominal aneurysm, assess for ischemic colitis

PAOP, Pulmonary artery occlusion pressure; *RAP,* right atrial pressure; *SvO$_2$,* mixed venous oxygen saturation.

GERIATRIC CONSIDERATIONS

The geriatric cardiac patient needs special considerations when planning and implementing care. Many older patients react differently and with more sensitivity to medications, procedures, and other modes of treatment. Some areas of special consideration include the following:

Medications
Great caution must be exercised when administering any medication to a geriatric patient, especially cardiac medications. Elderly persons may have greater sensitivity to these medications, they may not require the usual recommended dosage, or they may require more if they have been taking the medication in question for a long period of time. Monitor the patient closely for signs of drug effectiveness, adverse reactions, and possible interactions with other medications.

Procedures
The geriatric patient may need more information, support, and attendance during diagnostic or treatment procedures. Always having someone in attendance is a major consideration. It is also necessary to answer any and all questions to the extent needed for understanding and compliance. Frequent repetition and intentionality to reassessment in the elderly patient will emphasize the importance of teaching.

Surgery
Cardiac surgery is a major stress factor for anyone. The geriatric patient needs special attention to answer questions at the appropriate level of understanding and to provide the support for a very stressful, life-threatening procedure. Information and education are important, but be cautious of overwhelming the patient and causing greater stress.

Postoperative
The geriatric patient has special needs in the postoperative period. The aging patient has a natural physiological process of gradually diminished circulation. Anesthesia and a major surgical procedure add to this problem area and warrant careful monitoring and continuous assessment.

Family
It is imperative to have the involvement of family members or close friends. This can add a stabilizing factor that elderly patients need as they adjust to changes in treatment, activity, diet, medications, and ability to maintain activities of daily living.

Rehabilitation
Rehabilitation is important for any cardiac patient, whether after a myocardial infarction or after surgery. The geriatric patient needs extra encouragement to adhere to the set regimen to progress to maximum cardiac and vascular function.

CASE STUDY

Mr. S. was admitted to the emergency department (ED) by the emergency medical service with a complaint of sudden onset of substernal chest pain while he was mowing his lawn. The paramedics placed Mr. S. on oxygen at 2 L/min by nasal cannula. They started an 18-gauge intravenous (IV) line in his left antecubital area with normal saline at keep open rate. They gave Mr. S. aspirin and three sublingual nitroglycerin tablets every 5 minutes en route. Mr. S. states that his pain has gone from a 7, on a scale from 0 to 10, to a 3.

The ED nurse places Mr. S. on the cardiac monitor and notes that he is in sinus rhythm with frequent premature ventricular contractions (PVCs). The paramedic states that Mr. S. was diaphoretic, cool, and clammy on arrival of the emergency medical service at the scene. Mr. S. is warm and less clammy, although he is still quite pale. His blood pressure is 154/88 mm Hg, pulse is 95 beats per minute, and respiratory rate is 24 breaths per minute and nonlabored.

While awaiting the arrival of the ED physician to examine Mr. S., the nurse starts a second IV line, gives Mr. S. another nitroglycerin tablet, and proceeds to obtain a brief history from Mr. S.

Mr. S. is a 63-year-old white man, 220 lb, and he has been married for 41 years. He is hypertensive and diabetic, and he smokes 1½ packs of cigarettes per day. He is allergic to penicillin.

While the nurse is obtaining the history from Mr. S., the monitor alarms. She identifies the rhythm as ventricular fibrillation and begins cardiopulmonary resuscitation. The code team arrives, and Mr. S. is defibrillated with 200 J using the biphasic defibrillator. Following defibrillation, his rhythm is regular sinus with frequent PVCs. His blood pressure is 92/56 mm Hg, his pulse is thready, and he is diaphoretic. His pupils are 4 mm, equal and reactive. His respiratory rate is 16 breaths per minute and shallow, and his oxygen saturation is 92%. He has developed crackles in his lower and middle lung fields bilaterally. He is not fully awake at this time, but he is moving all his extremities. A 150-mg IV bolus of amiodarone is given over 10 minutes, and an infusion is started at 1 mg/min. Emergency laboratory tests and arterial blood gases are ordered, along with a 12-lead electrocardiogram (ECG). A request for an emergency consultation is placed to the cardiologist.

Mr. S.'s cardiac enzyme results return:

Creatine kinase (CK)	456 units/L
Creatine kinase–myocardial band (CK-MB)	52%
Troponin I	0.5 ng/mL
Troponin T	151 mcg/L

Electrolyte values are:

Sodium	143 mEq/L
Potassium	3.4 mEq/L
Chloride	109 mEq/L
Carbon dioxide	34 mEq/L
Glucose	354 mg/dL
Magnesium	1.5 mEq/L

Arterial blood gas values are:

pH	7.32
$PaCO_2$	49 mm Hg
PaO_2	77 mm Hg
Bicarbonate	24 mEq/L
SaO_2	92%

H&H:

Hemoglobin level	16.9 g/dL
Hematocrit	47.2%

A 12-lead ECG shows ST elevation in leads V_2, V_3, and V_4. Mr. S. is diagnosed with an acute anterior myocardial infarction. His oxygen is increased to 6 L/min by nasal cannula. Based on these assessment and study results, tissue plasminogen activator (t-PA) is administered.

Questions

1. What do Mr. S's cardiac enzyme values indicate about the time and extent of his myocardial infarction?
2. What would you expect his repeat troponin levels to be at the following times after his heart attack?
   a. At 8 hours
   b. At 12 hours
3. What complications may be anticipated for Mr. S. related to the infusion of t-PA? What parameters would the nurse need to monitor?
4. What assessments would indicate that the t-PA was effective?
5. What risk factors for CAD should be addressed before Mr. S.'s discharge to reduce his risk of another MI?

SUMMARY

This chapter focuses on the care of the patient with alterations in cardiovascular status. Geriatric patients are increasingly having medical and surgical interventions. They have even greater needs associated with the aging process (see box, "Geriatric Considerations"). The purpose of this chapter is to acquaint the critical care nurse with the problems and pathological conditions most commonly seen in the cardiovascular patient. This chapter is intended to provide a basic understanding of the cardiovascular patient that will facilitate sound clinical judgment in the planning of care that is holistic and incorporates a cooperative, interdisciplinary approach.

CRITICAL THINKING EXERCISES

1. You are taking care of a 58-year-old post-MI male patient readmitted to the unit because of recurrent chest pain, shortness of breath, and the need for intravenous nitroglycerin.
   a. Prioritize your actions at this time.
   b. What assessment findings regarding MI would concern you?
   c. What pertinent information from the patient's history would you want to obtain?
   d. What diagnostic tests do you anticipate?
2. Many patients now come into the hospital the same day that cardiac surgery is performed. Discuss methods for teaching patients effectively given this situation.
3. You are caring for a 63-year-old woman who has just returned to the cardiac care unit after PTCA and stent placement to the right coronary artery. Her proximal right coronary artery had a 90% occlusive lesion. She has her arterial sheath in place to the right femoral artery. She is receiving intravenous nitroglycerin and eptifibatide (Integrilin).
   a. What type of dysrhythmia would you anticipate if her right coronary artery were to reocclude?
   b. Prioritize your actions on her arrival.
   c. What type of assessment would you perform regarding the sheath?
4. A patient has been hospitalized three times in the past 2 months for chronic HF. What teaching and interventions can you implement to prevent rehospitalization after discharge?

REFERENCES

1. Adams JD, Garcia LM, Kern JA. Endovascular repair of the thoracic aorta. *Surgical Clinics of North America.* 2009;89(4):895-912
2. American Heart Association. *Minimally Invasive Heart Surgery.* Available at http://www.heart.org/HEARTORG/Conditions/HeartAttack/PreventionTreatmentofHeartAttack/Cardiac-Procedures-and-Surgeries_UCM_303939_Article.jsp#.T0BuyczgJPU; Accessed April 13, 2011.
3. American Heart Association. *Transmyocardial Revascularization.* Available at http://www.americanheart.org/presenter.jhtml?identifier=4782; Accessed April 13, 2011.
4. Antman EM, Morrow DA. ST-segment elevation myocardial infarction: management. In: Bonow RO. *Braunwald's Heart Disease: A Textbook of Cardiovascular Medicine.* 9th ed. Philadelphia: Saunders; 2011.
5. Braverman AC, Thompson RW, Sanchez LA. Diseases of the aorta. In: Bonow RO. *Braunwald's Heart Disease: A Textbook of Cardiovascular Medicine.* 9th ed. Philadelphia: Saunders; 2011.
6. Brusch JL. *Infective Endocarditis.* Available at http://emedicine.medscape.com/article/216650-overview; 2011. Accessed December 16, 2011.
7. Bunch TJ, Hayes DL, Friedman PA. Clinically relevant basics of pacing and defibrillation. In: Hayes DL, Friedman PA, eds. *Cardiac Pacing, Defibrillation and Resynchronization.* 2nd ed. West Sussex: Wiley-Blackwell; 2008.
8. Chatterjee NA, Fifer MA. Heart failure. In: Lilly LS, ed. *Pathophysiology of Heart Disease.* 5th ed. Philadelphia: Lippincott Williams & Wilkins; 2011.
9. Chernecky CC, Berger BJ. *Laboratory Tests & Diagnostic Procedures.* 6th ed. Philadelphia: Saunders; 2011.
10. Epstein AE, DiMarco JP, Ellenbogen KA, et al. ACC/AHA/HRS 2008. Guidelines for device-based therapy of cardiac rhythm abnormalities. *Circulation.* 2008;117:2820-2840.
11. Gulanick M, Myers J. *Nursing Care Plans.* 7th ed. St. Louis: Mosby; 2011.
12. Hobbs R, Boyle A. *Heart Failure.* Available at http://www.clevelandclinicmeded.com/medicalpubs/diseasemanagement/cardiology/heart-failure/; 2010.
13. Hu R, Stevenson WG, Strichartz GR, et al. Mechanics of cardiac arrhythmias. In: Lilly LS, ed. *Pathophysiology of Heart Disease.* 5th ed. Philadelphia: Lippincott Williams & Wilkins; 2011.
14. Isselbacher EM. Contemporary reviews in cardiovascular medicine: Thoracic and abdominal aortic aneurysms. *Circulation.* 2005;111:816-828.
15. Kandzari DE, Columbo A, Park S-J, et al. Revascularization for unprotected left main disease: evolution of the evidence basis to redefine treatment standards. *Journal of the American College of Cardiology.* 2009;54(17):1576-1588.
16. Kushner FG, Hand M, Smith SC Jr, et al. 2009 focused updates: ACC/AHA guidelines for the management of patients with ST-elevation myocardial infarction and ACC/AHA/SCAI guidelines on percutaneous coronary intervention: a report of the American College of Cardiology Foundation/American Heart Association Task Force on practice guidelines. *Journal of the American College of Cardiology.* 2009;54(23):2205-2241.
17. Lee CT, Dec GW, Lilly LS. The cardiomyopathies. In: Lilly LS, ed. *Pathophysiology of Heart Disease.* 5th ed. Philadelphia: Lippincott Williams & Wilkins; 2011.
18. Liang F, Creager MA. Diseases of the peripheral vasculature. In: Lilly LS, ed. *Pathophysiology of Heart Disease.* 5th ed. Philadelphia: Lippincott Williams & Wilkins; 2011.
19. McPherson JA. *Coronary Artery Atherosclerosis.* Available at http://emedicine.medscape.com/article/153647-overview; 2011. Accessed April 18, 2011.
20. Miller CA, O'Gara PT, Lilly LS. Valvular heart disease. In: Lilly LS, ed. *Pathophysiology of Heart Disease.* 5th ed. Philadelphia: Lippincott Williams & Wilkins; 2011.
21. Morrow DA, Boden WE. Stable Ischemic Heart Disease. In: Bonow RO: *Braunwald's Heart Disease: A Textbook of Cardiovascular Medicine.* 9th ed. Philadelphia: Saunders; 2011.
22. National Heart, Lung, and Blood Institute (NHLBI). National cholesterol education project: ATP III guidelines at-a-glance quick desk reference. Available at http://www.nhlbi.nih.gov/guidelines/cholesterol/atglance.pdf; 2001. Accessed December 16, 2011.

23. Newby LK, Douglas PS. Cardiovascular disease in women. In: Bonow RO: *Braunwald's Heart Disease: A Textbook of Cardiovascular Medicine.* 9th ed. Philadelphia: Saunders; 2011.

24. O'Connor RE, Brady W, Brooks SC. 2010 American Heart Association guidelines for cardiopulmonary resuscitation and emergency cardiovascular care science part 10: acute coronary syndromes. *Circulation.* 2010;122:787-817.

25. Ren Y, Lilly LS. Diseases of the pericardium. In: Lilly LS, ed. *Pathophysiology of Heart Disease.* 5th ed. Philadelphia: Lippincott Williams & Wilkins; 2011.

26. Rhee JW, Sabatine MS, Lilly LS. Acute coronary syndromes. In: Lilly LS, ed. *Pathophysiology of Heart Disease.* 5th ed. Philadelphia: Lippincott Williams & Wilkins; 2011.

27. Rhee JW, Sabatine MS, Lilly LS. Ischemic heart disease. In: Lilly LS, ed. *Pathophysiology of Heart Disease.* 5th ed. Philadelphia: Lippincott Williams & Wilkins; 2011.

28. Skidmore-Roth, L. *Mosby's 2011 Nursing Drug Reference.* 24th ed. St. Louis: Mosby; 2011.

29. Strom JB, Libby P. Atherosclerosis. In: Lilly LS, ed. *Pathophysiology of Heart Disease.* 5th ed. Philadelphia: Lippincott Williams & Wilkins; 2011.

30. Wann LS, Curtis AB, January CT, et al. 2011 ACCF/AHA/HRS focused update on the management of patients with atrial fibrillation. *Circulation.* 2011;123:104-123

31. Wiegand DLM. *AACN Procedure Manual for Critical Care.* 6th ed. St. Louis: Mosby; 2011.

32. Wilson W, Taubert KA, Gewitz M, et al. Prevention of infective endocarditis. *Circulation.* 2007;116:1736-1754.

33. Wright RS, Anderson JL, Adams CD, et al. 2011. ACCF/AHA focused update of the guidelines for the management of patients with unstable angina/non ST-elevation myocardial infarction: a report of the American College of Cardiology Foundation/American Heart Association Task Force on Practice Guidelines. *Journal of the American College of Cardiology.* 2011;57;(19):e215-e367.

Nervous System Alterations

Christina Stewart-Amidei, PhD, RN, CNRN, CCRN, FAAN
Deborah G. Klein, MSN, RN, APRN-BC, CCRN, FAHA

⊝volve WEBSITE

Many additional resources, including self-assessment exercises, are located on the Evolve companion website at
http://evolve.elsevier.com/Sole.

- Review Questions
- Mosby's Nursing Skills Procedures

- Animations
- Video Clips

INTRODUCTION

The central and peripheral nervous systems are responsible for producing consciousness and higher mental functions, movement, sensation, and reflex activity. When these structures are damaged, a person's ability to provide self-care and interact with the environment may be greatly altered. In this chapter, the pathophysiology, assessment, and nursing and medical management related to common neurological problems, such as increased intracranial pressure (ICP), head and traumatic brain injury (TBI), meningitis, status epilepticus (SE), cerebrovascular diseases, and spinal cord injury (SCI), are discussed.

ANATOMY AND PHYSIOLOGY OF THE NERVOUS SYSTEM

Cells of the Nervous System

The nervous system is composed of two types of cells, neurons and neuroglia. The *neuron,* or nerve cell, is the basic functional unit of the nervous system and serves as the transmitter of nerve impulses (Figure 13-1). Each neuron is unique in character, and its features are determined by its specific function. During nerve transmission, *dendrites* receive an electrical impulse from other neurons. The electrical impulse is transmitted along the *axon* of the neuron to the *synaptic knobs,* which release neurotransmitters into the synapse. Once in the synapse, the neurotransmitters bind to available receptor sites, usually on a nerve or muscle cell.

Neurotransmitter binding then propagates receptor membrane depolarization and continuation of impulse transmission.

Postsynaptic responses may be excitation or inhibition, depending on the type of neurotransmitter released. It is generally believed that each neuron releases the same neurotransmitter at its nerve terminals. Acetylcholine, norepinephrine, dopamine, serotonin, glutamate, gamma-aminobutyric acid (GABA), substance P, and endorphins are neurotransmitters associated with nervous system dysfunction.

Some axons are surrounded by a white, protein-lipid complex *(myelin)* that is formed by Schwann cells in the peripheral nervous system (PNS) and by oligodendrocytes in the central nervous system (CNS). Periodic constrictions along the axon are nonmyelinated; these areas are known as nodes of Ranvier, and they facilitate fast and efficient impulse conduction (see Figure 13-1). The speed of impulse conduction depends on both the thickness of the myelin and the distance between nodes.

Neuroglial cells (glia) constitute the supportive tissue of the CNS. These cells are approximately 5 to 10 times as numerous as neurons. Most primary CNS tumors originate from glial cells and are thus termed gliomas. Four types of glial cells exist, each with specific functions. *Microglia* act as phagocytic scavenger cells when nervous tissue is damaged. *Astrocytes* are star-shaped cells that play a critical role in transport of nutrients, gases, and waste products among neurons, the vascular system, and cerebrospinal fluid (CSF); formation of scar tissue in the brain; and function of the blood-brain barrier. *Oligodendrocytes* are responsible for myelin formation. *Ependymal* cells produce specialized glial tissue that forms the lining of the ventricles of the brain and the central canal of the spinal cord; they also play a role in production of CSF.

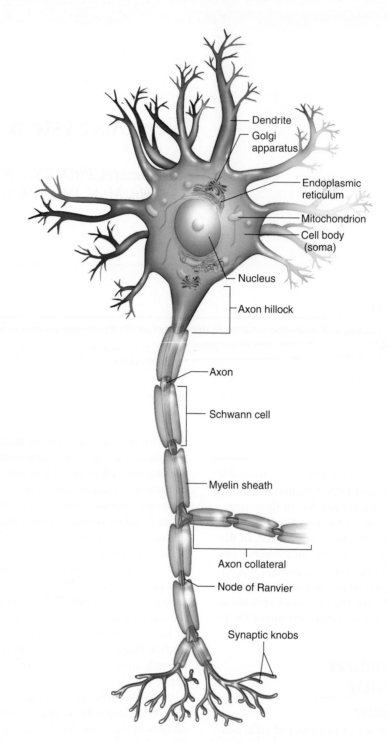

FIGURE 13-1 Structure of a typical neuron. (From Patton KT, Thibodeau GA, Douglas MM. *Essentials of Anatomy and Physiology*. St. Louis: Mosby; 2012.)

Cerebral Circulation

The cerebral circulation must provide sufficient blood to supply oxygen, glucose, and nutrients to the cerebral tissues. The brain does not have any energy stores and is dependent on aerobic metabolism. Therefore even a brief interruption in blood supply may result in significant ischemic tissue damage. The brain receives approximately 750 mL of blood per minute, or 15% to 20% of the total resting cardiac output.[9]

The blood supply of the brain arises from two major sets of arteries, the carotid arteries (anterior circulation) and the vertebral arteries (posterior circulation). Specifically, the left common carotid artery originates from the aortic arch, and the right common carotid artery originates from the innominate artery. The common carotid arteries then branch to form the external and internal carotid arteries. The external carotid artery supplies the face, scalp, and other extracranial structures. Each internal carotid artery terminates by dividing into anterior cerebral and middle cerebral arteries. The anterior cerebral artery and its branches supply the medial aspects of the motor cortex and the frontal lobes. The middle cerebral artery (MCA) comprises the principal blood supply of the frontal, temporal, and parietal lobes. Almost 90% of all strokes involve the MCA.

The paired vertebral arteries originate from the subclavian arteries and enter the skull through the foramen magnum. The vertebral arteries and their branches supply the upper spinal cord, medulla, and cerebellum before joining at the pons to form the basilar artery. The basilar artery sends branches to the cerebellum, medulla, pons, and internal ear. Then the basilar artery bifurcates and terminates as the posterior cerebral arteries, which serve the medial portions of the occipital and inferior temporal lobes.

These two arterial systems interconnect at the base of the brain via communicating arteries. The posterior communicating artery connects the internal carotid artery to the posterior cerebral artery, and the anterior communicating artery connects the two anterior cerebral arteries. This interconnection is known as the cerebral arterial circle (of Willis) at the base of the brain (Figure 13-2).

Cerebral veins, which do not have a muscle layer or valves, empty blood into venous sinuses located throughout the cranium. Since the venous sinuses play a role in absorption of CSF, they parallel the ventricular system rather than the arterial system, as in most other organs. The venous blood is emptied into the internal jugular vein and, ultimately, the superior vena cava, which returns the blood to the heart.

Cerebral Metabolism

Glucose is the brain's sole source of energy for cellular function. Because the brain is unable to store glucose, it requires a continuous supply of glucose to maintain normal brain metabolism. If the cerebral glucose level drops below 70 mg/dL, confusion may develop. Seizures may occur if the glucose level continues to decrease. Cellular damage develops when the brain glucose level drops to less than 20 mg/dL.

Aerobic metabolism is used to meet cerebral energy demands because anaerobic metabolism produces only a minimal amount of adenosine triphosphate (ATP). If the brain is deprived of oxygen, even for a few minutes, metabolism changes from aerobic to the less efficient anaerobic cellular metabolism, resulting in energy failure and neurological deficits.

Maintaining a constant *cerebral blood flow* (CBF) is essential to sustain normal cerebral metabolism. In the absence of adequate blood flow, cell membrane integrity is lost, allowing extracellular fluid to flow into the cell, causing edema. The extracellular environment becomes acidotic as a result of lactic acid production from anaerobic metabolism, and cellular damage ensues. Neurological manifestations occur owing to slowing of electrical activity. If an anoxic state lasts for 5 minutes or longer at normal body temperature, cerebral neurons are destroyed and cannot regenerate.[3]

A process called autoregulation ensures continuous CBF regardless of the mean arterial pressure (MAP). *Autoregulation* is defined as the ability of cerebral blood vessels to adjust their diameter to arterial pressure changes within the brain. If a rapid increase in MAP occurs, the cerebral vessels constrict to prevent excessive distention of the cerebral arteries. Conversely, if the MAP drops, the cerebral blood vessels dilate to maintain normal CBF and to prevent cerebral ischemia.

The cerebral vessels are also sensitive to the chemical regulators that maintain cerebral blood flow, such as the partial pressure of arterial carbon dioxide ($PaCO_2$) or oxygen (PaO_2), and the hydrogen ion concentration. Carbon dioxide is the most potent agent influencing CBF. When $PaCO_2$ is greater than 45 mm Hg, cerebral blood vessels vasodilate, increasing CBF. A low $PaCO_2$ causes the cerebral arteries to constrict, leading to decreased CBF and decreased tissue perfusion. Cerebral arteries are less sensitive to changes in PaO_2. When PaO_2 is less than 50 mm Hg, cerebral vessels dilate to increase CBF and oxygen delivery. If the PaO_2 is not raised, anaerobic metabolism begins, resulting in lactic acid accumulation. An increased hydrogen ion concentration further increases vasodilation to facilitate the removal of acidic end products from cerebral tissue.[3]

Blood-Brain Barrier System

The *blood-brain barrier system* protects the brain from toxic elements and disease-causing organisms that may circulate in the blood. The blood-brain barrier operates on the concept of tight junctions between adjacent cells and selective permeability that prevents the free movement of materials from the vascular bed into the brain. Typically, large molecules do not cross the blood-brain barrier, whereas small molecules cross easily. Water, carbon dioxide, oxygen, and glucose freely cross the cerebral capillaries. The movement of other substances into the brain is dependent on the chemical dissociation, lipid solubility, and protein-binding potential. Infections, tumors, and certain other disease states may also alter the blood-brain barrier.

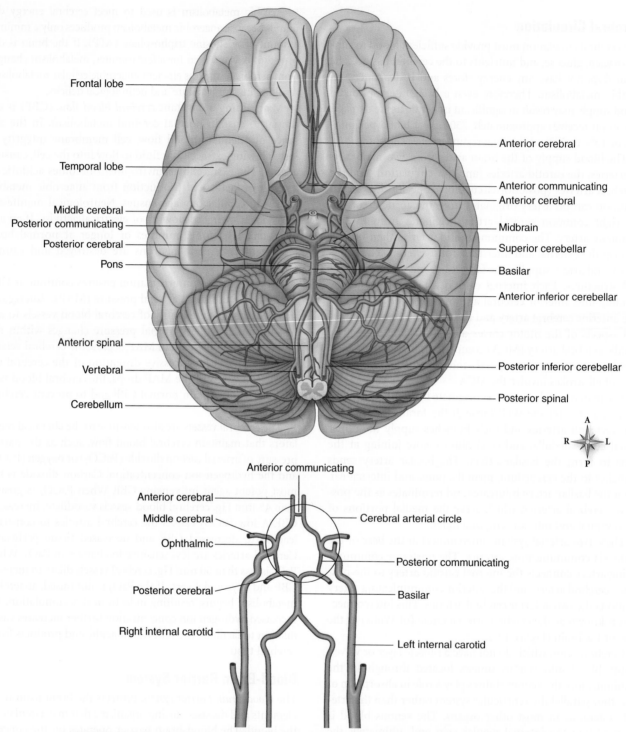

Frontal lobe

Temporal lobe

Middle cerebral
Posterior communicating
Posterior cerebral
Pons

Anterior spinal

Vertebral

Cerebellum

Anterior cerebral

Anterior communicating
Anterior cerebral

Midbrain

Superior cerebellar

Basilar

Anterior inferior cerebellar

Posterior inferior cerebellar

Posterior spinal

A
R — L
P

Anterior communicating

Anterior cerebral

Middle cerebral

Ophthalmic

Posterior cerebral

Right internal carotid

Cerebral arterial circle

Posterior communicating

Basilar

Left internal carotid

FIGURE 13-2 Arterial blood supply of the brain. The circle of Willis is formed by the two anterior cerebral arteries, joined to each other by the anterior communicating artery; arising from the internal carotid arteries, the posterior communicating arteries connect to the posterior cerebral arteries. (Modified from Patton KT, Thibodeau GA. *Anatomy and Physiology.* 7th ed. St. Louis: Mosby; 2010.)

Ventricular System and Cerebrospinal Fluid

The four *ventricles* of the adult brain are hollow spaces lined by ependymal cells. Specialized epithelium in the ventricular wall, called the *choroid plexus,* produce CSF. A smaller amount of CSF is secreted from the ependymal cells that line the ventricles, and the blood vessels of the meninges and the brain. CSF is continually secreted from these surfaces at about 500 mL per day, or about 20 mL per hour.[3] On average, 150 mL of CSF is contained in the ventricles and subarachnoid space. The CSF plays a role in metabolic function of the brain and provides a cushioning effect during head movement.

CSF flows from the two lateral ventricles into the third ventricle through the foramen of Monro. From the third ventricle, CSF flows through the aqueduct of Sylvius into the fourth ventricle. From there, the CSF flow is directed through the foramina of Luschka and Magendie into the cisterna and subarachnoid space (Figure 13-3). After circulating around the brain and spinal cord, CSF is reabsorbed into the venous sinuses of the brain through the arachnoid villi, which are dural projections from the arachnoid space.

FUNCTIONAL AND STRUCTURAL DIVISIONS OF THE CENTRAL NERVOUS SYSTEM

Meninges

Meninges cover the brain and spinal cord and consist of three layers: dura mater, arachnoid mater, and pia mater (see Figure 13-3). The *dura mater* is the outermost covering and has two layers. The outer surface adheres to the skull, and the inner layer produces prominent folds (falx cerebri, tentorium cerebelli, falx cerebelli) that subdivide the interior cranial cavity to support and protect the brain. The inner dura mater also covers the spine. The *arachnoid mater* is located inside the dura mater. It is a delicate, avascular layer that loosely encloses the brain and spine. The *pia mater* closely adheres to the brain's outer surface and contains a network of blood vessels. The pia mater surrounding the spinal cord is less vascular.

Actual or potential spaces exist between the meningeal layers. The epidural space is a potential space between the skull and the outer dura mater. The subdural space is between the dura mater and the arachnoid mater and is filled

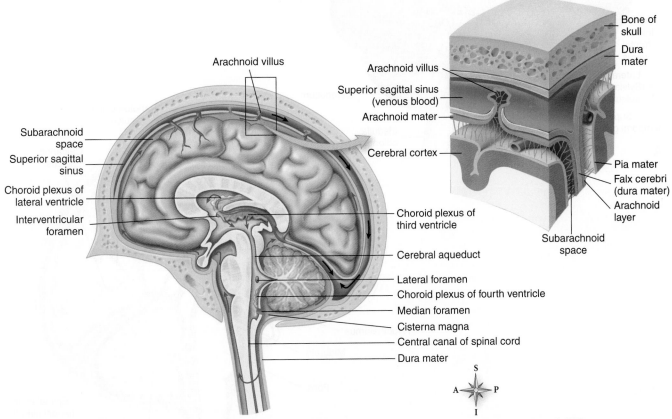

FIGURE 13-3 Flow of cerebrospinal fluid (CSF) circulation. Arrows represent the route of CSF. CSF is produced in the ventricles and returns to the venous circulation in the superior sagittal sinus. Note the meningeal layers (dura, arachnoid, and pia). (Modified from Patton KT, Thibodeau GA. *Anatomy and Physiology.* 8th ed. St. Louis: Mosby; 2013.)

with a small amount of lubricating fluid. The subarachnoid space, a considerable area between the arachnoid and pia mater, contains circulating CSF. In addition, the subarachnoid space has a vast network of arteries travelling through it.

Brain (Encephalon)

The brain is approximately 2% of body weight. Brain weight decreases with aging, primarily because of neuronal loss. The brain is divided into three major areas: the cerebrum, the brainstem, and the cerebellum.

Cerebrum

The *cerebrum* (Figure 13-4) is composed of the right and left cerebral hemispheres, basal ganglia and diencephalon. The cerebral hemispheres are separated by a deep longitudinal fissure. The *corpus callosum* consists of fibers that travel from one hemisphere to the other, providing intricate connections between the two hemispheres.

Individuals have a dominant hemisphere. The left hemisphere specializes in language for most individuals and dominates skilled and gesturing hand movements. The

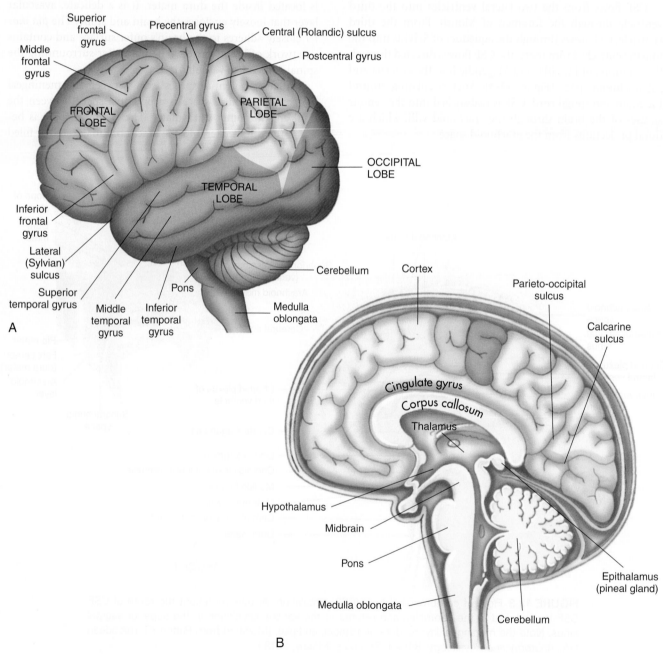

FIGURE 13-4 Cerebral hemispheres and structures of the brain. **A,** Lateral external view. **B,** Midsagittal view. (Modified from McCance KL, Huether SE. *Pathophysiology: The Biological Basis for Disease in Adults and Children.* 6th ed. St. Louis: Mosby; 2010.)

right hemisphere specializes in the perception of certain nonverbal auditory stimuli, such as music. Processing visual information and determining spatial relationships are also functions of the right hemisphere. Both sides of the brain communicate with each other to facilitate complex functions.

The surface of each hemisphere appears wrinkled because of the numerous raised areas, called *gyri* (see Figure 13-4). Each gyrus folds into another, causing the convoluted appearance and substantially increasing the surface area of the brain. The surface of the cerebral hemisphere is approximately six cells deep and is called the *cerebral cortex,* or gray matter. Beneath the cortex is a layer of white matter, consisting of mostly myelinated axons, which serve as association and projection pathways.

A *fissure,* or *sulcus,* is a separation in the cerebral hemisphere. The fissures serve as important divisions or landmarks (see Figure 13-4). The longitudinal fissure separates the cerebral hemispheres into left and right sections. The lateral, or Sylvian, fissure, divides the frontal and temporal lobes. The central, or Rolandic, fissure separates the frontal and the parietal lobes. The parieto-occipital fissure separates the occipital lobe from the parietal and temporal lobes.

The cerebrum is divided into lobes (see Figure 13-4). Each lobe has a specific function. Functions for each lobe (Table 13-1) guide assessment and facilitate localization of the patient's problem.

The *diencephalon,* on the inferior surface (see Figure 13-4), connects the brainstem to the cerebrum and the midbrain. It is divided into four paired regions: thalamus, hypothalamus, subthalamus, and epithalamus. The *thalamus* is the largest structure within the diencephalon and integrates all bodily sensations except smell. The thalamus assists in recognizing pain, touch, and temperature, and relays sensory information to the cerebrum. It also plays a role in emotions, arousal and alertness, and complex reflexes. The *hypothalamus* acts as a regulatory center for the autonomic nervous system (ANS). The general functions of the hypothalamus include temperature control, water balance, control of appetite and thirst, cardiovascular regulation, sleep-wake cycle, circadian rhythms, and sexual activity. The hypothalamus also controls the release of hormones from the pituitary gland.

Brainstem

The *brainstem* is at the central core of the brain and controls vital functions. The major divisions of the brainstem are the midbrain, pons, and medulla (see Figure 13-4). The *midbrain,* also known as the mesencephalon, is a short segment of brainstem lying between the diencephalon and the pons. It contains nuclei of cranial nerves III (oculomotor) and IV (trochlear). The midbrain relays impulses to and from the cerebrum and lower brainstem. It also serves as the center for auditory and visual reflexes. The *pons* is seated between the midbrain and the medulla. It contains nuclei of cranial nerves V (trigeminal), VI (abducens), VII (facial), and VIII (vestibulocochlear), and it connects the cerebellum to the brainstem. In conjunction with the medulla, the pons controls the rate and duration of respirations. The *medulla oblongata* is situated between the pons and the spinal cord. It contains nuclei of cranial nerves IX (glossopharyngeal), X (vagus), XI (accessory), and XII (hypoglossal). The medulla regulates the basic rhythm of respiration, rate and strength of the pulse, and vasomotor activity. In addition, neurons within the medulla regulate certain reflexes, including sneezing, swallowing, coughing, and vomiting.

Cerebellum

The *cerebellum* is located posterior to the brainstem (see Figure 13-4). It is connected to the brainstem at the pons, by three paired cerebellar peduncles. The peduncles receive input from the spinal cord and brainstem and send it to the cerebellar cortex. The functions of equilibrium, fine movement, muscle tone, balance, and coordination are mediated by the cerebellum.

Specialized Systems Within the Central Nervous System

The *limbic system* provides primitive control of emotional responses and arousal. Structures of the limbic system include the amygdala (reward and fear stimuli), hippocampus (long-term memory), cingulate gyrus (attention and cognition), and connections to the hypothalamus and thalamus. The reticular activating system (RAS) consists of diffuse fibers that begin in the lower brainstem and connect to various locations in cerebral cortex. The RAS controls arousal, the sleep-wake cycle, selective attention, and perceptual awareness. If the RAS is intact, a person is aware and attentive. When the RAS is impaired, the person experiences inattention, alterations in the

TABLE 13-1	FUNCTIONS OF THE CEREBRAL HEMISPHERES	
STRUCTURE	**FUNCTION**
Frontal lobes	Conscious thought, abstract thinking, judgment, voluntary movement on opposite side of the body; prefrontal areas are responsible for affect, memory, and concentration; motor expression of language in Broca area on the left side in most individuals
Parietal lobes	Processing, association, and interpretation of sensory information from opposite side of the body
Temporal lobes	Processing, association, and interpretation of auditory information; comprehension of language in Wernicke area on the left side in most individuals; medial portion is responsible for memory and social behavior
Occipital lobes	Visual processing and interpretation
Basal ganglia	Motor control of fine body movements

sleep-wake cycle, or decreased arousal, which is manifest as coma.

Spinal Cord

The *spinal cord* is surrounded by the vertebral column and meninges. It begins as an extension from the medulla and ends at the first lumbar vertebrae. The dura and arachnoid layer of the meninges surround the spinal cord and contain CSF.

The spinal cord has 31 segments: 8 cervical, 12 thoracic, 5 lumbar, 5 sacral, and 1 coccygeal (Figure 13-5). The spinal nerves, originating at each segment of the spinal cord, are part of the peripheral nervous system. They transmit information to and from the periphery to the spinal cord. These

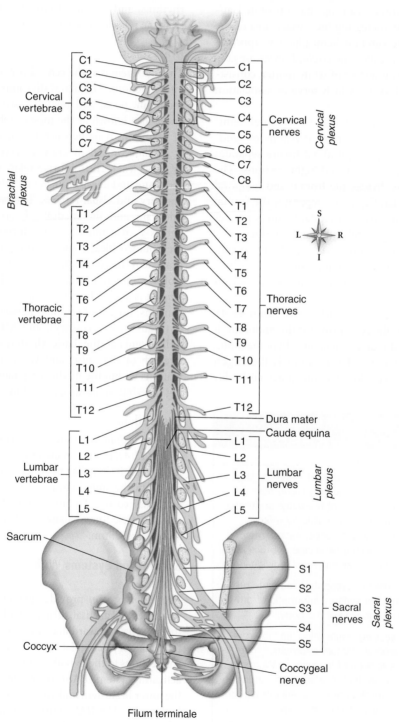

FIGURE 13-5 Spinal nerves and plexi as they relate to vertebral level. The names of the vertebrae are listed on the left, and the corresponding spinal nerves and plexi are listed on the right. (Modified from Patton KT, Thibodeau GA. *Anatomy and Physiology.* 7th ed. St. Louis: Mosby; 2010.)

nerves innervate the skin and musculature of most of the body. Each spinal nerve consists of a *dorsal root* (posterior) and *ventral root* (anterior). The dorsal roots convey afferent impulses (sensory input) into the spinal cord from skin segments that represent specific areas of the body known as *dermatomes*. The ventral roots carry efferent impulses (muscle signals) from the spinal cord to specific areas of the body known as myotomes. A dermatome and myotome chart traces the spinal nerves to their point of skin or muscle innervation and provides anatomical clues about level of injury or dysfunction (Figure 13-6).

The spinal nerves interconnect in three areas: the cervical, brachial, and lumbosacral plexuses. The *cervical plexus* includes spinal nerves C1 to C4 and innervates the muscles of the neck and shoulders. The phrenic nerve originates in this plexus and supplies the diaphragm. The *brachial plexus* comprises spinal nerves C4 to C8 and T1 and innervates the arms via the radial and ulnar nerves. The *lumbosacral plexus* is formed by spinal nerves L1 to L5 and S1 to S3. The femoral nerve arises from the lumbar plexus and the sciatic nerve from the sacral plexus, and both nerves innervate the legs (see Figure 13-5).

Cross-sectional size of the spinal cord varies by level, but structures remain the same at all levels. The H-shaped gray matter comprises the center of the cord. The anterior gray matter contains *sensory fibers* that convey sensory impulses from organs and muscles to the spinal cord. The posterior gray matter relays motor impulses from the spinal cord to skeletal muscles. The white matter of the cord consists of fibers that connect with gray matter, together comprising ascending (sensory) and descending (motor) pathways.

Peripheral Nervous System

The PNS is comprised of the 12 paired cranial nerves, 31 paired spinal nerves, and the ANS. The 12 pairs of *cranial nerves* originate in the brain and brainstem and exit from the cranial cavity. Cranial nerves have sensory or motor functions, or both. These nerves are primarily responsible for the innervation of structures in the head and neck. A summary

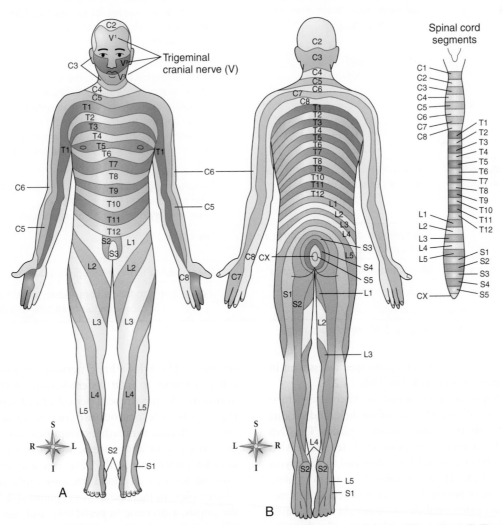

FIGURE 13-6 Dermatome distribution of spinal nerves. **A,** The front of the body's surface. **B,** The back of the body's surface. The inset illustrates the segments of the spinal cord connected with each of the spinal nerves associated with the sensory dermatomes shown in **A** and **B**. (Modified from Patton KT, Thibodeau GA. *Anatomy and Physiology.* 8th ed. St. Louis: Mosby; 2013.)

TABLE 13-2	THE CRANIAL NERVES AND ASSESSMENT IN THE CRITICALLY ILL PATIENT	
NERVE	**MAJOR FUNCTIONS**	**ASSESSMENT**
I—Olfactory (S)	Smell	Not assessed.
II—Optic (S)	Visual acuity	Assess gross ability to see.
III—Oculomotor (M)	Movement of eyes; pupillary constriction and accommodation	Evaluate pupil size (mm), shape, and equality with bright penlight in dimly lit room. Assess for direct and consensual reaction to light; rate as brisk, sluggish, or nonreactive.
IV—Trochlear (M)	Movement of eyes	Evaluate voluntary movement of eyes together—up, down, laterally and diagonally (tests CNs III, IV, and VI); In unconscious patients with stable cervical spine, assess *oculocephalic reflex* (doll's eye): turn the patient's head quickly from side to side while holding the eyes open. Note movement of eyes. The doll's eye reflex is present and cranial nerve intact if the eyes move bilaterally in the opposite direction of the head movement. Assess for nystagmus.
V—Trigeminal (S/M)	Chewing; sensation of scalp, face, teeth	Assess corneal reflex; observe for bilateral blink.
VI—Abducens (M)	Movement of eyes	See CN IV.
VII—Facial (M)	Facial expression; lacrimation, salivation; taste anterior tongue	Assess facial muscles for symmetry; if possible, ask patient to open eyes, arch eyebrows, smile, frown, and puff cheeks.
VIII—Auditory (S)	Hearing (cochlear) Equilibrium (vestibular)	Assess response to verbalization (gross hearing ability). In the unconscious patient, the caloric irrigation test is done to assess the *oculovestibular reflex* (may be more sensitive than the doll's eye): elevate the head of bed to 30 degrees to assess for intact tympanic membrane, irrigate the ear canal with cold water. Bilateral eye movement toward the irrigated ear indicates an intact reflex.
IX—Glossopharyngeal (S/M)	Swallowing; taste posterior tongue; general sensation pharynx	CNs IX and X evaluated together. Evaluate cough and gag reflex in response to suctioning the endotracheal tube and pharynx. Assess ability to manage oral secretions by swallowing.
X—Vagus (S/M)	Swallowing and laryngeal control; parasympathetic function	See CN IX.
XI—Spinal accessory (M)	Movement of head and shoulders	Assess ability to move/shrug shoulders and turn head.
XII—Hypoglossal (M)	Movement of tongue	If patient able to follow commands, assess ability to protrude and/or move tongue from side to side.

CN, Cranial nerve; *M,* motor; *S,* sensory; *S/M,* sensory and motor.

of the functions of the cranial nerves and their assessment in the critically ill patient is provided in Table 13-2.

The ANS comprises motor nerves to visceral effectors: cardiac muscle, smooth muscle, adrenal medulla, and various glands, including salivary, gastric, and sweat glands. The ANS controls visceral activities at an unconscious level. The ANS consists of the *sympathetic nervous system* and the *parasympathetic nervous system.* These parallel systems act to regulate visceral organs in opposing ways—one system stimulates effects whereas the other inhibits—to maintain homeostasis.

The *sympathetic nervous system* is known as the thoracolumbar system because the nerve fibers originate in the thoracic and lumbar regions of the spinal cord. This system contains a chain of ganglia located on both sides of the vertebrae. The sympathetic nervous system is sometimes called the *fight-or-flight* system because it is activated and dominates during stressful periods. Most sympathetic neurons release the neurotransmitter *norepinephrine* at the visceral effector. Sympathetic impulses cause vasoconstriction in the skin and viscera, vasodilation in the skeletal muscles, an increase in the heart rate and force of contraction, an increase in blood pressure (BP), dilation of the bronchioles, an increase in sweat gland activity, dilation of the pupils, a decrease in peristalsis, and contraction of the pilomotor muscles (gooseflesh).

The *parasympathetic nervous system* is known as the craniosacral system because the preganglionic fibers originate at certain cranial nerves and in the sacral spinal cord. The axons

GERIATRIC CONSIDERATIONS

- The effects of certain medications used to decrease intracranial pressure (osmotic and loop diuretics, barbiturates) should be closely monitored because of the older patient's decreased ability to absorb, metabolize, and/or excrete these drugs.
- Assessment of preexisting renal insufficiency and use of diuretics is necessary because the use of these drugs may place older patients at risk of hypokalemia or hyponatremia when they receive medications to reduce intracranial pressure.
- In the older patient, elevating the head of the bed to decrease intracranial pressure may compromise an already diminished cerebral blood flow. Continuous assessment of neurological function and/or cerebral perfusion pressure is necessary to prevent decreasing brain blood flow.

- Central cord syndrome is more common in the older population and may result from hyperextension of an osteoarthritic spine.
- Subdural hematomas are more common in the older population because as the brain atrophies with aging, it shrinks away from the dura and stretches bridging veins, which may easily tear. A large amount of blood can accumulate in the subdural space before the patient demonstrates overt signs and symptoms. Subtle mental status changes are often the first finding to appear and are easily misinterpreted as signs of normal aging.

are long, and ganglia are situated adjacent to or within specific organs. The parasympathetic system is dominant in nonstressful situations. It stimulates visceral activities associated with maintenance of normal functions. The effects of parasympathetic nervous system stimulation induce a return of systems to a normal state of functioning. All neurons within the parasympathetic nervous system release the neurotransmitter *acetylcholine* at the visceral effector.

Effects of Aging

Aging affects the nervous system in a variety of ways (see box, "Geriatric Considerations"). Loss of myelin and altered conduction may result in a decrease in reaction time of specific nerves. Cellular degeneration may result in a decreased speed and intensity of reflexes with an increased risk of injury. Decreased sensation may reduce the ability to taste, smell, see, and feel pain. Proprioception (one's position in space) is altered, resulting in an increased risk for falling. Hardening of the pupil sphincter may result in a decreased responsiveness to light, especially when moving from one level of lighting to another. Increased rigidity of the iris may result in decreased pupil size, with the need for more light for visual clarity. Altered motor functioning may result in physiological tremors, decreased neuromuscular control, change in posture, a shuffling gait, and a short stride, resulting in an increased risk for falls. Muscle atrophy may also be present.

Assessment

A thorough history provides information about the patient's condition. Ideally, the patient is the primary source of the historical data. If the patient is unable to give a history, family or friends should supply information related to symptoms, onset, progression, and chronology of the event. Comorbidities and contributing factors must also be considered. If pain is a presenting symptom, information must be obtained about the location, onset, type, duration, presence of other symptoms, and what makes the pain better or worse.

An initial baseline neurological assessment, along with ongoing assessments, assists in monitoring the patient's

condition and response to treatments and nursing interventions. When performing a neurological assessment, the critical care nurse focuses on mental status, level of consciousness (LOC), and cranial nerve, motor, and sensory function. Because many neurological changes represent life-threatening conditions that require emergent treatment, it is important for the nurse to immediately report adverse assessment findings to the physician.

! CLINICAL ALERT

Neurological Assessment

Perform the neurological assessment with the nurse who just cared for the patient. This ensures complete understanding of the prior documented assessment by the receiving nurse and quick recognition of neurological changes.

Mental Status

When assessing a patient's mental status, the critical care nurse tests consciousness (awareness of self and the environment) and cognition (the ability to produce a response), which includes expressive and receptive language, and memory.

The Glasgow Coma Scale (GCS; Figure 13-7) is a commonly used standardized tool that assesses consciousness and cognition.[22] The patient's ability to speak, open his eyes, and produce a motor response to verbal command or noxious stimuli is evaluated. A noxious stimulus may include firm pressure applied to the nail bed, a trapezium squeeze, supraorbital pressure, or sternal pressure. Noxious stimuli is applied only if the patient fails to respond to verbal stimuli. Care is taken to avoid injury when applying noxious stimuli.

The best response in each of the three categories of eye opening, verbal response, and motor response is scored, and the three scores are summed. GCS scores range from 3 (deep coma), to 15 (normal functioning). A GCS of 8 or less is consistent with coma. Several conditions limit application of the GCS, including medications and concurrent injuries, such as spinal cord injury (SCI). It is important to note that the GCS

Glasgow Coma Scale			
Eyes	Open	Spontaneously	4
		To verbal command	3
		To pain	2
		No response	1
Best motor response	To verbal command	Obeys	6
	To painful stimulus	Localizes pain	5
		Flexion-withdrawal	4
		Flexion-abnormal (Decorticate rigidity)	3
		Extension (Decerebrate rigidity)	2
		No response	1
Best verbal response		Oriented and converses	5
		Disoriented and converses	4
		Inappropriate words	3
		Incomprehensible sounds	2
		No response	1
Total			**3-15**

FIGURE 13-7 The Glasgow Coma Scale is a measure of consciousness based on eye opening, movement, and verbal responses. Each response is given a number, and the three scores are summed. Scores range from 3 to 15.

is a measure of consciousness and cognition, and does not replace neurological assessment of specific brain function.

Language

Fluency and spontaneity of speech, word-finding ability, and comprehension are language skills that are assessed. If intubated, the patient's ability to comprehend can be assessed by asking the patient to perform simple verbal commands such as pointing to the clock, blinking the eyes, or raising the right arm. Language skills may also be evaluated by asking the patient to write responses.

Language deficits are common in neurological disorders. *Expressive dysphasia* is a deficit in language output or speech production from a dysfunction in the dominant frontal lobe. It varies from mild word-finding difficulty to complete loss of both verbal and written communication skills. The inability to comprehend language and follow commands is called *receptive dysphasia*. Receptive dysphasia indicates dysfunction in the dominant temporal lobe. A nonintubated patient with receptive problems can speak spontaneously, but the verbal response does not follow the context of the conversation. An intubated patient may appear to be responsive, but is unable to follow simple verbal commands.

Memory

Both short- and long-term memory may be evaluated. *Short-term memory* is assessed by asking the patient to recall the names of three common words or objects (e.g., chair, clock, blue) after a 3-minute interval. *Long-term memory* is tested

by asking questions about the patient's distant past (e.g., birth place, year of birth, year of graduation from school, year of marriage). If intubated, the patient can write the answers.

Cranial Nerve Function

On initial baseline neurological assessment, all cranial nerves are assessed. Focused cranial nerve assessments may be conducted depending on anatomy involved. Table 13-2 presents assessments that can be done in patients who are critically ill, who often have a decreased LOC.

Pupil examination is the most critical component of cranial nerve assessment. Pupils are often assessed hourly for size, shape, equality, and response to light. Normal pupil diameter ranges from 1.5 to 6 mm. Measurement with a millimeter scale is the most reliable method of determining size and equality. Unequal pupils (*anisocoria*) occur normally in approximately 10% of the general population. Otherwise, inequality of pupils is a sign of a pathological process. Direct and consensual pupillary responses to light are assessed. A change in pupil reaction to light in one or both eyes is an important sign that may indicate increasing ICP or neurological deterioration. Hypoxia and medications may also influence pupillary size and reactivity to light.

Motor Function

The nurse assesses movement of all extremities, muscle strength, muscle tone and posture, and coordination. Muscle groups are assessed for symmetry. A more comprehensive assessment can be done if the patient is able to follow commands. If the patient is unable to follow commands, the nurse must assess motor response to noxious stimuli. Movement is assessed by asking the patient to move the extremities on command, or by observing while the patient moves around in bed. Muscle strength of the extremities is assessed and graded on a 5-point scale (Table 13-3). The grading is

TABLE 13-3	GRADING SCALE FOR MOTOR RESPONSES
NUMERIC RATING	**MOTOR RESPONSE**
0	Unable to lift the arm or leg to command, or in response to painful stimuli
1	Flicker of movement is felt or seen in the muscle(s) of the limb
2	Moves the limb, but unable to raise the extremity off the bed
3	Able to lift the extremity off the bed briefly, but does not have the strength to maintain the lift
4	Able to lift the extremity off the bed, but has difficulty resisting the examiner ("I am going to push your right arm/leg down, so try to prevent me from doing that")
5	Able to lift the extremity off the bed and maintain the position against resistance

TABLE 13-4	SPINAL NERVE INNERVATION (MYOTOMES) OF MAJOR MUSCLE GROUPS	
SPINAL NERVE	MUSCLE GROUP MOVEMENT	ASSESSMENT TECHNIQUE
C4-C5	Shoulder abduction	Shrug shoulders against downward pressure of examiner's hands
C5	Elbow flexion (biceps)	Arm pulled up from resting position against resistance
C7	Elbow extension (triceps) Thumb–index finger pinch	From the flexed position, arm straightened out against resistance Index finger held firmly to thumb against resistance to pull apart
C8	Hand grasp	Hand grasp strength evaluated
L2	Hip flexion	Leg lifted from bed against resistance
L3	Knee extension	From flexed position, knee extended against resistance
L4	Foot dorsiflexion	Foot pulled up toward nose against resistance
S1	Foot plantar flexion	Foot pushed down (stepping on the gas) against resistance

based on the ability to move muscle groups, hold a position against gravity, and maintain that position against resistance.

It is important to assess each limb, because differences between the right and left sides and upper and lower extremities can occur. In persons with spinal cord injury, individual muscle function by myotome (Table 13-4) is assessed to identify level of injury. *Hemiplegia* exists when one side of the patient's body is affected. *Paraplegia* exists when two of the same extremities are paralyzed.

In a conscious patient, checking for *arm drift* can detect subtle weakness. The patient is asked to close the eyes and stretch out the arms with palms up for 20 to 30 seconds. A downward drift of the arm or pronation of the palm on one side indicates subtle weakness in the involved extremity.

Muscle tone is assessed by taking each extremity through passive range of motion. Normal muscle tone shows slight resistance to range of motion. Flaccid muscles have diminished muscle tone, with no resistance to movement. Increased muscle tone is manifest as spasticity or rigidity.

Coordination of movement is under cerebellar control. It is assessed by asking the patient to perform rapid alternating movements, such as touching the finger to the nose or running the heel down the shin bilaterally. These tests require the patient to be able to follow verbal commands.

Abnormal posturing may be observed in unconscious patients with brain damage. These include flexion or extensor posturing (Figure 13-8). *Flexion posturing* involves rigid flexion and adduction of the arms, wrist flexion with clenched fists, and extension and internal rotation of the legs. It usually occurs secondary to damage of the corticospinal tract. *Extensor posturing* is the result of a midbrain or pons lesion. In this posture, the arms and legs are rigidly extended, and the feet are in plantar extension. The forearms may be pronated and abducted, and the wrists and fingers are flexed. Abnormal posturing can occur in response to noxious stimuli, such as suctioning or pain, or may be spontaneous. Different posturing may be noted on each side of the body.

Reflexes

There are three types of reflexes: deep tendon, superficial, and pathological. *Deep tendon reflexes* (DTRs) are obtained by a

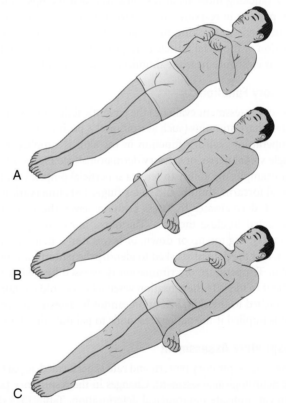

FIGURE 13-8 Abnormal motor responses. **A,** Flexion posturing. **B,** Extension posturing. **C,** Flexion posturing on right side and extension posturing on left side.

brisk tap of a reflex hammer on the tendons of a muscle group to elicit a motor response. The biceps reflex assesses spinal nerve roots C5-C6; brachioradialis, C5-C6; triceps, C7-C8; patellar, L2-L4; and Achilles tendon, S1-S2. DTRs are graded according to the response elicited: 0, no reflex; 1+, hypoactive; 2+, normal; 3+, increased but normal; 4+, very brisk, hyperreflexive, clonus. Alterations in DTRs may indicate damage of the spinal cord or brain. In spinal shock, DTRs are absent below the level of injury initially; return of DTRs signals resolution of spinal shock. Aging and metabolic factors, such as thyroid dysfunction or electrolyte abnormalities, may also affect DTRs.

Superficial reflexes are elicited by touching or stroking a specific area and observing the motor response. The corneal reflex is a superficial reflex, as are the palpebral, gag, abdominal, cremasteric, and anal reflexes.

Pathological reflexes are typically present at birth, disappear with maturing of the nervous system, then reappear as a consequence of impaired neurological function. The most common is the Babinski reflex. When the sole of the patient's foot is lightly stroked, the normal response is plantar flexion of the toes. A Babinski reflex is present when dorsiflexion of the great toe with fanning of the other toes is noted upon stimulation. In an adult, the presence of a Babinski reflex is a sign of an upper motor neuron lesion and damage to the corticospinal tract. Other pathological reflexes include the suck (sucking motions in response to touch the lips), snout (lip pursing in response to touching the lips), palmar (grasp in response to stroking the palm), and palmomental (contraction of the facial muscle in response to stimulation of the thenar eminence near the thumb) reflexes in adults.

Sensory Function

Sensory assessment evaluates the patient's ability to discriminate a sharp stimulus (such as a pinprick), position sense, and temperature. Sensory function in the skin is supplied by a single spinal nerve, or sensory dermatome (see Figure 13-6). For example, the ability to sense a superficial pinprick on the lateral forearm, thumb, and index finger tests innervation of the C6 dermatome. To assess position sense, the patient is instructed to close the eyes. The nurse moves the patient's thumb or big toe up or down, or leaves it in a neutral position, and the patient is asked to identify the pattern of movement. Temperature discrimination is assessed by asking the patient to identify the sensation when a hot or cold container is touched to the skin. Sensation cannot be assessed in coma but is implied if the patient responds to painful stimulation.

Respiratory Assessment

Assessing respiratory pattern and rate is performed as part of the neurological assessment. Changes in the respiratory pattern can indicate neurological deterioration. Table 13-5 describes abnormal respiratory patterns related to neurological dysfunction. However, these patterns are obscured in intubated and mechanically ventilated patients.

Hourly Assessment

The nurse assesses the neurological parameters based on ordered frequency (often hourly) and severity of the patient's condition. Reassessment is also done if changes are noted. Table 13-6 contains the components of an hourly neurological assessment for patients with increased ICP, head injury, or acute stroke. Focused assessments may be performed based on the patient's specific condition. All findings are documented per unit protocol, and abnormal findings are immediately reported to the physician.

TABLE 13-5	ANATOMICAL CORRELATES OF ABNORMAL RESPIRATORY PATTERNS IN NEUROLOGICAL DISORDERS
ABNORMAL PATTERN	**ANATOMICAL CORRELATE**
Cheyne-Stokes	Bilateral deep cerebral lesion or some cerebellar lesions
Central neurogenic hyperventilation	Lesions of the midbrain and upper pons
Apneustic	Lesions of the mid to lower pons
Cluster breathing	Lesions of the lower pons or upper medulla
Ataxic respirations	Lesions of the medulla

INCREASED INTRACRANIAL PRESSURE

A commonly encountered problem in the critical care setting is increased ICP. Many neurological problems are associated with increased ICP, such as brain injury and stroke. Sustained increases in ICP compound the extent of brain injury and can be life-threatening. Therefore it is important to assess and maintain ICP within normal limits.

Pathophysiology

The rigid cranial vault contains three types of noncompressible contents: brain tissue, blood, and CSF. The pressure exerted by the combined volumes of these three components is ICP. If the volume of any one of these three components increases, the volume of one or both of the other compartments must decrease proportionally, or an increase in ICP occurs (Monro-Kellie doctrine). This compensation is termed *compliance* (Figure 13-9). With adequate compliance, an increase in intracranial volume is compensated by displacement of CSF into the spinal subarachnoid space, displacement of blood into the venous sinuses, or both. The ICP remains normal despite increases in volume (flat part of curve). As compensatory mechanisms are exhausted, a small increase in volume leads to a large increase in ICP (steep part of curve).

As compliance decreases, ICP increases and CBF decreases. When CBF decreases, the brain becomes hypoxic, carbon dioxide levels increase, and acidosis occurs. In response to these changes, the cerebral blood vessels dilate to increase CBF. This compensatory response further increases intracranial volume, creating a vicious cycle that can be life-threatening (Figure 13-10).

Normal ICP ranges from 0 to 15 mm Hg. Increased ICP is defined as a pressure of 20 mm Hg or greater persisting for 5 minutes or longer, and is a life-threatening event. Sustained increases in ICP can lead to herniation, which occurs from shifting of brain tissue from an area of high pressure to

TABLE 13-6	COMPONENTS OF THE HOURLY NEUROLOGICAL ASSESSMENT FOR PATIENTS WITH INCREASED INTRACRANIAL PRESSURE, HEAD INJURY, OR ACUTE STROKE			
MENTAL STATUS	**FOCAL MOTOR**	**PUPILS**	**BRAINSTEM/CRANIAL NERVES**
Glasgow Coma Scale	Move all extremities	Size	Corneal reflex
Assesses level of conscious-ness, expressive language, ability to follow commands	Strength of all extremities (compare right and left sides)	Shape	Present: immediate blinking bilaterally
		Reaction to light (direct and consensual)	Diminished: blinking asymmetrically
	Motor response	Extraocular movements	Absent: no blinking
			Cough, gag, swallow reflex
			Observe for excessive drooling
			Observe for cough/swallow reflex

one of lower pressure. Herniation syndromes are classified as supratentorial (cingulate, central, and uncal herniation) or infratentorial (cerebellar tonsil herniation). These herniation syndromes are described in Table 13-7 and shown in Figure 13-11.

Along with MAP, the ICP determines cerebral perfusion pressure (CPP), which is the pressure required to perfuse the brain. CPP is calculated as the difference between MAP and ICP (CPP = MAP − ICP). The normal CPP in an adult is between 60 and 100 mm Hg and must be maintained at 70 mm Hg or greater in those with brain pathology. Any factor that decreases MAP and/or increases ICP decreases CPP. CPP determines CBF; therefore ischemia or infarction can occur if the CPP is inadequate. Measures to promote adequate CPP include lowering of increased ICP or, if this is not possible, increasing MAP to offset the effects of ICP on CPP. Often MAP will rise in the presence of increased ICP; lowering MAP in this circumstance may actually decrease CPP and should be prevented.[3,7]

Causes of Increased Intracranial Pressure

Factors that increase ICP are associated with increased brain volume, increased cerebral blood volume, and increased CSF.

Increased Brain Volume

The most common cause of increased brain volume is cerebral edema. Cerebral edema is an increase in the water content of the brain tissue; uncorrected, it may lead to increase in ICP. Cytotoxic edema and vasogenic edema are two categories of cerebral edema; they may occur independently or together. *Cytotoxic cerebral edema* is characterized by intracellular swelling of neurons, most often the result of hypoxia and hypo-osmolality. Hypoxia causes decreased ATP production, leading to the failure of the sodium-potassium pump.

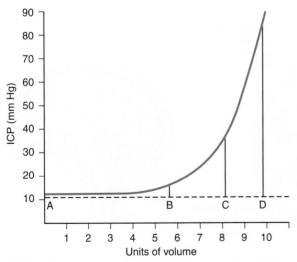

FIGURE 13-9 Intracranial pressure–volume curve. Between points *A* and *B*, intracranial compliance is present. Intracranial pressure (ICP) is normal, and increases in intracranial volume are tolerated without large increases in ICP. As compliance is lost, small increases in volume result in large and dangerous increases in ICP (points *C* and *D*).

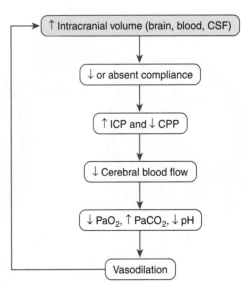

FIGURE 13-10 Pathophysiology flow diagram for increased intracranial pressure. *CPP,* Cerebral perfusion pressure; *ICP,* intracranial pressure; *PaCO₂,* partial pressure of arterial carbon dioxide; *PaO₂,* partial presure of arterial oxygen.

TABLE 13-7 HERNIATION SYNDROMES

SYNDROME	DEFINITION	SYMPTOMS
Cingulate	Shift of brain tissue from one cerebral hemisphere under the falx cerebri to the other hemisphere	No specific symptoms; may compromise cerebral blood flow
Central	Downward shift of cerebral hemispheres, basal ganglia, and diencephalon through the tentorial notch that compresses the brainstem	**Early** Decrease in LOC Motor weakness Cheyne-Stokes respiration Small, reactive pupils **Late** Coma Pupils dilated and fixed Abnormal flexion posturing, progressing to abnormal extensor posturing Unstable vital signs progressing to cardiopulmonary arrest
Uncal	Unilateral lesion forces uncus of temporal lobe to displace through the tentorial notch, compressing the midbrain Symptoms can progress rapidly	**Early** Decreased LOC Increased muscle tone Positive Babinski reflex Cheyne-Stokes respiration, progressing to central neurogenic hyperventilation Ipsilateral dilated pupil Weakness **Late** Pupils dilated and fixed Paralyzed eye movements Contralateral hemiplegia Decerebrate posturing Unstable vital signs progressing to cardiopulmonary arrest
Cerebellar tonsil	Displacement of cerebellar tonsils through foramen magnum, compressing the pons and medulla	Alterations in respiratory and cardiopulmonary function, rapidly progressing to cardiopulmonary arrest

LOC, Level of consciousness.

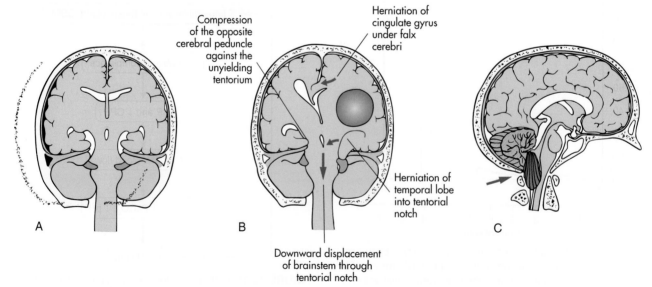

FIGURE 13-11 Herniation syndromes. **A,** Normal relationship of intracranial structures. **B,** Shift of intracranial structures *(red arrows)*. **C,** Downward herniation of the cerebellar tonsils into the foramen magnum *(red arrow)*. (From McCance KL, Huether SE. *Pathophysiology: The Biological Basis for Disease in Adults and Children.* 6th ed. St. Louis: Mosby; 2010.)

This allows sodium, chloride, and water to enter the cell while potassium exits. Cytotoxic edema is associated with brain ischemia or hypoxic events such as stroke or cardiac arrest. It is also seen with hypo-osmolar conditions including water intoxication and hyponatremia. *Vasogenic cerebral edema* occurs as a result of increased capillary permeability. With increased permeability, osmotically active substances (proteins) leak into the brain interstitium and draw water from the vascular system, leading to an increase in fluid in the extracellular space and consequently an increase in ICP. Brain injuries, brain tumors, meningitis, and abscesses are common causes of vasogenic cerebral edema.

Increased Cerebral Blood Volume

Several mechanisms increase cerebral blood volume. These include loss of autoregulation, physiological responses to decreased cerebral oxygenation, increased metabolic demand, and obstruction of venous outflow.

Within normal limits, the cerebral vasculature exhibits pressure and chemical autoregulation. Autoregulation provides a constant blood volume and CPP over a wide range of MAPs. Pathological states such as head injury or hypertension often lead to a loss of autoregulation. Without autoregulation, hyperemia may occur, leading to increased ICP.[9]

Decreased cerebral oxygenation leads to cerebral vasodilation in an attempt to improve oxygen delivery. Hypercapnia also causes vasodilation in the brain. Any factor that results in hypoxemia or hypercapnia, such as ineffective ventilation, airway obstruction, or endotracheal suctioning, can contribute to increased ICP.

CBF may increase to augment oxygen supply in response to increased metabolic demands. Several factors increase oxygen demands including fever, physical activity, pain, stimulation, and seizures.[9] Grouping nursing activities together (e.g., bathing, suctioning, turning), may also increase metabolic demands. Although sleep and rest are important, oxygen demands are higher during rapid eye movement (REM) sleep. Increases in ICP may be noted during any of these situations.

Obstruction of venous outflow results in increased cerebral blood volume and increases ICP. Hyperflexion, hyperextension, or rotation of the neck or tightly applied tracheostomy or endotracheal ties compress the jugular vein, inhibit venous return, and cause central venous engorgement. A tumor or abscess can compress the venous structures, causing an outflow obstruction. Mechanisms that increase intrathoracic or intraabdominal pressure also impair venous return (e.g., coughing, vomiting, posturing, isometric exercise, Valsalva maneuver, positive end-expiratory pressure, hip flexion).

Increased Cerebrospinal Fluid

Hydrocephalus, an increase in CSF, can increase ICP. Hydrocephalus may occur in any circumstance where CSF flow or absorption is blocked, such as subarachnoid hemorrhage or infection (meningitis, encephalitis), or when excess CSF is produced.

Assessment

A thorough neurological examination is performed with an emphasis placed on LOC and motor and cranial nerve function. Vital signs are part of the routine assessment. Hypertension is common early with increased ICP and represents a compensatory mechanism to augment CPP. Cushing triad is a late sign of increased ICP and consists of systolic hypertension with a widening pulse pressure, bradycardia, and irregular respirations. It often signifies irreversible damage.

Monitoring Techniques

Invasive monitoring of ICP, cerebral oxygenation, and other physiological parameters may be used to augment the clinical assessment.

Intracranial pressure monitoring. ICP monitoring is used to correlate objective data with the clinical picture and to determine cerebral perfusion. Monitoring is indicated for patients who have a GCS score between 3 and 8 due to a severe brain insult. It is used to assess response to therapy, such as after administering mannitol,[3] or to augment neurological assessment.

ICP monitoring systems are classified by location of device or type of transducer system. Devices can be placed in one of the ventricles, in the parenchyma, or in the subarachnoid, epidural, or subdural spaces (Figure 13-12). Each site has advantages and disadvantages (Table 13-8). Ventricular devices are most commonly used for monitoring because they also allow therapeutic interventions. A ventricular catheter system, also known as a ventriculostomy, may be connected to a drainage bag to drain CSF in a controlled manner to relieve increased ICP, or to remove blood products after subarachnoid hemorrhage. The ventricular catheter system allows continuous monitoring only, continuous CSF drainage only, or both monitoring and CSF drainage, depending on patient need.

The transducer system may be a microchip sensor device, fiberoptic catheter, or fluid-filled system.[3] The fluid-filled system is most often used for ICP monitoring. This system is similar to that used for hemodynamic monitoring with a few exceptions. The pressure tubing is flushed with sterile normal saline *without* preservatives because preservatives may damage brain tissue, and no pressurized fluid or flush system is used. The device is zero referenced, and the air-fluid interface is leveled with the foramen of Munro. The ICP waveform is observed on a channel on the bedside monitor. The mean ICP pressure is recorded.

Catheters with internal microchip sensors and fiberoptic catheters have the transducer built into the tip of the catheter. These devices only need to be zero referenced before insertion. They are connected via a cable to a stand-alone monitor provided by the manufacturer. Some monitors can be connected to the bedside monitor for an additional display of ICP and waveforms.[3]

ICP monitoring systems allow nurses to observe an ICP waveform pattern. The normal intracranial pulse waveform has three defined peaks of decreasing height that correlate with the arterial pulse waveform and are identified as P_1, P_2,

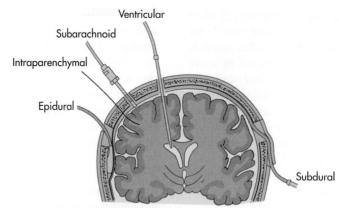

FIGURE 13-12 Intracranial pressure monitoring sites. (From Lewis SL, Dirksen SR, Heitkemper MM, et al. *Medical Surgical Nursing: Assessment and Management of Clinical Problems.* 8th ed. St. Louis: Mosby; 2011.)

and P_3 (Figure 13-13). P_1 (percussion wave) is fairly consistent in shape and amplitude; it represents the blood being ejected from the heart and correlates with cardiac systole. Extreme hypotension or hypertension produces changes in P_1. P_2 (tidal wave) represents intracranial brain bulk. It is variable in shape and is related to the state of compliance.

Decreased compliance exists when P_2 is equal to or higher than P_1. It also is helpful in predicting the risk for increases in ICP. P_3 (dicrotic wave) follows the dicrotic notch and represents closure of the aortic valve, correlating with cardiac diastole. Smaller peaks that follow the three main peaks vary among individual patients.[13]

TABLE 13-8   INTRACRANIAL PRESSURE MONITORING DEVICES

DEVICE	LOCATION	ADVANTAGES	DISADVANTAGES
Intraventricular catheter (ventriculostomy) or fiberoptic transducer	Lateral ventricle of non-dominant hemisphere; may be tunneled or bolted	Therapeutic or diagnostic removal of CSF to control ↑ ICP Good ICP waveform quality Accurate and reliable	Highest risk for infection; infection rate, 2%-5% Risk for hemorrhage Longer insertion time Rapid CSF drainage may result in collapsed ventricle CSF leakage around insertion site
Subarachnoid bolt or screw	Subarachnoid space	Inserted quickly Does not penetrate brain	Bolt can become occluded with clots or tissue, causing a dampened waveform CSF leakage may occur CSF drainage not possible
Epidural sensor or transducer	Between the skull and the dura	Least invasive Low risk of infection Low risk of hemorrhage Recommended in patients at risk for meningitis or other CNS infections	Indirect measure of ICP Less accurate and reliable CSF drainage not possible
Parenchymal fiberoptic catheter	1 cm into brain tissue	Inserted quickly Accurate and reliable Good ICP waveform quality	CSF drainage not possible Catheter relatively fragile Expensive

CNS, Central nervous system; *CSF,* cerebrospinal fluid; *ICP,* intracranial pressure.
Based on data from Bader MK, & Littlejohns L. (2010). *AANN Core Curriculum for Neuroscience Nursing* (5th edition). Glenview, IL: AANN; and American Association of Neuroscience Nurses. (2011). *Care of the Patient Undergoing Intracranial Pressure Monitoring/External Ventricular Drainage or Lumbar Drainage.* Glenview, IL: Author.

EVIDENCE-BASED PRACTICE

Positioning for Neurodynamic Stability

Problem

Increased intracranial pressure, decreased cerebral perfusion pressure, and decreased brain tissue oxygenation have been associated with poor outcomes following traumatic brain injury. Commonly used nursing interventions, such as head elevation and repositioning, may adversely affect these neurodynamic parameters.

Clinical Question

Is there an optimum position for patients with traumatic brain injury that promotes neurodynamic stability?

Evidence

Several groups of researchers have investigated the effect of body position on neurodynamics. Head elevation and repositioning are interventions nurses use to maximize systemic and cerebral oxygenation and protect skin while preventing other complications. Yet, head elevation to 30 degrees and 45 degrees and lateral positioning produced variable neurodynamic responses in severely brain-injured adults. Multiple neurodynamic measures were used to clarify understanding of these responses. Head elevation to at least 30 degrees significantly decreased ICP but also decreased CPP because of a decrease in mean arterial pressure. Lateral positioning, particularly to the left, with 15-degree head elevation was associated with an increase in ICP, a decrease in cerebral perfusion pressure, and a decrease in cerebral oxygenation, but not in all patients. Prone positioning has been reported to increase systemic oxygenation but is also associated with increased ICP and decreased CPP in some patients. Measurement of cerebral oxygenation provided additional data on neurodynamic response to routine nursing measures. Collectively, study findings suggest that responses to head elevation and repositioning are highly individualized and depend, in part, on cerebral autoregulatory integrity.

Implications for Nursing

No one position or degree of head elevation is optimal for patients with traumatic brain injury. Patient response to head elevation and position change must be carefully monitored, and when adverse changes are noted, alternative positions should be considered. The left lateral position, with or without head elevation, warrants the greatest attention. No single measure of neurodynamics is beneficial in monitoring response, so multimodality monitoring of response to head elevation and repositioning should be employed.

Level of Evidence

B—Well-designed controlled studies

References

Ledwith MB, Bloom S, Maloney-Wilensky E, Coyle B, Polomano, RC, & D. Effect of body position on cerebral oxygenation and physiologic parameters in patients with acute neurological conditions. *Journal of Neuroscience Nursing.* 2010;42(5), 280-287.

Nekludov M, Bellander BM, & Mire M. Oxygenation and cerebral perfusion pressure improved in the prone position. *Acta Anaesthesiologica Scandinavica.* 2006;50(8), 932-936.

Ng I, Lim J, & Wong HB. Effects of head posture on cerebral hemodynamics: Its influences on intracranial pressure, cerebral perfusion pressure, and cerebral oxygenation. *Neurosurgery.* 2004;54(3), 593-597.

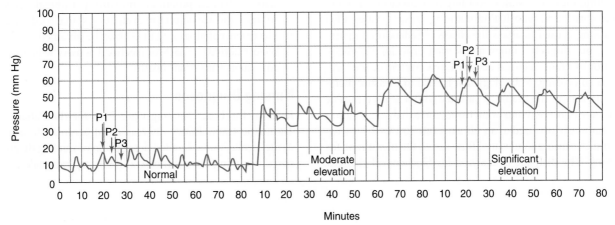

FIGURE 13-13 Intracranial pressure monitoring can be used to continuously measure ICP. The ICP tracing shows normal, elevated, and plateau waves. At high ICP the P$_2$ peak is higher than the P$_1$ peak, and the peaks become less distinct and plateau. (Modified from Lewis SL, Dirksen SR, Heitkemper MM, et al. *Medical Surgical Nursing: Assessment and Management of Clinical Problems.* 8th ed. St. Louis: Mosby; 2011.)

Cerebral oxygenation monitoring. Cerebral blood flow and brain oxygen utilization may be monitored by *jugular oxygen saturation* (S_jO_2). The technology is similar to mixed venous oxygen saturation (SvO_2) measured in the pulmonary artery. S_jO_2 is monitored via a fiberoptic catheter inserted retrogradely through the internal jugular vein into the jugular venous bulb. Placement of the catheter is verified by a neck x-ray. Oxygen saturation of venous blood is measured as it leaves the brain and provides a global measure of cerebral oxygenation. The normal value is 60% to 70%. Values less than 50% suggest cerebral ischemia. However, because the jugular vein drains only a portion of the brain, normal values do not ensure adequate perfusion to all brain areas.[7]

The *partial pressure of oxygen within brain tissue* ($PbtO_2$) can be measured by placing a monitoring probe directly into the brain white matter and attaching it to a stand-alone monitor. The probe may be inserted into the damaged portion of the brain to measure regional oxygenation, or inserted into an undamaged portion of the brain to measure global oxygenation. In a patient with traumatic brain injury, the goal of therapy is to maintain an adequate $PbtO_2$. Current studies recommend a $PbtO_2$ greater than 20 mm Hg. However, the science of brain tissue oxygenation is evolving, and target values may change. Values may also be device specific; therefore it is important to review the manufacturer's literature. Management of low $PbtO_2$ is directed at treating the underlying cause.[3,7,13,15]

Other physiological monitoring. Hemodynamic monitoring may be used to monitor fluid status and assist in maintaining adequate cerebral perfusion (see Chapter 8). Continuous monitoring of oxygen saturation via pulse oximetry (SpO_2), and of end-tidal carbon dioxide levels is useful to ensure adequate gas exchange in the neurological patient. Periodic arterial blood gas samples may also be obtained.

Continuous bedside electroencephalographic (EEG) monitoring provides a recording of electrical activity in the brain. The continuous EEG allows recording of brain electrical activity and correlation with ICP monitoring. In some cases, EEG monitoring is used to assess the effects of sedation and paralytic agents. Bispectral index monitoring provides a numeric indicator of brain electrical activity (see Chapter 5). Microdialysis is an evolving technology that is used to measure metabolic markers in the brain.[7] A catheter with a semipermeable membrane is inserted into brain tissue, and a dialysate solution is continuously perfused at an ultralow rate (0.1 to 0.5 microliters/min), causing solutes to diffuse across the membrane for sampling. The dialysate is analyzed for biochemical changes.

Data obtained from microdialysis can be used to adjust therapies and predict outcomes.

Diagnostic Testing

The initial baseline and ongoing *laboratory tests* obtained in a patient with increased ICP include:
- Arterial blood gases, SpO_2, end-tidal carbon dioxide
- Complete blood count, with an emphasis on hematocrit, hemoglobin, and platelets
- Coagulation profile including prothrombin time, international normalized ratio, and activated partial thromboplastin time, because brain injury may induce a coagulopathy
- Electrolytes, blood urea nitrogen, creatinine, liver function, and serum osmolality

Radiological studies and other diagnostic tests that may be performed on a patient with increased ICP include:
- Computed tomography (CT) scan (usually noncontrast) to assess the potential for a worsening intracranial mass effect
- Magnetic resonance imaging (MRI) to provide anatomical detail of pathology contributing to increased ICP
- Cerebral blood flow monitoring, in which a transcutaneous Doppler device (a noninvasive technology) measures the velocity of arterial flow and allows for the indirect monitoring of CBF at the bedside. Transcutaneous Doppler measurements are correlated with ICP values to assess patient response to treatment and nursing interventions. Monitoring is particularly useful to detect vasospasm in patients with a cerebral aneurysm. Vasospasm is noted by an increase in velocity.
- Evoked potential monitoring, which is a noninvasive procedure of applying sensory stimuli and recording the electrical potentials created. Each potential is recorded and stored in a computer, and an average curve is calculated. Brainstem auditory evoked potentials evaluate brainstem function and can be conducted on a conscious or unconscious patient, or even during surgery. Somatosensory evoked potentials measure peripheral nerve responses and are helpful in evaluating spinal cord function.
- Electroencephalogram (EEG) may be obtained to identify seizure activity or lack of electrical activity which may be consistent with brain death.

Nursing Diagnoses

Refer to the box, "Nursing Care Plan for the Patient with Traumatic Brain Injury, Increased Intracranial Pressure, or Acute Stroke," for a detailed description of nursing diagnoses, specific nursing interventions, and selected rationales.

◎ NURSING CARE PLAN

for the Patient with Traumatic Brain Injury, Increased Intracranial Pressure, or Acute Stroke

NURSING DIAGNOSIS

Decreased Intracranial Adaptive Capacity related to trauma/neurological illness

PATIENT OUTCOMES

Optimal cerebral perfusion

- GCS score >13, NIHSS score <4
- ICP <20 mm Hg, CPP >70 mm Hg
- Absence of new neurological deficit
- Vital signs within normal limits

NURSING INTERVENTIONS	RATIONALES
• Assess neurological status hourly	• Detect early changes indicative of increased ICP; change in pupil size or reaction, decrease in motor function, and CN impairment indicate worsening condition
• Monitor ICP and CPP; notify physician if ICP >20 mm Hg or CPP <70 mm Hg	• Ensure adequate cerebral perfusion
• Maintain airway; monitor SpO_2 and $EtCO_2$, or ABGs, for evidence of hypoxemia/hypercapnia; hyperoxygenate the patient before and after suctioning	• Ensure adequate cerebral perfusion; prevent cerebral vasodilation
• Monitor VS; be alert to changes in respiratory pattern, fluctuations in BP, bradycardia, widening pulse pressure	• Detect responses to increased ICP; however, these signs occur very late
• Maintain patient's head in a neutral position; maintain head-of-bed elevation that keeps ICP and CPP within normal ranges	• Facilitate cerebral venous drainage and prevent increased ICP
• Monitor fluid volume status; ensure precise delivery of IV fluids; administer osmotic diuretics as ordered	• Prevent fluid volume excess or deficit, both of which can affect ICP
• Evaluate patient's response to nursing interventions; space activities to avoid increases in ICP	• Prevent sustained elevations in ICP; ICP should return to normal values within 5 minutes of completion of activities
• Prevent increases in intrathoracic and intraabdominal pressure through proper positioning, avoiding coughing and Valsalva maneuver	• Facilitate cerebral venous drainage and prevent increased ICP
• If hyperthermic, administer treatments to reduce temperature to normal (or mild hypothermia) values	• Reduce cerebral metabolic demands
• Assess the need for medications (sedatives, analgesics, neuromuscular blockade, anticonvulsants); induce hypothermia as ordered	• Decrease cerebral metabolic demands and control ICP

NURSING DIAGNOSIS

Ineffective cerebral tissue perfusion related to increased ICP and decreased cerebral blood flow

PATIENT OUTCOME

Improved cerebral tissue perfusion

- VS WNL
- Adequate hemodynamic values
- Improved LOC, motor function

NURSING INTERVENTIONS	RATIONALES
• Assess neurological status hourly using GCS or NIHSS; monitor VS	• Assess for alterations in ICP
• Perform interventions to prevent and treat increased ICP	• Ensure adequate cerebral tissue perfusion
• Maintain blood pressure within desired range with prescribed medications; maintain IV fluid therapy	• Decreases in BP and hypovolemia may decrease cerebral perfusion pressure
• Monitor hemodynamic values to achieve and maintain prescribed parameters	• Provide objective assessment of fluid volume needs
• Administer calcium channel blockers (nimodipine), if ordered	• Reduce cerebral vasospasm

Continued

◎ NURSING CARE PLAN

for the Patient with Traumatic Brain Injury, Increased Intracranial Pressure, or Acute Stroke—cont'd

NURSING DIAGNOSIS

Impaired Gas Exchange related to decreased oxygen supply and increased carbon dioxide production secondary to decreased ventilatory drive

PATIENT OUTCOME

Optimal gas exchange
- $PaCO_2$ 35-40 mm Hg
- PaO_2 >80 mm Hg
- RR 12-20 breaths/min with normal depth/pattern
- Adventitious breath sounds absent
- LOC improved

NURSING INTERVENTIONS	RATIONALES
• Assess patient's RR, depth, and rhythm	• Assess adequacy of respiration; detect abnormal patterns
• Auscultate breath sounds every 1-4 hours	• Detect adventitious lung sounds
• Assess for signs of hypoxemia (confusion, agitation, restlessness, irritability)	• Identify need for oxygenation to prevent cerebral hypoxia
• Ensure a patent airway and assess the need for suctioning; hyperoxygenate the patient before and after suctioning	• Prevent cerebral hypoxia
• Monitor ABGs, SpO_2, and $EtCO_2$	• Assess adequate oxygenation and ventilation
• Turn every 2 hours, within the limits of patient's status	• Promote lung drainage and alveolar expansion

NURSING DIAGNOSIS

Risk for Imbalanced Fluid Volume related to fluids/medications administered; gastrointestinal suction; and development of complications (diabetes insipidus; SIADH; cerebral salt wasting)

PATIENT OUTCOME

Optimal fluid balance
- Adequate VS, hemodynamic values, and I&O
- Appropriate weight
- Moist mucous membranes

NURSING INTERVENTIONS	RATIONALES
• Weigh daily	• Monitor fluid volume status (all interventions)
• Monitor I&O hourly	
• Monitor laboratory results (electrolytes, serum and urine osmolality)	
• Assess skin and mucous membranes	
• Monitor VS and hemodynamic values	

NURSING DIAGNOSIS

Imbalanced Nutrition: Less than Body Requirements related to hypermetabolic state

PATIENT OUTCOME

Optimal nutrition
- Weight within normal range for patient
- Serum proteins and albumin within normal range
- Positive nitrogen balance

NURSING INTERVENTIONS	RATIONALES
• Implement early nutritional support	• Improve patient outcomes; reduce infection; promote healing
• Auscultate bowel sounds and monitor for abdominal distention	• Monitor bowel function; assess tolerance to nutritional support
• Weigh daily	• Monitor fluid volume and nutritional status
• Assess gastric tube feeding residual as ordered	• Prevent aspiration; neurological patients at increased risk

◎ NURSING CARE PLAN

for the Patient with Traumatic Brain Injury, Increased Intracranial Pressure, or Acute Stroke—cont'd

NURSING DIAGNOSES

Risk for Infection related to invasive techniques and devices; compromised immune system; and bacterial invasion caused by traumatic brain injury, pneumonia, or iatrogenic causes

PATIENT OUTCOME

Free of infection
- Normal WBCs
- Negative culture results
- VS WNL
- Absence of purulent drainage and other clinical indicators of infection
- Normothermia

NURSING INTERVENTIONS	RATIONALES
• Employ proper hand-washing technique before and after patient contact	• Hand washing is best strategy to prevent infection
• Use aseptic technique when performing invasive procedures and caring for catheters, tubes, and lines	• Prevent infection
• Assess VS, drainage, and skin for signs and symptoms of infection	• Detect signs of infection for early intervention
• Inspect cranial wounds for presence of erythema, tenderness, swelling, and drainage	• Detect signs of infection for early intervention
• Maintain a closed system for hemodynamic/ICP monitoring devices	• Prevent bacteria from entering systems and devices
• Monitor the results of CBC and cultures	• Assess for infection; guide treatment
• Assess and maintain adequate nutritional status	• Reduce risk for infection
• Administer antibiotics as ordered	• Treat infection

NURSING DIAGNOSIS

Disturbed thought processes related to impaired cerebral functioning

PATIENT OUTCOME

Optimal thought processes
- Improved attention, memory, and judgment
- Appropriate response with an improved level of orientation

NURSING INTERVENTIONS	RATIONALES
• Reorient frequently; place a clock or calendar within patient's view	• Provide reorientation to place and time
• Explain activities clearly and simply in a calm manner; allow adequate time for response	• Provide information; prevent anxiety
• Instruct the family in methods to deal with patient's altered thought processes	• Provide ongoing reorientation by all who interact with patient
• Maintain a consistent and fairly structured routine	• Facilitate reorientation
• Allow for frequent rest periods for the patient	• Promote energy conservation and recovery

NURSING DIAGNOSIS

Interrupted Family Processes related to situational crisis (patient's illness)

PATIENT OUTCOME

Family demonstrates effective adaptation to the situation
- Seek support
- Share concerns

NURSING INTERVENTIONS	RATIONALES
• Assess family structure; assess social, environmental, ethnic, and cultural relationships; role; and communication patterns	• Establish family structure as a baseline for determining interventions

Continued

NURSING CARE PLAN

for the Patient with Traumatic Brain Injury, Increased Intracranial Pressure, or Acute Stroke—cont'd

NURSING INTERVENTIONS	RATIONALES
• Establish open, honest communication and provide information	• Facilitate communication; meet family needs
• Assess knowledge regarding the patient's status and therapies; allow sufficient time for questions	• Identify knowledge deficits
• Acknowledge the family/significant other's involvement in patient care	• Promote family involvement; reduce family stress
• Provide opportunities to talk and share concerns in a private setting. Offer support and realistic hope	• Assist the family to develop realistic expectations
• Assess for ineffective coping (depression, substance abuse, withdrawal)	• Identify need for intervention and/or referral
• Encourage the family/significant other to schedule periods of rest or activity	• Provide support for family

ABG, Arterial blood gas; *BP,* blood pressure; *CBC,* complete blood count; *CN,* cranial nerve; *CPP,* cerebral perfusion pressure; *EtCO$_2$,* end-tidal carbon dioxide concentration; *GCS,* Glasgow Coma Scale; *ICP,* intracranial pressure; *I&O,* intake & output; *IV,* intravenous; *LOC,* level of consciousness; *NIHSS,* National Institutes of Health Stroke Scale; *PaCO$_2$,* partial pressure of arterial carbon dioxide; *PaO$_2$,* partial pressure of arterial oxygen; *RR,* respiratory rate; *SIADH,* syndrome of inappropriate antidiuretic hormone secretion; *SpO$_2$,* oxygen saturation via pulse oximetry; *VS,* vital signs; *WBC,* white blood cell count; *WNL,* within normal limits.
Based on data from Gulanick M, and Myers JL. (2011). *Nursing Care Plans: Diagnoses, Interventions, and Outcomes* (7th ed.). St. Louis: Mosby.

Management
Medical and Nursing Interventions (Nonsurgical)
The goal of management is to maintain an ICP of less than 20 mm Hg while maintaining the CPP above 70 mm Hg. The first task is to prevent an increase in ICP. If the ICP is elevated, therapy is instituted to decrease ICP and then identify the cause of increased ICP. Once the cause is discovered, management is centered on permanently decreasing the high ICP, maintaining CPP, maintaining the airway, providing ventilation and oxygenation, and decreasing the metabolic demands placed on the injured brain.

Nursing actions to manage intracranial pressure. The patient is positioned to minimize ICP and maximize CPP. Elevating the head of the bed to 30 degrees and keeping the head in a neutral midline position facilitates venous drainage and decreases the risk of venous obstruction. However, care must be taken to evaluate blood pressure response to head elevation.[19] Raising the head of the bed may decrease MAP, thereby decreasing CPP. Hemodynamically unstable patients may need to be cared for in a flat position. Patients with increased ICP can be turned from side to side. However, during any position change or change in elevation of the head of bed, it is imperative to monitor and document the patient's individualized cerebral and hemodynamic response. If the CPP does not return to the baseline value within 5 minutes after the position change, the patient must return to the position that maximized CPP.[19]

Because endotracheal suctioning is associated with hypoxemia, the patient should be suctioned only when necessary. The patient is preoxygenated with 100% oxygen before and between suction attempts, and for 1 minute after the procedure. Each suction attempt is limited to less than 10 seconds, with no more than two suction passes. The head is maintained in a neutral position during the suctioning procedure.

Several nursing activities are associated with increases in ICP. These include turning, repositioning, and hygiene measures. Elevated ICP resulting from nursing care is usually temporary, and the ICP should return to the resting baseline value within a few minutes. Sustained increases in ICP lasting longer than 5 minutes should be prevented. Spacing nursing care activities allows for rest between activities. If ICP pressure monitoring is available, the nurse directly monitors the ICP in response to care and other interventions.

Although many nurses believe that visitors should be limited for the patient with neurological pathology, family presence has been shown to decrease ICP. However, family members need to be cautioned to avoid excess stimulation of the patient or unpleasant conversations that may emotionally stimulate the patient (e.g., discussing prognosis, condition, deficits, restraints), because this can cause an elevation in ICP.[3] Assessing the patient's physiological response to visitors is an important nursing function.

Medical management. Medical management of increased ICP includes the following: adequate oxygenation and ventilation; cautious, limited use of hyperventilation; osmotic and loop diuretics; euvolemic fluid administration; maintenance of BP; and reduction of metabolic demands. Corticosteroids are useful for reducing cerebral edema associated with brain tumors and meningitis, but recent studies do not support administration of corticosteroids to reduce ICP associated with other intracranial conditions.[2,12]

Adequate oxygenation. The goal is to maintain a PaO$_2$ above 80 mm Hg and to ensure that oxygen delivery to the brain exceeds oxygen consumption. A PaO$_2$ below 50 mm Hg can precipitate increased ICP. For many patients with increased ICP, short-term management of the airway is accomplished by an endotracheal tube and mechanical ventilation. Positive end-expiratory pressure may be added to facilitate oxygenation; however, it must be used with extreme caution since it may prevent venous outflow and further increase ICP.[27] A tracheostomy tube may be required for long-term ventilatory management.[27] In addition, adequate hematocrit and hemoglobin levels are maintained to promote oxygenation.

Management of carbon dioxide. Hyperventilation decreases $PaCO_2$, which causes vasoconstriction of the cerebral arteries and a reduction of CBF. In the past, hyperventilation was commonly used to manage ICP. However, hyperventilation may cause neurological damage by decreasing cerebral perfusion. Hyperventilation is used to decrease ICP for short periods when acute neurological deterioration is occurring (i.e., herniation) and other methods to reduce ICP have failed. If the $PaCO_2$ level is purposefully lowered to less than 35 mm Hg for an extended period, oxygen delivery at the cellular level should be evaluated using a jugular bulb or cerebral tissue oxygen monitor.[7,12] It is recommended that the $PaCO_2$ be kept within a normal range, 35 to 45 mm Hg. Hyperventilation should also be avoided when providing manual ventilation via a bag-valve device.

Diuretics. Osmotic and loop diuretics are administered to reduce cerebral brain volume by removing fluid from the brain's extracellular compartment. *Osmotic diuretics,* such as mannitol or hypertonic saline (in solutions ranging from 1.5% to 24% normal saline)[18] draw water from the extracellular space to the plasma by creating an osmotic gradient, thereby decreasing ICP. The effects of decreasing ICP and increasing CPP occur within minutes of infusion. Side effects of osmotic diuretics include hypotension, electrolyte disturbances, and rebound increased ICP. If mannitol is used, the patient must have adequate intravascular volume to prevent hypotension and secondary brain injury. Mannitol is contraindicated in patients with acute kidney injury because it is not metabolized and is excreted unchanged in the urine. *Loop diuretics* (furosemide, torsemide, bumetanide, ethacrynic acid) decrease ICP by removing sodium and water from injured brain cells. These agents also decrease CSF formation (see Table 13-9).

Optimal fluid administration. Fluid administration is provided to optimize MAP, maintain intravascular volume, and normalize CPP. Normal saline solution (0.9%), an isotonic solution, is recommended for volume resuscitation. Hypotonic solutions are avoided to prevent an increase in cerebral edema. Strict measurement of intake and output while monitoring serum sodium, potassium, and osmolarity is required. The goal is to keep serum osmolality less than 320 mOsm/L.[12] If needed, colloids or blood products are administered to restore volume and maintain adequate hematocrit and hemoglobin levels. Hemodynamic monitoring may be used to optimize fluid administration.

Blood pressure management. BP must be carefully controlled in a patient with increased ICP. Usually the MAP is kept between 70 and 90 mm Hg. However, it is critical to monitor the ICP and MAP collectively to sustain an adequate CPP of at least 70 mm Hg.[3,12] Hypotension decreases CBF, which leads to cerebral ischemia. When hypotension occurs, or ICP cannot be reduced, manipulating the systolic BP with vasopressor drugs and fluids may be needed to achieve an adequate CPP.

Hypertension (>160 mm Hg systolic) can worsen cerebral edema by increasing microvascular pressure. However, hypertension may be necessary for adequate cerebral perfusion. If necessary, systolic BP is lowered with antihypertensive drugs such as labetalol. This beta-blocker decreases the sympathetic response and catecholamine release associated with neurological injury. Some antihypertensive agents (nitroprusside, nitroglycerin) and some calcium channel blockers (verapamil, nifedipine) cause cerebral vasodilation. This vasodilation increases CBF and causes increased ICP. Administration of these agents is avoided in patients with poor intracranial compliance. Nicardipine is a calcium channel blocker that does not affect cerebral vasculature and is very effective in providing faster and tighter control of BP than other antihypertensive agents.

Reducing metabolic demands. Several therapies may be required to reduce metabolic demands. These include temperature control, sedation, seizure prophylaxis, neuromuscular blockade, and barbiturate therapy.

Temperature control. Lowering body temperature to normal from a hyperthermic state or inducing hypothermia decreases cerebral metabolism, blood flow and volume, thereby decreasing ICP. Body temperature may be controlled noninvasively by using a cooling blanket or skin pads placed in direct contact with the skin (external cooling), or invasively using a catheter placed in a large vein (intravascular cooling). Target temperatures for induced hypothermia range from 34° C to 35° C and these temperatures are maintained for 24 to 72 hours. Induced hypothermia has many potential adverse effects, including coagulopathies and fluid and electrolyte disturbances (see Chapter 10).

Sedation. Patients are often sedated to lower increased ICP related to agitation, restlessness, or resistance to mechanical ventilation. Benzodiazepines are given for sedation and do not affect CBF or ICP. Propofol is a sedative-hypnotic agent that reduces cerebral metabolism and ICP. It is a short-acting drug with a rapid onset that is given by continuous infusion. Morphine or fentanyl can be administered for analgesia and sedation in a low-dose continuous infusion or in small frequent intravenous (IV) boluses. Refer to Chapter 5 for further information on comfort and sedation.

Seizure prophylaxis. Patients with brain disorders or injury are prone to seizures. Seizure activity is associated with high metabolic demands. Seizure prophylaxis is often initiated only in high-risk situations, because adverse effects can occur from prophylactic agents.

Neuromuscular blockade and barbiturate therapy. Neuromuscular blockade is considered for patients unresponsive to other treatments. Barbiturates are given selectively to reduce ICP refractory to other treatments. Pentobarbital is the most common agent used. Patients receiving neuromuscular blockade or barbiturate therapy require hemodynamic monitoring, mechanical ventilation, and intensive nursing management. Table 13-9 identifies drugs commonly used for patients with increased ICP.

TABLE 13-9	**PHARMACOLOGY**			

Frequently Used Medications in Nervous System Alterations

MEDICATION	ACTIONS/USE	DOSE/ROUTE	SIDE EFFECTS	NURSING IMPLICATIONS
Mannitol	Osmotic diuretic; pulls water from brain interstitium into plasma; used to treat ↑ ICP	0.5 to 1 g/kg IV over 5-10 minutes, then 0.25-2 g/kg IVP every 4-12 hours as needed depending on ICP, CPP, serum osmolality	Hypotension, dehydration, electrolyte disturbances, tachycardia Rebound edema	Neurological assessment every hour; monitor ICP, CPP, serum osmolality, electrolytes, ABGs, VS, I&O; check vial prior to use for crystals and shake or warm as needed; use an in-line filter to administer
Furosemide (Lasix)	Reduces cerebral edema by drawing sodium and water out of brain interstitium; used to treat cerebral edema	*Post cardiac arrest cerebral edema:* 40 mg IV over 1-2 minutes; if no response in 1 hour, increase to 80 mg or 0.5-1 mg/kg IV over 1-2 minutes; if no response, increase dose to 2 mg/kg	Ototoxicity, polyuria, electrolyte disturbances, gastric irritation, muscle cramps, hypotension, dehydration, embolism, vascular thrombosis	Monitor I&O, daily weights, electrolytes, ABGs, VS
Dexamethasone (Decadron)	Steroid that has a stabilizing effect on cell membrane; prevents destructive effect of oxygen free radicals; ↓ inflammation by suppressing white blood cells	*Cerebral edema:* 10-20 mg IV loading dose over 1 minute; 4-10 mg every 6 hours; reduce dose after 2-4 days; discontinue gradually over 5-7 days	Flushing, sweating, hypertension, tachycardia, thrombocytopenia, weakness, nausea, diarrhea, GI irritation/hemorrhage, fluid retention, poor wound healing, weight gain, hyperglycemia, muscle wasting, hypokalemia	↑ or ↓ effects of anticoagulants; ↓ effects of anticonvulsants; adjust dose of antidiabetic agents; ↑ effects of digitalis; monitor glucose, potassium, daily weights, VS; masks signs of infection; taper drug before discontinuing
Methylprednisolone (Solu-Medrol)	An adjunct to SCI management; improves blood flow to injury site facilitating tissue repair	30 mg/kg IV over 15 minutes; after 45 minutes, begin maintenance dose infusion of 5.4 mg/kg/hr for 23 hours	Same as dexamethasone	Same as dexamethasone
Labetalol (Normodyne; Trandate)	Nonselective beta-blocker to decrease BP	10-20 mg IVP over 2 minutes; may repeat with 40-80 mg IVP at 10 minute intervals until desired BP is achieved; do not exceed total dose of 300 mg After bolus, may give as continuous infusion at 2-8 mg/min	Hypotension; bradycardia; HF; bronchospasm; ventricular dysrhythmias; diaphoresis; flushing; somnolence; weakness/fatigue	Monitor BP, HR; I&O, daily weight; may ↓ glucose; may cause further hypotension with nitroglycerin; may potentiate with calcium channel blockers; adjust dosage of oral hypoglycemic medications
Enalapril (Vasotec)	ACE inhibitor to decrease BP; used to treat hypertension	0.625-1.25 mg IV every 6 hours over 5 min	Headache, hypotension, dysrhythmias, proteinuria, acute kidney injury, neutropenia, angioedema	Contraindicated in pregnancy; monitor BP frequently; assess labs: WBCs, electrolytes, renal and liver status; assess ECG rhythm, monitor for edema

TABLE 13-9   PHARMACOLOGY

Frequently Used Medications in Nervous System Alterations—cont'd

MEDICATION	ACTIONS/USE	DOSE/ROUTE	SIDE EFFECTS	NURSING IMPLICATIONS
Nicardipine (Cardene)	Calcium channel blocker, vasodilatory effect that lowers BP	*Severe hypertension:* 5 mg/hr continuous infusion, increase dose by 2.5 mg/hr every 15 minutes until desired BP is reached; not to exceed 15 mg/hr; when desired BP is reached, wean to 3 mg/hr; wean to off when continuous IV infusion is no longer required	Headache, confusion, hypotension, nausea and vomiting, and tachycardia; ECG changes (e.g., atrioventricular block, ST-segment depression, inverted T wave); may develop hypersensitivity reaction	Monitor BP continuously; lower doses and slower titration required for persons with heart failure or impaired hepatic or renal function
Phenytoin (Dilantin)	Depresses seizure activity by altering ion transport in motor cortex	*Status epilepticus:* 10-20 mg/kg IV in 0.9% NS only; administer over 20-30 minutes; do not exceed a total dose of 1.5 g; if seizure not terminated, consider other antiepileptic drugs, barbiturates, or anesthesia. Follow with maintenance dose of 100 mg IV over 2 minutes every 6 to 8 hours	Bradycardia, hypotension, nystagmus/ataxia; gingival hyperplasia; agranulocytosis; rash; Stevens-Johnson syndrome; lymphadenopathy; nausea; cardiac arrest; heart block	Slow rate if bradycardia, hypotension, or cardiac dysrhythmias occur; monitor ECG, BP, pulse, and respiratory function; dilute with 0.9% NS only; assess oral hygiene; assess for rash; monitor renal, hepatic, and hematological status; interacts with many drugs
Fosphenytoin (Cerebyx)	Depresses seizure activity by altering ion transport in motor cortex	*Status epilepticus loading dose:* 15-20 mg PE/kg IV (PE = phenytoin equivalent); each 100-150 mg PE over a minimum of 1 minute; if full effect is not immediate, may be necessary to use with benzodiazepine; maintenance dose 4-6 mg PE/kg/24 hours *Nonemergency loading dose:* 10-20 mg PE/kg; maintenance dose 4-6 mg PE/kg/24 hours	Transient ataxia, dizziness, headache, nystagmus, paresthesia, pruritus, somnolence, hypotension, bradycardia, heart block, respiratory arrest, ventricular fibrillation, tonic seizures, nausea/vomiting, lethargy, hypocalcemia, metabolic acidosis, rash	Slow infusion rate or temporarily stop infusion for bradycardia, hypotension, burning, itching, numbness, or pain along injection site; assess neurological, respiratory, and cardiovascular status; assess seizure activity; monitor renal, hepatic, and hematological status; interacts with many drugs
Levetiracetam (Keppra)	Mechanism of action unknown; may inhibit intracellular sodium influx in motor cortex; depresses seizure activity	500 mg IV BID, titrate by 1000 mg/day every 2 weeks for seizure control; max 3000 mg/day in divided doses	Suicidal ideation; muscle weakness; dizziness; psychosis; decreased RBCs, hemoglobin, hematocrit	Adjust dose with acute kidney injury; monitor CBC; monitor for adverse changes in mental status
Diazepam (Valium)	Depresses subcortical areas of CNS; antiepileptic, sedative-hypnotic; antianxiety; adjunct medication to depress seizure activity	*Status epilepticus:* 5-10 mg IV; give 5 mg over 1 minute. May be repeated every 10-15 minutes for a total dose of 30 mg; may repeat in 2-4 hours; or 0.2-0.5 mg/kg every 15-30 minutes for 2-3 doses; some specialists suggest 20 mg and titrate total dose over 10 minutes or until seizures stop; maximum dose in 24 hours is 100 mg	Respiratory depression; hypotension; drowsiness; lethargy; bradycardia; cardiac arrest	Monitor respiratory status, BP, HR; assess IV site for phlebitis and venous thrombosis

Continued

TABLE 13-9 PHARMACOLOGY

Frequently Used Medications in Nervous System Alterations—cont'd

MEDICATION	ACTIONS/USE	DOSE/ROUTE	SIDE EFFECTS	NURSING IMPLICATIONS
Lorazepam (Ativan)	Depresses subcortical areas of CNS; antiepileptic; sedative-hypnotic; antianxiety	*Status epilepticus:* 4 mg IV over 1 minute as initial dose; may repeat once in 10-15 minutes if seizure continues; or 0.05 mg/kg to a total of 4 mg; may repeat once in 10-15 minutes; do not exceed 8 mg in 12 hours	Airway obstruction; apnea; blurred vision; confusion; excessive drowsiness; hypotension; bradycardia; respiratory depression; somnolence	Same as diazepam
Pentobarbital sodium (Nembutal sodium)	Barbiturate; sedative; hypnotic agent; antiepileptic for control of increased ICP	100 mg IV initially; give over 2 minutes; additional doses in increments of 25-50 mg IV; give 50 mg over 1 minute; maximum dose 200-500 mg IV *Barbiturate coma:* loading dose 3-10 mg/kg over 3 minutes to 3 hours *Maintenance dose:* 1.5-2 mg/kg IV every 2 hours or an infusion of 0.5-3 mg/kg/hr; adjust to maintain pentobarbital blood level between 110 and 177 mmol/L (25-40 mg/dL) or ICP below 25 mm Hg	Hypotension; myocardial or respiratory depression; thrombocytopenia purpura Overdose: apnea, coma, cough reflex depression, flat EEG, hypotension, sluggish or absent reflexes, pulmonary edema	Monitor ICP, CPP, VS, and hemodynamic responses; monitor pentobarbital levels; patient response is variable
Nimodipine	Calcium channel blocker given to prevent vasospasm; reduces neurological deficits after SAH	60 mg PO every 4 hours for 21 days; start within 96 hours of SAH	Hypotension, peripheral edema, ECG abnormalities, nausea/vomiting, diarrhea, altered liver function, HF, cough, dyspnea	Assess neurological status; monitor VS, I&O, daily weights; watch for signs of HF

ABGs, Arterial blood gases; *ACE,* angiotensin converting enzyme; *BP,* blood pressure; *CBC,* complete blood count; *CNS,* central nervous system; *CPP,* cerebral perfusion pressure; *ECG,* electrocardiogram; *EEG,* electroencephalogram; *GI,* gastrointestinal; *HF,* heart failure; *HR,* heart rate; *I&O,* intake & output; *ICP,* intracranial pressure; *IV,* intravenous; *IVP,* intravenous push; *NS,* normal saline; *PO,* orally; *RBC,* red blood cells; *SAH,* subarachnoid hemorrhage; *SCI,* spinal cord injury; *VS,* vital signs; *WBC,* white blood cells.
Data from Gahart B., & Nazareno A. (2012). *2011 Intravenous Medications* (27th ed.). St. Louis: Mosby; and Skidmore-Roth, L. (2011). *Mosby's 2011 Nursing Drug Reference.* St. Louis: Mosby.

Surgical Interventions

Surgical intervention may be required to remove the source of a mass or lesion causing the increased ICP. Surgery may involve the removal of infarcted areas and hematomas (epidural, subdural, or intracerebral). Decompressive hemicraniectomy is occasionally performed for severe brain injury or large volume stroke. The cranial bone is removed and the dura is opened to create more space for edematous tissue. The nurse must be aware of the missing bone flap and protect the patient's brain from trauma.[11]

Psychosocial Support

Neurological insults usually occur without warning and may be severe. This places the family in a state of shock and disbelief. In addition, the patient has suffered an insult to the nervous system and may respond inappropriately or uncharacteristically, or may not be able to respond at all to the family.

Neurological insults cause uncertainty in the patient's physical and mental outcomes. The personality and mental changes associated with brain insults can be devastating to the family. Nurses support the family by providing information and psychosocial support to reduce their anxiety.

TRAUMATIC BRAIN INJURY

TBI is a common occurrence in the United States and is the leading cause of trauma-related deaths in persons younger than 45 years. Each year, 1.1 million TBIs occur, resulting in 50,000 immediate deaths and hospitalization of 235,000 individuals. Males are 1.5 times as likely as females to sustain a TBI. The highest incidences of TBI occur in children younger than 4 years and in persons aged 15 to 19 years. Survival after TBI is dependent on prompt emergency treatment and focused management of primary and secondary injuries.[8]

GENETICS

Neurotrauma: Injury and Recovery

Outcomes after brain injury are variable. Genetic variability contributes to both the pathophysiology of injury and responses to rehabilitation that affect recovery. For example, there are genes associated with risk-taking behavior and substance abuse that are associated with activities that result in traumatic brain injury (TBI).[6] Another genetic influence on the extent of injury is inherited variations in glutamate receptors. Glutamate is an excitatory neurotransmitter that is released in excess with TBI. Variations in receptor activity could alter injury cascades that contribute to severity of neuronal dysfunction.[4] A receptor with low reactivity may be less responsive to the overload of glutamate from injury, resulting in a lessened excitotoxic and inflammatory cascade and reduced cell damage. A third promising avenue of genomic investigation related to the extent of brain injury is polymorphisms in necrotic and apoptotic cascades. These are pathways that contribute to cell death. Two categories of enzymes that contribute to cell death are calpains and caspases. The calpains are implicated in necrosis, or induced cell death, by degrading the microtubules and microfilaments that form the architecture of the cell. Caspases are present in apoptotic or programmed cell death, interfering with repair of DNA. Genetic variations that are associated with the production or robustness of activity in these protein-destroying enzymes (i.e., proteases) are thought to contribute to the cascade of injury-initiated biochemistry after TBI.[4]

Inflammation is common after neurotrauma. It is not clear where the inflammatory response plays a beneficial or detrimental role for injured brain tissue.[5] Inflammation alters the blood-brain barrier and promotes cross talk in a variety of injury cascades. A diverse group of proteins modulate inflammation. Data from animal models suggest that variations in the regulation of cytokines, small proteins that turn on and turn off the inflammatory response, promote blood-brain barrier disruption and interfere with new neuron formation ("neurogenesis"), particularly in areas of the brain associated with memory (i.e., hippocampus) during recovery.[1] However, inflammatory factors released by microglia have essential roles in clearance of cell debris and toxic proteins, so it may be that some inflammatory gene variations promote protection of neurons and glial cells along with their repair.[5] Ongoing investigations continue to provide insight into the pathophysiology of inflammation as a sequela to brain injury. Understanding disease-relevant pathways has potential for discovering relevant diagnostic biomarkers as well as therapeutic intervention points.[7]

The gene most frequently investigated for its influence in recovery from TBI is the apolipoprotein E (APOE) gene. The presence of the APOE4 allele (or one copy of the gene) is associated with poorer outcomes and slower recovery rates in some studies.[3] There are also investigations linking APOE4 with susceptibility to post-TBI seizure disorders.[3] APOE is one of a family of compounds that transport lipids and lipid-soluble vitamins through the bloodstream and appears to contribute to cognition by promoting normal neuronal function. APOE variations on chromosome 19 have been implicated in neuronal repair after ischemia as well as injury.

The growth factor, brain-derived neurotrophic factor (BDNF), influences neuronal activity, function, and survival. Although genetic variations have not been implicated in manifestations of injury or trajectories of recovery, this protein is being investigated as treatment for spinal cord and brain injury. In laboratory studies, BDNF is being used to direct neuronal growth and neuronal replacement with stem cells to replace neurons after apoptosis or necrosis.[2,4]

These advances in understanding of the molecular basis of TBI pathology and recovery illustrate the challenges and promise of genetic contributions to complex conditions. Researchers predict that healthcare providers will use genetic information as a routine process to diagnose severity of brain injury and to individualize rehabilitation options.[3] Genomic approaches to modulating injury and enhancing recovery after TBI promise compelling and testable options for refining diagnosis and therapy.

References

1. Blaiss CA, Yu TS, Zhang G, Chen J, Dimchev G, Parada LF, et al. Temporally specified genetic ablation of neurogenesis impairs cognitive recovery after traumatic brain injury. Journal of Neuroscience. 2011;31(13), 4906-4916.
2. Bonne JF, Conners TM, Silverman WF, Kowalski DP, Lernay MA, Fischer I. Grafted neural progenitors integrate and restore synaptic connectivity across the injured spinal cord. Journal of Neuroscience. 2011;31(12), 4675-4686.
3. Conley YP, Alexander S, Genomic, transcriptomic, and epigenomic approaches to recovery after acquired brain injury. Physical Medicine and Rehabilitation. 2011;3(6 Suppl), S52-S58.
4. McAllister TW. Genetic factors modulating outcome after neurotrauma. Physical Medicine and Rehabilitation. 2010;2(12 Suppl 2), S241-S252.
5. Rivest S. The promise of anti-inflammatory therapies for CNS injuries and diseases. Expert Reviews in Neurotherapy. 2011;11(6), 783-786.
6. Silver JM, McAllister TW, Yudofsky SC. Textbook of Traumatic Brain Injury 2nd ed. Arlington, VA: American Psychiatric Publishing Inc.; 2011.
7. Zhang Z, Larner SF, Kobeissy F, Hayes RL, Wang KK. Systems biology and theranostic approach to drug discovery and development to treat traumatic brain injury. Methods in Molecular Biology. 2010;662:317-329.

Pathophysiology

Traumatic injury can result in damage to the scalp, skull, meninges, and brain, including neuronal pathways, cranial nerves, and intracranial vessels. The extent of TBI can range from mild to severe. Injuries may be open or closed. With an open injury, the scalp is torn or a fracture extends into the sinuses or middle ear. The meninges can also be penetrated.

A closed TBI occurs when there is no break in the scalp. Acceleration-deceleration is a common mechanism for TBI. With this injury, the movement of the head follows a straight line, and the moving head (acceleration) hits a stationary object (deceleration). Rotation or a twisting of the brain within the cranial vault adds to the insult. Genetics may play a role in both injury and recovery (see box, "Genetics").

Scalp Lacerations

Scalp lacerations are common in traumatic injury and are often associated with skull fracture. The scalp offers some resistance to compression and absorbs mild blows by distributing forces over the entire area of the scalp. The scalp is very vascular and can be the source of significant blood loss. The wound is cleansed, debrided, and inspected for a depressed skull fracture, then sutured closed. Inattention to these details can lead to infection.

Skull Fractures

The skull has high compressive strength and is somewhat elastic. After impact, there is an in-bending of the skull at the point of impact and an out-bending at the vertex. The area of out-bending of tensile stresses creates a fracture line that moves toward the base of the skull. There are several types of skull fractures—linear, depressed, and comminuted—and various locations of the fractures (Figure 13-14).

Linear skull fracture. A linear fracture is the most common type of skull fracture. This fracture usually does not lead to significant complications unless there is an extension

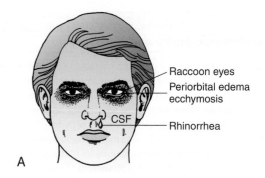
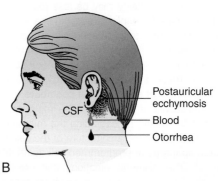

FIGURE 13-15 **A,** Raccoon eyes, rhinorrhea. **B,** Battle sign with otorrhea. (From Barker E. *Neuroscience Nursing: A Spectrum of Care.* 3rd ed. St. Louis: Mosby; 2008.)

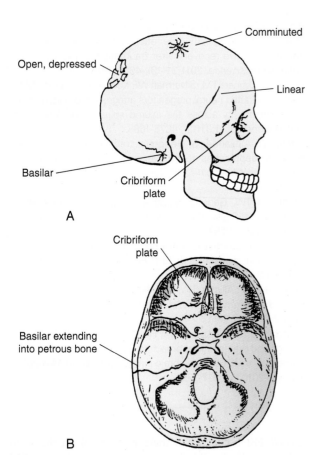

FIGURE 13-14 Skull fractures. **A,** Linear; open, depressed; basilar; and comminuted fractures. **B,** View of base of skull with fractures. (From Barker E. *Neuroscience Nursing: A Spectrum of Care.* 3rd ed. St. Louis: Mosby; 2008.)

of the fracture to the orbit, sinus, or across a vessel. When there is extension of the fracture, the patient is admitted for observation of signs of intracranial bleeding and epidural hematoma.

Linear fractures at the skull base are termed *basilar fractures.* This type of fracture is difficult to confirm on a skull x-ray study and is diagnosed by clinical presentation of the patient. Battle sign (bruising behind the ear) and the presence of "raccoon's eyes" (bilateral periorbital edema and bruising) may be indicative of a basilar skull fracture (Figure 13-15). Dural tears are very common with a basilar skull fracture and may lead to meningitis. Drainage of CSF from the nose (rhinorrhea), postnasal drainage, or drainage of CSF from the ear (otorrhea) may indicate a dural tear. When blood encircled by a yellowish stain is seen on a dressing or bed linen, it is called the *halo sign* and usually indicates CSF. If CSF is suspected in the drainage, a sample of the drainage is sent to the laboratory for analysis. In the event of a CSF leak, it is important to allow the CSF to flow freely. Nothing should be placed in the nose or ear, although small bandages under the nose or around the ear can be used to collect the drainage. The patient is instructed not to blow the nose. To avoid penetrating the brain as a result of the dural tear, tubes (e.g., gastric, suction catheters, endotracheal tubes) should be inserted through the mouth rather than through the nose.

Depressed skull fracture. A depressed skull fracture occurs when the outer table of the skull is depressed below the inner table of the surrounding intact skull. The dura may be intact, bruised, or torn. If the scalp is lacerated and dura is torn, there is direct communication between the brain and the environment, and meningitis can occur. In addition, the compressed and bruised brain beneath the depressed bone or bone lodged in brain parenchyma is the source of focal neurological deficit and may become a seizure focus.

Comminuted skull fracture. A comminuted skull fracture occurs from multiple linear fractures with a depressed area at the site of impact. The fracture radiates away from the impact site. Comminuted skull fracture is referred to as an "eggshell fracture" because of the appearance of the skull. Risks are similar to those occurring with a depressed fracture.

Brain Injury

TBI is classified as primary and secondary. Primary brain injury can be further divided into focal (contusions, hematomas, penetrating injuries) and diffuse lesions (diffuse axonal injury).

Primary brain injury. Primary brain injury is a direct injury that occurs to the brain from an impact. With impact, the semisolid brain moves around inside the skull. The area under the direct impact is injured (coup injury). Injury distal to the site of impact can occur as the brain moves inside the skull (contrecoup injury). The stretching, shearing, rotational, and tearing forces that result from impact interrupt normal neuronal pathways. Concussion, contusion, penetrating injuries, and diffuse axonal injury are all types of primary brain injury. Intracranial bleeding can occur as a complication of the primary injury. Secondary brain injury may occur because of biochemical consequences of the primary injury (Figure 13-16).

Concussion. Concussion occurs when a mechanical force of short duration is applied to the skull. This injury results in

the temporary failure of impulse conduction. The neurological deficits are reversible and are generally mild. Patients may lose consciousness for a few seconds at the time of injury, but lasting effects are not common.

Contusion. Contusion is the result of coup and contrecoup injuries, accompanied by bruising and bleeding into brain tissue. Lacerations of the cortical surface associated with contrecoup injuries may be greater than those seen directly under the point of impact. Signs and symptoms are variable, depending on location and extent of bleeding.

Diffuse axonal injury. A more global brain injury is diffuse axonal injury. With this injury, widespread white matter axonal damage occurs secondary to rotational and shearing forces. This type of injury is associated with disruption of axons in the cerebral hemispheres, diencephalon, and brainstem. This injury results in vasodilation and increased cerebral blood volume that precipitates increased ICP. Signs and symptoms are variable, and prognosis is poor.

Penetrating injury. Penetrating injuries are the result of low- or high-velocity forces such as gunshots, knives, or sharp objects. With this type of injury, there is a deep laceration of brain tissue and possible damage to the ventricular system. A low-velocity (stabbing) injury is limited to the tract of entry, and the greatest concern is bleeding and infection. A high-velocity (gunshot) injury causes extensive damage because of the entry of bone fragments at the site. In addition, because bullets spin irregularly, they create many paths and shock waves that cause extensive brain damage.

Hematoma. Acute hematomas can be life threatening. There are three types of hematomas: epidural, subdural, and intracerebral (Figure 13-17).

Epidural hematoma. Collection of blood in the potential space between the inner table of the skull and the dura causes an *epidural hematoma.* This hematoma is typically associated with a linear fracture of the temporal bone and results from the tearing of the middle meningeal artery. Arterial blood

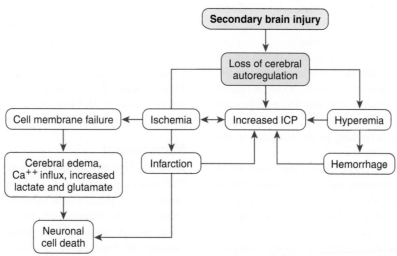

FIGURE 13-16 Pathophysiology of secondary brain injury. *Ca⁺⁺*, Calcium; *ICP*, intracranial pressure.

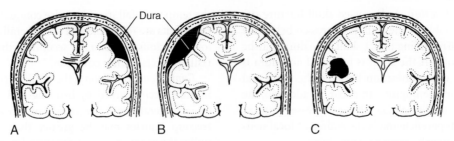

FIGURE 13-17 Types of hematomas. **A,** Subdural (takes on contour of brain). **B,** Epidural. **C,** Intracerebral. (From Barker E. *Neuroscience Nursing: A Spectrum of Care*. 3rd ed. St. Louis: Mosby; 2008.)

accumulates rapidly in this space. The patient typically experiences a brief loss of consciousness followed by a lucid period before neurological deterioration. The lucid period can last for a few hours to 48 hours. As the patient's condition deteriorates, the LOC decreases, contralateral deficits appear, and the pupil on the side of the lesion *(ipsilateral)* becomes fixed and dilated.

Subdural hematoma. Collection of blood in the subdural space causes a *subdural hematoma*. It occurs when a surface vein is torn around the cerebral cortex. There are three kinds of subdural hematomas: acute, subacute, and chronic. *Acute subdural hematoma* occurs within 48 hours of an injury. It is nearly always seen with cortical or brainstem injury and represents a mass lesion. The risk of death is high because of injury to brain tissue and the mass effect caused by an expanding hematoma. Surgical intervention occurring within 4 hours of injury improves mortality.[9] Symptoms of a *subacute subdural hematoma* occur anywhere from 48 hours to 2 weeks after an injury. The onset of symptoms is later because the hematoma grows slowly. A *chronic subdural hematoma* occurs as a result of a low-velocity impact. Symptoms occur from 2 weeks to several months after an injury. A higher incidence of chronic subdural hematomas is seen in the elderly, chronic alcohol abusers, or those taking anticoagulants, such as warfarin, or anti-platelet aggregants such as clopidogrel (Plavix), prasugrel (Effient), ticagrelor (Brilinta) or aspirin.[8] Because symptoms are often subtle, the diagnosis of chronic subdural hematoma is often missed.

Intracerebral hematoma. An intracerebral hematoma is a hemorrhage into brain tissue that creates a mass lesion. This lesion can occur anywhere in the brain. It can be caused by penetrating injuries, gunshot wounds, deep depressed skull fractures, stab wounds, or extension of a contusion. Signs and symptoms vary according to the location of the lesion and extent of hemorrhage.

Secondary brain injury. Secondary brain injury occurs as a consequence of the initial trauma and is characterized by an inflammatory response and release of cytokines from macrophages that cause increased vascular permeability of the blood vessel wall, leading to vasogenic cerebral edema. A series of biochemical events also contributes to the overproduction of free oxygen radicals that disrupt the cellular membrane, impair cellular metabolism, and cause neuronal

deterioration (see Figure 13-16). Decreased cerebral perfusion from numerous causes, hypoxia, infection, and/or fluid and electrolyte imbalances all contribute to secondary brain injury. These insults add to the degree and extent of cellular dysfunction after TBI, increase the extent of brain damage, and affect functional recovery. Proper management minimizes the effects of secondary brain injury.

Assessment

The GCS is used as a guide in assessing a patient with a TBI. The assessment is supplemented with a thorough neurological examination specific to the area of the brain involved. Assessment of airway and oxygenation status is essential to ensure adequate oxygenation and CBF. Abnormal respiratory patterns must be reported and documented because pattern changes usually indicate deterioration in neurological status. Additional assessment data include ICP, CPP, and hemodynamic monitoring. A patient with a TBI requires the same laboratory and diagnostic studies as a patient with increased ICP.

Nursing Diagnoses

The same nursing diagnoses are applicable for a TBI patient as for a patient with increased ICP (see box, "Nursing Care Plan for the Patient with Traumatic Brain Injury, Increased Intracranial Pressure, or Acute Stroke"). These diagnoses cover both primary and secondary head injuries. Additional nursing diagnoses include Impaired Swallowing, Disturbed Sensory Perception, Hyperthermia, Acute Pain, Decreased Cardiac Output, Risk for Constipation, Risk for Imbalanced Fluid Volume, Risk for Infection, Imbalanced Nutrition, Impaired Physical Mobility, Risk for Impaired Skin Integrity, and Impaired Verbal Communication.

Management
Medical (Nonsurgical) Interventions

The nonsurgical treatment of a patient with a TBI is the same as for a patient with increased ICP. The emphasis is on reducing ICP, maintaining the airway, providing oxygenation, maintaining cerebral perfusion, and preventing secondary TBI. Therapeutic hypothermia may be implemented to protect the injured brain.[12] Hypothermia decreases the cerebral metabolic rate and oxygen consumption, lowers levels of glutamate and interleukin-1β, decreases ICP, and increases CPP. Protecting the brain by using hypothermia may improve outcomes in persons with TBI.[22] Several strategies are available to induce hypothermia including external cooling systems, hypothermia blankets, endovascular or endonasal cooling devices, antipyretics, sponging with cold water, and applying ice packs. If available, monitoring the brain temperature to thermoregulate the patient is an optimal choice because the actual brain temperature may be higher than the blood temperature. The nurse should assess for adverse effects of hypothermia including dysrhythmias (atrial fibrillation), electrolyte imbalances, acidosis, shivering, and coagulopathies.

Nutritional support after TBI is essential. Hypermetabolism, accelerated catabolism, and excess nitrogen losses are responses to TBI. These responses result in depletion of energy stores, loss of lean muscle mass, reduced protein synthesis, loss of gastrointestinal mucosal integrity, and immune compromise. Nutritional support decreases susceptibility to infections, promotes wound healing, and facilitates weaning from mechanical ventilation.[22]

Surgical Interventions

Various surgical procedures exist to treat TBI. A depressed skull fracture may require surgery to elevate and repair or remove bone fragments. Acute subdural hematomas are usually evacuated via burr holes and epidural hematomas via craniotomy to prevent herniation. Penetrating wounds to the skull and brain may necessitate a craniotomy to explore the pathway of the missile, repair lacerations of intracranial vessels and brain tissue, remove bone fragments, or retrieve a foreign body such as a bullet.

Postoperative care is directed at the several interventions. Important goals are maintaining normal ICP and CPP, maintaining the airway and ventilation, preventing fluid and electrolyte imbalances, preventing complications of immobility, avoiding nutritional deficits, and reducing the incidence of infection.

The craniotomy dressing is assessed for drainage including color, odor, and amount. Once the dressing is removed, the incision is assessed for swelling, redness, drainage, and tenderness. Persistent CSF drainage from the wound after surgery may indicate a dural tear and may require a lumbar drain or ventriculostomy for several days to decrease pressure at the fistula site and to aid in healing. A craniotomy may be necessary to repair the dura if leakage persists. Patients with penetrating wounds to the brain are at high risk for the development of not only infections, but also brain abscesses.

ACUTE STROKE

Stroke is a major public health problem. It is the third leading cause of death in the United States, the most frequent cause of adult disability, and the leading cause of long-term care. Although most strokes are preventable by controlling major risk factors such as hypertension, more than 600,000 new strokes occur each year in the United States, and 185,000 have a recurrent stroke. More than 4 million people are stroke survivors.[25] Persons who have a stroke have a 10- to 20-fold increased risk of having another stroke. The cost of hospitalization, rehabilitation, long-term care, and lost wages from stroke is estimated at $57 billion annually. Stroke, also known as "brain attack," results in infarction of a focal area of the brain. Early recognition of the signs and symptoms is essential in order to preserve blood flow to the brain. A stroke should be assessed and treated as a life-threatening emergency because optimal early treatment improves long-term outcome.[20]

The hallmark of stroke is the sudden onset of focal neurological symptoms associated with changes in blood flow to the brain resulting from either a blockage of flow or hemorrhage. Stroke can present with maximal focal neurological deficits, or as stroke in evolution, in which symptoms evolve over several hours. The definition of stroke includes neurological deficits lasting 24 hours or longer. Although symptoms may completely resolve, CT or MRI will show evidence of permanent cerebral tissue damage.

Pathophysiology

Stroke occurs when the blood supply to the brain is disturbed by occlusion (ischemic) or hemorrhage. Brain cells survive only about 3 to 4 minutes when deprived of blood and oxygen. Normal CBF is 50 mL/100 g of brain tissue/min. When CBF drops to 25 mL/100 g/min, neurons become electrically silent but remain potentially viable for several hours. This region of brain is known as the ischemic penumbra (Figure 13-18). If CBF falls to less than the critical level of 10 mL/100 g/min, or the penumbra is not reperfused, irreversible damage occurs. A cascade of metabolic disturbances follows, including lactic acidosis production, glutamate release, depletion of ATP, and entry of sodium and calcium into the cells, leading to cytotoxic cerebral edema and mitochondrial failure.

Ischemic Stroke

Ischemic strokes are caused by large artery atherosclerosis, cardioembolic events (Figure 13-19), or small artery occlusive disease (lacunar stroke), or the cause is unknown

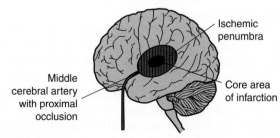

FIGURE 13-18 Proximal occlusion of left middle cerebral artery with infarction. Ischemic penumbra represents regional blood flow at about 25 mL/100 g/min. Ischemic penumbra is the area where acute therapies for stroke are targeted.

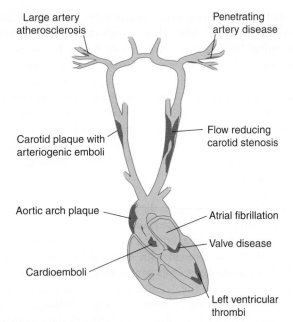

Large artery
atherosclerosis

Penetrating
artery disease

Carotid plaque with
arteriogenic emboli

Flow reducing
carotid stenosis

Aortic arch plaque

Atrial fibrillation

Valve disease

Cardioemboli

Left ventricular
thrombi

FIGURE 13-19 Common arterial and cardiac abnormalities causing ischemic stroke. (From Albers GW, Easton JD, Sacco RL, et al. Antithrombotic and thrombolytic therapy for ischemic stroke. *Chest.* 1998;114[suppl. 5]:683S-698S.)

(cryptogenic stroke). Approximately 85% of all strokes in the United States are ischemic.

Large artery atherosclerosis. Large artery atherosclerosis is the result of stenosis in the large arteries of the head and neck, caused by a cholesterol plaque or a thrombus superimposed on the plaque. Blood flow may be greatly reduced (stenosis), causing ischemia, or occluded completely, causing a stroke. Hypertension, diabetes, smoking, obesity, and hyperlipidemia are risk factors for this type of stroke.

Cardioembolic stroke. Low-flow states or stasis of blood within the cardiac chambers may result in blood clot formation. An embolism occurs when a blood clot or plaque fractures, breaks off, and travels to the brain. The most common causes of *cardioembolic stroke* are atrial fibrillation, rheumatic heart disease, acute myocardial infarction, endocarditis, mitral valve stenosis, and prosthetic heart valves. Because a cardiac abnormality is the source of the cerebral emboli, it is important to treat the underlying cardiac problem as well as the neurological problem.

Lacunar stroke. Lacunar strokes (small vessel occlusive disease) are caused by chronic hypertension, hyperlipidemia, obesity, and diabetes. These disease states cause lipid material to coat the small cerebral arteries within deep structures of the brain. This process leads to a thickening of the arterial walls, decreased blood flow, and ultimately a stroke. The characteristic locations of lacunar infarcts are the basal ganglia, subcortical white matter, thalamus, cerebellum, and brainstem. The recurrence rate of these strokes is about tenfold to twelvefold compared with other types of stroke. This type of stroke causes not only physical impairment, but also cognitive impairment such as vascular dementia. Patients can

have pure motor, pure sensory, or both motor and sensory features of stroke.

Cryptogenic stroke. The *cryptogenic* subtype refers to a stroke of unknown origin.

Hemorrhagic Stroke

Hemorrhagic strokes account for approximately 15% of all strokes in the United States. The most common causes of hemorrhagic stroke are primary intraparenchymal hemorrhage and ruptured vascular malformations, such as cerebral aneurysm or arteriovenous malformations (AVMs). Secondary causes include excessive anticoagulation (warfarin or heparin), inappropriate use of thrombolytics (recombinant tissue plasminogen activator [rt-PA]), vasopressor drugs, drug abuse (cocaine abuse), and coagulopathies.

Intraparenchymal hemorrhage. About 10% of strokes in the United States are intraparenchymal hemorrhages (bleeding into the brain substance), usually caused by uncontrolled hypertension. Another cause of intraparenchymal hemorrhage is cerebral amyloid angiopathy. This condition is the result of abnormal amyloid protein deposits in the cerebral blood vessels. As a result, the cerebral blood vessels become friable and therefore prone to spontaneous rupture, even in patients without hypertension.[16] When a blood vessel ruptures, the escaped blood forms a mass that displaces and compresses brain tissue. The severity of the symptoms is dependent on the location and amount of the hemorrhage. If the hemorrhage is large enough, herniation may result.

Ruptured cerebral aneurysm with subarachnoid hemorrhage. *Cerebral aneurysm* is a localized dilation of the cerebral artery wall that causes the artery to weaken and become susceptible to rupture. Most aneurysms develop at the bifurcation of large arteries at the base of the brain (circle of Willis). Patients with cerebral aneurysms are asymptomatic before the rupture unless they experience a warning "leak" or sentinel bleeding. The aneurysm commonly ruptures into the subarachnoid space of the basal cisterns and causes a *subarachnoid hemorrhage* (SAH). Bleeding into the subarachnoid space causes increased ICP, impaired cerebral autoregulation, reduced CBF, and irritation of the meninges. The bleeding generally stops through the formation of a fibrin plug and platelet aggregation within the ruptured artery.

After an aneurysm rupture, the patient can develop cardiac dysrhythmias, rebleeding, hydrocephalus, seizures, and cerebral vasospasm. Cardiac dysrhythmias occur as a result of sympathetic nervous system stimulation. Increased sympathetic tone can cause elevated T waves, prolonged QT intervals, and ST abnormalities. Rebleeding after the initial aneurysm rupture may occur before the aneurysm is secured. The mechanism causing the rebleeding is increased tension on the artery from hypertension, or normal breakdown of the clot, which occurs 7 to 10 days after the initial hemorrhage. Early endovascular or surgical intervention is recommended to prevent rebleeding.[4]

Hydrocephalus can occur after SAH through two mechanisms. Bleeding into the intraventricular space can block flow of CSF and cause acute obstructive hydrocephalus. As blood enters the subarachnoid space, an inflammatory response is triggered that causes fibrosis and thickening of the arachnoid villi, thereby preventing reabsorption of CSF and producing communicating hydrocephalus.

Seizures occurring within the first 12 hours after rupture are attributed to increased ICP or rebleeding of the aneurysm. Seizures occurring later are more likely due to ischemic damage secondary to vasospasm. Because of the adverse effects of medications, seizure prophylaxis is not recommended unless seizures occur beyond the first 12 hours after hemorrhage.

Cerebral vasospasm is a narrowing of arteries adjacent to the aneurysm that results in ischemia and infarction of brain tissue if it progresses. It is the leading cause of death after aneurysmal SAH. The usual period for vasospasm to occur can be anywhere between 3 and 14 days after the rupture. The exact mechanism for vasospasm is unknown, but some factors that contribute to vasospasm are structural changes in the adjacent cerebral arteries, denervation of adjacent arteries, generation of oxygen free radicals, and release of vasoactive substances (serotonin, catecholamines, prostaglandins) that initiate vasospasm, the inflammatory response, and calcium influx.

Arteriovenous malformation. An AVM is a congenital anomaly that forms an abnormal communication network between the arterial and venous systems in the brain. Arterial blood is directly shunted into the venous system without a capillary network. This predisposes the vessels to rupture into the ventricular system or subarachnoid space, causing SAH, or into the brain parenchyma, causing intracranial hemorrhage ICH. Impaired perfusion of the cerebral tissue adjacent to the AVM also occurs. The size and location of AVMs differ. Some AVMs do not hemorrhage, but rather cause varying degrees of ischemia, scarring of brain tissue with seizures, abnormal tissue development, compression, or hydrocephalus. AVMs are more prevalent in males and are commonly diagnosed after a patient has had a seizure. Headache is another common manifestation of AVM.

Assessment

Early identification of a stroke is imperative so rapid treatment can be initiated. The public must be educated on the symptoms of a brain attack because early intervention can minimize stroke deficit. Patients at high risk of stroke are taught risk reduction, the signs and symptoms of stroke, and to seek medical attention immediately (Box 13-1). Specialized stroke centers improve patient outcomes. The stroke center concept is designed to expedite evaluation and management of patients with suspected ischemic stroke, transient ischemic attack, or intracerebral hemorrhage. A stroke center is equipped with an emergency department (ED); a stroke team of physicians, nurses, and allied professionals with stroke-specific training; treatment protocols; emergent neuroradiology services; and access to neurosurgical services. Assessment in the ED includes an eyewitness description of symptoms, identification of the exact time symptoms started, and a neurological assessment.

BOX 13-1 SIGNS AND SYMPTOMS OF STROKE

- Weakness or numbness of one side of the body (face, arm, leg, or any combination of these)
- Slurred speech or an inability to comprehend what is being said
- Visual disturbance such as transient loss of vision in one or both eyes, double vision, or a visual field deficit
- Dizziness, incoordination, ataxia, or vertigo
- Sudden onset severe headache ("worst headache of my life")

The neurological examination includes evaluating mental status (LOC, arousal, orientation), cranial nerve function, motor strength, sensory function, neglect, coordination, and deep tendon reflexes. The National Institutes of Health Stroke Scale (Table 13-10) is used to assess the severity of the presenting signs and symptoms, especially if the patient is a candidate for thrombolytic therapy.

Assessment and stabilization of the airway, breathing, and circulation are a priority. Vital signs are monitored, generally every 15 minutes for the first 6 hours. BP elevations are common in these patients. Because reducing the BP can decrease blood flow and oxygenation to the ischemic brain tissue, a gradual 20% lowering of the BP is recommended to prevent enlargement of the infarcted area and worsening of the neurological deficit. The goal for ischemic stroke is to keep the systolic BP less than 220 mm Hg and the diastolic BP less than 120 mm Hg.[16] In hemorrhagic stroke, the goal is a MAP less than 130 mm Hg.[16] Monitoring the respiratory pattern is important because changes can indicate that the stroke is extending and more neurological damage is occurring. Hypoxemia after a stroke is common as a result of concurrent medical conditions such as aspiration, pneumonia, hypoventilation, atelectasis, and pulmonary embolism.[20] A baseline SpO_2 is obtained while the patient is breathing room air, and supplemental oxygen is provided when the SpO_2 is less than 95%. Cardiac assessment, including the presence of cardiac dysrhythmias, is important to determine whether the stroke was potentially caused by a cardioembolic event. IV access is obtained, and normal saline infusions are started; hypertonic solutions are avoided. Laboratory studies include electrolytes, cardiac enzymes, complete blood count, urinalysis, and coagulation studies. A serum glucose level is obtained because many patients who present with stroke are hyperglycemic. In addition, up to 20% of patients with stroke are diabetic.[20] Several studies indicate that individuals with hyperglycemia have poorer outcomes after stroke as compared with normoglycemic patients, even without a history of diabetes. The hyperglycemia seems to increase neuronal injury.[20]

Once the patient is transferred to the critical care unit, assessments are compared with the baseline assessments performed in the ED. Hemodynamic instability is common in an acute stroke because of cardiac disorders and the sympathetic

TABLE 13-10   NATIONAL INSTITUTES OF HEALTH STROKE SCALE

INSTRUCTIONS	SCALE		DEFINITION
1a. Level of Consciousness: The investigator must choose a response if a full evaluation is prevented by such obstacles as an endotracheal tube, language barrier, orotracheal trauma/bandages.	0 1 2 3	= = = =	**Alert;** keenly responsive. **Not alert;** but arousable by minor stimulation. **Not alert;** requires repeated stimulation to attend. **Responds** only with reflex motor or autonomic effects or totally unresponsive, flaccid, and areflexic.
1b. LOC Questions: The patient is asked the month and his/her age. The answer must be correct—there is no partial credit for being close.	0 1 2	= = =	**Answers** both questions correctly. **Answers** one question correctly. **Answers** neither question correctly.
1c. LOC Commands: The patient is asked to open and close the eyes and then to grip and release the nonparetic hand. Substitute another one-step command if the hands cannot be used.	0 1 2	= = =	**Performs** both tasks correctly. **Performs** one task correctly. **Performs** neither task correctly.
2. Best Gaze: Only horizontal eye movements will be tested. Voluntary or reflexive (oculocephalic) eye movements will be scored, but caloric testing is not done.	0 1 2	= = =	**Normal.** **Partial gaze palsy;** gaze is abnormal in one or both eyes. **Forced deviation,** or total gaze paresis not overcome by the oculocephalic maneuver.
3. Visual: Visual fields (upper and lower quadrants) are tested by confrontation, using finger counting or visual threat, as appropriate.	0 1 2 3	= = = =	**No visual loss.** **Partial hemianopia.** **Complete hemianopia.** **Bilateral hemianopia** (blind).
4. Facial Palsy: Ask—or use pantomime to encourage—the patient to show teeth or raise eyebrows and close eyes.	0 1 2 3	= = = =	**Normal** symmetrical movements. **Minor paralysis** (asymmetry on smiling). **Partial paralysis** (total or near-total paralysis of lower face). **Complete paralysis** of one or both sides.
5. Motor Arm: The limb is placed in the appropriate position: extend the arms (palms down) 90 degrees (if sitting) or 45 degrees (if supine). Drift is scored if the arm falls before 10 seconds. **5a.** Left arm **5b.** Right arm	0 1 2 3 4 UN	= = = = = =	**No drift;** limb holds position for 10 seconds. **Drift;** limb holds position, but drifts down before full 10 seconds. **Some effort against gravity;** limb cannot get to or maintain position, drifts down to bed, some effort against gravity. **No effort against gravity; limb falls.** **No movement.** **Amputation** or joint fusion.
6. Motor Leg: The limb is placed in the appropriate position: hold the leg at 30 degrees (always tested supine). Drift is scored if the leg falls before 5 seconds. **6a.** Left leg **6b.** Right leg	0 1 2 3 4 UN	= = = = = =	**No drift;** leg holds position for full 5 seconds. **Drift;** leg falls by the end of the 5-second period but does not hit bed. **Some effort against gravity;** leg falls to bed. By 5 seconds, has some effort against gravity. **No effort against gravity;** leg falls to bed immediately. **No movement.** **Amputation** or joint fusion
7. Limb Ataxia: The finger-nose-finger and heel-shin tests are performed on both sides with eyes open.	0 1 2 UN	= = = =	**Absent.** **Present in one limb.** **Present in two limbs.** **Amputation** or joint fusion.
8. Sensory: Sensation or grimace to pinprick when tested, or withdrawal from noxious stimulus in the obtunded or aphasic patient	0 1 2	= = =	**Normal;** no sensory loss. **Mild-to-moderate sensory loss;** feels pinprick is less sharp or is dull on the affected side; or there is a loss of superficial pain with pinprick, but aware of being touched **Severe to total sensory loss;** patient is not aware of being touched in the face, arm, and leg.

TABLE 13-10 NATIONAL INSTITUTES OF HEALTH STROKE SCALE—cont'd

INSTRUCTIONS	SCALE		DEFINITION
9. **Best Language:** Patient is asked to describe what is happening in the attached picture, to name the items on the attached naming sheet, and to read from the attached list of sentences. Comprehension is judged from responses here, as well as to all of the commands in the preceding general neurological exam.	0 1 2 3	= = = =	**No aphasia;** normal. **Mild-to-moderate aphasia;** some obvious loss of fluency or facility of comprehension, without significant limitation on ideas. **Severe aphasia;** all communication is through fragmentary expression; great need for inference, questioning, and guessing by the listener. **Mute, global aphasia;** no usable speech or auditory comprehension.
10. **Dysarthria:** An adequate sample of speech must be obtained by asking patient to read or repeat words from the attached list	0 1 2 UN	= = = =	**Normal.** **Mild-to-moderate dysarthria;** patient slurs some words; can be understood with some difficulty. **Severe dysarthria;** patient's speech is so slurred as to be unintelligible; or is mute/anarthric. **Intubated** or other physical barrier.
11. **Extinction and Inattention (formerly Neglect):** Sufficient information to identify neglect may be obtained during prior testing. If the patient has a severe visual loss preventing visual double simultaneous stimulation, and the cutaneous stimuli are normal, the score is normal.	0 1 2	= = =	**No abnormality.** **Visual, tactile, auditory, spatial, or personal inattention** or extinction to bilateral simultaneous stimulation in one of the sensory modalities. **Profound hemi-inattention or extinction to more than one modality;** does not recognize own hand or orients to only one side of space.

From National Institute of Neurological Disorders and Stroke at the National Institutes of Health. *NIH Stroke Scale.* www.ninds.nih.gov; 2003. Accessed July 25, 2011.

response; therefore assessment of the airway, vital signs, and fluid and electrolyte status continues to be a priority. Elderly patients with stroke often are dehydrated. Dehydration is caused by inadequate water intake, drowsiness, dysphagia, possible infection, diuretic use, and uncontrolled diabetes.[20] Dehydration after a stroke can cause an increased hematocrit and a reduced BP that can worsen the ischemic process.[16] In a patient with an acute stroke, neurological status, hemodynamic status, laboratory values, and cardiac function are monitored. Ongoing assessments are similar to those in patients with increased ICP. Patients with subarachnoid hemorrhage present differently than those with ischemic stroke. When arterial blood enters the subarachnoid space, its presence is irritating to the meninges. The patient may complain of a localized headache, stiff neck *(nuchal rigidity)*, pain

above and behind the eye, and photophobia. Patients with SAH are often anxious and agitated as a result of pain, altered LOC, and cognitive changes.[3] If conscious, the patient may complain of "the worst headache of my life." Vomiting and decreased LOC are commonly seen. Neurological assessment includes LOC, motor and sensory deficits, and pupillary response. Assessment findings may include mental status changes and subtle focal deficits to coma or severe neurological deficits.

Diagnostic Tests

Diagnostic tests are performed to differentiate ischemic from hemorrhagic stroke and to establish baseline parameters to monitor the effects of treatment.[20] Common diagnostic tests are summarized in Box 13-2.

BOX 13-2   DIAGNOSTIC TESTING FOR STROKE

Initial Diagnostic Testing
- Emergency CT scan without contrast
- 12-Lead electrocardiogram
- Review of time of onset and inclusion criteria for patients eligible for rt-PA, including NIHSS assessment
- **Complete blood count:** red blood cells, hemoglobin, hematocrit, platelet count
- **Coagulation studies:** prothrombin time, activated partial thromboplastin time, INR
- Serum electrolytes and glucose
- Urinalysis
- Troponin and cardiac enzymes, to rule out myocardial infarction

Additional Diagnostic Testing
- **MRI with diffusion and perfusion images:** detects ischemia, altered CBF, and cerebral blood volume
- **Arteriography:** detects shallow ulcerated plaques, thrombus, aneurysms, dissections, multiple lesions, AVMs, and collateral blood flow

- **MRA images:** detects carotid occlusion, intracranial stenosis or occlusions
- **CT perfusion images:** detects altered CBF and cerebral blood volume
- **CT angiography images:** detects carotid occlusion and intracranial stenosis or occlusions
- **Digital subtraction angiography:** detects carotid occlusion, and intracranial stenoses or occlusions
- **Doppler carotid ultrasound:** detects stenosis or occlusions of the carotid arteries
- **Transcranial Doppler ultrasound:** detects stenosis or occlusion of the circle of Willis, vertebral arteries, and basilar artery
- **Transthoracic echocardiogram:** detects cardioembolic abnormalities
- **Transesophageal echocardiogram:** detects cardioembolic abnormalities; more sensitive than transthoracic echocardiogram

---

AVMs, Arteriovenous malformations; *CBF,* cerebral blood flow; *CT,* computerized tomography; *INR,* international normalized ratio; *MRA,* magnetic resonance angiography; *MRI,* magnetic resonance imaging; *NIHSS,* National Institutes of Health Stroke Scale; *rt-PA,* recombinant tissue plasminogen activator.

Management
Nursing Diagnoses

A patient with stroke has similar nursing diagnoses as a patient with increased ICP and TBI. Refer to the "Nursing Care Plan for the Patient with Traumatic Brain Injury, Increased Intracranial Pressure, or Acute Stroke."

Ischemic Stroke

Thrombolytic candidates. Early thrombolysis is recommended when possible. rt-PA is the only approved therapy for acute ischemic stroke and must be given within 3 hours of symptom onset.[20] Administration after 3 hours has not shown to be beneficial and increases the risk for hemorrhagic transformation of the infarct. Unfortunately, only about 5% of eligible patients actually receive the treatment.[20] rt-PA does not affect the infarcted area, but by lysing the clot, it revitalizes the ischemic penumbra and improves overall neurological function. Careful assessment of patients potentially eligible for thrombolytic therapy must be made (Box 13-3).

Before the administration of rt-PA, two peripheral IV lines are inserted—one for the administration of rt-PA and one for fluids. Any catheters that are needed (e.g., urinary catheters, nasogastric tubes) are ideally placed before the administration of rt-PA to reduce the risk for bleeding. After the administration of rt-PA, invasive procedures may be performed; however, the risk of bleeding is higher. Anticoagulants, such as heparin or warfarin, and antiplatelet aggregates, such as aspirin, are withheld for 24 hours after administration of rt-PA to prevent bleeding complications.

Symptomatic hemorrhage is the most common complication after rt-PA administration, with an incidence of 6.4%.[20] The highest risk for hemorrhage is within the first 36 hours after administration. Hemorrhage usually occurs into the area of infarct; this is known as hemorrhagic transformation (HT). The incidence of HT may be reduced by ensuring rt-PA is given within 3 hours of symptom onset and maintaining the systolic BP at less than 185 mm Hg and the diastolic BP at less than 110 mm Hg. Antihypertensive agents are administered as needed to control the BP.

Signs and symptoms of intracerebral hemorrhage manifest as neurological deterioration, increased ICP, or cerebral herniation. If intracerebral hemorrhage is suspected, the rt-PA infusion is stopped, an emergency noncontrast CT scan of the head is obtained, and fresh frozen plasma or platelets are administered. Systemic bleeding can also occur. Signs and symptoms include hypotension, tachycardia, pallor, restlessness, or low back pain. Stool, urine, and gastric secretions are monitored for the presence of blood. IV sites and gums are monitored for signs of external bleeding. Baseline coagulation studies are compared with current studies.

Neurological assessment (LOC, language, motor and sensory testing, pupillary response) and vital signs are performed every 15 minutes for the first 2 hours, every 30 minutes for the next 6 hours, and every hour for 16 hours. Accurate intake and output are maintained. Continuous cardiac monitoring is done throughout the hyperacute phase (first 24 to 72 hours). Oxygen is given to maintain the SpO_2 at 95%. Pneumonia is a common complication after stroke; therefore frequent patient repositioning and nebulizer therapy may be indicated.[20]

Nonthrombolytic candidates. For a patient with stroke who is a not a candidate for thrombolytic therapy, interventions include neurological, respiratory, and cardiac assessments.

BOX 13-3 ADMINISTRATION OF TISSUE PLASMINOGEN ACTIVATOR FOR ACUTE ISCHEMIC STROKE

Inclusion Criteria
- Onset of stroke symptoms <3 hours
- Clinical diagnosis of ischemic stroke with a measurable deficit using the NIHSS
- Age >18 years
- CT scan consistent with ischemic stroke

Exclusion Criteria
- Stroke symptoms >3 hours of symptoms onset
- Rapidly improving minor or major stroke (i.e., transient ischemic attack)
- Evidence of intracerebral bleed including intraparenchymal subarachnoid hemorrhage or other pathological condition (neoplasm, AVM, or aneurysm on CT scan)
- Systolic BP >185 mm Hg or diastolic BP >110 mm Hg
- Glucose <50 mg/dL or >400 mg/dL
- Rapidly improving or deteriorating neurological signs or minor symptoms
- Recent myocardial infarction
- Seizure at the onset of stroke
- Active internal bleeding (e.g., urinary) within 21 days
- Arterial puncture at noncompressible site
- Known bleeding diathesis, including but not limited to:
  a. Current use of oral anticoagulants (e.g., warfarin) with prothrombin time of >15 seconds
  b. Administration of heparin within 48 hours preceding the onset of stroke and have an elevated aPTT at presentation
  c. Platelet count <100,000/microliter
- Lumbar puncture within 7 days; major surgery within 14 days

Administration
- rt-PA dosing: 0.9 mg/kg intravenously up to maximum of 90 mg
- Give bolus of 10% of total calculated dose intravenously over 1 minute
- Administer the remaining 90% over the next 60 minutes

aPTT, Activated partial thromboplastin time; *AVM,* arteriovenous malformation; *BP,* blood pressure; *CT,* computed tomography; *NIHSS,* National Institutes of Health Stroke Scale; *rt-PA,* recombinant tissue plasminogen activator.
Modified from the National Institute of Neurological Disorders and Stroke (NINDS) t-PA Stroke Study Group. (1995). Tissue plasminogen activator for acute ischemic stroke. *New England Journal of Medicine,* 333, 1581-1587; Activase (alteplase), Genentech, Inc., South San Francisco, CA, package insert.

These assessments and vital signs are performed every 1 to 2 hours during the first 24 hours after stroke. BP is controlled to prevent bleeding while maintaining an adequate CPP. For patients with uncontrolled hypertension, BP is managed carefully with IV medications including labetalol, nitroprusside, or nicardipine. Rapid drops in BP can cause further neurological deterioration by decreasing cerebral perfusion and extending the area of cerebral ischemia. Laboratory tests (complete blood count, chemistries, urinalysis, coagulations studies, cardiac enzymes) are performed to identify causes of the stroke.

Other interventions include the administration of medications to decrease ICP and maintenance of hemodynamic stability. The incidence of cerebral herniation peaks at about 72 hours after the stroke. Since hyperglycemia may exacerbate the extent of neurological injury, glycemic control is advocated (see Chapter 18). Hyponatremia due to cerebral salt wasting may occur; sodium and fluid replacement are necessary to maintain a normal sodium level.

Anticoagulants, such as warfarin, or antiplatelet aggregates, such as aspirin, combination aspirin/dipyridamole (Aggrenox), clopidogrel (Plavix), prasugrel (Effient), and ticagrelor (Brilinta) may be given for prevention of secondary stroke. Some patients require antihypertensive agents or antiepileptic medications. Maintaining adequate fluid balance is crucial to ensure proper hydration. Maintaining normothermia is important to reduce the metabolic needs of the brain. Hyperthermia may be the result of direct injury or bleeding into the hypothalamus, systemic infection, or drug-induced fever from antiepileptic medications. Aspiration precautions are implemented including elevating the head of the bed and maintaining nothing-by-mouth status until a swallow screening or formal study rules out dysphagia.

Other Ischemic Events

Transient ischemic attacks. A *transient ischemic attack* (TIA) is defined as the sudden onset of a temporary focal neurological deficit caused by a vascular event. During a TIA, a transient decrease in CBF occurs, but the patient does not experience any permanent deficits.

A TIA is commonly caused by stenosis of the carotid arteries. A common presentation of a TIA is amaurosis fugax (monocular blindness), a transient occlusion of the central retinal artery. Although symptoms of a TIA mimic those of stroke, by definition TIA symptoms last 24 hours or less.[20] Generally, patients with symptoms of TIA should receive a complete stroke workup to determine the cause of TIA. Patients may be managed with anticoagulants or antiplatelet therapy depending on the etiology of the symptoms.

It is important that persons with TIAs have preventive measures initiated to avoid stroke. Unfortunately, persons experiencing a TIA often ignore the symptoms because the symptoms are painless and short-lived, usually about 5 to 10 minutes. Within a year of having a TIA, many persons have a stroke and sustain permanent neurological deficits.

Patients experiencing TIAs with carotid stenosis are evaluated for carotid endarterectomy or carotid angioplasty and stenting. If a patient has carotid stenosis greater than 69% on the symptomatic side, carotid endarterectomy is recommended. Carotid angioplasty with stenting is also an accepted method of treating carotid stenosis for selected patients.

Hemorrhagic Stroke

Intraparenchymal stroke. Control of BP is important to prevent recurrent hemorrhage. The optimum threshold for BP is unknown. Elevations in BP are not usually treated unless the MAP is greater than 130 mm Hg, or the patient has a history of heart failure. If treatment is required, BP is lowered cautiously to prehemorrhage levels. Control of BP is important to prevent continued bleeding. Recombinant factor VIIa may be used to prevent extension of the hemorrhage, but is only effective if used within 6 hours of onset.

Medical assessment focuses on determining the size and location of the intracranial hemorrhage, and whether it is amenable to surgical intervention. Small clots usually resolve without surgery. In these instances, more aggressive BP management may be indicated. Surgery is considered in patients with hematomas larger than 3 cm or who are deteriorating neurologically, although the role of surgical intervention is controversial.[23] Comatose patients with large lesions usually have poorer outcomes, regardless of treatment.[16,20]

Subarachnoid Hemorrhage

Early diagnosis of the cause of SAH helps to guide treatment. Although a CT scan helps differentiate an aneurysm from an AVM, definitive diagnosis of an aneurysm is determined by digital subtraction or CT angiography. Early surgical or endovascular intervention (within 24 hours of admission) is recommended for patients in good neurological condition whose aneurysm is accessible by surgical or endovascular approaches. The goal is to secure the aneurysm before any episodes of rebleeding or vasospasm occur.[4]

Surgery for a cerebral aneurysm involves occluding the neck of the aneurysm with a metal clip; reinforcing the sac by wrapping the sac with muscle, fibrin foam, or solidifying polymer; or proximally ligating a feeding vessel. If the neck of the aneurysm is narrow and accessible, using a metal clip is desirable. When the neck of the aneurysm is too broad, reinforcing the aneurysmal sac is the goal of surgery. Proximal ligation may be preferred when the aneurysm is directly fed by the internal carotid artery. The disadvantage of this procedure is the potential for stroke should collateral circulation fail.

Interventional techniques such as endovascular therapy with coils or stents may be used to occlude the aneurysm. This therapy consists of navigating a microcatheter through the femoral artery to the aneurysm and placing platinum coils into the aneurysm sac or a stent to cover the opening. Thrombosis occurs, thus occluding the aneurysm from the feeder vessel. Both surgery and endovascular obliteration may be used for ruptured or unruptured aneurysms.

Patients with severe neurological compromise after a ruptured aneurysm may benefit from emergency ventriculostomy. The ventriculostomy assists in treating the hydrocephalus associated with the bleeding. The ventriculostomy also allows the clinician to monitor ICP and remove CSF to lower ICP if needed. However, where possible, ventriculostomy is not performed until after the aneurusym has been secured, because changing the ICP can contribute to rebleeding.

Management of BP is an important treatment of aneurysmal SAH.[4] Medications are administered to reduce BP before the aneurysm is secured to prevent rebleeding. After securing the aneurysm, blood pressure is allowed to rise to prevent vasospasm. If vasospasm occurs, blood pressure may be purposely increased with fluids and medications to augment CBF. Neurological status is assessed frequently by using the GCS and monitoring for focal deficits and pupillary changes. Temperature monitoring is important because persons with SAH often have a fever, which is associated with worse neurological outcome.[4] Elevation of the head of the bed may reduce ICP. A feeding tube may be required for nutritional support. Measures for venous thromboembolism prevention are initiated. Other important interventions include providing analgesia and bed rest.

Monitoring for signs of vasospasm is of paramount importance because early intervention results in better patient outcomes. Nimodipine, a neurospecific calcium channel blocker, reduces the incidence and severity of deficits associated with SAH.[4] The recommended dosage is 60 mg every 4 hours for 21 days. Vasospasm is often treated with volume expansion to increase CPP. The modalities used are hypervolemia and hypertension. Hypervolemia refers to increasing the blood volume by using crystalloids, colloids, albumin, plasma protein fraction, or blood. Systolic BP is maintained between 150 and 160 mm Hg (and sometimes higher). The increase in volume and BP forces blood through the vasospastic area at higher pressures. If the patient's BP cannot be maintained at the increased levels required, vasoactive infusions, such as dopamine, dobutamine, or phenylephrine (Neo-Synephrine), may be warranted.

Therapies for the treatment of symptomatic vasospasm include papaverine, nicardipine, and angioplasty. Intraarterial papaverine application increases the diameter of the vasospastic blood vessel and lasts less than 24 hours. Intraarterial administration of nicardipine (Cardene) is another option for treating vasospasm. Nicardipine, a calcium channel blocker, has a vasodilatory effect. The clinical indications for intraarterial nicardipine are similar to those for papaverine; however, nicardipine is effective for 2 to 5 days. Cerebral angioplasty is indicated for vasospasm when pharmacological therapy has failed. Risks of angioplasty include perforation or rupture, cerebral artery thrombosis, recurrent vasospasm, and transient neurological deficits.

Arteriovenous Malformation

Spontaneous bleeding from an AVM can occur into the ventricular system, intraparenchymal tissue, or subarachnoid space. Hemorrhage from an AVM is usually low-pressure bleeding, and the mortality from such a hemorrhage is lower than that from a ruptured aneurysm. The rebleeding rate is also much lower than that of an aneurysm. AVMs may also cause symptoms due to ischemia or act as a space-occupying lesion, similar to a tumor.

Treatment interventions for an AVM include embolization, surgery, radiotherapy, or a combination of all three. Surgery for removal of an AVM is done either as a single step or in multiple stages. Postoperatively, the major problem is breakthrough bleeding from cauterized vessels. Rapid increases in BP during recovery from anesthesia are to be avoided, and blood pressure must be tightly controlled for the first 48 hours after resection to prevent bleeding. Embolization is not a curative approach to the majority of AVMs, but rather is used as preparation for surgery. Embolization may occur in a single setting or may be staged in several procedures over days to weeks. Radiotherapy may be performed alone or for residual AVM after surgery; results are manifest over years.

Postoperative Neurosurgical Care

The postoperative care of a patient who has undergone a neurosurgical procedure involves frequent and ongoing hemodynamic, respiratory, metabolic, and neurological assessments. Neurological assessments are done every 15 to 30 minutes for the first 2 to 12 hours postoperatively, then every hour while the patient is in the critical care unit. Oxygenation and tissue perfusion are monitored. Chest x-rays, CT scans, EEGs, and other diagnostic tests may be necessary to monitor progress.

The position of the head of the bed depends on the specific surgical procedure, patient condition, and physician preference. Unless the patient is intubated, unconscious patients are never positioned flat because the tongue can slip backward and obstruct the airway. However, unconscious patients may be positioned in a lateral position with the head of the bed flat. The neck must always be maintained in a neutral position.

The most common postoperative complications include infection, cerebral hemorrhage, increased ICP, hydrocephalus, and seizures.[3] Intracerebral hemorrhage is detected by a decline in neurological status, signs of increasing ICP, and new or worsened focal deficits (i.e., hemiparesis/hemiplegia, aphasia). It is confirmed by CT scan. Treatment depends on CT findings and may require emergency surgery.

Hydrocephalus can develop any time during the postoperative course as a result of edema or bleeding into the subarachnoid space. Treatment may include placement of a ventriculostomy to drain CSF temporarily. If the hydrocephalus does not resolve, a surgical shunting procedure may be indicated to relieve the brain of excessive CSF.

Seizures can occur at any time but are most common within the first 7 days after surgery. Focal seizures in the form of twitching of selected muscles, particularly of the face and hand, are often seen. Patients may receive postoperative antiepileptic drugs, most commonly phenytoin, if concern for seizures is high. Serum phenytoin levels are monitored to maintain a therapeutic range.

SEIZURES AND STATUS EPILEPTICUS

A seizure is an abnormal electrical discharge in the brain caused by a variety of neurological disorders, systemic diseases, and metabolic disorders. Seizures consist of repetitive depolarization of hyperactive, hypersensitive cells that cause an altered state of brain function. Seizures are classified as either partial or generalized (Table 13-11). *Partial seizures* usually begin in one cerebral hemisphere and cause motor activity to be localized to one area of the body (e.g., arm, face). The seizure is classified as *simple partial* if consciousness remains intact, and *complex partial* if consciousness is impaired. *Generalized seizures* involve both cerebral hemispheres and cause altered consciousness and bilateral motor manifestations.

Pathophysiology of Status Epilepticus

When seizures occur in close proximity to each other, they have the potential to lead to a life-threatening medical emergency known as *status epilepticus* (SE). SE can occur with any type of seizure. By definition, SE is present when seizure activity lasts for 30 minutes or longer, or when two or more sequential seizures occur without full recovery of consciousness between seizures.[26] SE is more likely to occur with tonic-clonic seizures that have a specific causative factor than with idiopathic seizures. The most frequent precipitating factors for SE are irregular intake of antiepileptic drugs, withdrawal from habitual use of alcohol or sedative drugs, electrolyte imbalance, azotemia, head trauma, infection, and brain tumor.

Physiological changes that occur during SE are divided into two phases. During *phase 1*, cerebral metabolism is increased and compensatory mechanisms (increased CBF and catecholamine release) prevent cerebral damage from hypoxia or metabolic injury. However, these changes can lead to other problems. Hyperglycemia occurs from release of epinephrine and activation of hepatic gluconeogenesis. Hypertension occurs due to increase CBF. Hyperpyrexia results from excessive muscle activity and catecholamine release. Lactic acidosis occurs from anaerobic metabolism. Elevated epinephrine and norepinephrine levels and acidosis contribute to cardiac dysrhythmias. Autonomic dysfunction causes excessive sweating and vomiting, leading to dehydration and electrolyte loss.

Phase 2 begins 30 to 60 minutes after phase 1. Decompensation occurs because the increased metabolic demands cannot be met. This causes decreased CBF, systemic hypotension, increased ICP, and failure of cerebral autoregulation. The patient develops metabolic and respiratory acidosis from hypoxemia, and hypoglycemia from depleted energy stores. The lack of oxygen and glucose results in cellular injury. Pulmonary edema is common, and aspiration can occur from decreased laryngeal reflex sensitivity. Cardiac dysrhythmias and heart failure result from hypoxemia, hyperkalemia caused by increased muscle activity, and metabolic acidosis. Acute kidney injury may result from rhabdomyolysis and acute myoglobinuria. Myoglobin is released secondary to excessive muscle activity from prolonged skeletal muscle contraction and traumatic injury during the seizure.

Death from SE is more likely to occur when an underlying disease is responsible for the seizure, or from the acute illness that precipitated the seizure. Generalized seizures that last for 30 to 45 minutes can result in neuronal necrosis and permanent neurological deficits. Prompt diagnosis and treatment are

TABLE 13-11	CLASSIFICATION OF SEIZURES
TYPE	**SYMPTOMS**
I. Partial Simple (no loss of consciousness) Motor	"Jacksonian" march Movement of eye, head, and body to one side Stopping of movement or speech
Sensory or somatosensory	Tingling, numbness of body part Visual, auditory, olfactory, or taste sensations Dizzy spells
Autonomic	Pallor, sweating, flushing, piloerection, pupillary dilation
Psychic	Déjà vu ("already seen") Distortion of time sense Hallucinations Objects appearing small, large, or far away
Complex (alteration of consciousness); automatisms	Automatisms (lip smacking, picking with hands), wandering

II. Generalized
Absence
  Simple
  Atypical
	
	Staring spell lasting less than 15 seconds
	Staring spell with myoclonic jerks and automatisms

Myoclonic	Brief jerk of one or more muscle groups
Clonic	Repetitive jerking of muscle groups
Tonic	Stiffening of muscle groups
Tonic-clonic	Starts with the stiffening or tonic phase, followed by the jerking or clonic phase Unconsciousness Tongue biting Bowel and bladder incontinence
Atonic	Drop attack or abrupt loss of muscle tone

Modified from Barker, E. (2008). *Neuroscience Nursing: A Spectrum of Care* (3rd ed). St. Louis: Mosby.

important because seizure duration is an important prognostic factor.

Assessment

Assessment during SE incorporates the neurological, respiratory, and cardiovascular systems. Characteristics of the seizure and the neurological state before, between, and after seizures are important to monitor. Information to collect includes precipitating factors, preceding aura, type of movement observed, automatisms, changes in size of pupils or eye deviation, responsiveness to auditory or tactile stimuli, LOC throughout the seizure, urinary or bowel incontinence, behavior after the seizure, weakness or paralysis of extremities after the seizure, injuries caused by the seizure, and duration of the seizure.[3] Assessment of respirations and monitoring of SpO$_2$ are needed to ensure adequate oxygenation. Because decompensation can result in pulmonary edema, it is imperative to observe for the onset of fine basilar crackles. Suction equipment and oxygen should be readily available. Cardiac monitoring is necessary to assess for dysrhythmias. Hypoglycemia is an important cause of SE.

Bedside assessment of blood glucose is imperative in the initial assessment.

Diagnostic Tests

Laboratory studies for a patient with SE include serum electrolytes, liver function studies, serum medication levels, and blood and urine toxicology screens. Cardiac enzymes and arterial blood gases assist in assessing the effect of the seizure on other body systems. Patient monitoring includes ECG, EEG, noninvasive BP, and pulse oximetry.

Radiological studies are performed to rule out pathology that may be responsible for the episode of SE. These may include CT or MRI with contrast, or additional studies.

Management
Nursing Diagnoses

Nursing diagnoses that are relevant to the patient experiencing SE are as follows: ineffective tissue perfusion (cerebral and cardiopulmonary) related to continuous seizure activity or effects of antiepileptic medications; ineffective breathing pattern or impaired gas exchange related to hypoventilation; ineffective airway clearance related to underlying neurological problem and seizure activity; risk for trauma (oral and musculoskeletal) related to seizure activity; disturbed thought processes related to the postictal state; and deficient knowledge related to disease process, treatment, and necessary lifestyle changes.

Nursing and Medical Interventions

Management during SE includes maintaining a patent airway, providing adequate oxygenation, maintaining vascular access for the administration of medications and fluids, administering appropriate medications, and maintaining seizure precautions. A patent airway is facilitated by positioning appropriately; use of an oral/nasal airway or endotracheal tube may be necessary. Padded tongue blades are not to be inserted between the clenched teeth of a patient undergoing a seizure. Patients have inadvertently been injured from aspirating teeth that were loosened during forceful attempts to insert a padded tongue blade between their teeth. Suctioning is often needed to remove secretions that collect in the oropharynx. Supplemental oxygen is administered to improve oxygenation. Neuromuscular blocking agents may be used to facilitate intubation but will not be effective in halting neuronal firing; attention to seizure control is necessary, even when the patient is paralyzed. A nasogastric tube with intermittent suction may be needed to ensure that the airway is not compromised by aspiration.

Vascular access must be maintained to provide a route for the administration of medication. If unable to establish IV access, some antiepileptic medications can be administered rectally. The specific medication given to arrest the seizure depends on the type and duration of the seizure (see Table 13-9). It is essential to monitor BP and to administer volume replacement and vasoactive drugs if necessary. IV dextrose is administered unless the blood glucose level is known to be normal or high. Thiamine may also be given.

Seizure precautions are continued during SE. This includes padding the side rails on the patient's bed and making sure that the bed has full-length side rails. The bed is kept in a low position with side rails up, except when providing direct nursing care. If the patient is in a chair when a seizure begins, the patient is lowered to the floor and a soft object is placed under the patient's head. It is important to remove the patient's restrictive clothing and jewelry while always maintaining the patient's privacy. The patient should not be restrained because forceful tonic-clonic movements can traumatize the patient.

SE must be treated immediately. The nurse ensures a patent airway and maintains breathing and circulation. Medications are given using a sequential approach that progressively uses more potent medications to control the seizure. The first-line medication is a benzodiazepine, usually IV lorazepam (Ativan). If lorazepam fails to stop seizure activity within 10 minutes, or if intermittent seizures persist for longer than 20 minutes, phenytoin (Dilantin) or fosphenytoin (Cerebyx) may be administered.[26] Phenytoin is mixed only with normal saline, and it is stable in solution for only 20 minutes, thus making it impractical for IV piggyback administration. It may

be given slowly by IV push (25 to 50 mg/min, not to exceed 50 mg/min) after clearing the line with saline. Phenobarbital may be used as the an additional agent to control SE, but its utility in SE is lessened by the length of time required to achieve a therapeutic effect. Other drugs that have been used in SE include midazolam, pentobarbital, thiopental, propofol, and valproic acid.[26]

If SE continues despite phenytoin administration, propofol (Diprivan) is given. Propofol is a general anesthetic and sedative-hypnotic agent. Patients may require intubation and mechanical ventilation because inefficient ventilation may result. Pentobarbital may also be considered. Patients must be assessed for hypotension.

CENTRAL NERVOUS SYSTEM INFECTIONS

The brain and spinal cord are relatively well protected from infective agents by the bones of the skull and vertebral column, the meninges, and the blood-brain barrier. However, infective agents can enter the CNS through the air sinuses, middle ear, or blood. Penetrating injuries that disrupt the dura (e.g., basilar skull fractures, missile injuries, neurosurgical procedures) also increase the risk for infection. *Meningitis* (infection of the meninges) may be caused by bacteria, viruses, fungi, parasites, or other toxins. These infections are classified as acute, subacute, or chronic. The pathophysiology, clinical presentation, and management differ for each type of microorganism. Box 13-4 lists common organisms that cause meningitis.

Bacterial Meningitis

Bacterial meningitis is a neurological emergency and can lead to substantial morbidity and mortality.[6,17] Approximately

---

BOX 13-4 CAUSES OF MENINGITIS

Bacterial
- *Streptococcus pneumoniae* (pneumococcus)
- *Neisseria meningitidis* (meningococcus)
- *Haemophilus influenzae type B* (Hib)
- Staphylococci (*Staphylococcus aureus*)
- Gram-negative bacilli (*Escherichia coli, Enterobacter, Serratia*)

Viruses
- Echovirus
- Coxsackievirus
- Mumps
- Herpes simplex types 1 and 2
- St. Louis encephalitis
- Colorado tick fever
- Epstein-Barr
- West Nile
- Influenza types A and B

Fungal
- Histoplasmosis
- Candidiasis
- Aspergillosis

3000 cases occur in the United States each year, and more than 300 people die, with a significant fatality rate in adolescents.[17] Meningitis affects the very young, the very old, and immunosuppressed individuals. Because of its high mortality, vaccination against bacterial meningitis is recommended.

Pathophysiology

Bacterial meningitis is an infection of the pia mater and arachnoid layers of the meninges, and the CSF in the subarachnoid space. Bacteria gain access in one of three ways: (1) via the blood or through the spread of nearby infection, such as sinusitis; (2) CSF contamination through surgical procedures or catheters; or (3) through the skull. Airborne droplets passed from infected individuals through sneezing, coughing, or kissing, or droplets passed along through saliva and transmitted via drinks, cigarettes, or utensils, can occur. Bacteria enter through the choroid plexuses, multiply in the subarachnoid space, and irritate the meninges. An exudate forms that thickens the CSF and alters CSF flow through and around the brain and spinal cord, resulting in obstruction, interstitial edema, and further inflammation.

Assessment

The clinical assessment of adults with bacterial meningitis requires a thorough history and neurological assessment. Patients often are seen in the ED with an acute onset of symptoms (e.g., headache, fever, stiff neck, vomiting) that developed over 1 to 2 days. There may be a recent history of infection (ear, sinus, or upper respiratory), foreign travel, or illicit drug use. The clinical presentation often reveals signs of systemic infection including fever (temperature as high as 39.5° C), tachycardia, chills, and petechial rash. Initially the rash may be macular, but it progresses to petechiae and purpura, mainly on the trunk and extremities. Meningeal irritation produces a throbbing headache, photophobia, vomiting, and nuchal rigidity. A positive *Kernig sign* (pain in the neck when the thigh is flexed on the abdomen and the leg extended at the knee) and a positive *Brudzinski sign* (involuntary flexion of the hips when the neck is flexed toward the chest) may be present. The patient's condition can quickly deteriorate to hypotension, shock, and sepsis.

Assessment of the patient's LOC, motor response, and cranial nerves is performed. Confusion and decreasing LOC are evidence of cortical involvement. Focal neurological deficits may be seen including hemiparesis, hemiplegia, and ataxia as well as seizure activity and projectile vomiting. Irritation and damage to cranial nerves occur as a result of inflamed sheaths. As ICP increases, unconsciousness may occur.

Diagnostic Tests

The gold standard for the diagnosis of meningitis is examination of CSF, which may be obtained via lumbar puncture, or aspiration from a ventricular catheter. Diagnosis is also based on a nasopharyngeal smear and antigen tests. Blood and urine cultures are obtained before starting antibiotics. A CT scan, MRI, or both, may be beneficial in diagnosing bacterial meningitis to exclude other neurological pathological conditions such as cerebral edema, hydrocephalus, fractures, inner ear infection, or mastoiditis. However, scanning should not delay the lumbar puncture procedure if the patient has significant neurological deficits.[17]

Management

Nursing diagnoses. The following nursing diagnoses may be applicable to a patient with a CNS infection including bacterial meningitis: infection related to presence of bacteria, virus, or fungus within the CNS; risk for injury (seizures) related to cerebral irritation, focal edema, and/or inflammation; risk for ineffective cerebral tissue perfusion related to cerebral edema, increased ICP, and/or hydrocephalus; and acute pain related to meningeal irritation, increased ICP, or both.

Nursing and medical management. Antibiotics are started as soon as possible once the diagnosis is suspected because of the rapid progression of the disease process.[17] After administration of antibiotic therapy, the search begins for the offending organism based on patient history, physical examination, CSF cultures, and blood cultures. Droplet isolation is maintained for 24 hours after the initiation of antibiotic therapy. Unusual bacteria or other microorganisms are increasingly responsible for meningitis. Identification of the offending organism(s) may take time; final culture results may redirect treatment.

During the acute phase of bacterial meningitis, the patient requires close monitoring. Increased ICP may occur, requiring administration of mannitol or hypertonic saline, placement of a ventriculostomy catheter to drain CSF, or both. Patients are maintained on bed rest with the head of the bed elevated 30 to 40 degrees. IV antibiotic therapy is continued to treat the specific organism identified. IV corticosteroids may reduce mortality, hearing loss, and neurological sequelae in bacterial meningitis by decreasing meningeal inflammation.[6] Current practice guidelines recommend that dexamethasone (Decadron) 10 mg be initiated before or with the

Droplet Precautions for Meningitis

Haemophilus influenzae type B and *Neisseria meningitidis* are common bacteria that cause meningitis. These bacteria are easily spread by droplets generated by coughing, sneezing, or talking, or during invasive respiratory procedures. Any patient with suspected meningitis should be placed on droplet precautions. Once these bacteria are ruled out as the source of infection, or when 24 hours of effective antibiotic therapy has been instituted, droplet precautions may be discontinued.

ASSESSMENT	SIGNIFICANCE
Presence of fever, cough, meningeal signs	Provides evidence of active infection
Duration of antibiotic therapy specific to organism	Confirms adequacy of treatment before discontinuation of precautions
Visitor use of appropriate droplet precautions	Prevents spread from individuals who may be carriers or have been exposed before patient's hospitalization

first dose of antibiotics, and then every 6 hours for 4 days in adult patients with suspected bacterial meningitis.[6,17]

Patients are placed in a private room, and the lighting is dimmed. Seizure precautions are implemented. Fever is managed with antipyretics and cooling devices. As the acute inflammatory period subsides, the patient continues to require close monitoring to prevent secondary complications. These include seizures, increased ICP, syndrome of inappropriate antidiuretic hormone secretion, cerebral infarction, gastric bleeding, venous thromboembolism, pneumonia, and sepsis.

SPINAL CORD INJURY

Approximately 200,000 people in the United States are living with SCI. Each year, about 11,000 additional individuals sustain SCI. Most SCIs occur in individuals between the ages of 16 and 30 years.[10] The most common causes of SCI are motor vehicle crashes, falls, acts of violence (primarily gunshot wounds), sports injuries, and diving accidents.[10] TBI often occurs with SCI; therefore SCI should be considered a possibility in all unconscious patients.[21] Providing emergency intervention at the scene by skilled providers, decreasing transport time to the hospital, and implementing evidence-based SCI guidelines improve a patient's outcome.

Pathophysiology

SCI occurs with or without associated vertebral injury, resulting in complex and multifaceted biochemical changes in the spinal cord. An inflammatory reaction creates spinal cord edema, which compresses tissue as well as blood vessels. Cord edema can ascend or descend from the level of injury. Vascular changes also occur. Microscopic hemorrhages occur in the central gray matter of the spinal cord with extension into surrounding white matter. Hemorrhage exacerbates edema and further decreases blood flow, resulting in ischemia. If the ischemia is not reversed, axonal degeneration and conduction failure of the neurons occur. Eventually, cell death occurs with permanent loss of function (Figure 13-20).

SCI produces two types of shock. *Spinal shock* is an electrical silence of the cord below the level of injury that causes complete loss of motor, sensory, and reflex activity. It begins within minutes of an injury and lasts for 4 to 6 weeks. Often the permanence of injury is not known until spinal shock resolves. Resolution is signalled by return of deep tendon reflexes; rarely, motor or sensory function may return. *Neurogenic shock* occurs from disruption of autonomic pathways, resulting in temporary loss of autonomic function below the level of the injury. Sympathetic input is lost, causing vasodilation and distributive shock, which manifests as hypotension, bradycardia, and hypothermia. Bradycardia may be so severe that a temporary pacemaker is required. Duration of neurogenic shock is variable; resolution is signaled by return of sympathetic tone.

SCI can result in a complete or incomplete lesion (Figure 13-21). A *complete lesion* causes total, permanent loss of motor and sensory function below the level of injury. An incomplete lesion is more common and results in the sparing of some motor and sensory function below the level of injury. The three types of *incomplete lesions* are *central cord, anterior cord,* and *Brown-Séquard* syndromes. The clinical presentation of each syndrome is based on damage to spinal cord organization and crossing of tracts. Most patients with an incomplete lesion show a mixed pattern of motor and sensory function and have a potential for at least partial recovery.

Assessment
Airway and Respiratory Assessment

Assessment of respiratory and neurological status is the first assessment priority. Respiratory problems are common with cervical and thoracic SCI. Ineffective breathing patterns are caused by paralysis of the diaphragm or intercostal muscles, or both. Baseline arterial blood gases are obtained on admission. Ongoing assessment of the adequacy of the airway and ventilation, including continuous monitoring of SpO_2, is

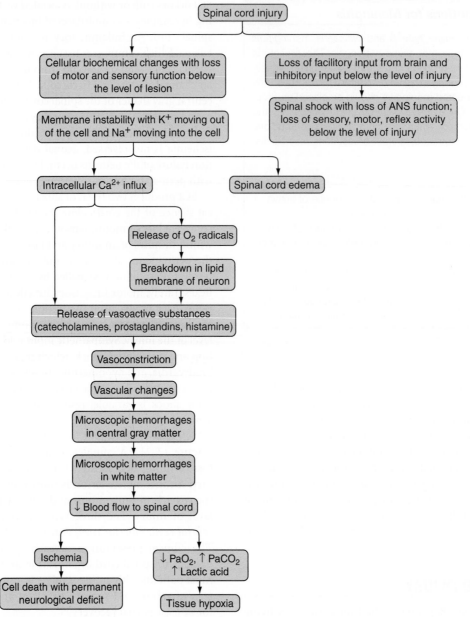

FIGURE 13-20 Pathophysiology flow diagram for spinal cord injury. *ANS*, Autonomic nervous system; *Ca²⁺*, calcium; *K⁺*, potassium; *Na⁺*, sodium; *O₂*, oxygen; *PaCO₂*, partial pressure of carbon dioxide in arterial blood; *PaO₂*, partial pressure of oxygen in arterial blood.

essential. Emergent treatment, including endotracheal intubation and mechanical ventilation, may be needed.

Respiratory impairment varies with the level and type of injury (complete or incomplete). Complete lesions are associated with the following:

C1-C3: ventilator dependency

C4-C5: phrenic nerve impairment that may be treated with a phrenic nerve pacemaker

Cervical injury below C5-T6: intact diaphragmatic breathing, with varying impairment of intercostal and abdominal muscle function

Those with incomplete spinal cord lesions present with varying degrees of respiratory impairment, depending on the level of the lesion and whether the respiratory muscles are impaired.

Neurological Assessment

All components of the neurological examination are performed on the patient with an SCI, with an emphasis on the motor, reflex, and sensory responses. An assessment of the major muscle groups (see Table 13-4) and sensory level (see Figure 13-6) is completed to determine the level of injury.

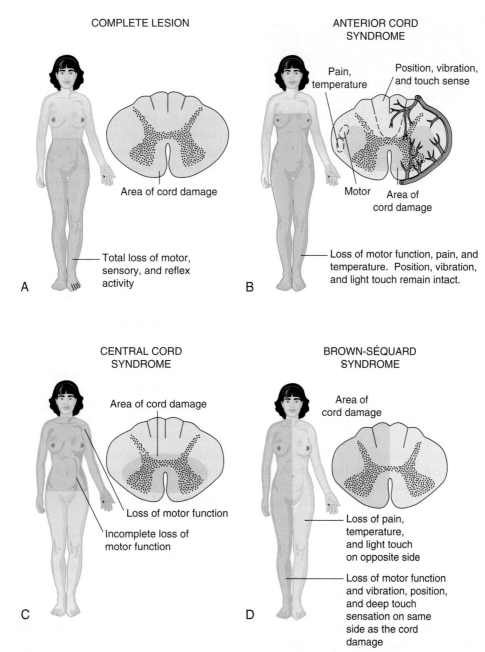

COMPLETE LESION

Area of cord damage

Total loss of motor, sensory, and reflex activity

A

ANTERIOR CORD SYNDROME

Pain, temperature

Position, vibration, and touch sense

Motor   Area of cord damage

Loss of motor function, pain, and temperature. Position, vibration, and light touch remain intact.

B

CENTRAL CORD SYNDROME

Area of cord damage

Loss of motor function

Incomplete loss of motor function

C

BROWN-SÉQUARD SYNDROME

Area of cord damage

Loss of pain, temperature, and light touch on opposite side

Loss of motor function and vibration, position, and deep touch sensation on same side as the cord damage

D

FIGURE 13-21 Common spinal cord syndromes. **A,** Complete lesion. **B,** Anterior cord syndrome. **C,** Central cord syndrome. **D,** Brown-Sequard syndrome. (Modified from Ignatavicius DD, Workman ML. *Medical-surgical Nursing: Patient-centered Collaborative Care.* 6th ed. Philadelphia: Saunders; 2010.)

Components of the hourly assessment for an SCI patient are reviewed in Table 13-12.

A patient with neurogenic shock (injury at T6 and above) is unable to regulate body temperature; body temperature accommodates to the environmental temperature. The inability to adequately autoregulate body temperature is called *poikilothermia.* Temperature should be closely monitored, and the patient should be kept warm with blankets at an appropriate room temperature to avoid hypothermia. Hyperthermia can occur quickly if the patient is excessively warmed.

Hemodynamic Assessment

Patients with an SCI are managed in a critical care unit for the first 7 to 14 days after injury to allow early detection and management of hemodynamic instability.[1,5] Decreases in heart rate may be associated with hypothermia and hypoxemia as well as neurogenic shock. Venous stasis occurs as a result of loss of vasomotor tone and paralysis, increasing the risk of venous thromboembolism.

TABLE 13-12 COMPONENTS OF THE HOURLY NEUROLOGICAL ASSESSMENT FOR PATIENTS WITH ACUTE SPINAL CORD INJURY

MOTOR	SENSATION
Respirations—rate, rhythm, effort	Pinprick (sharp, dull) all surfaces of body
Movement/strength bilaterally	Position sense
Shrug shoulders	Temperature all surfaces of body
Elbow flexion	
Elbow extension	
Bending wrists	
Touch thumb to index finger	
Hand grasp	
Lift leg off the bed	
Bend knee	
Extend knee	
Pull feet up	
Push feet down	

Bowel and Bladder Function

Spinal shock results in atony of the bowel and bladder. The bladder does not contract, and the detrusor muscle does not open. Urinary retention occurs and an indwelling urinary catheter is required to prevent damage to the bladder wall. Loss of peristaltic movement increases the risk of paralytic ileus. The patient may require gastrointestinal decompression and is assessed for return of bowel sounds, flatus, and bowel movement. A bowel program is initiated as soon as bowel sounds are present.

Skin Assessment

Because of impaired circulation and immobility, the patient with SCI is at risk of skin breakdown. A complete assessment of all skin surfaces is done every 4 hours. If halo traction or cervical tongs is used to stabilize a cervical fracture, the skin around pin sites and under traction devices is carefully inspected. Assessment includes observing the site for redness, swelling, drainage, and pain. If a cervical collar is in place, skin integrity is assessed with an emphasis on pressure points (occipital, chin, and sternal regions).

Psychological Assessment

A psychological assessment is important during the acute phase of SCI. Initially, the patient is concerned with surviving the injury and does not realize the extent of injury or disability. The patient's perceptions are also impaired by medications and the physiological effects of injury. Patients often experience denial, anger, and depression. As the patient gains insight into the situation, it is important for the nurse to include the patient in care planning and to give the patient choices, because feelings of powerlessness are common.

Family members also go through a similar experience. First they experience shock related to the injury itself and the seriousness of the patient's condition. During this time, family members need support and answers to their questions.[3] Consultation with a psychiatric or mental health nurse or a psychiatrist may be indicated.[1] Early involvement of the patient and family in plans for rehabilitation is also important.

Diagnostic Studies

Baseline laboratory studies include electrolytes, complete blood count, prothrombin time, partial thromboplastin time, platelet count, and arterial blood gases. Common diagnostic studies to confirm the extent of vertebral and cord injury include anteroposterior and lateral spine x-ray studies, chest x-ray studies, CT scan, MRI, and myelography. Somatosensory-cortical evoked potentials may be performed to see whether sensory pathways between the site of stimulation and the site of recording are intact.

Management
Nursing Interventions

Nursing interventions are focused on maintaining stabilization of the spinal alignment, preserving the airway and respiratory status, and preventing complications associated with immobility and the SCI (see box, "Nursing Care Plan for the Patient with Spinal Cord Injury"). Once neurogenic shock has resolved, the patient with a complete SCI above T6 must be observed for autonomic dysreflexia (Box 13-5).

◎ NURSING CARE PLAN

for the Patient with Spinal Cord Injury

NURSING DIAGNOSIS

Impaired Physical Mobility related to muscle weakness or paralysis and spinal immobilization

PATIENT OUTCOME

Consequences of immobility minimized
- Maintenance of vertebral alignment
- Absence of progressive neurological dysfunction
- Improved sensory, motor, and reflex function

NURSING INTERVENTIONS	RATIONALES
• Perform neurological assessments (motor, reflex, and sensory)	• Assess subtle changes indicating neurological deterioration or improvement
• Report progression of deficits from baseline (↑ difficulty with swallowing or coughing, respiratory stridor, sternal retraction, bradycardia, fluctuating BP, and ↑ motor and sensory loss at a higher level than the initial findings)	• Detect worsening of symptoms that indicate need for interventions (e.g., airway management and ventilation)
• Administer methylprednisolone as ordered	• Improve spinal cord function; decreases ischemia and prevents secondary cord injury
• Institute measures to prevent hazards of immobility: frequent repositioning, use of heel and elbow protectors, passive range of motion	• Promotes blood flow to lungs; minimizes risk for skin breakdown; prevents muscle breakdown
• Maintain halo or tong traction for immobilization	• Maintain alignment and prevent complications
• Perform pin care every 8 hours	• Prevent infection at the pin site
• If skeletal traction slips or is accidentally removed, maintain the patient's head in a neutral position	• Maintain alignment and prevent further damage
• Turn, lift, and transfer the patient with at least three people, with one at head to stabilize neck and to coordinate the move	• Proper turning keeps the spinal cord in alignment and prevents further trauma to the spinal cord

NURSING DIAGNOSIS

Ineffective Breathing Pattern related to hypoventilation secondary to paresis or paralysis of respiratory muscles

PATIENT OUTCOME

Adequate gas exchange
- Orientation
- $PaO_2 \geq 80$ mm Hg
- $PaCO_2 > 35$ to 45 mm Hg
- RR 12 to 20 breaths per minute with normal depth and pattern

NURSING INTERVENTIONS	RATIONALES
• Monitor respiratory rate, depth, vital capacity, oxygen saturation, ABGs	• Assesses oxygenation status; changes may indicate the need for assisted ventilation
• Monitor chest x-ray studies	• Assess worsening or improvement of status
• Monitor respiratory status, especially in a patient with cranial tongs or traction with a halo vest	• Ensure that the vest is not restricting diaphragmatic movement
• Assess for absent or adventitious breath sounds and inspect chest movement	• Assess adequacy of ventilation

NURSING DIAGNOSIS

Ineffective Airway Clearance related to decreased or absent cough reflex secondary to injury or depressant effect of some medications

PATIENT OUTCOME

Within 24 to 48 hours, airway clear
- Absence of adventitious breath sounds

Continued

◎ NURSING CARE PLAN

for the Patient with Spinal Cord Injury—cont'd

NURSING INTERVENTIONS	RATIONALES
• Monitor lung sounds every 1 to 4 hours	• Identify need for coughing and/or suctioning
• Suction airway as needed; provide oxygenation before and between suction attempts	• Clear airway of secretions; improve gas exchange
• Assess ability to cough and facilitate cough as needed	• Identify need for assistance in removing secretions
• Perform incentive spirometry every hour patient is able	• Promote expansion of lungs and facilitate secretion removal
• Turn and reposition patient every 2 hours; consider need for therapeutic bed (e.g., RotoRest)	• Mobilize secretions; reduce risk for pneumonia

NURSING DIAGNOSIS
Ineffective Thermoregulation related to inability of body to adapt to environmental temperature changes secondary to loss of autonomic innervation

PATIENT OUTCOME
Normothermia
• Within 2 to 4 hours of diagnosis, patient normothermic
• Normothermia maintained

NURSING INTERVENTIONS	RATIONALES
• Monitor temperature at least every 4 hours	• Assess need for intervention
• Assess for signs of ineffective thermoregulation (skin warm above level of injury or cool below; complaints of being too cold or warm, pilomotor erection)	• Identify need for intervention to maintain normothermia
• Implement measures to attain normothermia (warm or cool as indicated; adjust ambient room temperature)	• Maintain normothermia; prevent complications

NURSING DIAGNOSIS
Risk for Decreased CO related to relative hypovolemia secondary to neurogenic shock

PATIENT OUTCOME
Adequate CO
• Orientation to name, place, time
• SBP >90 mm Hg
• HR >50 beats per minute, ECG shows NSR

NURSING INTERVENTIONS	RATIONALES
• Monitor symptoms of low CO: hypotension, lightheadedness, confusion	• Identify low CO to provide prompt interventions
• Monitor hemodynamic measurements; administer fluids	• Provide objective data to guide and monitor treatment
• Continuously assess the ECG	• Identify dysrhythmias associated with low CO
• Implement measures to prevent orthostatic hypotension: change position slowly; antiembolic hose	• Prevent orthostatic hypotension

NURSING DIAGNOSIS
Imbalanced Nutrition: Less Than Body Requirements related to hypermetabolic state; decreased oral intake secondary; difficulty eating in prone position; fear of choking and aspiration; inability to feed self; and decreased gastrointestinal motility

PATIENT OUTCOME
Adequate nutrition
• Balanced nitrogen state
• Serum albumin 3.5 to 5.5 g/dL

NURSING INTERVENTIONS	RATIONALES
• Weigh the patient daily	• Assess fluid volume and nutritional status
• Attach NGT on low suction to prevent abdominal distention or aspiration	• Decompress the stomach; reduce risk of aspiration

◎ NURSING CARE PLAN

for the Patient with Spinal Cord Injury—cont'd

NURSING INTERVENTIONS	RATIONALES
• Maintain NPO until bowel sounds present	• Prevent complications associated with spinal shock
• Assess readiness for oral intake (bowel sounds present, passing flatus, or bowel movement)	• Assess resolution of spinal shock and return of GI function
• Perform a nutrition assessment	• Assess nutritional needs
• Give parenteral or enteral nutrition if ordered	• Maintain adequate nutrition
• Progress slowly from liquids to solids	• Assess tolerance to change in diet
• Give small, frequent feedings	• Prevent abdominal distention and less tiring

NURSING DIAGNOSIS

Ineffective Tissue Perfusion related to venous stasis and hypercoagulability from decreased vasomotor tone and immobility (see Chapter 14 for interventions).

PATIENT OUTCOME

• **Absence of venous thromboembolism**

NURSING DIAGNOSIS

Risk for Infection related to inadequate primary defenses (broken skin) secondary to immobilization and presence of invasive devices

PATIENT OUTCOME

Free of infection
• No infection at insertion site for tongs, surgical incision, IV catheter, urinary catheter
• Absence of pneumonia
• Negative culture results
• Normal WBCs

NURSING INTERVENTIONS	RATIONALES
• Perform pin, IV, and urinary catheter care	• Prevent infection
• Monitor WBCs	• Assess for infection
• Use sterile technique to change all dressings	• Prevent infection
• Use proper hand-washing techniques	• Prevent infection

NURSING DIAGNOSIS

Risk for Impaired Skin Integrity related to prolonged immobility

PATIENT OUTCOME

Skin remains intact

NURSING INTERVENTIONS	RATIONALES
• Assess the patient's skin every 4 hours; include area under the halo vest or cervical collar	• Assess potential for skin breakdown early
• Ensure that the patient's skin is clean and dry	• Prevent skin breakdown
• Pad the halo vest to decrease irritation and friction	• Prevent skin breakdown
• Turn the patient every 2 hours	• Increase circulation to prevent skin breakdown
• Consider need for therapeutic bed or other protective devices	• Prevent skin breakdown

NURSING DIAGNOSIS

Constipation related to neuromuscular impairment secondary to spinal shock, SCI

PATIENT OUTCOME

Soft, formed bowel movement within 48 hours of admission

NURSING INTERVENTIONS	RATIONALES
• Monitor for nausea, vomiting, abdominal distention, malaise, and the presence of a hard fecal mass on digital examination	• Assess constipation and fecal impaction
• Monitor the patient's bowel sounds	• Assess bowel function

Continued

◎ NURSING CARE PLAN

for the Patient with Spinal Cord Injury—cont'd

NURSING INTERVENTIONS	RATIONALES
• Administer stool softeners	• Promote adequate bowel movement
• Document the patient's bowel movements	• Assess effectiveness of bowel management program

NURSING DIAGNOSIS

Fear/Anxiety related to loss of motor and sensory function; immobilizing device to stabilize and align spine; lack of understanding of diagnostic tests and treatment; unfamiliar environment; financial concerns; and anticipated effect of SCI on lifestyle and roles

PATIENT OUTCOME

Reduced fear and anxiety
- Verbalization of feeling less anxious
- Usual sleep pattern
- Relaxed facial expression
- Healthy interaction with others

NURSING INTERVENTIONS	RATIONALES
• Assess for signs and symptoms of fear and anxiety (tense, insomnia)	• Assess need for intervention
• Implement measures to reduce fear and anxiety	• Assist in coping with changes and reduce anxiety
• Explain the need for frequent neurological checks	• Provide information to reduce anxiety
• Provide information concerning all nursing care	• Promote successful resolution of the crisis and establish a positive coping mechanism
• Assure the patient that staff members are nearby; provide a call signal that is adapted to meet the patient's needs; answer the call signal as soon as possible	• Assure that needs will be met; reduce anxiety
• Include the patient in planning care	• Provide a sense of control
• Encourage expressions of fear or questions	• Identify concerns; provide information to reduce anxiety

NURSING DIAGNOSIS

Powerlessness related to SCI

PATIENT OUTCOME

Verbalizing of increased control over activities

NURSING INTERVENTIONS	RATIONALES
• Encourage talking	• All facilitate communication and promote sense of control
• Include the patient in planning	
• Allow the patient to make choices	
• Display sensitivity toward events that could cause powerlessness	
• Encourage asking questions	

ABG, Arterial blood gas; *BP,* blood pressure; *CO,* cardiac output; *ECG,* electrocardiogram; *GI,* gastrointestinal; *HR,* heart rate; *IV,* intravenous; *NGT,* nasogastric tube; *NPO,* nothing by mouth; *NSR,* normal sinus rhythm; *PaCO₂*, partial pressure of arterial carbon dioxide; *PaO₂*, partial pressure of arterial oxygen; *RR,* respiratory rate; *SBP,* systolic blood pressure; *SCI,* spinal cord injury; *WBC,* white blood cell count.
Based on data from Baird MS, Keen JH, & Swearingen PL. (2005). *Manual of Critical Care Nursing* (5th ed.). St. Louis: Mosby; and Gulanick M, Myers JL. (2011). *Nursing Care Plans: Diagnoses, Interventions, and Outcomes* (7th ed.). St. Louis: Mosby.

Nursing and Medical Interventions

Maintaining a patent airway and respiratory function is a priority. Endotracheal intubation and mechanical ventilation are often required, especially in high cervical spine injuries. Care must be taken to prevent neck hyperextension during endotracheal intubation. Patients with complete cervical injury may be placed on a bed that provides side to side rotation (e.g., RotoRest, KCI) to optimize pulmonary function;

however, patients must be assessed for the risk of skin breakdown.

Immobilization of the spinal cord must occur at the scene to prevent further injury. A rigid cervical collar with supporting blocks on a rigid backboard is recommended.[1] Once the patient is hospitalized, external stabilization of a fracture or dislocation is often accomplished by cervical collar, skeletal traction (cervical tongs), a halo vest, or brace (Figure 13-22). The halo vest offers many advantages, such as easy access to

BOX 13-5 AUTONOMIC DYSREFLEXIA

Medical Emergency; Can Result in Stroke, Seizures, or Other Complications
- Occurs with injury at T6 or above, after spinal shock has resolved
- Characterized by exaggerated response of the sympathetic nervous system

Triggered by a Variety of Stimuli
- Bladder—kinked indwelling catheter, distention, infection, calculi, cystoscopy
- Bowel—fecal impaction, rectal examination, insertion of suppository
- Skin—tight clothing, irritation from bed linens, temperature extremes

Common Signs and Symptoms
- Sudden, severe, pounding headache
- Elevated, uncontrolled blood pressure
- Bradycardia
- Nasal congestion
- Blurred vision
- Profuse diaphoresis above the level of injury
- Flushing above the level of injury
- Pallor, chills, and pilomotor erection below the level of the injury
- Anxiety

Treatment
- Find and remove the cause of stimulation
- Elevate the head of bed
- Remain calm and supportive
- If symptoms persist, give vasodilators to decrease blood pressure
- Teach patient to recognize and report symptoms

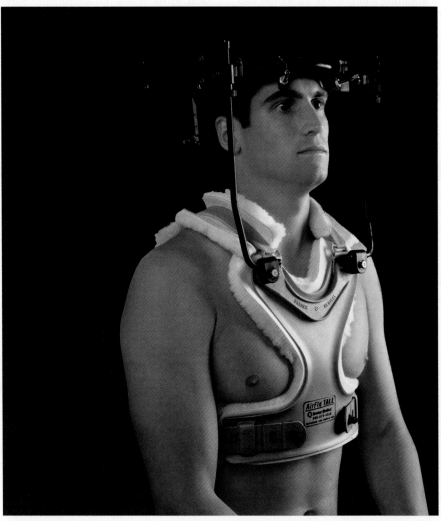

FIGURE 13-22 Halo vest. (Courtesy DePuy Spine, Inc., Raynham, Massachusetts.)

the neck for diagnostic procedures and surgery, early mobilization, and ambulation. Surgical stabilization of vertebral instability may be required and is usually performed within 24 hours of injury.

Maintaining perfusion to the spinal cord is crucial. The MAP should be maintained at 85 to 90 mm Hg for the first 7 days after the SCI. A systolic BP less than 90 mm Hg must be avoided, because hypotension contributes to secondary injury by decreasing spinal cord blood flow and perfusion, leading to ischemia and neurological deficit. Fluid volume administration and vasopressor drugs may be needed to sustain the BP.[24] However, vasopressor drug response can vary widely because of autonomic instability. A pulmonary artery catheter may be used to determine the need for fluids accurately.

Acute management of SCI often includes administration of glucocorticoids. Guidelines for the management of acute cervical spine and spinal cord injuries recommend treatment with high-dose methylprednisolone (Solu-Medrol), to be started within the first 8 hours of injury as an option for the patient with SCI (see Table 13-9).[1,5] The high-dose therapy requires astute monitoring for adverse effects.

During the first 72 hours after SCI, a nasogastric tube is inserted for gastric decompression until bowel sounds return. This also helps prevent vomiting and possible aspiration and improve pulmonary function. Stress ulcers can occur as a result of ischemia of gastric mucosa and excess gastric acid production. Administration of steroids also increases the risk of ulcer formation. Histamine (H_2)-antagonists or proton pump inhibitors are given to prevent stress ulcers. A bowel care program should be instituted as soon as bowel sounds return.

The skin must be kept clean and dry at all times. Various skin protection devices may be required, including therapeutic beds, mattress overlays, boots, and skin barrier creams. An indwelling urinary catheter is inserted immediately on admission to prevent bladder distention; an intermittent catheterization program is instituted upon resolution of spinal shock.

Because of the limited mobility of patients with SCIs, measures to prevent venous thromboembolism are started immediately on admission.[1,3] Intermittent pneumatic compression devices are commonly ordered. Heparin prophylaxis may be initiated if the risk of intramedullary or epidural hemorrhage into the spine is low. If the patient is not a candidate for anticoagulation, a vena cava filter may be considered; however, its effectiveness is controversial. Since metabolic demands are initially increased, adequate nutrition must also be provided.

Surgical Intervention

SCIs may require surgical intervention to achieve greater neurological recovery and restore spinal stability. Surgery is indicated for neurological deterioration, unstable fractures, cord compression in the presence of an incomplete injury, and gross spinal misalignment. Surgery may involve the placement of plates or rods, and a bone graft to fuse the spine. Depending on the injury, bone fragments may be removed, or the spine may need to be realigned. The issue of when surgery should be performed is controversial.[14] External immobilization devices, such as cervical traction or halo vest, may also be used.

CASE STUDY

Ms. J. is a 45-year-old patient who had a clipping of an aneurysm 5 days ago. At present, she is receiving mechanical ventilation and has a pulmonary artery catheter, arterial line, and ventriculostomy in place. Cerebral angiography performed today indicates that she is experiencing cerebral vasospasm. To reverse or overcome the vasospasm, she is started on oral nimodipine. Other treatments include fluid administration (hypervolemia) and medications to increase the blood pressure (hypertension).

Questions
1. When is a patient at greatest risk for developing vasospasm?
2. What effects does vasospasm have on cerebral function?
3. Discuss the benefits of administering nimodipine, and achieving hypervolemia and hypertension?
4. Explain the purpose of a ventriculostomy in this patient.

SUMMARY

Care of the patient with a neurological problem is challenging and complex. Knowledge of normal structure and function of the nervous system is essential to understand common disorders and injuries. Nurses must carefully consider how interventions affect patients. Skills in neurological assessment are important to learn because changes are often subtle. Nursing assessments and interventions that are tailored to each patient are essential to promote positive patient outcomes. In addition, many nervous system disorders affect multiple body systems and result in a prolonged recovery period. It is important for the nurse to provide comprehensive care that prevents the complications that can result from bed rest and immobility. Other disciplines need to be involved in the patient's care as soon as possible to assist in promoting rehabilitation, including physical therapists, occupational therapists, and speech therapists. The nurse is instrumental in getting consults for these services and coordinating the multiprofessional plan of care that improves outcomes for this patient population.

CRITICAL THINKING EXERCISES

1. You are caring for Mr. S., who has sustained a closed head injury from a motor vehicle crash. He has an intraventricular catheter for continuous measurement of intracranial pressure (ICP). His ICP has been stable at 13 mm Hg for the past 4 hours. The alarm on the monitor sounds because his ICP is now 20 mm Hg. What are your priority assessments and interventions at this time?

2. Many nurses believe that visiting should be restricted for neurological patients, especially those with head injuries. What assessments can you make to determine whether family visits are helpful or harmful to your patient?

3. What interventions can you teach families to assist in the care and rehabilitation of patients with prolonged unconsciousness after a head injury or cranial surgery?

4. Mr. B. is an 18-year-old patient who was admitted in generalized convulsive status epilepticus. Describe the appropriate nursing and medical interventions.

REFERENCES

1. American Association of Neurological Surgeons & Congress of Neurological Surgeons. Guidelines for the management of acute cervical spine and spinal cord injuries. *Neurosurgery.* 2002;50(3 suppl.).
2. Arabi YM, Haddad S, Tamim HM, et al. Mortality reduction after implementing a clinical practice guidelines-based management protocol for severe traumatic brain injury. *Journal of Critical Care.* 2010;25(2):190-195.
3. Bader MK, Littlejohns L. *AANN Core Curriculum for Neuroscience Nursing.* 5th edition. Glenview, IL: AANN; 2010.
4. Bederson JB, Connolly EJ, Batjer HH, et al. Guidelines for the management of aneurysmal subarachnoid hemorrhage: a statement for healthcare professionals from a special writing group of the Stroke Council, American Heart Association. *Stroke.* 2009;40(3):994-1025.
5. Berney S, Bragge P, Granger C, et al. The acute respiratory management of cervical spinal cord injury in the first 6 weeks after injury: a systematic review. *Spinal Cord.* 2011;49(1):17-29.
6. Brouwer MC, McIntyre P, de Gans J, et al. Corticosteroids for acute bacterial meningitis. *Cochrane Database of Systematic Reviews.* 2010;(9).
7. Cecil S, Chen PM, Callaway SE, et al. Traumatic brain injury: advanced multimodal neuromonitoring from theory to clinical practice. *Critical Care Nurse.* 2011;31(2):25-37.
8. Corrigan JD, Selassie AW, Orman JA. The epidemiology of traumatic brain injury. *Journal of Head Trauma Rehabilitation.* 2010;25(2):72-80.
9. Czosnyka M, Brady K, Reinhard M, et al. Monitoring of cerebrovascular autoregulation: facts, myths, and missing links. *Neurocritical Care.* 2009;10(3):373-386.
10. DeVivo MJ, Chen Y. Trends in new injuries, prevalent cases, and aging with spinal cord injury. *Archives of Physical Medicine & Rehabilitation.* 2011;92(3):332-338.
11. Diedler J, Sykora M, Blatow M, et al. Decompressive surgery for severe brain edema. *Journal of Intensive Care Medicine.* 2009;24(3):168-178.
12. Espinosa-Aguilar A, Reyes-Morales H, Huerta-Posada C, et al. Design and validation of a critical pathway for hospital management of patients with severe traumatic brain injury. *Journal of Trauma.* 2008;64(5):1327-1341.
13. Fan J, Kirkness C, Vicini P, et al. Intracranial pressure waveform morphology and intracranial adaptive capacity. *American Journal of Critical Care.* 2008;17(6):545-554.
14. Fehlings MG, Wilson JR, Dvorak MF, et al. The challenges of managing spine and spinal cord injuries: an evolving consensus and opportunities for change. *Spine.* 2010;35(21):S161-S165.
15. Helliwell R. Advances in brain tissue oxygen monitoring: using the Licox system in neurointensive care. *British Journal of Neuroscience Nursing.* 2009;5(1):22-24.
16. Hocker S, Morales-Vidal S, Schneck MJ. Management of arterial blood pressure in acute ischemic and hemorrhagic stroke. *Neurologic Clinics.* 2010;28(4):863-886.
17. Koedel U, Klein M, Pfister H. New understandings on the pathophysiology of bacterial meningitis. *Current Opinion in Infectious Diseases.* 2010;23(3):217-223.
18. Koenig MA, Bryan M, Lewin JL III, et al. Reversal of transtentorial herniation with hypertonic saline. *Neurology.* 2008;70(13):1023-1029.
19. Ledwith MB, Bloom S, Maloney-Wilensky E, et al. Effect of body position on cerebral oxygenation and physiologic parameters in patients with acute neurological conditions. *Journal of Neuroscience Nursing.* 2010;42(5):280-287.
20. Lukovits TG, Goddeau RJ. Critical care of patients with acute ischemic and hemorrhagic stroke: update on recent evidence and international guidelines. *Chest.* 2011;139(3):694-700.
21. Macciocchi S, Seel RT, Thompson N, et al. Spinal cord injury and co-occurring traumatic brain injury: assessment and incidence. *Archives of Physical Medicine & Rehabilitation.* 2008;89(7):1350-1357.
22. McNett MM, Gianakis A. Nursing interventions for critically ill traumatic brain injury patients. *Journal of Neuroscience Nursing.* 2010;42(2):71-79.
23. Morgenstern LB, Hemphill J III, Anderson C, et al. Guidelines for the management of spontaneous intracerebral hemorrhage: a guideline for healthcare professionals from the American Heart Association/American Stroke Association. *Stroke.* 2010;41(9):2108-2129.
24. Ploumis A, Yadlapalli N, Fehlings MG, et al. A systematic review of the evidence supporting a role for vasopressor support in acute SCI. *Spinal Cord.* 2010;48(5):356-362.
25. Roger VL, Go AS, Lloyd-Jones D, et al. Heart disease and stroke statistics—2011 update: a report from the American Heart Association. *Circulation.* 2011;123(4):e18-209.
26. Shearer P, Riviello J. Generalized convulsive status epilepticus in adults and children: treatment guidelines and protocols. *Emergency Medicine Clinics of North America.* 2011;29(1):51-64.
27. Young N, Rhodes J, Mascia L, et al. Ventilatory strategies for patients with acute brain injury. *Current Opinion in Critical Care.* 2010;16(1):45-52.

CHAPTER

14

Acute Respiratory Failure

Maureen A. Seckel, MSN, RN, APN, ACNS-BC, CCNS, CCRN

evolve WEBSITE

Many additional resources, including self-assessment exercises, are located on the Evolve companion website at http://evolve.elsevier.com/Sole.

- Review Questions
- Mosby's Nursing Skills Procedures

- Animations
- Video Clips

INTRODUCTION

Acute respiratory failure (ARF) occurs in many disease states. It may be the patient's primary problem or a complicating factor in other conditions. This chapter reviews the pathophysiology of ARF, several common causes, and the nursing care involved in the treatment of these patients.

ACUTE RESPIRATORY FAILURE

Definition

ARF is defined as a state of altered gas exchange in which the respiratory system fails in either oxygenation or carbon dioxide (CO_2) elimination. These failures are classified into one of two categories: type 1 hypoxemic or oxygenation failure, or type II hypercapnic or ventilatory failure. Hypoxemic or oxygenation failure is characterized by an abnormal arterial blood gas (ABG) value obtained with the patient breathing room air; partial pressure of oxygen (O_2) in arterial blood (PaO_2) is less than 60 mm Hg, and the partial pressure of carbon dioxide (CO_2) level ($PaCO_2$) is normal or low. Hypercapnic or ventilatory failure is characterized by a $PaCO_2$ of greater than 50 mm Hg with a pH of less than 7.30.[4] ARF differs from chronic respiratory failure in the length of time necessary for it to develop. ARF occurs rapidly over minutes to hours, with little time for physiological compensation. Chronic respiratory failure develops over time and allows the body's compensatory mechanisms to activate. ARF and chronic respiratory failure are not mutually exclusive. ARF may occur when a person who has chronic respiratory failure develops a sudden respiratory infection or is exposed to other types of stressors. This is referred to as acute-on-chronic respiratory failure. Obese individuals may also be at a greater risk for respiratory failure (see box, "Bariatric Considerations").

BARIATRIC CONSIDERATIONS

Several pathophysiological mechanisms may contribute to respiratory failure in obese individuals:

Hypoxemic Respiratory Failure
- Increase in PAO_2/PaO_2 gradient secondary to ventilation/perfusion imbalance associated with hyperperfusion and airway closure/collapse

Hypercapneic Respiratory Failure
- Decrease in compliance
- Increase in resistance
- Diminished respiratory strength
- Respiratory muscle fatigue
- Diaphragm dysfunction
- Altered ventilator pattern

Coexisting Conditions
- Sleep apnea-hypopnea syndrome
- Chronic obstructive pulmonary disease

Aggravating Conditions
- Supine position
- Rapid eye movement (REM) sleep

Adapted from Rabec C, Ramos P, Veale D. Respiratory complications of obesity. *Archivos de Bronconeumologia.*, 2011;47:252-261.

Pathophysiology

Failure of Oxygenation

Failure of oxygenation is present when the PaO_2 cannot be adequately maintained. Five generally accepted mechanisms that reduce PaO_2 and create a state of hypoxemia are (1) hypoventilation, (2) intrapulmonary shunting, (3) ventilation-perfusion mismatching, (4) diffusion defects, and (5) decreased barometric pressure (Figure 14-1). Decreased barometric pressure, which occurs at high altitudes, is not addressed in this text. Nonpulmonary conditions such as decreased cardiac output and low hemoglobin level may also result in tissue hypoxia.

Hypoventilation. In the normal lung, the partial pressure of alveolar O_2 (PAO_2) is approximately equal to the arterial O_2 (PaO_2). Alveolar ventilation refers to the amount of gas that enters the alveoli per minute. If the alveolar ventilation is reduced because of hypoventilation, the PAO_2 and the PaO_2 are reduced. Factors that may lead to hypoventilation include a drug overdose that causes central nervous system depression, neurological disorders that cause a decrease in the rate or depth of respirations, and abdominal or thoracic surgery leading to shallow breathing patterns secondary to pain on inspiration.

Hypoventilation also produces an increase in the alveolar CO_2 level because the CO_2 that is produced in the tissues is delivered to the lungs but is not released from the body.

Intrapulmonary shunting. In normally functioning lungs, a small amount of blood returns to the left side of the heart without engaging in alveolar gas exchange. This is referred to as the physiological shunt. If, however, a larger amount of blood returns to the left side of the heart without participating in gas exchange, the shunt becomes pathological and a decrease in the PaO_2 occurs.[4] The condition exists when areas of the lung that are inadequately ventilated are adequately perfused (see Figure 14-1). The blood, therefore, is shunted past the lung and returns unoxygenated to the left side of the heart. Causes of shunting include atrial or ventricular septal defects, atelectasis, pneumonia, and pulmonary edema.[3]

As the shunt worsens, the PaO_2 continues to decrease. This cause of hypoxemia cannot be effectively treated by solely increasing the fraction of inspired O_2 (FiO_2) because the increased oxygen is unable to reach the alveoli. Treatment is directed toward opening the alveoli and improving ventilation.

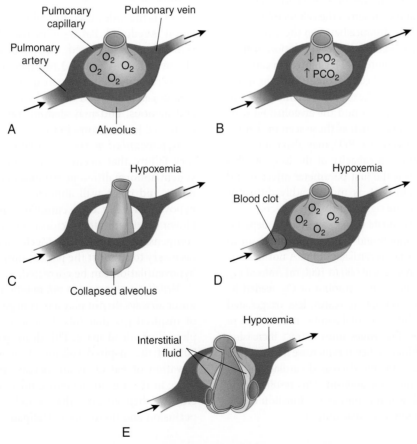

FIGURE 14-1 Pulmonary causes of hypoxemia. **A,** Normal alveolar-capillary unit. **B,** Hypoventilation causes an increased $PaCO_2$ and decreased PaO_2. **C,** Shunt. **D,** Ventilation-perfusion mismatch resulting from pulmonary embolus. **E,** Diffusion defect due to increased interstitial fluid.

Ventilation-perfusion mismatch. Gas exchange in the lungs is dependent upon the balance between ventilated areas of the lung (ventilation) receiving blood flow (perfusion). The rate of ventilation ($\dot{V}$) usually equals the rate of perfusion ($\dot{Q}$), resulting in a ventilation-to-perfusion ($\dot{V}/\dot{Q}$) ratio of 1.0. If ventilation exceeds blood flow, the $\dot{V}/\dot{Q}$ ratio is greater than 1.0; if ventilation is less than blood flow, the $\dot{V}/\dot{Q}$ ratio is less than 1. Both of these conditions are examples of $\dot{V}/\dot{Q}$ mismatch. In respiratory failure, $\dot{V}/\dot{Q}$ mismatch is the most common cause of hypoxemia and can often be corrected by increasing the FiO_2.[3] $\dot{V}/\dot{Q}$ mismatch can occur in conditions such as pneumonia or pulmonary edema when obstructed airways inhibit ventilation (and perfusion is normal), or in the case of pulmonary embolism when a clot in the pulmonary circulation obstructs perfusion.[3]

Diffusion defects. Diffusion is the movement of gas from an area of high concentration to an area of low concentration. In the lungs, O_2 and CO_2 move between the alveoli and the blood by diffusing across the alveolar-capillary membrane. The alveolar-capillary membrane has six barriers to the diffusion of O_2 and CO_2: surfactant, alveolar epithelium, interstitial fluid, capillary endothelium, plasma, and red blood cell membrane. Under normal circumstances, O_2 and CO_2 diffuse across the alveolar-capillary membrane in 0.25 seconds. The distance between an alveolus and a pulmonary capillary is usually only one or two cells thick. This narrowness of space facilitates efficient diffusion of O_2 and CO_2 across the cell membrane.

In respiratory failure, the distance between the alveoli and the capillaries may be increased by the accumulation of fluid in the interstitial space (see Figure 14-1). Changes in capillary perfusion pressure, leakage of plasma proteins into the interstitial space, and destruction of the capillary membrane contribute to the buildup of fluids around the alveolus. Fibrotic changes in the lung tissue itself, such as those seen in chronic obstructive pulmonary disease (COPD), may also contribute to a reduction in the diffusion capacity of the lung. As this capacity is reduced, PaO_2 is the first parameter affected and hypoxemia results. Because CO_2 is more readily diffusible than O_2, hypercapnia is a late sign of diffusion defects.

Low cardiac output. Adequate tissue oxygenation depends on a balance between O_2 supply and demand. The mechanism for delivering O_2 to the tissues is cardiac output. A normal cardiac output results in the delivery of 600 to 1000 mL/min of O_2, which generally exceeds the normal amount of O_2 needed by the tissues. If the cardiac output decreases, less oxygenated blood is delivered. To maintain normal aerobic metabolism in low cardiac output states, the tissues must extract increasing amounts of O_2 from the blood. When this increase in extraction can no longer compensate for the decreased cardiac output, the cells convert to anaerobic metabolism. This results in the production of lactic acid, which depresses the function of the myocardium and further lowers cardiac output.

Low hemoglobin level. Approximately 95% of the body's O_2 is transported to the tissues bound to hemoglobin. Each gram of hemoglobin can carry 1.34 mL of O_2 when all of its O_2 binding sites are completely filled. Oxygen saturation (SaO_2) refers to the percentage of O_2 binding sites on each hemoglobin molecule that are filled with O_2. The hemoglobin of a healthy person breathing room air is about 95% saturated. If a patient's hemoglobin level is less than normal, the O_2 supply to the tissues may be impaired and tissue hypoxia can occur. An alteration in hemoglobin function (i.e., carbon monoxide poisoning or sickle cell disease) can also decrease O_2 delivery to the tissues.

Tissue hypoxia. The final step in oxygenation is the use of O_2 by the tissues. Anaerobic metabolism occurs when the tissues cannot obtain adequate O_2 to meet metabolic needs. In addition, some conditions such as cyanide poisoning may leave the tissues unable to use O_2 despite normal O_2 delivery.[26] Anaerobic metabolism is inefficient and results in the accumulation of lactic acid. The point at which anaerobic metabolism begins to occur is not known and may vary with different organ systems. The effects of tissue hypoxia vary with the severity of the hypoxia but may result in cellular death and subsequent organ failure.

Failure of Ventilation

$PaCO_2$ is the index used to evaluate ventilation. When ventilation is reduced, $PaCO_2$ is increased (hypercapnia). When ventilation is increased, $PaCO_2$ is reduced (hypocapnia). Hypoventilation and $\dot{V}/\dot{Q}$ mismatching are the two mechanisms responsible for hypercapnia. Hypercapnia greatly increases cerebral blood flow. The patient may appear restless and anxious, and may demonstrate slurred speech and a decreased level of consciousness.

Hypoventilation. Hypoventilation is the cause of respiratory failure that occurs in patients with central nervous system abnormalities, neuromuscular disorders, drug overdoses, and chest wall abnormalities (see Figure 14-1). In hypoventilation, CO_2 accumulates in the alveoli and is not blown off. Respiratory acidosis occurs rapidly before renal compensation can occur. Mechanical ventilation may be necessary to support the patient until the initial cause of the hypoventilation can be corrected.

Ventilation-perfusion mismatch. Because the upper and lower airways do not play a part in gas exchange, the volume of inspired gas that fills these structures is referred to as physiologic dead space. This dead space is normally 25% to 30% of the inspired volume. A major mechanism for the elevation of $PaCO_2$ is an increase in the volume of dead space in relation to the entire tidal volume. Dead space increases when an area that is well ventilated has reduced perfusion and no longer participates in gas exchange.

Assessment

Respiratory assessment and evaluation of gas exchange are discussed in depth in Chapter 9. Assessment of the patient with ARF begins with the neurological system. Changes in mental status resulting from hypoxia and hypercapnia begin with anxiety, restlessness, and confusion and may progress to lethargy, severe somnolence, and coma.

The respiratory assessment continues with observing the rate, depth, and pattern of respiration. In response to hypoxemia, compensatory mechanisms produce tachypnea and an increase in tidal volume. As these compensatory mechanisms fail, respirations become shallow. A decrease in respiratory rate is an ominous sign. Use of accessory muscles and sternal retractions are a cause for concern as they indicate respiratory muscle fatigue. By auscultation, the nurse assesses the adequacy of airflow and the presence of adventitious breath sounds. The presence of a cough and the amount and characteristics of any sputum production are noted.

A thorough cardiac assessment provides information about the heart's ability to deliver O_2 to the tissues. The patient must be closely monitored for changes in blood pressure, heart rate, and cardiac rhythm. ARF initially causes tachycardia and increased blood pressure. As ARF progresses, it may lead to dysrhythmias, angina, bradycardia, hypotension, and cardiac arrest. The nurse should evaluate peripheral perfusion by assessing pulses for strength and bilateral equality. The skin is assessed for a decrease in temperature and the presence of cyanosis or pallor, which are additional indicators of poor perfusion.

The patient's nutritional status must be evaluated because this is an important factor in maintaining respiratory muscle strength. The nurse looks for recent weight loss, muscle wasting, nausea, vomiting, abdominal distention, and skin turgor quality.

It is important to assess the patient's psychosocial status. This includes identifying the patient's significant others and their role in the family structure. An understanding of the patient's educational level, socioeconomic background, spiritual beliefs, and cultural or ethnic practices is important in determining an educational plan for discharge and future self-care.

Serial chest x-rays and pulmonary function tests provide important assessment information. Laboratory studies that are essential for the patient with respiratory failure include the following: electrolytes, which determine adequate muscle function; hemoglobin and hematocrit to evaluate the blood's O_2 carrying capacity; and ABG measurements to assess gas exchange and acid-base balance. Noninvasive monitoring such as pulse oximetry (SpO_2) provides information about the patient's oxygenation, whereas continuous end-tidal CO_2 monitoring provides information about the patient's ventilation.

Effects of Aging

Many age-related factors increase the older adult's risk for developing ARF. Physiological changes may make identifying the signs and symptoms of ARF more difficult in the elderly. The most common early sign of hypoxemia in the elderly is a change in mental status, such as confusion or agitation. These changes are often mistaken for dementia or a normal sign of advancing age[21,46] (see box, "Geriatric Considerations").

GERIATRIC CONSIDERATIONS

PHYSIOLOGICAL CHANGES	NURSING IMPLICATIONS
Calcification of costal and sternal cartilage	Decreased chest wall mobility
Osteoporosis	Increased functional residual capacity and residual volume
Spinal degeneration	Decreased tidal volume, vital capacity, and forced expiratory volume
Kyphosis	Decreased chest wall mobility and restricted ventilation
Flattening of diaphragm	Increased work of breathing
Decline in muscle mass	Respiratory muscle fatigue
Diminished cough reflex	Ventilation/perfusion mismatch
Decreased mucociliary clearance	Early airway collapse
Decline in surfactant production	Increased risk of atelectasis and pneumonia
Decreased effectiveness of immune system	Increased susceptibility to infection
Thickening of alveolar-capillary membrane	Ventilation/perfusion mismatch
Decreased pulmonary blood flow	Ventilation/perfusion mismatch

Based on data from El Sohl AA, & Ramadan FH. Overview of respiratory failure in older adults. *Journal of Intensive Care Medicine.* 2006;21(6), 345-351; and Muir J, Lamia B, Molano C, & Cuvelier A. Respiratory failure in the elderly. *Seminars in Respiratory and Critical Care Medicine.* 2010;31(5), 634-646.

Because of age-related decreases in chemoreceptor and central nervous system function, older adults have a lower ventilatory response to hypoxia and hypercapnia. In addition, hypoxia in the elderly may not produce the same compensatory increases in heart rate, stroke volume, and cardiac output that are seen in younger adults. This may be due to preexisting cardiac disease or the effects of cardiac medications such as digoxin or beta-blockers. Increasing age can also lead to a slower response to O_2 therapy, making early identification and treatment of hypoxia essential in this population. Finally, normal PaO_2 levels decrease with age, but aging does not produce alterations in $PaCO_2$. For this reason hypercapnia and a falling pH are causes for concern.

Interventions

The goals of treating patients with ARF are fivefold and include (1) maintaining a patent airway, (2) optimizing O_2 delivery, (3) minimizing O_2 demand, (4) treating the cause of ARF, and (5) preventing complications.

Maintaining a Patent Airway

Some causes of acute respiratory failure such as COPD, cardiogenic pulmonary edema, pulmonary infiltrates in immunocompromised patients, and palliation in the terminally ill may be effectively treated with noninvasive positive-pressure ventilation (NPPV).[49] However, if a patient is unable to maintain a patent airway, intubation and mechanical ventilation may be required for treatment. (Refer to Chapter 9 for nursing care related to NPPV and mechanical ventilation.)

Optimizing O₂ Delivery

Optimizing O_2 delivery can be achieved in many ways, depending on the needs of the patient. The first is to provide supplemental O_2 via nasal cannula or face mask to maintain the PaO_2 above 60 mm Hg or the SaO_2 above 90%.[4] Higher PaO_2 values are indicated in cases of severe tissue hypoxia, low flow states, or deficiencies in O_2 carrying capacity.[3] If supplemental O_2 is ineffective in raising PaO_2 levels, noninvasive or invasive mechanical ventilation is indicated (see box, "Clinical Alert: Acute Respiratory Failure"). Patients are positioned for comfort and to enhance $\dot{V}/\dot{Q}$ matching. Some patients who are alert and dyspneic are able to oxygenate more effectively in the semi-Fowler to high Fowler position. Patients with unilateral lung disease should be positioned on their side with the better functioning "good" lung down. This allows gravity to perfuse the lung that has the best ventilation. Other methods to optimize O_2 delivery include red blood cell transfusion to ensure adequate hemoglobin levels to transport O_2, and enhancing cardiac output and blood pressure to deliver sufficient O_2 to the tissues.

Minimizing O₂ Demand

Decreasing the patient's O_2 demand begins with providing adequate rest. Unnecessary physical activity is avoided in the patient with ARF. Agitation, restlessness, fever, sepsis, and patient-ventilator dyssynchrony must be addressed because they all contribute to increased O_2 demand and consumption.

! CLINICAL ALERT

Acute Respiratory Failure

CONCERN	SYMPTOMS	NURSING ACTIONS
Respiratory muscle fatigue	Diaphoresis Nasal flaring Tachycardia Abdominal paradox Muscle retractions Intercostal Suprasternal Supraclavicular Central cyanosis	**Improve O₂ delivery:** Administer O_2 Ensure adequate cardiac output and blood pressure Correct low hemoglobin Administer bronchodilators **Decrease O₂ demand:** Provide rest Reduce fever Relieve pain and anxiety Decrease work of breathing Position patient for optimum gas exchange and perfusion Prepare for possible intubation and mechanical ventilation
Cerebral hypoxia and carbon dioxide narcosis from increased CO_2 retention	Lethargy Somnolence Coma Respiratory acidosis	Maintain airway patency Prepare for possible intubation and mechanical ventilation

Treating the Cause of ARF

While the patient's hypoxia is being treated, efforts must be made to identify and reverse the cause of the ARF. Specific interventions for acute respiratory distress syndrome (ARDS), COPD, asthma, pneumonia, and pulmonary embolism are detailed later in this chapter.

Preventing Complications

Finally, the critical care nurse must be alert to the potential complications that the patient with ARF may encounter. Preventive measures must be taken to prevent the complications of immobility, adverse effects from medications, fluid and electrolyte imbalances, development of gastric ulcers, and the hazards of mechanical ventilation.

Nursing Diagnoses

Several nursing diagnoses must be considered in the care of a patient with ARF and are discussed in the "Nursing Care Plan for a Patient with Acute Respiratory Failure." Expected outcomes include adequate organ and tissue oxygenation, and effective breathing and adequate gas exchange.

◎ NURSING CARE PLAN

*for a Patient with Acute Respiratory Failure**

NURSING DIAGNOSIS

Impaired Spontaneous Ventilation related to hypoventilation, respiratory muscle fatigue, bronchospasm, infection, inflammation, central nervous system depression

PATIENT OUTCOMES

Adequate ventilation

- Ventilatory demand decreased
- Respiratory distress absent
- Respirations unlabored at a rate of 12 to 16 breaths per minute
- Arterial blood gases WNL

NURSING INTERVENTIONS	RATIONALES
• Assess respiratory status every 1 to 2 hours, including breath sounds, breathing pattern, rate, depth, and rhythm respirations	• Assess for respiratory distress; changes in breath sounds may indicate fluid in the airways (crackles), accumulation of mucus (rhonchi), or airway obstruction (wheezes)
• Monitor for dyspnea and signs of respiratory distress	• Indicate worsening of condition
• Assess for restlessness or change in level of consciousness	• Assess for signs of hypoxemia
• Position patient in semi-Fowler position (45 degrees) or position in which breathing pattern is most comfortable	• Promote maximal air exchange and lung expansion
• If patient has lung pathology, position for maximal gas exchange; place the "good" lung down	• Increase perfusion to the good lung and facilitate gas exchange
• Assist with activities; provide patient with periods of rest	• Reduce oxygen consumption and demands
• Administer medications to increase airflow as prescribed; evaluate their effectiveness	• Decrease airway resistance secondary to bronchoconstriction
• Give oxygen therapy or maintain mechanical ventilation	• Correct hypoxemia
• Monitor ABGs	• Assess for worsening hypoxemia and/or increasing $PaCO_2$; assess response to treatments
• If patient is mechanically ventilated, sedate according to goals for patient; avoid oversedation	• Facilitate gas exchange and mechanical ventilation; oversedation prolongs time on mechanical ventilation and its associated risks

NURSING DIAGNOSIS

Risk for Ineffective Airway Clearance related to inability to cough, presence of endotracheal tube, thick secretions, fatigue.

PATIENT OUTCOMES

Effective airway clearance

- Airway clear of secretions
- Lung sounds clear

NURSING INTERVENTIONS	RATIONALES
• Assess lung sounds	• Rhonchi may be audible with accumulation of secretions
• Change patient's position every 2 hours	• Mobilize secretions
• Encourage patient to cough and deep breathe	• Improve lung capacity and facilitate gas exchange
• Suction (nasotracheal or endotracheal) as determined by patient assessment	• "As needed" suctioning prevents damage to the airway from the suctioning procedure
• Provide adequate humidification with supplemental oxygen or mechanical ventilation	• Prevent drying of secretions and facilitate secretion removal
• Assess amount, color, consistency of secretions	• Indicate need for humidification and/or signs of infection

*Please see Chapter 9 for Nursing Care Plan for the Mechanically Ventilated Patient.   *Continued*

◎ **NURSING CARE PLAN**

for a Patient with Acute Respiratory Failure—cont'd

NURSING DIAGNOSIS

Risk for Infection related to underlying illness/disease process, endotracheal intubation

PATIENT OUTCOMES

Absence of infection
- Normal temperature
- White blood cell count WNL
- Chest x-ray normal
- Negative cultures of sputum and bronchial aspirates

NURSING INTERVENTIONS	RATIONALES
• Monitor temperature every 4 hours, more frequently if elevated	• Fever may be first sign of infection
• Monitor white blood cell count	• Rising count indicates body's response to combat pathogens
• Assess amount, color, consistency of secretions	• Assess for infection
• Monitor results of cultures of sputum and/or bronchial specimens	• Assess need for antibiotic and appropriate antibiotic coverage
• Elevate the head of bed to at least 30 degrees	• Reduce the risk of aspiration and ventilator-associated pneumonia
• Provide oral care every 2 to 4 hours and as needed; brush teeth every 12 hours; consider chlorhexidine gluconate (0.12%) oral rinse every 12 hours	• Reduce bacterial growth and colonization of oropharyngeal secretions; promotes patient comfort

NURSING DIAGNOSIS

Anxiety related to inability to speak, situational crises, uncertainty, fear of death, and lack of control

PATIENT OUTCOMES

Anxiety decreased or absent
- Vital signs WNL
- Relaxed facial expression and body movements, and normal sleep patterns
- Usual perceptual ability and interactions with others

NURSING INTERVENTIONS	RATIONALES
• Monitor for signs of anxiety: increased heart rate, blood pressure, respiratory rate, muscle tension, inappropriate behaviors	• Anxiety is highly individualized response to life events; signs must be recognized to provide interventions
• Develop trusting relationship by using calm, consistent, and reliable behaviors	• Encourage communication and enhance feelings of safety
• Always introduce yourself and all unfamiliar persons to the patient and explain why they are there	• Uncertainty and lack of predictability contribute to feelings of anxiety
• Provide nurturing environment; allow the patient some control over decision making	• Increase sense of independence and normality
• Provide a means of communication (e.g., nonverbal, yes/no, picture charts, pencil/paper)	• Assist in meeting patient's needs and reduce anxiety
• Teach relaxation techniques (e.g., the use of slow rhythmic breathing during stressful periods)	• Enhance coping and improve physiological response
• Reassure patient of staff member's presence and prompt interventions as needed	• Assist in meeting needs and reducing anxiety
• Allow family member to remain at bedside to decrease isolation	• Provide a sense of security and familiarity; facilitate communication

◎ NURSING CARE PLAN

for a Patient with Acute Respiratory Failure—cont'd

NURSING DIAGNOSIS

Risk for Impaired Skin Integrity related to bed rest and altered metabolic state

PATIENT OUTCOMES

Skin intact

NURSING INTERVENTIONS	RATIONALES
• Assess skin every shift for areas of breakdown	• Identify problems and promote preventive interventions
• Keep patient's skin clean and dry	• Decrease the risk of skin breakdown
• Reposition every 2 hours; if unable to manually turn patient because of hemodynamic instability, consider continuous lateral rotation or kinetic therapy with pressure relief mattress with continued skin assessment every 2 hours	• Reduce pressure on bony prominences

NURSING DIAGNOSIS

Risk for Ineffective Family Coping related to knowledge deficits of family members

PATIENT OUTCOMES

Family integrity maintained

• Family members verbalize educational needs and fears
• Family members feel comfortable asking questions related to patient's prognosis

NURSING INTERVENTIONS	RATIONALES
• Assess family unit and coping behaviors	• Allow for anticipatory care and guidance to help family unit maintain support and coping strategies
• Assist family to identify roles to maintain family integrity	• Positive feedback from one family member can reinforce a behavior of another member
• Assist family members to verbalize fears and distress	• Promote effective communication
• Answer questions; explain procedures, equipment, changes in patient's condition, and outcomes to family members in a sensitive manner	• Establish a trusting relationship; reduce anxiety
• Inform family of resources available to them such as chaplain and psychiatric liaison	• Enhance the use of services that may assist family
• Initiate multiprofessional conferences with family to provide information and make decisions regarding ongoing treatment	• Establish trust with all health care team and encourages compliance with treatments

ABGs, Arterial blood gases; *HOB,* head of bed; *PaCO₂,* partial pressure of carbon dioxide in arterial blood; *WNL,* within normal limits.
Based on data from Gulanick M and Myers JL. *Nursing Care Plans: Diagnoses, Interventions, and Outcomes,* 7th ed. St. Louis: Mosby, 2011.

RESPIRATORY FAILURE IN ACUTE RESPIRATORY DISTRESS SYNDROME

Definition

ARDS was originally described in 1967 as an acute illness manifested by dyspnea, tachypnea, decreased lung compliance, and diffuse alveolar infiltrates on chest x-ray studies. The syndrome was observed in young adult patients after trauma who developed shock, required excessive fluid administration, or both. Autopsy results revealed that pathological heart and lung findings were similar to those described in infant respiratory distress syndrome.

In 1994, the American-European Consensus Conference recommended a definition of ARDS as a subset of acute lung injury. The definition included three criteria: PaO_2/FiO_2 ratio less than 200, bilateral infiltrates on chest x-ray, and pulmonary artery occlusion pressure (PAOP) less than 18 mm Hg or no clinical evidence of left atrial hypertension.[27]

The 1994 definition of ARDS was revised in 2012 by a multi-society consensus panel, and is termed the Berlin definition.[65a] Criteria for ARDS include 1) acute onset within one week of clinical insult; 2) bilateral pulmonary opacities not explained by other conditions; and 3) altered PaO_2/FiO_2 ratio. The PAOP requirement was removed from the definition. Severity is determined by the PaO_2/FiO_2 ratio, and PEEP or CPAP requirements of ≥ 5 cm H_2O: 1) Mild ARDS—201-300 mm Hg; 2) Moderate—101-200 mm Hg; and 3) Severe— ≤ 100 mm Hg.

Etiology

Several possible causes of ARDS are listed in Box 14-1, and are categorized into direct and indirect factors. However,

Direct Causes
- Aspiration of gastric contents
- Diffuse pneumonia
- Fat embolism
- Near-drowning
- Neurogenic pulmonary edema
- Oxygen toxicity
- Pulmonary contusion
- Multisystem trauma (chest and/or lung injury)
- Radiation (chest)

Indirect Causes
- Sepsis
- Multisystem trauma (without chest and/or lung injury)
- Cardiopulmonary bypass
- Anaphylaxis
- Disseminated intravascular coagulation
- Drug overdose
- Eclampsia
- Fractures, especially of the pelvis or long bones
- Leukemia
- Transfusion-related acute lung injury
- Pancreatitis
- Thrombotic thrombocytopenic purpura

certain risk factors have a higher associated frequency of ARDS, and the presence of two or more factors increases the risk. The most common risk factors or disease processes associated with ARDS are sepsis, pneumonia, trauma, and aspiration of gastric contents. These four risk factors are believed to account for approximately 85% of all ARDS cases, with sepsis being the most common cause. Approximately one third of hospitalized patients who aspirate gastric contents develop ARDS. In addition, critically ill patients with a history of chronic alcoholism are at an increased risk of developing ARDS. Other causes with significant incidences are multiple transfusions including fresh frozen plasma and platelets, fat embolism, ischemia reperfusion, and pancreatitis.[27] Acute lung injury (mild ARDS with Berlin definition) is the most common cause of mortality related to transfusions with an incidence of about 1 for every 5000 transfusions, and a mortality of 6% to 23%. The syndrome has been named TRALI (transfusion-related acute lung injury) with defined criteria.[38]

The mortality rate for patients with diagnosed ARDS has been improving over the last decade. The 28-day mortality rate is reported to be 25% to 30%.[71] In the Berlin definition, mortality is estimated based on ARDS severity: mild, 27%;

moderate, 32%; and severe, 45%.[65a] As more individuals survive ARDS, prevention of long-term disabilities must be a priority of care. One study of patients who survived ARDS revealed that although lung volume and pulmonary function were normal by 6 months, functional disability persisted 1 year after discharge.[29] Another study reported that nearly half of ARDS survivors had significant neurocognitive impairment and a decrease in quality of life that persisted for at least 2 years.[32]

Pathophysiology

ARDS is characterized by acute and diffuse injury to the lungs, leading to respiratory failure. It is a two-phase condition including the acute exudation response phase and the late phase of fibroproliferation. The acute response is a systemic inflammatory reaction secondary to direct or indirect lung injury. Initial injury causes damage to the pulmonary capillary endothelium, which activates massive aggregation of platelets and formation of intravascular thrombi. The platelets release serotonin and a substance that activates neutrophils. Other inflammatory factors such as endotoxin, tumor necrosis factor, and interleukin-1 are also activated. Neutrophil activation causes release of inflammatory mediators such as proteolytic enzymes, toxic O_2 products, arachidonic acid metabolites, and platelet-activating factors. The release of these mediators damages the alveolar-capillary membrane, which leads to increased capillary membrane permeability. Fluids, protein, and blood cells leak from the capillary beds into the alveoli, resulting in pulmonary edema. Pulmonary hypertension occurs secondary to vasoconstriction caused by the inflammatory mediators. The pulmonary hypertension and pulmonary edema lead to $\dot{V}/\dot{Q}$ mismatching. The production of surfactant is stopped, and the surfactant present is inactivated.[7,27]

During the acute phase of ARDS, damage to the alveolar epithelium and vascular endothelium occurs. The damaged cells become susceptible to bacterial infection and pneumonia. The lungs become less compliant, resulting in decreased ventilation. A right-to-left shunt of pulmonary blood develops, and hypoxemia refractory to O_2 supplementation becomes profound. The work of breathing increases.[7]

The late phase of ARDS is the fibroproliferation stage. As ARDS proceeds over time (greater than 24 to 48 hours), a fibrin matrix (hyaline membrane) forms. After approximately 7 days, fibrosis obliterates the alveoli, bronchioles, and interstitium. The lungs become fibrotic with decreased functional residual capacity and severe right-to-left shunting. The inflammation and edema become worse with narrowing of the airways. Resistance to airflow and atelectasis increase.

The inflammatory mediators responsible for lung damage also cause harm to other organs in the body, often resulting in multiple organ dysfunction syndrome. The pathophysiology of ARDS is outlined in Figure 14-2.

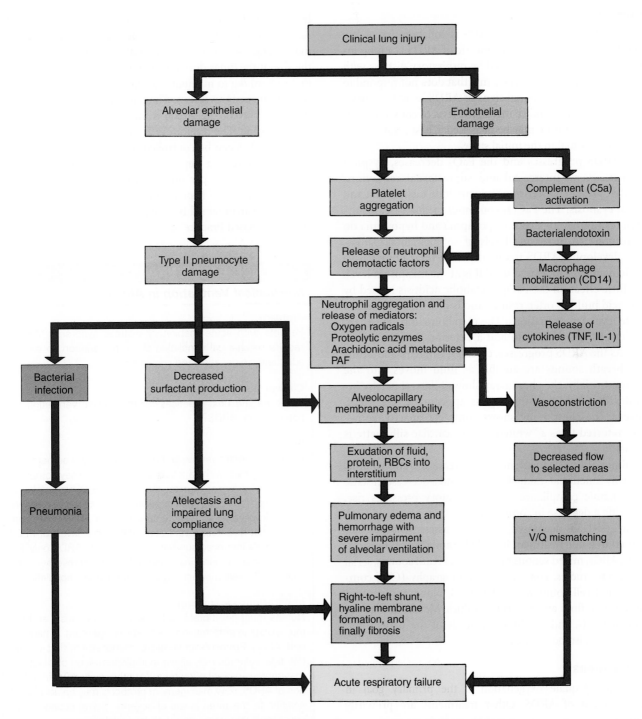

FIGURE 14-2 Pathogenesis of acute respiratory distress syndrome (ARDS). *TNF,* Tumor necrosis factor; *IL-1,* interleukin-1; *PAF,* platelet-activating factor; *RBCs,* red blood cells. (From McCance KL, Huether SE. *Pathophysiology: The Biologic Basis for Diseases in Adults and Children.* 6th ed. St. Louis: Mosby; 2010.)

Assessment

Assessment of a patient with ARDS is collaborative. A key clinical finding that is often diagnostic of ARDS is a lung insult (direct or indirect) followed by respiratory distress with dyspnea, tachypnea, and hypoxemia that does not respond to O_2 therapy and PEEP. Initial signs of ARDS include restlessness, disorientation, and change in the level of consciousness. Pulse and temperature may be increased. Chest x-ray studies are usually normal in the initial stage.

As ARDS progresses and the PaO_2 decreases, dyspnea becomes severe. Intercostal and suprasternal retractions are often present. Other signs may include tachycardia and central cyanosis. The $PaCO_2$ continues to decrease, resulting in respiratory alkalosis. Hypocapnia and hypoxemia do not respond to increasing levels of supplemental O_2. Patients developing ARDS frequently need their noninvasive supplemental O_2 increased until it is at the maximum level, with little effect on the PaO_2. Metabolic acidosis caused by lactic acid buildup often results, and is confirmed by serum lactate level determinations. The metabolic imbalances are a result of a low $\dot{V}/\dot{Q}$ ratio and a deteriorating PaO_2/FiO_2 ratio. As the ARDS progresses, crackles, rhonchi, and bronchial breath sounds are audible as fluid moves into the airways. Initially, the chest x-ray shows bilateral patchy infiltrates that have a "ground glass appearance." As ARDS worsens, the chest x-ray shows complete opacity, sometimes referred to as a "whiteout." The cardiac silhouette is normal.[62]

Pulmonary mechanics show a decrease in lung volume, especially functional residual capacity, and a decrease in static and dynamic compliance. Peak inspiratory pressures rise, indicating a decrease in compliance.

Once ARDS is diagnosed, important assessment data that are used to guide treatment include hemodynamic measurements, ABGs, mixed venous blood gases, breath sounds, serial chest x-ray studies, computerized tomography (CT), complete blood cell count with differential, blood and sputum cultures, and fluid and electrolyte values. Metabolic and nutritional needs, and psychosocial needs of the patient and family, must also be assessed.

Interventions

Achieving adequate oxygenation is the primary goal in the treatment of ARDS. Other treatments are primarily supportive.

Oxygenation

Patients with ARDS generally require intubation and mechanical ventilation. Selection of ventilator settings is based on lung-protective strategies that attempt to achieve adequate oxygenation while minimizing the risks of ventilator-associated complications. Lung-protective strategies consist of low tidal volume (V_T), low end-inspiratory plateau pressure, FiO_2 at nontoxic levels (less than 0.60), and positive end-expiratory pressure (PEEP) (Table 14-1). Large clinical studies have shown reduced mortality and complications with the use of low V_T. The target V_T recommended is 6 mL/kg of predicted ideal

body weight (calculated from sex and height) (see Table 14-1). Actual body weight should not be used. The body weight may change secondary to accumulation of body fluid, but the size of the lungs does not change. The V_T may be reduced to 4 to 5 mL/kg to maintain the end-inspiratory plateau pressure at 30 cm H_2O or less. These lower volumes and plateau pressures prevent the alveoli from overdistending and minimize shearing. The respiratory acidosis that occurs secondary to the low V_Ts can be controlled by increasing the ventilator respiratory rate in a stepwise manner generally to an upper limit of 35 breaths per minute. The $PaCO_2$ should be kept within a permissive hypercapnia range of 50 to 70 mm Hg, and the pH maintained between 7.30 and 7.45[3,22,27] (see box, "Evidence-Based Practice").

TABLE 14-1 MECHANICAL VENTILATION PROTOCOL FOR ACUTE RESPIRATORY DISTRESS SYNDROME (NHLBI, NIH)

Definition:
1. Acute onset
2. PaO_2/FiO_2 ≤300 mm Hg, ALI (Berlin definition mild ARDS); PaO_2/FiO_2 ≤200, ARDS (Berlin definition moderate to severe ARDS) (referred to as P/F ratio)
3. Bilateral (patchy, diffuse, or homogeneous) infiltrates consistent with pulmonary edema
4. No clinical evidence of left atrial hypertension

Ventilator Setup and Adjustment:
1. Calculate predicted body weight (PBW)
   Males   = 50.0 + 2.3 (height [inches] − 60)
   Females = 45.5 + 2.3 (height [inches] − 60)
2. Select any ventilator mode
3. Set initial V_T to 8 mL/kg PBW
4. Reduce V_T by 1 mL/kg at intervals ≤2 hours until V_T = 6 mL/kg PBW
5. Set initial rate to approximate baseline VE (not >35 breaths/min)
6. Adjust V_T and RR to achieve pH and plateau pressure goals

Oxygenation Goal: PaO_2 55-80 mm Hg or SpO_2 88%-95%
Lower PEEP/higher FiO_2 Recommendations:

FiO_2	0.3	0.4	0.4	0.5	0.5	0.6	0.7	0.7
PEEP cm H_2O	5	5	8	8	10	10	10	12
FiO_2	0.7	0.8	0.9	0.9	0.9	1.0		
PEEP cm H_2O	14	14	14	16	18	18-24		

Higher PEEP/lower FiO_2 Recommendations:

FiO_2	0.3	0.3	0.3	0.3	0.3	0.4	0.4	0.5
PEEP	5	8	10	12	14	14	16	16
FiO_2	0.5	0.5-0.8	0.8	0.9	1.0	1.0		
PEEP	18	20	22	22	22	24		

Plateau Pressure Goal: ≤30 cm H_2O
Check Pplat, at least every 4 hours and after each change in PEEP or V_T
1. **If Pplat >30 cm H_2O:** decrease V_T by 1-mL/kg steps (minimum, 4 mL/kg)
2. **If Pplat <25 cm H_2O:** V_T <6 mL/kg, increase V_T by 1 mL/kg until Pplat >25 cm H_2O or V_T = 6 mL/kg
3. **If Pplat <30 cm H_2O and breath stacking occurs:** may increase V_T in 1-mL/kg increments (maximum, 8 mL/kg)

pH Goal: 7.30-7.45
Acidosis Management: (pH <7.30)
1. **If pH 7.15-7.30:** Increase RR until pH >7.30 or $PaCO_2$ <25 mm Hg (maximum RR, 35 breaths/min)
2. **If pH <7.15:** Increase RR to 35 breaths/min; V_T may be increased in 1-mL/kg steps until pH >7.15 (Pplat target may be exceeded).
Alkalosis Management: (pH >7.45)
1. Decrease ventilator breaths/min rate if possible

I:E Ratio Goal: Duration of inspiration ≤ duration of expiration

ALI, Acute lung injury; *ARDS,* acute respiratory distress syndrome; *FiO_2,* fraction of inspired oxygen; *H_2O,* water; *I:E,* inspiration-to-expiration ratio; *$NaHCO_3$,* sodium bicarbonate; *NHLBI,* National Heart, Lung, and Blood Institute; *NIH,* National Institutes of Health; *PaO_2,* partial pressure of oxygen in arterial blood; *$PaCO_2$,* partial pressure of carbon dioxide in arterial blood; *Pplat,* peak plateau pressure; *PEEP,* positive end-expiratory pressure; *P/F,* PaO_2/FiO_2 (oxygenation index); *RR,* respiratory rate; *SaO_2,* arterial oxygen saturation; *SpO_2,* arterial oxygen saturation via pulse oximeter; *VT,* tidal volume; *VE,* minute ventilation.
Adapted from the NIH NHLBI *ARDS Clinical Network Mechanical Ventilation Protocol Summary.* Retrieved on May 27, 2012, from http://www.ardsnet.org/system/files/Ventilator%20Protocol%20Card.pdf.

Patients with ARDS require significant support to achieve and maintain arterial oxygenation. High levels of FiO_2 may be required for short periods while aggressively working to reduce the FiO_2 to the lowest level that maintains the PaO_2 above 60 mm Hg. To prevent O_2 toxicity, the goal is to maintain the PaO_2 with levels of FiO_2 at 0.60 or below.

Ventilatory support typically includes PEEP to restore functional residual capacity, open collapsed alveoli, prevent collapse of unstable alveoli, and improve arterial oxygenation.[22] The National Heart, Lung, and Blood Institute ARDS network developed a protocol for PEEP application based on amount of FiO_2 requirements (see Table 14-1). Studies have shown that higher PEEP resulted in improved survival without increase in the incidence of pneumothorax in ARDS patients only; decreased mortality was not seen in patients with acute lung injury.[8]

When using high levels of PEEP, the nurse must assess for potential adverse effects. PEEP increases intrathoracic pressure, potentially leading to decreased cardiac output. Excessive pressure in stiff lungs increases peak inspiratory and plateau pressures, which may result in barotrauma and pneumothorax. Treatment of a pneumothorax requires prompt insertion of a chest tube. A patient receiving high levels of PEEP therapy should be monitored every 2 to 4 hours, and after every adjustment in the PEEP setting, for changes in respiratory status such as increased respiratory rate, worsening adventitious breath sounds, decreased or absent breath sounds, decreased SpO_2, and increasing dyspnea.

A few unconventional modes of mechanical ventilation are used to treat ARDS when patients are unable to be oxygenated with standard modes of ventilation. These modes include high-frequency oscillatory ventilation; pressure-controlled, inverse-ratio ventilation; and airway pressure release ventilation. These modes often improve alveolar ventilation and arterial oxygenation while decreasing the risk of lung injury. None have been successful enough to be considered standard therapy (see Chapter 9).

Sedation and Comfort

Patients with ARDS routinely receive sedation to promote comfort and sleep/rest, alleviate anxiety, prevent self-extubation or harm, and ensure adequate ventilation. A major adverse effect of undersedation is breathing dyssynchrony between the patient and ventilator. Ventilator dyssynchrony causes inadequate gas exchange and increases the patient's risk for ventilator-induced lung injury.[24,44]

Oversedation can also lead to long-term sequelae such as delirium. The amount of sedation used must be monitored carefully to achieve predetermined end points or goals (see Chapter 5). Sedation goals are based on the patient's response to therapy and are determined through a collaborative effort between the physician, clinical pharmacist, and the critical care nurse. Regular assessment and documentation of response to therapy with a validated sedation assessment scale along with a validated delirium assessment scale are essential.[34,58]

Therapeutic paralysis with a neuromuscular blocking agent may be required to completely control ventilation and promote adequate oxygenation. Patients who require unconventional modes of mechanical ventilation often need neuromuscular blockade because these modes are uncomfortable for the patient and provide an unnatural means of respiration.[10] Use of neuromuscular blocking agents require careful consideration and monitoring because of the increased risk of prolonged myopathy (see Chapter 5). However, a recent article showed that early administration of neuromuscular blocking agents in patients with severe ARDS improved survival, increased the time off the ventilator, and did not increase muscle weakness in this subset population.[55]

Prone Positioning

Patients with ARDS who do not respond to standard treatment may benefit from prone positioning. Turning the patient to the prone position (*proning*) alters the $\dot{V}/\dot{Q}$ ratio by shifting perfusion from the posterior bases of the lung to the anterior portion with improved ventilation. Proning also removes the weight of the heart and abdomen from the lungs, facilitates removal of secretions, improves oxygenation, and enhances recruitment of airways.[63,67] Proning should be considered when the PaO_2/FiO_2 ratio falls below 100, other lung recruitment strategies have been maximized, and/or the pulmonary status continues to deteriorate. Once turned to the prone position, the optimal duration of therapy is up to 24 hours daily, with therapy continuing until the improvement in oxygenation is maximized.[4,67]

Turning the patient to the prone position is a cumbersome procedure requiring involvement of several healthcare professionals to ensure the patient's safety. Care must be taken to prevent dislodging the ETT and other tubes and lines. Several commercial devices are available to assist in turning the patient such as the Vollman Prone Positioner (Hill-Rom Services Corp.) and specialized proning beds.

Potential complications from the prone position are gastric aspiration, peripheral nerve injury, pressure ulcers, corneal ulceration, and facial edema. Gastric tube feedings are turned off for 1 hour or aspirated before turning the patient to reduce the risk of aspiration. Proper body alignment must be maintained while the patient is in the prone position to decrease the risk of nerve damage. Pillows and foam support equipment are used to prevent overextension or flexion of the spine and reduce weight-bearing on bony prominences. Protective pads are used at the shoulders, iliac crest, and knees to decrease alterations in skin integrity and peripheral nerve damage. To avoid peripheral nerve injury and contractures of the shoulders, the arms are positioned carefully and repositioned often. A moisture barrier is applied to the patient's entire face to protect the skin from the massive amount of drainage from the mouth and nose. Absorbent pads, an emesis basin, or both, can be placed to capture the excessive oral and nasal drainage. The eyes must be protected to prevent direct ocular pressure caused by facial edema. The eyes are lubricated and taped shut to prevent corneal drying and abrasions.[67]

Fluids and Electrolytes

Conservative fluid management, including diureis, is the goal for patients with ARDS, resulting in reduced mortality, improved lung function, shorter length of mechanical ventilation, and fewer critical care unit days.[27,59] Patients who are hypotensive or hypovolemic should however, receive aggressive fluid resuscitation until the condition has resolved. The use of colloids along with diuretics has been shown to be effective in hypoproteinemic patients only.[28,69]

Nutrition

The goal of nutritional support is to provide adequate nutrition to meet the patient's level of metabolism and reduce morbidity[17] (see Chapter 6). Several studies have evaluated the effects of a specialized enteral nutritional formula enriched with eicosapentaenoic acid (EPA), gamma-linolenic acid (GLA), and elevated antioxidants (EPA/GLA) in the treatment of ARDS. The studies have demonstrated reduced mortality, improved oxygenation secondary to reduced pulmonary inflammation, and fewer days of mechanical ventilation.[56]

Pharmacological Treatment

Despite clinical studies of various medications, no pharmacological agents are considered standard therapy for ARDS. Furosemide with albumin is advocated when the patient's protein level is low. The combination has resulted in improved oxygenation and reduced time receiving mechanical ventilation. Corticosteroids administration should be considered in patients with severe ARDS and before day 14.[59,64] Studies with inhaled nitric oxide have not shown improvements in survival or duration of mechanical ventilation; however, it is used as rescue therapy for severe refractory hypoxemia. The early use of cisatracurium, a neuromuscular blocking agent, during the first 48 hours in patients with severe ARDS may improve some some outcomes.[55] Several new and different drugs are being studied, including statins and granulocyte-macrophage colony-stimulating factor.[59]

Psychosocial Support

The onset of ARDS and its long recovery phase result in stress and anxiety for both the patient and the family. The patient may also experience feelings of isolation and dependence because of the length of the recovery phase. Healthcare team members must always remember to provide a warm, nurturing environment in which the patient and family can feel safe. A therapeutic environment includes taking the time to explain procedures, equipment, changes in the patient's condition, and outcomes to the patient and family members. Allowing the patient to participate in the planning of care and to verbalize fears and questions may help reduce stress and anxiety. In the intubated patient, communication is impaired, which increases the patient's sense of isolation. The isolation and accompanying depression can be minimized by encouraging a family member to stay with the patient and displaying personal items from home, such as photographs of loved ones.

ACUTE RESPIRATORY FAILURE IN CHRONIC OBSTRUCTIVE PULMONARY DISEASE

Pathophysiology

COPD is a progressive disease characterized by airflow limitations that are not fully reversible. These airflow limitations are associated with an abnormal inflammatory response to noxious particles or gases.[47] COPD is characterized by a mixture of small airway disease (obstructive bronchiolitis) and parenchymal destruction (emphysema). COPD is a preventable disease with treatment goals of decreasing symptoms and reducing exacerbations. Its incidence and impact on chronic morbidity and mortality are increasing. COPD is the fourth leading cause of death in the United States after cardiac disease, cancer, and stroke. The primary cause of COPD is tobacco smoke, and smoking cessation is the most effective intervention to reduce the risk of developing COPD and stop disease progression.[47] Other contributing factors to the development of COPD include air pollution, occupational exposure to dust or chemicals, and the genetic abnormality alpha$_1$-antitrypsin deficiency.[20]

The primary pathogenic mechanism in COPD is chronic inflammation, which may be both direct injury to the airway and also lead to systemic effects.[53] Exposure to inhaled particles leads to airway inflammation and injury. The body repairs this injury through the process of airway remodeling, which causes scarring, narrowing, and obstruction of the airways. Destruction of alveolar walls and connective tissue results in permanent enlargement of air spaces. Increased mucus production results from enlargement of mucus-secreting glands and an increase in the number of goblet cells. Areas of cilia are destroyed, contributing to the patient's inability to clear thick, tenacious mucus. Structural changes in the pulmonary capillaries thicken the vascular walls and inhibit gas exchange. Systemic inflammation also causes direct effects on peripheral blood vessels and may be a concomitant factor in the association of cardiovascular disease in these patients. Table 14-2 outlines the physiological changes that result from COPD.

ARF can occur at any time in the patient with COPD. These patients normally have little respiratory reserve, and any condition that increases the work of breathing worsens V̇/Q̇ mismatching. Common causes of ARF in patients with COPD are acute exacerbations, heart failure, dysrhythmias, pulmonary edema, pneumonia, dehydration, and electrolyte imbalances.

Assessment

The hallmark symptoms of COPD are dyspnea, chronic cough, and sputum production. The diagnosis is confirmed by postbronchodilator spirometry that documents irreversible airflow limitations.[47] These pulmonary function tests show an increase in total lung capacity and a reduction in forced expiratory volume over 1 second (FEV_1). Functional residual capacity is increased as a result of air trapping.

TABLE 14-2   PATHOLOGICAL AND PHYSIOLOGICAL CHANGES IN CHRONIC OBSTRUCTIVE PULMONARY DISEASE

PATHOLOGICAL CHANGES	PHYSIOLOGICAL CHANGES
Mucus hypersecretion	Sputum production
Ciliary dysfunction	Retained secretions Chronic cough
Chronic airway inflammation	Expiratory airflow limitation
Airway remodeling	Terminal airway collapse Air trapping Lung hyperinflation
Thickening of pulmonary vessels	Poor gas exchange with hypoxemia and hypercapnia Pulmonary hypertension Cor pulmonale (right ventricular enlargement and heart failure)

By the time the characteristic physical findings of COPD are evident on physical examination, a significant decline in lung function has occurred. The chest will be overexpanded, or barrel-shaped, because the anteroposterior diameter increases in size. Respiration may include the use of accessory muscles and pursed-lip breathing. Clubbing of the fingers indicates long-term hypoxemia. Lung auscultation usually reveals diminished breath sounds, prolonged exhalation, wheezing, and crackles. ABG results show mild hypoxemia in the early stages of the disease, and worsening hypoxemia and hypercapnia as the disease progresses. Over time, as a compensatory mechanism, the kidneys increase bicarbonate production and retention (metabolic alkalosis) in an attempt to keep the pH within normal limits.

Exacerbations of COPD often result in a change in the patient's baseline dyspnea and an increase in sputum volume. Changes in the character of the sputum may signal the development of a respiratory infection. Additional symptoms may include anxiety, wheezing, chest tightness, tachypnea, tachycardia, fatigue, malaise, confusion, fever, and sleeping difficulties. Wheezing indicates narrowing of the airways. Retraction of intercostal muscles may occur with inspiration, and exhalation is prolonged through pursed lips. The patient is generally more comfortable in the upright position. Tachycardia and hypotension may result from reduced cardiac output.

ABG monitoring is a sensitive indicator of the respiratory status of the patient with COPD. It is important to know the patient's baseline ABG values to detect changes that indicate ARF. The patient with COPD usually has baseline ABG results that show a normal pH, a moderately low PaO_2 in the range of 60 to 65 mm Hg, and an elevated $PaCO_2$ in the range of 50 to 60 mm Hg (compensated respiratory acidosis). When ARF ensues, the pH decreases, the $PaCO_2$ increases, and the PaO_2 often decreases, resulting in respiratory acidosis and tissue hypoxia. An additional indicator is a change in the patient's mental status and signals an immediate evaluation (see box, "Clinical Alert: Chronic Obstructive Pulmonary Disease").

❗ CLINICAL ALERT
Chronic Obstructive Pulmonary Disease

During an acute exacerbation of chronic obstructive pulmonary disease, the risk of death is highest in patients with a low PaO_2, respiratory acidosis, significant comorbidities, and the need for ventilatory support.

Interventions

Box 14-2 outlines the care of patients with stable COPD. These interventions should be individualized to reduce risk factors, manage symptoms, limit complications, and enhance the patient's quality of life. When a patient has an acute exacerbation, the goals of therapy are to provide support during the episode of acute failure, to treat the triggering event, and to return the patient to the previous level of functioning.

BOX 14-2   TREATMENT OF STABLE CHRONIC OBSTRUCTIVE PULMONARY DISEASE

- Reduce exposure to airway irritants
- Counseling/treatment for smoking cessation
- Remain in air-conditioned environment during times of high air pollution
- Influenza and pneumococcal vaccinations
- Inhaled bronchodilators (short-acting, long-acting, or combination)
- Inhaled glucocorticosteroids (for severe disease and repeated exacerbations)
- Pulmonary rehabilitation program with exercise training
- Long-term administration of oxygen more than 15 hours/day (for severe disease)

Oxygen

The most important intervention for acute exacerbation of COPD is to correct hypoxemia. O_2 should be administered to achieve a PaO_2 greater than 60 mm Hg or an SaO_2 greater than 90%.[47,53] However, delivering high concentrations of O_2 in an attempt to raise the PaO_2 above 60 mm Hg will not significantly raise the SaO_2 and may also blunt the COPD patient's hypoxic drive. This can diminish respiratory efforts and further increase CO_2 retention. Oxygen should be titrated slowly and incrementally along with reevaluation of arterial blood gases to monitor both O_2 and CO_2 levels.

Bronchodilator Therapy

Table 14-3 lists commonly administered bronchodilator agents. Short-acting, inhaled beta$_2$-agonists cause bronchial smooth muscle relaxation that reverses bronchoconstriction. They are primarily administered via a nebulizer or a metered-dose inhaler with a spacer. The dosage and frequency vary, depending on the delivery method and the severity of bronchoconstriction. Adverse effects are dose related and are more common with oral or intravenous administration compared with inhalation. Adverse effects include tachycardia, dysrhythmias, tremors, hypokalemia, anxiety, bronchospasm, and dyspnea. Beta$_2$-agonists should be administered cautiously in patients with cardiac disease. Long-acting beta$_2$-agonists are effective in controlling stable COPD, but their onset of action is too long to be useful in the rapid treatment of acute exacerbations. They are administered by inhalation using a metered-dose inhaler or dry powder inhaler.

Anticholinergics may also be administered to treat bronchoconstriction. They are indicated for patients who are not immediately responsive to tolerate beta$_2$-agonists and may be used in combination. The use of methylxanthines for acute exacerbation is controversial and requires the monitoring of trough blood levels to maintain therapeutic concentrations.[47] Cardiac side effects may be seen in addition to central nervous system stimulation that may lead to headache, restlessness, and seizures. The use of expectorants, mucolytic agents, and chest physical therapy has not been found to be effective in the management of COPD exacerbations.

Corticosteroids

Administration of oral or intravenous corticosteroids for a period of 7 to 10 days to decrease airway inflammation is beneficial in the management of an acute exacerbation of COPD.[47] Common adverse effects of steroid therapy include hyperglycemia and an increased risk of infection. There may also be an unexplained association between steroid use in the critically ill and the development of skeletal muscle neuromyopathy.

Antibiotics

Antibiotic therapy is recommended when dyspnea is accompanied by increased sputum volume and purulence, or if mechanical ventilation is needed. Infections are commonly caused by *Haemophilus influenzae*, *Streptococcus pneumoniae*, and *Moraxella catarrhalis*.[47] Multiple drug-resistant bacterial infections are common in COPD exacerbations, and antibiotic selection should be based on local bacterial resistance patterns and on sensitivity reports from sputum cultures.[52]

TABLE 14-3	**PHARMACOLOGY**	
Bronchodilators		
MEDICATION	**MECHANISM OF ACTION**	**ADVERSE EFFECTS/NURSING IMPLICATIONS**
Beta$_2$-agonists (short-acting) Albuterol Bitolterol Fenoterol Pirbuterol Terbutaline	Bronchial smooth muscle relaxation; relief of acute symptoms	Tremor, anxiety, bronchospasm, dyspnea, tachycardia, dysrhythmias, palpitations, hypertension, hypokalemia, throat irritation
Beta$_2$-agonists (long-acting) Salmeterol Formoterol	Bronchial smooth muscle relaxation; long-term prevention of symptoms	Same as for short-acting beta$_2$-agonists; do not use to treat acute exacerbations
Anticholinergics Ipratropium bromide Oxitropium bromide Tiotropium bromide	Inhibit action of acetylcholine, causing bronchial smooth muscle relaxation	Dry mouth, bitter taste, dizziness, bronchoconstriction, palpitations; lower incidence of tachycardia than beta$_2$-agonists; avoid contact with eyes
Methylxanthines Theophylline Aminophylline	Phosphodiesterase inhibitor	Tremor, tachycardia, dysrhythmias, CNS stimulation (headache, seizures, restlessness), nausea, vomiting; do not crush sustained-release capsules; monitor trough levels

CNS, Central nervous system.

Ventilatory Assistance

Patients with ARF from a COPD exacerbation benefit from early treatment with NPPV. Unlike invasive mechanical ventilation that requires insertion of an ETT or a tracheostomy, NPPV assists the patient's respiratory efforts by delivering positive airway pressure through a nasal, oronasal, or full face mask.

Contraindications to NPPV include respiratory arrest, hemodynamic instability, thick or copious secretions, a change in mental status or uncooperative, extreme obesity, burns, and head or facial trauma/surgery.[49] Studies on the use of NPPV in COPD exacerbations have shown a decrease in the need for intubation, lower mortality rates, a decreased critical care length of stay, and a decrease in the occurrence of health care–acquired pneumonia.[40,49]

Intubation and invasive mechanical ventilation are indicated in those patients who, despite aggressive therapy, develop significant mental status changes, severe dyspnea and respiratory muscle fatigue, respiratory acidosis, significant hypoxemia, or hypercapnia.

In the late stages of severe COPD, patients often report that their quality of life deteriorates because of severe activity limitations and comorbid conditions. Decisions regarding the use or avoidance of intubation, mechanical ventilation, cardiopulmonary resuscitation, and other forms of life support should be made by the patient in conjunction with the patient's family and physician before ARF occurs. Critical care nurses are in an ideal position to facilitate discussions about advance directives and to answer questions for the patient and significant others.

ACUTE RESPIRATORY FAILURE IN ASTHMA

Pathophysiology

Asthma is a chronic inflammatory disorder of the airways. The inflammation causes the airways to become hyperresponsive when the patient inhales allergens, viruses, or other irritants (Box 14-3). Episodic airflow obstruction results because these irritants cause bronchoconstriction, airway edema, mucus plugging, and airway remodeling[48,60] (Figure 14-3). Air trapping, prolonged exhalation, and $\dot{V}/\dot{Q}$ mismatching with an increased intrapulmonary shunt occur. The airflow limitations in asthma are largely reversible. When asthma is controlled, symptoms and exacerbations should be infrequent.

Assessment

Symptoms of asthma exacerbation are wheezing, dyspnea, chest tightness, and cough, especially at night or in the morning. The

---

BOX 14-3 ASTHMA TRIGGERS

Inhalant Allergens
- Animals
- House-dust mites
- Cockroaches
- Indoor fungi
- Outdoor allergens

Occupational Exposure
- Organic and inorganic dusts
- Chemical agents
- Fumes

Irritants
- Tobacco smoke
- Indoor/outdoor pollution
- Fumes: perfumes, cleaning agents, sprays

Other Factors Influencing Asthma Severity
- Viral respiratory infections
- Rhinitis/sinusitis
- Gastroesophageal reflux disease
- Exercise
- Sensitivity: aspirin, other nonsteroidal antiinflammatory drugs, sulfites
- Topical and systemic beta-blockers

---

patient initially hyperventilates, producing respiratory alkalosis. As the airways continue to narrow, it becomes more difficult for the patient to exhale. Peak expiratory flow readings will be less than 50% of the patient's normal values. The lungs become overinflated and stiff, which further increases the work of breathing. Nursing assessment will reveal tachypnea, tachycardia, pulsus paradoxus greater than 25 mm Hg, agitation, possible use of accessory muscles, and suprasternal retractions. A severe asthma exacerbation, previously referred to as status asthmaticus, occurs when the bronchoconstriction does not respond to bronchodilator therapy, and ARF ensues. The patient experiences fatigue from the severe dyspnea, cough, and increased work of breathing. Hypercapnia, hypoxia, and respiratory acidosis develop, and cardiac output decreases as a result of a decreased venous return that is related to increased intrathoracic pressures (see box, "Clinical Alert: Asthma").

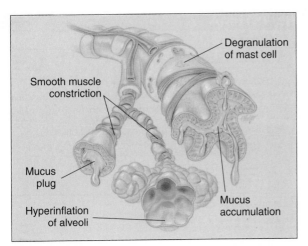

FIGURE 14-3 Airway obstruction caused by asthma. Bronchial asthma: thick mucus, mucosal edema, and smooth muscle spasm causing obstruction of small airways. (From McCance KL, Huether SE. *Pathophysiology: The Biologic Basis for Diseases in Adults and Children.* 6th ed. St. Louis: Mosby; 2010.)

! CLINICAL ALERT

Asthma

Signs of impending acute respiratory failure in a patient with severe asthma include:
- Breathlessness at rest and the need to sit upright
- Speaking in single words; unable to speak in sentences or phrases
- Lethargy or confusion
- Paradoxical thoracoabdominal movement
- Absence of wheezing ("silent chest") indicating no air movement and respiratory muscle fatigue
- Bradycardia
- Respiratory acidosis and hypoxemia with $PaCO_2$ higher than 45 mm Hg and PaO_2 less than 60 mm Hg

Interventions

Mild exacerbations of asthma can be managed by the patient at home with the use of short-acting beta$_2$-agonists to treat bronchoconstriction (see Table 14-3). Treatment of acute, severe exacerbations of asthma requires O_2 therapy, repeated administration of rapid-acting inhaled bronchodilators, and systemic steroid administration (Table 14-4). Most patients respond well to treatment, but some may need intubation and mechanical ventilation. Because of severe airflow obstruction, these patients are at risk for developing dynamic lung hyperinflation (auto-PEEP), lung injury from barotrauma, and hemodynamic compromise.[9] Precise management of mechanical ventilation is required to enhance outcomes and prevent complications. In cases that are refractory to standard treatment, oxygenation may be improved by delivering a mixture of helium and O_2 (heliox) to the lungs. Because helium is less dense than O_2, it enhances gas flow through the constricted airways and may improve oxygenation.[9]

During a patient's recovery from a severe asthmatic event, the critical care nurse should focus efforts on teaching the patient asthma management techniques because patient and family education is essential for achieving asthma control. Persons with asthma are taught how to implement environmental controls to prevent symptoms, understand the differences between medications that relieve and control symptoms, properly use inhaler devices, and monitor their level of asthma control.[48] A written action plan and goals of treatment mutually determined by the patient and the healthcare provider helps patients to achieve asthma control and assists with early identification and treatment of exacerbations.

ACUTE RESPIRATORY FAILURE RESULTING FROM PNEUMONIA

Definition and Etiology

Pneumonia is the leading cause of death from infection in the United States and a common cause of acute respiratory failure.[43,50,68] Pneumonia is a lower respiratory tract infection with a variety of risk factors. Classification of the pneumonia is important because of the likely organism and treatment (Table 14-5). Populations that are at increased risk include the elderly, alcoholics, tobacco smokers, and those with lung or heart disease, head injury, malignancies, renal or liver failure, diabetes mellitus, splenic dysfunction, or any conditions with immunosuppression.

TABLE 14-4	EMERGENCY TREATMENT OF SEVERE ASTHMA	
THERAPY	**PURPOSE**	**GOALS**
Oxygen via nasal cannula or face mask	Correct hypoxemia	Maintain SpO_2 ≥90%
Inhaled rapid-acting beta$_2$-agonists via nebulizer (continuous); followed by intermittent on-demand therapy	Relieve airway obstruction caused by bronchoconstriction	Achieve PEF >70% of predicted or personal best; normalizing/improving ABGs; respiratory rate <30 breaths/min without use of accessory muscles
Inhaled anticholinergics (added to beta$_2$-agonist therapy)	Relieve bronchoconstriction	Relieve sensation of dyspnea; patient able to complete full sentences without breathlessness
Systemic corticosteroids (orally or intravenous)	Reverse airway inflammation	Improve lung sounds; prevent intubation

ABGs, Arterial blood gases; *PEF,* peak expiratory flow; *SpO$_2$,* arterial oxygen saturation by pulse oximetry.

TABLE 14-5	PNEUMONIA DEFINITIONS AND COMMON INFECTIOUS CAUSES	
PNEUMONIA	**CRITERIA**	**LEADING INFECTIOUS CAUSES**
Community-acquired pneumonia (CAP)	Pneumonia that develops outside the hospital in patients who have either not been hospitalized or living in a long-term care facility for more than 2 weeks	*Streptococcus pneumoniae* *Haemophillus influenzae* *Mycoplasma pneumoniae* *Chlamydophila pneumonia* *Legionella*
Healthcare-acquired pneumonia (HCAP)	Develops in patients who were hospitalized in an acute care hospital for 2 or more days within 90 days of the infection; resided in a long-term care facility; received intravenous antibiotic therapy, chemotherapy, or wound care within the past 30 days; or had hemodialysis at a hospital or clinic	*Staphylococcus aureus* *Pseudomonas aeruginosa* *Enterobacter species* *Acinetobacter baumannii* *Klebsiella pneumoniae* *Escherichia coli* *Candida* species *Klebsiella oxytoca* Coagulase-negative staphylococci *Enterococcus* species
Hospital-acquired pneumonia (HAP)	Pneumonia that develops in hospitalized patients which occurs more than 48 hours after hospital admission excluding any infection incubating at the time of admission	
Ventilator-associated pneumonia (VAP)	Pneumonia that develops in patients which develops 48 hours or more after intubation	

Based on data from Mandell LA, Wunderkink RG, Anzueto A, Bartlett JG, et al. Infectious disease society of America/American thoracic society concensus guidelines on the management of community-acquired pneumonia in adults. *Clinical Infectious Disease,* 2007;44, S27-S72; Hidron AL, Edwards JR, Patel J, Horan TC, et al. Antimicrobial-resistant pathogens associated with healthcare-associated infections: annual summary of data reported to the national healthcare safety network at the centers for disease control and prevention, 2006-2007. *Infection Control and Hospital Epidemiology,* 2008;29(11), 996-1011.

Pathophysiology

For pneumonia to occur, enough organisms must accumulate in the lower respiratory tract to overwhelm the patient's normally competent defense mechanisms. The lower respiratory tract is usually a sterile environment and protected by the filtration, warming and filtering of air through the upper airway, closure of the epiglottis, cough and sneezing reflexes, mucocilliary clearance, and alveolar macrophages. The major routes of entry for these organisms include aspiration of gastric or oropharyngeal secretions, inhalation of aerosols or particles, and hematogenous spread from another infected site into the lungs. The normal bronchomucociliary clearance mechanism is overwhelmed by the organism, causing a large influx of phagocytic cells along with exudate into the airways and alveoli. This inflammatory response leads to a ventilation perfusion mismatch resulting in dyspnea, hypoxemia, fever, and leukocytosis.[7]

The pathogens responsible for pneumonia vary depending on the type (community versus hospital-acquired) and are also based on the environmental factor or cause[30,42] (see Table 14-5). The pathogens include bacterial, viral, and fungal causes along with multidrug-resistant organisms, such as methicillin-resistant *Staphylococcus aureus* (MRSA). The most common bacterial causes of CAP are *streptococcus* and *pneumococcus* infection. Pneumococcal pneumonia, is preventable by receiving the pneumococcal vaccination[12] (Table 14-6). The most common viral cause is influenza. The influenza vaccine has been shown to reduce the incidence of pneumonia by 53%, and routine vaccination annually is recommended for all persons older than 6 years in the United States.[11,50] The composition of the vaccine changes yearly based on projected viruses for that season. As an example, influenza A or H1N1 vaccine was added to the 2010 vaccination in response to the 2009 H1N1 pandemic. Fungal causes of pneumonia are uncommon unless the patient is immunocompromised.

Assessment

The clinical presentation for pneumonia commonly includes fever, cough, purulent sputum, hemoptysis, dyspnea, tachypnea, pleuritic chest pain, and abnormal breath sounds. Elderly patients may present with nonspecific symptoms such as confusion, weakness, lethargy, or change in appetite.[51] Recommended diagnostic studies include a chest x-ray which may show new or progressive infiltrates. Pretreatment blood and sputum cultures should be obtained without delaying implementation of antibiotic therapy. Urinary antigen tests for *Legionella pneumophila* and streptococcus pneumonia may also be obtained.[42] Abnormal laboratory results include an elevated white blood cell count and arterial blood gases demonstrating hypoxemia and hypocapnia.[7]

TABLE 14-6   PNEUMOCCAL VACCINE RECOMMENDATIONS FOR PREVENTION OF PNEUMOCOCCAL DISEASE

- All persons between 19 and 64 years old by risk group (single dose)
- All persons 65 years of age or older (single dose if not previously received, or second dose with waiting period of 5 years between doses if received previously as high risk)

RISK GROUP	UNDERLYING MEDICAL INDICATION
Immunocompetent	Chronic heart disease (excluding hypertension)
	Chronic lung disease
	Diabetes mellitus
	Cerebrospinal fluid leaks
	Cochlear implants
	Alcoholism
	Chronic liver disease (includes cirrhosis)
	Cigarette smoking
Functional or anatomical asplenia	Sickle cell disease or other hemoglobinopathies
	Asplenia, spenic dysfunction, or splenectomy
Immunocompromised	Congenital or acquired
	Human immunodeficiency virus infection
	Chronic renal failure
	Hemotological and generalized malignancies
	Treatment with immunosuppressive drugs (including long-term systemic corticosteroids or radiation therapy)
	Solid organ transplantation

Modified from the Centers for Disease Control and Prevention. Updated recommendations for prevention of invasive pneumococcal disease among adults using the 23-valent pneumococcal polysaccharide vaccine. *MMWR. Morbidity and Mortality Weekly Report,* 2010;59:1102-1106.

The Centers for Medicare & Medicaid Services defined core performance measure for pneumonia that are collected by all U.S. hospitals and publicly reported at www.hospitalcompare.hhs.gov. These core measures include: (1) the first dose of antibiotics is given within 6 hours of arrival to the hospital; (2) the correct antibiotic is given; (3) blood cultures are obtained within 24 hours for all patients admitted to an ICU, with blood cultures drawn in the ED before antibiotics are given; (4) smoking cessation advice given to the patient is documented; and (5) pneumococcal and influenza vaccines are administered to appropriate candidates.

VENTILATOR-ASSOCIATED PNEUMONIA

Ventilator-associated pneumonia (VAP) is a preventable hospital-acquired infection with high morbidity and mortality. Crude mortality varies from 10% to 40% and reaches as high as 76% if the disease is caused by high-risk pathogens.[1] Ventilated patients who develop VAP have higher mortality rates and longer length of stays for both the ICU and hospital.[5] The risk for developing VAP is highest during the first 5 days of ventilation.[37] Recently reported VAP rates ranged from 0.5 cases per 1000 ventilator days in respiratory ICUs to 10.7 cases per 1000 ventilator days in burn units.[19]

Pathophysiology

The pathogenesis of VAP is depicted in Figure 14-4. Patients with an ETT are at increased risk for aspiration secondary to the natural anatomical barrier of the glottis being violated. The ETT is inserted into the trachea past the vocal cords,

thereby holding the glottis in the open position and compromising its ability to prevent aspiration.[1] Sources of exogenous pathogens include contamination from healthcare personnel, ventilator and respiratory equipment, and the biofilm coating on the ETT.

Assessment

Clinical criteria for the diagnosis of VAP include a new or progressive pulmonary infiltrate along with fever, leukocytosis, and purulent tracheobronchial secretions. Cultures can be obtained via bronchoscopy, protected-specimen brush, or endotracheal aspirate, and results are reported in either quantitative or semiquantitative terms. Diagnosis is complicated by a lack of sensitive and specific criteria; there is no gold standard. Over 1500 hospitals nationally report VAP rates using the National Healthcare Safety Network (NHSN) surveillance criteria. This includes the presence of a new or persistent lung density seen on chest x-rays with two or more of the following: temperature of more than 38.5° C or less than 36.5° C, leukocyte count of more than 11,000 cells/microliter or less than 5000 cells/microliter, and the presence of purulent endotracheal secretions.[1,13] The clinical pulmonary infection score (CPIS) may also aid in diagnosis. This score combines clinical, radiographic, physiological (PaO_2/FiO_2 ratio), and microbiological information into a numerical value that predicts the presence or absence of pneumonia (Table 14-7).[1,23]

Because of the difficulty in accurately diagnosing VAP based on existing criteria, the NHSN has proposed new surveillance for ventilator-associated events, which includes VAP. Proposed changes to surveillance criteria for adult patients receiving traditional ventilation are summarized in Figure 14-5. As these

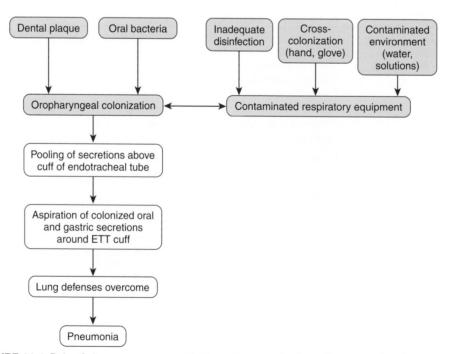

FIGURE 14-4 Role of airway management in the pathogenesis of ventilator-associated pneumonia.

TABLE 14-7   MODIFIED CLINICAL PULMONARY INFECTION SCORE

CPIS POINTS	0	1	2
Tracheal secretions	Rare	Abundant	Abundant and purulent
Chest x-ray infiltrates	No infiltrate	Diffuse	Localized
Temperature (°C)	≥36.5 and ≤38.4	≥38.5 and ≤38.9	≥39 or ≤36
Leukocyte count (per microliter)	≥4000 and ≤11,000	<4000 or >11,000	<4000 or >11,000 + band forms ≥500
PaO_2/FiO_2 ratio (mm Hg)	>240 or ARDS		≤240 and no evidence of ARDS
Microbiology	Negative		Positive

Score each section and determine total points. A score of more than 6 at baseline or after incorporating the Gram stains or culture results is suggestive of pneumonia.

ARDS, Acute respiratory distress syndrome; *CPIS,* clinical pulmonary infection score; *FiO_2,* fraction of inspired oxygen; *PaO_2,* partial pressure of oxygen in arterial blood.

From Fartoukh M, Maitre B, Honore S, Cerf C, Zahar JR, & Brun-Buisson C. Diagnosing pneumonia during mechanical ventilation: The clinical pulmonary infection score revisited. *American Journal of Respiratory and Critical Care Medicine,* 2003;*168,* 173-179.

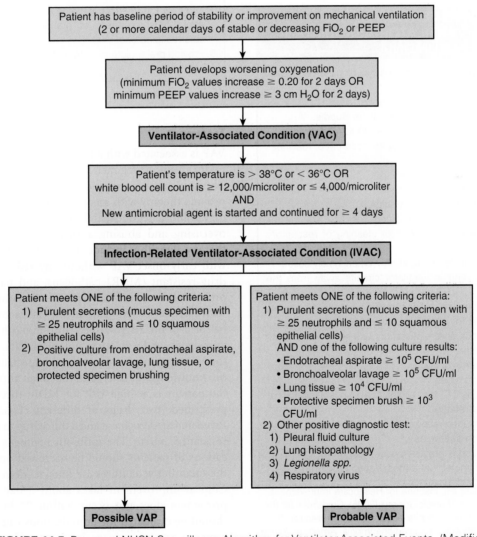

FIGURE 14-5 Proposed NHSN Surveillance Algorithm for Ventilator-Associated Events. (Modified from Centers for Disease Control and Prevention. *Improving Surveillance for Ventilator-Associated Events in Adults,* 2012. Retrieved May 28, 2012 from http://www.cdc.gov/nhsn/PDFs/vae/CDC_VAE_CommunicationsSummary-for-compliance_20120313.pdf.)

criteria are evolving at time of publication, the reader is encouraged to monitor the NHSN website for updated information.

Interventions

The interventions for VAP are aimed at prevention and treatment. The prevention of VAP is a major focus of many recent safety initiatives and focuses on modification of risk factors. The Institute for Healthcare Improvement proposed a "bundle of care" for mechanically ventilated patients. Bundles are evidence-based interventions grouped together to improve outcomes. Five strategies are included in the ventilator bundle: elevation of head of bed (HOB) to at least 30 degrees, daily awakening ("sedation vacation") with assessment of the need for mechanical ventilation, prophylaxis for stress ulcers, prophylaxis for deep venous thrombosis, and daily oral care with chlorhexidine.[2,33] Strategies for prevention of VAP are summarized in Box 14-4, and an example of an oral care protocol is described in Box 14-5

BOX 14-4   PREVENTION OF VENTILATOR-ASSOCIATED PNEUMONIA

1. Effective infection control measures including staff education and hand hygiene
2. Conduct surveillance of ICU infections.
3. Implement components of IHI Ventilator Bundle.
   - Maintain head-of-bed elevation at 30 to 45 degrees.
   - Sedation interruptions and daily assessment of readiness to wean from ventilator
   - Deep vein thrombosis prophylaxis
   - Peptic ulcer disease prophylaxis
   - Daily oral care with chlorohexidine
4. Prevent transmission of microorganisms.
   - Use sterile water for use in or cleaning of respiratory equipment.
   - Change the ventilator circuit only when visibly soiled.
   - Drain condensate in ventilator circuits away from the patient.
   - Do not instill normal saline into ETT.
5. Modify host risk for infections: prevent aspiration.
   - Avoid intubation and reintubation, use noninvasive ventilation if possible.
   - Intubate patients orally.
   - Use orogastric tubes.
   - If available, use ETT that allows continuous aspiration of subglottic secretions.
   - Use sedation and weaning protocols.
6. Other prevention strategies
   - Enteral nutrition is preferred over parenteral.
   - Develop and implement a mobilization program.

ETT, Endotracheal tube; *IHI,* Institute for Healthcare Improvement. Modified from American Thoracic Society. (2005). Guidelines for the management of adults with hospital-acquired, ventilator-acquired pneumonia, and healthcare-associated pneumonia. *American Journal of Respiratory and Critical Care Medicine, 171,* 388-416; Institute of Healthcare Improvement. (2010). *Protecting 5 million lives from harm. Getting started kit: Prevent ventilator-associated pneumonia how-to guide.* Retrieved May 22, 2011, from www.ihi.org.

BOX 14-5   EXAMPLE OF AN ORAL CARE PROTOCOL

Equipment
1. Oral suction catheter
2. Soft toothbrush or suction-toothbrush
3. Toothettes, oral swab or suction-swab
4. 1.5% Hydrogen peroxide mouth rinse or toothpaste
5. Water-based mouth moisturizer
6. Oral chlorhexidine gluconate (0.12%) rinse
7. Suction source and tubing

Interventions
1. Assess intubated patients every 2 hours, before repositioning or deflating the endotracheal tube, and as needed to determine the need for removal of oropharyngeal secretions. Suction as needed.
2. Brush teeth, gums and tongue twice a day using a soft pediatric or adult toothbrush with toothpaste or cleaning solution.
3. Swab oral chlorhexidine gluconate (0.12%) over all oral surfaces for 30 seconds twice a day; suction excess.
4. Avoid brushing teeth or oral intake for 2 hours after chlorhexidine use.
5. Provide oral moisturizing to oral mucosa and lips every 2 to 4 hours.

Treatment

VAP is associated with a high risk of mortality if an appropriate antibiotic regimen is not started in a timely manner.[1] The guidelines for antibiotic use have two major goals: to provide therapy with an appropriate and adequate empirical antibiotic regimen, and to achieve the first goal without overusing and abusing antibiotics. The initial antibiotic therapy algorithm includes two groups of patients: patients with early-onset VAP without any risk factors for multidrug-resistant (MDR) pathogens, and patients with late-onset VAP or risk factors for MDR pathogens.[30] Patients with early-onset VAP without any risk factors for MDR may be placed on narrow-spectrum monotherapy based on knowledge of local microbiological data. Patients at risk for MDR pathogens require broad-spectrum therapy based on knowledge of the local hospital antibiogram. When the patient is at high risk for MDR, three antibiotics are prescribed: two drugs of different classes active against *Pseudomonas aeruginosa* and a third drug to treat methicillin-resistant *S. aureus.* The antibiotic regimens for both classifications of patients should be narrowed once the results of the quantitative cultures are known *(deescalation therapy).* Clinical improvement takes about 3 days. If clinical improvement does not occur within 72 hours, the patient should be evaluated for noninfectious causes of the symptoms or extrapulmonary infections. If a patient receives an appropriate antibiotic regimen, the duration of therapy can be reduced to 7 to 8 days versus the traditional 14 to 21 days.[1,57]

ACUTE RESPIRATORY FAILURE RESULTING FROM PULMONARY EMBOLISM

Definition/Classification

An embolus is a clot or plug of material that travels from one blood vessel to another smaller vessel. The clot lodges in the smaller vessel and obstructs blood flow. An embolus in the pulmonary vasculature is called a pulmonary embolism (PE). The embolus may be a clot that has broken off from a deep vein thrombosis (DVT), a globule of fat from a long bone fracture, septic vegetation, or an iatrogenic catheter fragment. In pregnancy, amniotic fluid can be the cause of a PE. Most PEs originate from DVT of the lower extremities. PE and DVT are the two components of the disease process known as venous thromboembolism (VTE).[54]

PE is classified in several different ways. An initial classification may be acute or chronic. An acute PE occurs quickly and either responds to treatment, or death occurs. A chronic PE initially responds to treatment but then reoccurs. In chronic PE, small clots continue to develop and travel to the pulmonary vascular bed after treatment. Chronic PE is typically caused by a coagulopathy. A PE is also classified based on the amount of pulmonary vascular occlusion: massive, submassive, or nonmassive.[54] A massive PE obstructs 50% or more of the pulmonary vasculature or two or more lobar arteries. The clinical presentation of a massive PE may include syncope, hypotension, extreme hypoxemia, or cardiac arrest.[18,41] A *submassive* PE is usually noted on an echocardiogram as right ventricular dysfunction without hemodynamic instability. A *nonmassive* PE is not associated with right ventricular dysfunction.

Etiology

The three main mechanisms that favor the development of VTE, often referred to as Virchow triad, are (1) venous stasis, or a reduction in blood flow; (2) altered coagulability of blood; and (3) damage to the vessel walls. Specific causes of VTE are listed in Box 14-6.

Acute PE remains a cardiovascular emergency and has a high mortality rate. PE is the third highest cause of hospital mortality and is considered to be the leading cause of preventable hospital deaths in the United States. The Centers for Medicare & Medicaid Services has noted DVT and PE following total knee or hip replacements as a *never event*; an avoidable medical error.[45] Critically ill patients are also at high risk for VTE, and DVT prophylaxis is a part of the IHI ventilator bundle. PE is also the leading cause of maternal death after delivery. It occurs in 2 of every 100,000 live births.[61]

Pathophysiology

When an embolus completely or partially occludes the pulmonary artery or one of its branches, a mechanical obstruction impedes forward flow of blood. The pulmonary circulation has an enormous capacity to compensate for a PE. This compensatory mechanism results from the lung

---

BOX 14-6   RISK FACTORS FOR VENOUS THROMBOEMBOLISM

Hereditary
- Antithrombin deficiency
- Protein C deficiency
- Protein S deficiency
- Factor V Leiden
- Activated protein C resistance
- Dysfibrinogenemia
- Plasminogen deficiency

Acquired
- Reduced mobility
- Advanced age
- Cancer
- Acute medical illness
- Major surgery
- Trauma
- Spinal cord injury
- Pregnancy and postpartum
- Polycythemia vera
- Antiphospholipid antibody syndrome
- Oral contraceptives
- Hormone replacement therapy
- Heparins
- Chemotherapy
- Obesity
- Central venous catheterization
- Immobilizer or cast

Modified from Tapson VF. Acute pulmonary embolism. *New England Journal of Medicine*, 2008;358(10), 1037-1052.

---

vasculature that is necessary to accommodate increased blood flow during exercise, and it is the reason many patients do not initially decompensate from a massive PE. After an embolus lodges in the pulmonary vasculature, blood flow to the alveoli beyond the occlusion is eliminated. The result is a lack of perfusion to ventilated alveoli, an increase in dead space, a $\dot{V}/\dot{Q}$ mismatch, and a decrease in CO_2 tension in the embolized lung zone. Gas exchange cannot occur. Reaction to the mechanical obstruction causes the release of a number of inflammatory mediators such as prostaglandin, serotonin, and histamine. The ensuing inflammation causes constriction of bronchi and surrounding blood vessels.[7]

Constriction in the terminal airways of the nonperfused lung zones results in alveolar shrinking and an increase in the work of breathing. The reduction in blood flow to the alveoli also results in hypoxia for the type II pneumocytes, which are responsible for the production of surfactant. Although the effects are not seen for 24 to 48 hours, the decrease in surfactant results in an unequal gas distribution, an increase in the work of breathing, and a stiffening and collapse of the alveoli. Ventilation is then shifted away from these units, thus worsening the $\dot{V}/\dot{Q}$ mismatch. Atelectasis and shunting transpire as a result of the release of serotonin from the platelets that surround the clot. The result is peripheral airway constriction, which often involves functioning alveoli. In this situation, perfusion with inadequate ventilation occurs.[18,41,65]

The entire process may lead to pulmonary hypertension and an increase in right ventricular workload to maintain pulmonary blood flow. The right ventricle increases in size, causing a leftward shift of the septum. As the process continues, it can lead to decreased left ventricular filling and output. The patient may develop right and left ventricular failure, leading to decreased cardiac output and shock.[7]

The overall prognosis after a PE depends on two main factors. The first is the patient's underlying disease state before the PE, and the second is the appropriate diagnosis and treatment. Appropriate anticoagulation decreases mortality to less than 5%.[54,65]

Assessment

Dyspnea, hemoptysis, and chest pain have been called the "classic" signs and symptoms for a PE, but the three signs and symptoms actually occur in less than 20% of cases.[65] A PE should be suspected in any patient who has unexplained cardiorespiratory complaints and has any risk factors for VTE. A relatively common symptom of PE is the sudden onset of dyspnea. The patient may also be especially apprehensive or anxious, with a feeling of impending doom. Syncope, defined as a loss of consciousness lasting at least 2 minutes, is the presenting symptom in 10% to 15% of patients with a PE. Other common signs and symptoms of PE are chest wall tenderness, chest pain aggravated by deep inspiration, tachypnea, decreased SpO_2, tachycardia, cough, crackles, wheezing, and hemoptysis. Additional signs and symptoms that may occur are an accentuated pulmonic component of the second heart sound (S2), new-onset atrial fibrillation, fever, new-onset reactive airway disease (adult onset asthma), cyanosis, and diaphoresis.[41,54,65] Approximately 79% of patients with PE have positive evidence of DVT in their legs.

Diagnosis

D-Dimer Assay

D-Dimers are fibrin degradation products or fragments produced during fibrinolysis. The D-dimer assay is a sensitive but nonspecific test to diagnose a PE. A negative D-dimer assay has about 90% sensitivity for ruling out a PE in young patients with no comorbidities. A positive D-dimer assay can occur in a number of other conditions such as infection, cancer, surgery, pregnancy, heart failure, or kidney failure.[54,65]

Ventilation-Perfusion Scan

A V̇/Q̇ scan is a noninvasive scintigraphic lung scan that calculates pulmonary airflow and blood flow. A V̇/Q̇ scan may detect dead space from impaired perfusion of ventilated alveoli. Results of V̇/Q̇ scans are reported as low, medium, or high probability.[65]

Duplex Ultrasonography

Duplex ultrasonography is a noninvasive imaging study useful in detecting lower extremity DVT. It has a high sensitivity and specificity for DVT in the leg above the knee, but is not accurate in detecting DVT in pelvic vessels or small vessels in the calf.[54,61]

High-Resolution Multidetector Computed Tomography Angiography

High-resolution multidetector CT angiography (MDCTA; spiral CT) has become the preferred tool for detecting a PE. It is highly accurate for direct visualization of large emboli in the main and lobar pulmonary arteries. MDCTA does not always visualize small emboli in distal vessels, but a pulmonary angiogram has the same limitation.[65]

Magnetic Resonance Imaging

Magnetic resonance imaging has a sensitivity and specificity comparable to that of spiral CT, but it is rarely used to diagnose PE in critically ill patients.

Pulmonary Angiogram

A pulmonary angiogram is considered the gold standard for detecting a PE. It provides direct anatomical visualization of the pulmonary vasculature. Pulmonary angiography is an invasive procedure consisting of catheterization of the right side of the heart with contrast medium injected through the catheter into the pulmonary vascular system. MDCTA is replacing pulmonary angiography as the standard because it is noninvasive and has a high level of sensitivity and specificity.[54]

Prevention

The best therapy for VTE and subsequent PE is prevention.[25,31] Evidence-based strategies for prevention of VTE include the following. (1) Assess patients on hospital admission and routinely throughout their hospital stay for risk of VTE. The nurse, physician, and other members of the multiprofessional team need to review daily both risk and use of VTE prophylaxis. All critically ill patients should receive prophylaxis treatment. (2) It is recommended that patients at high risk for bleeding use mechanical prophylaxis with graduated compression stockings, intermittent pneumatic compression devices, or both, until the risk for bleeding has been resolved. When using these devices, it is imperative to ensure that they are applied correctly and removed for only short periods each day. (3) Patients at moderate risk for developing VTE should receive either low-dose unfractionated heparin or low–molecular weight heparin. (4) Low–molecular weight heparin is recommended for patients at high risk for VTE. (5) The nurse should implement a mobilization regimen for the patient, with the goal of maximizing the patient's mobility.[31] Box 14-7 outlines some nursing interventions to prevent VTE.

BOX 14-7 NURSING MEASURES TO PREVENT VENOUS THROMBOEMBOLISM

Assess Patient on Admission to Unit for Risk for VTE and Anticipate Prophylaxis Orders

Review Daily with Healthcare Team
- Current VTE risk factors
- Necessity for central venous catheter
- Current VTE prophylaxis
- Risk for bleeding
- Response to treatment

Implement Prescribed Prophylactic Regimen
- Pharmacological (according to risk level)
  - *Moderate-risk:* low-dose unfractionated heparin, low–molecular weight heparin, or fondaparinux
  - *High-risk:* low–molecular weight heparin, fondaparinux, or oral vitamin K antagonist
- Nonpharmacological (mechanical) (patient at high risk for bleeding or in conjunction with pharmacological prophylaxis)
  - Graduated compression stockings and/or intermitted pneumatic compression device

Document Implementation Tolerance, and Complications, of Prophylaxis

Assess Extremities on a Regular Basis
- Pain/tenderness
- Unilateral edema
- Erythema
- Warmth

Implement a Mobility Program

Monitor for Low-Grade Fever

Encourage Fluids to Prevent Dehydration;
- Administer IV Fluids as Prescribed; Maintain Accurate Intake and Output Records

Avoid Adjusting the Knee Section of the Bed or Using Pillows Under Knees

Provide Patient Education Regarding Prevention

DVT, Deep vein thrombosis; *IV,* intravenous; *VTE,* venous thromboembolism.

Treatment

Thrombolytic therapy is indicated for a patient with a massive PE who is in cardiogenic shock or has hypotension unless absolute contraindications are present. Thrombolytics may also be considered for a patient who is hemodynamically stable but has signs and symptoms of reduced right ventricular function.[36] Thrombolytic regimens with short infusion times are recommended. Of the four fibrinolytic drugs available—streptokinase, urokinase, t-PA (alteplase), and r-PA (reteplase)—alteplase has the shortest infusion times and is the most widely used agent.[65,66]

Parenteral anticoagulation therapy is recommended for the treatment of an acute PE and in conjunction with thrombolytic therapy in massive PE.[31,54,65] Anticoagulants do not dissolve the existing clot, but allow the fibrinolytic system to function decreasing the thromboembolic burden. Oral anticoagulation with warfarin may also be initiated concurrently on day 1, and overlap therapy should continue until the international normalized ratio (INR) is in the therapeutic range for at least 2 days. It is essential that the critical care nurse regularly monitor the laboratory values and to assess the patient for any signs or symptoms of bleeding or heparin-induced thrombocytopenia (HIT). The nurse must be attuned to major bleeding, such as intracranial or retroperitoneal hemorrhage, and minor bleeding. Heparin-induced thrombocytopenia is a well-known complication of low–molecular weight heparin and unfractionated heparin. It is caused by antibodies that activate platelets and leads to thrombocytopenia.[61] Direct thrombin inhibitors such as argatroban or lepirudin are alternatives in patients who have developed or have a history of HIT.

Catheter embolectomy or local intraembolic thrombolytic therapies are reserved for patients who have contraindications to thrombolytic therapy. Surgical embolectomy is rarely used and involves manual removal of the thrombus from the pulmonary artery. The patient must be placed on a cardiopulmonary support system during the procedure.[65]

Vena cava filters may be placed in the inferior vena cava to prevent recurrence of PE by preventing clots from migrating from the lower extremities. Two types of filters are available: permanent and temporary retrievable. Permanent vena cava filters are rarely used and have a number of associated complications. Temporary retrievable vena cava filters are used to prevent PE in patients who have contraindications for anticoagulation therapy, major bleeding during anticoagulation therapy, or have recurring PE. These devices can be removed by a minimally invasive technique under fluoroscopy.[65]

Other treatments are focused on maintaining the airway, breathing, and circulation. Supplemental O_2 may be administered to maintain SaO_2 at more than 90%. If the location of the PE is known, positioning the patient with the "good" lung in the dependent position is warranted. Analgesics are given to alleviate pain and anxiety. If the patient is hemodynamically unstable, inotropic or vasopressor support may be required.

ACUTE RESPIRATORY FAILURE IN ADULT PATIENTS WITH CYSTIC FIBROSIS

Definition

Cystic fibrosis (CF) is a genetic disorder (see box, "Genetics") resulting from defective chloride ion transport. The mutation in chloride transport causes the formation of mucus with little water. The thick, sticky mucus obstructs the glands of the lungs, pancreas, liver, salivary glands, and testes, causing organ dysfunction. Although CF is a multisystem disease, it has the greatest effect on the lungs. The thick mucus narrows the airways and reduces airflow. The constant presence of thick mucus provides an excellent breeding ground for bacteria, leading to chronic lower respiratory tract bacterial infection, chronic bronchitis, and dilatation of the bronchioles. The mucus-producing cells in the lungs increase in number and size over time. Respiratory complications of CF include pneumothorax, arterial erosion, hemorrhage, chronic bacterial infection, and respiratory failure.[35]

GENETICS

Cystic Fibrosis: A Heritable Disorder with Pulmonary and Gastrointestinal Complications

Cystic fibrosis (CF) is a lifelong disorder that may lead to critical illness. The basic pathological abnormality in this disease is a defect in a protein that forms part of the ion channel that transports chloride across epithelial cell membranes on mucosal surfaces. The defective protein is a result of a variation in the *CFTR* gene on chromosome 7.[1] There are more than 1500 variations in this gene. All of them cause some degree of alteration in the construction and function of the chloride ion channel in epithelial cells, typically resulting in reduced chloride transport across epithelial cell membranes in mucus secreting organs.[1]

Organs and tissues most profoundly affected by the defective chloride ion channels are in the pancreas, intestines, lungs, sweat glands, and vas deferens. As a result of defects in the chloride ion channel, there is reduced secretion of chloride and increased reabsorption of sodium and water across epithelial cells. This leads to synthesis of thick mucus. Thick mucus in the respiratory and gastrointestinal tracts, the pancreas, the sweat glands, and other tissues is difficult to clear and interferes with normal organ function. For example, mucus production in the lungs interferes with gas exchange, leading to chronic hypoxemia. Mucus production in the gastrointestinal tract blocks intestinal fluids, resulting in gastrointestinal obstruction. Thick mucus is also more likely to colonize microorganisms, contributing to infection and inflammation with subsequent adverse and irreversible changes in these organs.[1]

The degree of impairment in the chloride ion channel varies as a result of differences in the protein coded by the *CTFR* gene. For example, the most common genetic variation among patients diagnosed with CF, prevents the CTFR protein from folding properly so that the chloride pump does not reach the cell surface. A different genetic defect, less common and associated with less severe symptoms, results in a functional pump but one with a "sticky" gate that disturbs the ability of the epithelial cell to secrete chloride.[5]

Abnormalities are typically not seen unless CFTR function is less than 10%.[3] Those patients with the most severe symptoms have less than 1% CFTR activity and manifest the full spectrum of disease involvement including pancreatic insufficiency; recurrent, severe pulmonary infections; gastrointestinal obstruction; and congenital absence of the vas deferens.[3]

CF is the most common lethal disease inherited by the white population. One in 22 people of European heritage carry one gene for CF.[2] CF is an autosomal recessive disease, which means that both parents must be a carrier of variant *CFTR* genes or have the disease in order for their children to inherit the gene variation that causes CF. Because so many individuals in the United States are symptomless carriers of CF (estimated at more than 10 million people), genetic testing for all couples who are at high risk for being a carrier because of their ethnicity or family history is recommended.[3,4] In general, testing is performed on just one future parent initially; if that person is a carrier, then the other future parent is tested to calculate the risk that their children will have CF. It is not possible to test for all 1300 variations of the *CFTR* gene in a single genetic test. Testing typically looks for 32 to 70 common mutations.[3] Therefore a negative screen does not guarantee that a child will not have CF. A child with CF usually has the same mutation as the carrier parent. If a family has a known uncommon variant, then specific testing for that polymorphism can be performed.

Symptoms of CF are most often manifested in infancy and early childhood by a persistent cough with mucus production that is frequently colonized with bacteria; by loose, bulky stools; and by failure to thrive. Those with milder disease may not have CF diagnosed until adolescence or early adulthood. The presence of aspermia or male infertility is an indication to the clinician to include CF as a diagnostic possibility. In addition to genotyping, tests of pancreatic function and nasal potential-difference measurements are used to diagnose CF. Diagnosis by sweat testing is also used because the defect in chloride ion channels leads to salty secretions. About 1000 new cases of CF are diagnosed in the United States annually.[2]

If CF genetic testing shows both parents are carriers, genetic counseling is strongly recommended by healthcare providers. When both parents have a *CFTR* variant, as with any autosomal disorder, there is a 1-in-4 chance with each pregnancy that the child will have CF.[1,3] Remember, many variants of CF are not included in the typical genetic test, manifestations of CF can be mild, and not all parents will perceive the diagnosis of CF as a serious disorder. In addition, genetic testing and counseling may not be covered by insurance companies. Thus the healthcare provider needs to individualize the approach to advising persons seeking CF genetic testing. The Cystic Fibrosis Foundation has

Cystic Fibrosis: A Heritable Disorder with Pulmonary and Gastrointestinal Complications—cont'd

links to information as well as support groups when CF is a potential or actual condition in a family.[2] Because of improved treatments over the past four decades, the average life span of a child with diagnosed CF has increased from 10 to 36 years.[1] Genomic science is also offering new strategies for treatment.

Therapies for CF have traditionally focused on alleviating symptoms. However, genomic science has resulted in a line of research to identify small molecules that correct the different defects in *CFTR*. Currently, a new drug is in phase 1 testing (in humans). This drug, VX-770, is designed to "prop open" chloride channels characterized by a specific genetic variation (i.e., the G551D mutation).[5] This milestone provides new hope for people who have CF in terms of providing treatment to prevent permanent, irreversible pathology. Active research programs in several academic centers continue to pursue a cure.

References
1. Boucher RC, Knowles MR, Yankasker JR, Cystic Fibrosis. In Mason RJ, Brouaddus VC, Martin TR, King TE, Schraufnagel DE, Murray JF, & Nadal JA (Eds). *Murray and Nadel's Textbook of Respiratory Medicine* (5th edition pp. 985-1022) Philadelphia: Saunders; 2010.
2. Cystic Fibrosis Foundation. (updated February, 2011). *About Cystic Fibrosis.* http://www.cff.org/AboutCF/. Accessed February 12, 2012.
3. Lashley FR. *Essentials of Clinical Genetics in Nursing Practice.* New York: Springer; 2007.
4. National Institutes of Health. (2011). *Cystic Fibrosis.* Retrieved July 15, 2011 from http://ghr.nlm.nih.gov/condition/cystic-fibrosis. Accessed July 15, 2011.
5. Welsh MJ. Targeting the basic defect in cystic fibrosis. *New England Journal of Medicine.* 2010;363:2056-2057.

Etiology

CF affects primarily whites but is occasionally seen in other races. For many years, CF was considered a disease of children. Because of significant improvements in care, most people with CF are now living into the third decade of life or longer, and 40% of CF patients are older than 18 years.[16] The diagnosis of CF is typically made early in life (70% by age 1 year), but a few patients receive a diagnosis of CF as adults. A sweat test is the typical diagnostics tool for CF in children. Patients who do not receive a diagnosis until adulthood generally present with respiratory problems and have fewer other systems involved. Many of these patients have a normal or borderline sweat test result. They generally have a better prognosis.

Interventions

Respiratory failure is the cause of death for more than 80% of patients with CF.[39] As the disease process progresses, patients develop increased ventilator requirements, air trapping, and respiratory muscle weakness. All of these conditions are complicated by chronic bacterial infections that can quickly become overwhelming. In the past, mechanical ventilation was not considered a treatment option because patient outcomes were poor. During the last 20 years, the standard of care for ARF in CF has been revisited because of improved ventilator modalities, more aggressive pharmacological therapy, and the option of lung transplantation. Lung transplantation provides the opportunity for a tremendous improvement in the quality of life, but acute exacerbations of respiratory failure must be overcome during the wait for a transplant.

The three cornerstones of care for a patient with CF are antibiotic therapy, airway clearance, and nutritional support. Any patient with CF who is admitted to a critical care unit in ARF must have these three issues addressed immediately.

Antibiotic Therapy

A frequent cause of respiratory failure is pneumonia. Antibiotic selection is based on the patient's most recent sputum bacterial isolates. *P. aeruginosa* is the most common pathogen found in adult patients with CF. Patients with CF are at high risk of having MDR bacterial isolates. They require higher doses of antibiotics and shorter dosing intervals than other patients because of differences in the volume of drug distribution and the rate of elimination.

Airway Clearance

Mucolytic agents are routinely administered to facilitate clearance of mucus. Recombinant human DNase (Pulmozyme) is the drug of choice. It decreases the viscosity of sputum by catalyzing extracellular DNA into smaller fragments. Chest physiotherapy is used to increase airway clearance. Bronchodilators are routinely prescribed and administered before chest physiotherapy to increase airway clearance.

Nutritional Support

Enteral nutrition with pancreatic enzyme supplements, if needed, is started early in the course of treatment.[16,35]

Ventilatory Support

If ventilator support is necessary, noninvasive mechanical ventilation is the first line of therapy. Endotracheal intubation with mechanical ventilation is the next step. The goal of mechanical ventilation is the same as with any patient with ARF. Adult patients with CF are at high risk for pneumothorax and massive hemoptysis. The critical care nurse must be aware of these life-threatening complications, constantly monitoring for them, and respond quickly.

CASE STUDY

Mrs. P. is a 57-year-old woman admitted to the critical care unit after a motor vehicle crash. She sustained multiple long bone fractures and a chest contusion, and experienced an episode of hypotension in the emergency department. She received 3 units of red blood cells and 2 L of intravenous fluid in the emergency department. Within 12 hours she became short of breath with an increase in respiratory rate requiring high levels of supplemental oxygen. She was electively intubated and placed on volume-control mechanical ventilation with a positive end-expiratory pressure (PEEP) of 5 cm H_2O. A continuous intravenous sedation infusion was started. The decision was made to titrate the infusion to keep her calm and comfortable. During the next 8 hours, her oxygen saturation by pulse oximetry (SpO_2) steadily deteriorated, and the high-pressure alarms on the ventilator activated frequently. The nurse noted steadily rising peak airway pressures. The fraction of inspired oxygen (FiO_2) had to be increased to 0.80 and the PEEP increased to 14 cm H_2O to maintain her partial pressure of oxygen in arterial blood (PaO_2) at 60 mm Hg. Her chest x-ray study showed bilateral infiltrates with normal heart size. A pulmonary artery catheter was inserted with an initial pulmonary artery occlusion pressure of 14 mm Hg. The sedation infusion required frequent upward titrations to maintain the desired goal of light sedation. The diagnosis of acute respiratory distress syndrome (ARDS) was made.

During the next 6 hours, Mrs. P. steadily became more hypoxemic. She was changed to pressure-controlled ventilation with a PEEP of 20 cm H_2O. The FiO_2 had to be increased to 1.0 (100%) to maintain a PaO_2 of greater than 60 mm Hg. She was extremely restless, with tachycardia, diaphoresis, and a labile SaO_2. The decision was made to start a neuromuscular blocking agent with sedation. During the next few hours her general condition continued to deteriorate. Her SaO_2 ranged from 85%

to 87%. Her chest x-ray findings were worse and revealed a complete *whiteout*. The nurses and physicians decided to turn her to the prone position in an effort to improve oxygenation. An hour after turning her to the prone position, her SpO_2 began to slowly rise. After 2 hours in the prone position, her SpO_2 stabilized at 93%. Slowly, the FiO_2 was decreased to 0.60, with a stable SpO_2 of 92%. After 18 hours she was returned to the supine position. Her SpO_2 decreased to 90% and it remained stable. She was weaned off the neuromuscular blocking agent, and the sedation level was reduced to reach a goal of calm and comfortable.

Mrs. P. slowly improved over the next week. Her ventilator settings were changed from pressure-control to assist-control then to pressure support (PS). The PEEP level was decreased to a physiological level. The sedation was interrupted on a daily basis for weaning parameters and spontaneous breathing trial. On the seventh day, she was extubated and the following day transferred to the general orthopedic nursing unit on 4 liters of oxygen per nasal cannula.

Questions
1. Identify the risk factors Mrs. P. had for developing ARDS.
2. The American-European Consensus Conference recommended three criteria for diagnosing ARDS in the presence of a risk factor. List the criteria.
3. Explain the use of the high PEEP and the nursing monitoring responsibilities.
4. Explain the rationale for the use of sedation and neuromuscular blocking agents and what nursing interventions should occur when using these agents.
5. Explain the rationale for placing the patient in the prone position and what nursing interventions should occur before and after turning a patient to the prone position.

SUMMARY

ARF is a disorder that can affect all segments of the population, from young trauma patients to elderly persons with long-standing pulmonary disease. Patients in the critical care areas are at high risk of ARF. The critical care nurse must be constantly alert to signs of impending respiratory failure.

Changes in respiratory rate and character, breath sounds, and blood gas values must be closely evaluated. Frequent position changes, good pulmonary hygiene, and careful attention to nutritional status all contribute to maintaining a patient's respiratory system and preventing ARF.

CRITICAL THINKING EXERCISES

1. Mr. R. is a 66-year-old man who has smoked 1.5 packs of cigarettes a day for 40 years (60 pack-years). He is admitted with an acute exacerbation of COPD. His baseline ABGs drawn in the clinic 2 weeks ago showed: pH, 7.36; $PaCO_2$, 55 mm Hg; PaO_2, 69 mm Hg; bicarbonate, 30 mEq/L; SaO_2, 92%. In the critical care unit, Mr. R. has coarse crackles in his left lower lung base and a mild expiratory wheeze bilaterally. His cough is productive of thick yellow sputum. His skin turgor is poor; he is febrile, tachycardic, and tachypneic. Currently, Mr. R.'s ABGs while receiving O_2 at 2 L/min via a nasal cannula are: pH, 7.32; $PaCO_2$, 64 mm Hg; PaO_2, 50 mm Hg; bicarbonate, 30 mEq/L; SaO_2, 86%.

   a. What is your interpretation of Mr. R.'s baseline ABGs from the clinic?

   b. What is the probable cause of Mr. R.'s COPD exacerbation, and what treatment is indicated at this time?

   c. What ABG changes would indicate that Mr. R.'s respiratory status is deteriorating?

2. Ms. T. is a 41-year-old woman admitted to the critical care unit and mechanically ventilated for acute asthma. She was extubated yesterday and will be transferred out of the critical care unit tomorrow. What are the important points you must cover in your teaching with Ms. T.?

3. Mr. B. has just been intubated for ARF. Currently, he is agitated and very restless. What risks are associated with Mr. B.'s agitation? What nursing actions are indicated in this situation?

4. Mr. C., age 27 years, was hospitalized 3 days ago after fracturing his femur in a snow-skiing accident. He has just been admitted to the critical care unit with a PE and is orally intubated and receiving mechanical ventilation. What actions would you take to decrease Mr. C.'s risk of developing VAP?

REFERENCES

1. American Thoracic Society. Guidelines for the management of adults with hospital-acquired, ventilator-acquired pneumonia, and healthcare-associated pneumonia. *American Journal of Respiratory and Critical Care Medicine.* 2005;171:388-416.
2. Aragon D, Sole ML. Implementing best practice strategies to prevent infection in the ICU. *Critical Care Nursing Clinics of North America.* 2006;18(4):441-452.
3. Arbour RA. Nursing management: respiratory failure and acute respiratory distress syndrome. In: Lewis SL, Dirksen SR, Heitkemper MM, et al, eds. *Medical-Surgical Nursing: Assessment and Management of Clinical Problems.* 8th ed., pp. 1744-1764. St. Louis: Mosby; 2011.
4. Baumgartner L. Acute respiratory failure and acute lung injury. In: Carlson KK, ed. *AACN Advanced Critical Care Nursing.* St. Louis: Saunders; 2009.
5. Bonten MJ. Ventilator-associated pneumonia: preventing the inevitable. *Healthcare Epidemiology.* 2011;52(1):115-121.
6. Brar NK, Niederman MS. Management of community-acquired pneumonia. *Therapeutic Advances in Respiratory Disease.* 2011;5(1):61-78.
7. Brashers VL. Alterations of pulmonary function. In: McCance KL, Brashers VL, Neal V, eds. *Pathophysiology: The Biologic Basis for Diseases in Adults and Children.* 6th ed., pp. 1266. 1323. St. Louis: Mosby; 2010.
8. Briel M, Meade M, Mercat A, et al. Higher vs lower positive end-expiratory pressure in patients with acute lung injury and acute respiratory distress syndrome. *Journal of the American Medical Association.* 2010;302(9):865-873.
9. Burns SM. Ventilating patients with acute severe asthma: What do we really know? *AACN Advanced Critical Care.* 2006;17(2):186-193.
10. Burton S, Alexander E. Avoiding the pitfalls of ensuring the safety of sustained neuromuscular blockade. *AACN Advanced Critical Care.* 2006;17(3):239-243.
11. Centers for Disease Control and Prevention. Update: recommendations of the advisory committee on immunization practices (ACIP) regarding use of CSL seasonal influenza vaccine (AFluria) in the United States during 2010. 11. *Morbidity and Mortality Weekly Reports.* 2010;59(31):989-992.
12. Centers for Disease Control and Prevention. Updated recommendations for prevention of invasive pneumococcal disease among adults using the 23-valent pneumococcal polysaccharide vaccine (PPSV23). *Morbidity and Mortality Weekly Report.* 59(34):1102-1106.
13. Centers for Disease Control and Prevention. Guidelines for preventing health-care associated pneumonia, 2003. Recommendation of CDC and the healthcare infection control practices advisory committee. *MMWR Morbidity and Mortality Weekly Report.* 2004;53(RR03):1-36.

14. Centers for Disease Control and Prevention. *Frequently Asked Questions about SARS.* http://www.cdc.gov/sars/about/faq.pdf; 2005. Accessed February 12, 2012.

15. Centers for Disease Control. Deaths from chronic obstructive pulmonary disease: United States, 2000. 2005. *MMWR Morbidity and Mortality Weekly Report.* 2008;57(45):1229-1232.

16. Cystic Fibrosis Foundation. *CF Care Guidelines.* http://www.cff.org/treatments/CFCareGuidelines/; 2011. Accessed May 22, 2011.

17. DeMichele SJ, Wood SM, Wennberg AK. A nutritional strategy to improve oxygenation and decrease morbidity in patients who have acute respiratory distress syndrome. *Respiratory Care Clinics of North America.* 2006;12(4):547-566.

18. Dressler DK. Coagulopathies. In: Carlson KK, ed. *AACN Advanced Critical Care Nursing.* pp. 995-1017. St. Louis: Saunders; 2009.

19. Edwards JR, Peterson KD, Banerjee S, et al. Healthcare Safety Network (NHSN) report, data summary for 2006 through 2008; issued December 2009. *American Journal of Infection Control.* 2009;37(10):783-805.

20. Eisner MD, Anthonisen N, Coultas D, et al. An official American Thoracic Society public policy statement: novel risk factors and the global burden of chronic obstructive pulmonary disease. *American Journal of Respiratory and Critical Care Medicine.* 2010;182:693-718.

21. El Sohl AA, Ramadan FH. Overview of respiratory failure in older adults. *Journal of Intensive Care Medicine.* 2006;21(6):345-351.

22. Esan A, Hess D, Raoof S, et al. Severe hypoxemic respiratory failure: part 1-ventilatory strategies. *Chest.* 2010;137(5):1203-1216.

23. Fartoukh M, Maitre B, Honore S, et al. Diagnosing pneumonia during mechanical ventilation: the clinical pulmonary infection score revisited. *American Journal of Respiratory and Critical Care Medicine.* 2003;168:173-179.

24. Fuchs EM, Von Reuden K. Sedation management in the mechanically ventilated critically ill patient. *AACN Advanced Critical Care.* 2008;19(4):421-432.

25. Geerts WH, Bergqvist D, Peneo GF, et al. Prevention of venous thromboembolism. *Chest.* 2008;133(6):381S-453S.

26. Hall J. Respiratory insufficiency: pathophysiology, diagnosis, oxygen therapy. In: Hall J, ed. *Guyton and Hall Textbook of Medical Physiology.* Philadelphia: Saunders; 2011.

27. Harman EM. Acute respiratory distress syndrome. In: Franklin C, Talavera F, Rice TD, et al, eds. *eMedicine* (from Medscape). www.emedicine.medscape.com/article/161539; 2010. Accessed August 30, 2010.

28. Heresi GA, Arroliga AC, Weidemann HP, et al. Pulmonary artery catheter and fluid management in acute lung injury and the acute respiratory distress syndrome. *Clinics of Chest Medicine.* 2006;27(4):627-635.

29. Herridge MS, Cheung AM, Taney MS, et al. One-year outcomes in survivors of the acute respiratory distress syndrome. *New England Journal of Medicine.* 2003;348(8):683-693.

30. Hidron AL, Edwards JR, Patel J, et al. Antimicrobial-resistant pathogens associated with healthcare-associated infections: annual summary of data reported to the national healthcare safety network at the centers for disease control and prevention, 2006. 2007. *Infection Control and Hospital Epidemiology.* 2008;29(11):996-1011.

31. Hirsch J, Guyatt G, Albers GW, et al. Executive summary antithrombotic and thrombolytic therapy. American College of Chest Physicians Evidence-Based Clinical Practice Guidelines. 8th ed. *Chest.* 2008;133(6 suppl.):71S-105S.

32. Hopkins RO, Weaver LK, Collingridge D, et al. Two-year cognitive, emotional, and quality-of-life outcomes in acute respiratory distress syndrome. *American Journal of Respiratory and Critical Care Medicine.* 2005;171:340-347.

33. Institute of Healthcare Improvement. *Protecting 5 Million Lives from Harm. Getting Started Kit: Prevent Ventilator-associated Pneumonia How-to Guide.* http://www.ihi.org/knowledge/Pages/Tools/HowtoGuidePreventVAP.aspx; 2010. Accessed February 12, 2012.

34. Jacobi J, Fraser GL, Coursin DB, et al. Clinical practice guidelines for the sustained use of sedatives and analgesics in the critically ill patient. *Critical Care Medicine.* 2002;30(1):119-141.

35. Kaufman JS. Nursing management. Obstructive pulmonary diseases. In: Lewis SL, Dirksen SR, Heitkemper MM, et al, eds. *Medical-Surgical Nursing: Assessment and Management of Clinical Problems.* 8th ed., pp. 587-640. St. Louis: Mosby.

36. Kearon C, Kahn SR, Agnelli G, et al. Antithrombotic therapy for venous thromboembolic disease. *Chest.* 2008;133(6):454S-545S.

37. Kollef MH. What is ventilator-associated pneumonia and why is it important? *Respiratory Care.* 2005;50(6):714-721.

38. Kyle DM. Blood conservation and blood component replacement. In: Carlson KK, ed. *AACN Advanced Critical Care Nursing.* pp. 969-994. St. Louis: Saunders; 2009.

39. Liou TG, Adler FR, Cox DR, et al. Lung transplantation and survival in children with cystic fibrosis. *New England Journal of Medicine.* 2007;357(21):2143-2152.

40. Majid A, Hill NS. Noninvasive ventilation for acute respiratory failure. *Current Opinion in Critical Care.* 2005;11(1):77-81.

41. Malone MJ. Nursing management: lower respiratory problems. In: Lewis SL, Dirksen SR, Heitkemper MM, et al, eds. *Medical-Surgical Nursing: Assessment and Management of Clinical Problems.* 8th ed., pp. 545-586. St. Louis: Mosby; 2011.

42. Mandell LA, Wunderkink RG, Anzueto A, et al. Infectious diseases society of America/American Thoracic Society consensus guidelines on the management of community-acquired pneumonia in adults. *Clinical Infectious Diseases.* 2007;4:S27-S72.

43. Mehta RM, Niederman MS. Acute infectious pneumonia. In: Irwin RS, Rippe JM, eds. *Irwin and Rippe's Intensive Care Medicine.* 6th ed., pp. 823-847. Philadelphia: Lippincott Williams & Wilkins; 2008.

44. Mellott KG, Grap MJ, Munro CL, et al. Patient-ventilator dyssynchrony: clinical significance and implications for practice. *Critical Care Nurse.* 2009;29(6):41-55.

45. Miller A. Hospital reporting and "never events". http://www.medicarepatientmanagement.com/issues/04-03/mpmMJ09-NeverEvents.pdf; 2009. Accessed February 12, 2012.

46. Muir J, Lamia B, Molano C, et al. Respiratory failure in the elderly. *Seminars in Respiratory and Critical Care Medicine.* 2010;31(5):634-646.

47. National Heart, Lung, and Blood Institute, World Health Organization. *Global Initiative for Chronic Obstructive Lung Disease (GOLD) Global Strategy for the Diagnosis, Management and Prevention of Chronic Obstructive Pulmonary Disease.* http://www.goldcopd.org/uploads/users/files/GOLD_Report_2011_Jan21.pdf; 2011. Accessed February 12, 2012.

48. National Heart, Lung, and Blood Institute. *Global Initiative for Asthma (GINA) Global Strategy for Asthma Management and Prevention.* http://www.ginasthma.org/uploads/users/files/GINA_Report_2011.pdf; 2011. Accessed February 12, 2012.

49. Nava S, Hill N. Non-invasive ventilation in acute respiratory failure. *Lancet.* 2009:374:250-259.

50. Niederman M. Community-acquired pneumonia: the U.S. perspective. *Seminars in Respiratory and Critical Care Medicine.* 2009;30(2):179-188.

51. Niederman M. In the clinic; community-acquired pneumonia. *Annals of Internal Medicine.* 2009;151(7):ITC4-2-ITC4-14.

52. Nseir S, Pompeo C, Calvestri B, et al. Multiple-drug-resistant bacteria in patients with severe acute exacerbation of chronic obstructive pulmonary disease: prevalence, risk factors and outcome. *Critical Care Medicine.* 2006;34(12):2959-2966.

53. Nussbaumer-Ochsner Y, Rabe KF. Systemic manifestations of COPD. *Chest.* 2011;139(1):165-173.

54. Ouellette DR, Setnik G, Beeson MS, et al. Pulmonary embolism. In *eMedicine.* http://emedicine.medscape.com/article/300901-overview; 2011. Accessed February 12, 2012.

55. Papazian L, Forel J, Gacouin A, et al. Neuromuscular blockers in early acute respiratory distress syndrome. *New England Journal of Medicine.* 2010;363(12):1107-1116.

56. Pontes-Arruda A, DeMichele S, Seth A, et al. The use of an in-flammation-modulating diet in patients with acute lung injury or acute respiratory distress syndrome: a meta-analysis of outcome data. *Journal of Parenteral and Enteral Nutrition.* 2008;32(6):596-605.

57. Porzecanski I, Bowton DL. Diagnosis and treatment of ventila-tor-associated pneumonia. *Chest.* 2006;130:597-604.

58. Pun B, Dunn J. The sedation of critically ill adults: part 1: assessment. *American Journal of Nursing.* 2007;107(7):40-48.

59. Raoof S, Goulet K, Esan A, et al. Severe hypexmic respiratory failure: part 2-nonventilatory strategies. *Chest.* 2010;137(6);1437-1448.

60. Reddel HK, Taylor R, Bateman ED, et al. An official American Thoracic Society/European respiratory society statement: asthma control and exacerbations. *American Journal of Respiratory and Critical Care Medicine.* 2009;180:59-99.

61. Shaughnessy K. Massive pulmonary embolism. *Critical Care Nurse.* 2007;27(1):39-50.

62. Siela, D. Chest radiograph evaluation and interpretation. *AACN Advanced Critical Care.* 2008;19:444-473.

63. Sud A, Friedrick JO, Taccone P, et al. Prone ventilation reduces mortality in patients with acute respiratory failure and severe hypoxemia: systemic review and meta-analysis. *Intensive Care Medicine.* 2010;36(4):585-599.

64. Tang BM, Craig JC, Eslick GD, et al. Use of corticosteroids in acute lung injury and acute respiratory distress syndrome: a systematic review and meta-analysis. *Chest.* 2009;37(5):1594-1603.

65. Tapson VF. Acute pulmonary embolism. *The New England Journal of Medicine.* 2008;358(10):1037-1052.

65a. The ARDS Definition Task Force. Acute respiratory distress syndrome: the Berlin definition. *Journal of the American Medical Association.* 2012;307:2526-2533.

66. Todd JL, Tapson VF. Thrombolytic therapy for acute pulmo-nary embolism: a critical appraisal. *Chest.* 2009;135(5):1321-1329.

67. Vollman KM, Powers J. Pronation therapy. In: Wiegand DL, ed. *AACN Procedure Manual for Critical Care.* 6th ed., pp. 129-149. St. Louis: Mosby; 2011.

68. Vollman KM, Sole ML. Endotracheal tube and oral care. In: Wiegand DL, ed. *AACN Procedure Manual for Critical Care.* 6th ed., pp. 31-38; 2011.

69. Waterer GW, Rello J, Wunderink RG. Management of commu-nity-acquired pneumonia in adults. *American Journal of Respiratory and Critical Care Medicine.* 2011;183:157-164.

70. Weidenmann HP, Wheeler AP, Bernard GR, et al. National heart, lung, and blood institute acute respiratory distress syndrome (ARDS) clinical trial network. Comparison of two fluid-management strategies in acute lung injury. *New England Journal of Medicine.* 2006;354(24):2564-2575.

71. Zambon M, Vincent J. Mortality rates for patients with acute lung injury/ARDS have decreased over time. *Chest.* 2008;133(5):1120-1127.

15

Acute Kidney Injury

Kathleen Kerber, MSN, RN, ACNS-BC, CCRN

ℯvolve WEBSITE

Many additional resources, including self-assessment exercises, are located on the Evolve companion website at http://evolve.elsevier.com/Sole.

- Review Questions
- Mosby's Nursing Skills Procedures
- Animations
- Video Clips

INTRODUCTION

The kidney is the primary regulator of the body's internal environment. With sudden cessation of renal function, all body systems are affected by the inability to maintain fluid and electrolyte balance and eliminate metabolic waste. Renal dysfunction is a common problem in the critical care unit with nearly two thirds of patients experiencing some degree of renal dysfunction.[19,36] The most severe cases requiring renal replacement therapy have a reported mortality of 50% to 60%.[19,37]

Acute kidney injury (AKI) is the internationally recognized term for renal dysfunction in acutely ill patients.[2,8,34] In contrast to acute renal failure, AKI encompasses the range of renal dysfunction from mild impairment to complete cessation of renal function. Acute kidney injury that progresses to chronic renal failure is associated with increased morbidity and mortality, and reduced quality of life.[11] Nurses play a pivotal role in promoting positive outcomes in patients with AKI. Recognition of high-risk patients, preventive measures, sharp assessment skills, and supportive nursing care are fundamental to ensure delivery of high-quality care to these challenging and complex patients. In this chapter, the pathophysiology, assessment, and collaborative management of AKI are discussed.

REVIEW OF ANATOMY AND PHYSIOLOGY

The kidneys are a pair of highly vascularized, bean-shaped organs that are located retroperitoneally on each side of the vertebral column, adjacent to the first and second lumbar vertebrae. The right kidney sits slightly lower than the left kidney because the liver lies above it. An adrenal gland sits on top of each kidney and is responsible for the production of aldosterone, a hormone that influences sodium and water balance. Each kidney is divided into two regions: an outer region, called the *cortex,* and an inner region, called the *medulla.*

The *nephron* is the basic functional unit of the kidney. A nephron is composed of a renal corpuscle (glomerulus and Bowman's capsule) and a tubular structure, as depicted in Figure 15-1. Approximately 1 to 3 million nephrons exist in each kidney. About 85% of these nephrons are found in the cortex of the kidney and have short loops of Henle. The remaining 15% of nephrons are called *juxtamedullary nephrons* because of their location just outside the medulla. Juxtamedullary nephrons have long loops of Henle and, along with the vasa recta (long capillary loops), are primarily responsible for concentration of urine.

The kidneys receive approximately 20% to 25% of the cardiac output, which computes to 1200 mL of blood per minute. Blood enters the kidneys through the renal artery, travels through a series of arterial branches, and reaches the glomerulus by way of the afferent arteriole (*afferent* meaning to carry toward). Blood leaves the glomerulus through the efferent arteriole (*efferent* meaning to carry away from), which then divides into two extensive capillary networks called the *peritubular capillaries* and the *vasa recta.* The capillaries then rejoin to form venous branches by which blood eventually exits the kidney via the renal vein. The glomerulus is a cluster of minute blood vessels that filter blood. The glomerular walls

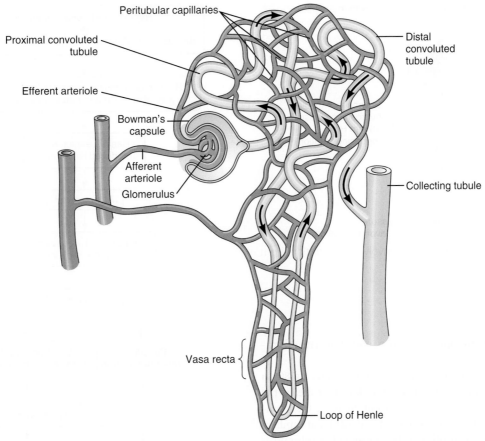

FIGURE 15-1 Anatomy of the nephron, the functional unit of the kidney. (From Banasik J. Renal function. In Copstead L, Banasik J, eds. *Pathophysiology*. 4th ed. Philadelphia: Saunders. 2010.)

BOX 15-1	**FUNCTIONS OF THE KIDNEY**

- Regulation of fluid volume
- Regulation of electrolyte balance
- Regulation of acid-base balance
- Regulation of blood pressure
- Excretion of nitrogenous waste products
- Regulation of erythropoiesis
- Metabolism of vitamin D
- Synthesis of prostaglandin

are composed of three layers: the endothelium, the basement membrane, and the epithelium. The epithelium of the glomerulus is continuous with the inner layer of Bowman's capsule, the sac that surrounds the glomerulus. Bowman's capsule is the entry site for filtrate leaving the glomerulus.[25]

The kidneys perform numerous functions that are essential for the maintenance of a stable internal environment. The following text provides a brief overview of key roles the kidneys perform in maintaining homeostasis. Box 15-1 lists functions of the kidney.

Regulation of Fluid and Electrolytes and Excretion of Waste Products

As blood flows through each glomerulus, water, electrolytes, and waste products are filtered out of the blood across the glomerular membrane and into Bowman's capsule, to form what is known as *filtrate*. The glomerular capillary membrane is approximately 100 times more permeable than other capillaries. It acts as a high-efficiency sieve and normally allows only substances with a certain molecular weight to cross. Normal glomerular filtrate is basically protein free and contains electrolytes, including sodium, chloride, and phosphate, and nitrogenous waste products, such as creatinine, urea, and uric acid, in amounts similar to those in plasma.[16,25] Red blood cells, albumin, and globulin are too large to pass through the healthy glomerular membrane.

Glomerular filtration occurs as a result of a pressure gradient, which is the difference between the forces that favor filtration and the pressures that oppose filtration. Generally, the capillary hydrostatic pressure favors glomerular filtration, whereas the colloid osmotic pressure and the hydrostatic pressure in Bowman's capsule oppose filtration (Figure 15-2). Under normal conditions, the capillary hydrostatic pressure

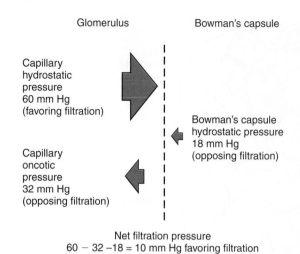

Glomerulus   Bowman's capsule

Capillary hydrostatic pressure 60 mm Hg (favoring filtration)

Bowman's capsule hydrostatic pressure 18 mm Hg (opposing filtration)

Capillary oncotic pressure 32 mm Hg (opposing filtration)

Net filtration pressure
60 − 32 −18 = 10 mm Hg favoring filtration

FIGURE 15-2 Average pressures involved in filtration from the glomerular capillaries.

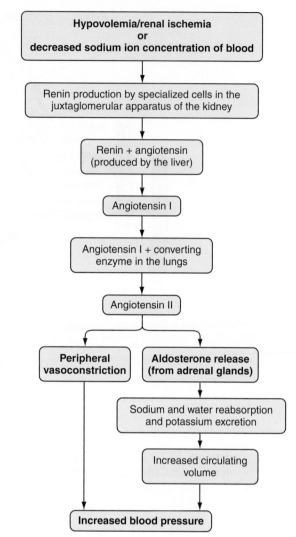

Hypovolemia/renal ischemia
or
decreased sodium ion concentration of blood

Renin production by specialized cells in the juxtaglomerular apparatus of the kidney

Renin + angiotensin (produced by the liver)

Angiotensin I

Angiotensin I + converting enzyme in the lungs

Angiotensin II

Peripheral vasoconstriction

Aldosterone release (from adrenal glands)

Sodium and water reabsorption and potassium excretion

Increased circulating volume

Increased blood pressure

FIGURE 15-3 Renin-angiotensin-aldosterone cascade.

is greater than the two opposing forces, and glomerular filtration occurs.

At a normal glomerular filtration rate (GFR) of 80 to 125 mL/min, the kidneys produce 180 L/day of filtrate. As the filtrate passes through the various components of the nephron's tubules, 99% is reabsorbed into the peritubular capillaries or vasa recta. Reabsorption is the movement of substances from the filtrate back into the capillaries. A second process that occurs in the tubules is secretion, or the movement of substances from the peritubular capillaries into the tubular network. Various electrolytes are reabsorbed or secreted at numerous points along the tubules, thus helping to regulate the electrolyte composition of the internal environment.

Aldosterone and antidiuretic hormone (ADH) play a role in water reabsorption in the distal convoluted tubule and collecting duct. Aldosterone also plays a role in sodium reabsorption and promotes the excretion of potassium. Eventually, the remaining filtrate (1% of the original 180 L/day) is excreted as urine, for an average urine output of 1 to 2 L/day.

Regulation of Acid-Base Balance

The kidneys help to maintain acid-base equilibrium in three ways: by reabsorbing filtered bicarbonate, producing new bicarbonate, and excreting small amounts of hydrogen ions (acid) buffered by phosphates and ammonia.[17] The tubular cells are capable of generating ammonia to help with excretion of hydrogen ions. This ability of the kidney to assist with ammonia production and excretion of hydrogen ions (in exchange for sodium) is the predominant adaptive response by the kidney when the patient is acidotic. When alkalosis is present, increased amounts of bicarbonate are excreted in the urine and cause the serum pH to return toward normal.

Regulation of Blood Pressure

Specialized cells in the afferent and efferent arterioles and the distal tubule are collectively known as the *juxtaglomerular*

apparatus. These cells are responsible for the production of a hormone called *renin,* which plays a role in blood pressure regulation. Renin is released whenever blood flow through the afferent and efferent arterioles decreases. A decrease in the sodium ion concentration of the blood flowing past the specialized cells (e.g., in hypovolemia) also stimulates the release of renin. Renin activates the renin-angiotensin-aldosterone cascade, as depicted in Figure 15-3, which ultimately results in angiotensin II production. Angiotensin II causes vasoconstriction and release of aldosterone from the adrenal glands, thereby raising blood pressure and flow and increasing sodium and water reabsorption in the distal tubule and collecting ducts.

Effects of Aging

The most important renal physiological change that occurs with aging is a decrease in the GFR. After age 40 years, renal blood flow gradually diminishes at a rate of 10% per decade.[28] With advancing age, there is also a decrease in renal mass, the number of glomeruli, and peritubular density.[5]

Serum creatinine levels may remain the same in the elderly patient even with a declining GFR because of decreased muscle mass and hence decreased creatinine production.

The ability to concentrate and dilute urine is impaired as well, due to an inability of the renal tubules to maintain the osmotic gradient in the medullary portion of the kidney. This tubular change affects the countercurrent mechanism, significantly altering sodium conservation, especially if a salt-restricted diet is being followed. Other tubular changes include a diminished ability to excrete drugs, including radiocontrast dyes used in diagnostic testing, which necessitates a decrease in drug dosing to prevent nephrotoxicity. Many medications, including antibiotics require dose adjustments as kidney function declines. Drug databases are available for appropriate dosing.

Age-related changes in renin and aldosterone levels also occur that can lead to fluid and electrolyte abnormalities. Renin levels are decreased by 30% to 50% in the elderly, resulting in less angiotensin II production and lower aldosterone levels. Together these can cause an increased risk of hyperkalemia (with possible cardiac conduction abnormalities), a decreased ability to conserve sodium, and a tendency to develop volume depletion and dehydration. The aging kidney is also slower to correct an increase in acids, causing a prolonged metabolic acidosis and the subsequent shifting of potassium out of cells and worsening hyperkalemia. There is a slight increase in ADH production with aging, but an associated decreased responsiveness to ADH may exacerbate volume depletion and dehydration.[28]

PATHOPHYSIOLOGY OF ACUTE KIDNEY INJURY

Definition

Acute kidney injury is defined as the sudden decline in kidney function causing disturbances in fluid, electrolyte, and acid-base balance because of a loss in small solute clearance and decreased glomerular filtration rate.[10] The cardinal features of AKI are azotemia and oliguria. Azotemia refers to increases in blood urea nitrogen and serum creatinine. Oliguria is defined as urine output less than 0.5 mL/kg/hr. Two international consensus groups have worked to define and stage AKI based on serum creatinine levels and urine output. The Acute Dialysis Quality Initiative (ADQI) created the RIFLE classification system.[2] The RIFLE criteria are shown in Figure 15-4. This staging system identifies five levels with three grades of severity (risk, injury, and failure) and two outcomes (loss and end-stage renal disease). Each grade of severity is based on changes from baseline serum creatinine level or urine output over time. The Acute Kidney Injury Network (AKIN) identified three stages that correspond to the RIFLE system (risk, injury, and failure) but assess changes over 48 hours (Table 15-1).[27]

The Kidney Disease Improving Global Outcomes (KDIGO) is an international program of the National Kidney Foundation. In 2012, the KDIGO Clinical Practice Guidelines for Acute Kidney Injury were published that focus on the prevention, recognition, and management of AKI.[24] These guidelines combine both RIFLE and AKIN criteria to define and diagnose AKI (see Table 15-1).[19]

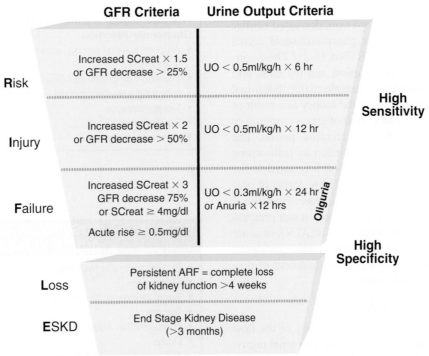

FIGURE 15-4 RIFLE classification system. *ARF,* Acute renal failure; *GFR,* glomerular filtration rate; *SCreat,* serum creatinine; *UO,* urine output. Note: The RIFLE classification system was developed before the terminology was changed from *acute renal failure* to *acute kidney injury.* (From Bellomo R, Ronc C, Kellum J, et al. Acute renal failure-definition outcome measures, animal models, fluid therapy and information technology needs: The Second International Consensus Conference of the Acute Dialysis Quality Initiative [ADHQI] Group, *Critical Care.* 2004;8[4]:R204-R212.)

TABLE 15-1 ACUTE KIDNEY INJURY NETWORK STAGING

STAGE	CRITERIA
1	Creatinine increases >0.3 mg/dL or more than or equal to 150%-200% (1.5-2.0 times baseline) >12 hours Urine output <0.5 mL/kg/hr for more than 6 hours
2	Creatinine increase 2-3 times baseline Urine output <0.5 mL/kg/hr for more than 12 hours
3	Creatinine increase 3 times baseline or >4 mg/dL with acute rise of 0.5 mg/dL Urine output <0.3 mL/kg/hr × 24 hours, or anuria for 12 hours

From Mehta RL, Kellum JA, Shah SV, Molitoris BA, Ronco C, Warnock DG & Acute Kidney Injury Network. (2007). Acute Kidney Injury Network: report of an initiative to improve outcomes in acute kidney injury. *Critical Care*, 11(2), R31.

Etiology

The etiology of AKI in critically ill patients is often multifactorial and develops from a combination of hypovolemia, sepsis, medications, and hemodynamic instability.[10] Sepsis is the most common cause of AKI.[37] The etiology of AKI is classified as either prerenal, postrenal, or intrarenal. Classification depends on where the precipitating factor exerts its pathophysiological effect on the kidney.

Prerenal Causes of Acute Kidney Injury

Conditions that result in AKI by interfering with renal perfusion are classified as *prerenal*. Most prerenal causes of AKI are related to intravascular volume depletion, decreased cardiac output, renal vasoconstriction, or pharmacological agents that impair autoregulation and GFR (Box 15-2).[8] These conditions reduce the glomerular perfusion and the GFR, and the kidneys are hypoperfused. For example, major abdominal surgery can cause hypoperfusion of the kidney as a result of blood loss during surgery, or as a result of excess vomiting or nasogastric suction during the postoperative period. The body attempts to normalize renal perfusion by reabsorbing sodium and water. If adequate blood flow is restored to the kidney, normal renal function resumes. Most forms of prerenal AKI can be reversed by treating the cause. However, if the prerenal situation is prolonged or severe, it can progress to intrarenal damage, acute tubular necrosis (ATN), or acute cortical necrosis.[23] Implementation of preventive measures, recognition of the condition, and prompt treatment of prerenal conditions are extremely important.

Postrenal Causes of Acute Kidney Injury

Acute kidney injury resulting from obstruction of the flow of urine is classified as *postrenal*, or obstructive renal injury. Obstruction can occur at any point along the urinary system (Box 15-3). With postrenal conditions, increased intratubular pressure results in a decrease in the GFR and abnormal nephron function. The presence of hydronephrosis on renal

BOX 15-2 PRERENAL CAUSES OF ACUTE KIDNEY INJURY

Intravascular Volume Depletion
- Hemorrhage
- Trauma
- Surgery
- Intraabdominal compartment syndrome
- Gastrointestinal loss
- Renal loss
- Diuretics
- Osmotic diuresis
- Diabetes insipidus
- Volume shifts
- Burns

Vasodilation
- Sepsis
- Anaphylaxis
- Medications
  - Antihypertensives
  - Afterload reducing agents
- Anesthesia

Decreased Cardiac Output
- Heart failure
- Myocardial infarction
- Cardiogenic shock
- Dysrhythmias
- Pulmonary embolism
- Pulmonary hypertension
- Positive-pressure ventilation
- Pericardial tamponade

Pharmacological Agents that Impair Autoregulation and Glomerular Filtration
- Angiotensin-converting enzyme inhibitors in renal artery stenosis
- Inhibition of prostaglandins by nonsteroidal antiinflammatory drug use during renal hypoperfusion
- Norepinephrine
- Ergotamine
- Hypercalcemia

BOX 15-3 POSTRENAL CAUSES OF ACUTE KIDNEY INJURY

- Benign prostatic hypertrophy
- Blood clots
- Renal stones or crystals
- Tumors
- Postoperative edema
- Drugs
  - Tricyclic antidepressants
  - Ganglionic blocking agents
- Foley catheter obstruction
- Ligation of ureter during surgery

ultrasound or a postvoid residual volume greater than 100 mL is suggestive of postrenal obstruction. The location of the obstruction in the urinary tract determines the method by which the obstruction is treated and may include bladder catheterization, ureteral stenting, or the placement of nephrostomy tubes.

Intrarenal Causes of Acute Kidney Injury

Conditions that produce AKI by directly acting on functioning kidney tissue (either the glomerulus or the renal tubules) are classified as *intrarenal.* The most common intrarenal condition is ATN.[8] This condition may occur after prolonged ischemia (prerenal), exposure to nephrotoxic substances, or a combination of these. Ischemic ATN usually occurs when perfusion to the kidney is considerably reduced. The renal ischemia overwhelms the normal autoregulatory defenses of the kidneys and thus initiates cell injury that may lead to cell death. Some patients have ATN after only several minutes of hypotension or hypovolemia, whereas others can tolerate hours of renal ischemia without having any apparent tubular damage

Nephrotoxic agents (particularly aminoglycosides and radiographic contrast media) damage the tubular epithelium as a result of direct drug toxicity, intrarenal vasoconstriction, and intratubular obstruction. AKI does not occur in all patients who receive nephrotoxic agents; however, predisposing factors such as advanced age, diabetes mellitus, and dehydration enhance susceptibility to intrinsic damage.[13,33] Other intrarenal causes of AKI are listed in Box 15-4.

Multiple mechanisms are involved in the pathophysiology of ATN. Figure 15-5 is a detailed schematic of some of the mechanisms that play a role in the ATN cascade resulting in a reduced GFR. Mechanisms include alterations in renal hemodynamics, tubular function, and tubular cellular metabolism.

Decreases in cardiac output, intravascular volume, or renal blood flow activate the renin-angiotensin-aldosterone cascade. Angiotensin II causes further renal vasoconstriction and decreased glomerular capillary pressure, resulting in a decreased GFR. The decreased GFR and renal blood flow lead to tubular dysfunction. In addition, administration of medications that cause vasoconstriction of the renal vessels can precipitate ATN, including nonsteroidal antiinflammatory drugs, angiotensin-converting enzyme inhibitors, angiotensin receptor blockers, cyclosporine, and tacrolimus.[8,23] Endogenous substances that have been implicated in both causing and maintaining renal vessel vasoconstriction include endothelin-1, prostaglandins, adenosine, angiotensin II, and nitric oxide. A deficiency of renal vasodilators (prostaglandins, atrial natriuretic peptide, and endothelium-derived nitric oxide) has also been implicated.[8]

The renal tubules in the medulla are very susceptible to ischemia. The medulla receives only 20% of the renal blood flow but is very sensitive to any reduction in blood flow. When the tubules are damaged, necrotic endothelial cells and other cellular debris accumulate and can obstruct the lumen of the tubule. This intratubular obstruction increases the intratubular pressure, which decreases the GFR and leads to tubular dysfunction. In addition, the tubular damage often produces alterations in the tubular structure that permit the glomerular filtrate to leak out of the tubular lumen and back into the plasma, resulting in oliguria.[8]

Ischemic episodes result in decreased energy supplies, including adenosine triphosphate (ATP). Oxygen deprivation results in a rapid breakdown of ATP. The proximal tubule is very dependent on ATP, which explains why it is the most commonly injured portion of the renal tubule. Without ATP, the sodium-potassium ATPase of the cell membrane is not able to effectively transport electrolytes across the membrane. This leads to increased intracellular calcium levels, free

---

BOX 15-4   INTRARENAL CAUSES OF ACUTE KIDNEY INJURY

Glomerular, Vascular, or Hematological Problems
- Glomerulonephritis (poststreptococcal)
- Vasculitis
- Malignant hypertension
- Systemic lupus erythematosus
- Hemolytic uremic syndrome
- Disseminated intravascular coagulation
- Scleroderma
- Bacterial endocarditis
- Hypertension of pregnancy
- Thrombosis of renal artery or vein

Tubular Problem (Acute Tubular Necrosis or Acute Interstitial Nephritis)
- Ischemia
- Causes of prerenal azotemia (see Box 15-2)
- Hypotension from any cause

- Hypovolemia from any cause
- Obstetric complications (hemorrhage, abruptio placentae, placenta previa)
- Medications (see Box 15-5)
- Radiocontrast media (large volume; multiple procedures)
- Transfusion reaction causing hemoglobinuria
- Tumor lysis syndrome
- Rhabdomyolysis
- Miscellaneous: heavy metals (mercury, arsenic), paraquat, snake bites, organic solvents (ethylene glycol, toluene, carbon tetrachloride), pesticides, fungicides
- Preexisting renal impairment
- Diabetes mellitus
- Hypertension
- Volume depletion
- Severe heart failure
- Advanced age

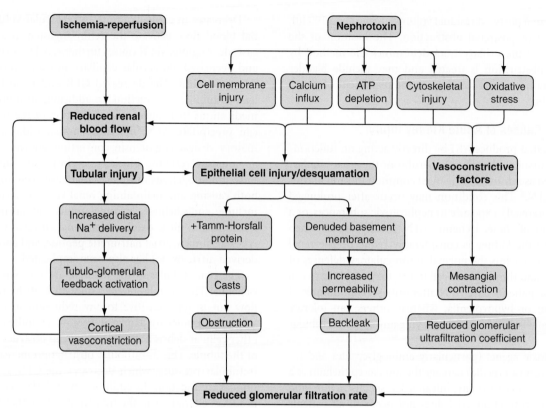

FIGURE 15-5 Schematic of loss of glomerular filtration seen in ischemic and nephrotoxic acute tubular necrosis. *ATP,* adenosine triphosphate; *Na+,* sodium. (From Woolfson R, Hillman K. Causes of acute renal failure. In Johnson R, Feehally, eds. *Comprehensive Clinical Nephrology.* 2nd ed. London: Mosby. 2003.)

radical formation (which produces toxic effects), and breakdown of phospholipids. Cellular edema occurs and further decreases renal blood flow, damages the tubules, and ultimately leads to tubular dysfunction and oliguria.[8]

Contrast-induced nephropathy. Though the administration of contrast is generally considered safe for the individual with normal kidney function, contrast-induced nephropathy (CIN) is the third leading cause of AKI in the hospitalized patient[3,21] (see box, "Evidence-Based Practice"). *Contrast-induced nephropathy* is defined as the sudden, rapid deterioration of kidney function resulting from parenteral contrast administration in the absence of another clinical explanation.[21] Contrast-induced kidney injury is diagnosed by an increase in serum creatinine of 25% or more, or a value of 0.5 mg/dL or more, occurring within 48 to 72 hours following the administration of contrast.[33] Urine output usually remains normal; however, in severe cases oliguria may be seen.

Two pathological mechanisms contribute to the development of contrast-induced AKI. The first mechanism is by the direct toxic effect of the contrast media on the cells lining the renal tubule.[31,33] The second mechanism of injury is the result of reduced medullary blood flow.

Contrast media is suspected to initiate vasodilation of renal blood vessels followed by an intense and persistent vasoconstriction.[8] Oxygen delivery to the renal cells is reduced, precipitating cell injury. In addition, contrast agents stimulate the influx of extracellular calcium, which may lead to a loss of medullary autoregulation as well as a direct toxic effect on the renal tubules.[33] Patients with chronic renal insufficiency are at the greatest risk for developing CIN.[8] Other risk factors include diabetes, dehydration, advancing age, heart failure, ongoing treatment with nephrotoxic drugs, and vascular disease.[3,33]

Reduced medullary blood flow from cholesterol embolism or atheromatous emboli are common causes of AKI after an interventional radiology procedure. Any arterial angiographic procedure, such as cardiac catheterization, can dislodge atheromatous emboli, which can lodge in small renal arteries and produce an occlusion of the vessel, ischemia, and tubular dysfunction. A decline in renal function typically occurs over a period of 3 to 8 weeks, rather than the rapid decline seen with CIN. Patients also typically have evidence of embolization to other areas of the body, including the skin (digital necrosis and gangrene), central nervous system (stroke, blindness), or gastrointestinal system (pancreatitis).

EVIDENCE-BASED PRACTICE

Acute Kidney Injury Related to Contrast Media

Problem

Contrast-induced nephropathy is the third leading cause of AKI in hospitalized patients and is associated with significant patient morbidity, prolongation of hospital stays, and increased healthcare costs. Critically ill patients are at increased risk for contrast-induced nephropathy because of hemodynamic instability, volume depletion, multiple organ dysfunction, and the use of nephrotoxic medications. Critically ill diabetic patients receiving radiological contrast have multiple risk factors for contrast-induced nephropathy. Preventive measures are needed to reduce the risk of contrast-induced nephropathy in high risk populations.

Clinical Question

What are the most effective interventions for preventing contrast-induced AKI?

Evidence

Many studies have been conducted to evaluate interventions to reduce the risk of contrast-induced nephropathy; however, results have been inconsistent. Hydration is the intervention that has demonstrated benefit in most randomized controlled trials. Data are controversial on which intravenous fluid is best for hydration. Although isotonic saline has been identified as effective, intravenous administration of a 154 mEq/L solution of sodium bicarbonate has been proposed as an effective method of hydration that offers additional protection from the alkalinizing properties of contrast agents.

The PREVENT Trial compared the ability of sodium bicarbonate plus N-acetylcysteine (NAC) versus sodium chloride plus NAC to prevent contrast-induced nephropathy in 382 diabetic patients with impaired renal function undergoing coronary or endovascular angiography or interventions.[2] The findings of this trial indicated hydration with sodium bicarbonate was not superior to hydration with sodium chloride in preventing contrast-induced nephropathy in the study population.

The CIN Consensus Working Panel recommends that adequate intravenous volume expansion with isotonic crystalloid (normal saline [0.9%], 1.0-1.5 mL/kg/hr) for 3 to 12 hours before the procedure and continue for 6 to 24 hours afterward can lessen the probability of contrast-induced nephropathy in patients at risk.[3]

Implications for Nursing

The findings of this study support current recommendations for the use of normal saline for hydration. High-risk hospitalized patients can begin intravenous hydration 12 hours before the procedure, and the infusion can be continued for at least 6 to 12 hours afterward. For outpatients, especially those with risk factors for contrast-induced nephropathy, intravenous hydration can be started 3 hours before the procedure and continued for 6 or more hours afterwards. The recommended fluid administration rate is 1 mL/kg/hr.[1] In some circumstances, the physician may request a rate of 2 mL/kg/hr for the first 2 hours followed by a rate of 1 mL/kg/hr.[1] Ongoing clinical trials will determine additional preventive strategies in hopes of reducing the incidence of contrast-induced nephropathy. Nurses must assist in identifying patients at risk for contrast-induced nephropathy and advocating for early and adequate hydration.

Level of Evidence

B—Controlled studies with consistent results

References

1. Ellis J & Cohan R. Prevention of contrast-induced nephropathy: an overview. *Radiologic Clinics North America*, 2009;47, 801-811.
2. Lee S, Kim W, Kim Y, Park S, Park D, Yun S, Lee J, Kang S, Lee C, Park S. Preventive strategies of renal insufficiency in patient with diabetes undergoing intervention or arteriography (the PREVENT trial). *American Journal of Cardiology*, 2011;107(10), 1447-1452.
3. Kellum J, Lamiere N, Aspelin P, Barsoum R, Burdman E, Goldstein S, et al. (2012). KDIGO Clinical practice guidelines for acute kidney injury. *Kidney International*, 2(1) (Supp.l) S1-138.

Course of Acute Kidney Injury

The patient with AKI progresses through three phases of the disease process: the initiation phase, the maintenance phase, and the recovery phase.[31]

Initiation Phase

The initiation phase is the period that elapses from the occurrence of the precipitating event to the beginning of the change in urine output. This phase spans several hours to 2 days, during which time the normal renal processes begin to deteriorate, but actual intrinsic renal damage has not yet occurred. The patient is unable to compensate for the diminished renal function and exhibits clinical signs and symptoms that reflect the chemical imbalances. Renal dysfunction is potentially reversible during the initiation phase.

Maintenance Phase

During the maintenance phase, intrinsic renal damage is established, and the GFR stabilizes at approximately 5 to 10 mL/min. Urine volume is usually at its lowest point during the maintenance phase; however, patients may be nonoliguric, with urine outputs greater than 400 mL in 24 hours. This phase usually lasts 8 to 14 days, but it may last up to 11 months. The longer a patient remains in this stage, the slower the recovery and the greater the chance of permanent renal damage. Complications resulting from uremia, including hyperkalemia and infection, occur during this phase.

Recovery Phase

This phase is the period during which the renal tissue recovers and repairs itself. A gradual increase in urine output and an improvement in laboratory values occur. Some patients may experience diuresis during this phase. This diuresis reflects excretion of salt and water accumulated during the maintenance phase, the osmotic diuresis induced by filtered urea and other solutes, and the administration of diuretics to enhance salt and water elimination.[8] However, with early and aggressive use of dialytic therapy, many patients are maintained in a relative "dry" or volume-depleted state and do have a large post-ATN diuresis. Recovery may take as long as 4 to 6 months.

ASSESSMENT

Patient History

Obtaining a thorough patient history is important. Renal-related symptoms provide valuable clues to assist the clinician in focusing the assessment. For example, dysuria, frequency, incontinence, nocturia, pyuria, and hematuria can be indicative of urinary tract infection. The history provides clues about medical conditions that predispose the patient to AKI, including diabetes mellitus, hypertension, immunological diseases, and any hereditary disorders, such as polycystic disease. The medical record is reviewed to elicit additional risk factors, such as hypotensive episodes or any surgical or radiographic procedures performed. Information regarding exposure to potential nephrotoxins is extremely important. Common nephrotoxins include antibiotics such as aminoglycosides. Risk factors for development of aminoglycoside nephrotoxicity include volume depletion, prolonged use of the drug (>10 days), hypokalemia, sepsis, preexisting renal disease, high trough concentrations, concurrent use of other nephrotoxic drugs, and older age.[31] Symptoms of AKI are usually seen about 1 to 2 weeks after exposure. Because of this delay, the patient must be questioned about any recent medical visits (clinic or emergency department) for which an aminoglycoside may have been prescribed. In addition, a history of over-the-counter medication use, including nonsteroidal antiinflammatory medications, is important. Box 15-5 lists medications that are associated with AKI.

Vital Signs

Changes in blood pressure are common in AKI. Patients with kidney injury from prerenal causes may be hypotensive and tachycardic as a result of volume deficits. ATN, particularly if associated with oliguria, often causes hypertension. Patients may hyperventilate as the lungs attempt to compensate for the metabolic acidosis often seen in AKI. Body temperature may be decreased (as a result of the antipyretic effect of the uremic toxins), normal, or increased (as a result of infection).

> ### BOX 15-5 COMMON NEPHROTOXIC MEDICATIONS
>
> - Aminoglycosides
> - Amphotericin B
> - Penicillins
> - Acyclovir
> - Vancomycin
> - Pentamidine
> - Rifampin
> - Cephalosporins
> - Cyclosporine
> - Tacrolimus
> - Methotrexate
> - Cisplatin
> - Fluorouracil (5-FU)
> - Nonsteroidal antiinflammatory drugs (NSAIDs)
> - Angiotensin-converting enzyme (ACE) inhibitors
> - Angiotensin receptor blockers (ARBs)
> - Interferon
> - Indinavir
> - Ritonavir
> - Adefovir

Physical Assessment

The patient's general appearance is assessed for signs of *uremia* (retention of nitrogenous substances normally excreted by the kidneys) such as malaise, fatigue, disorientation, and drowsiness. The skin is assessed for color, texture, bruising, petechiae, and edema. The patient's hydration status is also carefully assessed. Current and admission body weight and intake and output information are evaluated. Skin turgor, mucous membranes, breath sounds, presence of edema, neck vein distention, and vital signs (blood pressure and heart rate) are all key indicators of fluid balance. An oliguric patient with weight loss, tachycardia, hypotension, dry mucous membranes, flat neck veins, and poor skin turgor may be volume depleted (prerenal cause). Weight gain, edema, distended neck veins, and hypertension in the presence of oliguria suggest an intrarenal cause. Table 15-2 summarizes the systemic manifestations of AKI according to body system and also lists the pathophysiological mechanisms involved.

Evaluation of Laboratory Values

Alteration in renal function is associated with changes in serum and urine laboratory values. The serum creatinine level is often used to evaluate kidney function. Creatinine is a by-product of muscle metabolism and is produced at a relatively constant rate, then cleared by the kidneys. With stable kidney function, creatinine production and excretion are fairly equal, and serum creatinine levels remain constant. When kidney function decreases, creatinine levels rapidly rise, indicating a decline in function or a decrease in the GFR. The serum

TABLE 15-2	SYSTEMIC MANIFESTATIONS OF ACUTE KIDNEY INJURY	
SYSTEM	**MANIFESTATION**	**PATHOPHYSIOLOGICAL MECHANISM**
Cardiovascular	Heart failure	Fluid overload and hypertension
	Pulmonary edema	↑ Pulmonary capillary permeability
		Fluid overload
		Left ventricular dysfunction
	Dysrhythmias	Electrolyte imbalances (especially hyperkalemia and hypocalcemia)
	Peripheral edema	Fluid overload
		Right ventricular dysfunction
	Hypertension	Fluid overload
		↑ Sodium retention
Hematological	Anemia	↓ Erythropoietin secretion
		Loss of RBCs through GI tract, mucous membranes, or dialysis
		↓ RBC survival time
		Uremic toxins' interference with folic acid secretion
	Alterations in coagulation	Platelet dysfunction
	↑ Susceptibility to infection	↓ Neutrophil phagocytosis
Electrolyte imbalances	Metabolic acidosis	↓ Hydrogen ion excretion
		↓ Bicarbonate ion reabsorption and generation
		↓ Excretion of phosphate salts or titratable acids
		↓ Ammonia synthesis and ammonium excretion
Respiratory	Pneumonia	Thick tenacious sputum from ↓ oral intake
		Depressed cough reflex
		↓ Pulmonary macrophage activity
	Pulmonary edema	Fluid overload
		Left ventricular dysfunction
		↑ Pulmonary capillary permeability
Gastrointestinal	Anorexia, nausea, vomiting	Uremic toxins
		Decomposition of urea releasing ammonia that irritates mucosa
	Stomatitis and uremic halitosis	Uremic toxins
		Decomposition of urea releasing ammonia that irritates oral mucosa
	Gastritis and bleeding	Uremic toxins
		Decomposition of urea releasing ammonia that irritates mucosa, causing ulcerations and increased capillary fragility
Neuromuscular	Drowsiness, confusion, irritability, and coma	Uremic toxins produce encephalopathy
		Metabolic acidosis
		Electrolyte imbalances
	Tremors, twitching, and convulsions	Uremic toxins produce encephalopathy
		↓ Nerve conduction from uremic toxins
Psychosocial	Decreased mentation, decreased concentration, and altered perceptions	Uremic toxins produce encephalopathy
		Electrolyte imbalances
		Metabolic acidosis
		Tendency to develop cerebral edema
Integumentary	Pallor	Anemia
	Yellowness	Retained urochrome pigment
	Dryness	↓ Secretions from oil and sweat glands
	Pruritus	Dry skin
		Calcium and/or phosphate deposits in skin
		Uremic toxins' effect on nerve endings
	Purpura	↑ Capillary fragility
		Platelet dysfunction
	Uremic frost (rarely seen)	Urea or urate crystal excretion
Endocrine	Glucose intolerance (usually not clinically significant)	Peripheral insensitivity to insulin
		Prolonged insulin half-life from ↓ renal metabolism
Skeletal	Hypocalcemia	Hyperphosphatemia from ↓ excretion of phosphates ↓
		↓ GI absorption of vitamin D
		Deposition of calcium phosphate crystals in soft tissues

GI, Gastrointestinal; *RBC,* red blood cell.

> ## ! CLINICAL ALERT
> ### *Serum Creatinine*
>
> The same serum creatinine level can reflect very different glomerular filtration rates in patients because of differences in muscle mass. For example, a 25-year-old man weighing 220 lb with a serum creatinine level of 1.2 mg/dL has an estimated glomerular filtration rate of 133 mL/hr (normal), whereas a 75-year-old woman weighing 121 lb with the same serum creatinine level of 1.2 mg/dL has an estimated glomerular filtration rate of 35 mL/hr (markedly decreased).

creatinine level should not be the only measure used to assess kidney function (see box, "Clinical Alert: Serum Creatinine"). When evaluating the serum creatinine level, it is helpful to review past values to determine whether an elevated level is due to an acute insult or a progressive loss of renal function. If past creatinine levels are not available, it is often difficult to distinguish acute from chronic kidney failure.

Although the serum blood urea nitrogen (BUN) level is also used to evaluate kidney function, the BUN level is not a reliable indicator of kidney function because the rate of protein metabolism (urea is a by-product of protein metabolism) is not constant. Extrarenal factors including dehydration, a high-protein diet, starvation, blood in the gastrointestinal tract, corticosteroids, and fever all can elevate the BUN level. For example, when a patient has gastrointestinal bleeding, the blood in the gut breaks down and results in an increased protein load and hence an elevated BUN level.

The *BUN/creatinine ratio* provides useful information. The normal BUN/creatinine ratio is 10:1 to 20:1 (e.g., BUN level, 20 mg/dL, and creatinine level, 1.0 mg/dL). If the ratio is greater than 20:1 (e.g., BUN level, 60 mg/dL, and creatinine level, 1.0 mg/dL), problems other than kidney failure should be suspected. In prerenal conditions, an increased BUN/creatinine ratio is typically noted. There is a decrease in the GFR and hence a drop in urine flow through the renal tubules. This allows more time for urea to be reabsorbed from the renal tubules back into the blood. Creatinine is not readily reabsorbed; therefore the serum BUN level rises out of proportion to the serum creatinine level. A normal BUN/creatinine ratio is present in ATN, where there is actual injury to the renal tubules and a rapid decline in the GFR. Hence urea and creatinine levels both rise proportionally from increased reabsorption and decreased clearance.[8]

Assessment of the urine is important in the evaluation of AKI. Historically, timed 24-hour urine collections have been used to evaluate GFR or creatinine clearance. Timed urine collections are cumbersome and time-consuming, and are susceptible to multiple errors in collection. To measure creatinine clearance accurately, the nurse and patient must rigidly adhere to the following procedure:

1. The patient empties his or her bladder, the exact time is recorded, and the specimen is discarded.
2. All urine for the next 24 hours is saved in a container and stored in a refrigerator.
3. Exactly 24 hours after the start of the procedure, the patient voids again, and the specimen is saved.
4. The serum creatinine level is assessed at the end of 24 hours.
5. The 24-hour urine collection is sent to the laboratory for testing. (Urine can also be obtained from an indwelling urinary catheter.)

Urinary *creatinine clearance* is calculated with the following formula:

$$U_c \times V/P_c = C_{cr}$$

U_c = concentration of creatinine in the urine
V = volume of urine per unit of time
P_c = concentration of creatinine in the plasma
C_{cr} = creatinine clearance

Creatinine clearance is an estimate of GFR and is measured in mL/min. Thus, given the following set of patient data,

U_c = 175 mg/100 mL
V = 288 mL/1440 min (24 hours = 1440 min)
P_c = 17.5 mg/100 mL

the patient's creatinine clearance would be calculated as follows:

$$\frac{175 \text{ mg}/100 \text{ mL} \times 288 \text{ mL}/1440 \text{ min}}{17.5 \text{ mg}/100 \text{ mL}} = 2 \text{ mL/min}$$

Because a normal creatinine clearance is about 84 to 138 mL/min, the clinician recognizes this patient's creatinine clearance as being consistent with severe renal dysfunction.

If a reliable 24-hour urine collection is not possible, the Cockcroft and Gault formula may be used to determine the creatinine clearance from a serum creatinine value[23,26]:

$$C_{cr} = \frac{(140 - \text{Age [yr]}) \times (\text{Lean body weight [kg]})}{72 \times \text{Serum creatinine (mg/dL)}}$$

For women, the calculated result is multiplied by 0.85 to account for the smaller muscle mass as compared to men.

Analysis of urinary sediment and electrolyte levels is helpful in distinguishing among the various causes of AKI. Urine is inspected for the presence of cells, casts, and crystals. In prerenal conditions, the urine typically has no cells but may contain hyaline casts. Casts are cylindrical bodies that form when proteins precipitate in the distal tubules and collecting ducts. Postrenal conditions may present with stones, crystals, sediment, bacteria, and clots from the obstruction. Coarse, muddy brown granular casts are classic findings in ATN.[8] Microscopic hematuria and a small amount of protein may also be seen on a random urine specimen. If a 24-hour urine specimen is collected, microalbumin levels are usually less than 30 mg/L, but vary with many factors such as age, activity, and infection.

Urine electrolyte levels help to discriminate between prerenal causes and ATN. The nurse obtains urine samples (often called spot urine levels) for electrolyte determinations before diuretics are administered because these drugs alter the urine results for up to 24 hours. Urinary sodium concentrations of less than 10 mEq/L are seen in prerenal conditions, as the kidneys attempt to conserve sodium and water to compensate for the hypoperfusion state. Urine sodium concentrations are greater than 40 mEq/L in

ATN as a result of impaired reabsorption in the diseased tubules.[8]

The fractional excretion of sodium (FE_{Na}) is a useful test for assessing how well the kidney can concentrate urine and conserve sodium. To determine the FE_{Na}, the following formula is used:

$$FE_{Na} = \frac{(\text{Urine sodium}) (\text{Serum creatinine}) \times 100}{(\text{Urine creatinine}) (\text{Serum sodium})}$$

In prerenal conditions, the FE_{Na} is less than 1%, whereas ATN presents with a FE_{Na} of greater than 1%.[8,11] Table 15-3 summarizes laboratory data useful in differentiating among the three categories of AKI.

Urine specific gravity and osmolality have a limited role in the diagnosis of AKI, especially in older adults, because the body's ability to concentrate urine decreases with age (see box, "Geriatric Considerations").[5,29] In general, prerenal conditions cause concentrated urine (high specific gravity and osmolality), whereas intrinsic azotemia causes dilute urine (low specific gravity and osmolality). The volume of urine output is also not a good indicator of renal function. Although patients with nonoliguric AKI excrete large volumes of fluid with little solute, they still have renal dysfunction and azotemia. In an older adult, assessment parameters are modified when assessing for acute renal failure.

TABLE 15-3 LABORATORY FINDINGS USEFUL IN DIFFERENTIATING CAUSES OF ACUTE KIDNEY INJURY

TYPE OF ACUTE KIDNEY INJURY	SPECIFIC GRAVITY	URINE OSMOLALITY	URINE SODIUM	MICROSCOPIC EXAMINATION	BUN/CR RATIO	FE_{NA}
Prerenal	>1.020	>500 mOsm/L	<10 mEq/L	Few hyaline casts possible	Elevated	<1%
Intrarenal	1.010	<350 mOsm/L	>20 mEq/L	Epithelial casts, red blood cell casts, pigmented granular casts	Normal	>1%
Postrenal	Normal to 1.010	Variable	Normal to 40 mEq/L	May have stones, crystals, sediment, clots, or bacteria	Normal	>1%

BUN, Blood urea nitrogen; *CR*, creatinine; *FE_{Na}*, fractional excretion of sodium.

GERIATRIC CONSIDERATIONS

Management of Acute Kidney Injury

- Older adults are at increased risk for AKI related to comorbidities such as diabetes mellitus, hypertension, and from polypharmacy. Commonly prescribed classes of medications that have adverse effects on renal blood flow are nonsteroidal antiinflammatory drugs and angiotensin-converting enzyme inhibitors.[31]
- The aging kidney is more susceptible to nephrotoxic and ischemic injury. Monitor drug dosages carefully, adjust drug dosages for underlying renal insufficiency, and use nephrotoxic agents judiciously.
- The primary risk factor for contrast-induced nephropathy is a preexisting decline in renal function, which places the elderly patient at risk. Monitor radiographic contrast media usage closely, using only as necessary. Maintain adequate hydration if radiographic contrast media must be used.
- Older adults are prone to developing volume depletion (prerenal conditions) because of a decreased ability to concentrate urine and conserve sodium. Volume status is difficult to assess because of altered skin turgor and decreased skin elasticity, decreased baroreceptor reflexes, and mouth dryness caused by mouth breathing. Be sure fluids are easily within reach of older adults not on fluid restriction. Offer fluids frequently if not on fluid restriction (diminished thirst response and may not feel thirsty). Provide intravenous fluids to maintain adequate hydration as prescribed.
- Urinary indices are of limited value in assessment of older adults because of impaired ability to concentrate urine.

- Older patients tend to exhibit uremic symptoms at lower levels of serum blood urea nitrogen and creatinine than do younger patients. The typical signs and symptoms of AKI may be attributed to other disorders associated with aging, thus delaying prompt diagnosis and treatment.
- Atypical signs and symptoms of uremia may be seen, such as an unexplained exacerbation of well-controlled heart failure, unexplained mental status changes, or personality changes.
- Older adults often have poor nutritional status before AKI and require early and adequate nutrition.
- Older adults have special needs in regard to renal replacement therapies. They may need dialysis or continuous renal replacement therapy earlier than younger patients, because they become symptomatic with lower serum creatinine and blood urea nitrogen levels. They are at an increased risk for vascular access problems secondary to diabetes mellitus and peripheral vascular disease. Keep ultrafiltration rate less than 1 L/hr because decreased cardiac reserve and autonomic dysfunction make ultrafiltration difficult.
- Supply supplemental oxygen if needed to offset the hypoxemia that often develops at the start of dialysis. Monitor for increased risk of complications associated with systemic heparinization, including subdural hematomas from falls and gastritis.
- Older adults are more prone to infection because of a compromised immune system. Use meticulous technique for all procedures. Avoid indwelling urinary catheters especially if the patient is anuric; use intermittent catheterization as necessary.

TABLE 15-4	INVASIVE DIAGNOSTIC PROCEDURES FOR ASSESSING THE RENAL SYSTEM	
PROCEDURE	**PURPOSE**	**POTENTIAL PROBLEMS**
Intravenous pyelography	To visualize the renal parenchyma, calyces, renal pelvis, ureters, and bladder to obtain information regarding size, shape, position, and function of the kidneys	Hypersensitivity reaction to contrast media Acute kidney injury
Computed tomography	To visualize the renal parenchyma to obtain data regarding the size, shape, and presence of lesions, cysts, masses, calculi, obstructions, congenital anomalies, and abnormal accumulations of fluid	Hypersensitivity reaction to contrast media (if used)
Renal angiography	To visualize the arterial tree, capillaries, and venous drainage of the kidneys to obtain data regarding the presence of tumors, cysts, stenosis infarction, aneurysms, hematomas, lacerations, and abscesses	Hypersensitivity reaction to contrast media Hemorrhage or hematoma at the catheter insertion site Acute kidney injury
Renal scanning	To determine renal function by visualizing the appearance and disappearance of the radioisotopes within the kidney; also provides some anatomical information	Hypersensitivity reaction to contrast media
Renal biopsy	To obtain data for making a histological diagnosis to determine the extent of the pathology, the appropriate therapy, and the possible prognosis	Hemorrhage Postbiopsy hematoma

DIAGNOSTIC PROCEDURES

Various diagnostic procedures are used to evaluate renal function. Noninvasive diagnostic procedures are usually performed before any invasive diagnostic procedures are conducted. Noninvasive diagnostic procedures that assess the renal system are radiography of the kidneys, ureters, and bladder (KUB), renal ultrasonography, and magnetic resonance imaging (MRI). A KUB x-ray delineates the size, shape, and position of the kidneys. It may also detect abnormalities such as calculi, hydronephrosis (dilatation of the renal pelvis), cysts, or tumors. Renal ultrasound is helpful in evaluating for obstruction, which is manifest by hydronephrosis or hydroureter (dilatation of the ureters). Ultrasound can also document the size of the kidneys, which may be helpful in differentiating acute from chronic renal conditions. The kidneys are often small (<10 cm) in chronic kidney disease. Real-time ultrasound is used during renal biopsy and during placement of percutaneous nephrostomy tubes (often placed for hydronephrosis). MRI provides anatomical information about renal structures.

Invasive diagnostic procedures for assessing the renal system include intravenous pyelography, computed tomography, renal angiography, renal scanning, and renal biopsy.[3] These procedures are summarized in Table 15-4.

As for all diagnostic procedures, the nurse instructs the patient, assists with the procedures, and monitors the patient after the procedure. When workup is done for AKI, it is also important to assess for allergies to contrast media and provide appropriate fluids to the patient to maintain hydration before and after the procedures. Urinary output is closely monitored after the procedure.

NURSING DIAGNOSES

Nursing care of the patient with acute kidney injury is complex. Multiple nursing diagnoses must be dealt with in these often critically ill patients. The Nursing Care Plan for the Patient with Acute Kidney Injury (see box) addresses nursing diagnoses, patient outcomes, and interventions.

◎ NURSING CARE PLAN

for the Patient with Acute Kidney Injury

NURSING DIAGNOSIS
Excess Fluid Volume related to sodium and water retention and excess intake

PATIENT OUTCOMES
Stable fluid balance
- Body weight within 2 lb of dry weight
- Intake and output balanced; bilateral breath sounds clear; vital signs normal

NURSING INTERVENTIONS	RATIONALES
• Obtain daily weights	• Weight gain is best indicator of fluid gain
• Maintain accurate intake and output records	• Identify imbalances
• Monitor respiratory status, including respiratory rate and crackles	• Assess volume overload
• Assess heart rate, blood pressure, and respiratory rate	• Hypertension, tachycardia, and tachypnea indicate volume overload
• Administer all fluids and medications in the least amount of fluid possible	• Minimize intake
• Monitor blood and urine laboratory tests	• Levels are altered in acute kidney injury

NURSING DIAGNOSIS
Risk for Infection related to depressed immune response secondary to uremia and Impaired Skin Integrity

PATIENT OUTCOMES
Absence of infection
- Infection is absent
- Patient is afebrile
- WBC count and differential are normal
- All cultures are negative

NURSING INTERVENTIONS	RATIONALES
• Monitor WBC count and culture results	• Detect infection early
• Monitor temperature	• Fever may indicate infection
• Avoid invasive equipment whenever possible, such as indwelling urinary catheters and central lines	• Prevent infection
• Use good hand-washing technique	• Prevent infection
• Use aseptic technique for all procedures	• Prevent infection
• Perform pulmonary preventive techniques (turn, cough, deep breathing)	• Mobilize secretions to prevent pneumonia
• Assess potential sites of infection (urinary, pulmonary, wound, intravenous catheters)	• Detect early signs of infection

NURSING DIAGNOSIS
Imbalanced Nutrition: Less Than Body Requirements related to uremia, altered oral mucous membranes, and dietary restrictions

PATIENT OUTCOMES
Adequate nutritional and caloric intake
- Body weight at patient's baseline
- Energy level appropriate
- Verbalizes comfort of oral cavity and ability to taste food normally

NURSING INTERVENTIONS	RATIONALES
• Monitor body weight and caloric intake daily	• Identify deficits in nutritional intake and response to nutritional therapy
• Collaborate with dietitian about nutritional needs	• Provide optimal nutritional support
• Provide diet with essential nutrients but within restrictions	• Prevent nutritional deficits; prevent electrolyte imbalances and fluid overload
• Provide oral hygiene every 2 to 4 hours	• Minimize dryness of oral mucosa and promote patient comfort
• Remove noxious stimuli from room	• Reduce nausea, vomiting, and anorexia

Continued

⊚ **NURSING CARE PLAN**

for the Patient with Acute Kidney Injury—cont'd

NURSING DIAGNOSIS
Anxiety related to diagnosis, treatment plan, prognosis, and unfamiliar environment

PATIENT OUTCOME
Anxiety levels reduced
• Effective coping mechanisms
• Participation in treatment plan

NURSING INTERVENTIONS	RATIONALES
• Monitor for signs of anxiety: tachycardia, muscle tension, inappropriate behaviors	• Recognize anxiety
• Explain all procedures; provide calm, relaxing environment	• Reduce anxiety by providing factual information
• Implement measures to reduce fear and anxiety	• Facilitate relaxation
• Allow patient to make choices	• Promote feelings of control to reduce anxiety
• Assess for ineffective coping (depression, withdrawal)	• Assess need for counseling and/or medications
• Administer antianxiety medications as prescribed	• Reduce anxiety

NURSING DIAGNOSIS
Deficient Knowledge related to disease process and therapeutic regimen

PATIENT OUTCOME
Adequate knowledge of disease and treatment
• Patient and family have sufficient, accurate information related to condition to be informed participants in the care

NURSING INTERVENTIONS	RATIONALES
• Provide specific, factual information on acute kidney injury, impact on the patient, and treatment plan	• Knowledge will enhance patient understanding
• Encourage patient and family to ask questions	• Promote increased knowledge
• Encourage patient and family members to participate in care	• Facilitate self-care management

WBC, White blood cell.
Based on data from Gulanick M and Myers JL. *Nursing Care Plans: Diagnoses, Interventions, and Outcomes,* 7th ed. St. Louis: Mosby; 2011.

NURSING INTERVENTIONS

Accurate measurement of intake and output and determination of daily weights are two vital nursing interventions. A urine meter or other type of accurate measuring device is essential for recording urinary output. Normal urine output is 0.5 to 1 mL/kg/hr. Oral fluid intake must also be carefully monitored. Fluid intake levels are often restricted to the amount of urine output in a 24-hour period plus insensible losses (approximately 600 to 1000 mL/day).[38] Administration of intravenous fluids as prescribed before procedures in which radiocontrast media will be given is critical.[13]

Assessment of daily weights is one of the most useful noninvasive diagnostic tools. The daily weight is used to validate intake and output measurements. A 1-kg gain in body weight is equal to a 1000-mL fluid gain. Weight should be obtained at the same time each day with the same scale. Many critical care beds have built-in scales, which simplify the procedure. When the patient is weighed, the nurse ensures that the scale is properly calibrated and that the same number of bed linens and pillows are weighed with the patient each time. The nurse must recognize signs and symptoms of fluid volume overload, which can lead to pulmonary edema and severe respiratory distress (see box, "Clinical Alert: Fluid Volume Overload").

❗ **CLINICAL ALERT**
Fluid Volume Overload

Signs and symptoms of fluid volume overload include hypertension, edema, crackles, dyspnea, neck vein distention, weight gain, increased pulmonary artery pressures, decreased urine output, decreased hematocrit, and presence of an S_3 heart sound.

Infection is the most common and serious complication of AKI and accounts for up to 75% of deaths in patients with AKI.[8] Nurses play a key role in preventing infections. Indwelling urinary catheters should not routinely be inserted, because they increase the risk of infection, and many patients remain oliguric for 8 to 14 days. Strict aseptic technique with all intravenous lines (central and peripheral), including temporary access devices used for dialysis, is also of extreme importance, both at the time of insertion and during daily maintenance.

Another important role of the nurse in preventing AKI, as well as delaying its progression, is monitoring trough drug levels. Nurses are responsible for scheduling and obtaining the trough blood levels at the appropriate times to ensure accurate results. Drug dosage adjustments must be made to prevent accumulation of the drug and toxic side effects. For example, aminoglycoside doses are based on drug levels and the patient's estimated creatinine clearance. If the drug level is too high, either the dose of the aminoglycoside can be kept constant and the interval between doses increased, or the interval can be kept constant and the dose is decreased. A trough level is drawn just before the next dose is given and is an indicator of how the body has cleared the drug.

MEDICAL MANAGEMENT OF ACUTE KIDNEY INJURY

Prerenal Causes

Acute kidney injury from prerenal conditions is usually reversible if renal perfusion is quickly restored; therefore early recognition and prompt treatment are essential. However, prevention of prerenal conditions is just as important as early recognition and aggressive management. Prompt replacement of extracellular fluids and aggressive treatment of shock may help prevent AKI. Hypovolemia is treated in various ways, depending on the cause. Blood loss may necessitate blood transfusions, whereas patients with pancreatitis and peritonitis are usually treated with isotonic solutions such as normal saline. Hypovolemia resulting from large urine or gastrointestinal losses often requires the administration of a hypotonic solution, such as 0.45% saline. Patients with cardiac instability usually require positive inotropic agents, antidysrhythmic agents, preload or afterload reducers, or an intraaortic balloon pump. Hypovolemia from intense vasodilation may require vasoconstrictor medications, isotonic fluid replacement, and antibiotics (if the patient has sepsis) until the underlying problem has been resolved. Invasive hemodynamic monitoring with a central venous catheter or pulmonary artery catheter may be considered in the management of fluid balance.

Postrenal Causes

Postrenal obstruction should be suspected whenever a patient has an unexpected decrease in urine volume. Postrenal conditions are usually resolved with the insertion of an indwelling bladder catheter, either transurethral or suprapubic.

Occasionally, a ureteral stent may have to be placed if the obstruction is caused by calculi or carcinoma.

Intrarenal Causes: Acute Tubular Necrosis

Common interventions for the patient with ATN include drug therapy, dietary management such as protein and electrolyte restrictions, management of fluid and electrolyte imbalances, and renal replacement therapies such as intermittent hemodialysis or continuous renal replacement therapy (CRRT).

Considering the detrimental impact of AKI, nurses must focus on efforts aimed at prevention. The most important preventive strategies include identification of patients at risk and elimination of potential contributing factors. Aggressive treatment must begin at the earliest sign of renal dysfunction.

In general, maintenance of cardiovascular function and adequate intravascular volume are the two key goals in the prevention of AKI. Box 15-6 summarizes important measures for preventing AKI.

Pharmacological Management

Diuretics. Diuretic therapy in the treatment of patients with AKI is controversial. In clinical practice, diuretics may be used to manage volume overload. Although it is believed

---

BOX 15-6 MEASURES TO PREVENT ACUTE KIDNEY INJURY

Avoid Nephrotoxins
- Use iso-osmolar radiocontrast media (e.g., iodixanol)
- Limit contrast volume to <100 mL
- Use antibiotics cautiously with appropriate dose modification
- Monitor drug levels (aminoglycosides)
- Stop certain medications (NSAIDs, ACE inhibitors, ARBs) before high-risk procedures

Optimize Volume Status Before Surgery or Invasive Procedures
- Aim for urinary output >40 mL/hr
- Keep mean arterial pressure >80 mm Hg
- Hydrate with normal saline before and after procedures requiring radiocontrast media
- Hold diuretics day before and day of procedure

Reduce Incidence of Nosocomial Infections
- Use indwelling urinary catheters judiciously
- Remove indwelling urinary catheters when no longer needed
- Use strict aseptic technique with all intravenous lines

Implement Tight Glycemic Control in the Critically Ill

Aggressively Investigate and Treat Sepsis

ACE, Angiotensin-converting enzyme; *ARBs,* angiotensin receptor blockers; *NSAIDs,* nonsteroidal antiinflammatory drugs.

that diuretics increase renal blood flow and GFR (thereby increasing urine output), and reduce tubular dysfunction and obstruction, evidence suggests that they may cause excess diuresis and renal hypoperfusion, compromising an already insulted renal system.[8] Diuretics may increase the risk of AKI from volume depletion when they are given before procedures requiring radiological contrast media or if the patient is hypovolemic. Adequate hydration before administration of diuretics is essential. The widespread use of diuretics is currently being discouraged.[8,10]

If diuretic therapy is implemented, a loop diuretic is commonly ordered. Large doses of furosemide are often needed to induce diuresis. This may lead to excessive diuresis and volume depletion. High doses of furosemide have been associated with deafness, which may become permanent.[8]

Mannitol, an osmotic diuretic often used in AKI caused by rhabdomyolysis, increases plasma volume and is believed to protect the kidney by minimizing postischemic swelling. Patients may be at risk for the development of pulmonary edema due to the rapid expansion of intravascular volume triggered by mannitol.

Dopamine. The role of dopamine is controversial in the treatment of AKI. Low-dose dopamine continues to be ordered for patients with AKI despite numerous studies that fail to show any benefit. Dopamine in low doses (1 to 3 mcg/kg/min) may cause a transient increase renal blood flow and GFR by stimulating the dopaminergic receptors in the kidney.[10] However, there is broad consensus that dopamine is potentially harmful and its use for renal perfusion should be avoided.[8,10,18]

N-Acetylcysteine. Multiple studies have been conducted using prophylactic *N*-acetylcysteine (Mucomyst) in patients at risk of contrast-induced AKI. *N*-Acetylcysteine, an antioxidant, in conjunction with intravenous fluids has been thought to reduce the incidence of contrast-induced AKI. The mechanism of action is unclear, but *N*-acetylcysteine is thought to act by scavenging oxygen free radicals or enhancing the vasodilatory effects of nitric oxide.[13,33] Prophylactic administration of *N*-acetylcysteine (600 mg orally twice a day on the day before and on the day the contrast is given), along with hydration (half-normal [0.45%] saline at 1 mL/kg/hr overnight before procedure) is hypothesized to reduce the amount of acute renal damage in high-risk patients undergoing procedures requiring contrast agents.[13,24,33] However, current data on the administration of acetylcysteine remains inconclusive.[13,33]

Fenoldopam. Another agent that is postulated to protect against contrast-induced AKI is fenoldopam, a dopamine-1 receptor agonist (DA-1). Fenoldopam (Corlopam) acts as a vasodilator of peripheral arteries (reducing blood pressure) and as a potent renal vasodilator (increasing renal blood flow). It is six times more potent than dopamine in increasing renal blood flow, especially to critical regions in the renal medulla. Fenoldopam is given via intravenous infusion several hours before the contrast agent is given and is continued for a minimum of 4 hours after the procedure. Ongoing studies are focused on the use of fenoldopam in the prevention of

contrast-induced nephropathy; however, no consistent outcome has been noted.[13,18,33]

Miscellaneous agents. Multiple miscellaneous agents have been administered in an attempt to attenuate the course of AKI. None, however, has consistently proved effective. Many of these drugs are administered in an attempt to improve renal blood flow through vasodilation (atrial natriuretic peptide, endothelin-1 receptor antagonists, prostaglandin E_1), prevent accumulation of intracellular calcium as occurs in ischemic azotemia (calcium channel blockers), protect renal tubule cells during ischemia (glycine, magnesium adenosine triphosphate dichloride) or stimulate renal cell regeneration (epidermal growth factor, growth hormone, insulin-like growth factor). Many of these agents and numerous others have shown beneficial results in experimental models, but results are inconsistent in the clinical setting.

Prostaglandin E_1 has a vasodilatory effect and has been shown in small studies to counteract the vasoconstriction from radiocontrast media that may cause AKI in high-risk patients. Administration of an intravenous sodium bicarbonate solution before and after the procedure is also thought to prevent CIN. It is speculated that alkalinizing the urine may reduce the nephrotoxic potential of the radiocontrast media in the renal capillaries or tubules. However, trials comparing administration of normal saline with sodium bicarbonate solutions are inconclusive.[8,13,24] Ongoing studies are being conducted on a variety of agents in the prevention and treatment of AKI.[3,8,10]

Pharmacological management considerations. Drug therapy for the patient with AKI poses a challenge because two thirds of all drugs or their metabolites are eliminated from the body by the kidneys. Substantial alterations in drug dosages are often necessary to prevent toxic levels and adverse reactions. Assessment of renal function by creatinine clearance is often used to assist with drug dosing. The pharmacokinetic characteristics of the drug to be given, the route of elimination, and the extent of protein binding are also considered. Clinical pharmacists assist in determining optimum drug dosages for critically ill patients.

Many drugs are removed by dialysis, and extra doses are often required to avoid suboptimal drug levels. Drugs that are primarily water soluble, such as vitamins, cimetidine, and phenobarbital should be administered after dialysis. Drugs that become bound to proteins or lipids or are metabolized by the liver, such as phenytoin, lidocaine, and vancomycin, are not removed by dialysis and can be given at any time.[8] Box 15-7 is a partial list of drugs that are removed by dialysis and should be administered after dialysis.

Dietary Management

Dietary management in patients with AKI is important. Energy expenditure in catabolic patients with acute kidney injury is much higher than normal. Dialysis also contributes to protein catabolism. The loss of amino acids and water-soluble vitamins in the dialysate solution constitutes another drain on the patient's nutritional stores. The overall goal of dietary management for acute kidney injury is provision of

BOX 15-7   COMMON DRUGS REMOVED BY HEMODIALYSIS*

- Aminoglycosides (gentamicin, tobramycin)
- Aspirin
- Cephalosporins (including cefoxitin and ceftazidime)
- Cimetidine
- Enalapril
- Erythromycin
- Folic acid
- Isoniazid
- Lisinopril
- Lithium carbonate
- Metformin
- Methyldopa
- Metoprolol
- Nitroprusside
- Penicillins (piperacillin, penicillin G)
- Phenobarbital
- Procainamide
- Quinidine
- Ranitidine
- Sulfonamides (sulfamethoxazole, sulfisoxazole)
- Trimethoprim-sulfamethoxazole
- Water-soluble vitamins

*If possible, hold daily doses until after dialysis; supplemental doses may be required for many of these agents.

adequate energy, protein, and micronutrients to maintain homeostasis in patients who may be extremely catabolic. Nutritional recommendations include the following[9]:

- Caloric intake of 25 to 35 kcal/kg of ideal body weight per day
- Protein intake of no less than 0.8 g/kg. Patients who are extremely catabolic should receive 1.5 to 2.0 g/kg of ideal body weight per day—75% to 80% of which contains all the required essential amino acids.
- Sodium intake of 0.5 to 1.0 g/day
- Potassium intake of 20 to 50 mEq/day
- Calcium intake of 800 to 1200 mg/day
- Fluid intake equal to the volume of the patient's urine output plus an additional 600 to 1000 mL/day

In addition, patients undergoing dialysis usually receive multivitamins, folic acid, and occasionally an iron supplement to replace the water-soluble vitamins and other essential elements lost during dialysis. If the patient is unable to ingest or tolerate an adequate oral nutritional intake, enteral feedings or total parenteral nutrition are prescribed. Nutritional support must supply the patient with sufficient nonprotein glucose calories, essential amino acids, fluids, electrolytes, and essential vitamins. Adequate nutrition not only prevents further catabolism, negative nitrogen balance, muscle wasting, and other uremic complications, but also enhances the patient's tubular regenerating capacity, resistance to infection, and ability to combat other multisystem dysfunctions. The physician may also prescribe early renal replacement therapy to treat the increased fluid volume the patient receives from enteral or total parenteral nutrition.

Management of Fluid, Electrolyte, and Acid-Base Imbalances

Fluid imbalance. Volume overload is managed by dietary restriction of salt and water and administration of diuretics. In addition, dialysis or other renal replacement therapies may be indicated for fluid control. These modalities are discussed later in this chapter.

Electrolyte imbalance. Common electrolyte imbalances in AKI are listed in the box, "Laboratory Alert," along with their "critical" values and the significance of the laboratory alert. The nurse immediately notifies the physician once a critical laboratory value is known. Hyperkalemia is common in AKI, especially if the patient is hypercatabolic. Hyperkalemia occurs when potassium excretion is reduced as a result of the decrease in GFR. Sudden changes in the serum potassium level can cause dysrhythmias, which may be fatal. Figure 15-6 shows the electrocardiographic changes commonly seen in hyperkalemia.

Three approaches are used to treat hyperkalemia: (1) reduce the body potassium content, (2) shift the potassium from outside the cell to inside the cell and (3) antagonize the membrane effect of the hyperkalemia. Only dialysis and administration of cation exchange resins (sodium polystyrene sulfonate [Kayexalate]) actually reduce plasma potassium levels and total

! LABORATORY ALERT

Acute Kidney Injury

LABORATORY TEST	CRITICAL VALUE	SIGNIFICANCE
Potassium (K^+)	>6.6 mEq/L	**Hyperkalemia:** potential for heart blocks, asystole, ventricular fibrillation; may cause muscle weakness, diarrhea, and abdominal cramps
Sodium (Na^+)	≤110 mEq/L	**Hyponatremia:** potential for lethargy, confusion, coma, or seizures; may cause nausea, vomiting, and headaches
Total calcium (Ca^{++})	<7.0 mg/dL	**Hypocalcemia:** potential for seizures, laryngospasm, stridor, tetany, heart blocks, and cardiac arrest; may see positive Chvostek or Trousseau sign
Magnesium (Mg^{++})	>3.0 mg/dL	**Hypermagnesemia:** potential for bradycardia and heart blocks, lethargy, coma, hypotension, hypoventilation, and weak-to-absent deep tendon reflexes

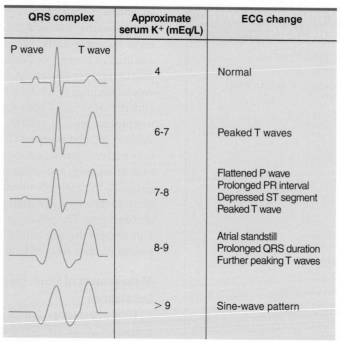

QRS complex	Approximate serum K+ (mEq/L)	ECG change
P wave T wave	4	Normal
	6-7	Peaked T waves
	7-8	Flattened P wave Prolonged PR interval Depressed ST segment Peaked T wave
	8-9	Atrial standstill Prolonged QRS duration Further peaking T waves
	> 9	Sine-wave pattern

FIGURE 15-6 Electrocardiographic (ECG) changes seen in hyperkalemia. (From Weiner D, Linas S, Wingo C. Disorders of potassium metabolism. In Feehally J, Floege J, Johnson R, eds. *Comprehensive Clinical Nephrology*. Philadelphia: Mosby. 2007.)

body potassium content in a patient with renal dysfunction. In the past, sorbitol has been combined with sodium polystyrene sulfonate powder for administration. The concomitant use of sorbitol with sodium polystyrene sulfonate has been implicated in cases of colonic intestinal necrosis and therefore this combination is not recommended.[22] Other treatments only "protect" the patient for a short time until dialysis or cation exchange resins can be instituted. Table 15-5 summarizes medications used in the treatment of hyperkalemia. Commonly prescribed treatments for hyperkalemia consists of the following[32]:

- Calcium gluconate, 10 mL of a 10% solution given intravenously over 5 minutes
- Regular insulin, 10 units given intravenously with glucose (50 mL of 50% dextrose) intravenously
- Albuterol 10 to 20 mg given by nebulized inhalation over 15 minutes
- Sodium bicarbonate, 50 mEq/L given intravenously in patients with severe acidosis with pH less than 7.2 or serum HCO_3^- less than 15 mEq/L

Hyponatremia generally occurs from water overload. However, as nephrons are progressively damaged, the ability to conserve sodium is lost, and major salt-wasting states can develop, causing hyponatremia. Hyponatremia is treated with fluid restriction, specifically restriction of free water intake. Alterations in the serum calcium and phosphorus levels occur frequently in AKI as a result of abnormalities in excretion, absorption, and metabolism of the electrolytes. Mild degrees of hypermagnesemia are common in AKI secondary to decreased renal excretion.

Acid-base imbalance. Metabolic acidosis is the primary acid-base imbalance seen in AKI. Box 15-8 summarizes the etiology and the signs and symptoms of metabolic acidosis in AKI. Treatment of metabolic acidosis depends on its severity. In mild metabolic acidosis, the lungs compensate by excreting carbon dioxide. Patients with a serum bicarbonate level of less than 15 mEq/L and a pH of less than 7.20 are usually treated with intravenous sodium bicarbonate. The goal of treatment is to raise the pH to a value greater than 7.20. Rapid correction of the acidosis should be avoided, because tetany may occur as a result of hypocalcemia. The pH determines how much ionized calcium is present in the serum; the more acidic the serum, the more ionized calcium is present. If the metabolic acidosis is rapidly corrected, the serum ionized calcium level decreases as the calcium binds with albumin and other substances such as phosphate and sulfate. For this reason, intravenous calcium gluconate may be prescribed. Renal replacement therapies also may correct metabolic acidosis because it removes excess hydrogen ions, and bicarbonate is added to the dialysate and replacement solutions.

Renal Replacement Therapy

Renal replacement therapy is the primary treatment for the patient with AKI. The decision to initiate renal replacement therapy is a clinical decision based on the fluid, electrolyte, and metabolic status of each patient. Renal replacement therapy options include intermittent hemodialysis, CRRT, or peritoneal dialysis.

TABLE 15-5   PHARMACOLOGY

Medications to Treat Hyperkalemia

MEDICATION	ACTION/USE	DOSAGE/ROUTE	SIDE EFFECTS	NURSING IMPLICATIONS
Sodium polystyrene sulfonate (Kayexalate)	↑ Fecal excretion of potassium by exchanging sodium ions for potassium ions	*Oral:* 15 g 1-4 times daily by mouth *Rectal:* 30-50 g via enema every 6 hours	Constipation, hypokalemia, hypernatremia, nausea and vomiting, fecal impaction in the elderly	Available as a powder or suspension Mix powder with full glass of liquid and chill to increase palatability Do not mix oral powder with orange juice Do not mix with sorbitol
Furosemide (Lasix)	↑ Renal excretion of potassium	*Oral:* 20-80 mg daily twice a day *IV:* 20-40 mg/dose every 6-12 hours *Continuous infusion:* 10-40 mg/hr	Orthostatic hypotension, hypokalemia, urinary frequency, dizziness, ototoxicity	Administer IV dose over several minutes; ototoxicity is associated with rapid administration Assess for allergy to sulfonylurea before giving Monitor for dehydration, hypokalemia, hypotension Diuretics only work if the patient is nonoliguric
Insulin/ dextrose	Shifts potassium temporarily from the extracellular fluid (blood) into the intracellular fluid; the dextrose helps prevent hypoglycemia	*IV:* 10 units regular insulin and 50 mL of 50% dextrose IV push	Hyperglycemia, hypoglycemia, hypokalemia	If the serum glucose is >300 mg/dL, the physician may order only the insulin
Sodium bicarbonate	Shifts potassium temporarily from the extracellular fluid (blood) to the intracellular fluid	*IV:* 50 mEq/L IV push	Hypernatremia, hypokalemia, pulmonary edema	Do not mix with any other medications to prevent precipitation Helpful if patient has a severe metabolic acidosis
Albuterol	Adrenergic agonist ↑ plasma insulin concentration; shifts potassium to intracellular space	*Inhalation:* 10-20 mg over 10 minutes *IV:* 0.5 mg over 15 minutes	Tachycardia, angina, palpitations, hypertension, nervousness, irritability	Note that the dose used is much higher than that used in treating pulmonary conditions Use concentrated form (5 mg/mL) so the volume to be inhaled is minimized
Calcium gluconate	Electrolyte replacement	*IV:* 10 mL of 10% solution IV push over 5 minutes	Bradycardia, hypotension, syncope, necrosis if infiltrated	Has no effect on actually lowering serum potassium Will see almost immediate effect on ECG appearance Be sure IV is patent; prevent extravasation

ECG, Electrocardiogram; *IV,* intravenous.

BOX 15-8   METABOLIC ACIDOSIS IN ACUTE KIDNEY INJURY

Etiology

- Inability of kidney to excrete hydrogen ions; decreased production of ammonia by the kidney (normally assists with hydrogen ion excretion)
- Retention of acid end-products of metabolism, which use available buffers in the body; inability of kidney to synthesize bicarbonate

Signs and Symptoms

- Low pH of arterial blood (pH <7.35)
- Low serum bicarbonate
- Increased rate and depth of respirations to excrete carbon dioxide from the lungs (compensatory mechanism); known as Kussmaul's respiration
- Low $PaCO_2$
- Lethargy and coma if severe

$PaCO_2$, Partial pressure of carbon dioxide in arterial blood.

Definition. *Dialysis* is defined as the separation of solutes by differential diffusion through a porous or semipermeable membrane that is placed between two solutions. The various dialysis methods are distinguished by the type of semipermeable membrane and the two solutions that are used.

Indications for dialysis. The most common reasons for initiating dialysis in AKI include acidosis, hyperkalemia, volume overload, and uremia. Dialysis is usually started early in the course of the renal dysfunction before uremic complications occur. In addition, dialysis is may be started for fluid management when total parenteral nutrition is administered in patients with impaired renal function.[7]

Principles and mechanisms. Dialysis therapy is based on two physical principles that operate simultaneously: diffusion and ultrafiltration. *Diffusion* (or clearance) is the movement of solutes such as urea from the patient's blood to the dialysate cleansing fluid, across a semipermeable membrane (the hemofilter). Substances such as bicarbonate may also cross in the opposite direction, from the dialysate through the semipermeable membrane into the patient's blood. Movement of solutes across the semipermeable membrane depends on the following:

- The amount of solutes on each side of the semipermeable membrane; typically, the patient's blood has larger amounts of solutes such as urea, creatinine, and potassium
- The surface area of the semipermeable membrane (the size of the hemofilter)
- The permeability of the semipermeable membrane
- The size and charge of the solutes
- The rate of blood flowing through the hemofilter
- The rate of dialysate cleansing fluid flowing through the hemofilter

Ultrafiltration is the removal of plasma water and some low–molecular weight particles by using a pressure or osmotic gradient. Ultrafiltration is primarily aimed at controlling fluid volume, whereas dialysis is aimed at decreasing waste products and treating fluid and electrolyte imbalances.[6]

Vascular access. An essential component of all the renal replacement therapies is adequate, easy access to the patient's bloodstream. Various types of vascular access devices (Figures 15-7 and 15-8) are used for hemodialysis: percutaneous venous catheters, arteriovenous fistulas, and arteriovenous grafts.

Temporary percutaneous catheters are commonly used in patients with AKI because they can be used immediately. The typical catheter has a single or double lumen and is designed only for short-term renal replacement therapy during acute situations. Though these catheters can be inserted into the subclavian, jugular, or femoral veins, the femoral site is discouraged because it carries an increased risk of infection.[30] The subclavian site should also be avoided in patients with advanced kidney disease because of the risk of subclavian vein stenosis.[30] Routine replacement of hemodialysis catheters to prevent infection is not recommended.[30] The decision to remove or replace the catheter is based on clinical need and/or signs and symptoms of infection.[30] Occasionally a percutaneous tunneled

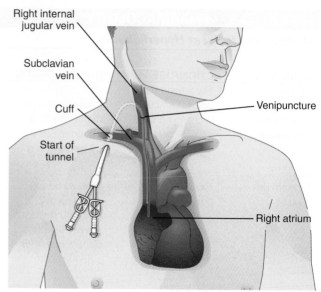

FIGURE 15-7 Central venous catheter used for hemodialysis. (From Headley CM. Acute kidney injury and chronic kidney disease. In Lewis SL, Dirksen SR, Heitkemper MM, et al, eds. *Medical-Surgical Nursing: Assessment and Management of Clinical Problems.* 8th ed. St. Louis: Mosby, 2011.)

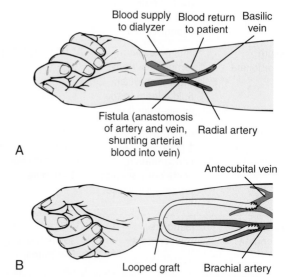

FIGURE 15-8 Hemodialysis access devices. **A,** Arteriovenous fistula. **B,** Arteriovenous graft. (From Headley CM. Acute kidney injury and chronic kidney disease. In Lewis SL, Dirksen SR, Heitkemper MM, et al, eds. *Medical-Surgical Nursing: Assessment and Management of Clinical Problems.* 8th ed. St. Louis: Mosby, 2011.)

catheter is placed if the patient needs ongoing hemodialysis. These catheters are usually inserted in the operating room or in an interventional radiology area. Examples of tunneled hemodialysis catheters include the Permacath and Tesio twin catheters.

An *arteriovenous fistula* is an internal, surgically created communication between an artery and a vein. The most frequently created fistula is the Brescia-Cimino fistula, which involves anastomosing the radial artery and cephalic vein in a side-to-side or end-to-side manner. The anastomosis permits blood to bypass the capillaries and to flow directly from the artery into the vein. As a result, the vein is forced to dilate to accommodate the increased pressure that accompanies the arterial blood. This method produces a vessel that is easy to cannulate but requires 4 to 6 weeks before it is mature enough to use.

Arteriovenous grafts are created by using different types of prosthetic materials. Most commonly, polytetrafluoroethylene (Teflon) grafts are placed under the skin and are surgically anastomosed between an artery (usually brachial) and a vein (usually antecubital). The graft site usually heals within 2 to 4 weeks.

Nursing care of arteriovenous fistula or graft. The nurse must protect the vascular access site. An arteriovenous fistula or graft should be auscultated for a bruit and palpated for the presence of a thrill or buzz every 8 hours. The extremity that has a fistula or graft must never be used for drawing blood specimens, obtaining blood pressure measurements, or administering intravenous therapy or intramuscular injections. Such activities produce pressure changes within the altered vessels that could result in clotting or rupture. The nurse must alert other healthcare personnel of the presence of the fistula or graft by posting a large sign at the head of the patient's bed that indicates which arm should be used. The presence and strength of the pulse distal to the fistula or graft are evaluated at least every 8 hours. Inadequate collateral circulation past the fistula or graft may result in loss of this pulse. The physician is notified immediately if no bruit is auscultated, no thrill is palpated, or the distal pulse is absent.

Nursing care of percutaneous catheters. Strict aseptic technique must be applied to any percutaneous catheter placed for dialysis. Transparent, semipermeable polyurethane dressings are recommended because they allow continuous visualization for assessment of signs of infection.[30] Replace transparent dressings on temporary percutaneous catheters at least every 7 days and no more than once a week for tunneled percutaneous catheters unless the dressing is soiled or loose.[30] Monitor the catheter site visually when changing the dressing or by palpation through an intact dressing. Tenderness at the insertion site, swelling, erythema or drainage should be reported to the physician. To prevent accidental dislodging, minimize manipulation of the catheter. The catheter is not used to administer fluids or medications or to sample blood unless a specific order is obtained to do so. Dialysis personnel may instill medication in the catheter to maintain patency, and clamp the catheter when not in use.

Hemodialysis. Intermittent hemodialysis is the most frequently used renal replacement therapy for treating AKI. Hemodialysis consists of simply cleansing the patient's blood through a hemofilter by the use of diffusion and ultrafiltration. Water and waste products of metabolism are easily removed. Hemodialysis is efficient and corrects biochemical disturbances quickly. Treatments are typically 3 to 4 hours long and are performed in the critical care unit at the patient's bedside. Patients with AKI may be hemodynamically unstable and unable to tolerate intermittent hemodialysis. In those instances, other methods of renal replacement therapy such as peritoneal dialysis or CRRT are considered.

Complications. Several complications are associated with hemodialysis. Hypotension is common and is usually the result of preexisting hypovolemia, excessive amounts of fluid removal, or excessively rapid fluid removal.[15] Other factors that contribute to hypotension include left ventricular dysfunction from preexisting heart disease or medications, autonomic dysfunction resulting from medication or diabetes, and inappropriate vasodilation resulting from sepsis or antihypertensive drug therapy. Dialyzer membrane incompatibility may also cause hypotension.

Dysrhythmias may occur during dialysis. Causes of dysrhythmias include a rapid shift in the serum potassium level, clearance of antidysrhythmic medications, preexisting coronary artery disease, hypoxemia, or hypercalcemia from rapid influx of calcium from the dialysate solution.

Muscle cramps may occur during dialysis, but they occur more commonly in chronic renal failure. Cramping is thought to be caused by ischemia of the skeletal muscles resulting from aggressive fluid removal. The cramps typically involve the legs, feet, and hands and occur most often during the last half of the dialysis treatment.

A decrease in the arterial oxygen content of the blood can occur in patients undergoing hemodialysis. Usually the decrease ranges from 5 to 35 mm Hg (mean, 15 mm Hg) and is not clinically significant except in the unstable critically ill patient. Several theories have been offered to explain the hypoxemia, including leukocyte interactions with the hemofilter and a decrease in carbon dioxide levels, resulting from either an acetate dialysate solution or a loss of carbon dioxide across the semipermeable membrane.

Dialysis disequilibrium syndrome often occurs after the first or second dialysis treatment or in patients who have had sudden, large decreases in BUN and creatinine levels as a result of the hemodialysis. Because of the blood-brain barrier, dialysis does not deplete the concentrations of BUN, creatinine, and other uremic toxins in the brain as rapidly as it decreases those substances in the extracellular fluid. An osmotic concentration gradient established in the brain allows fluid to enter until the concentration levels equal those of the extracellular fluid. The extra fluid in the brain tissue creates a state of cerebral edema for the patient, which results in severe headaches, nausea and vomiting, twitching, mental confusion, and occasionally seizures. The incidence of dialysis disequilibrium syndrome may be decreased by the use of shorter, more frequent dialysis treatments.

Infectious complications associated with hemodialysis include vascular access infections and hepatitis C. Vascular access infections are usually caused by a break in sterile technique, whereas hepatitis C is usually acquired through transfusion.

Hemolysis, air embolism, and hyperthermia are rare complications of hemodialysis. Hemolysis can occur when the patient's blood is exposed to incorrectly mixed dialysate solution or hypotonic chemicals (formaldehyde and bleach). An air embolism can occur when air is introduced into the bloodstream through a break in the dialysis circuit. Hyperthermia may result if the temperature control devices on the dialysis machine malfunction. Complications of hemodialysis are summarized in Box 15-9.

Nursing care of the patient. The patient receiving hemodialysis requires specialized monitoring and interventions by the critical care nurse. Laboratory values are monitored and abnormal results reported to the nephrologist and dialysis staff. The patient is weighed daily to monitor fluid status. On the day of dialysis, dialyzable (water-soluble) medications are not given until after treatment. The dialysis nurse or pharmacist can be consulted to determine which medications to withhold or administer. Supplemental doses are administered as ordered after dialysis. Administration of antihypertensive agents is avoided for 4 to 6 hours before treatment, if possible. Doses of other medications that lower blood pressure (narcotics, sedatives) are reduced, if possible. The percutaneous catheter, fistula, or graft is assessed frequently; unusual findings such as loss of bruit, redness, or drainage at the site must be reported. After dialysis, the patient is assessed for signs of bleeding, hypovolemia, and dialysis disequilibrium syndrome.

Continuous renal replacement therapy. CRRT is a continuous extracorporeal blood purification system managed by the bedside critical care nurse. It is similar to conventional intermittent hemodialysis in that a hemofilter is used to facilitate the processes of ultrafiltration and diffusion. It differs in that CRRT provides a slow removal of solutes and water as compared to the rapid removal of water and solutes that occurs with intermittent hemodialysis.

Indications. The clinical indications for CRRT are similar to those for intermittent hemodialysis, including volume overload, hyperkalemia, acidosis, and uremia. It is frequently selected for patients with AKI because of the ability to provide a gentle correction of uremia and fluid imbalances while minimizing hypotension. CRRT modalities have also been thought to absorb many of the interleukins associated with inflammation and sepsis.[4,7,20]

Principles. The first CRRT systems were introduced in the 1970s. The extracorporeal circuit consisted of an arterial access catheter, hemofilter, and venous return catheter. The patient's blood pressure determined the flow rate through the circuit. Arteriovenous systems are no longer used because of therapy limitations related to patient dependent blood flow and concern for complications related to arterial cannulation. Venovenous circuits are currently the standard for renal replacement therapy.[1] Improvements in dual-lumen venous catheters, mechanical blood pumps, and user-friendly renal replacement therapy cassette circuits and monitors have increased the safety and efficiency of venovenous replacement therapies. In venovenous therapy, two venous accesses or a dual-lumen venous catheter are used. Blood is pulled from the access port of the dual-lumen dialysis catheter or one of two single-lumen venous catheters by the negative pressure gradient created by a blood pump. The blood travels through the hemofilter and returns to the patient via the return port of the dual-lumen venous dialysis catheter or a second venous catheter (Figure 15-9).

There are four types of continuous venovenous replacement therapies:
1. Slow continuous ultrafiltration (SCUF)
2. Continuous venovenous hemofiltration (CVVH)
3. Continuous venovenous hemodialysis (CVVHD)
4. Continuous venovenous hemodiafiltration (CVVHDF)
Table 15-6 outlines the various CRRT modalities.

Slow continuous ultrafiltration (SCUF) is also known as isolated ultrafiltration and is used to remove plasma water in cases of volume overload. SCUF can remove 3 to 6 liters of ultrafiltrate per day. Solute removal is minimal and therefore is not indicated for patients with conditions requiring removal of uremic toxins and correction of acidosis.

Continuous venovenous hemofiltration (CVVH) is used to remove fluids and solutes through the process of convection, which is the transfer of solutes across the semipermeable membranes of the hemofilter. As plasma moves across the membrane (ultrafiltration), it carries solute molecules. Increasing the volume of plasma water that crosses the hemofilter membranes increases the amount of solute removed. Replacement solution is added to replenish plasma water and electrolytes lost because of the high ultrafiltration rate. Replacement solutions typically are commercially prepared and contain electrolytes and a bicarbonate or lactate base. Calcium and magnesium are two electrolytes not present in bicarbonate-based replacement solutions because they will form precipitates. These two electrolytes must be administered separately. Replacement solutions can be administered before the hemofilter (predilution) or after the hemofilter (postdilution).

Continuous venovenous hemodialysis (CVVHD) is similar to CVVH in that ultrafiltration removes plasma water. It differs in

---

BOX 15-9   COMPLICATIONS OF DIALYSIS

- Hypotension
- Cramps
- Bleeding/clotting
- Dialyzer reaction
- Hemolysis
- Dysrhythmias
- Infections
- Hypoxemia
- Pyrogen reactions
- Dialysis disequilibrium syndrome
- Vascular access dysfunction
- Technical errors (incorrect dialysate mixture, contaminated dialysate, or air embolism)

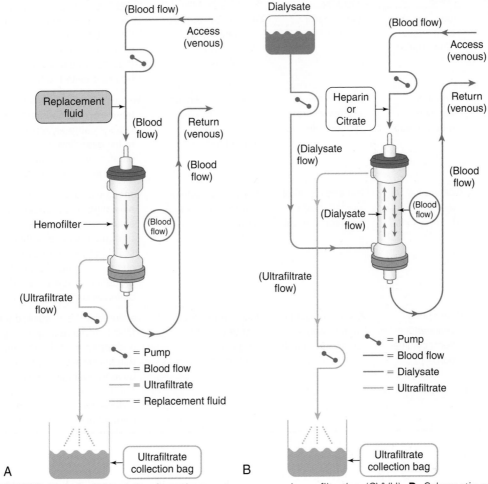

FIGURE 15-9 A, Schematic of continuous venovenous hemofiltration (CVVH). **B,** Schematic of continuous venovenous hemodialysis (CVVHD). (From Urden L, Stacy K, Lough M, eds. *Thelan's Critical Care Nursing: Diagnosis and Management.* 5th ed. St. Louis: Mosby, 2005.)

that dialysate solution is added around the hemofilter membranes to facilitate solute removal by the process of diffusion. Since the dialysate solution is constantly refreshed around the hemofilter membranes, the solute clearance is greater with this therapy and therefore can be used to treat both volume overload and azotemia.

Continuous venovenous hemodiafiltration (CVVHDF) combines ultrafiltration, convection, and dialysis to maximize fluid and solute removal. It is useful for the management of volume overload associated with high solute removal requirements.

Automated devices are currently marketed to facilitate the delivery of the different CRRT therapies (Figure 15-10).

Anticoagulation. The efficiency of the hemofilter can decline over time or fail suddenly because of clogging or clotting. Clogging results from the accumulation of protein and blood cells on the hemofilter membrane.[4] Filter clotting is the result of progressive loss of the hollow fibers within the hemofilter.[4] CRRT requires some form of intervention to prevent clogging and clotting. Hourly normal saline flushes may be used to extend the life of the hemofilter.

During CRRT, the patient's blood comes in contact with extracorporeal circuit and activates the coagulation cascade. Heparin is used frequently in CRRT to inhibit coagulation and extend the life of the hemofilter. However, heparin may be contraindicated if there is a risk of bleeding and heparin-induced thrombocytopenia.

An alternative to heparin during CRRT is citrate.[12,14,35] Citrate chelates calcium in the serum and inhibits activation of the coagulation cascade.[15] Systemic anticoagulation is minimal because the liver quickly converts citrate to bicarbonate. Citrate is infused into the circuit above the filter. Close monitoring of serum ionized calcium levels and calcium replacement through a separate venous line are required. Metabolic alkalosis is a concern with this therapy. Bicarbonate-based replacement solutions should not be used.

Nursing care. The critical care nurse is responsible for monitoring the patient receiving CRRT. In many critical care units, the CRRT system is set up by the dialysis staff but is maintained by critical care nurses with additional training. The patient's hemodynamic status is monitored hourly, including fluid intake and output. Temperature is monitored

TABLE 15-6 CONTINUOUS RENAL REPLACEMENT THERAPIES

ABBREVIATION	NAME	PURPOSE	VASCULAR ACCESS REQUIRED	DESCRIPTION
SCUF	Slow continuous ultrafiltration	Fluid removal	Dual-lumen venous catheter or two large venous catheters	Venous blood is circulated through a hemofilter and returned to the patient through a venous catheter: ultrafiltrate (fluid removed) is collected in a drainage bag as it exits the hemofilter
CVVH	Continuous venovenous hemofiltration	Fluid and some uremic waste product removal	Dual-lumen venous catheter or two large venous catheters	Venous blood is circulated through a hemofilter and returned to the patient through a venous catheter; replacement fluid is used to increase flow through the hemofilter; ultrafiltrate (fluid removed) is collected in a drainage bag as it exits the hemofilter
CVVHD	Continuous venovenous hemodialysis	Fluid and maximal uremic waste product removal	Dual-lumen venous catheter or two large venous catheters	Venous blood is circulated through a hemofilter (surrounded by a dialysate solution) and returned to the patient through a venous catheter; replacement solution may be used to improve convection; ultrafiltrate (fluid and waste products removed) is collected in a drainage bag as it exits the hemofilter
CVVHDF	Continuous venovenous hemodiafiltration	Maximal fluid and uremic waste product removal	Dual-lumen venous catheter or two large venous catheters	Venous blood is circulated through a hemofilter (surrounded by a dialysate solution) and returned to the patient through a venous catheter; replacement solution is used to maintain fluid balance; ultrafiltration (fluid and waste products removed) is collected in a drainage bag as it exits the hemofilter

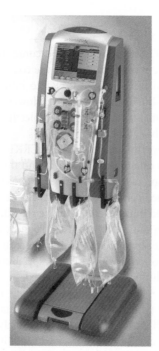

FIGURE 15-10 Prismaflex continuous renal replacement therapy system. (Courtesy Gambro, Lakewood, CO.)

because significant heat can be lost when blood is circulating through the extracorporeal circuit. Specialized devices to warm the dialysate or replacement fluid or to rewarm the blood returning to patient are available.

Ultrafiltration volume is assessed hourly, and appropriate replacement fluid is administered. The hemofilter is assessed every 2 to 4 hours for clotting (as evidenced by dark fibers or a rapid decrease in the amount of ultrafiltration without a change in the patient's hemodynamic status). If clotting is suspected, the system is flushed with 50 to 100 mL of normal saline and observed for dark streaks or clots.[12] If present, the system may have to be changed. Results of serum chemistries, clotting studies, and other tests are monitored. The CRRT system is frequently assessed to ensure filter and lines are visible at all times, kinks are prevented, and the blood tubing is warm to the touch. The ultrafiltrate is assessed for blood (pink-tinged to frank blood), which is indicative of membrane rupture. Sterile technique is performed during vascular access dressing changes.

Peritoneal dialysis. Peritoneal dialysis is the removal of solutes and fluid by diffusion through a patient's own semipermeable membrane (the peritoneal membrane) with a dialysate solution that has been instilled into the peritoneal cavity. The peritoneal membrane surrounds the abdominal cavity and lines the organs inside the abdominal cavity. This renal replacement therapy is not commonly used for the treatment of AKI because of its comparatively slow ability to alter biochemical imbalances.

Indications. Clinical indications for peritoneal dialysis include acute and chronic kidney injury, severe water intoxication, electrolyte disorders, and drug overdose. Advantages of peritoneal dialysis include easy and rapid assembly of the equipment, relatively inexpensive cost, minimal danger of acute electrolyte imbalances or hemorrhage, and easily individualized dialysate solutions. In addition, automated peritoneal dialysis systems are available. Disadvantages of peritoneal dialysis include that it is time intensive, requiring at least 36 hours for a therapeutic effect to be achieved; biochemical disturbances are corrected slowly; access to the peritoneal cavity is sometimes difficult; and the risk of peritonitis is high.

Complications. Although rare, many complications can result from peritoneal dialysis. Complications can be divided into three categories: mechanical problems, metabolic imbalances, and inflammatory reactions. Potential complications resulting from mechanical problems include perforation of the abdominal viscera during insertion of the catheter, poor drainage in or out of the abdominal cavity as a result of catheter blockage, patient discomfort from the pressure of the fluid within the peritoneal cavity, and pulmonary complications as a result of the pressure of the fluid in the peritoneal cavity. Metabolic imbalances include hypovolemia and hypernatremia from excessively rapid removal of fluid, hypervolemia from impaired drainage of fluid, hypokalemia from the use of potassium-free dialysate, alkalosis from the use of an alkaline dialysate, disequilibrium syndrome from excessively rapid removal of fluid and waste products, and

hyperglycemia from the high glucose concentration of the dialysate. Inflammatory reactions include peritoneal irritation produced by the catheter and peritonitis from bacterial infection.

Peritonitis is the most common complication of peritoneal dialysis therapy and is usually caused by contamination in the system. Aseptic technique must occur when handling the peritoneal catheter and connections. Peritonitis is manifested by abdominal pain, cloudy peritoneal fluid, fever and chills, nausea and vomiting, and difficulty in draining fluid from the peritoneal cavity.

OUTCOMES

With appropriate nursing and medical interventions, expected outcomes for the patient with AKI include:

- Fluid balance and hemodynamic status are stable.
- Body weight is within 2 lb of dry weight.
- Vital signs are stable and are consistent with baseline.
- Skin turgor is normal, and oral mucosa is intact and well hydrated.
- Serum laboratory values and arterial blood gas results are within normal limits.
- Infection is absent.
- Nutritional intake is adequate for the maintenance of the desired weight.
- The patient and family members are able to participate in the patient's care and are able to make informed decisions.

CASE STUDY

Mr. K.G. is a thin 60-year-old man admitted to the hospital for cardiac catheterization for recurrent angina. Past medical history includes hypertension, type 2 diabetes mellitus, and a previous myocardial infarction 2 years ago. Current medications are metformin (Glucophage), glipizide (Glucotrol), enteric-coated aspirin (Ecotrin), and lisinopril (Zestril). Laboratory tests on admission revealed the following: normal electrolyte levels; blood urea nitrogen (BUN), 40 mg/dL; and serum creatinine, 2.0 mg/dL. A complete blood cell count and urinalysis were unremarkable. Mr. K.G. receives intravenous fluids at 20 mL/hr on the morning of the procedure. He successfully undergoes the catheterization and returns to the telemetry unit. The day after the procedure, Mr. K.G.'s urine output decreases to less than 10 mL/hr. Mr. K.G. is given a fluid bolus of normal saline without any increase in urine output. Furosemide is administered intravenously, with a slight increase in urine output to 15 mL/hr for several hours. Laboratory studies reveal the

following: potassium, 5.9 mEq/L; BUN, 70 mg/dL; serum creatinine, 7.1 mg/dL, and carbon dioxide total content, 16 mEq/L. The next day Mr. K.G. has 2+ edema and basilar crackles, and he complains of feeling short of breath. A preliminary diagnosis of AKI is made.

Questions

1. What are possible factors predisposing Mr. K.G. for AKI?
2. What laboratory studies assist in the diagnosis of AKI? Describe expected results for a patient with acute tubular necrosis.
3. What medical interventions do you anticipate for Mr. K.G.?
4. What interventions could have been taken before Mr. K.G.'s cardiac catheterization to possibly prevent his AKI?
5. Discuss the advantages and disadvantages of using diuretic therapy in patients with AKI.

◼ SUMMARY

The patient with AKI poses many clinical challenges for healthcare personnel. Many of these patients have multisystem failure and require intensive and aggressive care. In addition, the development of AKI is an event that often

catches the patient and family unprepared. Nurses play a pivotal role in promoting positive patient outcomes through prevention, sharp assessment skills, and supportive nursing care.

CRITICAL THINKING EXERCISES

1. Identify two strategies that the critical care nurse can use to help prevent AKI.
2. Describe physical examination and laboratory findings that may be seen in patients with prerenal AKI.
3. Describe patients who are at high risk for contrast-induced nephropathy and discuss medical and nursing interventions that may be used to decrease their risk.

4. You are caring for a patient with AKI postoperatively. The cardiac monitor demonstrates tall, tented T waves and a PR interval of 0.26 seconds.
   a. What electrolyte imbalance do you suspect?
   b. What medical interventions do you anticipate?
   c. Describe the mechanism of action for each medical intervention.
5. What are common indications for initiating dialysis in patients with AKI?

REFERENCES

1. Astle S. Continuous renal replacement therapies. In Wiegand D, ed. *AACN Procedure Manual for Critical Care.* 6th ed. Philadelphia: Saunders. 2011:1018-1032.
2. Bellomo R, Ronco C, Kellum J, et al. Acute renal failure-definition, outcome measures, animal models, fluid therapy and information technology needs: the Second International Consensus Conference of the Acute Dialysis Quality Initiative (ADQI) Group, *Critical Care.* 2004;8(4):R204-R212.
3. Boswell W, Jadvar H, Palmer S. Diagnostic kidney imaging. In Brenner BM, Levine SA, eds. *Brenner and Rector's The Kidney.* 8th ed. Philadelphia, PA: Saunders. 2007;839-914.
4. Boyle M, Baldwin I. Understanding the continuous renal replacement therapy circuit for acute renal failure support. *AACN Advanced Critical Care.* 2010;21(4):367-375.
5. Choudhury D, Levi M. Aging and kidney disease. In Brenner BM, Levine SA, eds. *Brenner and Rector's The Kidney.* 8th ed. Philadelphia, PA: Saunders. 2007;681-701.
6. Chrysochoou G, Marcus R, Sureshkumar K, et al. Renal replacement therapy in the critical care unit. *Critical Care Nursing Quarterly.* 2008;31(4):282-290.
7. Chung K, Juncos L, Wolf S, et al. Continuous renal replacement therapy improves survival in severely burned military casualties with acute kidney injury. *The Journal of Trauma.* 2008;64(2): S179-S187.
8. Clarkson M, Friedlewald J, Eustace J, et al. Acute kidney injury. In Brenner BM, Levine SA, eds. *Brenner and Rector's The Kidney.* 8th ed. Philadelphia, PA: Saunders. 2007;943-986.
9. Curhan GC, Mitch WE. Diet and kidney disease. In Brenner BM, Levine SA, eds. *Brenner and Rector's The Kidney.* 8th ed. Philadelphia, PA: Saunders. 2007;1817-1847:2.
10. Dennen P, Douglas I, Anderson R. Acute kidney injury in the intensive care unit: an update and primer for the intensivist. *Critical Care Medicine.* 2010;38(1):261-275.
11. Dirkes S. Acute kidney injury: not just acute renal failure anymore? *Critical Care Nurse.* 2011;31(1):37-50.
12. Dirkes S, Hodge K. Continuous renal replacement therapy in the adult intensive care unit: history and current trends. *Critical Care Nurse.* February Supplement. 2008;8-27.
13. Ellis J, Cohan R. Prevention of contrast-induced nephropathy: an overview. *Radiologic Clinics North America.* 2009;47: 801-811.
14. Faybik P, Hetz H, Mitterer G, et al. Regional citrate anticoagulation in patients with liver failure supported by a molecular adsorbent recirculating system. *Critical Care Medicine.* 2011;39(2):273-279.
15. Goldberg S, Vijayan A. Renal replacement therapy. In Koleff M, Bedient T, Isakow W, et al, eds. *The Washington Manual of Critical Care.* Philadelphia: Lippincott, Williams & Wilkins. 2008;304-309.
16. Gong R, Dworkin L, Brenner B, et al. The renal circulation and glomerular ultrafiltration. In Brenner BM, Levine SA, eds. *Brenner and Rector's The Kidney.* 8th ed. 2007;91-129.
17. Hamm L, Nakhoul N. Renal acidification. In Brenner BM, Levine SA, eds. *Brenner and Rector's The Kidney.* 8th ed. Philadelphia, PA: Saunders. 2007;248-279.
18. Himmelfarb J, Joannidis M, Molitoris B, et al. Evaluation and initial management of acute kidney injury. *Clinical Journal of American Society of Nephrology.* 2008;3:962-967.
19. Hoste E, Schurgers M. Epidemiology of acute kidney injury: how big is the problem? *Critical Care Medicine.* 2008;36 (4 Suppl.):S146-S151.
20. Ishihara S, Ward J, Tasaki O, et al. Cardiac contractility during hemofiltration in an awake mode of hyperdynamic endotoxemia. *The Journal of Trauma.* 2009;67(5):1055-1061.
21. Katzberg R, Lamba R. Contrast-induced nephropathy: after intravenous administration: fact or fiction? *Radiologic Clinics of North America.* 2009;47:789-900.
22. U.S. Food and Drug Administration. *Kayexalate (Sodium Polystyrene Sulfonate) Powder [Safety –Medwatch Fact Sheet].* (January 2011). www.fda.gov/safety/medwatch/safetyinformation/ucm186845.htm; 2011 Accessed May 15, 2011.
23. Kellum J. Acute kidney injury. *Critical Care Medicine.* 2008;36(4 Suppl.):S141-S145.
24. Kellum J, Lamiere N, Aspelin P, et al. KDIGO Clinical practice guidelines for acute kidney injury. *Kidney International.* 2012;2(1 Suppl.):S1-138.
25. Klouche K, Amigues L, Deleuse S, et al. Preventive strategies of renal insufficiency in patients with diabetes undergoing intervention or arteriography (the PREVENT trial). *American Journal of Cardiology.* 2011;107(10):1447-1452.
26. Madsen K, Nielsen S, Tisher C. Anatomy of the kidney. In Brenner BM, Levine SA, eds. *Brenner and Rector's The Kidney.* 8th ed. Philadelphia, PA: Saunders. 2007;25-90.
27. Martin R. Acute kidney injury. *AACN Advanced Critical Care.* 2010;21(4):350-356.
28. Mehta R, Kellum J, Shah S, et al. Acute Kidney Injury Network: report of an initiative to improve outcomes in acute kidney injury. *Critical Care.* 2007;11(2):R31.

29. Miller A. Urinary function. In *Nursing for Wellness in Older Adults*. 5th ed. Urinary function. Philadelphia: Lippincott, Williams & Wilkins. 2009;390-416.

30. O'Grady N, Alexander M, Burns L, et al. Healthcare Infection Control Practices Advisory Committee. Guidelines for the prevention of intravascular catheter-related infections 2011. http://www.cdc.gov/hicpac/pdf/guidelines/bsi-guidelines-2011. pdf; 2011 Accessed March 3, 2012.

31. Ostermann M, Chang R. Acute kidney injury in the intensive care unit according to RIFLE. *Critical Care Medicine*. 2007;35(8):1837-1843.

32. Pannu N, Nadim M. An overview of drug-induced acute kidney injury. *Critical Care Medicine*. 2008;36(4 Suppl.): S216-S223.

33. Shingarev R, Allon M. A physiologic-based approach to treatment of acute hyperkalemia. *American Journal of Kidney Diseases*. 2010;56(3):578-584.

34. Solomon R. Contrast-induced acute kidney injury. *Radiologic Clinics of North America*. 2009;47:783-788.

35. Srisawat N, Hoste E, Kellum J. Modern classification of acute kidney injury. *Blood Purification*. 2010;29:300-307.

36. Tillman J. Heparin versus citrate for anticoagulation in critically ill patients treated with continuous renal replacement therapy. *Nursing in Critical Care*. 2009;14(4):191-197.

37. Uchino S, Bellomo R, Goldsmith D, et al. An assessment of the RIFLE criteria for acute renal failure in hospitalized patients. *Critical Care Medicine*. 2006;34(7):1913-1917.

38. Uchino S, Kellum J, Bellomo R, et al (2005). Acute renal failure in critically ill patients: a multinational, multicenter study. *Journal of the American Medical Association*. 2005;294(7): 813-818.

CHAPTER

16

Hematological and Immune Disorders

Patricia B. Wolff, MSN, RN, ACNS-BC, AOCNS
Jill T. Dickerson, MSN, RN, CNS-MS, FNP-BC, CWON
Marthe J. Moseley, PhD, RN, CCNS

⊖volve WEBSITE

Many additional resources, including self-assessment exercises, are located on the Evolve companion website at
http://evolve.elsevier.com/Sole.

- Review Questions
- Mosby's Nursing Skills Procedures

- Animations
- Video Clips

INTRODUCTION

Hematological and immunological functions are necessary for gas exchange, tissue perfusion, nutrition, acid-base balance, protection against infection, and hemostasis. These complex, integrated responses are easily disrupted. Because most critically ill patients experience some abnormalities in hematological and immune function, this chapter provides a general overview of the pertinent anatomy and physiology of these organ systems and the typical alterations in red blood cells (RBCs), immune activity, and coagulation function. Table 16-1 defines key terms used in this chapter in describing hematological and immunological disorders. Guidelines are also presented for assessment and nursing care strategies needed by novice critical care nurses caring for patients at risk for these disorders.

REVIEW OF ANATOMY AND PHYSIOLOGY

Hematopoiesis

Hematopoiesis is defined as the formation and maturation of blood cells. The primary site of hematopoietic cell production is the bone marrow; however, secondary hematopoietic organs that participate in this process include the spleen, liver, thymus, lymphatic system, and lymphoid tissues. Negative feedback mechanisms within the body induce the bone marrow's pluripotent hematopoietic stem cells to differentiate into one of the three blood cells (Figure 16-1): erythrocytes (RBCs), leukocytes (white blood cells [WBCs]), or thrombocytes (platelets).[10]

In infancy, most bones are filled with blood-forming red marrow; in adulthood, productive bone marrow is found in the vertebrae, skull, mandible, thoracic cage, shoulder, pelvis, femora, and humeri.[16] The hematopoietic and immunological organs and their key functions are summarized in Figure 16-2.

Effects of Aging

Aging affects several aspects of both hematological and immune systems. For example, elderly individuals have a greater risk of infection related to alterations in immunoglobulin levels. Changes in bone marrow reserve, immune function, lean body mass, hepatic function, and renal function contribute to the challenges of caring for this rapidly expanding, vulnerable population. These changes and implications are described in the Geriatric Considerations feature.

Components and Characteristics of Blood

Blood was recognized as being essential to life as early as the 1600s, but the specific composition and characteristics of blood were not defined until the twentieth century. Blood has four major components: (1) a fluid component called plasma, (2) circulating solutes such as ions, (3) serum proteins, and (4) cells. Plasma comprises about 55% of blood volume and is the transportation medium for important serum proteins such as albumin, globulin, fibrinogen, prothrombin, and plasminogen. The hematopoietic cells comprise the remaining 45% of blood volume. Characteristics of blood and potential alterations that may be encountered in critically ill patients are shown in Table 16-2.[16]

460

TABLE 16-1   HEMATOLOGY-IMMUNOLOGY KEY TERMS

TERM	DEFINITION
Active immunity	A term used when the body actively produces cells and mediators that result in the destruction of the antigen
Anemia	A reduction in the number of circulating red blood cells or hemoglobin that leads to inadequate oxygenation of tissues; subtypes named by etiology (e.g., aplastic anemia means "without cells") or by cell appearance (e.g., macrocytic anemia has large cells)
Antibody	Immune globulin, created by specific lymphocytes, and designed to immunologically destroy a specific foreign antigen
Anticoagulants	Factors inhibiting the clotting process
Antigen	Any substance that is capable of stimulating an immune response in the host
Autoimmunity	Situation in which the body abnormally sees self as nonself, and an immune response is activated against those tissues
Bone marrow transplant	Replacement of defective bone marrow with marrow that is functional; described in transplant terms of the source (e.g., autologous comes from self, and allogeneic comes from another person)
Cellular immunity	Production of cytokines in response to foreign antigen
Coagulation pathway	A predetermined cascade of coagulation proteins that are stimulated by production of the platelet plug, and occurs progressively, producing a fibrin clot; there are two pathways (intrinsic and extrinsic) triggered by different events that merge into a single list of events leading to a fibrin clot; clotting may be initiated by either or both pathways
Coagulopathy	Disorder of normal clotting mechanisms; usually used to describe inappropriate bleeding more often than excess clotting, but can refer to either one
Cytokines	Cell killer substances, or mediators secreted by white blood cells; when secreted by a lymphocyte, also called lymphokine, and secretions from monocytes are called monokines
Disseminated intravascular coagulation	Disorder of hemostasis characterized by exaggerated microvascular coagulation and intravascular depletion of clotting factors, with subsequent bleeding; also called consumption coagulopathy
Ecchymosis	Blue or purplish hemorrhagic spot on skin or mucous membrane; round or irregular, nonelevated
Epistaxis	Bleeding from the nose
Erythrocyte	Red blood cell
Fibrinolysis	Breakdown of fibrin clots that naturally occurs 1-3 days after clot development
Hemarthrosis	Blood in a joint cavity
Hematemesis	Bloody emesis
Hematochezia	Blood in stool; bright red
Hematoma	Raised, hardened mass indicative of blood vessel rupture and clotting beneath the skin surface; if subcutaneous, appears as a blue-purple or purple-black area; may occur in spaces such as pleural or retroperitoneal area
Hematopoiesis	Development of the early blood cells (erythrocytes, leukocytes, thrombocytes), encompassing their maturation in the bone marrow or lymphoreticular organs
Hematuria	Blood in the urine
Hemoglobinuria	Hemoglobin in the urine
Hemoptysis	Coughing up blood from the airways or lungs
Hemorrhage	Copious, active bleeding
Hemostasis	A physiological process involving hematological and nonhematological factors to form a platelet or fibrin clot to control the loss of blood
Human immunodeficiency virus	A retrovirus that transcribes its RNA-containing genetic material into DNA of the host cell nucleus; this virus has a propensity for the immune cells, replacing the RNA of lymphocytes and macrophages, causing an immunodeficient state
Humoral immunity	Production of antibodies in response to foreign proteins
Immunocompromised	Quantitative or qualitative defects in white blood cells or immune physiology; defect may be congenital or acquired and involve a single element or multiple processes; immune incompetence leads to lack of normal inflammatory, phagocytic, antibody, or cytokine responses

Continued

TABLE 16-1   HEMATOLOGY-IMMUNOLOGY KEY TERMS—cont'd

TERM	DEFINITION
Immunoglobulin	A specific type of antibody named by its molecular structure (e.g., immunoglobulin A or immunoglobulin against cytomegalovirus)
Leukocyte	General word encompassing white blood cells; made up of three major subtypes: granulocytes (neutrophils, basophils, eosinophils), lymphocytes, and monocytes
Lymphoreticular system	Cells and organs containing immunologically active cells
Macrophage	Differentiated monocyte that migrates to lymphoreticular tissues of the body
Melena	Blood pigments in stool; dark or black
Menorrhagia	Excessive bleeding during menstruation
Neutropenia	Serum neutrophil count lower than normal; predisposes patients to infection
Passive immunity	A situation in which antibodies against a specific disease are transferred from another person
Petechiae	Small, red or purple, nonelevated dots indicative of capillary rupture, often located in areas of increased pressure (e.g., feet or back), or on the chest and trunk
Primary immunodeficiency	Congenital disorders in which some part of the immune system fails to develop
Procoagulants	Factors enhancing clotting mechanisms
Purpura	Large, mottled bruises
Reticulocytes	Slightly immature erythrocytes able to continue some essential functions of red blood cells
Secondary or acquired immunodeficiency	Immune disorder resulting from factors outside the immune system and involving the loss of a previously functional immune defense
Thrombocyte	Platelet
Thrombocytopenia	Serum platelet count less than normal; predisposes individuals to bleeding as a result of inadequate platelet plugs
Thrombosis	Creation of clots; usually refers to excess clotting
Tissue anergy	Absence of a "wheal" tissue response to antigens and evidence of altered antibody capabilities
Tolerance	The body's ability to recognize self as self and therefore mount a rejection response against nonself, but not itself
Transfusion	Intravenous infusion of blood or blood products

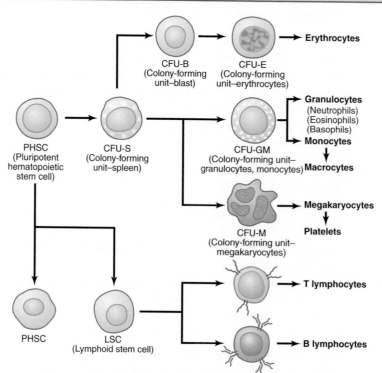

FIGURE 16-1 Formation of the multiple different blood cells from the original pluripotent hematopoietic stem cell (PHSC) in the bone marrow. (From Hall J. *Guyton and Hall Textbook of Medical Physiology*. 12th ed. Philadelphia: Saunders. 2011.)

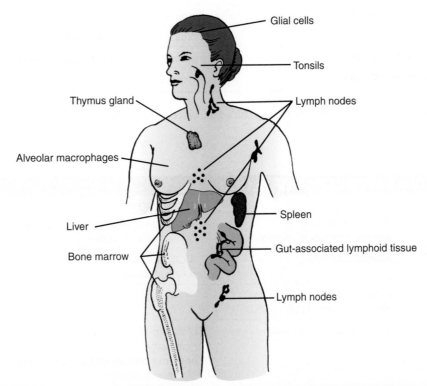

FIGURE 16-2 Hematopoietic organs and their function. (Modified from Black JM, Hawks JH, eds. *Medical-Surgical Nursing: Clinical Management for Positive Outcomes*. 8th ed. Philadelphia: Saunders. 2009.)

Organ	Key Functions
Bone marrow	Site of production for all hematopoietic cells.
Liver	The liver produces clotting factors, produces bile from RBC breakdown, and detoxifies many substances in the blood; its proper functioning is essential for normal hemostasis and metabolism. The liver filters and stores blood in addition to its many other metabolic functions.
Lymph nodes	Storage site for lymphocytes. Part of the continuous lymphatic system that filters foreign matter.
Spleen	The spleen is a highly vascular organ involved in the production of lymphocytes; the filtering and destruction of erythrocytes; the filtering and trapping of foreign matter, including bacteria and viruses; and the storage of blood. Although it is not necessary for survival, the spleen plays an important role in hemostasis and protection against infection.
Thymus gland	The thymus gland and lymph nodes are also part of the hematopoietic system; they are primarily involved in immunological functions.
Tonsils, glial cells, alveolar macrophages, gut-associated lymphoid tissue	Lymphoid tissue responsive to antigens passing the initial barrier defenses, and possessing some inflammatory properties.

GERIATRIC CONSIDERATIONS

AGE-RELATED CHANGES	IMPLICATIONS
Decreased percentage of marrow space occupied by hematopoietic tissue	Ineffective erythropoiesis, especially after blood loss
Decreased number of T cells produced	Delayed hypersensitivity
Decreased T-cell function	Increased incidence of infection
Appearance of autoimmune antibodies	Increased risk of autoimmune disorders
Increased IgA and decreased IgG levels	Increased prevalence of infection

IgA, Immunoglobulin A; *IgG,* immunoglobulin G.
From Thames D. Infection. In Meiner SE, *Gerontologic Nursing.* 4th ed. St. Louis: Mosby. 2011.

TABLE 16-2 CHARACTERISTICS OF BLOOD

CHARACTERISTIC	NORMAL	ALTERATIONS
Color	*Arterial:* bright red *Venous:* dark red or crimson	Hypochromic (light color) in anemia Lighter color in dilution
pH	*Arterial:* 7.35-7.45	<7.35: acidosis >7.45: alkalosis
Specific gravity	*Plasma:* 1.026 *Red blood cells:* 1.093	— —
Viscosity	3.5-4.5 times that of water	Loss of plasma volume or increased cell production increases viscosity Abnormal immunoglobulin such as multiple myeloma increases viscosity
Volume	*Plasma volume:* 45 mL/kg *Cell volume:* 30 mL/kg *Average male:* about 5000 mL	Fat tissue contains little water, so total blood volume best correlates to lean body mass Women have more fat, and therefore blood volume is usually lower than in men Plasma volume rises with progression of pregnancy Volume increases with immobility and decreases with prolonged standing; may be result of changes in pressure in glomerulus and glomerular filtration rate Blood volume highest in neonate and lowest in elderly Lack of nutrients causes decreased red blood cell and plasma formation Increased environmental temperature increases blood volume

Hematopoietic Cells

Erythrocytes

Erythrocytes (RBCs) are flexible biconcave disks without nuclei whose primary function is to be an oxygen-carrying molecule called hemoglobin. This physiological configuration permits RBCs to travel at high speeds and to navigate small blood vessels, exposing more surface area for gas exchange. In each microliter of blood, there are approximately 5 million RBCs.[16]

RBCs are generated from precursor stem cells under the influence of a growth factor called *erythropoietin. Erythropoietin* is secreted by the kidney in response to a perceived decrease in perfusion or tissue hypoxia. Maturation of RBCs takes 4 to 5 days, and their life span is about 120 days. *Reticulocytes* are immature RBCs that may be released when there is a demand for RBCs that exceeds the number of available mature cells. Reticulocytes are active but less effective than mature cells and circulate about 24 hours before maturing. The spleen and liver are important for removal and clearance of senescent RBCs.[4]

The RBC transports *hemoglobin,* whose function is the transport of oxygen and carbon dioxide. Hemoglobin binds with oxygen in the lungs and transports it to the tissues. The rate of erythrocyte production increases when oxygen transport to tissues is impaired, and it decreases when tissues are hypertransfused or exposed to high oxygen tension. The oxygen affinity for hemoglobin is modulated primarily by the concentration of 2,3-diphosphoglycerate (2,3-DPG) and depends on the blood pH and body temperature. Erythrocytes are also vital in the maintenance of acid-base balance because they transport carbon dioxide away from the tissues.[12]

Platelets

Platelets, or *thrombocytes,* are the smallest of the formed elements of the blood. A normal platelet count ranges from 150,000 to 400,000 per microliter of blood. Platelets are created by hematopoietic stem cells in response to hormonal stimulation. Platelets have a life span of 8 to 12 days, but they may be used more rapidly if there are many vascular injuries or clotting stimuli. Two thirds of the platelets circulate in the blood. The spleen stores the remaining third and may become enlarged if excess or rapid platelet removal occurs. In patients who have had a splenectomy, 100% of the platelets remain in circulation.[3,8]

Platelets are the first responders in the clotting response, and they form a platelet plug that temporarily repairs an injured vessel. Platelets also release mediators necessary for completion of clotting. Mediators include histamine and serotonin, which contribute to vasospasm; adenosine diphosphate, which assists platelet adhesion and aggregation; and calcium and phospholipids, which are necessary for clotting.[8,24] During circulation, platelets also adhere to roughened or sheared surfaces, such as blood vessel walls or indwelling catheters.

Leukocytes

Leukocytes (WBCs) are larger and less numerous than RBCs, and they have nuclei. The average number of WBCs ranges from 5000 to 10,000 per microliter of blood in the adult. Leukocytes are derived from hematopoietic stem cells that are stimulated by a triggering mechanism within the immunological response. Cells vary in appearance, function, storage site, and life span. Specific characteristics of cell development and life cycle are shown in Table 16-3.

Leukocytes are released into the bloodstream for transport to the tissues, where they perform specific functions.[11] WBCs play a key role in the defense against infectious organisms and foreign antigens. They produce and transport factors such as antibodies that are vital in maintaining immunity. Numbers of WBCs are increased in circumstances of inflammation, tissue injury, allergy, or invasion with pathogenic organisms. Their numbers are diminished in malnutrition, advancing age, and immune diseases.[26]

WBCs are classified according to their structure (granulocytes or agranulocytes), function (phagocytes or immunocytes), and affinity for certain dyes. The *granulocytes* (or *polymorphonuclear leukocytes*) include neutrophils, basophils, and eosinophils, and all function in phagocytosis.[6] The *agranulocytes* consist of *monocytes* (phagocytes) and *lymphocytes* (immunocytes).[9]

TABLE 16-3 OVERVIEW OF LEUKOCYTES

CELL TYPE	CHARACTERISTICS	DEVELOPMENT AND MIGRATION	LIFE SPAN
GRANULOCYTES			
Polymorphonuclear leukocytes (polys)	Large granules and horseshoe-shaped nuclei that differentiate and become multilobed	Mature in the bone marrow. Maturing granulocytes that are no longer dividing, accumulate as a reserve in the bone marrow. Normally about a 5-day supply in the bone marrow	Average of 12 hours in the circulation. About 2 to 3 days in the tissues
Neutrophils	Have small, fine, light pink or lilac acidophilic granules stained and a segmented, irregularly lobed, purple nucleus		4 days
Band neutrophils	Bands less well defined, because they are slightly immature forms of the same cell	Normally takes about 14 days for development	
Eosinophils	Have large, round granules that contain red-staining basic mucopolysaccharides and multilobed purple-blue nuclei		Unknown
Basophils	Coarse blue granules conceal the segmented nucleus. Granules contain histamine, heparin, and acid mucopolysaccharides		Unknown

Continued

TABLE 16-3	OVERVIEW OF LEUKOCYTES—cont'd		
CELL TYPE	CHARACTERISTICS	DEVELOPMENT AND MIGRATION	LIFE SPAN
	AGRANULOCYTES		
Lymphocytes	Small cells with a large, round, deep-staining, single-lobed nucleus and very little cytoplasm Cytoplasm slightly basophilic and stains pale blue	T lymphocytes constantly circulate, following a path from the blood to the lymphatic tissue, through the lymphatic channels, and back to the blood through the thoracic duct B lymphocytes largely noncirculating; remain mainly in the lymphoid tissue and may differentiate into plasma cells	Life span varies Small populations of memory lymphocytes survive for many years Most T lymphocytes of the peripheral lymphatic tissue recirculate about every 10 hours Mature plasma cells have a survival rate of about 2 to 3 days
Monocytes	Large cells with a prominent, multishaped nucleus that is sometimes kidney shaped Chromatin in the nucleus looks like lace, with small particles linked together like strands Blue-gray cytoplasm filled with many fine lysozymes that stain pink with Wright stain	Monocytes spend less time in the bone marrow pool than granulocytes	Circulation about 36 hours After the monocyte is transformed into macrophage in the tissues, life span ranges from months to years

Granular leukocytes

Neutrophils. Neutrophils are the most numerous of the granulocytes, constituting 54% to 62% of the WBC differential count.[9] The *differential count* measures the percentage of each type of WBC present in the venous blood sample. These cells are further broken down into segmented neutrophils, in which filaments in the cell give the nuclei an appearance of having lobes, and band neutrophils, which are immature and have a thicker or U-shaped nucleus. Normally, segmented neutrophils make up the majority of WBCs, whereas band neutrophils constitute only about 3% to 5%.[3] The phrase *a shift to the left* refers to an increased number of "bands," or band neutrophils, compared with mature neutrophils on a complete blood count (CBC) report. This finding generally indicates an acute bacterial infectious process that draws on the WBC reserves in the bone marrow and causes less mature forms to be released. Likewise, a *shift to the right* indicates an increased number of circulating mature cells and may be associated with liver disease, Down syndrome, and megaloblastic and pernicious anemia.[3]

The survival time of neutrophils is short. Once released from the bone marrow, they circulate in the blood less than 24 hours before migrating to the tissues, where they live another few days. When serious infection is present, neutrophils may live only hours as the neutrophils phagocytize infectious organisms.[9] Because of this short life span, drugs that affect rapidly multiplying cells (e.g., chemotherapeutic agents) quickly decrease the neutrophil count and alter the patient's ability to fight infection.

Eosinophils. Eosinophils are larger than neutrophils and make up 1% to 3% of the WBC count.[3,9] They are important in the defense against allergens and parasites, and are thought to be involved in the detoxification of foreign proteins. Eosinophils are found largely in the tissues of the skin, lung, and gastrointestinal tract. Eosinophils respond to chemotactic mechanisms triggering them to participate in phagocytosis, but they also contain bactericidal substances and lysosomal enzymes that aid in the destruction of invading organisms.[9]

Basophils. The third type of granulocyte is the basophil, which has large granules that contain heparin, serotonin, and histamine. Basophils participate in the body's inflammatory and allergic responses by releasing these substances. Basophils, which constitute up to 0.75% of the WBC differential, play an important role in acute systemic allergic reactions and inflammatory responses.[9]

Nongranular leukocytes (agranulocytes)

Monocytes. Monocytes are the largest of the leukocytes and constitute only 3% to 7% of the WBC differential.[3] Once they migrate from the bloodstream into the tissues, monocytes mature into tissue macrophages, which are powerful phagocytes. In the lung, these tissue macrophages are known as alveolar macrophages; in the liver, they are Kupffer cells; in connective tissue, they are histiocytes. In addition to *phagocytosis,* ("eating" large foreign particles and cell fragments), macrophages are vital in the phagocytosis of necrotic tissue and debris. Like eosinophils, macrophages contain lysosomal enzymes and bactericidal substances. When activated by antigens, macrophages secrete substances called monokines that act as chemical communicators between the cells involved in the immune response. Although monocytes may circulate for only 36 hours, they can survive for months or even years as tissue macrophages.[9]

Lymphocytes. In the adult, approximately 25% to 33% of the total WBCs are lymphocytes.[3] Lymphocytes circulate in and out of tissues and may live days or years, depending on their type. They contribute to the body's defense against microorganisms, but they are also essential for tumor immunity (surveillance for abnormal cells), delayed hypersensitivity reactions, autoimmune diseases, and foreign tissue rejection. Lymphocytes are responsible for specific immune responses and participate in two types of immunity: *humoral immunity,* which is mediated by B lymphocytes; and *cellular immunity,* which is mediated by T lymphocytes. B lymphocytes, or B cells, originate in the bone marrow and are also thought to mature there. B cells perform in antibody production. T cells are produced in the bone marrow, but they migrate to the thymus for maturation; then most travel and reside in lymphoid tissues throughout the body. They live longer than B cells and participate in long-term immunity. The natural killer cell is a third type of lymphocyte thought to be a differentiated form of the T lymphocyte. It is responsible for surveillance and destruction of virus-infected and malignant cells. T-cell functions include delayed hypersensitivity, graft rejection, graft-versus-host reaction, defense against intracellular organisms, and defense against neoplasms.[9]

Immune Anatomy

Immune activity involves an integrated, multilevel response against invading pathogens. It requires both WBCs of the hematopoietic system and the secondary hematopoietic organs, also termed the *lymphoreticular system.* The lymphoreticular system consists of lymphoid tissue, lymphatic channels and nodes, and phagocytic cells, which engulf and process foreign materials (see Figure 16-2).

The body's ability to resist and fight infection is termed *immunity.* Our bodies are constantly exposed to normal and unusual microorganisms that are capable of causing disease. The healthy person's immune system recognizes potential pathogens and destroys them before tissue invasion can occur; however, the person with a dysfunctional immune system is at risk of overwhelming, life-threatening infection.

Immune Physiology

The immune response protects the body from disease by recognizing, processing, and destroying foreign invaders. It aids in the removal of damaged cells and defends the body against the proliferation of abnormal or malignant cells.

The recognition and destruction of nonself molecules called *antigens* are the key triggering activities of the immune system. Microorganisms (e.g., bacteria, viruses, fungi, and parasites), abnormal or mutated cells, transplanted cells, nonself protein molecules (e.g., vaccines), and nonhuman molecules (e.g., penicillin) can act as antigens. These antigens are detected by the body as foreign, or nonself, and are destroyed by immunological processes. The body's response to an antigen is determined by factors such as genetics, amount of antigen, and route of exposure. In autoimmunity, the body abnormally sees self as nonself and an immune response is activated against those tissues. Autoimmunity can result from injury to tissues, infection, or malignancy, although in many cases the cause is not known. An example of an autoimmune disease is systemic lupus erythematosus.[15]

An intact and healthy immune system consists of both natural (nonspecific) defenses and acquired (specific) defenses. The nonspecific defenses are the first line of protection and include the processes of inflammation and phagocytosis. When nonspecific mechanisms fail to protect the body from invasion, the specific defenses of humoral and cellular immunity are put into action. *Active immunity* is a term used when the body actively produces cells and mediators that result in the destruction of the antigen. *Passive immunity* is that which is transferred from another person (e.g., maternal antibodies transferred to the newborn through the placenta).[22]

Nonspecific Defenses

The body's nonspecific defenses consist of the physical and chemical barriers to invasion, the protective and repairing processes of inflammation and phagocytosis, and other substances that stimulate the body to fight back. The body's first line of defense against infection consists of physical and chemical barriers.

Epithelial surfaces. The epithelial surfaces are those that are exposed to the environment. Intact skin and mucous membranes provide a protective covering; they also secrete substances that have antimicrobial effects. For example, sweat glands produce a lysozyme, an antimicrobial enzyme; and sebaceous glands secrete sebum, which has antimicrobial and antifungal properties. The skin constantly exfoliates, a process that sloughs off bacterial and chemical hazards. These same epithelial surfaces are colonized by "normal" bacterial flora that protect the body from microorganisms by occupying space on the epithelium, preventing pathogen attachment.

Epithelial surfaces also have unique physical and chemical properties protecting them from pathogen invasion. For example, mucus and cilia work together to trap and remove harmful substances in the respiratory tract. The motility of the intestines maintains an even distribution of bacterial flora, thereby preventing overgrowth or invasion of pathogens, and promotes evacuation of harmful microbes. Chemical barriers to pathogenic entry include the unique pH of the skin and mucosa of the gastrointestinal and urinary tracts. This pH inhibits the growth of many microorganisms. Immunoglobulin A (IgA, also called *secretory IgA*) and phagocytic cells are biological factors present in respiratory and gastrointestinal secretions. They are essential for destruction of particular pyogenic bacteria.[9,19]

Inflammation and phagocytosis. The second line of defense involves the processes of inflammation and phagocytosis. Inflammation is initiated by cellular injury, is necessary for tissue repair, and is harmful when uncontrolled. When cellular injury occurs, a process called *chemotaxis* generates both a mediator and a neutrophil response. Mediator substances (histamine, serotonin, kinins, lysosomal enzymes, prostaglandin, platelet-activating factor, clotting factors, and complement proteins) are released at the site of injury. These mediators cause vasodilation, increase blood flow, induce capillary permeability, and promote chemotaxis and phagocytosis by neutrophils. Inflammatory symptoms such as redness, heat, pain, and swelling are sequelae of these responses. *Complement* proteins enhance the antibody activity, phagocytosis, and inflammation.[9,19]

Neutrophils are attracted to and migrate to areas of inflammation or bacterial invasion, where they ingest and kill invading microorganisms by phagocytosis. The inflammatory response is a rapid process initiated by granulocytes and macrophages, with granulocytes arriving within minutes of cellular injury. Once phagocytes have been attracted to an area by the release of mediators, a process called *opsonization* occurs, in which antibody and complement proteins attach to the target cell and enhance the phagocyte's ability to engulf the target cell. Once the bacteria have been engulfed, they are killed and digested within the cell by lysosomal enzymes. Exudate formation at the inflammatory site has three functions: dilute the toxins produced, deliver proteins and leukocytes to the site, and carry away toxins and debris.[9]

When infectious organisms escape the local phagocytic responses, they may be engulfed and destroyed in a similar fashion by the tissue macrophages within the lymphoreticular organs. The portal circulation of the spleen and liver filters the majority of blood, where infectious organisms can be removed before infecting the tissues. In the lymphatic system, pathogenic substances are filtered by the lymph nodes and are phagocytized by tissue macrophages. Here they may also stimulate immune responses by the lymphoid cells.

Other nonspecific defenses. Another nonspecific defensive activity is the release of cytokines and chemokines from WBCs, and are either proinflammatory, antinflammatory, or both. These naturally occurring biological response modifiers, which include interleukins (ILs), tumor necrosis factor, colony-stimulating factors, monoclonal antibodies, and interferons (IFNs), mediate various interactions between immune system cells.[19] At least 30 human ILs have been identified. An example of an interleukin is IL-1. IL-1 is a proinflammatory cytokine that increases body temperature in infection (endogenous pyrogen), thereby inhibiting the growth of temperature-sensitive pathogens. IL-1 also activates phagocytes and lymphocytes, and acts as a growth factor for many cells. The IFNs have antitumor and antiviral activity and include 20 subtypes of IFN-alpha, 2 subtypes of IFN-beta, and IFN-gamma. Through recombinant DNA technology, IFNs and other naturally occurring substances can be produced synthetically for the treatment of many disorders. IFNs, colony-stimulating factors, and monoclonal antibodies are some examples of biological therapies currently approved for the treatment of certain malignant disorders.[1]

Specific Defenses
Specificity refers to the finding that an immune response stimulates cells to develop immunity for a specific antigen. Two types of specific immune responses exist: humoral immunity and cell-mediated immunity. They are not mutually exclusive but act together to provide immunity.

Humoral immunity. Humoral immunity is mediated by B lymphocytes and involves the formation of antibodies (immunoglobulins) in response to specific antigens that bind to their receptor sites. Antigen binding activates B-lymphocyte differentiation into plasma cells that produce specific antibodies in response to those antigens. Five classes of immunoglobulins exist: IgG, IgM, IgA, IgE, and IgD. The clinical features and abnormalities associated with these immunoglobulins are described in Table 16-4.[19]

Once antibodies have been synthesized and released, they bind to their specific antigen and form an antigen-antibody complex that activates phagocytosis and complement proteins. This humoral response is regulated by the activity of T lymphocytes. Helper T cells promote B-lymphocyte activity and the production of antibodies, whereas suppressor T cells downgrade the humoral response.

The body generates both primary and secondary humoral responses. In the *primary response,* antigens that have evaded the nonspecific defenses are engulfed and processed by macrophages. The macrophages then present the processed antigens to the lymphocytes, which proliferate, differentiate, and produce antibodies. In this first exposure, antibodies of the IgM subtype appear first and predominate, whereas IgG immunoglobulins appear later. During this primary response, the immunoglobulins develop an immunological memory for antigens. When any subsequent exposure to the antigen occurs, a quicker, stronger, and longer-lasting IgG-mediated *secondary response* occurs. IgG antibodies predominate and may be detectable in the serum for decades.[19]

Cell-mediated immunity. Cellular immunity is mediated by the T lymphocyte. Cell-mediated immunity is a more delayed reaction than the humoral response and can occur only when in direct contact with sensitized lymphocytes. It is important in viral, fungal, and intracellular infections and is the mechanism involved in transplant rejection and recognition of neoplastic cells.

Cell-mediated immunity is initiated by macrophage recognition of nonself foreign materials. The macrophages trap, process, and present such materials to T lymphocytes, which then migrate to the site of the antigen, where they complete antigen destruction. Once contact is made with a specific antigen, the T lymphocyte differentiates into helper/inducer T cells, suppressor T cells, and cytotoxic killer cells. Although these T cells are microscopically identical, they can be distinguished by proteins present on the cell surface called clusters of differentiation (CDs). Helper T cells (also known as T4 cells because they carry a CD4 marker) enhance the

TABLE 16-4   IMMUNOGLOBULINS

ANTIBODY	DESCRIPTION	NORMAL VALUE
IgG	Most abundant immunoglobulin Major influence with bacterial disease Crosses the placenta Coats microorganisms to enhance phagocytosis Activates complement	75% of total 500-1600 mg/dL
IgM	Primary Ig response to antigen, with levels increased within 7 days of exposure Present mostly in intravascular space Causes antigenic agglutination and cell lysis via complement activation	10% of total 60-280 mg/dL
IgA	Found on mucosal surfaces of respiratory, GI, and GU systems preventing antigen adherence Influential with bacteria and some viral organisms First antibody formed with exposure to antigen but rapidly diminishes as IgG increases Does not cross the placenta, but passes to newborn through colostrum and breast milk Deficiency caused by congenital autosomal dominant or recessive disease or related to anticonvulsant use Deficiency (<5 mg/dL) manifests as chronic sinopulmonary infection	15% of total 90-450 mg/dL
IgD	Activates B lymphocytes to plasma cells, which are the key immunoglobulin-producing cells	1% of total 0.5-3.0 mg/dL
IgE	Attaches to mast cells and basophils on epithelial surfaces and enhances release of histamine and other vasoactive mediators responsible for the "wheal flare" reaction Important for allergic responses, inflammatory reactions, and parasitic infections	0.002% of total 0.01-0.04 mg/dL

GI, Gastrointestinal; *GU,* genitourinary; *Ig,* immunoglobulin.

humoral immune response by stimulating B cells to differentiate and produce antibodies.[11] Suppressor T cells downgrade and suppress the humoral and cell-mediated responses. The ratio of helper to suppressor T cells is normally 2:1, and an alteration in this ratio may cause disease.[3] For example, a depressed ratio (a decrease of helper T cells in relation to suppressor T cells) is found in acquired immunodeficiency syndrome (AIDS), whereas a higher ratio (a decrease in suppressor T cells in relation to helper T cells) is a feature of an autoimmune disease. Cytotoxic or killer T cells (CD8 marker) participate directly in the destruction of antigens by binding to and altering the intracellular environment, which ultimately destroys the cell. Killer cells also release cytotoxic substances into the antigen cell that cause cell lysis. Killer T cells additionally provide the body with immunosurveillance capabilities that monitor for abnormal cells or tissue. This mechanism is responsible for the rejection of transplanted tissue and the destruction of single malignant cells.[25]

Hemostasis

Hemostasis is a physiological process involving platelets, blood proteins (clotting factors), and the vasculature. This process involves the formation of blood clots to stop bleeding from injured vessels, and natural anticoagulant and fibrinolytic systems to limit clot formation. Many substances are released during tissue destruction, including collagen, proteases, and bacterial endotoxins, that may activate the clotting system. The three physiological mechanisms known to trigger clotting in the body are tissue injury, vessel injury, and the

presence of a foreign body in the bloodstream. When one of these trigger factors is present, a series of physical events occurs that results in a fibrin clot.

Although the events of hemostasis are sequential, they require integration of components from the hematopoietic and coagulation systems. Within seconds after injury, platelets are attracted and adhere to the site of injury. The activated platelets then undergo changes in shape to expose receptors on their surfaces. RBCs increase the rate of platelet adherence by facilitating migration of platelets to the site and by liberating adenosine diphosphate, which enables platelets to stick to the exposed tissue (collagen). The exposed receptors on the activated platelet surfaces are capable of binding fibrinogen, an essential component underlying platelet aggregation. Serotonin and histamine are released by the adhered platelets and cause immediate constriction of the injured vessel to lessen bleeding. Vasoconstriction is followed by vasodilation, bringing the necessary cellular products of the inflammatory response to the site. With minor vessel injury, *primary hemostasis* is temporarily achieved with platelet plugs, usually within seconds. During *secondary hemostasis,* the platelet plug is solidified with fibrin, an end product of the coagulation pathway, and requires several minutes to reach completion (Figure 16-3).[18,21]

Coagulation Pathway

The classic theory of coagulation is viewed as occurring through two distinct pathways, *intrinsic* and *extrinsic,* which share a common "final" pathway, formation of insoluble

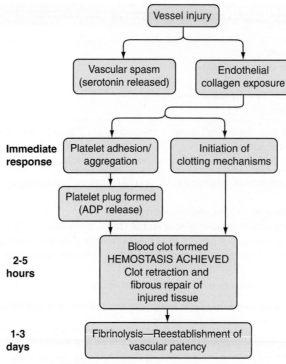

FIGURE 16-3 Coagulation physiology.

fibrin (Figure 16-4). It is now known that the classic cascade theory of coagulation illustrates what occurs in vitro. In vivo, the primary activator of the coagulation cascade occurs via the extrinsic pathway. The intrinsic pathway serves to amplify the coagulation cascade.[17,18,21]

Both pathways begin with an initiating event and have a cascade sequence of clotting factor activation precipitated by a preceding reaction. The soluble clotting factors become insoluble fibrin. When blood is exposed to subendothelial collagen or is "injured," factor XII is activated, which initiates coagulation via the *intrinsic pathway*. In the *extrinsic pathway*, tissue injury precipitates release of a substance known as tissue factor, which activates factor VII. Factor VII is key in initiating blood coagulation, and the two pathways intersect at the activation of factor X.[18,21] Both coagulation pathways illustrate a *final common pathway* of clot formation, retraction, and fibrinolysis.

The coagulation factors are plasma proteins that circulate as inactive enzymes, and most are synthesized in the liver. Vitamin K is necessary for synthesis of factors II, VII, IX, and X, and protein C and protein S (anticoagulation factors). Thus liver disease and vitamin K deficiency are commonly associated with impaired hemostasis.[4,8]

Coagulation Antagonists and Clot Lysis

Activation of the clotting factors, inhibition of these activated clotting factors, and production of circulating anticoagulant proteins maintain the balance of the coagulation processes. Normal vascular endothelium is smooth and intact, thereby preventing the collagen exposure that initiates the intrinsic

clotting pathway. Rapid blood flow dilutes and disperses clotting factors. Clotting factors that are not contained within a formed clot are filtered and removed from circulation by the liver. Several plasma proteins, including antiplasmin and antithrombin III, are present to localize clotting at the site of injury. When coagulation protein levels are deficient, clotting may become inappropriately widespread, such as in disseminated intravascular coagulation (DIC). The most potent anticoagulant forces are the fibrin threads, which absorb 85% to 90% of thrombin during clot formation, and antithrombin III, which inactivates thrombin that is not contained within the clot. Heparin, which is produced in small quantities by basophils and tissue mast cells, acts as a potent anticoagulant. Heparin combines with antithrombin III to increase the effectiveness of the latter greatly. This complex removes several of the activated coagulation factors from the blood.[8]

Once blood vessel integrity has been restored via hemostasis, blood flow must be reestablished. This goal is accomplished by the fibrinolytic system, by which clots are broken down (lysed) and removed. *Fibrinolysis* occurs 1 to 3 days after clot formation and is mediated by plasmin, an enzyme that digests fibrinogen and fibrin (Figure 16-5). The plasma protein plasminogen is the inactive form of plasmin. It is incorporated into the blood clot as the clot forms, and it cannot initiate clot lysis until it is activated. Substances capable of activating plasminogen include tissue plasminogen activator, thrombin, fibrin, factor XII, lysosomal enzymes, and urokinase.[8] Thrombin and plasmin are key for the balance between coagulation and lysis. Fibrinolysis is active within the microcirculation, where it maintains the

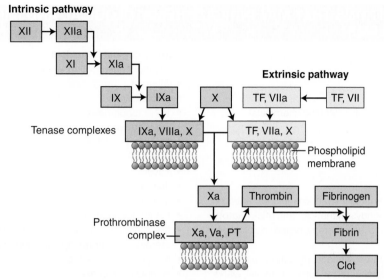

Intrinsic pathway

Extrinsic pathway

Tenase complexes

Phospholipid
membrane

Prothrombinase
complex

FIGURE 16-4 Coagulation cascade. (From McCance KL. Structure and function of the hemato-logical system. In McCance KL, Huether SE, eds. *Pathophysiology: The Biologic Basis for Disease in Adults and Children.* 6th ed. St. Louis: Mosby. 2010.)

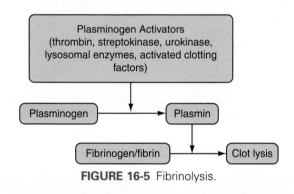

FIGURE 16-5 Fibrinolysis.

patency of the capillary beds. Larger vessels contain less plasminogen activator, a characteristic that may predispose them to clot formation.

When plasmin digests fibrinogen, fragments known as *fibrin split products,* or *fibrin degradation products,* are produced and function as potent anticoagulants. In cases of excessive clotting and clot lysis, these fibrin split products contribute to the coagulopathy. Fibrin split products are not normally present in the circulation but are seen in some hematological disorders as well as with thrombolytic therapy.

NURSING ASSESSMENT OF HEMATOLOGICAL AND IMMUNOLOGICAL FUNCTION

An understanding of both normal and disrupted hematological and immunological system activities is paramount to good assessment skills and use of therapeutic interventions. Nursing assessment involves evaluation of risk factors for hematological and immunological alterations, assessment of

the patient's complaints, performance of a focused physical examination, and interpretation of pertinent laboratory tests.

Past Medical History

A complete health history includes an assessment of prior medical and surgical problems, allergies, medication or homeopathic remedy use, and family history. Conditions that may indicate hematological or immunological disorders are noted in Box 16-1.

Evaluation of Patient Complaints and Physical Examination

The nurse inspects the patient's general appearance and assesses for signs of fatigue, acute illness, or chronic disease. The most common manifestations of either hematological or immunological disease include indicators of altered oxygenation, bleeding or clotting tendencies, and infection or accentuated immunological activity. The most important assessment parameters for detection of anemia, bleeding, and infection are shown in Table 16-5. Transplantation may be indicated for a variety of hematological or immunological disorders (Box 16-2).

Diagnostic Tests

Hematological or immunological abnormalities can usually be diagnosed by using the patient's clinical profile in conjunction with a few key laboratory tests. The most invasive microscopic examinations of the bone marrow or lymph nodes are reserved for circumstances when laboratory tests are inconclusive or when an abnormality in cellular maturation is suspected (e.g., aplastic anemia, leukemia, or lymphoma).

The first screening diagnostic tests performed to detect hematological or immunological dysfunction are a complete blood count (CBC) with differential and a coagulation

BOX 16-1 CONDITIONS THAT MAY INDICATE HEMATOLOGICAL AND IMMUNOLOGICAL PROBLEMS*

Hematological Disorders

- Alcohol consumption, excess
- Allergies
- Anemia of any kind
- Benzene exposure (gasoline, dry cleaning chemicals)
- Blood clots
- Delayed wound healing
- Excess bleeding
- Jaundice
- Liver disease
- Medications: allopurinol, antibiotics, anticoagulants, anticonvulsants, antidiabetics, antidysrhythmics, antiinflammatory agents, aspirin derivatives, chemotherapy, histamine blockers
- Neoplastic disease
- Pertinent surgical procedures: hepatic resection, partial or total gastric resection, splenectomy, tumor removal, valve replacement
- Pesticide exposure
- Previous transfusion of blood or blood products
- Poor nutrition
- Radiation: occupational, environmental
- Recurrent infection
- Renal disease
- Substance abuse

Immunological Disorders

- Alcohol consumption, excess
- Allergies
- Anorexia
- Bone tenderness
- Delayed wound healing
- Diabetes mellitus
- Diarrhea
- Fever
- Joint pain
- Liver disease
- Lymphadenopathy
- Medications: antibiotics, antiinflammatory agents, corticosteroids, chemotherapy, immunosuppressives
- Nausea and vomiting
- Neoplastic disease
- Night sweats
- Pertinent surgeries: hepatic resection, lung resection, small bowel resection, splenectomy, tumor removal
- Pesticide exposure
- Poor nutrition
- Previous transfusion of blood or blood products
- Radiation: occupational, environmental
- Recurrent infections
- Renal disease
- Sexual practices
- Substance abuse
- Weight loss

*This chart does not correlate specific risks with particular disease conditions, because many overlap. History information should be supplemented with physical examination and laboratory test information.

TABLE 16-5 PHYSICAL ASSESSMENT FOR HEMATOLOGICAL AND IMMUNE DISORDERS

BODY SYSTEM	ANEMIA	BLEEDING	INFECTION*
Neurological	Difficulty concentrating Dizziness Fatigue Somnolence Vertigo	*Bleeding into brain (cerebrum, cerebellum)*: alteration in level of consciousness, focal deficits such as unequal pupils or motor movement, headache *Bleeding into potential spaces*	*Encephalitis:* confusion, lethargy, difficulty arousing, headache, visual difficulty/photosensitivity, nausea, hypertension *Meningitis:* lethargy and somnolence, confusion, nuchal rigidity
Head/neck	Headache Tinnitus	*Bleeding into eye:* visual disturbances, frank hemorrhagic conjunctiva, bloody tears *Bleeding into nasopharyngeal area:* nasal stuffiness, epistaxis *Oral bleeding:* petechiae of buccal mucosa or gums, hemorrhagic oral lesions *Bleeding into subcutaneous tissue of head or neck:* enlarged, bruised areas, raccoon's eyes, bruising	*Conjunctivitis:* reddened conjunctiva, excess tearing of eye, puslike exudates from eye, blurred vision, swelling of eyelid, eye itching *Otitis media:* earache, difficulty hearing, itching inner ear, ear drainage *Sinusitis:* discolored nasal mucus, nasal congestion, face pain, eye pain, blurred vision *Oropharyngeal:* oral ulcerations or plaques, halitosis, reddened gums, abnormal papillae of the tongue, sore throat, difficulty swallowing *Lymphadenitis:* swollen neck lymph glands, tender lymph glands, a lump left when patient swallows

TABLE 16-5   PHYSICAL ASSESSMENT FOR HEMATOLOGICAL AND IMMUNE DISORDERS—cont'd

BODY SYSTEM	ANEMIA	BLEEDING	INFECTION*
Pulmonary	Air hunger Anxiety Dyspnea Tachypnea	*Alveolar bleeding:* crackles on breath sound assessment, alveolar fluid on x-ray, low oxygen saturation *Upper airway bleeding (e.g., trachea or bronchi):* hemoptysis *Pleural space bleeding:* decreased breath sounds, unequal chest excursion	*Bronchitis:* persistent cough, sputum production, gurgles in upper airways, wheezes in upper airways, hypoxemia and/or hypercapnia *Pneumonia:* chest discomfort pronounced with inspiration, persistent cough, sputum production, diminished breath sounds, crackles or gurgles, asymmetrical chest wall movement, labored breathing, nasal flaring with breathing, hypoxemia *Pleurisy:* chest discomfort pronounced with inspiration, sides of chest more painful, usually unilateral discomfort, splinting with deep breaths
Cardiovascular	Clubbing of digits Heart murmur Hypotension Nail beds pale and slow capillary refill Peripheral pulses weak and thread Tachycardia	*Pericardial bleeding:* dyspnea, chest discomfort, hypotension, narrow pulse pressure, muffled heart sounds, increased jugular venous distention *Vascular bleeding:* visible blood, hematoma, or bruising of subcutaneous tissue	*Myocarditis:* dysrhythmias, murmurs or gallops, elevated jugular venous pulsations, weak thready pulses, hypotension, point of maximal impulse shifted laterally *Pericarditis:* constant aching discomfort in the chest unrelieved by rest or nitrates; pericardial rub; muffled heart sounds
Gastrointestinal	Abdominal pain Constipation Splenic enlargement, tenderness	*Upper GI bleeding:* hematemesis, vomiting (coffee ground appearance) *Lower GI bleeding:* melena *Hepatic or splenic rupture:* acute abdominal pain; abdominal distention, rapid onset hypotension with ↓ hematocrit and hemoglobin *Hemorrhagic pancreatitis:* acute abdominal pain, abdominal distention, hypotension with ↓ hematocrit and hemoglobin	*Gastritis:* nausea, vomiting within 30 minutes of eating, heme-positive emesis, gastric pain that is initially improved by eating *Infectious diarrhea:* greater than six loose stools per day, clay-colored or foul-smelling stools, abdominal cramping or distention *Cholelithiasis/pancreatitis:* epigastric pain, intolerance to high-fat meal, clay-colored stools, nausea and vomiting, hyperglycemia, hypocalcemia, ↓ albumin, ↑ lipase and amylase *Hepatitis:* jaundice, right upper quadrant discomfort, hepatomegaly, elevated transaminases and bilirubin, fatty food intolerances, nausea and vomiting, diarrhea
Genitourinary		Bladder spasms with distended bladder Hematuria	*Urethritis:* painful urination, difficulty urinating, genitourinary itching *Cystitis:* small frequent urination, feeling of bladder fullness *Nephritis:* flank discomfort, oliguria, protein in urine *Vaginitis:* itching or vaginal discharge
Musculoskeletal	Muscle fatigue Muscle weakness	Altered joint mobility Painful or swollen joints Warm, painful, swollen muscles	*Arthritis:* joint discomfort, swollen and warm joints *Myositis:* aching muscles, weakness
Dermatological	Cyanosis Jaundice (hemolytic anemia) Pallor Poor skin turgor Skin cool to touch	Bleeding from line insertion sites, puncture wounds, skin tears Ecchymoses Petechiae	*Superficial skin infection:* rashes, itching, raised and/or discolored skin lesions, open-draining skin lesions *Cellulitis:* redness, warmth and swelling of subcutaneous tissue area, radiating pain from area toward middle of body
Hematological/ immunological			*Bacteremia:* Positive blood culture

*Signs and symptoms presented in this chart are unique features of each process and do not include the common constitutional signs and symptoms seen with all infections such as fever, chills, malaise, leukocytosis, positive tissue culture for microorganisms, or increased erythrocyte sedimentation rate.

GI, Gastrointestinal.

BOX 16-2 HEMATOPOIETIC STEM CELL TRANSPLANTATION

Indications

A hematopoietic stem cell transplant (HSCT) may be considered treatment for a variety of hematological or immunological diseases in which the stem cells do not function properly: abnormal RBC production (sickle cell disease), hematological malignancies (leukemia, lymphoma, myeloma, myelodysplastic syndrome), lack of normal blood cell production (aplastic anemia), and immune system disorders (severe combined immunodeficiency syndrome). Transplant of stem cells may help to correct the underlying physiological problem. HSCT is classified by the source of the donor stem cells, which include: bone marrow transplantation (BMT), peripheral blood stem cell transplantation (PBSCT), or umbilical cord blood.

Categories

Allogeneic transplant: patient receives stem cells from a sibling, parent, or unrelated donor (not immunologically identical)

Autologous transplant: patient receives his/her own stem cells after treatment with chemotherapy or radiation

Syngeneic transplant: patient receives stem cells from his/her identical twin (immunologically identical match)

Mini-transplant: lower doses of chemotherapy or radiation are administered in preparation for transplant

Tandem transplant: high dose chemotherapy and transplant given in two sequential courses

Tissue Typing

Proteins on the surface of leukocytes, called human leukocyte antigens (HLAs), are present on both donor and recipient cells. HLA-matching between donor and recipient is critically important for determining an appropriate donor. If the donor's cells are not an adequate match, they will recognize the patient's organs and tissues as foreign, and destroy them—known as graft-versus-host disease (GVHD). Additionally, the patient's immune system may recognize the donor stem cells as foreign

and destroy them—known as graft rejection. The higher the number of matching HLA antigens, the greater the chance the transplant will be successful.

Complications

Patients receiving HSCT are susceptible to severe infections, due to their profoundly immunocompromised state resulting from disease; bone marrow ablation in preparation for transplant, and use of the immunosuppressive therapy posttransplant to prevent GVHD and graft rejection. Engraftment occurs after the transplant when stem cells repopulate the bone marrow and are able to reconstitute the immune system. Complications may occur at any time during the HSCT continuum: preengraftment to day 30 posttransplant; early after engraftment, usually from day 30 to 100; and late after transplantation, more than 100 days posttransplant of donor stem cells.

Complications may include bacterial, fungal, protozoal, or viral infections; bleeding; sepsis; GVHD (acute or chronic); hepatic veno-occlusive disease (weight gain, painful hepatomegaly, and jaundice); and respiratory complications. Short-term side effects include nausea, vomiting, fatigue, anorexia, mucositis, alopecia, and skin reactions. Potential long-term risks related to the pretransplant chemotherapy and radiation include: infertility, cataracts, new cancers, and damage to major organs.

References

1. Antin JH, Raley DY. *Manual of Stem Cell & Bone Marrow Transplantation.* Cambridge, UK: Cambridge University Press. 2009.
2. National Cancer Institute, National Institutes of Health. *Bone Marrow Transplantation and Peripheral Blood Stem Cell Transplantation: Questions and Answers.* http://www.cancer.gov/cancertopics/factsheet/Therapy/bone-marrow-transplant; Accessed December 21, 2011.
3. Soiffer RJ. *Hematopoietic Stem Cell Transplantation.* Totowa, NJ: Springer Science & Business Media. 2009.

profile. The CBC evaluates the cellular components of blood.[3,6] The CBC reports the total RBC count and RBC indices, hematocrit, hemoglobin, WBC count and differential, platelet count, and cell morphologies. A summary of common hematological diagnostic laboratory tests with their normal values, and general implications of abnormal findings, is shown in Table 16-6 (RBCs and WBCs) and Table 16-7 (coagulation).

SELECTED ERYTHROCYTE DISORDERS

Many pathological conditions affect the erythrocytes, ranging from mild anemias to life-threatening RBC lysis. A decrease in functional RBCs with a resulting oxygenation deficit is termed *anemia* and is a common problem in critically ill patients. *Polycythemia*, a disorder in which the number of circulating RBCs is increased, is seen less often but can affect

hypoxic patients (e.g., chronic obstructive pulmonary disease). It leads to increased blood viscosity and thrombotic complications.

Anemia
Pathophysiology

The term *anemia* refers to a reduction in the number of circulating RBCs or hemoglobin, which leads to inadequate oxygenation of tissues. Although symptoms vary depending on the type, cause, or severity of anemia, the basic clinical findings are the same. As oxygenation delivery is decreased, tissues become hypoxic and 2,3-DPG increases causing hemoglobin to release oxygen. Blood flow is redistributed to areas where oxygenation is most vital, such as the brain, heart, and lungs. Anemia is described as mild, moderate, or severe, based on symptoms, irrespective of actual RBC serum values. Patients are able to adjust and compensate to

TABLE 16-6 FUNCTIONS AND NORMAL VALUES OF BLOOD CELLS

TEST	REASON EVALUATED	NORMAL VALUE	ALTERATIONS
RBCs			
Erythrocyte (RBC)	Respiration Oxygen transport Acid-base balance	5 million/microliter	↑ Polycythemia, dehydration ↓ Anemia, fluid overload, hemorrhage
Mean corpuscular volume (MCV)	Average size of each RBC reflects maturity	80-100/femtoliter	Nutrition deficiency cause ↑ ↓ Iron deficiency
Mean corpuscular hemoglobin (MCH)	Average amount of hemoglobin in each RBC	26-34 pg	↓ Disorders of hemoglobin production
Mean corpuscular hemoglobin concentration (MCHC)	Average concentration of hemoglobin within a single RBC	31%-38%	↓ Cell has hemoglobin deficiency
Reticulocyte count	Immature RBCs released when sudden ↑ demand	1%-2% of total RBC count	↑ Recent blood loss or with chronic hemolysis
Serum folate	Amount of available vitamin for RBC development	95-500 mcg/mL	↓ Malnutrition or folic acid deficiency
Serum iron level	Iron stores within the body	40-160 mcg/dL	↓ Inadequate iron intake or inadequate absorption (e.g., gastric resection)
Total iron binding capacity (TIBC)	Reflection of liver function and nutrition	250-400 mcg/dL	↓ Chronic illness (infection, neoplasia, cirrhosis)
Ferritin level	Precursor to iron reflective of body's ability to create new iron stores	15-200 ng/mL	↓ Levels demonstrate inability to regenerate iron stores and hemoglobin
Transferrin level	Protein that binds to iron for removal or recirculation after RBCs are hemolyzed	200-400 mg/dL	↓ Excess hemolysis
Haptoglobin level	Protein that binds with heme for removal or recirculation after RBCs are hemolyzed	40-240 mg/dL	↓ Excess hemolysis
WBCs			
Leukocytes (WBCs)	Inflammatory and immune responses Defend against infection, foreign tissue	4500-11,000/microliter	↑ Inflammation, tissue necrosis, infection, hematological malignancy ↓ Bone marrow depression (radiation, immune disorders), chronic disease
Granular Leukocytes			
Neutrophils	Polymorphonuclear neutrophils Phagocytosis of invading organisms	50%-70% of WBCs	↑ Inflammation, infection, surgery, myocardial infarction ↓ Aplastic anemia, hepatitis, some pharmacological agents
Eosinophils	Defend against parasites; detoxification of foreign proteins Phagocytosis	1%-5% of WBCs	↑ Allergic attacks, autoimmune diseases, parasitic infections, dermatological condition ↓ Stress reactions, severe infections
Basophils	Release heparin, serotonin, and histamine in allergic reactions; inflammatory response	0%-1% of WBCs	↑ Postsplenectomy, hemolytic anemia, radiation, hypothyroidism, leukemia, chronic hypersensitivity ↓ Stress reactions
Nongranular Leukocytes			
Monocytes	Mature into macrophages; phagocytosis of necrotic tissue, debris, foreign particles	1%-8% of WBCs	↑ Bacterial, parasitic, and some viral infections, chronic inflammation ↓ Stress reactions
Lymphocytes	Defend against microorganisms	20%-40% of WBCs	↑ Bacterial and viral infections, lymphocytic leukemia ↓ Immunoglobulin deficiency

Continued

TABLE 16-6   FUNCTIONS AND NORMAL VALUES OF BLOOD CELLS—cont'd

TEST	REASON EVALUATED	NORMAL VALUE	ALTERATIONS
B lymphocytes	Humoral immunity and production of antibodies	270-640/microliter	↑ Bacterial and viral infections, lymphocytic leukemia ↓ Immunoglobulin deficiency, stress
T lymphocytes	Cell-mediated immunity	500-2400/microliter	↓ Chemotherapy, immunodeficiencies, HIV disease, end-stage renal disease, immunosuppressive drugs
Platelets Thrombocytes (platelets)	Blood clotting; hemostasis	150,000-400,000/microliter	↑ Polycythemia vera, postsplenectomy, certain cancers ↓ Leukemia, bone marrow failure, disseminated intravascular coagulation, hemorrhage, hypersplenism, radiation exposure, large foreign bodies in blood (e.g., aortic balloon pump), hypothermia, hyperthermia, severe infection

HIV, Human immunodeficiency virus; *pg,* picograms; *RBCs,* red blood cells; *WBCs,* white blood cells.

TABLE 16-7   COAGULATION PROFILE STUDIES

TEST	NORMAL VALUE	COMMENTS
Lee-White clotting time	6-12 minutes	Nonspecific for clotting abnormalities
Activated partial thromboplastin time (APTT)	<35 seconds	Used to monitor heparin therapy and detect bleeding tendencies, hemorrhagic disorders ↑ Anticoagulation therapy, liver disease, vitamin K deficiency, DIC
Prothrombin time (PT)	10-15 seconds 1.0-1.2 INR	Evaluates extrinsic pathway; used to monitor oral anticoagulant therapy ↑ Warfarin therapy, liver disease, vitamin K deficiency, obstructive jaundice
Thrombin time (TT)	9-13 seconds	Detect fibrinogen abnormalities, monitor heparin therapy ↑ Fibrinogen abnormalities, multiple myeloma, cirrhosis of liver, heparin therapy
Fibrinogen level	150-400 mg/dL	↓ DIC and fibrinogen disorders ↑ Acute infection, hepatitis, or with oral contraceptive use
Fibrin degradation products (FDPs)	<10 mcg/mL	Evaluates hematological disorders ↑ DIC, fibrinolysis, thrombolytic therapy
Fibrin D-dimer	0-0.5 mcg/mL	Presence diagnostic for DIC
Platelet count	150,000-400,000/microliter	Measures number of circulating platelets ↓ Thrombocytopenia
Platelet aggregation test	3-5 minutes	Measures platelet adherence ability Prolonged in von Willebrand disease, acute leukemia, idiopathic thrombocytopenic purpura, liver cirrhosis, aspirin use
Bleeding time	1-4 minutes	Evaluates platelet function ↑ Thrombocytopenia and aspirin therapy
Calcium	9-11 mg/dL	↓ Massive transfusions of stored blood

DIC, Disseminated intravascular coagulation; *Hgb,* hemoglobin; *INR,* international normalized ratio.

lower RBC levels when the condition is chronic or slow in onset.

Anemia is classified by its origin or by the microscopic appearance of the RBCs. Hematologists generally use the microscopic classifications (e.g., microcytic, hypochromic), but critical care nurses can best plan their nursing care by using the etiological classifications. Causes of anemia include (1) blood loss (acute or chronic), (2) impaired production, (3) increased RBC destruction, or (4) a combination of these.[6] Iron deficiency anemia is the most common type of anemia.[6] The types of anemia are described in Table 16-8.

TABLE 16-8 ANEMIAS

	MARROW FAILURE TO PRODUCE RBCS		SICKLE CELL ANEMIA (HEMOLYTIC SUBTYPE)	VITAMIN B₁₂ DEFICIENCY	FOLIC ACID DEFICIENCY	IRON DEFICIENCY
	APLASTIC ANEMIA	HEMOLYTIC ANEMIA				
Pathophysiology	Disorder or bone marrow toxin damages the erythrocyte precursors, leading to ↓ RBC production	Stimulus causes extrasplenic destruction of the RBC, leading to hemolyzed RBC fragments in the circulating bloodstream; cell fragments blood viscosity and slow blood flow, leading to ischemia and/or infarction. Extrasplenic hemolysis also leads to ↑ levels of circulating bilirubin and unbound iron	Presence of abnormal hemoglobin causes RBCs to assume a sickle or crescent shape. Sickling alters the blood viscosity, leading to microvascular occlusion; sickling crisis leads to hypoxia, thrombosis, and infarction in tissues and organs	Pernicious anemia is caused by decreased gastric production of HCl and intrinsic factor that play a role in vitamin B₁₂ absorption	Malabsorption of dietary folic acid resulting from the lack of intake or absorption	Body's iron stores inadequate for RBC development; Hgb-deficient RBCs result

Etiology			SICKLE CELL ANEMIA	VITAMIN B₁₂ DEFICIENCY	FOLIC ACID DEFICIENCY	IRON DEFICIENCY
	APLASTIC ANEMIA	HEMOLYTIC ANEMIA				
	Disorders: Bone metastases **Drugs:** Chemotherapy agents Antiretroviral agents **Toxic exposures:** Radiation to long bones	**Abnormal RBC membrane or hemoglobin:** Anemia of liver or renal disease Hereditary RBC shape disorders Paroxysmal nocturnal hemoglobinuria Porphyria Sickle cell disease G6PD deficiency Thalassemias **Immune reaction:** Autoimmune hemolytic syndrome: BMT hemolytic transfusion reaction Autoimmune diseases **Physical damage to RBC:** Blunt trauma Extracorporeal circulation Prosthetic heart valves Thermal injury **Unknown:** Diabetes mellitus IgA deficiency Illicit drug stimulants: cocaine Ovarian cyst Snake or spider bite	Hereditary hemolytic anemia caused by abnormal amount of hemoglobin S in relation to hemoglobin A	Familial incidence related to autoimmune response with gastric mucosal atrophy Higher incidence in autoimmune disorders: SLE, myxedema, Graves disease Common in Northern Europeans; rare in children, black and Asian populations Occurs postoperatively with gastric surgery	Common in infants, adolescents, pregnant and lactating women, alcoholic patients, older adults, cancer, intestinal disease (jejunitis, small bowel resection), prolonged anticonvulsants and estrogens, excessive cooking of foods	10%-30% of all American adults; primarily from dietary deficiency Also in pregnant and lactating women, infants, adolescents Malabsorption such as diarrhea, gastric resection, blood loss, or intravascular hemolysis

Disorders: Immune suppression Postorthotopic liver transplant status Pregnancy Vitamin B₁₂ deficiency Viral infection: EBV, CMV **Drugs:** Anticonvulsants Antidysrhythmics Antiinflammatory agents Chloramphenicol Quinines **Toxic exposures:** Benzene Arsenic Herbicides/insecticides Lacquers Paint thinners Radiation exposure Toluene (glue)

Continued

TABLE 16-8 ANEMIAS—cont'd

	MARROW FAILURE TO PRODUCE RBCS	APLASTIC ANEMIA	HEMOLYTIC ANEMIA	SICKLE CELL ANEMIA (HEMOLYTIC SUBTYPE)	VITAMIN B$_{12}$ DEFICIENCY	FOLIC ACID DEFICIENCY	IRON DEFICIENCY
Nursing Implications	Monitor diet and medications that interfere with marrow production of cells[13]	High risk of infection and bleeding: implement bleeding precautions Administer transfusions cautiously; exposure to antigens may enhance rejection if BMT is required later	Begin plasma reinfusion at a rate of 25 mL/hour for 15 minutes, then to 100 mL/hour Assess for hypersensitivity Assess for fluid shifts into the interstitial spaces during infusion or within 6-12 hours after infusion Monitor for vomiting, pain at infusion site, diarrhea	Incurable, although severity remains consistent throughout lifetime Children who do not have pain managed effectively can develop maladaptive coping Life expectancy prolonged as a result of more effective supportive care Common cause of death is intracranial thrombosis or hemorrhage	Lifetime treatment requires ongoing patient teaching Heart failure prevention Special oral hygiene Monitor for persistent neurological deficits	**Foods high in folic acid:** beef, liver, peanut butter, red beans, oatmeal, asparagus, broccoli	Monitor for allergic reactions to iron Give oral supplements with straw to prevent staining teeth; causes skin irritation and iron deposits
Clinical Presentation	→ Production of cells in the earliest phase: bone marrow resulting in low RBC count Signs and symptoms are those common in profound anemia	Symptoms of infection, bleeding, and anemia occur simultaneously; earliest symptoms usually the result of WBC dysfunction Platelet production abnormalities lead to bleeding symptoms within 7-10 days followed by symptoms of anemia	Rapid hemolysis of RBCs leads to spleen uptake with enlarged and tender spleen; metabolism of RBCs often leads to excess bilirubin with jaundice and itching	Hyperviscosity and poor perfusion (e.g., altered mentation, hypoxemia, abdominal cramping); sickled cells removed from circulation, causing enlarged and tender spleen; long-term sickling and thrombosis causes → joint mobility, gut dysfunction, cardiac failure, and risk for stroke	Inhibited growth of all cells: anemia, leukopenia, thrombocytopenia Demyelination of peripheral nerves to spinal cord Triad: weakness, sore tongue, paresthesias	Similar to vitamin B$_{12}$ deficiency but without neurological symptoms Signs: poor oxygenation, dizziness, irritability, dyspnea, pallor, headache, oral ulcers, tachycardia	Classic: "pica" (desire to eat nonfood items), ice or dirt cravings Symptoms of cardiovascular/respiratory compromise: hypoxia, fatigue, headache, cracks in mouth corners, smooth tongue, paresthesias, neuralgias

Diagnostic Tests

CBC used as screening test; Bone marrow aspiration and biopsy confirm maturation failure	Reticulocytes usually ≥4% total; RBC count; ↑ Total bilirubin; ↑ Direct bilirubin; ↓ Transferrin; ↓ Haptoglobin	Hemoglobin electrophoresis abnormality	Schilling test; Hgb and RBC ↓; MCV ↑; MCHC ↓; WBC ↓; Platelets ↓; LDH ↑	Macrocytosis; Serum folate <4 mg/dL; Abnormal platelet appearance; ↑ Reticulocyte count	↓ Hct and Hgb; ↑ Iron level with ↑ binding capacity; ↓ Ferritin level; ↓ RBC with hypochromia and microcytes; ↓ MCHC

Management

Erythropoietin per dosing guidelines (Procrit, Aranesp); Eliminate cause; Bone marrow stimulants may be tried early; Corticosteroids; Immunosuppressive agents if suspected autoimmune process; Chelating (iron binding) agents; Limit transfusions when possible to ↓ risk of rejection; Allogeneic BMT	Staphylococcal protein A is capable of trapping IgG complexes that are thought to cause RBC autoantibodies; If autoantibodies are present, give immunosuppressive agents; Administer antiplatelet medications (e.g., salicylic acid)	Administer large volumes of IV fluids to dilute viscous blood; Oxygen therapy reduces sickling; Treat infections early with fluids and antibiotics; Sickling causes extreme pain (result of ischemia); narcotics may be required; Gene transplants used experimentally	Vitamin B_{12} 30 mcg IM or deep SC for 5-10 days then 100-200 micrograms IM or deep SC every month	Folic acid 0.25-1 mg/day PO	Ferrous sulfate 325 mg PO TID and ascorbic acid to aid absorption

BMT, Bone marrow transplant; CMV, cytomegalovirus; 2,3-DPG, 2,3-diphosphoglycerate; EBV, Epstein-Barr virus; G6PD, glucose-6-phosphate dehydrogenase; Hct, hematocrit; Hgb, hemoglobin; IM, intramuscularly; IV, intravenously; LDH, lactate dehydrogenase; MCHC, mean corpuscular hemoglobin concentration; MCV, mean corpuscular volume; PO, orally; RBC, red blood cell; SC, subcutaneously; SLE, systemic lupus erythematosus; TID, three times a day; WBC, white blood cell.

Assessment and Clinical Manifestations

Signs and symptoms of anemia begin gradually and initially include fatigue, weakness, and shortness of breath.[6,23] Signs and symptoms are related to three physiological effects of reduced RBCs: (1) decreased circulating volume caused by loss of RBC mass, (2) decreased oxygenation of tissues resulting from reduced hemoglobin binding sites, and (3) compensatory mechanisms implemented by the body in its attempt to improve tissue oxygenation. Decreased circulating volume is manifested by clinical findings reflective of low blood volume (e.g., low right atrial pressure) and the effects of gravity on the lack of volume (e.g., orthostasis). Tissue hypoxia from inadequate oxygen delivery results in compensatory activities, including an increased depth and rate of respiration to increase oxygen availability, tachycardia to increase oxygen delivery, and the shunting of blood away from nonvital organs to perfuse the vital organs.[6,23] Inadequate oxygenation of the tissues leads to organ dysfunction.

In addition to the general symptoms of anemia, unique disorders have their own classic clinical features. The patient with aplastic anemia may have bruising, nosebleeds, petechiae, and a decreased ability to fight infections. These effects result from thrombocytopenia and decreased WBC counts, which occur when the bone marrow fails to produce blood cells. Assessment of the patient with hemolytic anemia may reveal jaundice, abdominal pain, and enlargement of the spleen or liver. These findings result from the increased destruction of RBCs, their sequestration (abnormal distribution in the spleen and liver[4]), and the accumulation of breakdown products. Patients with sickle cell anemia may have joint swelling or pain, and delayed physical and sexual development. In crisis, the sickle cell patient often has decreased urine output, peripheral edema, and signs of uremia because renal tissue perfusion is impaired as a result of sluggish blood flow.

Laboratory findings in anemia include a decreased RBC count and decreased hemoglobin and hematocrit values. The reticulocyte count is usually increased, indicating a compensatory increased RBC production with release of immature cells. Patients with hemolytic anemia also have an increased bilirubin level. In sickle cell disease, a stained blood smear reveals sickled cells. In aplastic anemia, the reticulocyte, platelet, RBC, and WBC counts are decreased because the marrow fails to produce any cells.

Nursing Diagnoses

Nursing diagnoses of the anemic patient may include the following:

- Decreased cardiac output related to decreased circulating blood volume
- Altered tissue perfusion, impaired gas exchange, or both, related to decreased or dysfunctional RBCs or hemoglobin
- Risk for fluid volume excess or deficit related to fluid replacement or hemorrhage
- Impaired skin integrity related to inadequate perfusion and tissue hypoxia

- Pain related to tissue ischemia and microvascular occlusion
- Risk for infection related to bone marrow failure and low WBC count
- Risk for injury related to transfusions

Medical Interventions

Medical treatment of anemia includes identification and removal of causative agents or conditions, supplemental oxygen, blood component therapy, and cardiovascular system support. In anemia associated with blood loss, initial treatment is restoration of blood volume with intravenous administration of volume expanders (crystalloid or colloid) and/or transfusion of packed red blood cells. Erythropoietin products are given to stimulate RBC production. For certain types of anemia, cause-specific interventions may be indicated. Splenectomy may be performed for hemolytic anemia, and bone marrow transplantation may be preferred for refractory aplastic anemia. In sickle cell disease, oxygenation and correction of dehydration are important for the prevention or reversal of erythrocyte sickling.

Nursing Interventions

Nursing management of anemia is based on a continuous, thorough nursing assessment and the prescribed medical treatment. Physical assessment is vital; monitoring of vital signs, the electrocardiogram, hemodynamics, heart and lung sounds, and peripheral pulses assists the nurse in the assessment of tissue perfusion and gas exchange. Tachycardia and orthostatic hypotension are important signs that indicate that the patient's cardiovascular system is not adequately compensating for the anemia. Mental status, urine output, and skin color or temperature are important general indicators of tissue perfusion. Pain management and comfort measures are instituted as needed. Scrupulous skin care is given to prevent tissue breakdown, and the patient is monitored closely for signs of infection. For patients at risk of further blood loss, bleeding precautions are instituted. Interventions for patients at risk of bleeding or infection are listed later in this chapter.

Laboratory results, such as the CBC, are carefully monitored.[4] Other vital nursing interventions include the following: promotion of rest and oxygen conservation; careful administration of blood components, drug therapy, and intravenous fluids; and monitoring of the patient's responses to the therapy. The desired goal of treatment and nursing intervention is optimal tissue perfusion, oxygenation, and gas exchange.

WHITE BLOOD CELL AND IMMUNE DISORDERS

Many pathological conditions can be classified as WBC or immune disorders. They may involve the WBCs themselves or other complementary immune processes. The immune system can fail to develop properly, lose its ability to react to invasion by pathogens, overreact to harmless antigens, or turn immune functions against self. Regardless of the cause, WBC and immune disorders or their treatments suppress the mechanisms needed for inflammation and combating infection. Because the clinical features and complications are similar among a variety of disorders, this first section addresses general causes, signs and symptoms, and management of immunological suppression. This is followed by in-depth descriptions of specific WBC and immune disorders.

The Immunocompromised Patient
Pathophysiology

The *immunocompromised* patient is one with defined quantitative or qualitative defects in WBCs or immune physiology. The defect may be congenital or acquired, and may involve a single element or multiple processes. Regardless of the cause, the physiological outcome is immune incompetence, with lack of normal inflammatory, phagocytic, antibody, or cytokine responses. Immune incompetence is often asymptomatic until pathogenic organisms invade the body and create infection. Infection is the leading cause of death in the immunocompromised patient.

Assessment and Clinical Manifestations

The nursing diagnosis *risk for infection* is frequently documented in critically ill patients and is the primary clinical problem for those with immune compromise. A detailed database containing the patient's history, physical examination findings, and laboratory studies is paramount for rapid detection of infection.

Immunocompromise in the critically ill is caused by many factors. In addition to existing immunodeficiency diseases and life-threatening illness, immune defenses are altered by invasive procedures, inadequate nutrition, and the presence of opportunistic pathogens. Many of the drugs and treatments administered in critical care can also depress the patient's immune system. The patient's medical and social history, current medications, and risk factors for infection are evaluated. Risk factors for immune compromise are described in Table 16-9. Immunosuppressed patients do not respond to infection with typical signs and symptoms of inflammation (see box, "Clinical Alert: Infection in Immunocompromised Patients").

TABLE 16-9 RISK FACTORS FOR INFECTIONS IN THE IMMUNOCOMPROMISED PATIENT

PATIENT CHARACTERISTICS	PHYSIOLOGICAL MECHANISM OF RISK OF INFECTION
Host Characteristics	
Alcoholism	↓ Neutrophil activity Hepatic/splenic congestion also slows phagocytic response
Abuse of intravenous drugs	Chronic altered barrier defense leads to reduced WBCs and slowed phagocytic responses Constant viral exposure may also alter T-cell function
Aging	Slowed phagocytosis: bacterial infection, more rapid dissemination of infection Slowed macrophage activity—more fungal infection, more visceral infection Atrophy of thymus: ↑ risk of viral illness ↓ Antigen-specific immunoglobulins: diminished immune memory
Frequent hospitalizations	Frequent exposure to environmental organisms other than own normal flora Potential exposure to resistant organisms Potential exposure to other people's organisms via equipment, supplies, transport, person-to-person exposure
Malnutrition	*Inadequate WBC count:* infection ↓ *Neutrophil activity:* bacterial infection, at risk of infection *Impaired phagocytic function:* bacterial infection *Impaired integumentary/mucosal barrier:* general infection risk ↓ *Macrophage mobilization:* ↑ risk of fungal or rapidly disseminating infection ↓ *Lymphocyte function:* ↑ risk of viral and opportunistic infection Thymus and lymph node atrophy with iron deficiency
Stress	Induces ↑ release of adrenal hormones (cortisol), which causes ↓ circulating eosinophils and lymphocytes
Immune Defects and Disorders	
Lymphopenia	↓ Antibody response to previous exposed antigens ↓ Recognition and destruction of viral and opportunistic organisms
Macrophage dysfunction/destruction	Altered response to fungi Inadequate antigen-antibody response Greater potential for visceral infection

Continued

TABLE 16-9   RISK FACTORS FOR INFECTIONS IN THE IMMUNOCOMPROMISED PATIENT—cont'd

PATIENT CHARACTERISTICS	PHYSIOLOGICAL MECHANISM OF RISK OF INFECTION
Neutropenia	Inadequate neutrophils to combat pathogens (especially bacterial)
Splenectomy	Inability to recognize and remove encapsulated bacteria (e.g., streptococcus) Compromised reticuloendothelial system and ↓ antibodies lead to frequent and early bacteremia
Disease Processes	
Burns	Physiological stressor thought to ↓ phagocytic responses Altered barrier defenses allowing pathogen entry Protein loss through skin leads to malnutrition-related immunocompromise
Cancer	Structural disruption may lead to bone marrow or lymphatic abnormalities Certain cancers have specific immune defects (e.g., diminished phagocytic activity or T-cell defects) Radiation therapy destroys lymphocytes and causes shrinkage of lymphoid tissue Chemotherapy causes ↓ lymphocytes and alters the proliferation and differentiation of stem cells
Cardiovascular disease	Inadequate tissue perfusion slows WBC response to tissue with pathogenic organism
Diabetes mellitus	↓ Numbers of neutrophils Hyperglycemia causes ↓ phagocytic activity and immunoglobin defects Vascular insufficiency leads to slowed phagocytic response to pathogens Neuropathy and glycosuria predisposes person to ↓ bladder emptying and urinary tract infections
Gastrointestinal disease	↓ Bowel motility allows normal flora to translocate across the gastrointestinal wall to the bloodstream
Hepatic disease	↓ Neutrophil count
Infectious diseases	↓ Phagocytic activity Hypermetabolism with infection accelerates phagocytic cell use and death Certain viral and opportunistic infections ↓ bone marrow production of WBCs
Pulmonary disease	Inadequate oxygenation suppresses neutrophil activity
Renal disease	↓ Neutrophil activity caused by uremic toxins ↓ Immunoglobulin activity
Traumatic injuries	Altered barrier defenses allowing pathogen entry Type of infection dependent on source and severity of injury (e.g., soil contamination, water contamination, skin flora)
Medication/Treatment	
Antibiotics	Normal flora destroyed and enhanced resistant organism growth, fungal superinfection
Immunosuppressive agents and corticosteroids	↓ Phagocytic activity Altered T-cell recognition of pathogens, especially viral ↓ Interleukin-2 production leads to increased risk of malignancy ↓ IgG production Lack of immune memory to recall antibodies to previously encountered pathogens
Invasive devices	Altered barrier defenses allowing pathogen entry, especially skin organisms
Surgical procedures/wounds	Normal flora may be translocated by surgical procedure Altered barrier defenses caused by surgical entry Stress of surgery and anesthetic agents reduce neutrophil activity
Transfusion of blood products	Risk of transfusion-transmitted infections undetected by donor screening: cytomegalovirus, hepatitis, human immunodeficiency virus Exposure to foreign antigens in blood products causes T-lymphocytic immune suppression and increases risk of infection

IgG, Immunoglobulin G; *WBC,* white blood cell.

! CLINICAL ALERT

Infection in Immunocompromised Patients

Immunocompromised patients do not have typical signs and symptoms of infection.

- Erythema, swelling, and exudate formation are usually not evident.
- Symptoms of infection may be absent, masked, or present atypically.
- Fever is considered the cardinal and sometimes only symptom of infection. However, some patients with infection may not have a fever.
- Patients are also more likely to describe pain at the site of infection, although physical inflammatory signs may be absent.

Laboratory results that reflect leukopenia, low CD4 counts, and decreased immunoglobulin levels may demonstrate disorders of immune components.[6] A common test of the humoral (antibody) response to antigens is a skin test with intradermal injection of typical pathogens capable of initiating an antibody response. Absence of a "wheal" tissue response to the antigens (called tissue anergy) is evidence of altered antibody capabilities.

Nursing Diagnoses

The patient with compromised immune system function is most likely to have one of the following nursing diagnoses: risk for infection, altered protection, or hyperthermia.

Medical Interventions

Medical therapy is directed at reversing the cause of the immune dysfunction and preventing infectious complications. In *primary immunodeficiencies,* B-cell and T-cell defects are treated with specific replacement therapy or bone marrow transplantation. IgG blood levels of less than 300 mg/dL warrant immunoglobulin infusion. Gene replacement therapy may soon be a realistic curative treatment option for some disorders. In *secondary immunodeficiencies,* the underlying causative condition is treated. For example, malnutrition is corrected, or doses of immunosuppressive medications are adjusted.

Additional risk factors for infection are carefully monitored and avoided when possible. Invasive lines pose the most common risk for iatrogenic infection; lines should be kept to a minimum and managed with meticulous sterile technique.

Administration of prophylactic antimicrobial agents during the period of highest risk of infection is common. For example, patients receiving bone marrow–suppressing cancer chemotherapy receive broad-spectrum antimicrobials during the time of their lowest WBC count. Patients who have human immunodeficiency virus (HIV) infection or are recovering from organ transplantation have defined CD4 or immune suppression levels that place them at risk of specific infections.[14] Depending on predetermined criteria, these patients can receive antimicrobial prophylaxis against infections with herpes simplex, *Candida albicans, Pneumocystis jiroveci,* Mycobacterium avium-intracellulare, *Mycobacterium tuberculosis,* and cytomegalovirus.

Nursing Interventions

Nursing interventions focus on protecting the patient from infection. It has been proposed that a protective environment could reduce the risk of infection. Research studies support the use of high-efficiency particulate air (HEPA) filtration of air and laminar airflow in single-patient rooms for prevention of infection with airborne microorganisms. Comparative studies of isolation precautions and careful infection control practices, such as hand washing with an antimicrobial soap, do not demonstrate any added advantage to isolation techniques.

Nurses should diligently ensure adequate hygiene measures that include general bathing with antimicrobial soaps, oral care, and perineal care. Hand washing is paramount for staff, patients, and visitors. Nursing staff members play an important role in limiting breaks in skin integrity and ensuring sterile technique when procedures are unavoidable.

General health promotion of adequate fluid, nutrition, and sleep are important in bolstering the patient's defenses against infection. Dietary restriction, such as prohibiting raw fruits and vegetables, is controversial and not standardized.[7] For a more comprehensive list of nursing interventions, consult the "Nursing Care Plan for the Immunocompromised Patient" (see box).

⊚ **NURSING CARE PLAN**

for the Immunocompromised Patient

NURSING DIAGNOSIS

Risk for Infection related to immunocompromise or immunosuppression; invasive procedures; and presence of opportunistic pathogens.

PATIENT OUTCOMES

Patient remains free of infection

- Absence of fever, redness, swelling, pain, and heat
- WBC and differential, urinalysis, and cultures within normal limits
- Chest x-ray study without infiltrates
- Absence of adventitious breath sounds

NURSING INTERVENTIONS	RATIONALES
• Establish baseline assessment with documented history, physical examination, and laboratory study results	• Establish trends to guide and monitor treatment
• Follow universal precautions, including hand hygiene	• Decrease risk of infection
• Plan nurses' assignments to reduce the possibility of infection spread between patients	• Decrease spread of infection
• Be careful handling secretions/excretions that are known to be infected	• Prevent cross-contamination
• Monitor visitors for any recent history of communicable diseases	• Prevent infection
• Clean all multipurpose equipment (e.g., oximeter probes, non-invasive BP cuffs, bed scale slings, electronic thermometers) between patient use	• Prevent cross-contamination
• Assess patient for signs/symptoms of infection	• Accurate and timely interventions improve patient outcomes
• Monitor vital signs with temperature at least every 4 hours; any elevation in temperature is reported and investigated; rectal temperatures are not recommended	• Assess for infection
• Monitor laboratory results: WBC and differential, blood, urine, sputum, wound, and throat cultures; report abnormal results	• Assess for infection
• Note the presence of chills, tachycardia, oliguria, or altered mentation that may indicate sepsis; report subtle changes to physician	• Assess for infection
• Encourage incentive spirometry, changes of position every 1-2 hours	• Prevent atelectasis
• Avoid breaks in the skin and mucous membranes; change position every 2 hours, avoid wetness, provide skin lubricants and moisture barriers, provide meticulous oral and bathing hygiene	• Maintain intact skin—the first line of defense
• Use strict aseptic technique for dressing changes	• Prevent infection
• Avoid stopcocks in IV systems, use closed injection of site systems	• Stopcocks can harbor bacteria and are a source entry for any infectious agent
• Limit invasive devices/procedures when possible	• Decrease risk for infection
• Use private room, limit visitors, limit fresh flowers and standing water	• Fresh flowers have a potential to introduce pathogenic organisms
• Ensure that sleep needs are being met	• Enhance resistance to infection and aid in healing
• Control glucose levels	• Hyperglycemia compromises phagocytic activity
• Change oxygen setups with humidification (e.g., nasal cannula) every 24 hours	• Prevent bacterial growth
• Obtain cultures for first fever (38.0° C; temperature taken twice 4 hours apart), or new fever (38.3° C) after 72 hours on an antimicrobial regimen:	• Determine site of infections and pathogens for proper antimicrobial treatment
• Blood cultures from two different sites	
• Blood cultures from existing venous/arterial access devices	
• Urine culture	
• Sputum culture, if obtainable	
• Stool culture, if obtainable	
• Culture of open lesions or wounds	

◎ NURSING CARE PLAN

for the Immunocompromised Patient—cont'd

NURSING INTERVENTIONS	RATIONALES
• Administer antimicrobial therapy as ordered; perform antimicrobial peak and trough levels as ordered	• Treat infection and assess effectiveness of antibiotics
• Be alert to superinfection with fungal flora any time 7-10 days after initiation of antibiotics	• Assess complication of antibiotic therapy; oral or topical nystatin may be indicated

NURSING DIAGNOSIS

Risk for Impaired Skin Integrity and altered oral mucous membranes related to immobility, invasive devices and procedures, dehydration, malnutrition, and immunosuppression

PATIENT OUTCOMES

Skin and mucous membranes intact
• Absence of signs of pressure areas, breakdown, lesions, excoriation
• Skin turgor and moisture of mucous membranes adequate

NURSING INTERVENTIONS	RATIONALES
• Assess skin and mucous membranes every shift for pressure, breakdown, lesions, and excoriation	• Assess for complications
• Monitor incisions, IV and venipuncture sites, axillae, perineal areas for redness, swelling, pain, heat	• Signs of infection may not be obvious
• Provide meticulous skin care; keep skin clean, dry, and lubricated	• Prevent infection
• Provide frequent mouth care with nonirritating solutions and soft-bristled brush	• Maintain moisture of mucous membranes
• Turn/reposition the patient at least every 2 hours; evaluate need for therapeutic beds/mattresses	• Prevent skin breakdown
• Treat any pressure ulcers or areas of breakdown promptly; consult with wound care specialist	• Prevent further complications; obtain advice from wound experts
• Maintain adequate hydration and optimal nutritional status	• Decrease risk for skin breakdown

NURSING DIAGNOSIS

Altered Nutrition (less than body requirements) related to NPO status; anorexia, nausea/vomiting; and painful oral mucosa

PATIENT OUTCOMES

Optimal nutritional status maintained
• Adequate caloric and protein intake
• Ideal/stable body weight
• Laboratory values remain within normal limits (total protein, serum albumin, electrolytes, hemoglobin, and hematocrit)

NURSING INTERVENTIONS	RATIONALES
• Assess baseline nutritional status: height and weight (BMI), weight loss or gain, laboratory values; presence of weakness, fatigue, infection, or other signs of malnutrition	• Obtain baseline assessment
• Obtain dietary consult to determine nutrients/intake required[13]; administer enteral/parenteral nutritional therapy as ordered and observe response	• Optimize nutritional therapy to reduce risks
• Establish food preferences; encourage meals from home and provide relaxed atmosphere during meals.	• Tailor nutritional support based on patient's preferences
• Determine deterrents to adequate intake: fasting (NPO) status, presence of anorexia, nausea, vomiting, stomatitis	• Assess risks for decreased nutrition
• Monitor daily weight, laboratory values, protein and caloric intake, I&O	• Monitor status
• Encourage small, frequent, high-calorie and high-protein meals	• Promote adequate intake
• Provide meticulous mouth care before and after meals	• Maintain oral mucosa and facilitate oral intake
• Administer antiemetics as needed, 30 minutes before meals	• Encourage adequate intake

BMI, Body mass index; *BP,* blood pressure; *HEPA,* high-efficiency particulate air; *I&O,* intake and output; *IV,* intravenous; *NPO,* nothing by mouth; *WBC,* white blood cell.

Based on data from Gulanick M and Myers JL. *Nursing Care Plans: Diagnoses, Interventions, and Outcomes,* 7th ed. St. Louis: Mosby; 2011.

Several patient outcomes are desired as a result of nursing interventions. These include absence of fever, negative cultures, and normal laboratory test results. Both family members and patients should be able to verbalize strategies to control infection risks.

Neutropenia

Pathophysiology

Neutropenia is defined as an absolute neutrophil count of less than 1500 cells/microliter of blood. Neutropenia may occur as a result of inadequate production or excess destruction of neutrophils. Patients with low neutrophil counts are predisposed to infections because of the body's reduced phagocytic ability.[6,9] Neutropenia is classified based on the patient's predicted risk for infection: mild (1000 to 1500 cells/microliter), moderate (500 to 1000 cells/microliter), and severe (<500 cells/microliter).[6]

Assessment and Clinical Manifestations

The nurse must obtain a thorough medical and social history to identify risk factors for neutropenia. Common causes include acute or overwhelming infections, radiation, exposure to chemicals and drugs, or other disease states (Box 16-3).

There are no specific signs or symptoms of a low neutrophil count, although many patients describe fatigue or malaise that coincides with the drop in counts and precedes infectious signs and symptoms. This lack of a clear pattern of symptoms makes it essential to evaluate the patient carefully for risk factors for neutropenia. The patient is also monitored for clinical findings consistent with infection.

Every body system is examined for physical findings of infection. Typical signs may not be evident. Pain such as sore throat or urethral discomfort may be indicative of an infected site. Areas of heavy bacterial colonization (e.g., oral mucosa, perineal area, and venipuncture and catheter sites) have the highest risk of infection; however, the most common clinical infections are sepsis and pneumonia. Additional signs or symptoms of systemic infection include a rise in temperature from its normal set point, chills, and accompanying tachycardia.

The diagnostic test indicated when neutropenia is suspected is the WBC count with differential. The differential demonstrates the percentage of each type of WBC circulating in the bloodstream. The absolute neutrophil count is calculated by multiplying the total WBC count (without a decimal point) times the percentages (with decimal points) of polymorphonuclear leukocytes (polys; also called segs or neutrophils) and bands (immature neutrophils), as follows.

$$WBC \times (segs + bands) \times 100$$

This gives a number that is translated into the categories of mild, moderate, or severe neutropenia.

Nursing Diagnoses

The specific nursing diagnosis related to all patients with neutropenia is risk for infection.

Medical Interventions

Medical treatment of neutropenia is aimed at preventing and treating infection while reversing the cause of neutropenia. Patients with anticipated neutropenia, such as those receiving antineoplastic or antiretroviral therapy, may be administered bone marrow growth factors. Also known as *colony-stimulating factors* (CSFs), these agents enhance bone marrow regeneration of the granulocyte (G-CSF), macrophage (M-CSF), or both cell lines (GM-CSF).[5,6,15]

BOX 16-3 CAUSES OF NEUTROPENIA

Malnutrition
- Vitamin B deficiency
- Calorie deficiency
- Iron deficiency
- Protein deficiency

Health States
- Addison disease
- Anaphylactic shock
- Anorexia nervosa
- Brucellosis
- Chronic fever
- Chronic illness
- Cirrhosis
- Diabetes mellitus
- Elderly status
- Hypothermia
- Infectious diseases (any severe bacterial or viral): mononucleosis, measles, mumps, influenza
- Renal trauma

Medications
- Alcohol
- Alkylating agents (antineoplastic and immunosuppressive; e.g., cyclophosphamide)
- Allopurinol (Zyloprim)
- Anticonvulsants (e.g., phenytoin)
- Antidysrhythmics (e.g., procainamide, quinidine)
- Antimicrobials (e.g., aminoglycosides, chloramphenicol, sulfonamides, trimethoprim-sulfamethoxazole)
- Antiretroviral agents (e.g., zidovudine)
- Antitumor antibiotics (e.g., bleomycin, doxorubicin [Adriamycin])
- Arsenic
- Phenothiazines (e.g., prochlorperazine)

Prophylactic antiinfective agents may be ordered to prevent infection, and potent broad-spectrum antimicrobial agents are ordered when there is evidence of infection. In sepsis accompanying neutropenia, granulocyte transfusions are occasionally used to supplement phagocytosis.

Nursing Interventions

Nursing care of patients with neutropenia is the same as for all immunocompromised patients (see "Nursing Care Plan for the Immunocompromised Patient"). Desired patient outcomes related to medical and nursing interventions include absence of infection, negative cultures, and an absolute neutrophil count of 1500 cells/microliter or higher.

Malignant White Blood Cell Disorders: Leukemia, Lymphoma, and Multiple Myeloma
Pathophysiology

Malignant diseases involving WBCs are termed leukemia, lymphoma, and plasma cell neoplasm (multiple myeloma). They are differentiated by the cell type affected and by the stage of cell development when malignancy occurs. Regardless of the specific neoplastic disorder, a deficiency of functional WBCs is a common problem. The unique pathophysiological and clinical characteristics of these disorders are described in Table 16-10. Despite normal serum cell counts, WBC activity is always impaired, and infection is the most common complication of all these disorders.

TABLE 16-10	MALIGNANT WHITE BLOOD CELL DISORDERS	
LEUKEMIA	**LYMPHOMA**	**MULTIPLE MYELOMA**
Pathophysiology		
Cancer involving any of the WBCs during the early phase of maturation within the bone marrow	Cancer affects the lymphocytes after their bone marrow maturation, when they reside within the lymph node	Cancer involves the mature and differentiated immunoglobulin-producing macrophage called a plasma cell; the malignancy is primarily manifested by excess abnormal immunoglobulin
Classification		
Excess proliferation of immature cells is termed *acute* leukemia Excess proliferation of mature cells is termed *chronic* leukemia Leukemias are further classified according to whether they originate in the lymphocyte cell line or are nonlymphocytic	Hodgkin and non-Hodgkin subtypes have more subclassifications denoting the maturity of the cell involved and aggressiveness of the malignancy	Disease is classified as limited or extensive depending on the plasma viscosity, bone manifestations, presence of hypercalcemia, and renal involvement
Risk Factors		
Chromosomal abnormalities Viral infection Radiation Herbicides/pesticides Benzene/toluene Immunosuppressive therapy (e.g., high-dose steroids or posttransplant immunosuppressives)	Chromosomal abnormalities Alkylating agents Viral infection Radiation Herbicides/pesticides Benzene/toluene Immunosuppressive therapy (e.g., high-dose steroids or posttransplant immunosuppressives) Alkylating agents Autoimmune disease	Older age Male gender African American descent Chronic hypersensitivity reactions Autoimmune diseases
Clinical Manifestations		
Fever *Constitutional symptoms:* fatigue, malaise, weakness, night sweats Easy bruising and bleeding from mucous membranes such as gums Bone pain	Enlarged >2 cm, nontender lymph node(s) Usually immovable, and irregularly shaped Masses in body cavities or other organs (e.g., peritoneal cavity, lungs)	*Thrombotic events:* deep vein thrombosis, pulmonary embolism, cerebral infarction Bone pain Renal failure

Continued

TABLE 16-10	MALIGNANT WHITE BLOOD CELL DISORDERS—cont'd	
LEUKEMIA	**LYMPHOMA**	**MULTIPLE MYELOMA**
Acute Complications		
Leukostasis	Airway obstruction	Hyperviscosity
Disseminated intravascular coagulation	Superior vena cava syndrome	Renal failure
Tumor lysis syndrome	Bowel obstruction	Hypercalcemia
	Neoplastic tamponade	
	Pleural effusion	
Staging		
All patients are viewed as having systemic disease, or late-stage disease	Classified by the number of lymph nodes involved, the number of lymph node groups, whether involved nodes are only above the diaphragm or on both sides of the diaphragm, and how many extranodal sites are involved	Disease is classified as limited when there are only elevated abnormal immunoglobin levels; described as extensive when there are bone lesions, hypercalcemia, or renal dysfunction
Diagnostic Tests		
CBC shows either ↓ WBCs or large number of immature WBCs (blasts), ↓ RBCs, ↓ platelets	Lymph node biopsy	Bence-Jones protein in urine
	CT scans	Immunoglobulin electrophoresis
	Chemistry: alkaline phosphatase	Plasma viscosity
Bone marrow aspiration and biopsy		
Medical Management		
Systemic chemotherapy	Radiation therapy for single node or node group if above diaphragm for control or remission	Systemic chemotherapy only provides average of 14-36 months remission
BMT	Radiation used if palliation of tumor is goal of therapy	BMT or "double" BMT may increase survival
	Systemic chemotherapy for multinode involvement, aggressive tumor subtypes	Radiation therapy used to palliatively treat bone lesions
	Autologous BMT for patients with high risk of relapse	
	Allogeneic BMT for patients with residual disease, especially involving bone marrow	
Nursing Care Issues		
Infection control practices	Infection control practices	Infection control practices
Bleeding precautions	Edema management	Safe mobility
	Monitoring for lymphoma masses compressing body organs	Thrombosis precautions
		Aspiration precautions if hypercalcemic

BMT, Bone marrow transplant; *CBC,* complete blood count; *CT,* computed tomography; *RBCs,* red blood cells; *WBCs,* white blood cells.

Assessment and Clinical Manifestations

Malignant hematological diseases have common risk factors such as genetic mutations (see box, "Genetics"), viral infection (especially retroviral), radiation, carcinogens, benzene derivatives, pesticides, and T-lymphocyte immune suppression (e.g., high-dose steroids, immunosuppressives after transplantation). Other risk factors that are unique to the specific malignancy are included in Table 16-10.

Assessment findings common to all malignant WBC disorders involve alterations in the immunological response to injury or microbes. As in other disorders affecting WBC

function, minimized inflammatory reactions and response to pathogens are typical. Fever is particularly difficult to interpret because it may be a manifestation of the disease process or may accompany an infectious complication. General signs and symptoms such as fatigue, malaise, myalgias, activity intolerance, and night sweats are nonspecific indicators of immune disease. Each malignant WBC disorder is also associated with signs and symptoms representative of the cell line and location of the malignancy. For example, bone pain is common in multiple myeloma, whereas lymph node enlargement is more representative of lymphoma.[1] When

GENETICS

Factor V Leiden: An Inherited Clotting Disorder

There are many hereditary blood coagulation disorders. Some inherited disorders cause increased bleeding such as hemophilia. Other inherited disorders result in increased clotting or thrombophilia. The most common thrombophilic disorder with a genetic connection is factor V Leiden. This disorder is named after the city of Leiden, The Netherlands, where it was first identified in 1994. It is an autosomal dominant condition, present in 2% to 15% of the general population.[2,4]

Factor V is one of the proteins in the clotting cascade. Factor V Leiden is a variation in this protein caused by a single nucleotide polymorphism (SNP)—a substitution of adenine for guanine in the F5 gene on the long arm of chromosome 1.[6] This SNP changes the 506th amino acid of factor V from arginine to glutamine. The substitution of glutamine at this site increases the stability of factor V, resulting in prolonged clotting action. Normally, activated protein C inactivates factor V by cleaving it at three sites. When glutamine is present at the 506th amino acid site, activated protein C cannot inactivate factor V. When factor V remains active, it promotes overproduction of another clotting cascade protein, thrombin, leading to excess fibrin generation and clot formation.[6] Thus factor V Leiden is resistant to activated protein C. Once the coagulation process begins in someone with the Leiden variant of factor V, coagulation turns "off" more slowly than in someone with normal factor V.[1]

The clinical presentation of factor V Leiden varies. Many individuals with the factor V Leiden allele never develop thrombosis. The most common manifestation is venous thromboembolism (VTE), usually in the deep veins of the legs. The risk for increased thrombosis can also lead to pregnancy loss and placental abruption. In carriers of factor V Leiden, the risk of recurrent VTE is 2.5 times greater than in those patients without the mutation.[3] When two copies of the Leiden variant (homozygous) are inherited, the risk of thrombosis increases 30 to 80 times that of the general population; homozygosity may also present with a more catastrophic clotting event.[4] The presence of risk factors for VTE, such as immobility, injury, cancer, or other procoagulant conditions coexisting with thrombophilic disorders has synergistic effects in the clotting cascade. Therefore individuals with the Leiden allele are at an even higher risk for thrombosis with comorbid thrombophilic conditions

Treatment of an initial VTE in individuals with factor V Leiden follows the same guidelines for any first episode of VTE.[1] Long-term oral anticoagulation is considered for those individuals with recurrent VTE, multiple thrombophilic disorders, or coexistent risk factors. Heparin or low–molecular weight heparin prophylaxis may be used in women to prevent pregnancy loss.[7]

The diagnosis of factor V Leiden is made after global coagulation tests (protime, activated partial thromboplastin time, thromboplastin time, and fibrinogen) are completed.[5] Factor V Leiden can be assayed either by using a coagulation screening test (activated protein C resistance assay) or by DNA analysis of the F5 gene. Factor V Leiden testing should be performed in the following situations: a first VTE before 50 years of age; an unprovoked VTE; a history of recurrent VTE; a VTE at unusual sites such as cerebral, mesenteric, portal, or hepatic veins; VTE during pregnancy; a first VTE in an individual with a first-degree relative with VTE before 50 years of age; or in women with unexplained fetal loss after 10 weeks gestation.[5]

Although the factor V Leiden allele is fairly common, heterozygosity for the factor V Leiden variant results in only a small increased risk for thrombosis, and therefore routine genetic screening is not recommended. Clarification of the factor V Leiden genetic status may be indicated for at-risk relatives considering pregnancy, hormonal contraception, or hormone replacement therapy and with recurrent VTE. The challenges of sharing the potential for increased risk of VTE and genetic status is one of the ethical challenges of genomic medicine.

References

1. Anderson JA, Weitz JI. Hypercoagulable states. *Clinics in Chest Medicine*. 2010;31(4):659-673.
2. Coppola A, Tufano A, Cerbone AM, et al. Inherited thrombophilia: implications for prevention and treatment of venous thromboembolism. *Seminars in Thrombosis and Hemostasis*. 2009;35(7):683-694.
3. Kyrle PA, Rosendaal FR, Eichinger S. Risk assessment for recurrent venous thrombosis. *Lancet*. 2010;376(9757):2032-2039.
4. Lashley FR. *Clinical Genetics in Nursing Practice*. 3rd ed. New York: Springer. 2006.
5. Margetic S. Diagnostic algorithm for thrombophilia screening. *Clinical Chemistry and Laboratory Medicine*. 2010;48 (Suppl 1):S27-S39.
6. Pajic, T. (2010). Factor V Leiden and FII 20210 testing in thromboembolic disorders. *Clinical Chemistry and Laboratory Medicine*. 48 Suppl 1, S79-87.
7. Slusher KB. Factor V Leiden: a case study and review. *Dimensions in Critical Care Nursing*. 2010;29(1):6-10.

symptoms overlap into more than one component of the immune system, it may be difficult to differentiate between these disorders.

The critical care nurse must be aware of unique oncological emergencies associated with these malignant diseases. Oncological emergencies may be the consequence of the cancer itself or a specific treatment plan (see Table 16-10). These complications are more likely to precipitate admission to the critical care unit and are associated with significant morbidity and mortality.

Nursing Diagnoses

The nursing diagnoses associated with hematological malignancies have some variation with each disorder. Common nursing diagnoses include risk for infection, altered tissue perfusion related to anemia, and risk for injury (bleeding).

Medical Interventions

Each major subtype of hematological malignancy has slightly different presenting symptoms, prognostic variables, and treatment implications. The treatment plan is based on the stage of the definitive diagnosis established by histopathology.

Therapy commonly includes chemotherapy and biotherapy. Bone marrow transplantation is used in selected cases. Surgery may be performed to establish a pathological diagnosis by excisional or incisional biopsy, but has no other significant role in the management of hematological malignancies. Radiation may be used to treat lymphoma when the disease is limited to single nodes or node groups.

The complexity of treatment is noted in the following examples. Leukemia is considered a *systemic* disease at diagnosis. Treatment of acute leukemia requires a complex chemotherapy treatment plan called *induction* chemotherapy, and is associated with a period of severe cytopenia that requires supportive care and transfusion therapy. The management of chronic myelogenous leukemia has been improved with the development of imatinib mesylate (Gleevec), an oral agent that results in high remission rates. The management of chronic lymphocytic leukemia has seen major changes with the availability of newer agents. Multiple myeloma therapy involves careful staging and a choice of induction chemotherapy plans, leading to autologous stem cell transplantation for most patients. Radiation therapy is used palliatively to control the pain associated with bone lesions. Because of the rapid application of the advances in molecular biology, there has been a dramatic improvement in remission and cure rates for most hematological malignancies.

Nursing Interventions

The care of patients with hematological malignancies is similar to that for all immunocompromised patients; however, specialized management of cancer therapies must be incorporated into the individual care plan. Oncology nursing references for chemotherapy administration guidelines, management of acute therapy–related nausea and vomiting, and oncological treatment modalities are available from the Oncology Nursing Society (ONS).

SELECTED IMMUNOLOGICAL DISORDERS

Primary Immunodeficiency

In primary immunodeficiency, the dysfunction exists in the immune system. Most primary immunodeficiencies are congenital disorders related to a single gene defect. The onset of symptoms may occur within the first 2 years of life, or in the second or third decade of life. These defects of the immune system typically result in frequent or recurrent infections, and sometimes may predispose the affected individual to unusual or severe infections.[19] Disorders are grouped by their immunological disruption.

Secondary Immunodeficiency

Secondary or acquired immunodeficiency is the result of factors outside the immune system, not related to a genetic defect, and involves the loss of a previously functional immune defense system. AIDS is the most notable secondary immunodeficiency disorder caused by an infection. Aging, dietary insufficiencies, malignancies, stressors (emotional, physical), immunosuppressive therapies, and certain diseases such as diabetes or sickle cell disease are additional examples of conditions that may be associated with acquired immunodeficiencies. Risk factors for infections in immunocompromised patients are described in Table 16-9.

Acquired Immunodeficiency Syndrome and Human Immunodeficiency Virus

Pathophysiology. HIV is a retrovirus that transcribes its RNA-containing genetic material into the DNA of the host cell nucleus by using an enzyme called reverse transcriptase.[14] HIV causes AIDS by depleting helper T cells, CD4 cells, and macrophages.[2]

Seroconversion is manifested by the presence of HIV antibodies and usually occurs 2 to 4 weeks after the initial infection.[14] Symptoms associated with seroconversion include flulike symptoms such as fever, sore throat, headache, malaise, and nausea, and they usually last 1 to 2 week.[6] This seroconversion is followed by a decrease in the HIV antibody titer as infected cells are sequestered in the lymph nodes. The earlier stages of HIV infection may last as long as 10 years and may produce few or no symptoms, although viral particles are actively replacing normal cells. This phenomenon is evident through the decreasing CD4 cell counts as the disease progresses.[6] As the CD4 cell count decreases, the patient becomes more susceptible to opportunistic infections, malignancies, and neurological disease. AIDS is the final stage of HIV infection. Figure 16-6 shows the progression of disease and common clinical manifestations. It is estimated that 99% of untreated HIV-infected individuals will progress to AIDS.[6] Treatment with combined antiviral drug regimens are controlling the progression to AIDS; AIDS is now considered, for many infected individuals, a chronic disease.

HIV is transmitted through exposure to infected body fluids, blood, or blood products.[14] Common modes of transmission include rectal or vaginal intercourse with an infected person; intravenous drug use with contaminated equipment; transfusion with contaminated blood or blood products; and accidental exposure through needlesticks, breaks in the skin, gestation, or childbirth (from mother to fetus). Risk of transmission is more likely when the infected person has advanced disease, although transmission of HIV can occur at any time or stage of infection. Since the 1980s, all blood products have been screened for HIV, hepatitis virus, and human T-cell lymphotrophic virus. The risk of HIV transmission to healthcare workers is low.

Assessment and clinical manifestations. The initial phase of HIV disease may be asymptomatic, or it may manifest as an acute seroconversion syndrome with symptoms similar to those of mononucleosis. This is followed by asymptomatic disease as HIV progressively destroys immune cells, which leads to AIDS.[14] AIDS is defined by the presence of a CD4 count that is less than 200/microliter and the presence of an indicator condition[6] (see Figure 16-6).

Diagnosis of HIV infection is made by the presence of one of the core antigens of HIV or the presence of antibodies to

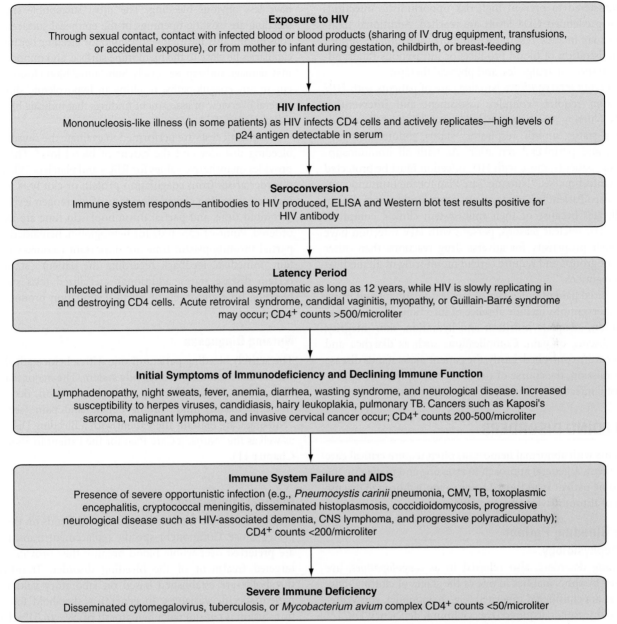

Exposure to HIV

Through sexual contact, contact with infected blood or blood products (sharing of IV drug equipment, transfusions, or accidental exposure), or from mother to infant during gestation, childbirth, or breast-feeding

HIV Infection

Mononucleosis-like illness (in some patients) as HIV infects CD4 cells and actively replicates—high levels of p24 antigen detectable in serum

Seroconversion

Immune system responds—antibodies to HIV produced, ELISA and Western blot test results positive for HIV antibody

Latency Period

Infected individual remains healthy and asymptomatic as long as 12 years, while HIV is slowly replicating in and destroying CD4 cells. Acute retroviral syndrome, candidal vaginitis, myopathy, or Guillain-Barré syndrome may occur; CD4$^+$ counts >500/microliter

Initial Symptoms of Immunodeficiency and Declining Immune Function

Lymphadenopathy, night sweats, fever, anemia, diarrhea, wasting syndrome, and neurological disease. Increased susceptibility to herpes viruses, candidiasis, hairy leukoplakia, pulmonary TB. Cancers such as Kaposi's sarcoma, malignant lymphoma, and invasive cervical cancer occur; CD4$^+$ counts 200-500/microliter

Immune System Failure and AIDS

Presence of severe opportunistic infection (e.g., *Pneumocystis carinii* pneumonia, CMV, TB, toxoplasmic encephalitis, cryptococcal meningitis, disseminated histoplasmosis, coccidioidomycosis, progressive neurological disease such as HIV-associated dementia, CNS lymphoma, and progressive polyradiculopathy); CD4$^+$ counts <200/microliter

Severe Immune Deficiency

Disseminated cytomegalovirus, tuberculosis, or *Mycobacterium avium* complex CD4$^+$ counts <50/microliter

FIGURE 16-6 Human immunodeficiency virus (HIV) pathophysiology. *CMV,* Cytomegalovirus; *CNS,* central nervous system; *ELISA,* enzyme-linked immunosorbent assay; *TB,* tuberculosis.

HIV. Core antigens are tested through protein electrophoresis. HIV antibodies are detected by enzyme-linked immunosorbent assay (ELISA) and are confirmed by the Western blot test and polymerase chain reaction (PCR).[3] Positive antibody test results are accurate for the presence of HIV infection, although a negative test result does not rule out HIV infection. Additional laboratory findings in AIDS may include an abnormal helper-to-suppressor ratio (<1.0), leukopenia, and thrombocytopenia.

Nursing diagnoses. Nursing care of the patient with AIDS is complex, and nursing diagnoses depend on the particular clinical manifestations of the disease. Nursing diagnoses for these patients may include risk for infection, impaired tissue integrity, altered nutrition, activity intolerance, and pain.

Medical interventions. Medical treatment consists of primary control of HIV invasion of CD4 cells through antiretroviral therapy. Antiretroviral medications are categorized as nucleoside reverse transcriptase inhibitors, nonnucleoside reverse transcriptase inhibitors, and protease inhibitors. The specific agents used and the strategies of combination therapy are a rapidly changing science that would be quickly outdated if included in this text.

Equally important to quality of life are prevention and management of opportunistic infections. Antimicrobials are administered to prevent high-risk opportunistic infections when predefined CD4 levels are reached. Additional treatment may include respiratory support, nutritional support, administration of blood products or intravenous fluids, administration of analgesics, and physical therapy.

Nursing interventions. Nursing care of patients with HIV infection requires complex assessment and intervention skills. Nursing assessment includes evaluation of the neurological status, mouth, respiratory status, abdominal symptoms, and peripheral sensation. As with all immunosuppressed patients, those with HIV infection must be protected from infection (see "Nursing Care Plan for the Immunocompromised Patient"). These patients provide additional clinical challenges because of their multisystem clinical complications. For unclear reasons, persons with HIV infection have a higher propensity for adverse drug reactions than other patient groups and require careful monitoring of all medication regimens.

Desired patient outcomes of medical treatment and nursing interventions include absence of infection, adequate oxygenation, adequate nutrition and hydration, skin integrity, and absence of pain. Complications such as diarrhea and seizures are controlled. Lastly, the patient understands disease transmission, the course of the disease, symptoms of opportunistic infections, treatments, and medications.

BLEEDING DISORDERS

Patients with abnormal hemostasis often require critical care treatment. A general approach to assessing and managing the bleeding patient is addressed before a more thorough discussion of thrombocytopenia and DIC.

The Bleeding Patient
Pathophysiology
Bleeding disorders, also referred to as *coagulopathies,* are caused by abnormalities in one of the stages of clotting. Disorders are considered inherited (e.g., hemophilia, von Willebrand disease) or acquired (e.g., vitamin K deficiency, DIC).[17] Coagulopathies induce bleeding manifestations, and many care principles are universal. This section addresses the universal care of patients with disorders of coagulation.

Assessment and Clinical Manifestations
A patient with abnormal bleeding requires a careful medical and social history. It is important to assess for medical disorders and medications known to interfere with platelets, coagulation proteins, or fibrinolysis. Disruptions in hemostasis commonly occur with renal disease, hepatic or gastrointestinal disorders, and malnutrition. Medications that may alter hemostasis include aminoglycosides, anticoagulants, antiplatelet agents, cephalosporins, histamine blockers, nitrates, sulfonamides, sympathomimetics, and vasodilators.

The physical examination is extremely important. Although many patients with bleeding disorders demonstrate active bleeding from body orifices, mucous membranes, and open lesions or intravenous line sites, equal numbers of patients have less obvious bleeding. The most susceptible sites for bleeding are existing openings in the epithelial surfaces. Mucous membranes have a low threshold for bleeding because the capillaries lie close to the membrane surface, and minor injury may damage and expose vessels. Substantial blood loss can occur in any coagulopathy, resulting in hypovolemic shock. A general overview of assessment findings that indicate bleeding is included in Table 16-5.

Diagnostic tests are performed to evaluate the cause of the bleeding disorder and the extent of blood loss.[6] The CBC provides quantitative values for RBCs and platelets. When the disorder arises from coagulation protein or clot lysis abnormalities, screening coagulation tests of fibrinogen level, prothrombin time, and partial thromboplastin time are usually ordered. Point-of-care tests for hemoglobin, hematocrit, and partial thromboplastin time are important resources to obtain immediate feedback regarding the patient's status. In certain disease states, additional specialized tests such as bleeding time and levels of fibrin degradation products are monitored.

Nursing Diagnoses
The actively bleeding patient or one with a hemostatic disorder can have bleeding in any body system. The major diagnoses include risk for bleeding, altered protection, decreased tissue perfusion, fluid volume deficit, and pain (see box, "Nursing Care Plan for the Patient with a Bleeding Disorder" as well as the "Nursing Care Plan for the Patient in Shock" in Chapter 11).

Medical Interventions
Medical treatment for bleeding patients depends on the suspected cause. Component-specific replacement transfusions are preferred over whole blood because they provide more targeted treatment of the bleeding disorder. Transfusion thresholds are established based on laboratory values and patient-specific variables. In general, a threshold for RBC transfusion is considered a hematocrit of 28% to 31%, based on the patient's cardiovascular tolerance (see box, "Evidence-Based Practice"). If angina or orthostasis is present, a higher threshold may be maintained. The threshold for transfusing platelets is usually between 20,000 and 50,000/microliter. Cryoprecipitate is usually infused if the fibrinogen level is less than 100 mg/dL.[3] Fresh frozen plasma is used to correct a prolonged prothrombin time and partial thromboplastin time or a specific factor deficiency.[3] A summary of blood product components, clinical indications, and nursing implications is included in Table 16-11.

When the cause of bleeding is unknown or multifactorial, nonspecific interventions aimed at stopping bleeding are used. These include local and systemic procoagulant medications and therapies. Local therapies to stop bleeding are used when systemic anticoagulation is necessary for treatment of another health condition (e.g., myocardial infarction, ischemic stroke, or pulmonary embolism). Local procoagulants act by direct tissue contact and initiation of a surface clot.

◎ NURSING CARE PLAN

for the Patient with a Bleeding Disorder

NURSING DIAGNOSIS

Altered tissue perfusion related to abnormal clotting, hypotension, and/or anemia

PATIENT OUTCOMES

Adequate perfusion maintained and damage to vital organs prevented

- Vital signs and hemodynamic stability, values within normal limits
- Normal mental status
- Arterial blood gas results within normal limits
- Urine output >30 mL/hr
- Skin warm with normal color for the patient
- Adequate peripheral pulses

NURSING INTERVENTIONS	RATIONALES
• Monitor hemodynamic parameters, vital signs, ABGs, I&O, and laboratory results	• Assess hemodynamic status to provide baseline
• Assess for and report signs of altered perfusion	• Assess for blood loss
• Provide good skin and oral care	• Promote circulation
• Evaluate vital signs for orthostatic changes	• Assess for blood loss
• Ensure no administration of rectal medications, IM injections, or flossing of teeth	• Prevent disruption in skin and mucous membranes
• Recognize signs and symptoms of subcutaneous bleeding (e.g., oozing, ecchymoses, hematomas)	• Assess for bleeding disorders
• Note increased girth of limbs or abdomen. Mark anatomical area for consistency of measurement	• Assess for bleeding into limbs and/or abdomen
• Elevate any limb that is bleeding	• Reduce blood flow to the area to prevent further blood loss
• Administer blood components as ordered and monitor for adverse effects	• Treat etiology of bleeding disorder
• Administer selective vasoconstrictor agents (e.g., vasopressin) as ordered	• Promote vasoconstriction and decrease bleeding
• Administer procoagulants (e.g., somatostatin, estrogen) as ordered	• Promote clotting and decrease bleeding
• Administer topical hemostatic agents if indicated	• Decrease bleeding from skin lesions

Based on data from Gulanick M and Myers JL. *Nursing Care Plans: Diagnoses, Interventions, and Outcomes,* 7th ed. St. Louis: Mosby; 2011.

EVIDENCE-BASED PRACTICE

Red Blood Cells Transfusion

Problem

Transfusion of red blood cells (RBCs) is not a benign procedure. It is associated with complications, including transfusion reactions and acute lung injury. Determining clinical indicators for transfusion, including thresholds, is important.

Clinical Question

What are outcomes associated with RBC transfusions? What clinical indicators and thresholds should be used to trigger transfusion orders?

Evidence

The meta-analysis conducted by Murad and colleagues evaluated 37 studies that were of mixed quality. They found that massive transfusion substantially reduced the risk of death in the trauma population. However, when massive transfusion was not indicated (e.g., surgery), transfusion was associated with an increased risk for death (not statistically significant) and a three-fold increased risk of developing acute lung injury.[2] *Cochrane Reviews* evaluated 17 trials of transfusion given by triggers versus clinical judgment. The researchers found that restrictive transfusions based on triggers significantly reduced the risk for infection, and no differences between groups on mortality, complications, and lengths of stay.[1] The Consensus Group of 15 experts reviewed data from 494 published articles and then rated appropriateness of transfusion in many scenarios. This group did not support transfusion if the hemoglobin was 10 g/dL or higher. Most supported transfusion when the hemoglobin fell below 8 g/dL. Transfusion when the hemoglobin is between 8 and 10 g/dL needs to be based on comorbidities of the patient (such as cardiac disease). They concluded that many areas related to transfusion practices need further study.[3]

Continued

EVIDENCE-BASED PRACTICE

Red Blood Cells Transfusion—cont'd

Implications for Nursing

With the exception of the trauma patient who requires massive transfusion, administration of RBCs is associated with a higher risk for acute lung injury and mortality. More restrictive use of transfusion therapy is recommended, with most experts not recommending a transfusion unless the hemoglobin falls below 8 g/dL. The patient's underlying comorbidities must be considered in decision making. Nurses must monitor serial hemoglobin levels and assess patients for signs and symptoms related to lower hemoglobin and hematocrit levels. If transfusion is suggested at a higher threshold, nurses should discuss rationale with the physician.

Level of Evidence

A—Meta-analysis

References

1. Carless PA, Henry DA, Carson JL, et al. Transfusion thresholds and other strategies for guiding allogeneic red blood cell transfusion. *Cochrane Database of Systematic Reviews.* 2010;10:Art. No. CD002042.
2. Murad MH, Stubbs JR, Gandhi MJ, et al. The effect of plasma transfusion on morbidity and mortality: a systematic review and meta-analysis. *Transfusion.* 2010;50:1370-1383.
3. Shander A, Fink A, Javidroozi M, et al. International Consensus Conference on Transfusion Outcomes Group. Appropriateness of allogeneic red blood cell transfusion: the international consensus conference on transfusion outcomes. *Transfusion Medicine Review.* 2011;25:232-246.

TABLE 16-11 SUMMARY OF BLOOD PRODUCTS AND ADMINISTRATION

BLOOD COMPONENT	DESCRIPTION	ACTIONS	INDICATIONS	ADMINISTRATION	COMPLICATIONS
Whole blood	RBCs, plasma, and stable clotting factors	Restores oxygen-carrying capacity and intravascular volume	Symptomatic anemia with major circulating volume deficit Massive hemorrhage with shock	Donor and recipient must be ABO compatible and Rh compatible Use microaggregate filter *Rate of infusion:* usually 2-4 unit/hour but more rapid in cases of shock	Hemolytic reaction Allergic reaction Hypothermia Electrolyte disturbances Citrate intoxication Infectious diseases
RBCs	RBCs centrifuged from whole blood	Restores oxygen-carrying capacity and intravascular volume	Symptomatic anemia when patient is at risk for fluid overload Acute hemorrhage	Donor and recipient must be ABO and Rh compatible Use microaggregate filter *Rate of infusion:* 2-4 unit/hour but more rapid in cases of shock	Infectious diseases Hemolytic reaction Allergic reaction Hypothermia Electrolyte disturbances Citrate intoxication
Leukocyte-poor cells or washed RBCs	RBCs from which leukocytes and plasma proteins have been reduced	Restores oxygen-carrying capacity and intravascular volume	Symptomatic anemia with patient history of repeated, febrile, nonhemolytic transfusion reactions Acute hemorrhage	Donor and recipient must be ABO and Rh compatible Use microaggregate filter *Rate of infusion:* 2-4 units/hour but more rapid in cases of shock	Allergic reaction Hemolytic reaction Hypothermia Electrolyte disturbances Citrate intoxication Infectious diseases

TABLE 16-11   SUMMARY OF BLOOD PRODUCTS AND ADMINISTRATION—cont'd

BLOOD COMPONENT	DESCRIPTION	ACTIONS	INDICATIONS	ADMINISTRATION	COMPLICATIONS
Fresh frozen plasma	Plasma rich in clotting factors with platelets removed	Replaces clotting factors	Deficit of coagulation factors as in DIC, liver disease, and massive transfusions Major trauma with signs/symptoms of hemorrhage	Donor and recipient must be ABO compatible, but not necessary to be Rh compatible *Rate of infusion:* 10 mL/min	Allergic reaction Febrile reactions Circulatory overload Infectious diseases
Platelets	Removed from whole blood	Increases platelet count and improves hemostasis	Thrombocytopenia Platelet dysfunction (prophylactically for platelet counts 10,000-20,000/ microliter), evidence of bleeding with platelet count <50,000/microliter	Do not use microaggregate filter; component filter obtained from blood bank ABO testing not necessary unless contaminated with RBCs but is usually done Usually give 6 units at one time	Infectious diseases Allergic reactions Febrile reactions
Cryoprecipitate antihemophilic factor	Coagulation factor VIII with 250 mg of fibrinogen and 20%-30% of factor XIII	Replaces selected clotting factors	Hemophilia A, von Willebrand disease Hypofibrinogenemia Factor XIII deficiency Massive transfusions	Repeat doses may be necessary to attain satisfactory serum level *Rate of infusion:* approximately 10 mL of diluted component per minute	Allergic reactions Infectious diseases
Albumin	Prepared from plasma	Expands intravascular volume by increasing oncotic pressure	Hypovolemic shock Liver failure	Special administration set Rate of infusion: over 30-60 minutes	Circulatory overload Febrile reaction
Granulocytes	Prepared by centrifugation or filtration leukopheresis, which removes granulocytes from whole blood	Increases the leukocyte level	Decreased WBCs usually from chemotherapy or radiation	Must be ABO compatible and Rh compatible *Rate of infusion:* 1 unit over 2-4 hours; closely observe for reaction	Rash Febrile reaction Hepatitis
Plasma proteins	Pooled from human plasma	Expands intravascular volume by increasing oncotic pressure	Hypovolemic shock	ABO compatibility not necessary *Rate of infusion:* over 30-60 minutes	Circulatory overload Febrile reaction

DIC, Disseminated intravascular coagulation; *RBCs,* red blood cells; *WBCs,* white blood cells.

Systemic procoagulant medications may be used judiciously to enhance vasoconstriction (e.g., vasopressin), enhance clot formation (e.g., somatostatin), or prevent fibrinolysis (e.g., aminocaproic acid). Each agent has significant adverse effects that must be considered before implementation. All may enhance clot production and induce thrombotic vascular or neurological events. They may be contraindicated when the patient has simultaneous procoagulant risk factors.

Nursing Interventions

Patients with bleeding disorders often have multisystem manifestations. Administration of fluids and blood products is a priority nursing intervention that requires careful consideration of the patient's specific coagulation defect. When the patient's blood does not clot because of thrombocytopenia, administration of RBCs before platelets will result in RBC loss from disrupted vascular structures.

Additional nursing interventions specific to the patient with a coagulopathy include the following: weigh dressings to assess blood loss, assess fluids for occult blood, observe for oozing and bleeding from skin and mucous membranes, and leave clots undisturbed. Precautions such as limiting invasive procedures, including indwelling urinary catheters or rectal temperature measurement, are also important.

Thrombocytopenia
Pathophysiology

A quantitative deficiency of platelets is termed *thrombocytopenia.* By definition, this is a platelet count of less than 150,000/microliter.[3,21] A value of 30,000/microliter is considered critically low, and spontaneous bleeding may occur.[3] Fatal hemorrhage is a great risk when the count is less than 10,000/microliter.[20] The pathophysiology may be related to decreased production of platelets by the bone marrow, increased destruction of platelets, or sequestration of platelets (abnormal distribution).[21,23]

Assessment and Clinical Manifestations

Many critical care therapies and medications interfere with platelet production or life span and cause thrombocytopenia. A thorough medical, social, and medication history can help to identify factors that may cause thrombocytopenia (Box 16-4). Heparin-induced thrombocytopenia (HIT) can occur and is described in Box 16-5.[6,21]

Clinically, the patient with thrombocytopenia presents with petechiae, purpura, and ecchymoses, with oozing from mucous membranes. The patient may also have melena, hematuria, or epistaxis.

Nursing Diagnoses

Patients with thrombocytopenia have many of the nursing diagnoses listed in care of the bleeding patient. Additional diagnoses include potential for bleeding and altered body image related to petechiae and ecchymoses (see box, "Clinical Alert: Bleeding Disorders").

BOX 16-4   CAUSES OF THROMBOCYTOPENIA

Bone Marrow Suppression
- Aplastic anemia
- Burns
- Cancer chemotherapy
- Exposure to ionizing radiation
- Nutritional deficiency (vitamin B_{12}, folate)

Interference with Platelet Production (Other than Nonspecific Marrow Suppression)
- Alcohol
- Histamine$_2$-blocking agents
- Histoplasmosis
- Hormones
- Thiazide diuretics

Platelet Destruction Outside the Bone Marrow
- Artificial heart valves
- Cardiac bypass machine
- Heat stroke
- Heparin
- Infections: severe or sepsis
- Large-bore intravenous lines
- Intraaortic balloon pump
- Splenic sequestration of platelets
- Sulfonamides
- Transfusions
- Trimethoprim-sulfamethoxazole

Immune Response Against Platelets
- Idiopathic thrombocytopenic purpura
- Mononucleosis
- Thrombotic thrombocytopenic purpura
- Vaccinations
- Viral illness

Interference with Platelet Function
- Aminoglycosides
- Catecholamines: epinephrine, dopamine
- Cirrhosis
- Dextran
- Diabetes mellitus
- Diazepam
- Digitoxin
- Hypothermia
- Loop diuretics
- Malignant lymphomas
- Nonsteroidal antiinflammatory agents
- Phenothiazines
- Phenytoin
- Salicylate derivatives
- Sarcoidosis
- Scleroderma
- Systemic lupus erythematosus
- Thyrotoxicosis
- Tricyclic antidepressants
- Uremia
- Vitamin E

BOX 16-5 HEPARIN-INDUCED THROMBOCYTOPENIA

Definition

Two types of heparin-induced thrombocytopenia (HIT) have been identified. Type I HIT is a nonimmunological response to heparin treatment, and it is thought to occur from an interaction between heparin and circulating platelets causing direct agglutination of platelets. It is usually self-limiting. Type II HIT is a severe immune-mediated drug reaction that can occur in any patient who has received heparin. Heparin binds to platelet factor 4 (PF4), forming an antigenic complex on the surface of the platelets. Some patients develop an antibody to this complex. The antibody stimulates removal of platelets by splenic macrophages, and thrombocytopenia develops. The primary complication of HIT is not bleeding, but thrombosis.

Risks

Up to 50% of patients who receive unfractionated heparin develop antibodies. However, the risk for developing Type II HIT is low, ranging from 0.5% to 5%.

Complications

Complications of Type I HIT are those associated with a low platelet count. Type II HIT is more severe, and its major complications are thromboembolic in nature. These include deep vein thrombosis, pulmonary embolism, myocardial infarction, thrombotic stroke, arterial occlusion in limbs, and disseminated intravascular coagulation.

Diagnosis

HIT usually develops 5 to 10 days after initiation of heparin therapy; however, rapid-onset HIT can occur within the first hours after heparin exposure. In Type I HIT, the platelet count does not usually fall below 100,000/microliter; no laboratory tests are required. Type II HIT is suspected if the platelet count drops below 100,000/microliter, or more than 50% from baseline values. Heparin-PF4 antibody testing assists in confirmation of Type II HIT. However, results may not be known rapidly, and treatment should start if HIT is suspected.

Treatment

Type I HIT is usually self-limiting. Type II HIT is treated by discontinuing all heparin products, including heparin flushes and heparin-coated infusion catheters. Treatment focuses on administration of drugs that inhibit thrombin formation or cause direct thrombin inhibition: lepirudin (Refludan), bivalirudin (Angiomax), or argatroban (Novastan). Treatment with warfarin, low–molecular weight heparin, aminocaproic acid, and platelets is avoided because these agents may exacerbate the prothrombotic state.

From Rizoli S, Aird WC. Thrombocytopenia. In Vincent JL, Abraham E, Moore FA, et al, eds. *Textbook of Critical Care.* 6th ed. Philadelphia: Saunders. 2011; Warkentin TE. Heparin-induced thrombocytopenia. *Hematology/Oncology Clinics of North America.* 2007;21:589-607.

! CLINICAL ALERT

Bleeding Disorders

All body surfaces should be inspected for overt bleeding such as bruising or petechiae that indicate subcutaneous bleeding. Internal bleeding is more difficult to recognize because bleeding may occur even without a known injury, and symptoms are often subtle.

Medical Interventions

Medical treatment of thrombocytopenia includes infusions of platelets. Patients who require multiple platelet transfusions should be evaluated for single-donor platelet products, which permit administration of 6 to 10 units of platelets with exposure to the antigens of only one person. For every unit of single-donor platelets, the platelet count should increase by 5000 to 10,000/microliter.[7] Patients who receive many platelet transfusions can become refractory, or alloimmunized, to the many different platelet antigens and may only benefit from receiving platelets that are a match for the patient's human leukocyte antigen (HLA) type. After multiple platelet transfusions, febrile and allergic transfusion reactions are common but can be reduced by administration of acetaminophen and diphenhydramine before transfusion.

Thrombopoietin, a platelet stimulating cytokine, is being investigated as an alternative to platelet transfusion. Some thrombocytopenias are autoimmune induced and

may respond to filtration of antibodies via plasmapheresis or immune suppression with corticosteroids. When the spleen is enlarged and tender and these other supportive therapies are unsuccessful, splenectomy can alleviate the autoimmune reaction.

Nursing Interventions

Nursing interventions for the patient with thrombocytopenia are similar to those listed for the bleeding patient. The nurse must recognize and limit factors that can deplete or shorten the life span of platelets. For example, high fever and high metabolic activity (e.g., seizures) prematurely destroy platelets.

Desired patient outcomes include adequate tissue perfusion, skin integrity, prompt recognition and treatment of bleeding, and absence of pain.

Disseminated Intravascular Coagulation
Pathophysiology

DIC is a serious disorder of hemostasis characterized by exaggerated microvascular coagulation, depletion of clotting factors, and subsequent bleeding.[16] Because clotting factors are used up in the abnormal coagulation process, this disorder is also termed consumption coagulopathy.

The clinical course of DIC ranges from an acute, life-threatening process to a chronic, low-grade condition. Sepsis is the most common cause of acute DIC.[21,24] Acute DIC develops rapidly and is the most serious form of acquired coagulopathy. With chronic DIC, the patient may have more subtle clinical and laboratory findings.

Whatever the initiating event in DIC, procoagulants that cause diffuse, uncontrolled clotting are released. The intrinsic or extrinsic pathways are activated by release of tissue factor, from either endothelial damage (intrinsic) or direct tissue damage (extrinsic). Large amounts of thrombin are produced, resulting in the deposition of fibrin in the microvasculature, the consumption of available clotting factors, and the stimulation of fibrinolysis.

Clotting in the microvasculature of the patient with DIC causes organ ischemia and necrosis. The skin, lungs, and kidneys are most often damaged. Thrombophlebitis, pulmonary

embolism, cerebrovascular accident, gastrointestinal bleeding, and renal failure may result from thrombosis. In addition, microvasculature thrombosis may result in cyanosis of the fingers and toes, purpura fulminans, or infarction and gangrene of the digits or tip of the nose or penis.[23]

The fibrinolysis that ensues results in the release of fibrin degradation products, which are potent anticoagulants that interfere with thrombin, fibrin, and platelet activity. RBCs are damaged as they try to pass through the blocked capillary beds; the damage to RBCs causes excess hemolysis. The lack of available clotting factors coupled with the anticoagulant forces results in an inability to form clots when needed and predisposes the patient with DIC to hemorrhage (Figure 16-7).

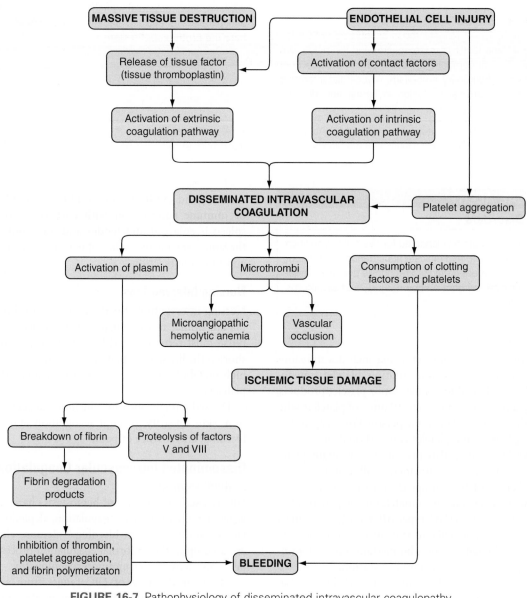

FIGURE 16-7 Pathophysiology of disseminated intravascular coagulopathy.

Assessment and Clinical Manifestations

DIC is always a secondary complication of excessive clotting stimuli and may be triggered by vessel injury caused by disease states, tissue injury, or a foreign body in the bloodstream. Sepsis, multisystem trauma, and burns are the main risk factors for DIC and also provide the most significant stimuli for the clotting cascade.[6] Recognition of potential risk factors and conscientious monitoring of the high-risk patient can permit early intervention. A summary of common risk factors for DIC is included in Table 16-12.

Clinically, the patient with DIC first develops microvascular thrombosis. Thrombosis leads to organ ischemia and necrosis that may be manifested as changes in mental status, angina, hypoxemia, oliguria, or nonspecific hepatitis. Cyanosis and infarction of the fingers and toes as well as infarction of the tip of the nose may occur if the DIC is severe. After a thrombotic phase of hours to a few days, depletion of clotting factors and clot lysis cause excessive bleeding. Early signs may include occult blood in the stool, emesis, and urine. Capillary fragility and depleted clotting factors often appear early as mucosal or subcutaneous tissue bleeding seen as gingival bleeding, petechiae, or ecchymoses. Overt bleeding ranges from mild oozing from venipuncture sites to massive hemorrhage from all body orifices. Occult bleeding into body cavities, such as the peritoneal and retroperitoneal spaces, may be detected by vital sign changes or other classic signs of blood loss.[6,21]

Diagnosis of DIC is made based on recognition of pertinent risk factors, clinical symptoms, and the results of laboratory studies. Evidence of factor depletion in the form of thrombocytopenia and low fibrinogen levels is seen in the early phase; however, definitive diagnosis is made by evidence of excess fibrinolysis detectable by elevated fibrin degradation products, an increased D-dimer level, or a decreased antithrombin III level.[6,21] Altered laboratory values in DIC are noted in the box, "Laboratory Alert: Disseminated Intravascular Coagulation."

⚠ LABORATORY ALERT
Disseminated Intravascular Coagulation

TEST	NORMAL VALUE	ALTERATION
Platelet count	150,000-400,000/ microliter	Decreased
Prothrombin time	11-16 seconds	Prolonged
Activated partial thromboplastin time	30-45 seconds	Prolonged
Thrombin time	10-15 seconds	Prolonged
Fibrinogen	150-400 mg/dL	Decreased
Fibrin degradation products	<10 mcg/mL	Increased
Antithrombin III	>50% of control (plasma)	Decreased
D-Dimer assay	<100 mcg/L	Increased
Protein C	71%-142% of normal activity	Decreased
Protein S	61%-130% of normal activity	Decreased

Nursing Diagnoses

The patient with DIC is likely to have multiple system involvement that encompasses both thrombotic and hemorrhagic manifestations. Nursing diagnoses may include altered tissue perfusion, fluid volume deficit, impaired skin integrity, and pain.

Medical Interventions

Medical treatment of DIC is aimed at identifying and treating the underlying cause, stopping the abnormal coagulation, and controlling the bleeding. Correction of hypotension, hypoxemia, and acidosis is vital, as is treatment of infection if it is the triggering factor. If the cause is obstetrical, evacuation

TABLE 16-12	CAUSES OF DISSEMINATED INTRAVASCULAR COAGULATION
CAUSE	**EXAMPLES**
Infections	Bacterial (especially gram-negative), fungal, viral, mycobacterial, protozoan, rickettsial
Trauma	Burns; crush or multiple injuries; snakebite; severe head injury
Obstetrical	Abruptio placentae, placenta previa, amniotic fluid embolism, retained dead fetus, missed abortion, eclampsia, hydatidiform mole, septic abortion
Hematological/immunological disorders	Transfusion reaction, transplant rejections, anaphylaxis, acute hemolysis, transfusion of mismatched blood products, autoimmune disorders, sickle cell crisis
Oncological disorders	Carcinomas, leukemias, metastatic cancer
Miscellaneous	Extracorporeal circulation, pulmonary or fat embolism, anoxia, acidosis, hyperthermia or hypothermia, hypovolemic shock, ARDS, sustained hypotension, shock

ARDS, Acute respiratory distress syndrome.
From Marti-Carvajal AJ, Simancas D, Cardona AF. Treatment for disseminated intravascular coagulation in patients with acute and chronic leukemia. *The Cochrane Database of Systematic Reviews.* 2011;15(6):CD008562.

of the uterus for retained fetal tissue or other tissue must be performed. Blood volume expanders and crystalloid intravenous fluids, such as lactated Ringer solution or normal saline, are given to counteract hypovolemia caused by blood loss.

Blood component therapy is used in DIC to replace deficient platelets and clotting factors and to treat hemorrhage. Platelet infusions are usually necessary because of consumptive thrombocytopenia. Administration of platelets is the highest priority for transfusion because they provide the clotting factors needed to establish an initial platelet plug from any bleeding site. Fresh frozen plasma is administered for fibrinogen replacement. It contains all clotting factors and antithrombin III; however, factor VIII is often inactivated by the freezing process, thus necessitating administration of concentrated factor VIII in the form of cryoprecipitate.[6,21,23] Transfusions of packed RBCs are given to replace cells lost in hemorrhage.

Heparin is a potent thrombin inhibitor and may be administered, in low doses, to block the clotting process that initiates DIC. Heparin is given to prevent further clotting and thrombosis that may lead to organ ischemia and necrosis. Although heparin's antithrombin activity prevents further clotting, it may increase the risk of bleeding and may cause further problems. Its use is controversial when it is administered to patients with DIC.[6,23]

Other pharmacological therapy in DIC includes the administration of synthetic antithrombin III, which also inhibits thrombin.[6,21] Antithrombin III concentrates may shorten the course of the disease and may increase the survival rate. Administration of aminocaproic acid (Amicar) inhibits fibrinolysis by interfering with plasmin activity. Fibrinolytics should be given only if other treatments have been unsuccessful and hemorrhage is life-threatening, as there is no clear evidence of the risk versus benefit with their use.[6]

Nursing Interventions

Nursing care of the patient with DIC is aimed at the prevention and recognition of thrombotic and hemorrhagic events. Continuous assessment for complications facilitates prompt and aggressive interventions. Psychosocial support of the patient and family is very important. Few patients who survive DIC are without some functional deficit caused by ischemia or hemorrhage.

Pain relief and promotion of comfort are important nursing priorities. The location, intensity, and quality of the patient's pain are assessed, along with the patient's response to discomfort. The nurse is conscientious not to enhance vasoconstriction, because it contributes to tissue ischemia and its associated discomfort. Relief of discomfort also reduces oxygen consumption, which is important for these patients with limited circulatory flow. Pain medication is offered as ordered and before painful procedures. Positioning, with support and proper body alignment and frequent changes, also enhances the patient's level of comfort.

Coagulation laboratory studies are carefully monitored for evidence of disease resolution. As fewer clots are created, the platelet count and fibrinogen level are among the first laboratory tests to return to normal. The fibrin degradation products and D-dimer levels fall, and antithrombin III levels rise, as fibrinolysis slows. Other coagulation tests are less sensitive and are not usually assessed.

The main desired outcomes for the patient with DIC include adequate oxygenation, adequate tissue perfusion, absence of bleeding, and skin integrity. Absence of pain and effective coping are additional expected outcomes.

CASE STUDY

Mr. F. is a 62-year-old man with acute myelogenous leukemia diagnosed 15 months ago. He received induction (high dose) chemotherapy, which resulted in disease remission. He received additional chemotherapy over the next 4 months, and underwent an allogeneic peripheral blood stem cell transplant (identical-matched donor; his sister). He was started on standard immunosuppressive drugs to prevent graft-versus-host disease (GVHD). Forty-three days after his transplant, Mr. F. was diagnosed with acute GVHD (skin changes on arms and palms of hands). During a routine follow-up visit, Mr. F. complains of mucositis and xerostomia, photosensitivity, dry and irritated eyes, joint pain, a rash on his arms, and an 8-lb weight loss since his last visit 1 month ago.

Questions
1. What risk factors are associated with developing chronic GVHD?
2. What are possible signs and symptoms of chronic GVHD?
3. What is the priority of care for the patient experiencing chronic GVHD?
4. What are key nursing interventions for the patient with chronic GVHD?

SUMMARY

All critically ill patients have the potential for hematological or immunological dysfunction. A thorough understanding of normal anatomy and physiology provides the critical care nurse with a basis on which a comprehensive assessment and treatment approach can be built. Because nurses play a key role in the outcome of patients with serious alterations in the hematological and immune systems, this knowledge is critical and has great impact on the well-being of patients.

CRITICAL THINKING EXERCISES

1. What disorders in critical care are associated with anemia?
2. Why is the critical care unit often a dangerous place for the immunosuppressed patient?
3. How can therapeutic choices such as interventions and medications worsen the hematological or immunological compromise of critically ill patients?
4. What criteria are to be used for prioritization of nursing and medical interventions for the bleeding patient?

REFERENCES

1. Cady J, Jackowski JA. Cancer. In Lewis SL, Dirksen SR, Heitkemper MM, et al, eds. *Medical-Surgical Nursing: Assessment and Management of Clinical Problems.* 8th ed. St. Louis: Mosby. 2011;260-300.
2. Centers for Disease Control and Prevention. Diagnoses of HIV Infection and AIDS in the United States and Dependent Areas, 2009. *HIV Surveillance Report,* Volume 21 http://www.cdc.gov/hiv/surveillance/resources/reports/2009report/index.htm; 2011 Accessed December 20, 2011.
3. Chernecky CC, Berger BJ. *Laboratory Tests and Diagnostic Procedures.* 5th ed. Philadelphia: Saunders. 2008.
4. Croghan A, Heitkemper MM. Nursing management: liver, pancreas, and biliary tract problems. In Lewis SL, Dirksen SR, Heitkemper MM, et al, eds. *Medical-Surgical Nursing: Assessment and Management of Clinical Problems.* 8th ed. St. Louis: Mosby. 2011;1058-1102.
5. Darmon M, Azoulay E. Management of neutropenic cancer patients. In Vincent JL, Abraham E, Moore FA, et al, eds. *Textbook of Critical Care.* 6th ed. Philadelphia: Saunders. 2011;1141-1144.
6. Ferri FF. *Ferri's Clinical Advisor: Instant Diagnosis and Treatment.* Philadelphia: Mosby. 2011.
7. Gulanick M, Myers JL. *Nursing Care Plans: Diagnosis, Interventions, and Outcomes.* 7th ed. St. Louis: Mosby. 2011.
8. Hall JE. Hemostasis and blood coagulation. In Hall JE, ed. *Guyton and Hall Textbook of Medical Physiology.* 12th ed. Philadelphia: Saunders. 2011;451-461.
9. Hall JE. Resistance of the body to infection: I. Leukocytes, granulocytes, the monocyte-macrophage system, and inflammation. In Hall JE, ed. *Guyton and Hall Textbook of Medical Physiology.* 12th ed. Philadelphia: Saunders. 2011;423-432.
10. Hall JE. Red blood cells, anemia, and polycythemia. In Hall JE, ed. *Guyton and Hall Textbook of Medical Physiology.* 12th ed. Philadelphia: Saunders. 2011;413-422.
11. Hall JE. Resistance of the body to infection: II. Immunity and the allergy innate immunity. In Hall JE, ed. *Guyton and Hall Textbook of Medical Physiology.* 12th ed. Philadelphia: Saunders. 2011;433-444.
12. Hall JE. Transport of oxygen and carbon dioxide in blood and tissue fluids. In J. E. Hall *Guyton and Hall Textbook of Medical Physiology.* 12th ed. Philadelphia: Saunders. 2011;495-504.
13. Jubelirer SJ. The benefit of the neutropenic diet: fact or fiction? *Oncologist.* 2011;16(5):704-707.
14. Kwong J, Bradley-Springer L. Infection and human immunodeficiency virus infection. In Lewis SL, Dirksen SR, Heitkemper MM, et al, eds. *Medical-Surgical Nursing: Assessment and Management of Clinical Problems.* 8th ed. St. Louis: Mosby. 2011;235-259.
15. Lewis SL. Genetics, altered immune responses, and transplantation. In Lewis SL, Dirksen SR, Heitkemper MM, et al, eds. *Medical-Surgical Nursing: Assessment and Management of Clinical Problems.* 8th ed. St. Louis: Mosby. 2011;206-234.
16. Marti-Carvajal AJ, Simancas D, Cardona AF. Treatment for disseminated intravascular coagulation in patients with acute and chronic leukemia. *Cochrane Database Syst Rev.* 2011;15(6):CD008562.
17. Olah Z, Bereczky Z, Szarvas M, et al. Coagulation: cascade! *Lancet.* 2011;378(9792):740.
18. Patton KT, Thibodeau GA. (2010). Blood. In Patton KT, Thibodeau GA, eds. *Anatomy & Physiology.* 7th ed. St. Louis: Mosby. 2010;582-610.
19. Patton KT, Thibodeau GA. (2010). Immune system. In Patton KT, Thibodeau GA, eds. *Anatomy & Physiology.* 7th ed. St. Louis: Mosby. 2010;723-759.
20. Rizoli S, Aird WC. Thrombocytopenia. In Vincent JL, Abraham E, Moore FA, et al, eds. *Textbook of Critical Care.* 6th ed. Philadelphia: Saunders. 2011;78-80.
21. Rizoli S, Aird WC. Coagulopathy. In Vincent JL, Abraham E, Moore FA, et al, eds. *Textbook of Critical Care.* 6th ed. Philadelphia: Saunders. 2011;81-83.
22. Roberts D. Nursing management: arthritis and connective tissue diseases. In Lewis SL, Dirksen SR, Heitkemper MM, et al, eds. *Medical-Surgical Nursing: Assessment and Management of Clinical Problems.* 8th ed. St. Louis: Mosby. 2011;1641-1679.
23. Rome SI. Nursing management: hematologic problems. In Lewis SL, Dirksen SR, Heitkemper MM, et al, eds. *Medical-Surgical Nursing: Assessment and Management of Clinical Problems.* 8th ed. St. Louis: Mosby. 2011;661-713.
24. Rome SI. Nursing assessment: hematologic system. In Lewis SL, Dirksen SR, Heitkemper MM, et al, eds. *Medical-Surgical Nursing: Assessment and Management of Clinical Problems.* 8th ed. St. Louis: Mosby. 2011;642-660.
25. Schonder KS, Weber RJ, Fung JJ, et al. Clinical use of immunosuppressants. In Vincent JL, Abraham E, Moore FA, et al, eds. *Textbook of Critical Care.* 6th ed. Philadelphia: Saunders. 2011;1308-1316.
26. Thames, D. Infection. In Meiner SE, ed. *Gerontologic Nursing.* St. Louis: Mosby. 2011;283-292.
27. Warkentin TE. Heparin-induced thrombocytopenia. *Hematology/Oncology Clinics of North America.* 2007;21:589-607.

CHAPTER

17

Gastrointestinal Alterations

Katherine F. Alford, MSN, RN, CCRN, PCCN

⊖volve WEBSITE

Many additional resources, including self-assessment exercises, are located on the Evolve companion website at
http://evolve.elsevier.com/Sole.
- Review Questions
- Mosby's Nursing Skills Procedures

- Animations
- Video Clips

INTRODUCTION

Body cells require water, electrolytes, and nutrients (carbohydrates, fats, and proteins) to obtain the energy necessary to fuel body functions. The primary function of the alimentary tract (oropharyngeal cavity, esophagus, stomach, and small and large intestine) and accessory organs (pancreas, liver, and gallbladder) is to provide the body with a continual supply of nutrients. In addition, food must move through the system at a rate slow enough for digestive and absorptive functions to occur, but also fast enough to meet the body's needs. Meeting these goals requires the appropriate and timely movement of nutrients through the gastrointestinal (GI) tract *(motility)*, the presence of specific enzymes to break down nutrients *(digestion)*, and the existence of transport mechanisms to move the nutrients into the bloodstream *(absorption)*. Each part is adapted for specific functions, including food passage, storage, digestion, and absorption. This chapter provides a brief physiological review of each section of the GI system and a general assessment of the GI system. This provides the foundation for the discussion of the GI disorders most commonly encountered in the critical care setting: acute upper GI bleeding, acute pancreatitis, and liver failure. The remainder of the chapter reviews the pathophysiology of each disorder, nursing and medical assessments, nursing diagnoses, nursing and medical interventions, and patient outcomes. Complete nursing plans of care for select nursing diagnoses are provided; these serve as valuable summaries of the most common patient care problems and collaborative interventions.

REVIEW OF ANATOMY AND PHYSIOLOGY

Gastrointestinal Tract

The anatomical structure of the GI system is shown in Figure 17-1. It comprises the alimentary canal (beginning at the oropharynx and ending at the anus) and the accessory organs (pancreas, liver, and gallbladder) that empty their products into the canal at certain points. A review of the anatomy of the gut wall is provided as an introduction to this section because it is the foundation for the understanding of absorption of nutrients and GI protective mechanisms.

Gut Wall

The GI tract begins in the esophagus and extends to the rectum. It is composed of multiple tissue layers.

Mucosa. The innermost layer, the mucosa, is the most important physiologically. This layer is exposed to food substances, and it therefore plays a role in nutrient metabolism. The mucosa is also protective. The cells in this layer are connected by tight junctions that produce an effective barrier against large molecules and bacteria. They also protect the GI tract from bacterial colonization. The goblet cells in the mucosa secrete mucus, which provides lubrication for food substances and protects the mucosa from excoriation.

Gastric mucosal barrier. In the stomach, the special architecture of cells of the mucosa and the mucus that is secreted are known as the *gastric mucosal barrier*. This physiological barrier is impermeable to hydrochloric acid, which is normally secreted in the stomach, but it is permeable to other

502

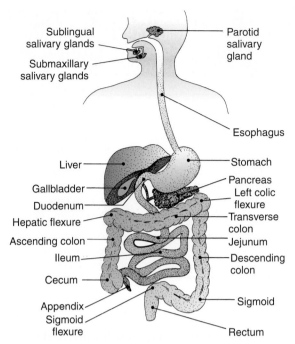

Sublingual salivary glands
Submaxillary salivary glands
Parotid salivary gland
Esophagus
Liver
Stomach
Gallbladder
Pancreas
Duodenum
Left colic flexure
Hepatic flexure
Transverse colon
Ascending colon
Jejunum
Ileum
Descending colon
Cecum
Appendix
Sigmoid
Sigmoid flexure
Rectum

FIGURE 17-1 The gastrointestinal system.

BOX 17-1   SWALLOWING STAGES

Oral: Voluntary
- Initiation of the swallowing process, usually stimulated by a bolus of food in the mouth near the pharynx

Pharyngeal: Involuntary
- Passage of food through the pharynx to the esophagus

Esophageal: Involuntary
- Promotes passage of food from the pharynx to the stomach

substances, such as salicylates, alcohol, steroids, and bile salts. The disruption of this barrier by these types of substances is thought to play a role in ulcer development. In addition, these cells have a special feature—they regenerate rapidly—that explains how disruptions in the mucosa can be quickly healed.

Submucosa. The second layer of the gut wall, the submucosa, is composed of connective tissue, blood vessels, and nerve fibers. The muscular layer is the major layer of the wall. The serosa is the outermost layer.

Beneath the mucosa, submucosa, and muscular layer are various nerve plexuses that are innervated by the autonomic nervous system. Disturbances in these neurons in a given segment of the GI tract cause a lack of motility.

Oropharyngeal Cavity

Mouth. Food substances are ingested into the oral cavity primarily by the intrinsic desire for food called *hunger.* Food in the mouth is initially subject to mechanical breakdown by the act of chewing *(mastication).* Chewing of food is important for digestion of all foods, but particularly for digestion of fruits and raw vegetables, because they require the cellulose membranes around their nutrients to be broken down. The muscles used for chewing are innervated by the motor branch of the fifth cranial nerve.

Salivary glands. Saliva is the major secretion of the oropharynx and is produced by three pairs of salivary glands: submaxillary, sublingual, and parotid. Saliva is rich in mucus, which lubricates food. Salivary amylase, a starch-digesting

enzyme, is also secreted. Stimuli such as sight, smell, thoughts, and taste of food stimulate salivary gland secretion. Parasympathetic stimulation promotes a copious secretion of watery saliva. Conversely, sympathetic stimulation produces a scant output of thick saliva. The normal daily secretion of saliva is 1200 mL.

Pharynx. Swallowing is a complex mechanism involving oral (voluntary), pharyngeal, and esophageal stages. It is made more complex because the pharynx serves several other functions, the most important of which is respiration. The pharynx participates in the function of swallowing for only a few seconds at a time to aid in the propulsion of food, which is triggered by the presence of fluid or food in the pharynx. Box 17-1 outlines the three broad stages of swallowing.

Esophagus

Once fluid or food enters the esophagus, it is propelled through the lumen by the process of *peristalsis,* which involves the relaxation and contraction of esophageal muscles that are stimulated by the bolus of food. This process occurs repeatedly until the food reaches the lower esophageal sphincter, which is the last centimeter of the esophagus. This area is normally contracted and thus prevents reflux of gastric contents into the esophagus, a phenomenon that would damage the lining by gastric acid and enzymes. Waves of peristalsis cause this sphincter to relax and allow food to enter the stomach. Mucosal layers in the esophagus secrete mucus, which protects the lining from damage by gastric secretions or food and also serves as a lubricant.

Stomach

The stomach is located at the distal end of the esophagus. It is divided into four regions: the *cardia,* the *fundus,* the *body,* and the *antrum* (Figure 17-2). The muscular walls form multiple folds that allow for greater expansion of the stomach. The opening at the distal end of the stomach opens into the small intestine and is surrounded by the pyloric sphincter. The motor functions of the stomach include storing food until it can be accommodated by the lower GI tract, mixing food with gastric secretions until it forms a semifluid mixture called *chyme,* and slowly emptying the chyme into the small

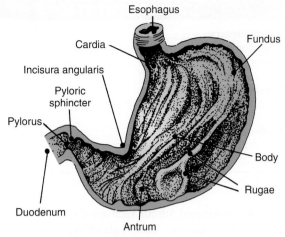

FIGURE 17-2 The stomach.

TABLE 17-2	ELECTROLYTE AND ACID-BASE DISTURBANCES ASSOCIATED WITH THE GASTROINTESTINAL TRACT
FLUID LOSS	**IMBALANCES**
Gastric juice	Metabolic alkalosis Potassium deficit Sodium deficit Fluid volume deficit
Small intestine juice/large intestine juice (recent ileostomy)	Metabolic acidosis Potassium deficit Sodium deficit Fluid volume deficit
Biliary or pancreatic fistula	Metabolic acidosis Sodium deficit Fluid volume deficit

TABLE 17-1	GASTRIC SECRETIONS
GLAND/CELLS	**SECRETION**
Cardiac gland	Mucus
Pyloric gland	Mucus
Fundic (gastric) gland	Mucus
Mucous neck cells	Mucus
Parietal cells	Water Hydrochloric acid Intrinsic factor
Chief cells	Pepsinogen Mucus

intestine at a rate that allows for proper digestion and absorption. Motility is accomplished through peristalsis. The pyloric sphincter at the distal end of the stomach prevents duodenal reflux.

Gastric secretions are produced by mucus-secreting cells that line the inner surface of the stomach and by two types of tubular glands: oxyntic (gastric) glands and pyloric glands. Table 17-1 summarizes the major gastric secretions.

An oxyntic gland is composed of three types of cells: mucous neck cells; peptic, or chief, cells; and oxyntic, or parietal cells. *Mucous cells* secrete a viscid and alkaline mucus that coats the stomach mucosa, thereby providing protection and lubrication for food transport. *Parietal cells* secrete hydrochloric acid solution, which begins the digestion of food in the stomach. Hydrochloric acid is very acidic (pH, 0.8). Stimulants of hydrochloric acid secretion include vagal stimulation, gastrin, and the chemical properties of chyme. Histamine, which stimulates the release of gastrin, also stimulates the secretion of hydrochloric acid. Current drug therapies for ulcer disease use H_2-histamine receptor blockers that block the effects of histamine and therefore hydrochloric acid stimulation. The acidic environment of the stomach

promotes the conversion of pepsinogen, a proteolytic enzyme secreted by gastric chief cells, to pepsin. Pepsin begins the initial breakdown of proteins. Pepsin is active only in a highly acidic environment (pH less than 5); therefore hydrochloric acid secretion is essential for protein digestion.

An essential protein secreted only by the stomach's parietal cells is *intrinsic factor*. Intrinsic factor is necessary for the absorption of vitamin B_{12} in the ileum. Vitamin B_{12} is critical for the formation of red blood cells (RBCs), and a deficiency in this vitamin causes anemia.

The stomach also secretes fluid that is rich in sodium, potassium, and other electrolytes. Loss of these fluids via vomiting or gastric suction places the patient at risk for fluid and electrolyte imbalances and acid-base disturbances (Table 17-2).

Small Intestine

The segment spanning the first 10 to 12 inches of the small intestine is called the *duodenum.* This anatomical area is physiologically important because pancreatic juices and bile from the liver empty into this structure. The duodenum also contains an extensive network of mucus-secreting glands called *Brunner's glands.* The function of this mucus is to protect the duodenal wall from digestion by gastric juice. Secretion of mucus by Brunner's glands is inhibited by sympathetic stimulation, which leaves the duodenum unprotected from gastric juice. This inhibition is thought to be one of the reasons why this area of the GI tract is the site for more than 50% of peptic ulcers.

The segment spanning the next 7 to 8 feet of the small intestine is called the *jejunum,* and the remaining 10 to 12 feet comprise the *ileum.* The opening into the first part of the large intestine is protected by the *ileocecal valve,* which prevents reflux of colonic contents back into the ileum.

The movements of the small intestine include mixing contractions and propulsive contractions. The chyme in the

TABLE 17-3 PANCREATIC ENZYMES AND THEIR ACTIONS

ENZYME	ACTION
Trypsin*	Digests proteins
Chymotrypsin*	Digests proteins
Carboxypolypeptidase*	Digests proteins
Ribonuclease	Digests proteins
Deoxyribonuclease	Digests proteins
Pancreatic amylase	Digests carbohydrates
Pancreatic lipase	Digests fats
Cholesterol esterase	Digests fats

*Activated only after it is secreted into the intestinal tract.

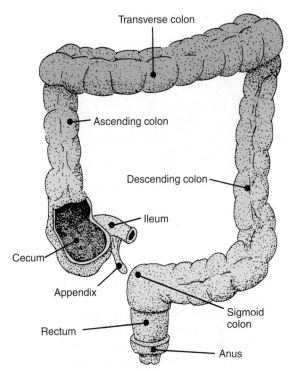

FIGURE 17-3 The intestinal system.

small intestine takes 3 to 5 hours to move from the pylorus to the ileocecal valve, although this activity is greatly increased after meals. Digestion and absorption of foodstuffs occur primarily in the small intestine. The anatomical arrangement of villi and microvilli in the small intestine greatly increases the surface area in this part of the intestine and accounts for its highly digestive and absorptive capabilities. Located on the entire surface of the small intestine are small pits called *crypts of Lieberkühn*, which produce intestinal secretions at a rate of 2000 mL per day. These secretions are neutral in pH and supply the watery vehicle necessary for absorption.

In the small intestine, digestion of carbohydrates, fats, and proteins begins with degradation by pancreatic enzymes that are secreted into the duodenum. Pancreatic juice contains enzymes necessary for digesting all three major types of food: proteins, carbohydrates, and fats (Table 17-3). It also contains large quantities of bicarbonate ions, which play an important role in neutralizing acidic chyme that is emptied from the stomach into the duodenum. Pancreatic juice is primarily secreted in response to the presence of chyme in the duodenum.

The small intestine also handles water, electrolyte, and vitamin absorption. Up to 10 L of fluid enters the GI tract daily, and fluid composition of stool is only about 200 mL. Sodium is actively reabsorbed in the small intestine. In the ileum, chloride is absorbed and sodium bicarbonate is secreted. Potassium is absorbed and secreted in the GI tract. Vitamins, with the exception of B_{12}, and iron are absorbed in the upper part of the small bowel. Vitamin B_{12} is absorbed in the terminal ileum in the presence of intrinsic factor.

Large Intestine

The large intestine, or colon, is anatomically divided into the ascending colon, transverse colon, descending colon, and rectum (Figure 17-3). The functions of the colon are absorption of the water and electrolytes from the chyme and storage of fecal material until it can be expelled. The proximal half of the colon performs primarily absorptive activities, whereas the distal half performs storage activities. The characteristic contractile activity in the colon is called *haustration*; it propels fecal material through the tract. A mass movement moves feces into the rectal vault, and then the urge to defecate is elicited. The mucosa of the large intestine is lined with crypts of Lieberkühn, but the cells contain very few enzymes. Rather, mucus is secreted, and this protects the colon wall against excoriation and serves as a medium for holding fecal matter together.

Accessory Organs
Pancreas

The pancreas is located in both upper quadrants of the abdomen, with the *head* in the upper right quadrant and the *tail* in the upper left quadrant. The head and tail are separated by a midsection called the *body of the pancreas* (Figure 17-4). Because the pancreas lies retroperitoneally, it cannot be palpated; this characteristic explains why diseases of the pancreas can cause pain that radiates to the back. In addition, a well-developed pancreatic capsule does not exist, and this may explain why inflammatory processes of the pancreas can freely spread and affect the surrounding organs (stomach and duodenum).

The pancreas has both *exocrine* (production of digestive enzymes) and *endocrine* (production of insulin and glucagon) functions. The cells of the pancreas, called *acini*, secrete the major pancreatic enzymes essential for normal digestion (see Table 17-3). Trypsinogen and chymotrypsinogen are secreted in an inactive form so autodigestion of the gland does not occur. Bicarbonate is also secreted by the pancreas

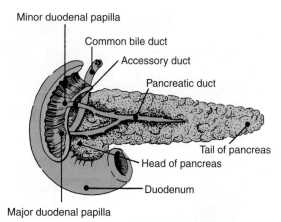

FIGURE 17-4 The pancreas.

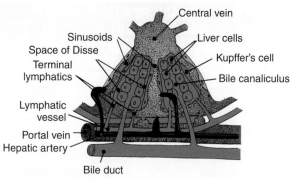

FIGURE 17-5 The normal liver lobule.

BOX 17-2   FUNCTIONS OF THE LIVER

Vascular Functions
- Blood storage
- Blood filtration

Secretory Functions
- Production of bile
- Secretion of bilirubin
- Conjugation of bilirubin

Metabolic Functions
- Carbohydrate metabolism
- Fat metabolism
- Protein metabolism
- Synthesis of prothrombin (factor I), fibrinogen (factor II), and factors VII, IX, and X
- Removal of activated clotting factors
- Detoxification of drugs, hormones, and other substances

Storage Functions
- Blood
- Glucose
- Vitamins (A, B_{12}, D, E, K)
- Fat

and plays an important role in enabling the pancreatic enzymes to work to break down foodstuffs. After breakdown by pancreatic enzymes, food is further digested by enzymes in the small intestine and is absorbed into the bloodstream. The presence of acid in the stomach stimulates the duodenum to produce the hormone secretin, which stimulates pancreatic secretions. Protein substances in the duodenum stimulate the production of cholecystokinin.

The endocrine functions of the pancreas are accomplished by groups of alpha and beta cells that compose the islets of Langerhans. *Beta cells* secrete insulin, and *alpha cells* secrete glucagon. Both are essential to carbohydrate metabolism. When beta cells are affected by disease, blood glucose levels can increase.

The exocrine and endocrine functions of the pancreas are essential to digestion and carbohydrate metabolism, respectively. Therefore pancreatic dysfunction can predispose the patient to malnutrition and accounts for many clinical problems (see Chapters 6 and 16).

The pancreatic response to low-flow states (decreased cardiac output), or hypotension, is often ischemia of the pancreatic cells. This ischemia is thought to play a role in the release of cardiotoxic factors (myocardial depressant factor), which decrease cardiac output. Pancreatic ischemia can also result in acute pancreatitis, which is discussed later in the chapter.

Liver

The liver is the largest internal organ of the body; it is located in the right upper abdominal quadrant. The basic functional unit of the liver is the liver lobule (Figure 17-5). Hepatic cells are arranged in cords that radiate from the central vein into the periphery. Blood from portal arterioles and venules empties into channels called *sinusoids*. Lining the walls of the sinusoids are specialized phagocytic cells called *Kupffer's cells*. These cells remove bacteria and other foreign material from the blood.

The liver has a rich blood supply. It receives blood from both the hepatic artery and the portal vein, which drains structures of the GI tract. The blood supplied to the liver by these two vessels accounts for approximately 25% of the cardiac output.

The liver performs more than 400 functions. The following discussion of hepatic functions is based on the classification by Guyton and Hall,[12] and includes vascular, secretory, metabolic, and storage functions. These actions are summarized in Box 17-2.

Vascular functions

Blood storage. Resistance to blood flow (hepatic vascular resistance) in the liver is normally low. Any increase in pressure in the veins that drain the liver causes blood to accumulate in the sinusoids, which store up to 400 mL of blood. This blood volume serves as a compensatory mechanism in cases of hypovolemic shock; blood from the liver is shunted into the circulation to increase blood volume.

Blood filtration. Kupffer's cells that line the sinusoids cleanse the blood of bacteria and foreign material that have been absorbed through the GI tract. These cells are extremely phagocytic and thus normally prevent almost all bacteria from reaching the systemic circulation.

Secretory functions

Bile production. The secretion of bile is a major function of the liver. Bile is composed of water, electrolytes, bile salts, phospholipids, cholesterol, and bilirubin. Approximately 500 to 1000 mL of bile is produced daily. Bile salts emulsify fats and foster their absorption. The bile salts are reabsorbed in the terminal portion of the ileum and are then transported back to the liver, where they can be used again. Bile travels to the gallbladder via the common bile duct, where it is stored and concentrated.

Bilirubin metabolism. Bilirubin, a physiologically inactive pigment, is a metabolic end product of the degradation of hemoglobin (Hgb). Bilirubin enters the circulation bound to albumin and is *unconjugated*. This portion of the bilirubin is reflected in the *indirect* serum bilirubin level. Accumulation of unconjugated bilirubin is toxic to cells. In the liver, bilirubin is *conjugated* with glucuronic acid. Conjugated bilirubin is soluble and excreted in bile. Some conjugated bilirubin returns to the blood and is reflected in the *direct* serum bilirubin level.

Excess bilirubin accumulation in the blood results in *jaundice*. Jaundice has several categories including hepatocellular, hemolytic, and obstructive. Hemolytic jaundice results from increased RBC destruction, such as that resulting from blood incompatibilities and sickle cell disease. Viral hepatitis is the most common cause of hepatocellular jaundice (jaundice caused by hepatic cell damage). Cirrhosis and liver cancer also decrease the liver's ability to conjugate bilirubin. Obstructive jaundice is usually caused by gallbladder disease such as gallstones.

Metabolic functions

Carbohydrate metabolism. The liver plays an important role in the maintenance of normal blood glucose concentration. When the concentration of glucose increases to greater than normal levels, it is stored as glycogen (*glycogenesis*). When blood glucose levels decrease, glycogen stored in the liver is split to form glucose (*glycogenolysis*). If blood glucose levels decrease to less than normal and glycogen stores are depleted, the liver can make glucose from proteins and fats (*gluconeogenesis*).

Fat metabolism. Almost all cells in the body are capable of lipid metabolism; however, the liver metabolizes fats so rapidly that it is the primary site for these functions. The liver is also the primary site for the conversion of excess carbohydrates and proteins to triglycerides.

Protein metabolism. All nonessential amino acids are produced in the liver. Amino acids must be deaminated (cleared of ammonia) to be used for energy by cells, or converted into carbohydrates or fats. Ammonia is released and removed from the blood by conversion to urea in the liver. The urea that is secreted by the liver into the bloodstream is excreted by the kidneys.

With the exception of gamma globulins, the liver also produces all plasma proteins in the blood. The major types of plasma proteins are albumins, globulins, and fibrinogen.

Albumin maintains blood oncotic pressure and prevents plasma loss from the capillaries. *Globulins* are essential for cellular enzymatic reactions. *Fibrinogen* helps to form blood clots.

Production and removal of blood clotting factors. The liver synthesizes fibrinogen (factor I); prothrombin (factor II); and factors VII, IX, and X. Vitamin K is essential for the synthesis of other clotting factors. The liver also removes active clotting factors from the circulation and therefore prevents clotting in the macrovasculature and microvasculature.

Detoxification. Drugs, hormones, and other toxic substances are metabolized by the liver into inactive forms for excretion. This process is usually accomplished by conversion of the fat-soluble compounds to water-soluble compounds. They can then be excreted via the bile or the urine. Genetics play a role in detoxification (see box, "Genetics").

Storage, synthesis, and transport of vitamins and minerals. The liver plays a central role in the storage, synthesis, and transport of various vitamins and minerals. It functions as a storage depot principally for vitamins A, D, and B_{12}, where up to 3-, 10-, and 12-month supplies, respectively, of these nutrients are stored to prevent deficiency states.

Gallbladder

The gallbladder is a saclike structure that lies beneath the right lobe of the liver. Its primary function is the storage and concentration of bile. The gallbladder holds approximately 70 mL of bile. Bile salts are secreted into the duodenum when nutrients are ingested. The gallbladder is connected to the duodenum via the common bile duct. Bile flow is controlled by contraction of the gallbladder and relaxation of the sphincter of Oddi, which is located at the junction of the common bile duct and the duodenum. Contraction of the gallbladder is controlled by hormonal (*cholecystokinin*) and central nervous system signals and is initiated by the presence of food in the duodenum. Bile salts emulsify fats and also assist in the absorption of fatty acids.

Neural Innervation of the Gastrointestinal System

Functions of the GI system are influenced by neural and hormonal factors. The autonomic nervous system exerts multiple effects. Parasympathetic cholinergic fibers, or drugs that mimic parasympathetic effects, stimulate GI secretion and motility. Sympathetic stimulation, or drugs with adrenergic effects, tends to be inhibitory. Parasympathetic and sympathetic fibers also innervate the gallbladder and the pancreas. Other neural regulators of gastric secretions are stimulated by sight, smell, and thoughts of food and by the presence of food in the mouth. In this phase (cephalic), the brain centers reflexively cause parasympathetic stimulation of gastric secretions by chief and parietal cells.

Hormonal Control of the Gastrointestinal System

The GI tract is considered to be the largest endocrine organ in the body. Hormones that influence GI function include those produced by specialized cells in the GI tract and those produced by other endocrine organs (pancreas and gallbladder).

GENETICS

Cytochrome P450 Enzymes and the Patient's Response to Drugs

More than half of prescription drugs and many over-the-counter and herbal agents are metabolized by enzymes to either convert a prodrug to an active form, or to change an active drug to an inactive metabolite before elimination. Drug-metabolizing enzymes common to both the liver and intestine are the cytochrome P450 (CYP) enzymes. This name reflects their red coloration (*cytochrome* means "colored cell" and results from a heme molecule in the enzyme structure) and the wavelength of light absorbed in mass spectrography (450 nanometers).[6] The CYP enzymes have important genetic variations that affect patient responses to many drugs.[7]

Three main cytochrome families are involved in drug metabolism in humans: CYP1, CYP2, and CYP3. Each of these superfamilies is further subdivided into subfamilies and isoforms; about 13 isoforms play a part in the metabolism of commonly used drugs. In addition to metabolizing drugs, CYP enzymes are used to transform procarcinogens, alcohol, fatty acids, prostaglandins, and hormones (both endogenous and exogenous). They also contribute to detoxifying food. The activity of nearly all the CYP enzymes are affected by foods, temperature (e.g., fever, hypothermia), pH, drugs, and other environmental factors.[9] The subfamilies in the CYP2 enzymes and their isoforms have polymorphisms that have been extensively studied and linked to variations in patient responses to drugs. Typically the polymorphism is a single nucleotide polymorphism (SNP, pronounced "snip") that leads to altered enzyme activity. A single change in the base pairs of the gene coding for this enzyme results in a change in either the quantity or effectiveness of the CYP2D6 ("D" designates the subfamily and "6" designates the isoform).

The CYP2D6 enzyme affects metabolism of more than 25% of prescription drugs.[10] Since each person inherits two genes—two alleles—for this genetic product, both the variation and the combined allele products contribute to drug metabolism. For example, the CYP2D4 (subfamily D, isoform 4) has more than 120 variations.[10] Functionally, these polymorphisms result in phenotypic poor, intermediate, extensive, and ultrafast metabolizers. Extensive metabolizers are considered normal or "wild type." Poor and intermediate metabolizers have less enzymatic activity, causing high serum drug concentrations with standard doses, or therapeutic failure when a prodrug is not converted to an active form. About 10% of white Europeans, and as many as 50% of Asians, may inherit alleles resulting in a slow metabolic response. Ultrafast metabolizers change drugs more quickly than normal, resulting in metabolism that leads to low drug levels and reduced effects despite administration of a therapeutic dose. Populations with a North African inheritance have more ultrafast metabolic alleles compared to other people.

Enzymes in the CYP2D4 family affect metabolism of some beta-blockers, several antidysrhythmics, antiplatelet agents, many antipsychotics, and drugs that use serotonin receptors.[2] Clopidogrel is a prodrug that requires activation via several CYP 450 enzymes in order to reduce platelet activity; reduced drug effectiveness is associated with reduced CYP effectiveness in preventing cardiovascular events. Increased incidence of bradycardia from some beta-blockers and lengthening of the QTc interval with antipsychotics use, including haloperidol, has been linked to CYP2D6 deficiency.[1,2] Drug-induced liver injury is also associated with inherited immune and liver enzyme activity.[3]

The CYP2D6 enzymes have specific clinical implications for the patient receiving codeine. Patients with inherited low CYP2D6 enzymatic activity, poor metabolizers, cannot convert codeine to its active form, and so codeine provides no pain relief. Increasing the dose or frequency of administration will not change this response.[9] Alternatively, individuals who inherit a genotype that results in extensive metabolism experience a quick conversion of codeine into its active form, causing unanticipated central nervous system effects such as euphoria or hallucinations that are not generally associated with codeine use.

Of all the drugs metabolized by CYP enzymes, the most commonly used family is CYP3; more specifically, CYP3A4. Although CYP3A4 does not have any known polymorphisms, there may be variations that precede the coding section of this gene that influence its activity. Areas that precede a gene and influence its expression or ability to generate proteins are promoter or inhibitor regions that "turn on" or "turn off" genes, respectively.[2,7]

Clinical observations support the laboratory genotyping for the CYP families as well as other metabolizing enzymes. Reports of "fast" and "slow" metabolizers have appeared for about 50 years in the literature.[7] The potential for clinical genotyping has some advantages over clinical observations. It can limit trial-and-error dosing and avoid adverse complications and undesirable effects from a dose that is too high or inadequate given an individual's ability to metabolize a drug. Results of genotyping can be obtained within 6 to 8 hours and are not affected by underlying disease or coadministration of other drugs. Genotype does not change, so it need be done only once.

This study of genetic variation and its effects on pharmaceuticals is called *pharmacogenetics* or *pharmacogenomics*. Pharmacogenetics specifically refers to the study of individual genetic variability or biochemical and other differences between individuals that influence one person's response to medication. Pharmacogenomics is the study of the whole genome and higher proteins (e.g., RNA, enzymes, and drug receptors) and focuses on how differences within the individual work together to create a response to medications.

Other genetic variations contribute to altered drug absorption, distribution, metabolism, and elimination. However, genetic variation is only one factor that affects therapeutic response and predisposition to adverse drug reactions. Genotyping is being used in clinical settings to guide drug therapy in oncology, cardiology and psychiatry.[5] For example, carbazapine is useful for a variety of neurological conditions but has a potentially lethal adverse drug reaction of toxic epidermal necrosis (TEN). The presence of a human leukocyte antigen (HLA) variation is highly associated with and contributes to both TEN and its milder pathology of Stevens-Johnson syndrome. Because this particularly HLA variation is common in Asian populations, it is common for clinicians to test for the mutation in Japan before starting carbazapine.[3,4,5] Though pharmacogenomic testing is less common in the United States, the test is commercially available.[5]

Pharmacogenetics is also improving drug design and clinical evaluation strategies.[6] Genomic information is helping to determine therapeutic approaches and better decision-making tools for efficacy.[8] These advances contribute to improving treatment response while avoiding complications of therapy. Critical care practitioners' awareness of pharmacogenomics contribute to patient safety in drug selection, administration, and monitoring.

GENETICS

Cytochrome P450 Enzymes and the Patient's Response to Drugs—cont'd

References

1. Daly AK. Drug-induced liver injury: past, present and future. *Pharmacogenomics*. 2010;11(5):607-611.
2. Empey PE. Genetic predisposition to adverse drug reactions in the intensive care unit. *Critical Care Medicine*. 2010;38(6 Suppl):S106-116.
3. Frueh FW, Amur S, Mummaneni P, et al. Pharmacogenomic biomarker information in drug labels approved by the United States food and drug administration: prevalence of related drug use. *Pharmacotherapy*. 2008;28(8):992-998.
4. Frueh FW. Real-world clinical effectiveness, regulatory transparency and payer coverage: three ingredients for translating pharmacogenomics into clinical practice. *Pharmacogenomics*. 2010;11(5):657-660.
5. Green ED, Guyer MS. Charting a course for genomic medicine from base pairs to bedside. *Nature*. 2011;470(7333):204-213.
6. Human Cytochrome P450 (CYP) Allele Nomenclature Committee 2009. http://www.cypalleles.ki.se/cyp2d6.htm; Accessed May 25, 2011.
7. Lashley FR. *Clinical Genetics in Nursing Practice*. 3rd ed. New York: Springer. 2006.
8. Lander ES. Initial impact of the sequencing of the human genome. *Nature*. 2011;470(7333):187-197.
9. Zhou SF, Liu JP, Chowbay B. Polymorphism of human cytochrome P450 enzymes and its clinical impact. *Drug Metabolism Review*. 2009;41(2):89-295.
10. Zhou SF. Polymorphism of human cytochrome P450 2D6 and its clinical significance: part II. *Clinical Pharmacokinetics*. 2009;48(12):761-804.

GI hormones modulate motility, secretion, absorption, and maturation of GI tissues. Table 17-4 summarizes the common GI hormones and their actions.

Blood Supply of the Gastrointestinal System

Blood supply to organs within the abdomen is referred to as the *splanchnic circulation*. The GI system receives the largest single percentage of the cardiac output. Approximately one third of the cardiac output supplies these tissues. The superior and inferior mesenteric and celiac arteries supply the stomach, small and large intestines, pancreas, and gallbladder. The liver has a dual blood supply and receives part of its blood supply from the hepatic artery. Circulation to the GI system is unique in that venous blood draining the system empties into the portal vein, which then perfuses the liver. The portal vein supplies approximately 70% to 75% of liver blood flow.

Because of the large percentage of cardiac output that perfuses the GI tract, the GI tract is a major source of blood flow during times of increased need, such as during exercise or as a compensatory mechanism in hemorrhage. Conversely, prolonged occlusion or hypoperfusion of a major artery supplying the GI tract can lead to mucosal ischemia and eventually necrosis. Necrosis of intestinal villi can destroy the GI tract's barrier to harmful toxins and bacteria. These bacteria can then enter the blood supply and cause septic shock.

Geriatric Considerations

Several changes occur in the GI system as a result of the aging process. Changes include decreased salivation, alterations in taste, delayed esophageal and bowel emptying, increased bowel emptying, decreased gastric secretions, and altered drug metabolism. The three most common gastrointestinal disorders seen in the elderly are functional bowel disorders such as irritable bowel syndrome, peptic ulcer disease, and neoplasms. It is important to note that upper abdominal discomfort in the elderly patient may be associated with coronary artery disease.[26] The box, "Geriatric Considerations," highlights these changes and related nursing implications.[20]

TABLE 17-4   ACTIONS OF GASTROINTESTINAL HORMONES

ACTION	GASTRIN	CHOLECYSTOKININ	SECRETIN	GASTRIC INHIBITORY PEPTIDE
Acid secretion	Stimulates	Stimulates	Inhibits	Inhibits
Gastric motility	Stimulates	Stimulates	Inhibits	—
Gastric emptying	Inhibits	Inhibits	Inhibits	Inhibits
Intestinal motility	Stimulates	Stimulates	Inhibits	—
Mucosal growth	Stimulates	Stimulates	Inhibits	—
Pancreatic HCO_3^- secretion	Stimulates	Stimulates	Stimulates	0
Pancreatic enzyme secretion	Stimulates	Stimulates	Stimulates	0
Pancreatic growth	Stimulates	Stimulates	Stimulates	—
Bile HCO_3^- secretion	Stimulates	Stimulates	Stimulates	0
Gallbladder contraction	Stimulates	Stimulates	Stimulates	—

0, No effect; —, not yet tested; *HCO_3^-*, bicarbonate.

GERIATRIC CONSIDERATIONS

PHYSIOLOGICAL CHANGES	NURSING IMPLICATIONS
Salivation decreased, resulting in dry mouth	Mouth care is essential to keep mucous membranes moist.
Decreased sense of taste	Providing adequate nutrition to those taking oral feedings may be more difficult because food may not be as appealing.
Esophageal emptying delayed	Assess for dysphagia/difficulty in swallowing. The elderly patient might describe this with drinking a large amount of water with meals. The risk of aspiration is higher; elevate the head of the bed for feedings.
Gastric acid secretion decreased	This may result in anemia; anemia can lead to hypoxemia. Assess complete blood count, arterial blood gases, and pulse oximetry values.
Incidence of gallstones increased	Assess for signs and symptoms of cholecystitis; the patients may be at higher risk for complications of gallbladder disease such as pancreatitis.
Drug metabolism by liver impaired because blood flow decreases by almost half by age 85 years	Assess for drug toxicity; drug dosages may need to be reduced.
Delayed bowel emptying resulting in higher incidence of constipation.	Assess bowel function; patients may need extra fluids, fiber, stool softeners, or laxatives to facilitate bowel function. Provide assistance to facilitate toileting.
Increased bowel emptying resulting in diarrhea.	Assess bowel function. Assess for use of medications such as laxatives and nonsteroidal antiinflammatory drugs (NSAIDs) that may cause bowel disturbances.

GENERAL ASSESSMENT OF THE GASTROINTESTINAL SYSTEM

A comprehensive assessment of the abdomen includes a history, inspection, auscultation, percussion, and palpation. Mapping of the abdomen for descriptive purposes is usually performed by use of the four-quadrant method by drawing imaginary lines crossing at the umbilicus: right upper, right lower, left upper, and left lower. Symptoms such as pain may also be described by these landmarks.

History

An assessment of the GI system begins with a history, unless an emergency situation exists that requires immediate intervention. The patient is questioned about any past problems with indigestion, difficulty swallowing (dysphagia), pain on swallowing, nausea and vomiting, heartburn, belching, abdominal distention or bloating, diarrhea, constipation, or bleeding. Problems such as anorexia, fatigue, and headache also point to specific GI ailments and should be noted. All symptoms should be explored in terms of when the symptoms became apparent, any precipitating factors, what treatment was sought, factors that relieved or made the symptoms worse, and whether the symptom is current. A weight history is also important and includes usual and ideal body weight along with a history of fluctuations, acute weight loss, and interventions or treatments for weight loss.

Pain assessment is challenging. Pain receptors in the abdomen are less likely to be localized and are mediated by common sensory structures projected to the skin. Therefore distinguishing the pain of a peptic ulcer or cholecystitis from that of a myocardial infarction is often difficult. Abdominal pain is often caused by engorged mucosa, pressure in the mucosa, distention, or spasm. Visceral pain is likely to cause pallor, perspiration, bradycardia, nausea and vomiting, weakness, and hypotension. Increasing intensity of pain, especially after surgery or other intervention, is always significant and usually signifies complicating factors, such as inflammation, gastric distention, hemorrhage into tissue or the peritoneal space, or peritonitis. The nurse obtains a description of the location and the type of pain in the patient's own words.

A history of any GI surgical procedures, including the specific types and dates, should be discussed. A current list of medications is also important, because many drugs have GI side effects.

Inspection

General inspection of the abdomen focuses on the following characteristics: skin color and texture, symmetry and contour of the abdomen, masses and pulsations, and peristalsis and movement.

Skin Color and Texture

The nurse observes for pigmentation of skin (jaundice), lesions, discolorations, old or new scars, and vascular and hair patterns. General nutrition and hydration status may also be discerned.

Symmetry and Contour of Abdomen

The nurse notes the size and shape of the abdomen and the presence of visible protrusions and adipose distribution. Abdominal distention, particularly in the presence of pain, should always be investigated because it usually indicates trapped air or fluid within the abdominal cavity.

Masses and Pulsations

The nurse looks for any obvious abdominal masses, which are best seen on deep inspiration. Pulsations, if they are seen, usually originate from the aorta.

Peristalsis and Movement

Motility of the stomach may be reflected in movement of the abdomen in lean patients, and is a normal sign. However, strong contractions are abnormal and indicate the presence of disease.

Auscultation

Bowel sounds are high-pitched, gurgling sounds caused by air and fluid as they move through the GI tract. Bowel sounds are auscultated before palpation. However, auscultation after palpation can be done if no bowel sounds were heard to stimulate peristalsis.[2] Optimal positioning of the patient to relax the abdomen is performed before auscultation is begun. A supine position with the patient's arms at the sides or folded at the chest is usually recommended. Placing a pillow under the patient's knees also helps to relax the abdominal wall.

Bowel sounds are best heard with the diaphragm of the stethoscope and are systematically assessed in all four quadrants of the abdomen. The frequency and character of the sounds are noted. The frequency of bowel sounds has been estimated at 5 to 35 per minute, and the sounds are usually irregular. The amount of time for bowel sounds to be auscultated ranges from 30 seconds to 7 minutes. It is recommended that bowel sounds be assessed a minimum of 5 minutes before an assessment of absence of bowel sounds can be made.[2] Box 17-3 reviews common causes of increased and decreased bowel sounds as they relate to acute illness.

Vascular sounds such as bruits may also be heard, and they indicate dilated, tortuous, or constricted vessels. Venous hums are also normally heard from the inferior vena cava. A hum in the periumbilical region in a patient with cirrhosis indicates obstructed portal circulation. Peritoneal friction rubs may also be heard and may indicate infection, abscess, or tumor.

Percussion

Percussion is aimed at detecting fluid, gaseous distention, or masses. Because of the presence of gas within the GI tract, percussed tympany predominates. Solid masses are dull on percussion. Organ borders of the liver, spleen, and stomach may also be ascertained.

Palpation

Palpation is used to evaluate the major organs with respect to shape, size, position, mobility, consistency, and tension. Palpation is performed last because it often elicits pain or muscle spasm. Deep abdominal tenderness and rebound tenderness must be differentiated. Rebound tenderness occurs when pain is elicited after the examiner's hand is quickly released after deep palpation. Rigidity or guarding of the abdomen is also noted. Masses in the liver, spleen, kidneys, gallbladder, and descending colon can also be palpated. In palpating the gallbladder for the thin, elderly female patient, it is recommended that the clinician palpate the right lower abdominal quadrant in addition to the right upper abdominal quadrant.[26]

ACUTE GASTROINTESTINAL BLEEDING

Pathophysiology

GI bleeding results in high patient morbidity and medical care costs. Many causes of acute GI bleeding necessitate admission of a patient to the critical care unit. Box 17-4 reviews the most common causes of this emergency.

Peptic Ulcer Disease

Peptic ulcer disease is characterized by a break in the mucosa that extends through the entire mucosa and into the muscle layers, damaging blood vessels and causing hemorrhage or perforation into the GI wall (Figure 17-6).[16] Duodenal and gastric ulcers are the most common cause of peptic ulcer

---

BOX 17-3 CAUSES OF INCREASED AND DECREASED BOWEL SOUNDS

Causes of Decreased Bowel Sounds
- Peritonitis
- Gangrene
- Reflux ileus
- Surgical manipulation of bowel
- Late bowel obstruction

Causes of Increased Bowel Sounds
- Early pyloric or intestinal obstruction
- Bleeding ulcers or electrolyte disturbances
- Bleeding esophageal varices
- Diarrhea
- Subsiding ileus

BOX 17-4 CAUSES OF GASTROINTESTINAL BLEEDING

Causes of Upper Gastrointestinal Bleeding
- Duodenal ulcer
- Gastric ulcer
- Esophageal or gastric varices
- Mallory-Weiss tear

Causes of Lower Gastrointestinal Bleeding
- Polyps
- Inflammatory disease
- Diverticulosis
- Cancer
- Vascular ectasias
- Hemorrhoids

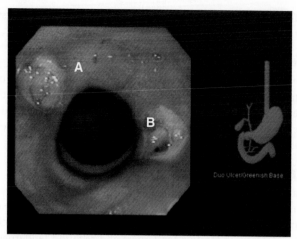

FIGURE 17-6 Duodenal ulcer. **A,** Duodenal ulcer. **B,** Deep ulceration in the duodenal wall extending as a crater through the entire mucosa and into the muscle layers. (Courtesy David Bjorkman, MD, University of Utah School of Medicine, Department of Gastroenterology. From Huether SE. Alterations of digestive function. In McCance KL, Huether SE, eds. *Pathophysiology: The Biologic Basis for Disease in Adults and Children.* 6th ed. St. Louis: Mosby. 2010.)

BOX 17-5   RISK FACTORS FOR PEPTIC ULCER DISEASE

- *Smoking:* stimulates acid secretion
- *Helicobacter pylori infection:* elevates levels of gastrin and pepsinogen, and releases toxins and enzymes promoting inflammation and ulceration
- *Habitual use of nonsteroidal antiinflammatory drugs:* inhibits prostaglandins
- Alcohol

BOX 17-6   CONTRIBUTING FACTORS TO ULCER FORMATION

- Increased number of parietal cells in the gastric mucosa
- Gastrin levels remain higher longer after eating
- Gastrin levels continue to stimulate secretion of acid and pepsin
- Feedback mechanism fails
- Rapid gastric emptying overwhelms buffering capacity
- Association of *Helicobacter pylori* with mucosal epithelial cell necrosis
- Decreased muscosal bicarbonate secretion

---

disease and the most common cause of upper GI bleeding. The ulcer in peptic ulcer disease is a crater surrounded by either acutely or chronically inflamed cells. Over time, the inflamed tissue is replaced by necrotic tissue, then by granulation tissue, and finally by scar tissue.

The secretion of acid is important in the pathogenesis of ulcer disease. Acetylcholine (a neurotransmitter), gastrin (a hormone), and secretin (a hormone) stimulate the chief cells, which stimulate acid secretion. Parietal cell mass in people with peptic ulcer disease is 1.5 to 2 times greater than in persons without disease. Risk factors for the development of peptic ulcer disease are noted in Box 17-5. Contributing factors in ulcer formation are noted in Box 17-6. Infection with *Helicobacter pylori* bacteria is a major cause of duodenal ulcers. Selected studies of GI function are noted in Table 17-5. Characteristics of gastric and duodenal ulcers are presented in Table 17-6.

Stress Ulcers

A stress ulcer is an acute form of peptic ulcer that often accompanies severe illness, systemic trauma, or neurological injury.[16] Ischemia is the prior etiology associated with stress ulcer formation. Ischemic ulcers develop within hours of an event such as hemorrhage, multisystem trauma, severe burns, heart failure, or sepsis.[16] The shock, anoxia, and sympathetic responses decrease mucosal blood flow leading to ischemia. Stress ulcers that develop as a result of burn injury are often called *Curling's ulcers.* Stress ulcers associated with severe head trauma or brain surgery are called *Cushing's ulcers.* The decreased mucosal blood flow and hypersecretion of acid caused by overstimulation of the vagal nuclei are associated with Cushing's ulcers.[16]

Administration of antacids and H_2-receptor blockers, and the suppression of vagal stimulation with anticholinergic drugs and proton pump inhibitors (PPI) are effective forms of therapy. These prophylactic measures are recommended by the Institute of Healthcare Improvement (IHI) as part of a "bundle" of best practices for care of the critically ill adult.[19]

Mallory-Weiss Tear

A Mallory-Weiss tear is an arterial hemorrhage from an acute longitudinal tear in the gastroesophageal mucosa and accounts for 10% to 15% of upper GI bleeding episodes. It is associated with long-term nonsteroidal antiinflammatory drug or aspirin ingestion and with excessive alcohol intake. The upper GI bleeding usually occurs after episodes of forceful retching. Bleeding usually resolves spontaneously; however, lacerations of the esophagogastric junction may cause massive GI bleeding, requiring surgical repair.

Esophageal Varices

In chronic liver failure, liver cell structure and function are impaired, resulting in increased portal venous pressure, called *portal hypertension* (see discussion of hepatic failure). As a result, part of the venous blood in the splanchnic system is diverted from the liver to the systemic circulation by the development of connections to neighboring low-pressure veins. This phenomenon is termed *collateral circulation.* The most common sites for the development of these collateral channels are the submucosa of the esophagus and rectum, the anterior abdominal wall, and the parietal peritoneum. Figure 17-7 shows a liver with collateral circulation. The

TABLE 17-5 SELECTED STUDIES OF GASTROINTESTINAL FUNCTION

TEST	NORMAL FINDINGS	CLINICAL SIGNIFICANCE
Stool studies	*Fat:* 2-6 g/24 hr	Steatorrhea can result from intestinal malabsorption or pancreatic insufficiency
	Occult blood: none	Positive tests associated with bleeding
Gastric acid stimulation	11-20 mEq/hr after stimulation	Increased with duodenal ulcers Decreased with gastric atrophy or gastric carcinoma
Glucose breath test or D-xylose	Negative for hydrogen or CO_2	May indicate intestinal bacterial overgrowth
Urea breath test	Negative for isotopically labeled CO_2	Presence of *Helicobacter pylori* infection

CO_2, Carbon dioxide.
Adapted from Huether SE. Structure and function of the digestive system. In McCance KL, Huether SE, *Pathophysiology: the biologic basis for disease in adults and children.* 6th ed. St. Louis: Mosby. 2010.

TABLE 17-6 CHARACTERISTICS OF GASTRIC AND DUODENAL ULCERS

CHARACTERISTICS	GASTRIC ULCER	DUODENAL ULCER
Incidence		
Age at onset	50-70 years	20-50 years
Family history	Usually negative	Positive
Gender (prevalence)	Equal in women and men	Equal in women and men
Stress factors	Increased	Average
Ulcerogenic drugs	Normal use	Increased use
Cancer risk	Increased	Not increased
Pathophysiology		
Abnormal mucus	May be present	May be present
Parietal cell mass	Normal or decreased	Increased
Acid production	Normal or decreased	Increased
Serum gastrin	Increased	Normal
Serum pepsinogen	Normal	Increased
Associated gastritis	More common	Usually not present
Helicobacter pylori	May be present (60%-80%)	Often present (95%-100%)
Clinical Manifestations		
Pain	Located in upper abdomen Intermittent Pain-antacid-relief pattern Food-pain pattern	Located in upper abdomen Intermittent Pain-antacid or food-relief pattern Nocturnal pain common
Clinical course	Chronic ulcer without pattern of remission and exacerbation	Pattern of remissions and exacerbations for years

From Huether SE. Alterations of digestive function. In McCance KL, Huether SE, *Pathophysiology: the biologic basis for disease in adults and children.* 6th ed. St. Louis: Mosby. 2010.

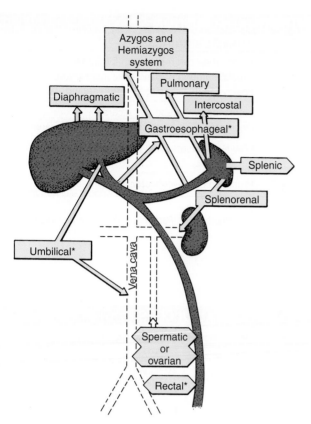

FIGURE 17-7 The liver and collateral circulation.
* Most common sites.

normal portal venous pressure is 2 to 6 mm Hg. As these veins experience increases in pressure, they become distended with blood, the vessels enlarge, and varices develop when the pressure increase exceeds 10 mm Hg. The varices tend to bleed when the portal venous pressures reach 12 mm Hg. The most common sites for the development of these varices are the esophagus and the upper portion of the stomach.

Assessment
Clinical Presentation
Patients manifest blood loss from the GI tract in several ways. Vomiting or drainage from a nasogastric tube that yields blood or coffee ground–like material is associated with upper GI bleeding. However, blood or coffee ground–like contents may not be present if bleeding has ceased, or arises beyond a closed pylorus. Upper GI bleeding commonly presents with *hematemesis,* which is bloody vomitus that is either bright red, indicating fresh blood; or has the appearance of coffee grounds, which results from older blood that has been in the stomach long enough for the gastric juices to act on it. Blood may also be passed via the colon. *Melena* is shiny, black, foul-smelling stool and results from the degradation of blood by stomach acids or intestinal bacteria. Bright red or maroon blood *(hematochezia)* is usually a sign of a lower GI source of bleeding, but can be seen when upper GI bleeding is massive (more than 1000 mL). GI blood loss is often occult, or

detected only by testing the stool with a chemical reagent (guaiac). Stool and nasogastric drainage can test positive with guaiac for up to 10 days after a bleeding episode. Hematemesis and melena indicate an episode of acute upper GI bleeding. Upper GI bleeding may also be accompanied by mild epigastric pain or abdominal distress. Pain is thought to arise from the acid bathing the ulcerated crater.

Finally, patients with acute upper GI bleeding may manifest clinical signs and symptoms of blood loss (see box, "Clinical Alert: Clinical Signs and Symptoms of Upper Gastrointestinal Bleeding"). Rapid assessment of the patient is undertaken to determine the seriousness of the bleeding, whether it is acute or chronic, and to assess hemodynamic stability. Patients with acute upper GI bleeding commonly have signs or symptoms of hypovolemic shock. Figure 17-8 describes the pathophysiology of acute upper GI bleeding.

> **! CLINICAL ALERT**
>
> *Clinical Signs and Symptoms of Upper Gastrointestinal Bleeding*
>
> - Hematemesis
> - Melena
> - Hematochezia
> - Abdominal discomfort
> - Signs and symptoms of hypovolemic shock
>   - Hypotension
>   - Tachycardia
>   - Cool, clammy skin
>   - Change in level of consciousness
>   - Decreased urine output
>   - Decreased gastric motility

Special care should be taken to assess comorbid conditions in the older adult. Conditions such as chronic hypertension or cardiovascular disease often mask signs of shock and make resuscitative attempts difficult.

Nursing Assessment
Initial evaluation of the patient with upper GI bleeding involves a rapid assessment of the severity of blood loss, hemodynamic stability and the necessity for fluid resuscitation, and frequent monitoring of vital signs and assessments of body systems for signs of hypovolemic shock. Changes in blood pressure and heart rate depend on the amount of blood loss, the suddenness of the blood loss, and the degree of cardiac and vascular compensation. Vital signs should be monitored at least every 15 minutes. As blood loss exceeds 1000 mL, the shock syndrome progresses, causing decreased blood flow to the skin, lungs, liver, and kidneys.

Hypotension is an advanced sign of shock. As a rule, a systolic pressure of less than 100 mm Hg, a postural decrease in blood pressure of greater than 10 mm Hg, or a heart rate of greater than 120 beats per minute reflects a blood loss of at least 1000 mL—25% of the total blood volume.

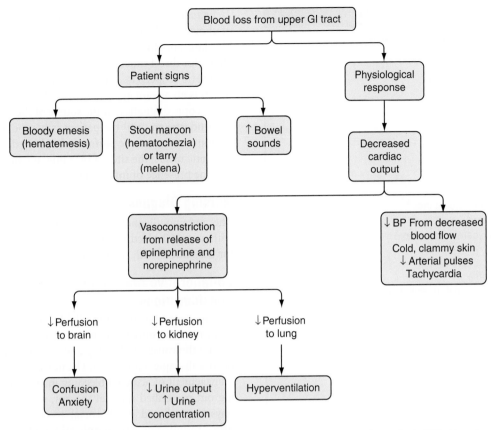

FIGURE 17-8 Pathophysiology flow diagram of acute upper gastrointestinal (GI) bleeding. *BP,* Blood pressure.

Hypertension is a common comorbid condition in those at risk of GI bleeding. In the chronically hypertensive patient, normal values for predicting perfusion no longer apply. Emphasis should be placed on other assessment findings, such as level of consciousness and urinary output. As blood pressure decreases, it can be assumed that more blood has been lost.

Rarely, a right atrial or pulmonary artery catheter is inserted to evaluate the patient's hemodynamic response to the blood loss. The electrocardiogram may also show ST-segment depression or flattening of the T waves, both of which indicate decreased coronary blood flow resulting in ischemia.

Abdominal assessment may reveal a soft or distended abdomen. Bowel sounds most often are hyperactive as a result of the sensitivity of the bowel to blood.

In addition to the physical examination, a history is taken to ascertain whether there have been previous episodes of bleeding or surgery for bleeding; a family history of bleeding; or a current illness or disease that may lead to bleeding, such as coagulopathies, cancer, and liver disease. Patterns of drug or alcohol ingestion and other risk factors are also assessed.

Medical Assessment

Laboratory studies. The common laboratory studies ordered for a patient with acute upper GI bleeding are listed in the box, "Laboratory Alert: Upper Gastrointestinal Bleeding."

Although a complete blood count is always ordered, the hematocrit (Hct) value does not change substantially during the first few hours after an acute bleeding episode. During this time, the severity of the bleeding must not be underestimated. Only when extravascular fluid enters the vascular space to restore volume does the Hct value decrease. This effect is further complicated by fluids and blood products that are administered during the resuscitation period. Platelet and white blood cell (WBC) counts may be increased, reflecting the body's attempt to restore homeostasis. An electrolyte profile is also ordered. Decreases in potassium and sodium levels are common as a result of the accompanying vomiting. Later, serum sodium levels may increase as a result of the loss of vascular volume. The glucose level is often increased related to the stress response. Increases in the blood urea nitrogen (BUN) and creatinine levels reflect decreased perfusion to the liver and kidneys, respectively. Liver function tests, clotting profiles, and serum ammonia levels are ordered to rule out preexisting liver disease. An arterial blood gas analysis is ordered to evaluate the patient's acid-base and oxygenation status. Respiratory alkalosis is common with GI bleeding as a result of the effects of the sympathetic nervous system on the lungs and patient anxiety. As shock progresses, the patient may develop metabolic acidosis as a result of anaerobic metabolism. Hypoxemia may also be present as a result of decreased circulating Hgb levels.

⚠ LABORATORY ALERT

Upper Gastrointestinal Bleeding

Complete Blood Count
Hemoglobin: Normal, then ↓
Hematocrit: Normal, then ↓
White blood cell count: ↑
Platelet count: Initially ↑ then ↓

Serum Electrolyte Panel
Potassium: ↓, then ↑
Sodium: ↑
Calcium: Normal or ↓
Blood urea nitrogen, creatinine: ↑
Ammonia: Possibly ↑
Glucose: Hyperglycemia common
Lactate: ↑

Hematology Profile
Prothrombin time, partial thromboplastin time: Usually ↑

Serum Enzyme Levels: ↓

Arterial Blood Gases
Respiratory alkalosis/metabolic acidosis

Gastric Aspirate for pH and Guaiac
Possibly acidotic pH
Guaiac positive

Endoscopy and barium study. Endoscopy is the procedure of choice for the diagnosis and treatment of active upper GI bleeding and for the prevention of rebleeding. Endoscopy allows for direct mucosal inspection with the use of a flexible, fiberoptic scope. The procedure can be done at the bedside, which is an advantage when caring for a critically ill patient. Endoscopic evaluation of the source of the bleeding is usually not undertaken until the patient is hemodynamically stable. Barium studies can be performed to help define the presence of peptic ulcers, the sites of bleeding, the presence of tumors, and the presence of inflammatory processes.

Nursing Diagnoses

The nursing diagnoses most commonly seen in patients with acute GI bleeding are found in the "Nursing Care Plan for the Patient with Acute Gastrointestinal Bleeding."

Collaborative Management: Nursing and Medical Considerations

The management of acute GI bleeding initially consists of treatment to restore hemodynamic stability followed by diagnosing the cause of bleeding and initiating specific and supportive therapies (Box 17-7). The nurse's role during the initial management of acute GI bleeding includes assessment, carrying out prescribed medical therapy, monitoring the patient's physiological and psychosocial responses to the interventions, monitoring for complications of the disease process

◎ NURSING CARE PLAN

for the Patient with Acute Gastrointestinal Bleeding

NURSING DIAGNOSIS
Fluid volume deficit related to decreased circulating blood volume

PATIENT OUTCOMES
Adequate circulating blood volume
• Hemorrhage controlled or resolved
• Preload indicators WNL
• Hct and Hgb levels stable
• I&O balanced

NURSING INTERVENTIONS	RATIONALES
• Monitor vital signs for hemodynamic instability and orthostatic changes	• Assess volume status
• Measure preload indicators: RAP, PAOP	• Assess volume status
• Monitor ECG, skin, urine output, amount and characteristics of GI secretions	• Monitor volume status and tissue perfusion
• Monitor response to blood and fluid replacement	• Assess response to treatment
• Monitor laboratory values: serial Hct, Hgb, BUN, potassium, sodium	• Assess acute bleeding
• Monitor bowel sounds	• Assess integrity and function of the gut
• Monitor for clinical manifestations of perforation: severe persistent abdominal pain; boardlike abdomen	• Assess for life-threatening complication
• Gastric lavage as ordered until clear	• May help to stop or reduce bleeding
• Administer medications and parenteral fluids	• Control bleeding and maintain fluid volume status
• Prepare for endoscopy, assist as necessary, and monitor for complications	• Assist in diagnosis of clinical problem; patients may not tolerate moderate sedation for GI procedures

◎ NURSING CARE PLAN

for the Patient with Acute Gastrointestinal Bleeding—cont'd

NURSING DIAGNOSIS

Altered tissue perfusion related to decreased circulating blood volume

PATIENT OUTCOMES

Adequate tissue perfusion

- Signs and symptoms of decreased perfusion absent: decreased sensorium, chest pain, renal failure
- Hemodynamics stable
- Urine output >30 mL/hr
- Skin warm and dry
- Bowel sounds WNL

NURSING INTERVENTIONS	RATIONALES
• Monitor for hypoperfusion and hemodynamic instability	• Prevent end-organ destruction
• Monitor vital signs every 15 minutes until stable	• Assess for hypovolemia and volume status
• Measure RAP, PAOP, cardiac output every hour until stable	• Assess volume status
• Monitor for tachycardia, chest pain, ST-segment elevation, diaphoresis, and cool/clammy extremities	• Assess for decreased cardiac output and decreased tissue perfusion
• Measure urine output every hour	• Monitor renal tissue perfusion
• Monitor level of consciousness	• Monitor tissue perfusion to the brain
• Assess bowel sounds	• Monitor tissue perfusion to the gut
• Monitor for elevated bilirubin	• Monitor liver dysfunction from hypoperfusion
• Notify the physician of changes and abnormalities	• Promote early intervention and prevent complications

NURSING DIAGNOSIS

Risk for fluid volume excess related to fluid overload from treatment regimen

PATIENT OUTCOMES

Normal volume status

- Respiratory pattern normal
- Lung congestion or pulmonary edema absent

NURSING INTERVENTIONS	RATIONALES
• Monitor hemodynamic response to fluid administration	• Monitor for fluid volume excess
• Monitor breath sounds at least every hour during fluid administration	• Monitor for pulmonary interstitial fluid collection, hypoxia, and fluid volume excess
• Monitor for restlessness or anxiety, dyspnea, tachycardia, coughing, crackles, frothy sputum, dysrhythmias, abnormal ABG results, blood pressure, increased RAP, jugular vein distention	• Assess signs and symptoms of fluid volume excess
• Record accurate I&O hourly	• Monitor fluid balance
• Document and report any abnormalities	• Maintain nurse-physician collaboration

ABG, Arterial blood gas; *BUN,* blood urea nitrogen; *ECG,* electrocardiogram; *GI,* gastrointestinal; *Hct,* hematocrit; *Hgb,* hemoglobin; *I&O,* intake and output; *PAOP,* pulmonary artery occlusion pressure; *RAP,* right atrial pressure; *WNL,* within normal limits.

BOX 17-7 MANAGEMENT OF UPPER GASTROINTESTINAL BLEEDING

Hemodynamic Stabilization
- Colloids
- Crystalloids
- Blood or blood products

Definitive and Supportive Therapies
- Gastric lavage
- Pharmacological therapies
  - Antacids

Definitive and Supportive Therapies—cont'd
- H₂-histamine blockers
- Proton pump inhibitors
- Mucosal barrier enhancers
- Endoscopic therapies
  - Sclerotherapy
  - Heater probe
  - Laser
- Surgical therapies

or treatment regimen, and providing supportive care. Patient and family support during the acute phase is a nursing priority. Explanations of the diagnostic tests, the medical therapies, and the critical care environment are extremely important nursing interventions.

Hemodynamic Stabilization

Patients who are hemodynamically unstable need to have immediate venous access (using large-bore intravenous [IV] catheters), and administration of fluid is started. Refer to Chapter 11 for management of hypovolemic shock. For the restoration of vascular volume, fluids are infused as rapidly as the patient's cardiovascular status allows and until the patient's vital signs return to baseline.

Patients who continue to bleed, or who have an excessively low Hct value (less than 25%) and have clinical symptoms, may be resuscitated with blood and blood products. The decision to use blood products is based on laboratory data and clinical examination. Blood is transfused to improve oxygenation (by increasing the number of RBCs) or to improve coagulation (by replacing platelets and plasma). The Hct value may not initially reflect actual blood volume during the first 24 to 72 hours after a hemorrhage and until vascular volume is restored. A reasonable goal for the management of blood transfusions is an Hct value of 30%, but this goal is individually determined for the patient based on clinical assessments. One unit of packed RBCs can be expected to increase the Hgb value by 1 g/dL and the Hct value by 2% to 3%, but this effect is influenced by the patient's intravascular volume status and whether the patient is actively bleeding. Careful monitoring for complications of blood transfusion therapy is also important. These complications include hypocalcemia, hyperkalemia, infection, increased ammonia levels, hypothermia, and anaphylactic reactions.

Gastric Lavage

Large-volume gastric lavage before endoscopy for acute upper gastrointestinal bleeding is safe and provides better visualization of the gastric fundus.[24] A large-bore nasogastric tube is inserted and is connected to suction. If lavage is ordered, 1000 to 2000 mL of room temperature normal saline is instilled via nasogastric tube and is then gently removed by intermittent suction or gravity until the secretions are clear. Iced lavage is used in some centers, although the evidence for this use is not well documented. After lavage, the nasogastric tube may be left in or removed. Nasogastric tubes left in place may increase hydrochloric acid secretion in the stomach and cause increased bleeding. Of all upper GI hemorrhages, 80% to 90% are self-limiting and stop with lavage therapy alone or on their own. The nurse must carefully document the nature of the nasogastric secretions or vomitus, such as the color, amount, and pH.

Pharmacological Therapy

Pharmacological agents are given to decrease gastric acid secretion or to reduce the effects of acid on the gastric mucosa.

The most common agents used include antacids, histamine antagonists (H_2-receptor blockers), proton pump inhibitors, and mucosal barrier enhancers. Antibiotics may also be ordered. Table 17-7 describes the treatments commonly used to decrease gastric acid secretion or reduce the effects of acid on the gastric mucosa.

Antibiotics. *H. pylori* infection is often associated with peptic ulcer disease. Triple-agent therapy with a proton pump inhibitor and two antibiotics for 14 days is the recommended treatment for eradication of *H. pylori*. The first-line treatment for *H. pylori* infection consists of a proton pump inhibitor (omeprazole, sesomeprazole, rabeprazole) and amoxicillin and clarithromycin (the two antibiotics).[27,29] In case first-line therapy fails, a bismuth-based quadruple therapy has been proven to be effective in 76% of patients. This second-line therapy consists of a PPI, bismuth, metronidazole, and a tetracycline. A 10-day course of levofloxacin may also be administered as a second-line therapy for *H. pylori* infections.[28]

Endoscopic Therapy

Endoscopy is the modality of choice for treatment of upper GI bleeding and several endoscopic therapies have been developed. Endoscopy is performed only after the patient is stabilized hemodynamically, but within 6 to 12 hours of presentation.[3] The advantage of endoscopic therapies is that they can be applied during the diagnostic procedure. *Sclerotherapy* involves injecting the bleeding ulcer with a necrotizing agent. The most common agents used are morrhuate sodium, ethanolamine, and tetradecyl sulfate. These agents work by traumatizing the endothelium, causing necrosis and eventual sclerosis of the bleeding vessel. Thermal methods of endoscopic therapy include use of the heater probe, laser photocoagulation, and electrocoagulation to tamponade the vessel. Endoclipping using band dilators and hemoclips may be used to provide hemostatis and to decrease the incidence of rebleeding.[8]

Because endoscopy is performed at the patient's bedside, the nurse assists with procedures and monitors for untoward effects. Maintenance of airway and breathing during endoscopic procedures is of major concern. Placement of the patient in a left lateral reverse Trendelenburg position helps to prevent respiratory complications. Other common complications of sclerotherapy include fever and oozing from the bleeding site.

Surgical Therapy

Surgery may be considered in patients who have massive GI bleeding that is immediately life-threatening, in patients who continue to bleed despite medical therapies, and in patients with perforation or unremitting pyloric obstruction. The purpose of emergency surgery in these situations is to prevent death from exsanguination. The patient is usually admitted to a critical care unit for initial management and stabilization in preparation for emergency surgery.

The most common reason for emergency surgery is massive rebleeding that occurs within 8 hours of admission.

TABLE 17-7 PHARMACOLOGICAL TREATMENTS TO DECREASE GASTRIC ACID SECRETION AND/OR REDUCE ACID EFFECTS ON GASTRIC MUCOSA

CLASSIFICATION, ACTION	MEDICATIONS	ADMINISTRATION
Histamine Blockers Block all factors that stimulate the parietal cells in the stomach to secrete hydrochloric acid	Cimetidine	300-1200 mg/day *IV push:* administer over not less than 5 minutes *Intermittent IV:* infuse over 15-20 minutes *IV infusion:* 100-1000 mL over 24 hours
	Famotidine	10-20 mg/day *IV push:* administer over 10 minutes Infuse piggyback over 15-30 minutes
	Nizatidine	150-300 mg/day Not available IV
	Ranitidine	150-300 mg/day *IV push:* administer over 5 minutes *Infuse piggyback:* over 15-20 minutes *IV infusion:* over 24 hours
Proton Pump Inhibitors Inhibit gastric acid secretion by specific inhibition of the hydrogen-potassium–adenosine triphosphatase enzyme system	Esomeprazole	20-40 mg/day *IV push:* administer over not less than 3 minutes *For intermittent infusion:* infuse over 15-30 minutes
	Lansoprazole	15-30 mg/day *IV administration:* infuse over 30 minutes
	Omeprazole	20-40 mg/day Not available IV
	Pantoprazole	40 mg/day *Infuse:* 10 mL solution over at least 2 minutes *Infuse:* 100 mL solution over at least 15 minutes
Mucosal Barrier Enhancers Reduce the effects of acid secretion; promotes healing	Sucralfate Colloidal bismuth	1 g 4 times a day 120 mg 4 times a day
Antacids Direct alkaline buffer to control the pH of the gastric mucosa	Aluminum hydroxide Calcium carbonate Magnesium hydroxide Magnesium oxide	500-1500 mg 3-6 times a day* 500-1500 mg as needed* Liquid: 2.5-7.5 mL up to 4 times a day* 400-800 mg/day*

*Often given every 1-2 hours to maintain gastric pH >5.
IV, Intravenous.
From Skidmore-Roth L. *Mosby's Drug Guide for Nurses.* 9th ed. St. Louis: Mosby. 2011.

Patients may also become surgical candidates if they continue to bleed despite aggressive medical intervention. Criteria for delayed surgery varies, but it is usually considered in patients who require more than 8 units of blood within a 24-hour period.

Impaired emptying of solids or liquids from the stomach into the small intestine (gastric outlet obstruction) may also necessitate surgical intervention. The major symptoms of obstruction include vomiting and continued pain that is localized in the epigastrium.

Surgical therapies for peptic ulcer disease include gastric resections (antrectomy, gastrectomy, gastroenterostomy, vagotomy), and combined operations to restore GI continuity (Billroth I, Billroth II) or to prevent complications of the surgery (vagotomy and pyloroplasty). An *antrectomy* may be performed for duodenal ulcers to decrease the acidity of

the duodenum by removing the antrum, which secretes gastric acid. A *vagotomy* decreases acid secretion in the stomach by dividing the vagus nerve along the esophagus. A *pyloroplasty* may be performed in conjunction with a vagotomy to prevent stomach atony, a common complication of the vagotomy procedure. A *Billroth I* procedure involves vagotomy, antrectomy, and anastomosis of the stomach to the duodenum. A *Billroth II* procedure involves vagotomy, resection of the antrum, and anastomosis of the stomach to the jejunum (Figure 17-9). A perforation can be treated by simple closure with the use of a patch to cover the gastric mucosal hole (omental patch) or by excision of the ulcer and suturing of the surrounding tissue.

Postoperative nursing care is focused on prevention and monitoring of potential complications. Fluid and electrolyte imbalances are common from loss of fluids during the

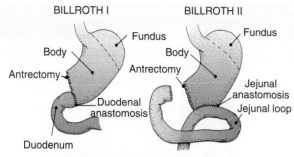

BILLROTH I

Fundus
Body
Antrectomy
Duodenal
anastomosis
Duodenum

BILLROTH II

Fundus
Body
Antrectomy
Jejunal
anastomosis
Jejunal loop

FIGURE 17-9 Billroth I and II procedures.

surgical procedure and drains that are left in place either to decompress the stomach (nasogastric tube) or to drain the surgical site. In addition, the GI system may not function normally after surgery, with resulting nausea, vomiting, ileus, or diarrhea. Provision of adequate nutrition is essential for proper wound healing. In cases of prolonged ileus after surgery, total parenteral nutrition may be considered. Monitoring for proper wound healing is also a nursing responsibility. Signs and symptoms of wound infection (erythema, swelling, tenderness, drainage, fever, increased WBC count) need to be documented and reported. A systemic infection may result from peritonitis in the case of perforation in which stomach or intestinal contents spill into the peritoneum. Postoperative rupture of the anastomosis may also lead to this complication.

Pain is also an important postoperative nursing concern. Abdominal incisions are associated with postoperative discomfort because of their anatomical location. Postoperative lung infections are also common in patients with abdominal incisions, because incisional pain impairs the ability to cough and breathe deeply.

Nursing Diagnoses

Several nursing diagnoses are associated with the postoperative care of the patient with upper GI bleeding. These diagnoses include risk for infection of wound, peritoneum, or both; altered nutrition; pain; fluid and electrolyte alterations; and impaired gas exchange.

Recognition of Potential Complications

Perforation of the gastric mucosa is the major GI complication of peptic ulcer disease. The nurse must be familiar with the signs and symptoms of acute perforation, which are reviewed in the box, "Clinical Alert: Acute Gastric Perforation." The most common signs of this complication are an abrupt onset of abdominal pain, followed rapidly by signs of peritonitis. Emergent surgery is indicated for treatment. Fluid and electrolyte resuscitation and treatment of any immediate complication is a priority. These patients almost always have

nasogastric tubes placed for gastric decompression. Broad-spectrum antibiotics are also usually prescribed before surgery. Antacids and histamine blockers may or may not be indicated, depending on the cause of the upper GI bleeding. Mortality rates for patients with perforations range from 10% to 40%, depending on the age and condition of the patient at the time of surgery.

> **! CLINICAL ALERT**
>
> *Acute Gastric Perforation*
>
> - Abrupt onset of severe abdominal pain
> - Abdominal tenderness
> - Boardlike abdomen
> - Usually absent bowel sounds
> - Leukocytosis
> - Presence of free air on x-ray study

Treatment of Variceal Bleeding

Bleeding esophageal or gastric varices are usually a medical emergency because they cause massive upper GI bleeding. The patient typically develops hemodynamic instability and signs and symptoms of shock. Often, the cause of the bleeding is unknown unless the patient has a history of cirrhosis or has previously bled from varices. Initial treatment of patients with esophageal or gastric varices is the same. Top priorities include hemodynamic stabilization and establishment of a patent airway. Gastric lavage may be used to clear the stomach and to document the amount of blood loss. Diagnosis of the cause of the bleeding through endoscopy is the next priority before definitive treatment for the varices can be started.

Somatostatin or Octreotide

Somatostatin or octreotide (a long-acting somatostatin) is commonly ordered to slow or stop bleeding. Early administration provides for stabilization before endoscopy. These drugs decrease splanchnic blood flow and reduce portal pressure, and have minimal adverse effects. Octreotide is given as an IV bolus of 50 to 100 mcg, followed by an infusion of 25 to 50 mcg/hr for up to 3 days. Patients must be monitored for both hypoglycemia and hyperglycemia.[13]

Vasopressin

Vasopressin (Pitressin) (Box 17-8) is a synthetic antidiuretic hormone. Vasopressin lowers portal pressure by vasoconstriction of the splanchnic arteriolar bed. Ultimately, it decreases pressure and flow in liver collateral circulation channels to decrease bleeding. However, vasopressin is not a first-line therapy because of its adverse effects.[14]

BOX 17-8   VASOPRESSIN (PITRESSIN) THERAPY

Mechanism of Action
- **Vasoconstrictor:** constricts the splanchnic vascular bed, contracts intestinal smooth muscle, and lowers portal vein pressure

Dose
- Given by intravenous (IV) route, although it may be given intra-arterially. IV infusion is started at 0.2-0.4 units/min, increased by 0.2 units/min each hour until hemorrhage is controlled, to a maximum dose of 0.9 units/min. (Drug may also be given by body weight: initial dose of 0.002-0.005 units/kg/minute IV titrated to a maximum dose of 0.01 units/kg/minute.)
- Vasopressin should be continued for at least 24 hours after bleeding is controlled. Wean slowly

Side Effects
- *Gastrointestinal:* cramping, nausea, vomiting, diarrhea
- *Cardiovascular:* dizziness, diaphoresis, hypertension, cardiac dysrhythmias, exacerbation of heart failure
- *Neurological:* tremors, headache, vertigo, decreased level of consciousness
- *Integumentary:* pallor, localized gangrene

Nursing Considerations
- Monitor for angina and dysrhythmias
- Infuse through a central line
- Assess serum sodium and neurological status
- Assess neurological status

From Gahart BL, Nazareno AR. *2011 Intravenous Medications: A Handbook for Nurses and Health Professionals.* 27th ed. St. Louis: Mosby.

Endoscopic Procedures

Sclerotherapy is another option in the treatment of bleeding varices. After the varices are identified, the sclerosing agent is injected into the varix and the surrounding tissue. Usually, several applications of the sclerosing agent several days apart are needed to decompress the bleeding varix.

Endoscopic band ligation is another treatment for varices.[35] Under endoscopy, a rubber band is placed over the varix. This treatment results in thrombosis, sloughing, and fibrosis of the varix.

Transjugular Intrahepatic Portosystemic Shunt

Transjugular intrahepatic portosystemic shunting (TIPS) is a nonsurgical treatment for recurrent variceal bleeding after sclerotherapy. Placement of the shunt is performed with the use of fluoroscopy. A stainless steel stent is placed between the hepatic and portal veins to create a portosystemic shunt in the liver and decrease portal pressure.[7] Decreasing portal pressure decreases pressure within the varix, thereby decreasing the risk for acute hemorrhage.

The role of TIPS in treating active hemorrhage uncontrolled by first-line therapy in patients who are good surgical candidates is not well-defined in clinical guidelines, and the choice remains up to the physician.[3] Approximately 10% to 20% of patients do not stop bleeding with endoscopic treatment combined with somatostatin infusion, whereas others rebleed in the first couple of days after cessation of the initial bleed. After a second unsuccessful endoscopic attempt, the TIPS procedure is used as a treatment option.

Esophagogastric Tamponade

If bleeding continues despite therapy, esophagogastric balloon tamponade therapy may provide temporary control of bleeding. Inflation of the balloon ports applies pressure to the vessels supplying the varices to decrease blood flow, thereby stopping the bleeding. Three types of tubes are used for tamponade: Sengstaken-Blakemore, Minnesota, and Linton tubes. The adult Sengstaken-Blakemore tube has three lumina: one for gastric aspiration, similar to that in a nasogastric tube; one for inflation of the esophageal balloon; and one for inflation of the gastric balloon (Figure 17-10). The Minnesota tube has an additional lumen that allows for aspiration of esophageal secretions. The Minnesota tube is commonly used because it allows for suction of secretions above and below the balloon. The Linton tube has a gastric balloon only, and lumens for gastric and esophageal suction; it is reserved for those with bleeding gastric varices.

Regardless of type, the balloon tip is inserted into the stomach, and the gastric balloon is inflated and clamped. The tube is then withdrawn slowly until resistance is met, so pressure is exerted at the gastroesophageal junction. Correct positioning and traction are maintained by using an external traction source, or a nasal cuff around the tube at the mouth or nose. External traction can be attached to a helmet or to the foot of the bed. Proper amounts of traction are essential because too little traction lets the balloon fall away from the gastric wall, resulting in insufficient pressure being placed on the bleeding vessels. Too much traction causes discomfort, gastric ulceration, or vomiting. If bleeding does not stop with inflation of the gastric balloon, the esophageal balloon is inflated and clamped (Sengstaken-Blakemore or Minnesota tube). Normal inflation pressure of the esophageal balloon is 20 to 45 mm Hg. Monitoring inflation pressures is important to prevent tissue damage.

The critical care nurse is responsible for maintaining balloon lumen pressures and patency of the system. The gastric balloon port placement below the gastroesophageal junction

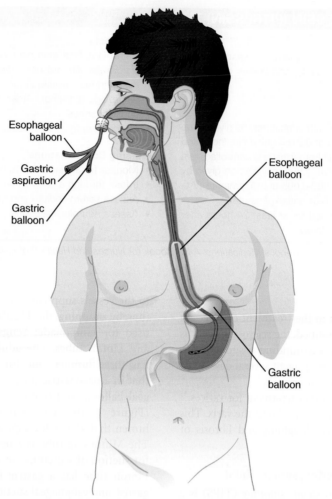

Esophageal
balloon

Gastric
aspiration

Gastric
balloon

Esophageal
balloon

Gastric
balloon

FIGURE 17-10 Sengstaken-Blakemore tube. (From Carlson KK, ed. *AACN: Advanced Critical Care Nursing.* Philadelphia: Saunders. 2009.)

must be confirmed by x-ray study. Ideally, the balloons are deflated every 8 to 12 hours to decompress the esophagus and gastric mucosa. The status of the bleeding varices can also be assessed at this time, and the nurse must be prepared for hematemesis during this procedure. It is crucial that the esophageal balloon be deflated before the gastric balloon is deflated, or else the entire tube will be displaced upward and occlude the airway.

Spontaneous rupture of the gastric balloon, upward migration of the tube, and occlusion of the airway are other possible complications that need to be assessed. Esophageal rupture may occur and is characterized by the abrupt onset of severe pain. In the event of either of these two life-threatening emergencies, all three lumina are cut and the entire tube is removed. For this reason, scissors are kept at the patient's bedside at all times. Endotracheal intubation is strongly recommended to protect the airway.

Other complications of esophagogastric tamponade include ulcerations of the esophageal or gastric mucosa. In addition, lesions can develop around the mouth and nose as a result of the traction devices. Frequent cleansing and

lubrication of these areas help to prevent skin breakdown. The nasopharynx requires frequent suctioning because of an increase in secretions and a decreased swallowing reflex. The nasogastric tube should also be irrigated at least every 2 hours to ensure patency and to keep the stomach empty. This measure helps to prevent aspiration, and also prevents accumulation of blood in the stomach, which is especially important in the patient with liver failure. Ammonia is a by-product of blood breakdown and cannot be detoxified by the patient with liver failure.

Surgical Interventions

Permanent decompression of portal hypertension is achieved only through surgical procedures that divert blood around the blocked portal system. These are called *portacaval shunts.* In these operations, a connection is made between the portal vein and the inferior vena cava that diverts blood flow into the vena cava to decrease portal pressure. Several variations of this procedure exist, including the end-to-side shunt and the side-to-side shunt (Figure 17-11). Other surgical techniques for reduction of portal pressure include splenorenal and mesocaval shunting.

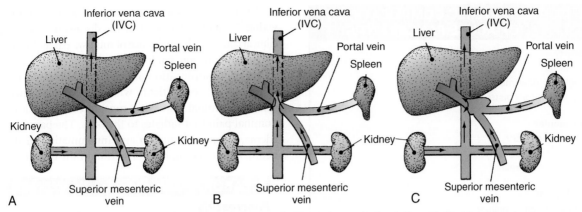

FIGURE 17-11 Types of portacaval shunts. **A,** Normal portal circulation. **B,** End-to-side shunt. **C,** Side-to-side shunt.

Surgical shunts decrease rebleeding but do not improve survival. The procedure is associated with a higher risk of encephalopathy and makes liver transplantation, if needed, more difficult. A temporary increase in ascites occurs after all of these procedures, and careful assessments and interventions are required in the care of this patient population (see the later discussion of hepatic failure).

Patient Outcomes

Expected patient care outcomes for each nursing diagnosis for the patient with acute GI bleeding are found in the "Nursing Care Plan for the Patient with Acute Gastrointestinal Bleeding."

ACUTE PANCREATITIS

Acute pancreatitis is an acute inflammatory disease of the pancreas. The intensity of the disease ranges from mild, in which the patient has abdominal pain and elevated blood amylase and lipase levels, to extremely severe, which results in multiple organ failure. In 85% to 90% of patients, the disease is self-limiting (mild acute pancreatitis), and patients recover rapidly. However, the disease can run a fulminant course and is associated with high mortality rates. Severe acute pancreatitis develops in 25% of patients with acute pancreatitis.[4] Management of patients with this severe form of the disease requires intensive nursing and medical care.

Pathophysiology

Acute pancreatitis is an inflammation of the pancreas with the potential for necrosis of pancreatic cells resulting from premature activation of pancreatic enzymes within the pancreas. It is one of the most common pancreatic diseases, with an incidence rate of 4.9 to 80 cases per 100,000 people per year.[22] Normally, pancreatic juices are secreted into the duodenum, where they are activated. These enzymes are essential to normal carbohydrate, fat, and protein metabolism. The most common theory regarding the development of pancreatitis is that an injury or disruption of pancreatic acinar cells allows leakage of the pancreatic enzymes into pancreatic tissue. The leaked enzymes (trypsin, chymotrypsin, and elastase) become activated in the tissue and start the process of *autodigestion*. The activated enzymes break down tissue and cell membranes, causing edema, vascular damage, hemorrhage, necrosis, and fibrosis.[17] These now toxic enzymes and inflammatory mediators are released into the bloodstream and cause injury to vessel and organ systems, such as the hepatic and renal systems. Acute pancreatitis starts as a localized pancreatic inflammation and is usually accompanied by a compensatory antiinflammatory response syndrome (CARS). Excessive CARS makes the patient susceptible to infections.[33] Box 17-9 reviews the major systemic complications of acute fulminating pancreatitis.

Acute pancreatitis has numerous causes (Box 17-10), but the most common are alcohol ingestion and biliary disease. Many medications may initiate acute pancreatitis as a result of either ingestion of toxic doses or a drug reaction. Pancreatitis resulting from blunt or penetrating abdominal trauma, or occurring after endoscopic exploration of the biliary tree, has also been reported.

Most patients with mild acute pancreatitis are treatable with a short period of bowel rest, simple IV hydration, and analgesia. Severe acute pancreatitis can be complicated by systemic inflammatory response syndrome. Thus the current therapy for acute pancreatitis has shifted to intensive hemodynamic and pulmonary management, nutrition support, infection control, and pharmacological treatments.[21]

Metabolic complications of acute pancreatitis include hypocalcemia and hyperlipidemia, which are thought to be related to the areas of fat necrosis. Hypocalcemia is a major complication and almost always indicates a more serious manifestation of acute pancreatitis. Various hormone imbalances, particularly parathyroid hormone imbalance, are also found in pancreatitis.

Assessment
History and Physical Examination

A diagnosis of acute pancreatitis is based on clinical examination and the results of laboratory and radiological tests (see box "Laboratory Alert: Pancreatitis"). Nurses conduct initial and ongoing assessments, monitor and report physical and laboratory data, and coordinate the multidisciplinary plan of care.

BOX 17-9 SYSTEMIC COMPLICATIONS OF ACUTE PANCREATITIS

Pulmonary
- Hypoxemia
- Atelectasis, pneumonia, pleural effusion
- Acute respiratory distress syndrome

Cardiovascular
- Hypovolemic shock
- Myocardial depression
- Cardiac dysrhythmias

Hematological
- Coagulation abnormalities
- Disseminated intravascular coagulation

Gastrointestinal
- Gastrointestinal bleeding
- Pancreatic pseudocyst
- Pancreatic abscess

Renal
- Azotemia
- Oliguria
- Acute renal failure

Metabolic
- Hypocalcemia
- Hyperlipidemia
- Hyperglycemia
- Metabolic acidosis

BOX 17-10 CAUSES OF ACUTE PANCREATITIS

- Biliary disease
  - Gallstones
  - Common bile duct obstruction
  - Post ERCP procedure
- Alcohol
- Traumatic injury of the pancreas
- Tumors of pancreatic ductal system or mestastatic
- Medications
  - Estrogen
  - Corticosteroids
  - Thiazide diuretics
  - Azathioprine
  - Sulfonamides
  - Furosemide
  - Pentamidine
  - Octreotide
- Heredity
- Hypercalcemia
- Hypertriglyceridemia
- Infections
- Idiopathic

ERCP, Endoscopic retrograde cholangiopancreatography.

Patients who present with organ failure at admission, or within 72 hours after onset of the disease, have a complicated clinical course with persistence of multisystem dysfunction. Multiorgan dysfunction syndrome triggers additional mechanisms that render translocation of bacteria manifesting as sepsis.[4]

In most cases, patients with acute pancreatitis develop severe abdominal pain.[16] It is most often epigastric or midabdominal pain that radiates to the back. The pain is caused by edema, chemical irritation and inflammation of the peritoneum, and irritation or obstruction of the biliary tract.[17]

! LABORATORY ALERT

Pancreatitis

Serum and urine amylase: ↑
Serum lipase: ↑
White blood cell count: ↑
Hematocrit: ↑ with dehydration; ↓ with hemorrhagic pancreatitis
Calcium: ↓
Potassium: ↓
Albumin: ↓
Glucose: ↑ with islet cell damage
Bilirubin, AST, LDH: ↑
Alkaline phosphatase: ↑ with biliary disease

AST, Aspartate transaminase; *LDH*, lactate dehydrogenase.

Nausea and vomiting are also common symptoms. They are caused by the hypermotility or paralytic ileus secondary to the pancreatitis or peritonitis. Abdominal distention accompanies the hypermotile bowel symptoms along with the accumulation of fluid in the peritoneal cavity.[17] This fluid contains enzymes and kinins that increase vascular permeability and dilate the blood vessels. Hypotension and shock occur from the intravascular volume depletion, which then causes myocardial insufficiency. Fever and leukocytosis are also symptoms of the inflammatory process.

Patients with more severe pancreatic disease may have ascites, jaundice, or palpable abdominal masses. Two rare signs that can be present with any disease associated with retroperitoneal hemorrhage include a bluish discoloration of the flanks (*Grey Turner's sign*) or around the umbilical area (*Cullen's sign*), indicative of blood in these areas.[25] Because of the increase in abdominal size, the abdominal girth is measured at least every 4 hours to detect internal bleeding (see box, "Clinical Alert: Signs and Symptoms of Acute Pancreatitis").

! CLINICAL ALERT

Signs and Symptoms of Acute Pancreatitis

- Pain
- Nausea and vomiting
- Fever
- Dehydration
- Abdominal guarding, distention
- Grey Turner's sign
- Cullen's sign

Diagnostic Tests

The diagnosis of acute pancreatitis is based on clinical findings, the presence of associated disorders, and laboratory testing. Pain associated with acute pancreatitis is similar to that associated with peptic ulcer disease, gallbladder disease, intestinal obstruction, and acute myocardial infarction. This similarity exists because pain receptors in the abdomen are poorly differentiated as they exit the skin surface. Because the clinical history, presenting signs and symptoms, and physical findings mimic many other GI and cardiovascular disorders, endoscopic and transabdominal ultrasound and computed tomography (CT) scans are performed in severe cases to determine the extent of involvement and the presence of complications.

Serum lipase and amylase tests are the most specific indicators of acute pancreatitis because as the pancreatic cells and ducts are destroyed, these enzymes are released. An elevated serum amylase level is a characteristic diagnostic feature. Amylase levels usually rise within 12 hours after the onset of symptoms and return to normal within 3 to 5 days. Serum lipase levels increase within 4 to 8 hours of clinical symptom onset and then decrease within 8 to 14 days. Serum trypsin levels are very specific for pancreatitis but may not be readily available. Urine trypsinogen-2 and urine amylase levels are also elevated. C-reactive protein level increases within 48 hours and is a marker of severity. The ratio of amylase clearance to creatinine clearance by the kidney can be diagnostic. Other conditions associated with increased serum amylase levels are listed in Box 17-11.[5]

Other common laboratory abnormalities associated with acute pancreatitis include an elevated WBC count resulting from the inflammatory process, and an elevated serum glucose level resulting from beta cell damage and pancreatic necrosis. Hypokalemia may be present because of associated vomiting. Hyperkalemia may be a systemic complication in the presence of acute renal failure. Hypocalcemia is common with severe disease and usually indicates pancreatic fat necrosis. Serum albumin and protein levels may be decreased as a result of the movement of fluid into the extracellular space. Increases in serum bilirubin, lactate dehydrogenase, and aspartate transaminase levels, and prothrombin time are common in the presence of concurrent liver disease. Serum triglyceride levels may increase dramatically and may be a causative factor in the development of the acute inflammatory process. Arterial blood gas analysis may show hypoxemia

and retained carbon dioxide levels, which indicate respiratory failure.

CT modalities and magnetic resonance imaging are also used to confirm the diagnosis. Contrast-enhanced computed tomography (CECT) reliably detects pancreatic necrosis located in the parenchyma. CECT is considered the gold standard for diagnosing pancreatic necrosis and for grading acute pancreatitis.[25] The Balthazar CT severity index is a scoring system that ranges from 0 to 10 and is obtained by adding the points attributed to the extent of the inflammatory process to the volume of pancreatic necrosis. A higher index is associated with increased severity of disease. Magnetic resonance imaging (MRI) can better detect necrosis in the peripancreatic collections. However, an acutely ill patient might not be able to tolerate this procedure.[33] Endoscopic retrograde cholangiopancreatography (ERCP) combines radiography with endoscopy and may assist in diagnosis.

Predicting the Severity of Acute Pancreatitis

Patients with acute pancreatitis can develop mild or fulminant disease. As a consequence, research has addressed criteria for predicting the prognosis of patients with acute pancreatitis. The early classification criteria were developed by Ranson[31] (Box 17-12), where the number of signs present

---

BOX 17-11 OTHER CONDITIONS ASSOCIATED WITH INCREASED SERUM AMYLASE LEVELS

- Salivary gland disease
- Renal insufficiency
- Diabetic ketoacidosis
- Intraabdominal disease (perforations, obstructions, aortic disease, peritonitis, appendicitis)
- Biliary tract disease
- Pregnancy
- Cerebral trauma
- Pneumonia
- Tumors
- Chronic alcoholism
- Burns
- Shock
- Gynecological disorders
- Prostatic disease

BOX 17-12 RANSON CRITERIA FOR PREDICTING SEVERITY OF ACUTE PANCREATITIS*

At Admission or on Diagnosis
- Age >55 years (>70)
- Leukocyte count >16,000/microliter (>18,000)
- Serum glucose level >200 mg/dL (>220)
- Serum LDH level >350 IU/L (>400)
- Serum AST level >250 IU/L

During Initial 48 Hours
- Decrease in hematocrit >10%
- Increase in blood urea nitrogen level >5 mg/dL (>2)
- Serum calcium level <8 mg/dL
- Base deficit >4 mEq/L (>5)
- Estimated fluid sequestration >6 L (>4)
- Partial pressure of arterial oxygen <60 mm Hg

*Criteria values for nonalcoholic acute pancreatitis differing from those in alcohol-related disease are in parentheses.
AST, Aspartate transaminase; *LDH,* lactate dehydrogenase.
Modified from Ranson JC. Risk factors in acute pancreatitis. *Hospital Practice.* 1985;20(4):69-73.

within the first 48 hours of admission directly relates to the patient's chance of significant morbidity and mortality. In Ranson's research, patients with fewer than three signs had a 1% mortality rate; those with three or four signs had a 15% mortality rate; those with five or six signs had a 40% mortality rate; and those with seven or more signs had a 100% mortality rate.

The Atlanta Classification has become accepted worldwide as the first clinically reliable classification system.[4] It defines severe acute pancreatitis as the presence of three or more of Ranson's criteria or a score of 8 or more with APACHE II (Acute Physiologic and Chronic Health Evaluation) criteria.[25] High severity-of-illness scores (APACHE III) and five or more Ranson criteria predict multiple complications or death.[31] Another scale used to predict multiorgan failure is the Sepsis-Related Organ Failure Assessment.[2]

Nursing Diagnoses

Actual or potential nursing diagnoses associated with acute pancreatitis or with systemic complications of the disease process are found in the "Nursing Care Plan for the Patient with Acute Pancreatitis."

NURSING CARE PLAN

for the Patient with Acute Pancreatitis

NURSING DIAGNOSIS
Fluid volume deficit related to loss of fluid into peritoneal cavity; dehydration from nausea and vomiting; fever; nasogastric suction; and defects in coagulation

PATIENT OUTCOMES
Adequate fluid volume
- Heart rate <100 beats/min
- PAOP WNL
- Urine output >30 mL/hr
- Extremities warm and dry
- Hct and Hgb values stable
- Absence of bleeding

NURSING INTERVENTIONS	RATIONALES
• Monitor hemodynamic status closely: VS, pulmonary artery pressures, I&O, and peripheral circulation	• Assess fluid volume status
• Administer replacement of fluid, blood, or blood products	• Maintain cardiac output and oxygen-carrying products; monitor response to treatment
• Monitor for signs and symptoms of hemorrhage, Hct and Hgb values, Cullen's sign, and Grey Turner's sign	• Assess bleeding in retroperitoneal and abdominal cavities
• Measure abdominal girth every 4 hours	• Assess intraabdominal bleeding
• Assess bladder pressure every 4 hours	• Assess for development of abdominal compartment syndrome

NURSING DIAGNOSIS
Pain related to interruption of blood supply to the pancreas; edema and distention of the pancreas; and peritoneal irritation

PATIENT OUTCOMES
Relief of pain

NURSING INTERVENTIONS	RATIONALES
• Perform a pain assessment, noting onset, duration, intensity, and location	• Establish baseline assessment
• Control pain with the drug of choice: (morphine) or equivalent analgesic	• Relieve pain, that may be severe
• Schedule pain medication to prevent severe pain episodes	• Provide adequate pain relief
• Differentiate pain from cardiac origin	• Release of myocardial depressant factor and a low cardiac output state increase risk of cardiac events
• Maintain bed rest restriction	• Promote comfort
• Position the patient to optimize comfort	• Relieve pain and promote comfort
• Administer sedation as needed	• Treat anxiety that may be associated with increased pain

NURSING CARE PLAN
for the Patient with Acute Pancreatitis—cont'd

NURSING DIAGNOSIS

Altered nutrition (less than body requirements) related to nausea and vomiting; depressed appetite; alcoholism; and impaired nutrient metabolism and altered production of digestive enzymes

PATIENT OUTCOMES
Adequate nutrition
- Positive nitrogen balance
- Serum albumin level WNL
- Weight stable

NURSING INTERVENTIONS	RATIONALES
• Assess nutritional status through clinical examination and laboratory analysis	• Establish baseline assessment
• Calculate caloric needs and compare intake	• Maintain adequate nutrition
• Consult dietician	• Ensure nutritional support to meet needs
• Provide adequate nutritional intake	• Ensure adequate calories to meet needs
• Administer enteral or TPN as ordered; monitor complications associated with administration	• Promote adequate nutrition (see Chapter 6)

NURSING DIAGNOSIS

Impaired Gas Exchange related to atelectasis; pleural effusions; acute respiratory distress syndrome; fluid overload; pulmonary embolus; and splinting from pain

PATIENT OUTCOMES
Adequate gas exchange
- PaO_2 >80 mm Hg
- $PaCO_2$ WNL or at baseline
- Pulmonary complications absent or resolved

NURSING INTERVENTIONS	RATIONALES
• Administer oxygen as prescribed	• Optimize oxygenation
• Monitor SpO_2 and ABGs	• Assess adequate gas exchange
• Auscultate breath sounds every 4 hours	• Assess signs of atelectasis or fluid overload
• Monitor the respiratory rate	• Tachypnea is early sign of respiratory compromise
• Administer vigorous pulmonary hygiene, coughing and deep breathing, and humidification therapy	• Reduce risk for atelectasis
• Note pulmonary secretions for amount, color, consistency, and presence of an odor	• Assess for pulmonary edema and pneumonia
• Administer analgesia to prevent pain caused by splinting	• Maintain normal depth of respiration and avoid atelectasis
• Reposition the patient frequently	• Maximize ventilation and perfusion and prevent pooling of secretions

NURSING DIAGNOSIS

Electrolyte imbalance related to prolonged nausea and vomiting; gastric suction; disease process; and therapeutic regimen

PATIENT OUTCOMES
Electrolyte and glucose values WNL

NURSING INTERVENTIONS	RATIONALES
• Monitor electrolytes and administer replacements according to unit protocol	• Assess status; ensure normal cellular environment and functions
• Monitor blood glucose level according to unit protocol; if using tight glucose control, monitor every hour	• Monitor response to treatment, prevent complications

ABG, Arterial blood gas; *GI*, gastrointestinal; *Hct*, hematocrit; *Hgb*, hemoglobin; *I&O*, intake and output; *PaCO₂*, partial pressure of carbon dioxide in arterial blood; *PaO₂*, partial pressure of oxygen in arterial blood; *PAOP*, pulmonary artery occlusion pressure; *SpO₂*, oxygen saturation via pulse oximetry; *TPN*, total parenteral nutrition; *VS*, vital signs; *WNL*, within normal limits.
Based on data from Gulanick M and Myers JL. *Nursing Care Plans: Diagnoses, Interventions, and Outcomes.* 7th ed. St. Louis: Mosby; 2011.

Medical and Nursing Interventions

Nursing and medical priorities for the management of acute pancreatitis include several interventions. Managing respiratory dysfunction is a high priority. Fluids and electrolytes are replaced to maintain or replenish vascular volume and electrolyte balance. Analgesics are given for pain control, and supportive therapies are aimed at decreasing gastrin release from the stomach and preventing the gastric contents from entering the duodenum.

Fluid Replacement

In patients with severe acute pancreatitis, some fluid collects in the retroperitoneal space and peritoneal cavity. Patients sequester up to one third of their plasma volume. Initially, most patients develop some degree of dehydration and, in severe cases, hypovolemic shock. Hypovolemia and shock are major causes of death early in the disease process. Fluid replacement is a high priority in the treatment of acute pancreatitis.

Fluid replacement helps to maintain perfusion to the pancreas and kidneys, reducing the potential for complications. The IV solutions ordered for fluid resuscitation are usually colloids or lactated Ringer's solution; however, fresh frozen plasma and albumin may also be given. IV fluid administration with crystalloids at 500 mL/hr is often required to maintain hemodynamic stability.[21] Vigorous IV fluid replacement at 250 to 300 mL/hr continues for the first 48 hours or a volume adequate to maintain a urine output of greater than or equal to 0.5 ml/kg body weight per hour.[2]

New Modalities

Surgical decompression of *abdominal compartment syndrome* (ACS), also referred to as intraabdominal hypertension (IAH), may be used to relieve retroperitoneal edema, fluid collections in the abdomen, ascites, ileus, and overaggressive use of fluid therapy in patients with severe acute pancreatitis. ACS is defined as intraabdominal pressure greater than 20 mmHg and new-onset organ failure. In severe acute pancreatitis, ACS is seen early in about 60% of patients and associated with multiple organ dysfunction.

Pentoxifylline has been shown to decrease inflammation, bacterial translocation, and infections.[33] It is a methylxanthine derivative that improves blood flow by increasing erythrocyte and leukocyte flexibility; it also stimulates production of cytokines. Clinical trials for off-label use in pancreatitis are underway.[32]

Critical assessments to evaluate fluid replacement include accurate monitoring of intake and output. A decrease in urine output to less than 50 mL/hr is an early and sensitive measure of hypovolemia and hypoperfusion.[4] Vital signs including blood pressure and heart rate are also sensitive measures of volume status. Expected patient outcomes must be individualized, but reasonable goals are maintenance of systolic blood pressure at greater than 100 mm Hg without an orthostatic decrease, a mean arterial pressure of greater than 60 mm Hg, and a heart rate of less than 100 beats/min. Warm extremities indicate adequate peripheral circulation.

Patients with severe manifestations of the disease may undergo pulmonary artery pressure monitoring to evaluate fluid status and response to treatment. The pulmonary artery occlusion pressure is the most sensitive measure of adequacy of volume status and left ventricular filling pressure. A pulmonary artery occlusion pressure between 11 and 14 mm Hg is a realistic goal for most patients with pancreatitis.

Patients with severe disease who do not respond to fluid therapy alone (i.e., hypotension continues) may need medications to support blood pressure (e.g., vasopressors). Patients with acute hemorrhagic pancreatitis may also need packed RBCs in addition to fluid therapy to restore intravascular volume.

Electrolyte Replacement

Hypocalcemia (serum calcium level less than 8.5 mg/dL) is a common electrolyte imbalance. It is associated with a high mortality rate. Calcium is essential for many physiological functions: catalyzing impulses for nerves and muscles, maintaining the integrity of cell membranes and vessels, clotting of blood, strengthening bones and teeth, and increasing contractility in the heart. A sign of hypocalcemia on the electrocardiogram is lengthening of the QT interval. Severe hypocalcemia (serum calcium level less than 6 mg/dL) may cause tetany, seizures, positive Chvostek's and Trousseau's signs, and respiratory distress. Patients with severe hypocalcemia should be placed on seizure precaution status, and respiratory support equipment should be available (e.g., oral airway, suction). The nurse is responsible for monitoring calcium levels, administering replacement, and monitoring the patient's response to any calcium given. Monitoring serum albumin levels is also important because true serum calcium levels can be evaluated only in comparison with serum albumin levels. The patient is also monitored for calcium toxicity. Symptoms include lethargy, nausea, shortening of the QT interval, and decreased excitability of nerves and muscles. Hypomagnesemia may also be present in hypocalcemia, and magnesium replacement may be required.

Potassium is another electrolyte that may need to be replaced early in the treatment regimen. Hypokalemia is associated with cardiac dysrhythmias, muscle weakness, hypotension, decreased bowel sounds, ileus, and irritability. Potassium must be diluted and administered via an infusion pump per unit protocol.

Hyperglycemia is not a common complication of acute pancreatitis because most of the pancreatic gland must be necrosed before the insulin-secreting islet cells are affected. More commonly, hyperglycemia is a result of the body's stress response to acute illness.

Nutrition Support

Nasogastric suction and "nothing by mouth" status were classic treatments for patients with acute pancreatitis to suppress pancreatic exocrine secretion by preventing the release

EVIDENCE-BASED PRACTICE

Early Enteral Nutrition

Problem

For many years patients with acute pancreatitis have been maintained with "nothing by mouth" orders to rest the pancreas. Total parenteral nutrition is often ordered to provide adequate nutrition, yet this therapy increases the risk for complications, including infection and hyperglycemia.

Clinical Question

What are the outcomes associated with early enteral feeding in acute pancreatitis compared to total parenteral nutrition? Is early enteral nutrition tolerated?

Evidence

Quan and colleagues reviewed the results of six randomized controlled trials of enteral versus parenteral nutrition. In these studies, patients were randomized to the type of nutrition. Meta-analysis found that enteral nutrition was associated with a significantly lower incidence of pancreatitis infection-related complications (infection, abscess, and necrosis), surgical interventions, and mortality. Parenteral nutrition was associated with a lower risk of non–infection related complications (acute respiratory distress syndrome, pancreatic cyst, diarrhea, and abdominal distention). They concluded that enteral nutrition was preferred over parenteral modalities. A systematic review by Spanier and coworkers of studies from a recent 10-year period found that early enteral nutrition was safe and well tolerated, and they advocated starting enteral feeding within 48 hours.

Implications for Nursing

These studies show support for early enteral nutritional support in patients with acute pancreatitis. Minimal adverse effects of enteral nutrition were reported. This intervention has the potential of reducing complications and length of stay.

Level of Evidence

A—Meta-analysis

References

1. Quan H, Wang X, Guo C. A meta-analysis of enteral nutrition and total parenteral nutrition in patients with acute pancreatitis. *Gastroenterology Research and Practice, epub, doi:10.1155/2011/698248.* 2011.
2. Spanier BWM, Bruno MJ, Mathus-Vliegen EMH. Enteral nutrition and pancreatitis: a review. *Gastroenterology Research and Practice, epub, doi:10.1155/2011/857949.* 2011.

of secretin from the duodenum. Normally, secretin, which stimulates pancreatic secretion production, is stimulated when acid is in the duodenum; therefore nasogastric suction has been a primary treatment. Nausea, vomiting, and abdominal pain may also be decreased with nasogastric suctioning. A nasogastric tube is also necessary in patients with ileus, severe gastric distention, and a decreased level of consciousness to prevent complications resulting from pulmonary aspiration.

Trends in nutritional management are changing. Early nutritional support may be ordered to prevent atrophy of gut lymphoid tissue, prevent bacterial overgrowth in the intestine, and increase intestinal permeability.[28] Immediate oral feeding in patients with mild acute pancreatitis is safe and may accelerate recovery.[9] Systematic reviews of early enteral nutrition for severe acute pancreatitis were done to evaluate its effectiveness and safety.[21,28] Early enteral nutrition appears effective and safe (see box, "Evidence-Based Practice").

Comfort Management

Pain control is a nursing priority in patients with acute pancreatitis not only because the disorder produces extreme patient discomfort, but also because pain increases the patient's metabolism and thus increases pancreatic secretions. The pain of pancreatitis is caused by edema and distention of the pancreatic capsule, obstruction of the biliary system, and peritoneal inflammation from pancreatic enzymes. Pain is often severe and unrelenting and is related to the degree of pancreatic inflammation.

A baseline pain assessment is performed early after the patient's admission and includes information about the onset, intensity, duration, and location (local or diffuse) of the pain. Analgesic administration is a nursing priority. Adequate pain control requires the use of IV opiates, often in the form of a patient-controlled analgesia (PCA) pump. In the case in which a PCA pump is not ordered, pain medications are administered on a routine schedule, rather than as needed, to prevent uncontrollable abdominal pain. Traditionally, opiate analgesics (e.g., morphine) were considered to cause spasm of the sphincter of Oddi and exacerbate pain; however, current research questions this practice.[35] Meperidine (Demerol) may be ordered in place of morphine if pancreatitis occurs secondary to gallbladder disease.[19] Insertion of a nasogastric tube connected to low intermittent suction may help ease pain. Patient positioning may also relieve some of the discomfort and should be facilitated by the nurse as the patient's hemodynamic status allows.

Pharmacological Intervention

Various pharmacological therapies have been researched in the treatment of acute pancreatitis. Drugs given to rest the pancreas have been studied, specifically anticholinergics, glucagon, somatostatin, cimetidine, and calcitonin, but these have not been shown to be effective. Prevention of stress ulcers is achieved through the use of histamine blockers and antacids.

Antibiotics have also been studied in the treatment of inflammation of the pancreas with the idea of preventing pancreatic pseudocysts or abscesses. It is not known whether antibiotics improve survival or merely prevent septic complications.[25] The role of prophylactic systemic antibiotics in acute pancreatitis is unsettled because studies evaluating the benefits and harms have produced disparate results.[18]

Treatment of Systemic Complications

Multisystemic complications of acute pancreatitis are related to the ability of the pancreas to produce many vasoactive substances that affect organs throughout the body. These complications are summarized in Box 17-9.

Pulmonary complications are common in patients with both mild and severe manifestations of the disease. Arterial hypoxemia, atelectasis, pleural effusions, ARDS, and pneumonia have been identified in many patients with acute pancreatitis. Accumulation of fluid in the peritoneum causes restricted movement of the diaphragm. Arterial oxygen saturation is continuously monitored, and arterial blood gases are assessed as needed. Treatment of hypoxemia includes supplemental oxygen and vigorous pulmonary hygiene, such as deep breathing, coughing, and frequent position changes. Some patients may need intubation to ensure adequate ventilation; others can be maintained with noninvasive ventilation modes. Pulmonary emboli have also been documented as a complication of acute pancreatitis. Careful fluid administration is necessary to prevent fluid overload and pulmonary congestion. Patients with severe disease may develop acute respiratory failure.

Close monitoring and management of other systemic complications of acute pancreatitis, such as coagulation abnormalities and hemorrhage, cardiovascular failure and dysrhythmias, and acute renal failure, are also important. Coagulation defects in acute pancreatitis are similar to disseminated intravascular coagulation, and are associated with a high mortality rate. The cardiac depression associated with acute pancreatitis may vary. The presence of hypovolemic shock is a grave presentation. Astute cardiovascular monitoring and volume replacement are required to reverse this serious complication. Impaired renal function has been documented in many patients.

GI complications of acute pancreatitis include pancreatic pseudocyst and abdominal abscess. A pseudocyst should be suspected in any patient who has persistent abdominal pain and nausea and vomiting, a prolonged fever, and an elevated serum amylase level. CT can be helpful in diagnosing the location and size of the pseudocyst. Signs and symptoms of an abdominal abscess include an increased WBC count, fever, abdominal pain, and vomiting. CT provides a definitive diagnosis. Early recognition and treatment of a pancreatic pseudocyst are important because this condition is associated with a high mortality rate.

Surgical Therapy

Pancreatic resection for acute necrotizing pancreatitis may be performed to prevent systemic complications of the disease process. In this procedure, dead or infected pancreatic tissue is surgically removed while preserving most of the gland.[25] A variety of surgical treatment modalities are currently available, including laparoscopic techniques.[4] The indication for surgical intervention is clinical deterioration of the patient despite conventional treatments, or the presence of peritonitis.

Surgery may also be indicated for pseudocysts; however, surgery is usually delayed because some pseudocysts resolve spontaneously. Surgical treatment of a pseudocyst can be performed through internal or external drainage, or needle aspiration. Acute surgical intervention may be required if the pseudocyst becomes infected or perforated.

Surgery may also be performed when gallstones are thought to be the cause of the acute pancreatitis. A cholecystectomy is usually performed.

Patient Outcomes

Expected outcomes for the patient with acute pancreatitis are found in the "Nursing Care Plan for the Patient with Acute Pancreatitis."

HEPATIC FAILURE

Chronic liver disease (CLD) or cirrhosis is the twelfth leading cause of death in the United States accounting for 29,165 deaths in 2007. However, recent data suggest liver-related mortality is higher than estimated by 121%, making it the eighth leading cause of death in the United States. End-stage liver disease (ESLD) is characterized as the deterioration of the patient from a compensated to an uncompensated state. Critically ill patients with ESLD have a mortality of about 50% to 100%.[30] Hepatic failure also results from chronic liver disease, in which healthy liver tissue is replaced by fibrotic tissue.[29] This form of liver failure is called *cirrhosis*. Finally, liver cells can be replaced by fatty cells or tissue and is known as *fatty liver disease.*

Pathophysiology

The normal liver architecture is pictured in Figure 17-5 and is characterized by a basic functional unit of the liver called a *lobule*. The liver lobule is uniquely made in that it has its own blood supply, which allows the liver cells (*hepatocytes*) to be exposed continuously to blood. Hepatic failure results when the liver is unable to perform its many functions (see Box 17-2). Liver failure results from necrosis or a decrease in the blood supply to liver cells. This problem is most often caused by hepatitis or inflammation of the liver.

Hepatitis

Hepatitis is an acute inflammation of the hepatocytes. This inflammation is accompanied by edema. As the inflammation progresses, blood supply to the hepatocytes is interrupted, causing necrosis and breakdown of healthy cells.

- Contact with:
  - Blood and blood products
  - Semen
  - Saliva
- Percutaneously through mucous membranes
- Direct contact with infected fluids or objects

! **CLINICAL ALERT**
Signs and Symptoms of Fulminant Hepatic Failure

- Hyperexcitability
- Insomnia
- Irritability
- Decreased level of consciousness, coma
- Convulsions
- Sudden onset of high fever
- Nausea and vomiting
- Chills
- Jaundice

Blood may back up in the portal system, causing *portal hypertension*.

Liver cells have the capacity to regenerate. Over time, liver cells that become damaged are removed by the body's immune system and are replaced with healthy liver cells. Therefore most patients with hepatitis recover and regain normal liver function.

Hepatitis is most often caused by a virus. Several hepatitis viruses have been identified: hepatitis A, B, C, D, E, and G. Researchers continue to study other viruses that may be associated with acute hepatitis. Modes of transmission are summarized in Box 17-13. Characteristics of hepatitis in terms of type, route of transmission, severity, and prophylaxis are presented in Table 17-8.

Assessment. Patients with hepatitis are often asymptomatic. In many patients, prodromal symptoms of anorexia, nausea, vomiting, abdominal pain, and fatigue may be present. Symptoms then progress to a low-grade fever, an enlarged and tender liver, and jaundice (see box, "Clinical Alert: Signs and Symptoms of Fulminant Hepatic Failure").[6]

Assessment of risk factors often assists in the diagnosis of hepatitis. Laboratory tests show elevated liver function tests. The diagnosis is confirmed by identifying antibodies specific to each type of hepatitis. Recovery from acute hepatitis usually occurs within 9 weeks for hepatitis A, and 16 weeks for hepatitis B. Hepatitis B, C, D, and G may progress to chronic forms.[16]

Nursing diagnoses. Many nursing diagnoses are associated with viral hepatitis. These include activity intolerance related to fatigue, fever, and flulike symptoms; altered nutrition (less than body requirements) related to loss of appetite, nausea, vomiting, and loss of liver metabolic functions; risk for infection related to loss of liver cell function for phagocytosis of bacteria; and risk for altered thought processes related to medications that require liver metabolism.

Medical and nursing interventions. No definitive treatment for acute inflammation of the liver exists. Goals for medical and nursing care include providing rest and assisting the patient in obtaining optimal nutrition. Most patients are cared for at home unless the disease becomes prolonged or

TABLE 17-8	**CHARACTERISTICS OF HEPATITIS**		
TYPE	**ROUTE OF TRANSMISSION**	**SEVERITY**	**PROPHYLAXIS**
Hepatitis A	Fecal-oral, parenteral, sexual	Mild	Hygiene, immune serum globulin, HAV vaccine, Twinrix*
Hepatitis B	Parenteral, sexual	Severe, may be prolonged or chronic	Hygiene, HBV vaccine, Twinrix*
Hepatitis C	Parenteral	Mild to severe	Hygiene, screening blood, interferon-alpha
Hepatitis D	Parenteral, fecal-oral, sexual	Severe	Hygiene, HBV vaccine
Hepatitis E	Fecal-oral	Severe in pregnant women	Hygiene, safe water
Hepatitis G	Parenteral, sexual	Unknown	Unknown

*A bivalent vaccine containing the antigenic components, a sterile suspension of inactivated hepatitis A virus combined with purified surface antigen of the hepatitis B virus.
HAV, Hepatitis A virus; *HBV*, Hepatitis B virus.
Adapted from Huether SE. Alterations of digestive function. In McCance KL, Huether SE, *Pathophysiology: The Biologic Basis for Disease in Adults and Children.* 6th ed. St. Louis: Mosby. 2010.

fulminant failure develops. Medications to help the patient rest or to decrease agitation must be closely monitored because most of these drugs require clearance by the liver, which is impaired during the acute phase.

Maintenance of the nutritional status of the patient is a nursing priority. Loss of appetite, nausea, and vomiting may persist for weeks. Nursing measures such as administration of antiemetics may be helpful. Small, frequent, palatable meals and supplements should be offered. Evaluation of nutritional status is ongoing and includes assessments of intake and output, daily weights, serum albumin level, and nitrogen balance. Patients must be instructed not to take any over-the-counter drugs that can cause liver damage. Box 17-14 lists common hepatotoxic drugs. Alcohol should be avoided.

Liver transplantation is the standard care of treatment for patients with progressive, irreversible acute or chronic liver disease for which there are no other medical or surgical options. The leading indication for liver transplantation is hepatitis C. (See Chapter 21 for more detail related to liver transplantation.)

Hepatitis can lead to acute hepatic failure. The clinical manifestations of this disorder are discussed in the sections on impaired metabolic processes and impaired bile formation and flow.

Special precautions must be taken to prevent spread of the virus when caring for the patient with hepatitis. These include the *universal precautions* while handling all items that are contaminated with the patient's body secretions, including patient care items such as thermometers, dishes, and eating utensils.

Several patient outcomes are expected after nursing and medical interventions. These include absence of pain, adequate nutrition, activity tolerance, absence of infection, and resolving/normal laboratory tests.

Cirrhosis

Cirrhosis causes severe alterations in the structure and function of liver cells. It is characterized by inflammation and liver cell necrosis that may be focal or diffuse. Fat deposits may also be present. The enlarged liver cells cause compression of the liver lobule and lead to increased resistance to blood flow and portal hypertension. Necrosis is followed by regeneration of liver tissue, but not in a normal fashion. Fibrous tissue is laid down over time, and this distorts the normal architecture of the liver lobule. These fibrotic changes are usually irreversible, resulting in chronic liver dysfunction. Table 17-9 characterizes the types of cirrhosis.

Fatty Liver

Fatty liver is an accumulation of excessive fats in the liver; it is morphologically distinguishable from cirrhosis. Alcohol abuse is the most common cause of this disorder. Other causes include obesity, diabetes, hepatic resection, starvation,

---

BOX 17-14	COMMON HEPATOTOXIC DRUGS

Analgesics
- Acetaminophen (Tylenol)
- Salicylates (aspirin)

Anesthetics
- Enflurane (Ethrane)
- Halothane (Fluothane)
- Methoxyflurane (Penthrane)

Anticonvulsants
- Phenytoin (Dilantin)
- Phenobarbital (Luminal)

Antidepressants
- Monoamine oxidase inhibitors
- Amitriptyline (Elavil)
- Doxepin (Sinequan)

Antimicrobial Agents
- Isoniazid
- Nitrofurantoin (Macrodantin)
- Rifampin
- Sulfonamides (sulfisoxazole acetyl [Gantrisin], silver sulfadiazine [Silvadene])
- Tetracycline

Antipsychotic Drugs
- Haloperidol (Haldol)
- Chlorpromazine (Thorazine)
- Fluphenazine (Prolixin)
- Prochlorperazine (Compazine)
- Promethazine (Phenergan)
- Thioridazine (Mellaril)

Cardiovascular Drugs
- Methyldopa (Aldomet)
- Quinidine sulfate

Hormonal Agents
- Antithyroid drugs
- Oral contraceptives
- Oral hypoglycemics (tolbutamide [Orinase], chlorpropamide [Diabinese])

Sedatives
- Chlordiazepoxide (Librium)
- Diazepam (Valium)

Others
- Cimetidine (Tagamet)

TABLE 17-9	CHARACTERISTICS OF TYPES OF CIRRHOSIS		
TYPE	**CAUSE**	**CONSEQUENCES**	**SEQUELAE**
Alcoholic (Laënnec's)	Long-term alcohol abuse	Fatty liver Fibrotic tissue replaces liver cells	Acetaldehyde, a toxic metabolite of alcohol ingestion, causes liver cell damage and death
Biliary	Long-term obstruction of bile ducts	Decrease in bile flow	Degeneration and fibrosis of the ducts
Cardiac	Severe long-term right-sided heart failure	Decreased oxygenation of liver cells	Cellular death
Postnecrotic	Exposure to hepatotoxins, chemicals, infection, or metabolic disorder	Massive death of liver cells	Development of liver cancer

and total parenteral nutrition. Damage caused by the fat deposits may result in liver dysfunction, failure, and death.

Assessment of Hepatic Failure
Presenting Clinical Signs

Initial clinical signs of hepatic failure are vague and include weakness, fatigue, loss of appetite, weight loss, abdominal discomfort, nausea and vomiting, and change in bowel habits.

As destruction in the liver progresses, the systemic effects of the disease become apparent. Impaired liver function results in loss of the normal vascular, secretory, and metabolic functions of the liver (see Box 17-2). The functional sequelae of liver disease are divided into three categories: (1) portal hypertension, (2) impaired liver metabolic processes, and (3) impaired bile formation and flow. These derangements and their clinical manifestations are summarized in Box 17-15.

BOX 17-15	CLINICAL SIGNS AND SYMPTOMS OF LIVER DISEASE

Cardiac
- Hyperdynamic circulation
- Portal hypertension
- Dysrhythmias
- Activity intolerance
- Edema

Dermatological
- Jaundice
- Spider angiomas
- Pruritus

Electrolytes
- Hypokalemia
- Hyponatremia (dilutional)
- Hypernatremia

Endocrine
- Increased aldosterone
- Increased antidiuretic hormone

Fluid Alterations
- Ascites
- Water retention
- Decreased volume in vascular space

Gastrointestinal
- Abdominal discomfort
- Decreased appetite
- Diarrhea
- Varices or gastrointestinal bleeding
- Malnutrition
- Nausea and vomiting

Hematological
- Anemia
- Impaired coagulation
- Disseminated intravascular coagulation

Immune System
- Increased susceptibility to infection

Neurological
- Hepatic encephalopathy

Pulmonary
- Dyspnea
- Hepatopulmonary syndrome
- Hyperventilation
- Hypoxemia
- Ineffective breathing patterns

Renal
- Hepatorenal syndrome

Portal hypertension. Portal hypertension causes two main clinical problems for the patient: hyperdynamic circulation and development of esophageal or gastric varices. Liver cell destruction causes shunting of blood and increased cardiac output. Vasodilation is also present, which causes decreased perfusion to all body organs, even though the cardiac output is very high. This phenomenon is known as *high-output failure* or *hyperdynamic circulation.* Clinical signs and symptoms are those of heart failure and include jugular vein distention, pulmonary crackles, and decreased perfusion to all organs. Initially, the patient may have hypertension, flushed skin, and bounding pulses. Blood pressure decreases and dysrhythmias are common. Increased portal venous pressure causes the formation of varices that shunt blood to decrease pressure. These varices can cause massive upper GI bleeding (see the earlier discussion of upper GI bleeding). Splenomegaly is also associated with portal hypertension.

Impaired metabolic processes. The liver is the most complex organ because it carries out many metabolic processes. Liver failure causes the following: altered carbohydrate, fat, and protein metabolism; decreased synthesis of blood clotting factors; decreased removal of activated clotting components; decreased metabolism of vitamins and iron; decreased storage functions; and decreased detoxification functions.

Altered carbohydrate metabolism may result in unstable blood glucose levels. The serum glucose level may increase to more than 200 mg/dL. This condition is termed *cirrhotic diabetes.* Altered carbohydrate metabolism may also result in malnutrition and a decreased stress response. Hypoglycemia may also be seen secondary to depletion of hepatic glycogen stores and decreased gluconeogenesis.[16]

Altered fat metabolism may result in a fatty liver. Fat is used by all cells for energy, and altered metabolism may cause fatigue and decreased activity tolerance in many patients. Alterations in skin integrity, which are common in chronic liver disease, are also thought to be related to this metabolic dysfunction. Bile salts are also not adequately produced, and this leads to an inability of fats to be metabolized by the small intestine. Malnutrition often results.

Protein metabolism, albumin synthesis, and serum albumin levels are decreased. Albumin is necessary for colloid oncotic pressure to hold fluid in the intravascular space and for nutrition. Low albumin levels are also thought to be associated with the development of ascites, a complication of hepatic failure. Globulin is another protein that is essential for the transport of substances in the blood. Fibrinogen is an essential protein that is necessary for normal clotting. A low plasma fibrinogen level, coupled with decreased synthesis of many blood clotting factors, predisposes the patient to bleeding. Clinical signs and symptoms range from bruising and nasal and gingival bleeding to frank hemorrhage. Disseminated intravascular coagulation may also develop.

Kupffer's cells in the liver play an important role in fighting infections throughout the body. Loss of this function predisposes the patient to severe infections, particularly sepsis caused by gram-negative bacteria.

The liver also removes activated clotting factors from the general circulation to prevent widespread clotting in the system. Loss of this function predisposes the patient to clot formation, and complications such as pulmonary embolus.

Decreased metabolism and storage of vitamins A, B_{12}, and D, and of iron, glucose, and fat predispose the patient to many nutritional deficiencies. The liver loses the function of detoxifying drugs, ammonia, and hormones. Loss of ammonia conversion to urea in the liver is responsible for many of the altered thought processes seen in liver failure, because ammonia is allowed to enter the central nervous system directly. These alterations range from minor sensory perceptual changes, such as tremors, slurred speech, and impaired decision making, to dramatic confusion or profound coma.

Hormonal imbalances are common in liver disease. The most important physiological imbalance is the activation of aldosterone and antidiuretic hormone, which contribute to some of the fluid and electrolyte disturbances commonly found in liver disease. Sodium and water retention and portal hypertension lead to a third spacing of fluid from the intravascular space into the peritoneal cavity *(ascites).* The resultant decrease in plasma volume causes activation of compensatory mechanisms in the body to release antidiuretic hormone and aldosterone. This situation causes further water and sodium retention. The *renin-angiotensin system* is also activated, which causes systemic vasoconstriction. The kidneys are most severely affected, and urine output decreases because of impaired perfusion. Sexual dysfunction is common in patients with liver disease, and this can lead to self-concept alterations. Dermatological lesions that occur in some patients with liver failure, called *spider angiomas,* are thought to be related to an endocrine imbalance. These vascular lesions may be venous or arterial and represent the progression of liver disease.

Impaired bile formation and flow. The liver's inability to metabolize bile is reflected clinically in an increased serum bilirubin level and a staining of tissue by bilirubin, or jaundice. Jaundice is generally present in patients with a serum bilirubin level greater than 3 mg/dL.

Nursing Diagnoses

The nursing diagnoses, actual and potential, can be derived from assessment data in a patient with liver failure (see box, "Nursing Care Plan for the Patient with Hepatic Failure").

◎ NURSING CARE PLAN

for the Patient with Hepatic Failure

NURSING DIAGNOSIS

Fluid volume deficit related to variceal hemorrhage; third spacing of peritoneal fluid (ascites); and coagulation abnormalities

PATIENT OUTCOMES

Adequate fluid volume
- Absence or resolution of bleeding
- Hct, Hgb, coagulation factors, protein, albumin values WNL
- Normal VS

NURSING INTERVENTIONS	RATIONALES
• See "Nursing Care Plan for the Patient with Acute Gastrointestinal Bleeding"	
• Monitor blood counts and coagulation function test results	• Assess for active bleeding and risk for bleeding from altered liver function
• Protect the patient from injury	• Volume deficits may cause lightheadedness and dizziness from poor perfusion to the brain
• Pad side rails and assist with activities of daily living	• Protect from injury
• Monitor for petechiae and bleeding from the IV site and mucous membranes	• Assess for bleeding
• Limit punctures for blood draws and IV lines	• Reduce risk of infection and bleeding from puncture sites
• Guaiac specimens	• Assess for occult bleeding
• Administer fluid and blood products as ordered, and monitor patient response	• Maintain fluid and blood volume
• Administer vitamin K and other coagulation products	• Promote normal coagulation

---

NURSING DIAGNOSIS

Altered nutrition (less than body requirements) related to altered liver metabolism of food nutrients; insufficient intake; impaired absorption of fat-soluble vitamins; and vitamin B_{12} deficiency

PATIENT OUTCOMES

Adequate nutrition
- Protein intake sufficient for liver regeneration
- BUN level WNL
- Liver function tests results WNL
- Serum albumin level WNL

NURSING INTERVENTIONS	RATIONALES
• Limit protein intake	• Reduce level of ammonia from inadequate protein metabolism
• Monitor serum BUN level	• Determine fluid volume status
• Administer vitamins synthesized by the liver: A, B, D, and K	• Replace essential vitamins
• Monitor nutritional status through serum albumin level and nitrogen balance	• Assess nutritional status
• Consider enteral feeding or TPN if oral intake is insufficient	• Promote normal nutritional status

Continued

◎ NURSING CARE PLAN

for the Patient with Hepatic Failure—cont'd

NURSING DIAGNOSIS

Ineffective Breathing Pattern and Impaired Gas Exchange related to dyspnea from ascites; and increased risk of pulmonary infections

PATIENT OUTCOMES

Effective breathing

- Effective lung expansion
- Dyspnea absent
- ABGs WNL

NURSING INTERVENTIONS	RATIONALES
• Administer oxygen as ordered according to clinical assessment	• Optimize oxygenation
• Monitor the patient's respiratory status	• Assess deteriorating pulmonary status
• Monitor ABGs for increasing $PaCO_2$ and decreasing PaO_2	• Recognize poor ventilatory efforts; guide treatment
• Encourage the patient to cough and deep breathe	• Mobilize pulmonary secretions, and reduce the risk of pulmonary compromise
• Administer sedatives and analgesics cautiously so as not to impair respiratory effort	• Drugs may not be cleared well when liver function is less than optimal
• Measure abdominal girth every 4 hours	• Assess ascites
• Monitor and restrict fluids and sodium, and administer diuretics as ordered	• Assess and manage ascites
• Assist with paracentesis as needed	• Relieve ascites

NURSING DIAGNOSIS

Altered thought processes related to impaired handling of ammonia; medications that require liver metabolism; and decreased perfusion states

PATIENT OUTCOMES

Normal thought processes

- Hepatic encephalopathy absent or resolved
- BUN level stable

NURSING INTERVENTIONS	RATIONALES
• Monitor ammonia levels and conduct ongoing neurological assessments	• The neurological assessment slowly returns to normal as ammonia levels return to normal
• Administer lactulose and neomycin, and monitor results	• Reduces ammonia levels
• Restrict protein intake	• Ammonia is a by-product of protein metabolism
• Reduce the risk of GI bleeding through antacid and H_2-histamine blocker administration	• Prevent bleeding and associated increase in ammonia levels
• Use sedatives and narcotics judiciously	• Drug metabolism is impaired in liver failure
• Prevent and treat infection, dehydration, and electrolyte or acid-base disturbances	• Reduce complications
• Reorient the patient and provide for safety during periods of impaired mentation	• High ammonia levels cause disorientation

ABG, Arterial blood gas; *BUN,* blood urea nitrogen; *GI,* gastrointestinal; *Hct,* hematocrit; *Hgb,* hemoglobin; *I&O,* intake and output; *IV,* intravenous; *PaCO₂,* partial pressure of carbon dioxide in arterial blood; *PaO₂,* partial pressure of oxygen in arterial blood; *TPN,* total parenteral nutrition; *VS,* vital signs; *WNL,* within normal limits.

Based on data from Gulanick M and Myers JL. *Nursing Care Plans: Diagnoses, Interventions, and Outcomes.* 7th ed. St. Louis: Mosby; 2011.

Medical and Nursing Interventions

Nursing and medical management of the patient with liver failure is aimed at supportive therapies and early recognition and treatment of complications associated with the disease process. Management of acute liver failure challenges the best skills of providers, intensivists, and nurses.[13]

Diagnostic Tests

Altered laboratory results in patients with liver disease (see box, "Laboratory Alert: Liver Failure") are a direct result of destruction of hepatic cells (liver enzymes) or of the effects of impaired liver metabolic processes.

Parenchymal tests such as liver biopsy can be performed to study the liver cell architecture directly. The liver is characteristically small and has a marked decrease in functioning hepatic cell structures. This characteristic allows for a definitive diagnosis of the cause of the hepatic failure. An ultrasound study may detect impaired bile flow.

! LABORATORY ALERT

Liver Failure

SERUM OR PLASMA	ALTERATION
Albumin	↓
Ammonia	↑
Bile Pigments	
Total bilirubin	↑
Direct or conjugated bilirubin	↑
Cholesterol	↑
Coagulation Tests	
Prothrombin time	Prolonged
Partial thromboplastin time	Prolonged
Enzymes	
APT	↑
AST	↑
ALT	↑
Urine	
Bilirubin	↑
Urobilinogen	↑

ALT, Alanine transaminase; *APT,* alkaline phosphatase; *AST,* aspartate transaminase.

Supportive Therapy

Hemodynamic instability and decreased perfusion to core organs are the end result of portal hypertension and hyperdynamic circulation. Invasive monitoring may be used in the critically ill patient, but it must be weighed in terms of the potential for infection in a patient with an impaired immune response. Administration of vasoactive drugs and fluids may be ordered to support blood pressure and kidney perfusion, which requires close monitoring by the nurse. Portal hypertension also predisposes the patient to esophageal and gastric varices, which have the potential to bleed.

The patient with liver failure is at risk for bleeding complications because of decreased synthesis of clotting factors. Patients with a prolonged prothrombin time and partial thromboplastin time and a decreased platelet count should be protected from injury through the use of padded side rails and assistance with all activity. Needlesticks should be kept to a minimum. Blood products may be ordered in severe cases. Antacids, proton pump inhibitors, or H$_2$-blockers are ordered to prevent gastritis and bleeding from stress ulcers.

Administration of all drugs metabolized by the liver must be restricted. The administration of such drugs could cause acute liver failure in a patient with chronic disease.

Support for the Failing Liver

Advances have been made in the development of artificial support of liver function, spurred on by the shortage of donor organs and the high incidence of mortality related to acute or chronic liver failure.[16] *Bioartificial liver devices* serve as a bridge to liver transplantation, or support liver function long enough to allow regeneration of normal liver function.[23] The bioartificial liver circulates the individual's blood around the outside of a system of hollow fibers packed with pig hepatocytes to allow toxins to be removed and nutrients to be replaced.[15]

Another type of support is the Molecular Adsorbents Recirculating System (MARS), an extracorporeal albumin dialysis technique that uses an albumin-impregnated membrane to remove both protein-bound and water-soluble toxins from the blood.[16] Cytokines are believed to play an important role in acute-on-chronic liver failure. Cytokines are cleared from plasma by both MARS and another system, the Fractionated Plasma Separation, Adsorption and Dialysis (Prometheus).[32] However, at present, neither of these treatments is able to change serum cytokine levels.

Treatment of Complications

Ascites. Impaired handling of salt and water by the kidneys and other abnormalities in fluid homeostasis predispose the patient to an accumulation of fluid in the peritoneum, or *ascites.* Ascites is problematic because as more fluid is retained, it pushes up on the diaphragm, thereby impairing breathing. Nursing assessment of respiratory rate, breath sounds, and pulse oximetry values is critical. Frequent monitoring of abdominal girth alerts the nurse to fluid accumulation. Abdominal girth should be measured at the level of the umbilicus. Positioning the patient in a semi-Fowler's position also allows for free diaphragm movement. Frequent deep-breathing and coughing exercises and changes in position are important to facilitate full/optimal breathing. Some patients may require elective

BOX 17-16   PHYSIOLOGICAL EFFECTS OF ABDOMINAL COMPARTMENT SYNDROME

Cardiovascular
- Decreased venous return
- Increased systemic vascular resistance and intrathoracic pressure
- Reduction in cardiac output

Respiratory
- Atelectasis
- Pneumonia
- Impaired ventilation
- Respiratory failure

Hepatic and Renal
- Decreased blood flow to liver and kidney
- Functional impairment of both organs

Gastrointestinal
- Impaired lymphatic, venous, and arterial flow
- Poor healing of anastomoses

Neurological
- Simultaneous increased intracranial pressure from both head trauma and intraabdominal hypertension

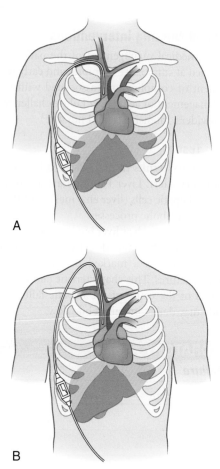

FIGURE 17-12 The Denver shunt. Percutaneous placement of both the venous and peritoneal catheters of a Denver Ascites Shunt. Venous catheter placement into the **A,** subclavian and **B,** internal jugular vein.

intubation until medical management of the ascites is accomplished. Ascites may also result in *abdominal compartment syndrome.* Box 17-16 lists the physiological that may occur with this complication.

Ascites is medically managed through bed rest, a low-sodium diet, fluid restriction, and diuretic therapy. Diuretics must be administered cautiously, however, because if the intravascular volume is depleted too quickly, acute renal failure may be induced. Close monitoring of the serum creatinine level, the BUN level, and urine output is important for the early detection of renal impairment. Careful monitoring of electrolyte balance, particularly serum potassium and sodium levels, is also important when diuretics are administered.

Paracentesis, in which ascitic fluid is withdrawn through percutaneous needle aspiration, is another medical therapy for ascites. Close monitoring of vital signs during this procedure is necessary, especially as fluid is withdrawn. Major complications include sudden loss of intravascular pressure (decreased blood pressure) and tachycardia. To prevent these complications, 1 to 2 L of fluid is generally withdrawn at one time. The amount, color, and character of peritoneal fluid obtained is documented. Often, a specimen of the fluid is sent to the laboratory for analysis. The patient's abdominal girth should be measured before and after the procedure. Albumin may be administered to increase colloid osmotic pressure and to decrease loss of fluid into the peritoneal cavity.

Peritoneovenous shunting is a surgical procedure used to relieve ascites that is resistant to other therapies. The LeVeen shunt is inserted by placing the distal end of a tube in the peritoneum and tunneling the other end under the skin into the jugular vein or superior vena cava. A valve that opens and closes according to pressure gradients allows ascitic fluid to flow into the superior vena cava. The patient's breathing normally triggers the valve. During inspiration, pressure increases in the peritoneum and decreases in the vena cava, thereby allowing fluid to flow from the peritoneum into the general circulation. Major complications of this therapy include hemodilution, shunt clotting, wound infection, leakage of ascitic fluid from the incision, and bleeding problems.

A variation of this procedure is use of the Denver shunt, which involves placement of a pump in addition to the peritoneal catheter (Figure 17-12).[5] Fluid is allowed to flow through the pump from the peritoneum into the general circulation at a uniform rate to increase blood volume and renal blood flow, retain nutrients and improve nutritional status, increase diuresis, improve mobility and respiration, and relieve massive, refractory ascites.

Portal systemic encephalopathy. Portal systemic encephalopathy, commonly known as *hepatic encephalopathy,* is a functional derangement of the central nervous system that causes altered levels of consciousness and cerebral manifestations ranging from confusion to coma. Impaired motor ability is also often present. *Asterixis,* a flapping tremor of the hand, is an early sign of hepatic encephalopathy that can be assessed by the nurse.

The exact cause of hepatic encephalopathy is unknown, but it is thought to be abnormal ammonia metabolism. Increased serum ammonia levels interfere with normal cerebral metabolism. In acute liver failure, signs and symptoms of this disorder may appear rapidly, whereas in chronic liver failure they often occur over time. Many conditions may precipitate the development of hepatic encephalopathy, including fluid and electrolyte and acid-base disturbances, increased protein intake, portosystemic shunts, blood transfusions, GI bleeding, and many drugs such as diuretics, analgesics, narcotics, and sedatives. Progression of hepatic encephalopathy can be divided into stages (Box 17-17).

Management of hepatic encephalopathy involves addressing precipitating factors such as infection, gastrointestinal bleeding, and electrolyte and acid-base imbalances.[1] Measures for decreasing ammonia production are necessary. Protein intake is limited to 20 to 40 g/day. Lactulose, neomycin, and metronidazole are medications that can be administered to reduce bacterial breakdown of protein in the bowel.

Lactulose is the first-line treatment for hepatic encephalopathy.[1] Lactulose creates an acidic environment in the bowel that causes the ammonia to leave the bloodstream and enter the colon. Ammonia is trapped in the bowel. Lactulose also has a laxative effect that allows for elimination of the ammonia. Lactulose is given orally or via a rectal enema.

Neomycin and metronidazole are second-line treatments for hepatic encephalopathy. Neomycin is a broad-spectrum antibiotic that destroys normal bacteria found in the bowel, thereby decreasing protein breakdown and ammonia production. Neomycin is given orally every 4 to 6 hours. This drug is toxic to the kidneys and therefore cannot be given to patients with renal failure. Daily renal function studies are monitored when neomycin is administered.[1] Metronidazole is given 500 mg to 1.5 g/day for 1 week. Metronidazole does not cause diarrhea and it is not nephrotoxic. Metronidazole may cause epigastric discomfort which may in turn result in poor compliance with long-term treatment.[24]

Restriction of medications that are toxic to the liver is another important treatment. All medications that are metabolized by the liver should be reviewed for their therapeutic effect. Consultation with the clinical pharmacist is warranted.

Nursing measures for protecting the patient with an altered mental status from harm are a priority. Many patients with hepatic encephalopathy need to be sedated to prevent them from doing harm to themselves or to others. Oxazepam (Serax), diazepam (Valium), or lorazepam (Ativan) must be used judiciously; however, these drugs are less dependent on liver function for excretion.

Hepatorenal syndrome. Acute renal failure that occurs with liver failure is called *hepatorenal syndrome.* The pathophysiology of this disorder is not well understood, but it is associated with end-stage cirrhosis and ascites, decreased albumin levels, and portal hypertension. Decreased urine output and an increased serum creatinine level usually occur acutely. The prognosis for the patient with hepatorenal syndrome is generally poor because therapies to improve renal function usually are ineffective. The goals of general medical therapies are to improve liver function while supporting renal function. Fluid administration and diuretic therapy are used to improve urine output. Medications that are toxic to the kidney are discontinued. Occasionally, hemodialysis is used to support renal function if there is a chance for an improvement in liver function. Because of the poor prognosis, it is appropriate for the critical care nurse to begin to address end-of-life decisions with the patient and family. This is done with consideration of the individual nurse's comfort level, as well as the organizational policy and family dynamics.

Hepatopulmonary syndrome. Hepatopulmonary syndrome is defined as the presence of hypoxia due to ventilation-perfusion mismatch, pulmonary capillary vasodilation, and limitation of oxygen diffusion in patients with ESLD. Current therapy for hepatopulmonary syndrome include oxygen, TIPS, and liver transplantation, with the latter as the definitive treatment to improve symptoms and survival.[1]

Patient Outcomes

Outcomes for the patient with liver failure are included in the "Nursing Care Plan for the Patient with Hepatic Failure."

BARIATRIC SURGERY

Although not a GI disorder, bariatric surgery is increasingly being done to treat morbid obesity. Morbid obesity is defined as a body mass index (BMI) of 40 kg/m² or higher, or 35 kg/m² and a documented comorbidity. Comorbidities include diabetes, hypertension, heart disease, and sleep apnea. Some morbidly obese individuals undergo bariatric surgery. These surgical patients may be cared for in the critical care unit or an acute care unit, depending on their acuity. See the box, "Bariatric Considerations," for nursing considerations related to bariatric surgery.

BARIATRIC CONSIDERATIONS

Bariatric surgery procedures have increased as a treatment for morbid obesity and those at-risk for obesity-related comorbidities. Gastric bypass and gastric banding are the most common surgical procedures.

Complications associated with bariatric surgery include pulmonary embolus, respiratory failure, stomal obstruction or stenosis, leaks from the anastomosis, wound infection, and bleeding. The most serious complication is an anastomotic leak, which is the most common cause of death. Symptoms of a leak are subtle and include increasing pain (back, left shoulder, abdomen, pelvis, or substernal pressure), hiccups, restlessness, and unexplained tachycardia or oliguria. Early mobility after surgery is important to prevent complications. However, it is important to have proper equipment and resources to prevent injury to both the patient and healthcare team members when attempting mobilization.

All obese patients, including those undergoing surgery, need to have appropriate equipment to facilitate safe patient care.

Equipment includes operating room tables that accommodate the higher weight of the patient and proper surgical instruments, and large-size stretchers, wheelchairs, bedside commodes, beds, scales, and bedside chairs. New bariatric beds facilitate movement of the patient to a sitting position.

Bariatric nursing has evolved into a nursing specialty. The National Association of Bariatric Nurses was formed to provide resources for those caring for bariatric patients (www.bariatricnurses.org). Their official publication is *Bariatric Nursing and Surgical Patient Care*, which provides a wealth of resources related to patient care management.

References

1. Barth MM, Jensen CE. Postoperative nursing care of gastric bypass patients. *American Journal of Critical Care*. 2006;15:378-387.
2. Burke LE, Wang J. Treatment strategies for overweight and obesity. *Journal of Nursing Scholarship*. 2011;43:368-375.

CASE STUDY

The critical care nurse receives a report from the emergency department of a patient to be admitted to the unit. Mr. G. is a 47-year-old man with a week-long history of severe abdominal pain that worsens with food intake. The pain is associated with nausea and vomiting. Mr. G. is oriented to person and place; however, he is disoriented to day and time and is described as "lethargic." A nasogastric tube and Foley catheter were placed and intravenous access was established in the emergency department.

Vital signs include the following: heart rate, 110 beats per minute; respirations, 30 breaths per minute; blood pressure, 104/56 mm Hg; and temperature, 38° C.

Laboratory values include the following: white blood cell count, 19,000/microliter; hematocrit, 38%; sodium, 148 mEq/L; potassium, 4.0 mEq/L; chloride, 114 mEq/L; blood urea nitrogen, 25 mg/dL; creatinine, 1.0 mg/dL; glucose, 180 mg/dL; amylase, 500 IU/L; and lipase, 600 IU/L.

Questions

1. What further data should the critical care nurse request from the nurse in the emergency department?
2. In addition to management of shock in Mr. G., what is another priority treatment?
3. What further assessment data would be valuable to the long-term management of this patient?

SUMMARY

Acute upper GI bleeding, acute pancreatitis, and liver failure account for potentially life-threatening emergencies that require careful and astute assessment and care by the critical care nurse and medical team. Priorities for care include initial assessments and resuscitation, diagnostic testing for making a definitive diagnosis, and prompt interventions for stabilizing or reversing the pathophysiological process and preventing complications. The nurse's scope of care includes ongoing assessments and monitoring, documentation and reporting of patient responses to diagnostic and treatment regimens, early detection of complications, and supportive care. Patient and family teaching of the critical care unit routine and all therapies instituted is also a priority. As appropriate, discharge teaching of the underlying pathological process and of the dietary, medication, and activity regimens may also be initiated in the ICU. Successful management of all these patient populations requires a collaborative effort of all disciplines.

CRITICAL THINKING EXERCISES

1. The nurse is caring for a patient who is admitted with acute abdominal pain and vomiting. His admission vital signs and laboratory values include the following:

Blood pressure	94/72 mm Hg
Heart rate	114 beats/min
Respiratory rate	32 breaths/min
Potassium	3.0 mEq/L
Calcium	7.0 mg/dL
Partial pressure of oxygen in arterial blood (PaO_2)	58 mm Hg
Oxygen saturation in arterial blood (SaO_2)	88%
Serum amylase	280 IU/L
Serum lipase	320 IU/L

   a. What is the suspected medical diagnosis?
   b. What are the priority nursing and medical interventions?

2. A 50-year-old patient is admitted with hematemesis and reports having dark stools for the past 12 hours. Which of the following admission data is the best indicator of the amount of blood lost:

Blood pressure	95/60 mm Hg (supine)
Heart rate	125 beats/min
Respiratory rate	28 breaths/min
Hematocrit	27%
Hemoglobin	14 g/dL

3. A 45-year-old business executive is admitted to the telemetry unit. He tells the nurse that he travels a lot for business and has recently returned from a trip to Mexico. During your initial assessment, he tells you that he is not married, and he relates stories about some of the women he has met and dated on his many trips. His history includes persistent abdominal pain, nausea with occasional vomiting, fatigue, and decreased appetite. Initial vital signs and laboratory results include the following:

Heart rate	70 beats/min
Urine	clear and dark yellow
Aspartate transaminase (AST)	20 IU/L
Alanine transaminase (ALT)	70 IU/L
Serum albumin	3.2 mg/dL
Total serum bilirubin	1.5 mg/dL

What is the most likely diagnosis, and what precautions should the nurse take while caring for this patient?

REFERENCES

1. Al-Khatafi A, Huang DT. Critical care management of patients with end-stage liver disease. *Critical Care Medicine.* 2011;39(5):1157-1166.
2. Baid H. A critical review of auscultating bowel sounds. *British Journal of Nursing.* 2009;18(18):1125-1130.
3. Beger HG, Rau BM. Severe acute pancreatitis: clinical course and management. *World Journal of Gastroenterology.* 2007;13(38):5043-5051.
4. Centers for Disease Control and Prevention. *Hepatitis Fact Sheets.* www.cdc.gov/hepatitis; 2011. Accessed November 20, 2011.
5. Chernecky CC, Berger BJ. *Laboratory Tests and Diagnostic Procedures.* 5th ed. Philadelphia: Saunders. 2008.
6. Constantin VD, Panar S, Ciofoaia VV, et al. Multimodal management of upper gastrointestinal bleeding caused by stress gastropathy. *Journal of Gastrointestinal and Liver Diseases.* 2009;18(3):279-284.
7. Dhamija N, Pousman R, Bajwa O, et al. Management of gastrointestinal bleeding. In Vincent J, Abraham E, Kochanek P, et al, eds. *Textbook of Critical Care.* 6th ed. Philadelphia: Saunders. 2011.
8. Dhillon A. Hepatorenal syndrome. In Vincent J, Abraham E, Kochanek P, et al, eds. *Textbook of Critical Care.* 6th ed. Philadelphia: Saunders. 2011.
9. Eckerwall GE, Tingstedt BB, Bergenzaum PE, et al. Immediate oral feeding in patients with mild acute pancreatitis is safe and may accelerate recovery: a randomized clinical study. *Clinical Nutrition.* 2007;85:S221-S229.
10. Gilbert D, Moellering R, Eliopoulos G, Sande M. *The Sandford Guide to Antimicrobial Therapy.* 37th ed. Sperry, VA: Antimicrobial Therapy Inc. 2007.
11. Guyton AC, Hall JE. *Textbook of Medical Physiology.* 12th ed. Philadelphia: Saunders. 2011.
12. Hojman H, Wai CJ, Nasraway SA. Gastrointestinal Hemorrhage. In Vincent J, Abraham E, Kochanek P, et al, eds. *Textbook of Critical Care.* 6th ed. Philadelphia: Saunders. 2011.
13. Hu WS. *Bioartificial liver.* http://hugroup.cems.umn.edu/Research/bal/BAL-howitworks.htm; 2007. Accessed November 2, 2007.
14. Huether SE. Alterations of digestive function. In McCance KL, Huether SE, eds. *Pathophysiology: The Biologic Basis for Disease in Adults and Children.* 6th ed. St. Louis: Mosby. 2010.
15. Huether SE. Structure and function of the digestive system. In McCance KL, Huether SE, eds. *Pathophysiology: The Biologic Basis for Disease in Adults and Children.* 6th ed. St. Louis: Mosby. 2010.
16. Institute of Healthcare Improvement. *Critical Care.* www.ihi.org/IHI/Topics/CriticalCare/; 2007. Accessed October 31, 2007.
17. Institute of Healthcare Improvement. *Implement the Ventilator Bundle: Peptic Ulcer Disease Prophylaxis.* http://www.ihi.org/knowledge/Pages/Changes/PepticUlcerDiseaseProphylaxis.aspx; 2011. Accessed November 20, 2011.

18. Jarvis C. *Physical Examination and Health Assessment*. 5th ed. Philadelphia: Saunders. 2008.

19. Jiang K, Chen XZ, Xia Q, et al. Early nasogastric enteral nutrition for severe acute pancreatitis: a systematic review. *World Journal of Gastroenterology*. 2007;13(39):5253-5260.

20. Jiang K, Chen XZ, Xia Q, et al. Early veno-venous hemofiltration for severe acute pancreatitis: a systematic review. *Chinese Journal of Evidence-Based Medicine*. 2007;7:121-134.

21. Kramer DJ. Liver transplantation. In Vincent J, Abraham E, Kochanek P, et al, eds. *Textbook of Critical Care*. 6th ed. Philadelphia: Saunders. 2011.

22. Lipsett PS. Acute pancreatitis. In Vincent J, Abraham E, Kochanek P, et al, eds. *Textbook of Critical Care*. 6th ed. Philadelphia: Saunders. 2011.

23. Longstreth GF, Thompson WG, Chey WD, et al. *Gastroenterology*. 2006;130:1480-1491.

24. Martinez-Camacho A, Fortune BE, Everson GT. Hepatic encephalopathy. In Vincent J, Abraham E, Kochanek P, et al, eds. *Textbook of Critical Care*. 6th ed. Philadelphia: Saunders. 2011.

25. O'Connor A, Gisbert J, O'Morain C. Treatment of *Helicobacter pylori* infection. *Helicobacter*. 2009;14(Suppl 1):46-51.

26. Rahimi RS, Rockey DD. Complications and outcomes in chronic liver disease. *Current Opinion in Gastroenterology*. 2011;27:204-209

27. Ranson JC. Risk factors in acute pancreatitis. *Hospital Practice*. 1985;20(4):69-73.

28. Skidmore-Roth L. *Mosby's Nursing Drug Reference*. 24th ed. St. Louis: Mosby. 2011.

29. Stadlbauer V, Krisper P, Aigner R, et al. Effect of extracorporeal liver support by MARS and Prometheus on serum cytokines in acute-on-chronic liver failure. *Critical Care*, 2006;10(6):R169.

30. Talukdar R, Vege SS. Early management of severe acute pancreatitis. *Current Gastroenterology Reports*. 2011;13:123-130.

31. Twinrix. *Hepatitis A Inactivated & Hepatitis B (Recombinant) Vaccine*. http://www.gsk.com/products/vaccines/ambirix.htm; 2012 Accessed December 3, 2012.

32. U.S. National Institutes of Health. *Pancreatitis Clinical Trials*. http://www.clinicaltrials.gov/ct2/results?term=pancreatitis; 2011. Accessed November 21, 2011.

33. Vincent J, Abraham E, Kochanek P, et al. *Textbook of Critical Care*. 6th ed. Philadelphia: Saunders. 2011.

34. Wendon J, Solis-Munoz P. Portal hypertension. In Vincent J, Abraham E, Kochanek P, et al, eds. *Textbook of Critical Care*. 6th ed. Philadelphia: Saunders. 2011.

35. Wu BW, Conwell DL. Acute pancreatitis part I: approach to early management. *Clinical Gastrology and Hepatology*. 2010;8(5):410-416.

36. Zagari RM, Bianchi-Porro G, Fiocca R, et al. Comparison of 1 and 2 weeks of omeprazole, amoxicillin and clarithromycin treatment for *Helicobacter pylori* eradication: the HYPER Study. *Gut*. 2007;56(4):475-479.

Endocrine Alterations

Jacqueline LaManna, MSN, ARNP-BC, ADM, CDE
Christina Stewart-Amidei, PhD, RN, CNRN, CCRN, FAAN

℮volve WEBSITE

Many additional resources, including self-assessment exercises, are located on the Evolve companion website at http://evolve.elsevier.com/Sole.

- Review Questions
- Mosby's Nursing Skills Procedures

- Animations
- Video Clips

INTRODUCTION

The endocrine glands form a communication network linking all body systems. Hormones from these glands control and regulate metabolic processes such as energy production, fluid and electrolyte balance, and response to stress. This system is closely linked to and integrated with the nervous system. In particular, the hypothalamus and pituitary gland play a major role in hormonal regulation. The hypothalamus manufactures and secretes several releasing or inhibiting hormones that are conveyed to the pituitary. The pituitary gland responds to these hormones by increasing or decreasing hormone secretion, thus regulating circulating hormone levels. This system is designed as a feedback control mechanism. Positive feedback stimulates release of a hormone when serum hormone levels are low. Negative feedback inhibits the release of hormones when serum hormone levels are high. Examples of how these feedback systems work to control circulating levels of cortisol are provided in Figure 18-1. This same feedback system also controls the secretion and inhibition of other hormones outside hypothalamic-pituitary control.

Changes in the Endocrine System in Critical Illness

The stress of critical illness provokes a significant response by the endocrine system. Excess glucose in the blood occurs as a result of release of *counterregulatory hormones* that promote hepatic gluconeogenesis and decreased peripheral utilization of glucose with resulting relative hypoinsulimemia. Adrenal insufficiency can occur as a result of insult or damage to the gland itself (primary) or because of dysfunction of the hypothalamus, pituitary, or both (secondary). Relative adrenal insufficiency may occur in critically ill patients whenever elevated cortisol levels are inadequate for the demand. Thyroid hormone balance is disrupted by changes in peripheral metabolism that cause a decrease in triiodothyronine (T_3) levels. Pituitary and hypothalamus dysfunction as a result of brain tumor, trauma, or surgery can cause significant fluid and electrolyte imbalances that complicate critical illness.

Disease States of the Endocrine System

Diseases involving the hypothalamus, the pituitary gland, and the primary endocrine organs (i.e., pancreas, adrenal glands, and thyroid gland) interfere with normal feedback mechanisms and the secretion of hormones. Crisis states occur when these diseases are untreated or undertreated, when the patient is stressed physiologically or psychologically, or as the result of many other factors.

This chapter describes both the endocrine response to critical illness, and the crises that occur as a result of imbalances of hormones from the pancreas, adrenal glands, thyroid gland, and posterior pituitary gland. For a summary of endocrine concerns for the older adult, see box, "Geriatric Considerations."

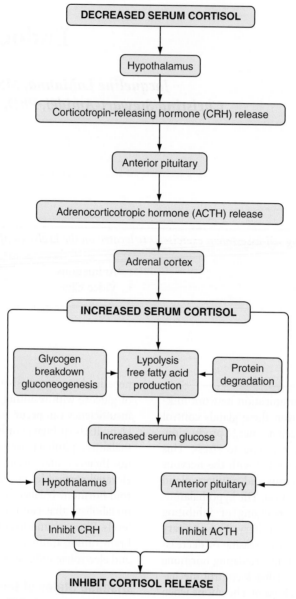

FIGURE 18-1 Feedback system for cortisol regulation.

GERIATRIC CONSIDERATIONS

Elderly patients present diagnostic and treatment challenges related to endocrine disorders. When critically ill, they are at increased risk for endocrine complications. Older adults have more comorbidities and take more medications that affect fluid and electrolyte balance. The presenting signs and symptoms of an endocrine disorder are frequently atypical and nonspecific, and the responses to dysfunction are blunted. Many of the compensatory mechanisms are lost with advanced age.

Pancreas

Over 25% of adults older than 65 years have diabetes, primarily type 2 diabetes.[6] Elderly persons are more prone to develop hyperosmolar hyperglycemic state. They are also at increased risk of being unaware of hypoglycemia. Elderly patients are more likely to have comorbid conditions, such as cardiac or renal disease, and to take medications that make them more reactive to electrolyte imbalances.[16] They are also slower to respond to treatments.

Adrenal

Utilization and clearance of cortisol decrease with age, resulting in increased serum cortisol levels. Cortisol secretion decreases because feedback systems are intact, leading to lower cortisol levels in the elderly. The absolute level of cortisol needed to maintain homeostasis is unknown. Poor nutrition and decreased albumin stores (one of cortisol's binding proteins) may compound the decline in cortisol availability and response.

Thyroid

Thyroid hormone levels decrease with age because of glandular atrophy and inflammation. Approximately 5% of people older than 60 years are affected by hypothyroidism. Detection of thyroid disease by assessment of signs or symptoms becomes more challenging. In addition, lower amounts of thyroid medication are needed as replacement, and adjustment of dosage must be slower to prevent potentially dangerous side effects. Elderly patients are less likely to tolerate urgent treatment with liothyronine sodium.

Older patients may not exhibit the typical signs of thyrotoxicosis. Anorexia, atrial fibrillation, apathy, and weight loss may already be present or misinterpreted. Goiter, hyperactive reflexes, sweating, heat intolerance, tremor, nervousness, and polydipsia are less commonly present. In the elderly, symptoms of thyroid storm may present as increasing angina or worsening congestive heart failure.

Pituitary

Decreased release of growth hormone leads to a decrease in lean body mass and increased blood glucose levels, leading to suppression of thyroid-stimulating hormone (thyrotropin), although usually not significantly. An increase in secretion of antidiuretic hormone occurs with advanced age and places the older person at risk of dilutional hyponatremia. Elderly patients are at greater risk of the syndrome of inappropriate antidiuretic hormone from any cause than are younger patients. Elderly patients can fail to recognize and respond to thirst, and therefore are at an increased risk for dehydration.

HYPERGLYCEMIA IN THE CRITICALLY ILL PATIENT

Critically ill patients are at high risk for hyperglycemia from many different stressors including their disease states, the illness-related hormonal responses to stress, and the critical care environment. Refer to Box 18-1 for risk factors associated with an increase in blood glucose levels.

Although stress-induced hyperglycemia is a normal physiological response related to the *fight-or-flight* mode, glucose elevation is associated with poor outcomes in hospitalized patients with and without a formal diagnosis of diabetes. Hyperglycemia in acutely ill patients has been linked to impaired immune function, cerebral ischemia, osmotic diuresis, poor wound healing, decreased erythropoiesis, increased hemolysis, endothelial dysfunction, increased thrombosis, vasoconstriction with resulting hypertension, decreased respiratory muscle function, neuronal damage, and impaired gastric motility.[7] Acute hyperglycemia during the course of illness has been associated with poor clinical outcomes, including mortality in

---

BOX 18-1   RISK FACTORS FOR THE DEVELOPMENT OF HYPERGLYCEMIA IN THE CRITICALLY ILL PATIENT

- Preexisting diabetes mellitus, diagnosed or undiagnosed
- Comorbidities such as obesity, pancreatitis, cirrhosis, hypokalemia
- Stress response release of cortisol, growth hormone, catecholamines (epinephrine and norepinephrine), glucagon, glucocorticoids, cytokines (interleukin-1, interleukin-6, and tumor necrosis factor)
- Aging
- Lack of muscular activity
- Relative insulin deficiency/insulin resistance
- Administration of exogenous catecholamines, glucocorticoids
- Administration of dextrose solutions, nutritional support
- Drug therapy such as thiazides, beta-blockers, highly active antiretroviral therapy, phenytoin, tacrolimus, cyclosporine

critically ill patients who have been treated for myocardial infarction, traumatic brain injury, burns, trauma, subarachnoid hemorrhage, and transplantation.[17]

Optimal glucose targets in critically ill patients are a matter of current debate. In 2001, Van den Berghe and colleaguespublished a landmark study showing that intensive insulin control of hyperglycemia in a critically ill surgical population decreased mortality and morbidity, including sepsis, acute kidney injury necessitating dialysis, blood transfusion requirements, and polyneuropathy.[26] Findings of this study led many hospitals to institute tight glycemic control protocols in critically ill patients as a standard of care. Subsequent studies conducted in broader populations have demonstrated higher rates of mortality in nonsurgical populations, and significantly higher rates of severe hypoglycemia, raising questions about the degree of glycemic control that should be attained in critically ill individuals.[9,18,25] In response, the American Diabetes Association and the American Association of Clinical Endocrinologists issued a joint statement on inpatient glycemic control. Current guidelines recommend an initial target glucose level of 180 mg/dL or less; targets of 140 to 180 mg/dL are appropriate for most critically ill patients. Lower targets may be desired for a select group of patients.[1,17] A summary of evidence to support this change in practice is discussed in this chapter.

Achieving Optimal Glycemic Control

To optimize patient safety, intravenous delivery using short-acting insulin as guided by an evidence-based protocol is the preferred method for treating hyperglycemia in critically ill patients (see box, "QSEN Exemplar").[1,7,17] These nurse-managed protocols include frequent glucose monitoring and insulin dosage adjustments based on patient-specific glucose targets. Frequent blood glucose monitoring is intended to ensure the appropriate insulin dosage and to minimize the incidence of hypoglycemia. The key elements for glycemic control protocols are described in Box 18-2. Effective protocols minimize complexity so there is less chance for error. Systems approaches are required to limit the patient risk associated with this complex therapy.[17] Computer decision support software is helpful in managing glucose control. Although strictly controlling insulin delivery is labor-intensive, these protocols reduce hospitalization costs secondary to fewer inpatient complications, reduce critical care and hospital lengths of stay, reduce ventilator days, and reduce charges for radiology, laboratory tests, and pharmaceuticals.[17]

The transition from intravenous to subcutaneous insulin therapy must be carefully timed to limit the risk for hyperglycemia. Most patients may be transitioned from intravenous to subcutaneous insulin when they are eating regular meals, or when their clinical conditions warrants transfer to a lower-intensity level of care.[17] Subcutaneous insulin should be administered 1 to 4 hours before discontinuation of the insulin infusion. It is recommended that the subcutaneous insulin regimen include basal and nutritional bolus insulin delivery in a dose equivalent to approximately 75% of the total daily

QSEN EXEMPLAR
Evidence-Based Practice and Quality Improvement

A critical care advanced practice registered nurse (APRN) attended a recent conference where findings of the NICE-SUGAR study were presented. The APRN's practice network used an intensive insulin protocol in all of its critical care units and progressive care units. The protocol was developed several years ago and used evidence provided by the Van den Berghe and colleagues trials to establish glucose targets. Following the conference, the APRN conducted a review of current literature on glycemic control of critically ill adults and additionally reviewed the most recent American Diabetes Association Clinical Practice Guidelines. The APRN noted discrepancies between current practice and the evidence and presented these findings at the critical care committee meeting. Committee members concurred that the current evidence and guidelines supported the need to amend practice, and formed a committee of stakeholders to evaluate network practice and revise the protocols using the FOCUS-PDSA approach to performance improvement. After multiple meetings, an initial draft of a revised protocol was developed and presented to appropriate physician and clinical groups. Necessary approvals were obtained, and an education program for providers, nurses, and affected disciplines such as pharmacy, nutrition, and laboratory services was developed and presented. The evidence supporting the revisions was emphasized. A formal implementation strategy was developed, and the revised protocol was introduced serially into each of the critical care units. The APRN worked with the quality and safety department to establish a follow-up monitoring plan. The APRN collected data continuously after the implementation and worked with the quality department to identify trends that suggested the need to modify the protocol. These findings were presented to appropriate parties, revisions made, and a continuous monitoring and reporting plan was established.

insulin infusion dose with the addition of a bolus correction scale.[17] Adjustments to this recommendation may be required if the patient is receiving enteral feedings, parenteral nutrition, or high-dose glucocorticoids. Insulin regimens that are composed exclusively of sliding scale insulin have been associated with poor patient outcomes.

Hypoglycemia as a Preventable Adverse Effect of Glucose Management

Intensive insulin therapy has been associated with a significant (sixfold) increase in the risk for an episode of severe hypoglycemia (glucose 40 mg/dL or less).[9] The increased incidence of hypoglycemia in critically ill patients is associated with a reduction or discontinuation of nutrition without adjustment of insulin therapy, such as the holding of parenteral or enteral feedings during diagnostic exams; a prior diagnosis of diabetes mellitus (DM); sepsis; and the use/change in dosage of inotropic drugs, vasopressor support, and glucocorticoid therapy.[7]

BOX 18-2   **KEY COMPONENTS OF A GLUCOSE MANAGEMENT PROTOCOL**

- Frequent plasma blood glucose measurements
- Concentration of insulin infusion (i.e., number of units of insulin mixed in quantity of normal saline)
- Initial intravenous insulin bolus dose if appropriate
- Table with titration for increasing or decreasing insulin infusion based on glucose level
- Interventions for:
  - Hypoglycemia, should it occur
  - When feeding is interrupted, either parenteral or enteral
  - When the patient is transported from the critical care unit for diagnostic testing
  - Discontinuing the intravenous insulin infusion
  - When the patient is transferred out of the critical care unit

Based on data from Moghissi ES, Korytkowski MT, DiNardo M, et al. American Association of Clinical Endocrinologists and American Diabetes Association consensus statement on inpatient glycemic control. *Diabetes Care.* 2009;32:1119-1131; Kitabchi AE, Umpierrez GE, Miles JM, et al. Hyperglycemic crisis in adult patients with diabetes. *Diabetes Care.* 2009;32:1335-1343.

Many episodes of hypoglycemia are preventable. The nurse must ensure that the glucose testing is accurate and consistent. Concurrent and shift-to-shift coordination and adjustment of all medical and nutritional therapies (including increasing, decreasing, or temporarily suspending any of them), is required to prevent hypoglycemia.

Hyperglycemia in the Critically Ill

Stress-induced hyperglycemia affects patients with and without a formal diagnosis of DM. In the critically ill, stress-induced hyperglycemia exacerbates the elevated glucose levels of patients with preexisting diabetes, predisposes them to an even higher incidence of complications and comorbidities, and impacts treatment for all disease states. Individuals with diabetes are hospitalized more frequently, are more prone to complications, and have longer hospital stays and higher hospital costs than patients without diabetes.[7] Therapy aimed at establishing euglycemic levels contributes to improved patient outcomes. Critically ill patients with diabetes are most effectively managed with insulin therapy regardless of their usual home self-management regimen.[17] Figure 18-2 and Table 18-1 provide a review of the insulin action profiles of a variety of insulin products and common insulin regimens. Additionally, Table 18-2 lists oral agents used in the management of type 2 diabetes presented by class along with information on injectable agents used to regulate blood glucose.

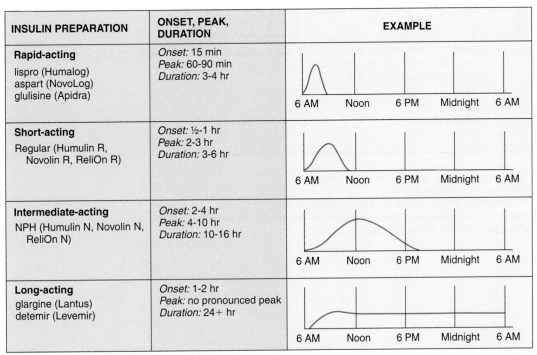

INSULIN PREPARATION	ONSET, PEAK, DURATION	EXAMPLE
Rapid-acting lispro (Humalog) aspart (NovoLog) glulisine (Apidra)	*Onset:* 15 min *Peak:* 60-90 min *Duration:* 3-4 hr	
Short-acting Regular (Humulin R, Novolin R, ReliOn R)	*Onset:* ½-1 hr *Peak:* 2-3 hr *Duration:* 3-6 hr	
Intermediate-acting NPH (Humulin N, Novolin N, ReliOn N)	*Onset:* 2-4 hr *Peak:* 4-10 hr *Duration:* 10-16 hr	
Long-acting glargine (Lantus) detemir (Levemir)	*Onset:* 1-2 hr *Peak:* no pronounced peak *Duration:* 24+ hr	

FIGURE 18-2 Commercially available insulin preparations showing onset, peak, and duration of action. (From Michel B. Nursing management of diabetes. In Lewis SL, Dirksen SR, Heitkemper MM, et al, eds. *Medical-Surgical Nursing: Assessment and Management of Clinical Problems.* 8th ed. St. Louis: Mosby. 2011.)

TABLE 18-1   COMMON INSULIN REGIMENS

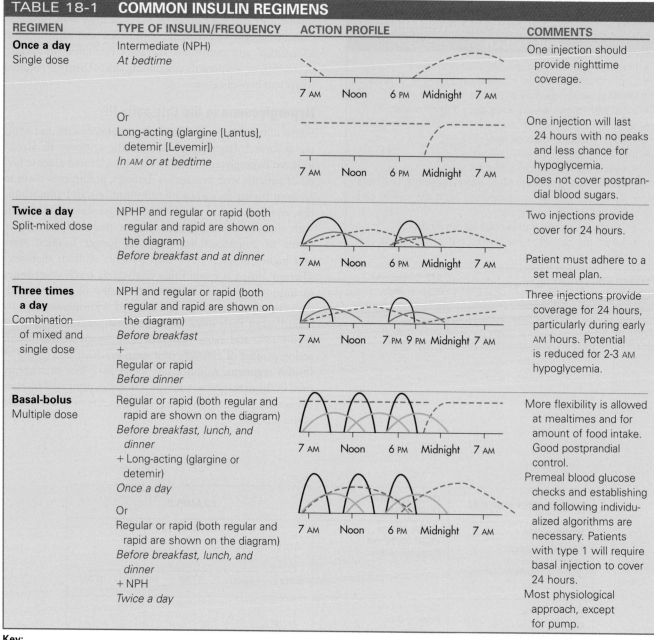

REGIMEN	TYPE OF INSULIN/FREQUENCY	ACTION PROFILE	COMMENTS
Once a day Single dose	Intermediate (NPH) *At bedtime*		One injection should provide nighttime coverage.
	Or Long-acting (glargine [Lantus], detemir [Levemir]) *In AM or at bedtime*		One injection will last 24 hours with no peaks and less chance for hypoglycemia. Does not cover postprandial blood sugars.
Twice a day Split-mixed dose	NPHP and regular or rapid (both regular and rapid are shown on the diagram) *Before breakfast and at dinner*		Two injections provide cover for 24 hours. Patient must adhere to a set meal plan.
Three times a day Combination of mixed and single dose	NPH and regular or rapid (both regular and rapid are shown on the diagram) *Before breakfast* + Regular or rapid *Before dinner*		Three injections provide coverage for 24 hours, particularly during early AM hours. Potential is reduced for 2-3 AM hypoglycemia.
Basal-bolus Multiple dose	Regular or rapid (both regular and rapid are shown on the diagram) *Before breakfast, lunch, and dinner* + Long-acting (glargine or detemir) *Once a day* Or Regular or rapid (both regular and rapid are shown on the diagram) *Before breakfast, lunch, and dinner* + NPH *Twice a day*		More flexibility is allowed at mealtimes and for amount of food intake. Good postprandial control. Premeal blood glucose checks and establishing and following individualized algorithms are necessary. Patients with type 1 will require basal injection to cover 24 hours. Most physiological approach, except for pump.

Key:

———————— Rapid-acting (lispro, aspart, glulisine) insulin.

———————— Short-acting (regular) insulin.

- - - - - - - - - Intermediate-acting (NPH) or long-acting (glargine, detemir) insulin.

From Michel B. Nursing management of diabetes. In Lewis SL, Dirksen SR, Heitkemper MM, eds. *Medical-Surgical Nursing: Assessment and Management of Clinical Problems.* 8th ed. St. Louis: Mosby. 2011.

TABLE 18-2   PHARMACOLOGICAL AGENTS USED IN THE MANAGEMENT OF DIABETES

CLASSIFICATION	ROUTE OF ADMINISTRATION	MECHANISM OF ACTION	SIDE EFFECTS
Sulfonylureas Glipizide (Glucotrol, Glucotrol XL) Glyburide (Micronase, DiaBeta, Glynase) Glimepiride (Amaryl)	Oral	Stimulates release of insulin from pancreatic beta cells; decreases glycogenesis and gluconeogenesis; enhances cellular sensitivity to insulin; agents are longer-acting	Hypoglycemia; weight gain; photosensitivity; cholestatic jaundice; use with caution in patients with hepatic or renal dysfunction
Meglitinides Repaglinide (Prandin) Nateglinide (Starlix)	Oral	Stimulates rapid, short-lived release of insulin from the pancreas; taken within 30 minutes of meal	Hypoglycemia; medication is held if no meal taken Weight gain
Biguanide Metformin (Glucophage, Glucophage XR, Fortamet, Riomet)	Oral	↓ Rate of hepatic glucose production; augments glucose uptake from tissues, especially muscles	Stomach upset—take with meals; Diarrhea; Lactic acidosis; medication held before IV contrast procedures and 48 hours after Withhold if creatinine ≥1.4 mg/dL in woman and ≥1.5 mg/dL in men or creatinine clearance <50 mL/min
α-Glucosidase Inhibitors Acarbose (Precose) Miglitol (Glyset)	Oral	Delays absorption of glucose from the GI tract; taken with first bite of food; withheld if meal missed	Flatulence; abdominal pain; diarrhea; avoid use in patients with chronic intestinal disorders; hypoglycemia treated with glucose only
Thiazolidinediones Pioglitazone (Actos) Rosiglitazone (Avandia)	Oral Administered at bedtime	↑ Glucose update in muscle; ↓ endogenous glucose production	Edema; contraindicated in Class III/IV congestive heart failure; hypoglycemia if used with insulin or sulfonylureas; weight gain; cardiovascular events such as myocardial infarction and stroke (Avandia: black box warning issued by FDA); increased risk of fracture in women; hepatic dysfunction – withhold if ALT >2.5 times upper limit of normal; Pioglitazone use for more than one year may be associated with increased risk for bladder cancer.
Dipeptidyl Peptidase-4 (DPP-4) Inhibitors Sitagliptin (Januvia) Saxagliptin (Onglyza)	Oral	Enhances incretin system; stimulates insulin release from pancreatic beta cells; ↓ hepatic glucose production	Upper respiratory tract infection; sore throat; GI upset; diarrhea; dose reduction for renal impairment; hypoglycemia (with sulfonylureas); hypersensitivity reactions (anaphylaxis, Stevens-Johnson Syndrome)
Incretin Mimetic Exenatide (Byetta) Liraglutide (Victoza)	Subcutaneous within 60 minutes of AM and PM meal; dose titrated	Stimulates release of insulin; ↓ glucagon secretion; ↑ satiety; ↓ gastric emptying (avoid in patients with gastroparesis); ↓ hepatic gluconeogenesis; used in treatment of type 2 DM	Hypoglycemia (with insulin-secreting agents); pancreatitis (may be fatal); nausea; vomiting; weight loss; diarrhea; headache (medullary thyroid cancer [Victoza])
Amylin Analog Pramlintide (Symlin)	Subcutaneous (abdomen or thigh)	Take with each significant carbohydrate-containing meal. ↓ glucagon secretion; ↑ satiety; ↓ gastric emptying; ↓ hepatic gluconeogenesis	Hypoglycemia, nausea; vomiting; decreased appetite; headache (May be used in type 1 and type 2 diabetes; held if no significant meal)
Combination Agents Variety of combinations available	Oral	Combine effects of each class	Combine side effects of all agents to obtain complete risk profiles. Combinations of sulfonylureas or meglitinides with other agents may increase the risk for hypoglycemia.

Adapted from Michel B. Nursing management of diabetes. In Lewis SL, Dirksen SR, Heitkemper MM, eds. *Medical-Surgical Nursing: Assessment and Management of Clinical Problems*. 8th ed. St. Louis: Mosby. 2011.

PANCREATIC ENDOCRINE EMERGENCIES

Review of Physiology

DM is a metabolic disease of glucose imbalance resulting from alterations in insulin secretion, insulin action, or both.[2] The number of people with DM has been increasing, with current incidence at more than 220 million worldwide.[27] The two most common types of DM are type 1 and type 2.

Type 1 DM is primarily caused by pancreatic islet beta cell destruction, resulting in an *absolute insulin deficiency* and a tendency to develop ketoacidosis. In most cases, type 1 diabetes is an autoimmune disorder. A subset of patients, primarily of African American or Asian ancestry, may experience a genetic but nonimmunological form of type 1 diabetes.[2]

Type 2 is the most common form of diabetes and results from the combination of insulin resistance and insulin

---

GENETICS

Type 2 Diabetes Mellitus: A Complex Disease with Complex Genetics

Type 2 diabetes mellitus (T2DM) is an example of a complex, multifactorial, polygenic disease. *Multifactorial* means that T2DM is a result of an interaction between genes, lifestyle, and the environment. *Polygenic* means that more than one gene is implicated in the development of this common, chronic disease. Other multifactorial and polygenic disorders that occur in adults include hypertension, atherosclerosis, many cancers, and manic-depressive psychosis.[3]

Environmental factors such as high caloric intake, physical inactivity, and obesity contribute to T2DM. Offspring of parents with T2DM have a 40% chance of being diagnosed with T2DM (a sixfold increase over the general population).[4] Over 40 genetic variations are identified as contributing to the clinical manifestation of T2DM. Initial investigations linked defects in pancreatic beta cell function to T2DM, explaining about 10% of T2DM heritability. These genetic findings suggest that insulin secretion rather than insulin resistance is the primary cause of T2DM.[2,3] More recently, genome-wide association studies (GWAS) suggest that intron or noncoding regions of the genome contribute to disturbances in fasting glucose, body mass index and dysplidemia—all traits associated with T2DM.[4] Experts suggest that each genetic variation contributes 5% to 10% toward genetic susceptibility for T2DM development.[4]

People with T2DM likely have pathological variations in multiple genes. They may also experience greater lifestyle and environmental hazards. The interaction between genes, lifestyle, and the environment in patients with diagnosed T2DM has been known for many decades. Specifically, a family history that includes diabetes combined with one's food intake, body weight (specifically, obesity), and low exercise is a strong predictor of T2DM. Genetic and environmental factors influence the onset and progression of diabetes in a number of ways; findings from investigations of risk factors for T2DM are summarized here.[4]

1. *Number of pancreatic beta cells that produce insulin.* Inheriting a greater number of beta cells may be protective despite a sedentary lifestyle, whereas few beta cells may result in early-onset or more severe T2DM. For example when the *CD-KN2A* gene overexpresses its protein product, pancreatic beta cell mass is reduced in mice.[4] Environmental toxins contribute to reduction in the number of pancreatic beta cells.

2. *Production of insulin.* The efficiency or effectiveness of insulin is influenced by genes such as *UBE2E2*, which increase insulin synthesis under stress. Toxic environmental agents and viruses also influence the synthesis and secretion of insulin.

3. *Secretion of insulin from the pancreatic beta cells.* Secretion is affected by genetic factors, food intake, and exercise. In a recent study, an overexpression of melatonin receptors (*MNR1B* variants) was associated with suppression of glucose-stimulated insulin secretion.[4]

4. *Insulin-signaling pathways that regulate the uptake of glucose by fat and muscle cells.* Genes influence the response of muscle and fat cells to insulin. The size and number of fat cells and skeletal muscle cells also influence insulin responsiveness.

5. *Control of fat metabolism and storage in the body.* Some genes influence fat absorption from the gastrointestinal tract and fat deposition in the body. Diet and exercise also influence the amount of fat intake and deposition.

The genetics of T2DM are complex. T2DM is not inherited in a clearly dominant or recessive manner. Though genetic polymorphisms that increase the risk for developing diabetes are becoming better characterized, new information is emerging about other genetic variations that reduce risk for T2DM. For example, in mitochondrial DNA, a variation in one haplogroup is significantly associated with resistance against T2DM.[4]

The American Diabetic Association recommends screening for diabetes onset every 3 years in individuals with a positive family history, and in all individuals older than 45 years.[1] Elucidating the genetics of T2DM helps to identify individuals at risk who may benefit from interventions before the disease develops. Taking and recording a family history will help to identify those at higher risk for diseases influenced by genetic factors.[3]

References

1. American Diabetic Association. Standards of medical care in diabetes. *Diabetes Care.* 2008;31(Suppl 1):S13-S54.
2. Lander ES. Initial impact of the sequencing of the human genome. *Nature.* 2011;470(7333):187-197.
3. Lashley FR. *Clinical Genetics in Nursing Practice.* 3rd ed. New York: Springer. 2006.
4. Park KS. The search for genetic risk factors of type 2 diabetes mellitus. *Diabetes Metabolism Journal.* 2011;35(1):12-22.

secretory defects.[2] The net result is a *relative insulin deficiency*. A combination of cardiovascular risk factors including hypertension, atherogenic dyslipidemia, and hyperglycemia comprise the *cardiometabolic risk syndrome* and significantly increases the risk of developing type 2 DM. The other causes of DM include insulin resistance during pregnancy (gestational DM), medications such as corticosteroids, genetic disorders such as cystic fibrosis, pancreatic damage, viruses, and disorders of the pituitary gland and adrenal gland.[2] Additionally, polycystic ovary syndrome is strongly associated with the development of obesity and insulin resistance and places a woman at significant risk for development of gestational diabetes and type 2 DM later in life.

Genetic factors have a strong role in the development of type 1 DM (see box, "Genetics"). For example, rates of type 1 DM are particularly high in Scandinavia. Genetic alterations may play a role in the development of type 2 DM and related conditions, such as obesity and the cardiometabolic risk syndrome. The incidence of type 2 DM in the United States is higher in Latinos, African Americans, Native Americans, Alaska Natives, Asian Americans, and Pacific Islanders.[2]

Normally, glucose transport into cells occurs by the process of facilitated diffusion using various glucose transport channel proteins.[24] Insulin is not required for glucose to enter cells in the liver, kidney tubules, central nervous system, retina, or intestinal mucosa; beta cells in the islets of Langerhans; or into erythrocytes. In response to increased levels of serum glucose, insulin is released from the pancreas by beta cells in the islets of Langerhans. Insulin promotes uptake of glucose by muscle, liver, and adipose cells and is integral in carbohydrate, protein, and lipid synthesis.[3] The physiological activity of insulin is summarized in Box 18-3.

Control of glucose levels and insulin secretion is affected by the pancreatic hormones glucagon, amylin, and somatostatin, as well as the gut-secreted incretin hormones such as glucagon-like peptide-1 (GLP-1).[3] Amylin is cosecreted by the pancreatic beta cells in response to glucose elevation in the postfed state and acts to suppress postprandial hepatic glucose output, delay gastric emptying, and promote satiety.[3] GLP-1 is produced by the small intestines in response to glucose entry into the gut following a meal. GLP-1 has actions similar to amylin and additionally promotes first-phase insulin release by the pancreas.[4] Circulating counterregulatory hormones including catecholamines, cortisol, glucagon, and growth hormone also are integral in blood glucose regulation. These hormones are released in response to decreased glucose levels and also as an element of the physiologic response to stress. Excretion of glucose by the renal tubules additionally plays a role in blood glucose regulation. Sodium-glucose cotransporter (SGLT-2) is a compound found in the proximal tubule of the nephron that is responsible for the majority of glucose excretion by the kidney. A new class of drugs called SGLT-2 inhibitors is being developed and will augment blood

> ### BOX 18-3 PHYSIOLOGICAL ACTIVITY OF INSULIN
>
> **Carbohydrate Metabolism**
> - Increases glucose transport across cell membrane in most cells including muscle and fat
> - Within liver and muscle, promotes glycogenesis, the storage form of glucose
> - Inhibits gluconeogenesis and glycogenolysis in the liver, thus sparing amino acids and glycerol for protein and fatty acid synthesis
>
> **Fat Metabolism**
> - Increases triglyceride synthesis
> - Increases fatty acid transport into adipose tissue
> - Inhibits lipolysis of triglycerides stored in adipose tissue
> - Stimulates fatty acid synthesis from glucose and other substrates
>
> **Protein Metabolism**
> - Increases amino acid transport across cell membrane of muscle and liver
> - Augments protein synthesis
> - Inhibits proteolysis

glucose control in people with type 2 diabetes by enhancing renal glucose excretion by limiting tubular reabsorption of glucose. The net result is a decrease in circulating levels of glucose.

Without insulin, glucose is unable to enter storage cells, and instead it accumulates in the blood and triggers a variety of physiological processes as the cells requiring insulin for glucose entry begin to starve. In contrast, levels of circulating insulin that exceed the body's requirement result in decreased serum glucose levels and changes in nervous system function including mental status, because glucose is the preferred substrate for the central nervous system.

Three common critical endocrine disorders associated with the pancreas are diabetic ketoacidosis (DKA), hyperosmolar hyperglycemic state (HHS), and hypoglycemia. An understanding of the normal physiology of insulin, as well as of the pathophysiology, critical assessments, and collaborative treatment regimens of the aforementioned disorders, is essential to the management and nursing care of these patients.

Effects of Aging

With aging, pancreatic endocrine function declines. Fasting glucose levels trend upward with age and glucose tolerance decreases. These changes are due to a combination of both decreased insulin production and increased insulin resistance, independent of any other coexisting disease states. Fifty percent of adults age 65 years and older have elevated blood glucose levels and are at increased risk for diabetes (prediabetes), and over one fourth of elders have glucose levels that meet diagnostic criteria for diabetes.[6]

Hyperglycemic Crises
Pathogenesis

DKA and HHS are endocrine emergencies. The underlying mechanism for both DKA and HHS is a reduction in the net effective action of circulating insulin coupled with a concomitant elevation of counterregulatory hormones (Figure 18-3). Together, this hormonal mix leads to increased hepatic and renal glucose production, but it prevents use of glucose in the peripheral tissues.

Historically, DKA was described as the crisis state in type 1 DM, whereas HHS was thought to occur in type 2 DM. Increasingly, DKA and HHS are seen concurrently in the same patient.[5]

Etiology of diabetic ketoacidosis. Numerous factors precipitate DKA (Box 18-4). Many patients present with DKA as the initial indication of previously undiagnosed type 1 DM. In the critically ill, the presence of coexisting autoimmune endocrine disorders of the thyroid and adrenal glands must be considered, especially in unstable patients with type 1 DM.[24] Additionally, the multiple endocrine changes that accompany pregnancy alter insulin needs that escalate rapidly in the second and third trimesters.[3] Pregnant women with type 1 DM are at increased risk for DKA. Signs and symptoms of DKA characteristically develop over a short period, and patients seek medical help early because of the associated symptoms.

The incidence of recurrent DKA is higher in females and peaks in the early teenage years. The risk of recurrent DKA is also higher in patients with DM diagnosed at an early age and in those of lower socioeconomic status. The causes of recurrent DKA are unclear but include physiological, psychosomatic, and psychosocial factors. Psychological problems complicated by eating disorders in younger patients with type 1 DM may contribute to 20% of recurrent DKA.[10]

Etiology of hyperosmolar hyperglycemic state. HHS is usually precipitated by inadequate insulin secretion or impaired action associated with rising glucose levels, and is more commonly seen in patients with who have type 2 DM or no prior history of DM.[10] Most patients who develop this condition are elderly, with decreased compensatory mechanisms to maintain homeostasis in hyperosmolar states. A major illness that mediates overproduction of glucose secondary to the stress response may contribute to the development of HHS. High-calorie parenteral and enteral feedings that exceed the patient's ability to metabolize glucose have induced HHS. Several medications are associated with the development of the disorder. The major etiological factors of HHS are included in Box 18-4.

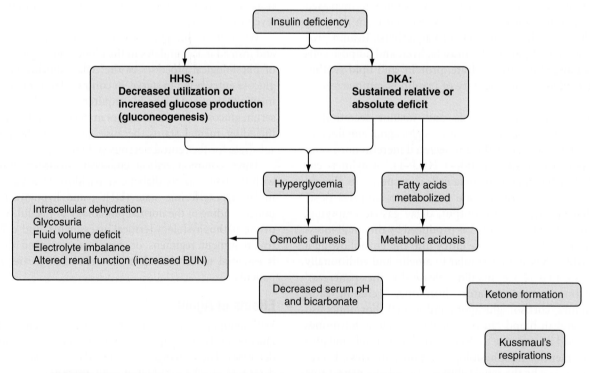

FIGURE 18-3 Pathophysiology of diabetic ketoacidosis (DKA) and hyperosmolar hyperglycemic state (HHS).

BOX 18-4 FACTORS LEADING TO DIABETIC KETOACIDOSIS AND HYPEROSMOLAR HYPERGLYCEMIC STATE

Common Factors

- *Infections:* pneumonia, urinary tract infection, sepsis, or abscess
- Omission of diabetic therapy or inadequate treatment
- New-onset diabetes mellitus
- *Preexisting illness:* cardiac, renal diseases
- *Major or acute illness:* MI, CVA, pancreatitis, trauma, surgery, renal disease
- *Other endocrine disorders:* hyperthyroidism, Cushing's disease, pheochromocytoma
- Stress
- High caloric parenteral or enteral nutrition

Medications

- Steroids (especially glucocorticoids)
- Beta-blockers
- Thiazide diuretics
- Calcium channel blockers
- Phenytoin
- Epinephrine
- Psychotropics, including tricyclic antidepressants
- Sympathomimetics
- Analgesics
- Cimetidine
- Calcium channel blockers
- Immunosuppressants
- Diazoxide
- Chemotherapeutic agents
- "Social drugs" such as cocaine, ecstasy

DKA-Specific Factors

- Malfunction of insulin pump
- Insulin pump infusion set site problems (infection, disconnection, catheter kinking or migration)
- Increased insulin needs secondary to insulin resistant states: pregnancy, puberty, before menstruation

HHS-Specific Factors

- Decreased thirst mechanism
- Difficult access to fluids (e.g., nursing home resident)

CVA, Cerebrovascular accident; *DKA*, diabetic ketoacidosis; *HHS*, hyperosmolar hyperglycemic state; *MI*, myocardial infarction.

Pathophysiology of Diabetic Ketoacidosis

Figure 18-4 details the intracellular and extracellular shifts that occur in both DKA and HHS. In both disorders, high extracellular glucose levels produce an osmotic gradient between the intracellular and extracellular spaces, causing fluid to translocate from cells.[10] This process is called *osmotic diuresis*. When serum glucose levels exceed the renal threshold (approximately 200 mg/dL), glucose is lost through the kidneys (*glycosuria*). As glycosuria and osmotic diuresis

progress, urinary losses of water, sodium, potassium, magnesium, calcium, and phosphorus occur. This cycle of osmotic diuresis causes increases in serum osmolality, further compensatory fluid shifts from the intracellular to the intravascular space, and worsening dehydration.

Typically, body water losses in DKA total 6 L.[24] The evolving hyperosmolarity further impairs insulin secretion and promotes a state of insulin resistance known as *glucose toxicity*.[3] The glomerular filtration rate in the kidney decreases in response to these severe fluid volume deficits. Decreased glucose excretion (causing increased serum glucose levels) and hemoconcentration result. The altered neurological status frequently seen in these patients is partially the result of cellular dehydration and the hyperosmolar state.

The absolute or relative insulin deficiency that precipitates DKA causes derangement of carbohydrate, protein, and fat metabolism.[10] Protein stores are depleted through the process of gluconeogenesis in the liver. Amino acids are metabolized into glucose and nitrogen to provide energy. Without insulin, the liberated glucose cannot be used, further increasing serum blood glucose and urine glucose concentrations and worsening osmotic diuresis. As nitrogen accumulates in the peripheral tissues, blood urea nitrogen (BUN) rises. Breakdown of protein stores also stimulates the shift of intracellular potassium into the extracellular serum (hyperkalemia). This additional circulating potassium may also be lost as a result of osmotic diuresis (hypokalemia). Serum electrolyte levels, particularly potassium, may be falsely elevated in relation to the actual intracellular level. Total body potassium deficits are common and must be considered in the overall management of DKA. Because of the fluid volume and potassium shifts, serum potassium values must be interpreted with caution in patients with DKA.[3]

The starvation state that accompanies DKA results in the breakdown of fat cells into free fatty acids.[10] The free fatty acids are released into the blood and are transported to the liver where they are oxidized into ketone bodies (beta-hydroxybutyrate) and acetoacetate. This leads to an increase in circulating ketone concentrations and further increases gluconeogenesis by the liver. Ketonuria and the accompanying rising glucose level contribute to osmotic diuresis. The ketoacids are transported to peripheral tissues where they are oxidized to acetone. Inadequate buffering of the excess ketone acids by bicarbonate results in metabolic acidosis as the ratio of carbonic acid to bicarbonate ions increases. As ketone and hydrogen ions accumulate and acidosis worsens, the respiratory system attempts to compensate for excess carbonic acid by "blowing off" carbon dioxide (CO_2), a weak acid. Kussmaul respirations, characterized by increases in the rate and depth of breathing, and an acetone ("fruity") breath odor are classic clinical signs of DKA associated with this compensatory process. In addition to ketonemia, patients with DKA may have an accumulation of lactic acid (lactic acidosis). The resulting dehydration may cause decreased perfusion to core organs, with consequent hypoxemia and worsening of the lactic acidosis.

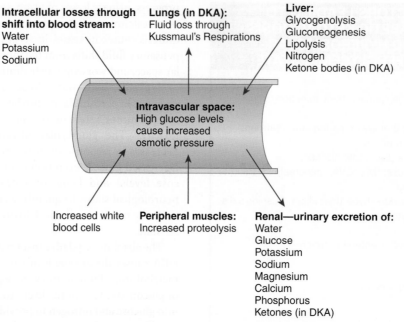

Intracellular losses through shift into blood stream:
Water
Potassium
Sodium

Lungs (in DKA):
Fluid loss through Kussmaul's Respirations

Liver:
Glycogenolysis
Gluconeogenesis
Lipolysis
Nitrogen
Ketone bodies (in DKA)

Intravascular space:
High glucose levels cause increased osmotic pressure

Increased white blood cells

Peripheral muscles:
Increased proteolysis

Renal—urinary excretion of:
Water
Glucose
Potassium
Sodium
Magnesium
Calcium
Phosphorus
Ketones (in DKA)

FIGURE 18-4 Intracellular/extracellular shifts in hyperglycemic crises. *DKA,* Diabetic ketoacidosis.

BOX 18-5 CALCULATION FOR ANION GAP

$$(Na^+ + K^+) - (Cl^- + HCO_3^-)$$

The normal value is 8 to 16 mEq/L. An elevated value indicates the accumulation of acids, such as is present in diabetic ketoacidosis.

Cl⁻, Chloride; *HCO₃⁻,* bicarbonate; *K⁺,* potassium; *Na⁺,* sodium.

Excess lactic acid results in an *increased anion gap* (increased body acids). Sodium, potassium, chloride, and bicarbonate are responsible for maintaining a normal anion gap, which is normally less than 16 mEq/L. Ketone accumulation causes an increase in the anion gap greater than 16 mEq/L. To calculate the anion gap, see Box 18-5.

Many enzymatic reactions within the body function only within a limited range of pH. As the patient becomes more acidotic and enzymes become less effective, body metabolism slows. This situation promotes further ketone formation, and acidosis worsens. The stress response associated with the progressing ketoacidosis state also contributes to metabolic alterations because the liver is stimulated by hormones (glucagon, catecholamines, cortisol, and growth hormones) to metabolize protein stores. The net result is an additional increase in serum glucose, nitrogen levels, and plasma osmolality. Some of these hormones also decrease the ability of cells to use glucose for ATP production and therefore compound the problem. The alterations in central nervous system function in DKA are thought to be influenced by the combination of acidosis and severe dehydration.

In summary, cells without glucose starve and begin to use existing stores of fat and protein to provide energy for body

processes (gluconeogenesis). Fats are metabolized faster than they can be stored, resulting in an accumulation of ketone acids, a by-product of fat metabolism in the liver. Ketone acids accumulate in the bloodstream, where hydrogen ions dissociate from the ketones and cause metabolic acidosis. The more acidotic the patient becomes, the less able the body is to metabolize these ketones.

Pathophysiology of Hyperosmotic Hyperglycemic State

The pathophysiology of HHS is similar to that of DKA. However, in HHS, there are significantly lower levels of free fatty acids, resulting in a lack of ketosis, but even higher levels of hyperglycemia, hyperosmolality, and severe dehydration (see Figure 18-3).[4] HHS is referred to by many different acronyms (Box 18-6).

Hyperglycemia results from decreased utilization of glucose, increased production of glucose, or both. The hyperglycemic

---

BOX 18-6 HHS AND OTHER SYNONYMOUS ACRONYMS

- *HHS:* Hyperosmolar hyperglycemic state
- *HHNC:* Hyperosmolar hyperglycemic nonketotic coma
- *HNS:* Hyperosmolar nonketotic state
- *HHNK:* Hyperosmolar hyperglycemic nonketosis
- *HHNS:* Hyperosmolar hyperglycemic nonketotic state/syndrome
- *HNKDC:* Hyperosmolar nonketotic diabetic coma
- *HONK:* Hyperosmolar nonketosis
- *HNAD:* Hyperglycemic nonacidotic diabetic coma

state causes an osmotic movement of water from a lesser concentration of solutes to a higher concentration of solutes. This results in expansion of the extracellular fluid volume and intracellular dehydration. The osmotic diuresis and resultant intracellular and extracellular dehydration in HHS are generally more severe than those found in DKA, because HHS generally develops insidiously over a period of weeks to months. Alterations in neurological status are common because of cellular dehydration. The typical total body water deficit is greater in HHS, approximately 9 L.[24] By the time these patients seek medical attention, they are profoundly dehydrated and hyperosmolar. As a result, the mortality rate of HHS is higher than that of DKA.

Most commonly, patients who develop HHS are older. They are also more likely to have other medical problems such as renal insufficiency, congestive heart failure, myocardial ischemia, and chronic lung disease that may limit the ability of providers to aggressively treat the condition,

particularly in regard to fluid resuscitation. Older adults that develop HHS are at very high risk for mortality.

Ketoacidosis is usually not seen in patients with HHS. It is believed that insulin levels in these patients are sufficient to prevent lipolysis and subsequent ketone formation.[4] The levels of glucose counterregulatory hormones that promote lipolysis are lower in patients with HHS than in those with DKA. However, persistence or worsening of the physiological stressor that precipitated the HHS episode may allow the hyperglycemia to progress to a state of extreme, insulin deficiency. Lipolysis occurs as a consequence of the severe insulin deficit, and ketoacidosis becomes superimposed upon the HHS.

Assessment

Clinical presentation. The presenting symptoms of DKA and HHS are similar (Table 18-3). Signs of DKA and HHS are related to the degree of dehydration present and the electrolyte

TABLE 18-3	MANIFESTATIONS OF DIABETIC KETOACIDOSIS AND HYPEROSMOLAR HYPERGLYCEMIC STATE	
	DIABETIC KETOACIDOSIS	HYPEROSMOLAR HYPERGLYCEMIC STATE
Pathophysiology	Relative or absolute insulin deficiency resulting in cellular dehydration and volume depletion, acidosis, and protein catabolism	Insulin deficiency resulting in dehydration and hyperosmolality
Health history	History of type 1 diabetes mellitus (DM) or use of insulin / Signs and symptoms of hyperglycemia before admission / Can also occur in type 2 DM in severe stress	History of type 2 DM signs and symptoms of hyperglycemia before admission / Occurs most frequently in elderly, with preexisting renal and cardiovascular disease
Onset	Develops quickly	Develops insidiously
Clinical presentation	Flushed, dry skin / Dry mucous membranes / ↓ Skin turgor / Tachycardia / Hypotension / Kussmaul's respirations / Acetone breath / Altered level of consciousness / Visual disturbances / Polydipsia / Nausea and vomiting / Anorexia / Abdominal pain	Flushed, dry skin / Dry mucous membranes / ↓ Skin turgor (may not be present in elderly) / Tachycardia / Hypotension / Shallow respirations / Altered level of consciousness (generally more profound and may include absent deep tendon reflexes, paresis, and positive Babinski's sign)
Diagnostics	↑ Plasma glucose (average: 675 mg/dL) / pH <7.30 / ↓ Bicarbonate / Ketosis / Azotemia / Electrolytes vary with state of hydration; often hyperkalemic / Plasma hyperosmolality (average: 330 mOsm/kg)	↑ Plasma glucose (usually >1000 mg/dL) / pH >7.30 / Bicarbonate >15 mEq/L / Absence of significant ketosis / Azotemia / Electrolytes vary with state of hydration; often hypernatremic / Plasma hyperosmolality (average: 350 mOsm/kg) / Hypotonic urine

imbalances. The osmotic diuresis occurring from hyperglycemia results in signs of increased thirst (polydipsia), increased urine output (polyuria), and dehydration. Increased hunger (polyphagia) may be an early sign. Elderly persons have a decreased sense of thirst, so this sign may not be observed in these patients. Signs of intravascular dehydration are common as the physiological processes continue.

Hyperglycemia and ketosis both contribute to delayed gastric emptying. Vomiting can occur, which further worsens total body dehydration. Patients also report symptoms of weakness and anorexia. Abdominal pain and tenderness are common presenting symptoms, particularly in DKA, and are associated with dehydration and underlying pathophysiology, such as pyelonephritis, duodenal ulcer, appendicitis, and metabolic acidosis. Pain associated with DKA usually disappears with treatment of dehydration. Significant weight loss occurs because of the fluid losses and an inability to metabolize glucose.

Altered states of consciousness range from restlessness, confusion, and agitation to somnolence and coma. Visual disturbances, especially blurred vision, are common in hyperglycemia. Generally, altered levels of consciousness are more pronounced in patients with HHS. This is related to the severity of hyperglycemia, serum hyperosmolality, and electrolyte disturbances. Seizures and focal neurological signs may also be present and often lead to misdiagnosis in patients with HHS.

In DKA, ketonuria and metabolic acidosis are seen. Nausea is an early sign of DKA and is thought to be a result of retained ketones. Kussmaul's respirations and an acetone breath odor additionally are clinical signs of ketosis. Later in the disease process, the respiratory status of the patient may be influenced by the neurological status, precipitating impaired breathing patterns and gas exchange. A decreased level of consciousness is also associated with the severe acidotic state (pH less than 7.15). The flushed face associated with DKA is the result of superficial vasodilation.

Laboratory evaluation. Numerous diagnostic studies are used to evaluate for the presence of DKA and HHS, to rule out other diseases, and to detect complications (see box, "Laboratory Alert: Pancreatic Endocrine Disorders"). In addition, cultures and testing are performed to determine any precipitating factors such as infection or myocardial infarction.

! LABORATORY ALERT

Pancreatic Endocrine Disorders

LABORATORY TEST*	CRITICAL VALUE	SIGNIFICANCE
Glucose	≥200 mg/dL (2 hours postprandial or random) ≥126 mg/dL (fasting)	Combined with symptoms, establishes diagnosis of diabetes mellitus
	>250 mg/dL	Suggestive of DKA; significantly higher in HHS
	<50 mg/dL	Hypoglycemia
Potassium	>6.0 mEq/L	Potential for heart blocks, bradydysrhythmias, sinus arrest, ventricular fibrillation, or asystole
	<3.0 mEq/L	Potential for ventricular dysrhythmias
Sodium	>150 mEq/L	May be a result of stress and dehydration
BUN	>20 mg/dL	Elevated due to protein breakdown and hemoconcentration
Bicarbonate	<20 mEq/L	Decreased in DKA due to compensation for acidosis
pH	<7.3	Decreased in DKA due to accumulation of acids
Osmolality	>330 mOsm/kg H_2O	Elevated in DKA relative to dehydration, higher in HHS
Phosphorus	<2.5 mg/dL	May result in impaired respiratory and cardiac functions
Magnesium	<1.3 mEq/L	Depleted by osmotic diuresis. May coincide with decreased potassium and calcium levels; may result in dysrhythmias
Beta-hydroxybutyrate	>3.0 mg/dL	Reflects blood ketosis in DKA

DKA, Diabetic ketoacidosis; *HHS*, hyperosmolar hyperglycemic state.
*Serum tests.

In DKA, an initial arterial blood gas analysis reflects metabolic acidosis (low pH and low bicarbonate level). The partial pressure of arterial carbon dioxide ($PaCO_2$) may also be low, reflecting the respiratory system's compensatory mechanism. Acidosis is subsequently monitored by venous pH, which correlates well with arterial pH but is easier to obtain and process. The severity of DKA is determined by the pH, bicarbonate level, ketone values, and the patient's mental status.[10] Severe acidosis is associated with cardiovascular collapse, which can result in death.

In HHS, the laboratory results are similar to those in DKA, but with four major differences: (1) the serum glucose concentration in HHS is generally significantly more elevated, (2) plasma osmolality is higher than in DKA and is associated with the degree of dehydration, (3) acidosis is not present or very mild compared with DKA, and (4) ketosis is usually absent or very mild in comparison with DKA.[10] Serum electrolyte concentrations may be low, normal, or elevated and generally are not reliable indicators of total body stores of electrolytes or water.

Nursing and Medical Interventions

Primary interventions in the treatment of DKA and HHS include respiratory support, fluid replacement, administration of insulin to correct hyperglycemia, replacement of electrolytes, correction of acidosis in DKA, prevention of complications, and patient teaching and support (see box, "Evidence-Based Practice").

Respiratory support. Assessment of the airway, breathing, and circulation is always the first priority in managing life-threatening disorders. Airway and breathing may be supported through the use of oral airways and oxygen therapy. In more severe cases, the patient may be intubated and placed on ventilatory support. Prevention of aspiration is accomplished by elevating the head of the bed. Nasogastric tube suction may be considered in a patient with impaired mentation who is actively vomiting.

Fluid replacement. Dehydration may have progressed to hypovolemic shock by the time of admission. Immediate intravenous (IV) access and rehydration need to be accomplished. In DKA, the typical water deficit approximates 100 mL/kg, and it may be as high as 200 mL/kg in HHS.[10] Monitoring for signs and symptoms of hypovolemic shock is a priority. Vital signs and neurological status are recorded at least every hour initially. Unstable patients require constant monitoring and recording of hemodynamic parameters at least every 15 minutes. Right atrial pressure or pulmonary artery pressure monitoring may also be instituted to evaluate fluid requirements and to monitor the

EVIDENCE-BASED PRACTICE

Tight Glycemic Control

Problem
Tight glycemic control has been advocated in critically ill patients. Issues and outcomes of achieving glycemic control need to be identified.

Clinical Question
What are the outcomes and issues associated with tight glycemic control in critically ill patients?

Evidence
Since the 2001 landmark study of Van den Berghe and colleagues demonstrated improved patient outcomes after initiation of tight glycemic control, most critical care units implemented protocols to achieve better glucose levels.[26] Many research studies have been conducted, and those cited in this box critically appraised recent evidenced—primarily from randomized controlled trials—on a variety of variables that have been studied. Findings of the NICE-SUGAR study raised important questions on the safety of tight glycemic targets in critically ill individuals.[1] The NICE-SUGAR trial included over 6000 critically ill patients, most of whom were mechanically ventilated. Those randomized to intensive control with glucose targets of 81 to 108 mg/dL experienced significantly higher 90-day mortality, primarily from cardiovascular causes, and higher rates of severe hypoglycemia than patients randomized to a target glycemic value of less than 180 mg/dL. Findings of a subsequent meta-analysis of 26 studies related to intensive glucose control in critically ill adults representing over 13,000 patients including those from the NICE-SUGAR trial concluded that intensive insulin therapy in critically ill patients does not reduce mortality and substantially increases the risk of serious hypoglycemia. But it may still provide specific benefit to surgical patients.[2] The degree of desired control remains a source of debate. Because significant hyperglycemia has been clearly associated with poor outcomes in the critically ill, current recommendations suggest that moderation of glucose targets to values between 140 and 180 mg/dL in critically ill patients should be maintained.

Implications for Nursing
Glycemic control has become a standard of practice within critical care settings. Nurses must be aware of protocols for achieving glycemic control and assist in ensuring that target glucose levels are achieved. Assessing patients for hypoglycemia is an essential nursing implication to prevent complications associated with treatment. Nurses will likely be involved in additional research over the next several years as protocols are refined based upon changing evidence.

Level of Evidence
A—Meta-analysis

References
1. NICE-SUGAR Study Investigators. Intensive verses conventional glucose control in critically ill patients. *New England Journal of Medicine*. 2011;360:1283-1297.
2. Griesdale DEG. Intensive insulin therapy and mortality among critically ill patients: a meta-analysis including NICE-SUGAR data, *Canadian Medical Association Journal*. 2009; 180:821-827.

patient's response to treatment. This is particularly true of patients with HHS, who tend to be elderly and have concurrent cardiovascular and renal disease. Accurate intake, hourly recording of urine output, and measurement of daily weight are also essential. Changes in mentation may also indicate a change in fluid status. Ongoing assessment of neurological status can alert the nurse to a change in mentation.

Normal saline (0.9% NS) is the fluid of choice for initial fluid replacement because it best replaces extracellular fluid volume deficits. Fluid replacement usually starts with an initial bolus of 1 L of 0.9% NS. This is followed by an infusion of 15 to 20 mL/kg during the first hour.[10] The effectiveness of fluid replacement is evaluated by hemodynamic status, intake and output, laboratory measures, and assessment of the patient's general physical condition, particularly mental status. IV fluids are rapidly infused until the patient's blood pressure and serum sodium level normalize. If the serum sodium is elevated or normal, IV fluid is changed to hypotonic saline (0.45% NS) and infused at slower rates to replace intracellular fluid deficits. When the plasma glucose level approaches 200 mg/dL, 5% dextrose is added to fluids to prevent hypoglycemia and assist in the resolution of ketosis.[10] The goal is to replace half of the estimated fluid deficit over the first 8 hours. The second half of the fluid deficit should be replaced during the next 16 hours of therapy so that the volume is restored in most patients within the first 24 hours of treatment.[10] Significant improvements in hyperglycemia may be seen with fluid resuscitation before initiation of insulin therapy. Hyperglycemia resolves more quickly than ketosis.

The goal of fluid resuscitation is normovolemia. Hypervolemia must be prevented, especially in patients with ischemic heart disease, heart failure, or acute kidney injury. Fluid overload from overaggressive fluid replacement can be prevented by monitoring breath sounds and performing cardiovascular assessments. Hemodynamic monitoring may be used to guide fluid resuscitation. Signs and symptoms of fluid overload are reviewed in Box 18-7. Rapid fluid administration may also contribute to cerebral edema, a complication associated with DKA. A rapid decrease in the plasma glucose level, combined with rapid fluid administration and concurrent insulin therapy (see next section), may lead to movement of water into brain cells, resulting in brain edema, which may be fatal.

Insulin therapy. Replacement of insulin is definitive therapy for DKA and HHS. Before starting insulin therapy, fluid replacement therapy must be underway and the serum potassium level must be greater than 3.3 mEq/L.[10] The goal is to restore normal glucose uptake by cells while preventing complications of excess insulin administration, such as hypoglycemia, hypokalemia, and hypophosphatemia. Hyperglycemic crises are commonly treated with IV insulin infusions because absorption is more predictable. An initial IV bolus of 0.1 units/kg of regular insulin is administered, followed by a continuous infusion of 0.1 units/kg per hour to achieve a steady decrease in serum glucose levels of 50 to 75 mg/dL per hour.[10] Initial insulin infusion rates of less than 0.1 units/kg per hour are typically insufficient to inhibit ketosis. Alternatively,

> **BOX 18-7**   **SIGNS AND SYMPTOMS OF FLUID OVERLOAD**
>
> - Tachypnea
> - Neck vein distention
> - Tachycardia
> - Crackles
> - Increased pulmonary artery occlusion or right atrial pressures
> - Declining level of consciousness in cerebral edema

patients with mild to moderate DKA may be treated with hourly subcutaneous injections of rapid-acting insulin using a titration scale.

Serum glucose levels are monitored every 1 to 2 hours using a consistent monitoring method. While receiving an intravenous insulin infusion, patients are generally allowed nothing by mouth. When glucose values are less than 200 mg/dL, insulin infusion rates may be decreased to 0.02 to 0.05 units/kg per hour and maintained to keep the glucose value in the range of 150 to 200 mg/dL.[10] Patients may be transitioned to subcutaneous insulin when the blood glucose is 200 mg/dL or less and when two of the following criteria are met: (1) venous pH is greater than 7.30, (2) serum bicarbonate level is greater than 15 mEq/L, and (3) calculated anion gap is 12 mEq/L or less.[10] Subcutaneous insulin therapy using a basal-bolus regimen that also includes an algorithm for correction doses of rapid acting insulin may be most appropriate for patients who are not receiving nutritional support in the form of enteral feedings or total parenteral nutrition. Glucose levels are monitored at least every 6 to 8 hours while a patient is receiving subcutaneous insulin.

In patients with HHS, insulin infusion rates may be decreased to 0.2 to 0.5 units/kg per hour when the glucose values reach 300 mg/dL.[10] Target glucose values of 200 to 300 mg/dL should be maintained until the patient's mental status improves, at which time the patient may be transitioned to subcutaneous insulin therapy.

It is important that serum glucose levels not be lowered too rapidly, not more than 50 to 75 mg/dL per hour, to prevent cerebral edema, which could result in seizures and coma. Any patient who exhibits an abrupt change in the level of consciousness after initiation of insulin therapy requires frequent blood glucose monitoring and protective steps instituted to prevent harm, such as seizure precautions. Treatment of acute cerebral edema usually involves administration of an osmotic diuretic (e.g., 20% mannitol solution).

Electrolyte management. Potassium, phosphate, chloride, and magnesium replacement may be required, especially during insulin administration. Osmotic diuresis in DKA and HHS results in total body potassium depletion ranging from 400 to 600 mEq. The potassium deficit may be greater in HHS. Insulin therapy will promote translocation of potassium into the intracellular space resulting in a further decrease in serum potassium levels.

The need for potassium therapy is based on serum laboratory results. In the absence of renal disease, insulin replacement and monitoring begins after the first liter of IV fluid has been administered, the serum potassium level is greater than 3.3 mEq/L, and the patient is producing urine. At that point, 20 to 30 mEq of potassium may be added to each liter of fluid administered. This may be augmented by additional doses of potassium as intermittent infusions.[10] Serum potassium levels should be maintained between 4 and 5 mEq/L during the course of therapy. In the event that the patient is admitted with hypokalemia, insulin therapy should be withheld until potassium values exceed 3.3 mEq/L.[10] The integrity of the IV site must be maintained to prevent extravasation. Electrocardiographic (ECG) monitoring for cardiac dysrhythmias and assessment of respiratory status is also important during potassium administration.

Total body phosphorus levels are also depleted by osmotic diuresis, but serum phosphate levels may remain in the normal range. Insulin therapy may cause further reductions in phosphate levels. Phosphate replacement occurs when there is associated respiratory or cardiac dysfunction. Potassium phosphate can be administered to treat part of the potassium deficit in a concentration of 20 to 30 mEq/L.[10] Phosphate replacement is used with extreme caution in patients with renal failure because these patients are unable to excrete phosphate and typically have underlying hyperphosphatemia.

Treatment of acidosis. Acidosis is a hallmark feature of DKA. However, multiple studies have shown that treatment with sodium bicarbonate is often not beneficial and may pose increased risk of hypoglycemia, cerebral edema, cellular hypoxemia secondary to decreased uptake of oxygen by body tissues, worsening hypokalemia, and development of central nervous system acidosis.[10] Therefore sodium bicarbonate is not routinely used to treat acidosis unless the serum pH is less than 6.9. Bicarbonate replacement is used only to bring the pH up to 7.0,

but not to normal levels. When administered, 100 mEq/L of bicarbonate may be added to 400 mL of sterile water with 20 mEq of KCl at a rate of 200 mL per hour until the venous pH exceeds 7.0.[10] Serum blood gas analysis is done frequently to assess for changes in pH, bicarbonate, anion gap, $PaCO_2$, and oxygenation status. Repeat infusions of the bicarbonate solution may be required every 2 hours until the pH exceeds 7.0. Once fluid and electrolyte imbalances are corrected and insulin is administered, the kidneys begin to conserve bicarbonate to restore acid-base homeostasis, and ketone formation ceases.

Patient and family education. A primary intervention to prevent DKA is patient education. Managing blood glucose levels with diet, exercise, and medication is a priority. Monitoring of hemoglobin A1c levels three to four times per year provides an indication of the patient's long-term control of blood glucose levels, changing insulin needs, and indications of psychosocial or behavioral factors that may impact control, including coping issues such as diabetes-related distress and depression.[1] The importance of a regular eating schedule, exercise, rest, sleep, and relaxation must be emphasized. Adjustments to the usual diabetic control regimen for illness is known as "sick day management," and all patients with diabetes and their families need to be instructed in this strategy for prevention of DM complications. Patients who go into DKA while on insulin pump therapy may require reeducation on pump features, insulin pump safety, management of pump failure, and troubleshooting abnormal glucose levels.

Patient Outcomes

Outcomes for a patient with DKA or HHS are included the nursing care plan (see box, "Nursing Care Plan for the Patient with Hyperglycemic Crisis").

◎ NURSING CARE PLAN

for the Patient with Hyperglycemic Crisis

NURSING DIAGNOSIS
Ineffective breathing pattern or impaired gas exchange related to acidosis (DKA), decreased level of consciousness

PATIENT OUTCOMES
Normal respiratory rate and pattern
- RR, 10-25 breaths/min
- Tidal volume >5 mL/kg
- ABG values WNL

NURSING INTERVENTIONS	RATIONALES
• Assess airway and breathing on admission and every 1-2 hours; correlate ABG/venous pH results with clinical examination	• Ability to protect airway and respiratory effort will stabilize as pH improves
• Assess for clinical signs of hypoxemia	• Impairment of ventilation may occur as a result of mental status or electrolyte changes
• Provide support as needed (e.g., airway, intubation, mechanical ventilation)	• Maintenance of oxygenation and ventilation are critical in maintaining cellular integrity and preventing worsening acidosis
• Assess neurological status every 1-2 hours	• Mental status changes may be first indication of hypoxemia and cerebral edema
• Prevent aspiration: elevate head of bed; NG tube for decompression may be needed	• Patients with altered level of consciousness are at higher risk for aspiration, and individuals with glycemic derangement are at higher risk for vomiting

Continued

NURSING CARE PLAN

for the Patient with Hyperglycemic Crisis—cont'd

NURSING DIAGNOSIS
Deficient fluid volume related to total body water loss secondary to osmotic diuresis, ketosis, increased lipolysis, and vomiting

PATIENT OUTCOMES
Adequate fluid volume status
- Normal serum glucose
- Hemodynamic stability: BP, HR, RAP, PAOP WNL
- Normal sinus rhythm
- Urine output >0.5 mL/kg/hr
- Balanced I&O
- Stable weight
- Warm, dry extremities
- Normal skin turgor
- Moist mucous membranes
- Serum osmolality and serum electrolyte levels WNL: sodium, potassium, calcium, phosphorus
- pH WNL

NURSING INTERVENTIONS	RATIONALES
• Assess fluid status: Vital signs every hour until stable I&O measurements every 1-2 hours Skin turgor, mucous membranes, thirst Consider insensible fluid losses Daily weight	• Provide clinical indications of hypovolemia and provide data for restoring cellular function
• Initiate fluid replacement therapy: Monitor for signs and symptoms of fluid overload Monitor effects of volume repletion Monitor neurological status closely	• Correct volume deficit and prevent/treat hypovolemic shock; neurological status should improve as electrolytes normalize Mental status changes may indicate cerebral edema if glycemic correction is too rapid
• Administer IV insulin infusion per hospital protocol; titrate therapy hourly based on glucose levels; provide a steady decrease in serum glucose levels; a decrease of 50 to 75 mg/dL per hour is desired	• Prevents cerebral edema and potentially dangerous electrolyte abnormalities
• Monitor glucose every hour via consistent method (serum or fingerstick capillary) during insulin infusion	• Assesses response to therapy and allows for immediate correction of glycemic abnormalities.
• Monitor for signs and symptoms of hypoglycemia	• Hypoglycemia may occur if the insulin dose is exceeds patient's needs
• Add dextrose to maintenance IV solutions once serum glucose level reaches 200 mg/dL in DKA and 300 mg/dL in HHS	• Prevents relative hypoglycemia and a decrease in plasma osmolality that may result in cerebral edema
• Monitor serum electrolyte levels (sodium, potassium, calcium, phosphorus); administer supplements according to protocols; assess causes of continuing electrolyte depletion such as diuresis, vomiting, NG suction	• Prevent complications of electrolyte imbalance; osmotic diuresis may result in increased excretion of potassium and hyponatremia; insulin therapy causes potassium and phosphate to shift to intracellular space
• Monitor pH	• pH is the best indicator of acidosis and response to treatment; acidosis will correct more slowly than hyperglycemia; correction of hyperglycemia without correction of ketosis may result in reoccurrence of DKA
• Administer bicarbonate only in severe acidosis (pH <6.9)	• Routine administration of bicarbonate has been associated with hypokalemia, hypoglycemia, cellular ischemia, cerebral edema, and CNS cellular acidosis

NURSING CARE PLAN

for the Patient with Hyperglycemic Crisis—cont'd

NURSING DIAGNOSIS

Risk for ineffective therapeutic management related to lack of knowledge of disease process, treatment regimen, complications, sick day management and/or ineffective coping

PATIENT OUTCOMES

Effective therapeutic management of diabetes

- Patient/family can describe the pathophysiology and causes of DKA and/or HHS; preventative interventions related to diet, exercise regimen, and medications; signs and symptoms of hypoglycemia and hyperglycemia; signs and symptoms of infections that require medical follow-up; sick day management; and emergency hypoglycemia management
- Patient/family can identify the patient's individual glucose targets
- Patient/family can demonstrate self–glucose monitoring and administration of oral hypoglycemic medications and/or insulin therapy according to glucose values

NURSING INTERVENTIONS	RATIONALES
• Assess patient/family's current diabetes self-management practices, ability to learn information, and psychomotor and sensory skills	• Allows for individualization of patient's plan of care to match physical, psychosocial and educational needs
• Implement a teaching program that includes information on pathophysiology and causes of DKA or HHS; diet and exercise restrictions; individualized target glucose values; signs and symptoms of hypoglycemia and hyperglycemia, including interventions; and signs and symptoms of infection and illness, including interventions	• Prevention of acute diabetes complications primarily rests with the patient and/or family who are capable and able to follow the self-management plan and act early on significant physiological changes
• Demonstrate methods for blood glucose monitoring; have the patient repeat the demonstration until proficient; if the patient takes insulin, demonstrate administration; for each skill, have the patient demonstrate abilities with repeat demonstration; review insulin pump use and abilities if used for treatment	• Regular glucose monitoring is essential for patient self-management; ensure that patient/family have the ability to perform these skills related to at-home monitoring, insulin delivery, and problem solving related to abnormal glucose findings before discharge
• Review administration of hypoglycemic medications and/or insulin, including dosage, frequency, action, duration, side effects, and situations when medication may need to be adjusted	• Patients and caregivers require a thorough knowledge of insulin therapy in order to optimize treatment; failure to adjust hypoglycemic medications to match changing glycemic demands may result in acute hyperglycemia or hypoglycemia
• Consult with clinical dietitian regarding disease-specific nutrition and diet needs	• Assist in identifying the appropriate diet based on the patient's condition and caloric needs
• Encourage patient to wear a form of identification for diabetes	• Assists in prompt recognition and treatment of complications should they occur
• Provide written materials for all content taught; provide means for the patient to get questions answered after discharge, and schedule follow-up diabetes self-management education after discharge	• Effective diabetes self-management education is a collaboration between the patient, family, and multiprofessional care providers; in the short term, diabetes self-management education improves glycemic control; regular reinforcement improves self-management outcomes

ABGs, Arterial blood gases; *BP*, blood pressure; *DKA*, diabetic ketoacidosis; *HHS*, hyperosmolar hyperglycemic state; *HR*, heart rate; *I&O*, intake and output; *IV*, intravenous; *NG*, nasogastric; *PaCO₂*, partial pressure of carbon dioxide in arterial blood; *PAOP*, pulmonary artery occlusion pressure; *RAP*, right atrial pressure; *RR*, respiratory rate; *WNL*, within normal limits.

Based on data from Gulanick M and Myers JL. *Nursing Care Plans: Diagnoses, Interventions, and Outcomes.* 7th ed. St. Louis: Mosby; 2011.

Hypoglycemia

Pathophysiology

A hypoglycemic episode is defined as a decrease in the plasma glucose level to less than 70 mg/dL and is sometimes referred to as *insulin shock* or *insulin reaction*. Glucose production falls behind glucose utilization, resulting in decrease in blood glucose. Because the brain is an obligate user of glucose, the first clinical sign of hypoglycemia is a change in mental status. A hypoglycemic event activates the sympathetic nervous system causing a rise in counterregulatory hormones, including glucagon, epinephrine, cortisol, and growth hormone. Those at highest risk for hypoglycemia are patients taking insulin, children and pregnant women with type 1 DM, patients with autonomic diabetic neuropathy, and elderly persons with type 1 or type 2 DM.

Hypoglycemia unawareness, also known as hypoglycemia-associated autonomic failure, is a term used to describe a diabetes-related condition where a patient does not recognize the onset of hypoglycemic signs and symptoms.[1] In this complication, the impairment of the autonomic nervous systems results in a blunted response to critically low glucose levels (see box, "Clinical Alert"). Patients with hypoglycemia unawareness may be asymptomatic while experiencing extremely low blood glucose levels. Patients who have other forms of autonomic neuropathy such as orthostasis, gastroparesis, erectile dysfunction, and cardiac autonomic neuropathy are at higher risk for this condition. Those at highest risk of hypoglycemia unawareness include the elderly because of their impeded stress responses and those with diminished mental function resulting from dementia, concurrent illness, or other factors. Patients taking beta-blockers are at risk of decreased awareness of signs of hypoglycemia because of the drug's impact on the sympathetic nervous system. The pathophysiological mechanisms associated with acute hypoglycemia and the associated central nervous system (CNS) and sympathetic symptoms are reviewed in Figure 18-5.

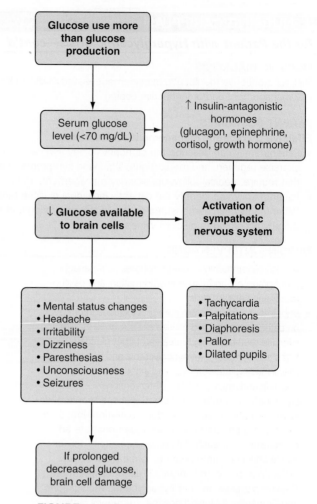

FIGURE 18-5 Pathophysiology of hypoglycemia.

> **! CLINICAL ALERT**
>
> ### *Hypoglycemic Unawareness*
>
> Some patients have hypoglycemia unawareness, and remain asymptomatic despite extremely low blood glucose levels. The elderly and those taking beta-blockers are at especially high risk.

Etiology

Patients receiving insulin therapy must be closely monitored for hypoglycemia when insulin requirements are decreased because of weight loss or renal insufficiency, when insulin doses are increased, when nondiabetes medications that may impact glycemia are prescribed or adjusted, or when injection sites are rotated from a hypertrophied area to one with unimpaired absorption. Additionally, patients who use oral agents that promote production and release of endogenous insulin, such as long-acting sulfonylureas, are at risk for hypoglycemia. Amylin and agents that act on incretin hormones (exenatide and gliptins) also increase the risk for a

hypoglycemic episode. Other causes of hypoglycemia in the hospitalized patient include insufficient caloric consumption because of a missed or delayed meal or snack, decreased intake because of nausea and vomiting, anorexia, and interrupted tube feedings or total parenteral nutrition. As a patient recovers from a stress event (infection illness, corticosteroid therapy, postpartum), the need for exogenous insulin decreases. Failure to adjust the insulin dose may precipitate hypoglycemia. Other major causes of hypoglycemia are reviewed in Box 18-8.

Severe hypoglycemia and hypoglycemia unawareness place a patient at risk for injury secondary to motor vehicle accidents, falls, and seizures. Patients with renal impairment or liver dysfunction are at particular risk for a severe hypoglycemic episode. Delayed degradation or excretion of hypoglycemic medications potentiates or prolongs the action of many diabetes medications. The resulting increase in circulating levels of active drug, including insulin, results in erratic glucose control. Close glucose monitoring and patient/family education on prevention, recognition, and treatment of hypoglycemia is critical in promoting safety in these very high-risk patients.

BOX 18-8   CAUSES OF HYPOGLYCEMIA

Excess Insulin or Oral Hypoglycemics
- Dose of insulin or oral hypoglycemics too high
- Islet cell tumors (insulinomas)
- Liver insufficiency or failure (impaired metabolism of insulin)
- Acute kidney injury (impaired inactivation of insulin)
- Autoimmune phenomenon
- Drugs that potentiate action of antidiabetic medications (propranolol, oxytetracycline, antibiotics)
- Sulfonylureas in elderly patients
- Amylin and incretin mimetic diabetes agents

Decreased Oral, Enteral, or Parenteral Intake

Underproduction of Glucose
- Heavy alcohol consumption
- Drugs: aspirin, disopyramide (Norpace), haloperidol (Haldol)
- Decreased production by liver
- Hormonal causes

Too Rapid Utilization of Glucose
- Gastrointestinal surgery
- Extrapancreatic tumor
- Increased or strenuous exercise

TABLE 18-4   SIGNS AND SYMPTOMS OF HYPOGLYCEMIA

DECREASE IN BLOOD SUGAR	
RAPID	**PROLONGED**
Activation of Sympathetic Nervous System	**Inadequate Glucose Supply to Neural Tissues**
Nervousness	Headache
Apprehension	Restlessness
Tachycardia	Difficulty speaking
Palpitations	Difficulty thinking
Pallor	Visual disturbances
Diaphoresis	Paresthesia
Dilated pupils	Difficulty walking
Tremors	Altered consciousness
Fatigue	Coma
General weakness	Convulsions
Headache	Change in personality
Hunger	Psychiatric reactions
	Maniacal behavior
	Catatonia
	Acute paranoia

Assessment

Clinical presentation. Common signs and symptoms of hypoglycemia are summarized in Table 18-4. Symptoms of hypoglycemia are categorized as (1) mild symptoms from autonomic nervous system stimulation that are characteristic of a rapid decrease in serum glucose levels, and (2) moderate symptoms reflective of an inadequate supply of glucose to neural tissues, associated with a slower, more prolonged decline in serum glucose levels.

With a rapid decrease in serum glucose levels, there is activation of the sympathetic nervous system, mediated by epinephrine release from the adrenal medulla. This compensatory fight-or-flight mechanism may result in symptoms such as tachycardia; palpitations; tremors; cool, clammy skin; diaphoresis; hunger; pallor; and dilated pupils. The patient may also report feelings of apprehension, nervousness, headache, tremulousness, and general weakness.

Slower and more prolonged declines in serum glucose levels result in symptoms related to an inadequate glucose supply to neural tissues *(neuroglycopenia)*. These include restlessness, difficulty in thinking and speaking, visual disturbances, and paresthesias. The patient may have profound changes in the level of consciousness, seizures, or both. Personality changes and psychiatric manifestations have been reported. Prolonged hypoglycemia may lead to irreversible brain damage and coma.

Laboratory evaluation. In most patients, the confirming laboratory test for hypoglycemia is a serum or capillary blood glucose level less than 70 mg/dL. Adults with a history of hypoglycemia unawareness, cognitively impaired elders, and older adults at high risk for falls may have higher target glucose ranges and an individualized protocol for management

of lower glucose values.[1] The glucose level should be checked in all high-risk patients with the aforementioned clinical signs before initiating treatment. It is important to know baseline values before treatment because patients who have experienced elevated glucose levels for some time may complain of hypoglycemia-like symptoms when their glucose levels are brought into normal range. In patients with a known history of DM, a thorough history of past experiences of hypoglycemia, including patient-specific associated signs and symptoms, is essential. It is important to identify the glucose level at which symptoms appear because this may vary with individuals. Additionally, renal function is evaluated in patients with long-standing diabetes who have a new history of recurrent hypoglycemia. Decreased renal function may result in impaired clearance of insulin and result in erratic glucose control in patients who are on short-acting insulins, long-acting insulins, or oral insulin secretagogues.

Nursing Diagnoses

The nursing diagnoses applicable to a patient with a hypoglycemic episode include the following:
- Unstable blood glucose related to excess circulating insulin as in relation to available plasma glucose
- Acute confusion related to decreased glucose delivery to the brain and nervous tissue
- Risk for injury (seizures and falls) related to altered neuronal function associated with hypoglycemia
- Deficient knowledge related to hypoglycemia: prevention, recognition, and treatment of hypoglycemia

Nursing and Medical Interventions

After serum or capillary glucose levels have been confirmed, carbohydrates must be replaced. The patient's neurological

BOX 18-9 TREATMENT OF HYPOGLYCEMIA

Mild Hypoglycemia

- Patient is completely alert. Symptoms may include pallor, diaphoresis, tachycardia, palpitations, hunger, or shakiness. Blood glucose is less than 70 mg/dL. Patient is able to drink.
- Treatment: 15 g of carbohydrate by mouth

Moderate Hypoglycemia

- Patient is conscious, cooperative, and able to swallow safely. Symptoms may include difficulty concentrating, confusion, slurred speech, or extreme fatigue. Blood glucose is usually less than 55 mg/dL. Patient is able to drink.
- Treatment: 20 to 30 g of carbohydrate by mouth

Severe Hypoglycemia

- Patient is uncooperative or unconscious. Blood glucose is usually less than 40 mg/dL or patient is unable to drink
- Treatment with intravenous access: 12.5 g of dextrose as $D_{50}W$
- Treatment without intravenous access: 1 mg of glucagon subcutaneously

$D_{50}W$, 50% dextrose in water.

BOX 18-10 SOURCES OF 15 GRAMS OF CARBOHYDRATES

- 4 oz sweetened carbonated beverage
- 4 oz unsweetened fruit juice
- 1 cup skim milk
- Glucose gels or tablets (follow manufacturer's instructions)
- 2 tablespoons raisins
- 4 or 5 saltine crackers
- 6 to 7 hard candies
- ½ roll of Life Savers type of candy

status and ability to swallow without aspiration determine the route to be used. Box 18-9 details a protocol for treatment of mild, moderate, and severe hypoglycemia. Common food substances that contain at least 15 g of carbohydrate are listed in Box 18-10. Glucose levels should be reassessed 15 minutes after treatment. If the blood glucose level remains lower than 70 mg/dL, treatment is repeated.

In the event of hypoglycemia, rapid-acting and short-acting insulin should be withheld temporarily. If the patient has an insulin pump, it should be suspended for moderate or severe hypoglycemia, but the infusion catheter should not be removed. The patient should determine whether to discontinue the infusion for mild hypoglycemia. Longer-acting basal insulins should typically not be withheld in patients on subcutaneous insulin therapy who are experiencing hypoglycemia, because this will increase the risk for both DKA in patients with type 1 diabetes and hyperglycemia in all insulin-treated patients with diabetes. Patients should be instructed to notify their diabetes care provider if two or more events of hypoglycemia are experienced within a week because the medication regimen may require adjustment.

Neurological assessments are done to detect any changes in cerebral function related to hypoglycemia. It is important to document baseline neurological status, including mental status, cranial nerve function, sensory and motor function, and deep tendon reflexes. There is a potential for seizure activity related to altered neuronal cellular metabolism during the hypoglycemic phase, so patients should be assessed for seizure activity. Descriptions of the seizure event and associated symptoms are important to note. Seizure precautions should be instituted, including padded side rails, oxygen, oral airway, and bedside suction, as well as removal of potentially harmful objects from the environment. Neurological status is the best clinical indicator of effective treatment for hypoglycemia.

Patient and family education about hypoglycemic episodes may also be appropriate in the critical care setting. The patient and family members need to be instructed on the causes, symptoms, treatment, and prevention of hypoglycemia. The relationship of carbohydrate intake, actions of insulin or oral hypoglycemic agents, excessive alcohol intake, and activity changes or exercise with hypoglycemia should be incorporated into the teaching plan. Instruction on the use of home blood glucose monitoring techniques, schedule, and pattern recognition may also be needed. Patients at risk for severe hypoglycemia should be prescribed a glucagon emergency kit, and family and significant regular contacts should be instructed in its use. The patient is encouraged to wear emergency medical identification and encouraged to perform a blood glucose test before driving. Patients at risk for nocturnal hypoglycemia are encouraged to store glucose gel at the bedside. Childbearing women with diabetes are at very high risk for hypoglycemia after delivery as the levels of insulin-resistant hormones drop quickly. Lactating women also may be at particular risk and may be encouraged to drink milk while nursing. Additionally, patients need to be instructed on the relationship between alcohol ingestion and hypoglycemia.

Patient Outcomes

Outcomes for a patient with a hypoglycemic episode include the following:

- Serum or capillary glucose levels within the patient's target range
- No acute signs and symptoms of hypoglycemia
- Mental status returned to baseline
- Absence of seizure activity
- Ability of the patient and family to identify causes of hypoglycemia, state symptoms of hypoglycemia, state type and amount of foods that may be used to treat hypoglycemia, and perform home blood glucose monitoring.

ACUTE AND RELATIVE ADRENAL INSUFFICIENCY

Etiology

Hypofunction of the adrenal gland results from either primary or secondary mechanisms that suppress secretion of cortisol, aldosterone, and androgens. Primary mechanisms, resulting in Addison's disease, are those that cause destruction of the adrenal gland itself. At least 90% of the adrenal cortex must be destroyed before clinical signs and symptoms appear. Primary disorders result in deficiencies of both glucocorticoids and mineralocorticoids. Primary adrenal insufficiency (AI) has a variety of causes including idiopathic autoimmune destruction of the gland, infection and sepsis, hemorrhagic destruction, and granulomatous infiltration from neoplasms, amyloidosis, sarcoidosis, or hemochromatosis.

Idiopathic autoimmune destruction of the adrenal gland is the most common cause of AI, accounting for 50% to 70% of cases. Autoimmune adrenal destruction may have a genetic component that leads to atrophy of the gland. Genetic adrenal disease may affect just the adrenal gland or be part of a constellation of autoimmune problems, such as autoimmune polyglandular disorder.[13] Young women with spontaneous premature ovarian failure are at increased risk of developing the autoimmune form of adrenal insufficiency.[13] In addition to sepsis, HIV infection and tuberculosis are significant infectious causes of AI.[12]

Secondary mechanisms that can produce adrenal insufficiency are those that decrease adrenocorticotropic hormone (ACTH) secretion, resulting in deficiency of glucocorticoids alone, because mineralocorticoids are not primarily dependent on ACTH secretion. Mechanisms that can produce secondary adrenal insufficiency include abrupt withdrawal of corticosteroids, pituitary and hypothalamic disorders, and sepsis. A more detailed listing of possible causes of primary and secondary adrenal insufficiency is given in Box 18-11.

The most common cause of acute adrenal insufficiency is abrupt withdrawal from corticosteroid therapy. Long-term corticosteroid use suppresses the normal *corticotropin-releasing hormone (CRH)-ACTH-adrenal feedback systems* (see Figure 18-1) and result in adrenal suppression. It is difficult to accurately predict the degree of adrenal suppression in patients receiving exogenous glucocorticoid therapy. Longer-acting agents such as dexamethasone are more likely to produce suppression than are shorter-acting corticosteroids such as hydrocortisone. Once corticosteroid use has been tapered off, it may take several months for these patients to resume normal secretion of corticosteroids. Thus it is important to be familiar with disorders that may be treated with corticosteroids, because the resulting adrenal suppression may prevent a normal stress response in these patients and may put them at risk of an adrenal crisis. Other drugs may contribute to adrenal

suppression. For example, administration of the drug etomidate to facilitate endotracheal intubation is associated with significant but temporary adrenal dysfunction and increased mortality.[23]

Infection, sepsis, or both are among the most common causes of adrenal insufficiency in the critical care setting.[14] The proinflammatory state commonly seen in critical illness is thought to produce AI by suppressing the hypothalamic-pituitary-adrenal axis. Glucocorticoid resistance and suppression of feedback mechanisms are postulated to contribute to low cortisol levels commonly seen in critical illness. Sepsis and septic shock can also cause thrombotic necrosis of the adrenal gland.[15] The concept of relative adrenal insufficiency has been debated for several years. The hypermetabolic state of critical illness may increase cortisol levels by as much as tenfold over baseline.[14] Patients with an inadequate physiological response to the demands of this hypermetabolic state have an increased mortality rate. The degree of response, how to best measure the response, and optimum treatment continue to be investigated.[11]

Review of Physiology

The manifestations of adrenal insufficiency result from a lack of adrenal cortical secretion of glucocorticoids (primarily

---

> **BOX 18-11** **CAUSES OF ADRENAL INSUFFICIENCY**
>
> **Primary**
> - *Autoimmune disease:* idiopathic and polyglandular
> - *Granulomatous disease:* tuberculosis, sarcoidosis, histoplasmosis, blastomycosis
> - Cancer
> - *Hemorrhagic destruction:* anticoagulation, trauma, sepsis
> - *Infectious:* meningococcal, staphylococcal, pneumococcal, fungal (candidiasis), cytomegalovirus
> - Acquired immunodeficiency syndrome
> - *Drugs:* ketoconazole, aminoglutethimide, trimethoprim, etomidate, 5-fluorouracil (suppress adrenals); phenytoin, barbiturates, rifampin (increase steroid degradation)
> - Irradiation
> - Adrenalectomy
> - Developmental or genetic abnormality
>
> **Secondary**
> - Abrupt withdrawal of corticosteroids
> - Pathology affecting the pituitary, such as tumors, hemorrhage, radiation, metastatic cancer, lymphoma, leukemia, sarcoidosis
> - Systemic inflammatory states: sepsis, vasculitis, sickle cell anemia
> - Postpartum pituitary hemorrhage (Sheehan's syndrome)
> - Trauma, especially head trauma, or surgery
> - Hypothalamic disorders

BOX 18-12 PHYSIOLOGICAL EFFECTS OF GLUCOCORTICOIDS (CORTISOL)

- *Protein metabolism:* promotes gluconeogenesis, stimulates protein breakdown, and inhibits protein synthesis
- *Fat metabolism:* ↑ lipolysis and free fatty acid production, promotes fat deposits in face and cervical area
- *Opposes action of insulin:* ↓ glucose transport and utilization in cells
- *Inhibits inflammatory response:*
  - Suppresses mediator release (kinins, histamine, interleukins, prostaglandins, leukotrienes, serotonin)
  - Stabilizes cell membrane and inhibits capillary dilation
  - ↓ Formation of edema
  - Inhibits leukocyte migration and phagocytic activity
- *Immunosuppression:*
  - ↓ Proliferation of T lymphocytes and killer cell activity
  - ↓ Complement production and immunoglobulins
- Circulating erythrocytes
- *Gastrointestinal effects:* ↑ appetite; increases rate of acid and pepsin secretion in stomach
- ↑ Uric acid excretion
- ↓ Serum calcium
- Sensitizes arterioles to effects of catecholamines; maintains blood pressure
- ↑ Renal glomerular filtration rate and excretion of water

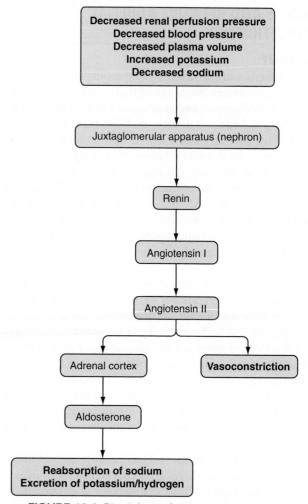

FIGURE 18-6 Physiology of aldosterone release.

cortisol), mineralocorticoids (primarily aldosterone), or both. The deficiency of glucocorticoids is especially significant because their influence on the defense mechanisms of the body and its response to stress makes them essential for life.

Cortisol is normally released in response to ACTH stimulation from the anterior pituitary gland (see Figure 18-1). ACTH is stimulated by CRH from the hypothalamus, which is influenced by circulating cortisol levels, circadian rhythms, and stress. Circadian rhythms affect ACTH and cortisol levels, creating peak levels of cortisol in the morning and the lowest levels around midnight. This normal diurnal rhythm can be overridden by stress. During stress, plasma cortisol may increase as much as 10 times its normal level. Release of cortisol increases the blood glucose concentration by promoting glycogen breakdown and gluconeogenesis in the liver, increases lipolysis and free fatty acid production, increases protein degradation, and inhibits the inflammatory and immune responses. Cortisol also increases sensitivity to catecholamines, producing vasoconstriction, hypertension, and tachycardia (Box 18-12).

Aldosterone is a mineralocorticoid synthesized in the adrenal cortex that regulates the body's electrolyte and water balance in the renal tubules. Secretion of aldosterone is regulated primarily by the renin-angiotensin-aldosterone system. Renin is an enzyme stored in the cells of the juxtaglomerular

apparatus (JGA) in the kidneys. It is released in response to stimulation of beta receptors on the JGA surface. Factors that stimulate the release of renin include low plasma sodium, increased plasma potassium levels, decreased extracellular fluid volume, decreased blood pressure, and decreased sympathetic nerve activity. Once released, renin cleaves angiotensinogen in the plasma to form angiotensin I. Angiotensin I is then converted to angiotensin II in the lungs under the influence of angiotensin-converting enzyme. Angiotensin II stimulates the secretion of aldosterone by the adrenal cortex while causing vasoconstriction of the arterioles. Aldosterone acts in the kidneys on the ascending loop of Henle, the distal convoluted tubule, and the collecting ducts to increase sodium ion reabsorption and to increase potassium and hydrogen ion excretion. Because reabsorption of sodium creates an osmotic gradient across the renal tubular membrane, antidiuretic hormone (ADH) is activated, causing water to be reabsorbed with sodium. The physiology of aldosterone release is summarized in Figure 18-6.

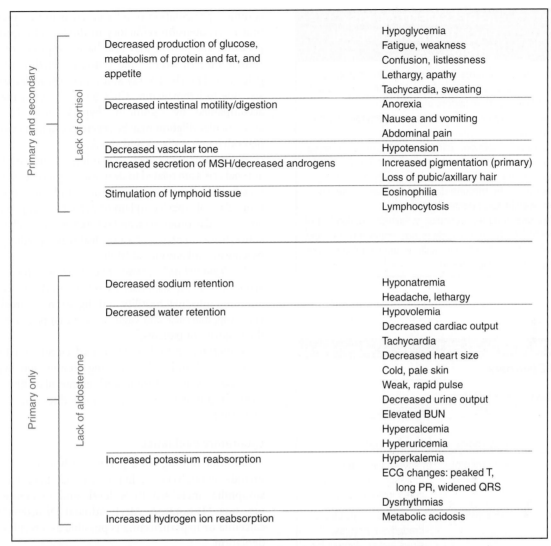

FIGURE 18-7 Pathophysiological effects of adrenal insufficiency. *BUN,* Blood urea nitrogen; *ECG,* electrocardiogram; *MSH,* melanocyte-stimulating hormone.

Pathophysiology

Adrenal crisis is a life-threatening absence of cortisol (glucocorticoid) and aldosterone (mineralocorticoid). A deficiency of cortisol results in decreased production of glucose, decreased metabolism of protein and fat, decreased appetite, decreased intestinal motility and digestion, decreased vascular tone, and diminished effects of catecholamines. If a patient with deficient cortisol is stressed, this deficiency can produce profound shock due to significant decreases in vascular tone caused by the diminished effects of catecholamines.[11,15]

Deficiency of aldosterone results in decreased retention of sodium and water, decreased circulating volume, and increased potassium and hydrogen ion reabsorption. These effects are seen in patients with underlying primary adrenal insufficiency but not secondary adrenal insufficiency, because aldosterone secretion is not primarily dependent on ACTH. A summary of pathophysiological effects of adrenal insufficiency can be found in Figure 18-7.

Assessment
Clinical Presentation

Adrenal crisis requires astute and rapid data collection. Box 18-13 identifies risk factors for adrenal crisis. Features of adrenal crisis are nonspecific and may be attributed to other medical disorders. Signs and symptoms vary (see Figure 18-6). Because this condition is a medical emergency, the diagnosis should be considered in any patient acutely ill with fever, vomiting, hypotension, shock, decreased serum sodium level, increased serum potassium level, or hypoglycemia (see box, "Laboratory Alert: Adrenal Disorders"). Specific system disturbances are widespread.

BOX 18-13 ASSESSMENT OF RISK FACTORS FOR ADRENAL CRISIS

Assess carefully for patients who are at risk, have predisposing factors, or have physical findings associated with chronic adrenal insufficiency. Risk factors include:

- *Drug history:* steroids in the past year, phenytoin, barbiturates, rifampin
- *Illness history:* infection, cancer, autoimmune disease, diseases treated with steroids, radiation to head or abdomen, human immunodeficiency virus–positive status
- *Family history:* autoimmune disease, Addison's disease
- *Nutrition:* weight loss, decreased appetite
- *Miscellaneous:* fatigue, dizziness, weakness, darkening of skin, low blood glucose that does not respond to therapy, salt craving (dramatic craving such as drinking pickle juice or eating salt from the shaker)

! LABORATORY ALERT

Adrenal Disorders

LABORATORY TEST	CRITICAL VALUE	SIGNIFICANCE
Serum		
Glucose	<50 mg/dL	Hypoglycemia
Cortisol	<10 mcg/dL	In severely ill patient or stressed patient, indicates insufficiency
Potassium	>6.6 mEq/L	Potential for heart blocks, bradydysrhythmias, sinus arrest, ventricular fibrillation, or asystole
	<3.0 mEq/L	Potential for ventricular dysrhythmias
Sodium	>150 mEq/L	May be a result of stress and dehydration
	<130 mEq/L	Due to lack of aldosterone
BUN	>20 mg/dL	↑ From protein breakdown and hemoconcentration
pH	<7.3	↓ From accumulation of acids and dehydration

BUN, Blood urea nitrogen.

Cardiovascular system. Cardiovascular signs and symptoms in adrenal crisis are related to hypovolemia (decreased water reabsorption), decreased vascular tone (decreased effectiveness of catecholamines), and hyperkalemia. The most common presentation of adrenal crisis in the intensive care unit is hypotension refractory to fluids and requiring vasopressors. The patient may also have symptoms of decreased cardiac output; weak, rapid pulse; dysrhythmias; and cold, pale skin. The chest x-ray study may show decreased heart size due to hypovolemia. Changes in the ECG may result if accompanied by significant hyperkalemia. Hypovolemia and vascular dilation may be severe enough in crisis to cause hemodynamic collapse and shock.

Neurological system. Neurological manifestations in adrenal crisis are related to decreases in glucose levels, protein metabolism, volume and perfusion, and sodium concentrations. Patients may complain of headache, fatigue that worsens as the day progresses, and severe weakness. They may also suffer from mental confusion, listlessness, lethargy, apathy, psychoses, and emotional lability.

Gastrointestinal system. The gastrointestinal signs and symptoms in adrenal crisis are related to decreased digestive enzymes, intestinal motility and digestion. Anorexia, nausea, vomiting, diarrhea, and vague abdominal pain are present in the majority of patients.[7]

Genitourinary system. Decreased circulation to the kidneys from diminished circulating volume and hypotension decreases renal perfusion and glomerular filtration rate. Urine output may decline and acute kidney injury may occur as a result.

Laboratory Evaluation

Laboratory findings in a patient with acute adrenal crisis include hypoglycemia, hyponatremia, hyperkalemia, eosinophilia, increased BUN level, and metabolic acidosis (see box, "Laboratory Alert: Adrenal Disorders"). Hypercalcemia or hyperuricemia is possible as a result of volume depletion.

The diagnosis of adrenal crisis is made by evaluating plasma cortisol levels. These levels vary diurnally in healthy individuals, but this pattern is lost in the critically ill, making the timing of the test unimportant. In crisis, plasma cortisol levels are less than 10 mg/dL. Differentiating between primary and secondary adrenal insufficiency is accomplished by evaluating serum ACTH levels. ACTH levels will be elevated in primary insufficiency and normal or decreased in secondary insufficiency.

The diagnosis of relative adrenal insufficiency is less clear. A "normal" cortisol level in a critically ill patient may actually be abnormal and indicate an inadequate response.[22] Because these tests are difficult to interpret, corticosteroid replacement should begin as soon as insufficiency is suspected. The technique for performing a cosyntropin (a synthetic ACTH) stimulation is outlined in Box 18-14. The test determines baseline levels as well as response to stimulation. A standard dose of 250 mcg cosyntropin is given, and the expected response is an increase in cortisol level of 7 to 9 mcg/dL from the baseline. A patient whose cortisol level does not increase

BOX 18-14	COSYNTROPIN STIMULATION TEST

Standard Method
- Obtain baseline serum cortisol level
- Administer cosyntropin, either 250 mcg or 1 mcg (low dose) IV
- Obtain serum cortisol level 30 and 60 minutes after cosyntropin

In emergency situations, may treat with dexamethasone (Decadron), 2 to 8 mg IV (will not interfere with cortisol levels)

Test Response
- *Expected response:* cortisol >20 mcg/dL, or increase from baseline of >9 mcg/dL
- *Primary aldosterone insufficiency:* a total level >20 mcg/dL and/or a change from baseline of >7 mcg/dL
- *Relative aldosterone insufficiency:* a change from baseline <9 mcg/dL regardless of baseline level

by this amount is deemed a nonresponder and has an increased risk of mortality.[11,19]

Nursing Diagnoses

The nursing diagnoses that may apply to a patient with adrenal crisis based on the assessment data include the following:
- Deficient fluid volume related to deficiency of aldosterone hormone (mineralocorticoid) and decreased sodium and water retention
- Ineffective tissue perfusion related to cortisol deficiency, resulting in decreased vascular tone and decreased effectiveness of catecholamines
- Disturbed thought processes related to decreased glucose levels, decreased protein metabolism, decreased perfusion, and decreased sodium levels
- Imbalanced nutrition (less than body requirements) related to cortisol deficiency and resultant decreased metabolism of protein and fats, decreased appetite, and decreased intestinal motility and digestion
- Deficient knowledge related to adrenal disorder: proper long-term corticosteroid management
- Activity intolerance related to use of endogenous protein for energy needs and loss of skeletal muscle mass as evidenced by early fatigue, weakness, and exertional dyspnea.

Nursing and Medical Interventions

Adrenal crisis requires immediate recognition and intervention if the patient is to survive. Primary objectives in the treatment of adrenal crisis include identifying and treating the precipitating cause, replacing fluid and electrolytes, replacing hormones, and educating the patient and family.

Fluid and Electrolyte Replacement

Fluid losses should be replaced with an infusion of 5% dextrose and NS until signs and symptoms of hypovolemia stabilize. This not only reverses the volume deficit but also provides glucose to minimize the hypoglycemia. The patient may need as much as 5 L of fluid in the first 12 to 24 hours to maintain an adequate blood pressure and urine output and to replace the fluid deficit.

Hyperkalemia frequently responds to volume expansion and glucocorticoid replacement and may require no further treatment. In fact, the patient may become hypokalemic during therapy and may require potassium replacement. The acidosis also usually corrects itself with volume expansion and glucocorticoid replacement. However, if the pH is less than 7.1 or the bicarbonate level is less than 10 mEq/L, the patient may require sodium bicarbonate.

Hormone Replacement

Initially, glucocorticoid replacement is the most important type of hormone replacement. If adrenal insufficiency has not been previously diagnosed and the patient's condition is unstable, dexamethasone phosphate (Decadron), 4 mg by IV push, then 4 mg every 8 hours, is given until the cosyntropin test has been done. This drug does not significantly cross-react with cortisol in the assay for cortisol and therefore can be administered to patients pending adrenal testing results.

Hydrocortisone sodium succinate (Solu-Cortef) is the drug of choice after diagnosis is confirmed by the cosyntropin test, because it has both glucocorticoid and mineralocorticoid activities in high doses. After a bolus dose, IV doses are administered for at least 24 hours or until the patient has stabilized. Cortisone acetate may be given intramuscularly if the IV route is not available.

Once the patient improves, the dose of hydrocortisone is decreased 10% to 20% daily until a maintenance dose is achieved. The patient can be switched to oral replacement once oral intake is resumed. At lower doses (less than 100 mg/day of hydrocortisone), a patient with primary adrenal insufficiency may also require mineralocorticoid replacement. Fludrocortisone, 0.05 to 0.2 mg daily is added. A nutritional consideration if the patient is experiencing excessive sweating or diarrhea is to increase sodium intake to 15 mEq/day. Table 18-5 describes the drugs used in the treatment of acute adrenal crisis.

Patient and Family Education

In a patient with known adrenal insufficiency and/or receiving corticosteroid therapy, adrenal crisis is preventable. Education of patients, family, and significant others is the key to prevention.

TABLE 18-5 PHARMACOLOGY
Medications Used to Treat Adrenal Crisis

MEDICATION	ACTION/USES	DOSAGE/ROUTE	SIDE EFFECTS	NURSING IMPLICATIONS
Hydrocortisone sodium succinate (Solu-Cortef)	Antiinflammatory and immunosuppressive effects Salt-retaining (mineralocorticoid) effects in high doses	Individualized: adrenal crisis: 100 mg IV bolus; 50-100 mg every 6-8 hours	Vertigo, headache, insomnia, menstrual abnormalities, fluid and electrolyte imbalance, hypertension, HF, peptic ulcers, nausea and vomiting, immunosuppression, impaired wound healing, increased serum glucose levels, cushingoid state	Institute prophylaxis against GI bleeding Be aware of multiple drug-drug interactions, especially with IV route: oral contraceptives, phenytoin, digoxin, phenobarbital, theophylline, insulin, anticoagulants, salicylates Avoid abrupt discontinuation Monitor serum glucose and electrolyte levels Watch for signs of fluid overload Observe for signs of infection (may be masked) Maintain adequate nutrition to avoid catabolic effects Provide meticulous mouth care
Cortisone acetate (Cortone)	Same as hydrocortisone	Individualized: adrenal crisis: 50 mg IM every 12 hours	Same as hydrocortisone	Same as for hydrocortisone
Dexamethasone (Decadron)	Has only glucocorticoid effects	Individualized doses PO, IM, IV	Same as hydrocortisone	Same as for hydrocortisone
Fludrocortisone acetate (Florinef)	Increases sodium reabsorption in renal tubules and increases potassium, water, and hydrogen loss	0.05-0.2 mg/day PO	Increased blood volume, edema, hypertension, HF, headaches, weakness of extremities	Assess for signs of fluid overload, HF Monitor serum sodium and potassium levels Use only in conjunction with glucocorticoids Restrict sodium intake if the patient has edema or fluid overload Not used to treat acute crisis; added as glucocorticoid dose is decreased

GI, Gastrointestinal; *HF,* heart failure; *IM,* intramuscular; *IV,* intravenous; *PO,* orally.

THYROID GLAND IN CRITICAL CARE
Review of Physiology

Thyroid hormones play a role in regulating the function of all body systems. Box 18-15 lists the physiological effects of thyroid hormones. The thyroid hormones thyroxine (T_4) and triiodothyronine (T_3) are secreted by the thyroid gland under the influence of the anterior pituitary gland via secretion of thyroid-stimulating hormone (TSH, also thyrotropin), which in turn is influenced by thyroid-releasing hormone (TRH, also called thyrotropin-releasing hormone) from the hypothalamus. Thyroid hormones are highly bound to globulin,

T_4-binding prealbumin, and albumin. Only the unbound (or free) fraction of the circulating hormone is biologically active. Regulation of these hormones occurs via positive and negative feedback mechanisms (Figure 18-8).

T_4 accounts for more than 95% of circulating thyroid hormones, but half of all thyroid activity comes from T_3. T_3 is five times more potent, acts more quickly, and enters cells more easily than T_4. T_3 is derived from conversion of T_4 in nonthyroid tissue. Certain conditions and drugs can block the conversion of T_4 to T_3, creating a potential thyroid imbalance. Possible causes for blocked conversion are listed in Box 18-16.

BOX 18-15 PHYSIOLOGICAL EFFECTS OF THYROID HORMONES

Major Effects
- ↑ Metabolic activities of all tissues
- ↑ Rate of nutrient use/oxygen consumption for ATP production
- ↑ Rate of growth
- ↑ Activities of other endocrine glands

Other Effects
- Regulate protein synthesis and catabolism
- Regulate body heat production and dissipation
- ↑ Gluconeogenesis and utilization of glucose
- Maintain appetite and gastrointestinal motility
- Maintain calcium metabolism
- Stimulate cholesterol synthesis
- Maintain cardiac rate, contractility, and output
- Affect respiratory rate, oxygen utilization, and carbon dioxide formation
- Affect red blood cell production
- Affect central nervous system affect and attention
- Produce muscle tone and vigor and provide normal skin constituents

BOX 18-16 FACTORS THAT BLOCK CONVERSION FROM THYROXINE TO TRIIODOTHYRONINE

- *Severe illness:* chronic renal failure, cancer, chronic liver disease
- Trauma
- Malnutrition, fasting
- *Drugs:* glucocorticoids, propranolol, propylthiouracil, amiodarone
- Radiopaque dyes
- Acidosis

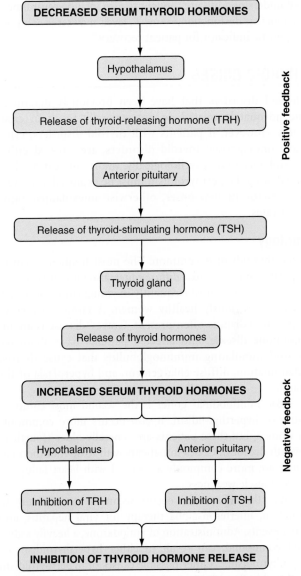

FIGURE 18-8 Feedback systems for thyroid hormone regulation.

Effects of Aging

With aging, thyroid function declines. Hypothyroidism occurs in the elderly, frequently with an insidious onset. The decrease in energy level; the feeling of being cold; the dry, flaky skin; and other signs are often mistakenly assumed to be part of aging, whereas they may be signs of decreased thyroid function. Thyroid function should be assessed in any elderly patient with a "sluggish" response to treatments.

Thyroid Function in the Critically Ill

During critical illness, stress-related changes occur in thyroid hormone balance. Initially, there is a decrease in plasma T_3 levels, known as *low T_3 syndrome* or *euthyroid sick syndrome.* These changes are thought to result from alterations in the peripheral metabolism of thyroid hormones, which may be an adaptation to severe illness in which the body attempts to reduce energy expenditure.[8] Generally, these changes are considered to be beneficial and do not require intervention. Within approximately 3 days, T_3 levels return to low-normal levels. In severe illness, T_3 levels may fail to normalize, and T_4 levels may also decrease.[19]

In the chronically critically ill, additional thyroid hormone changes occur. Both T_3 and T_4 levels are reduced as is TSH secretion. The changes in chronic critical illness are not well understood but are thought to also include central neuroendocrine dysfunction.[22] Low T_4 levels may serve as a poor prognostic indicator for patient recovery.

THYROID CRISES

Thyroid disorders that have been previously diagnosed and adequately treated do not generally result in crisis states. However, if patients with thyroid disorders, especially undiagnosed thyroid disorders, are stressed either physiologically or psychologically, the results can be life-threatening. Hyperthyroidism must be explored as a causative factor in new-onset, otherwise unexplained rapid heart rates.

Etiology

Hyperthyroidism is common. The most frequent form of hyperthyroidism is *toxic diffuse goiter,* also known as *Graves' disease.* It occurs most frequently in young (third or fourth decade), previously healthy women. A family history of hyperthyroidism is often present. Graves' disease is an autoimmune disease, and affected patients have abnormal thyroid-stimulating immunoglobulins that cause thyroid inflammation, diffuse enlargement, and hyperplasia of the gland.

Toxic multinodular goiter is the second most common cause of hyperthyroidism. It also occurs more commonly in women, but these patients are generally older (fourth to seventh decades). Crises in patients with toxic multinodular goiter are more commonly associated with heart failure or severe muscle weakness.

Hyperthyroidism also occurs secondary to exposure to radiation, interferon-alpha therapy for viral hepatitis, and other events. Administration of amiodarone, a heavily iodinated compound, can result in either hyperthyroidism or hypothyroidism.[20] Other possible causes of hyperthyroidism are listed in Box 18-17.

Low levels of thyroid hormones disrupt the normal physiology of most body systems. Hypothyroidism produces a hypodynamic, hypometabolic state. *Myxedema coma* is a magnification of these disruptions initiated by some type of stressor. This condition takes months to develop and should be suspected in patients with known hypothyroidism, with a surgical scar on the lower neck, or in those who are unusually sensitive to medications or narcotics.

The underlying causes of myxedema coma are those that produce hypothyroidism. Most cases occur either in patients with long-standing autoimmune disease of the thyroid (Hashimoto's thyroiditis) or in patients who have received surgical or radioactive iodine treatment for Graves' disease and have received inadequate hormone replacement.[23] Approximately 5% of adults have hypothyroidism as a result of a pituitary (secondary) or hypothalamic (tertiary) disorder. These and other less common causes of hypothyroidism are listed in Box 18-18.

BOX 18-17 CAUSES OF HYPERTHYROIDISM

Most Common
- Toxic diffuse goiter (Graves' disease)
- Toxic multinodular goiter
- Toxic uninodular goiter

Other Causes
- Triiodothyronine
- Exogenous iodine in patient with preexisting thyroid disease: exposure to iodine load from radiographic contrast dyes, medications (amiodarone)
- Thyroiditis (transient)
- Postpartum thyroiditis

Rare Causes
- Toxic thyroid adenoma—more common in the elderly
- Metastatic thyroid cancer
- Malignancies with circulating thyroid stimulators
- Pituitary tumors producing thyroid-stimulating hormone (thyrotropin)
- Acromegaly

Associated with Other Disorders*
- Pernicious anemia
- Idiopathic Addison's disease
- Myasthenia gravis
- Sarcoidosis
- Albright's syndrome

*The presence of these disorders in a patient in thyroid crisis increases the likelihood that the patient has underlying hyperthyroidism.

BOX 18-18 CAUSES OF HYPOTHYROIDISM

Primary Thyroid Disease
- Autoimmune (Hashimoto's thyroiditis)
- Radioactive iodine treatment of Graves' disease
- Thyroidectomy
- Congenital enzymatic defect in thyroid hormone biosynthesis
- Inhibition of thyroid hormone synthesis or release
- Antithyroid drugs
- Iodides
- Amiodarone
- Lithium carbonate
- Oral hypoglycemic agents
- Dopamine
- Idiopathic thyroid atrophy

Secondary (Pituitary) or Tertiary (Hypothalamus) Disease
- Tumors
- Infiltrative disease (sarcoidosis)
- Hypophysectomy
- Pituitary irradiation
- Head injury
- Strokes
- Pituitary infarction

Thyrotoxic Crisis (Thyroid Storm)
Pathophysiology

Thyroid storm occurs in untreated or inadequately treated patients with hyperthyroidism; it is rare in patients with normal thyroid gland function. The crisis is often precipitated by stress related to an underlying illness, general anesthesia, surgery, or infection. Thyroid hormones play a major role in regulating most body systems. Uncontrolled hyperthyroidism produces a hyperdynamic, hypermetabolic state that results in disruption of many major body functions, and without treatment, death may occur within 48 hours. The specific mechanism that produces thyroid storm is unknown but includes high levels of circulating thyroid hormones, an enhanced cellular response to those hormones, and hyperactivity of the sympathetic nervous system. Thyroid hormones normally increase the synthesis of enzymes that stimulate cellular mitochondria and energy production. When excess thyroid hormones are present, the increased activity of these enzymes produces excessive thermal energy and fever. It is believed that the rapidity with which hormone levels rise may be more important than the absolute levels.

Assessment

Clinical presentation. The excess thyroid hormone activity of hyperthyroidism affects the body in many ways. Box 18-19 gives signs associated with progressive hyperthyroidism. Common findings in patients with thyroid storm, their significance, and the actions nurses can take to address each of these findings are listed in Table 18-6.

BOX 18-19   PROGRESSIVE SIGNS OF HYPERTHYROIDISM

- *Cardiovascular:* Increased heart rate and palpitations. Hyperthyroidism may present as sinus tachycardia in a sleeping patient or as atrial fibrillation with a rapid ventricular response.
- *Neurological:* Increased irritability, hyperactivity, decreased attention span, and nervousness. In an elderly patient, these signs may be masked, and depression or apathy may be present.
- *Temperature intolerance:* Increased cold tolerance; heat intolerance; fever; excessive sweating; and warm, moist skin. Older patients may naturally lose their ability to shiver and may be less comfortable in the cold.
- *Respiratory:* Increased respiratory rate, weakened thoracic muscles, and decreased vital capacity are evident.
- *Gastrointestinal:* Increased appetite, decreased absorption (especially of vitamins), weight loss, and increased stools. Diarrhea is not common. Elderly patients may be constipated.
- *Musculoskeletal:* Fine tremors of tongue or eyelids, peripheral tremors with activity, and muscle wasting are noted.
- *Integumentary:* Thin, fine, and fragile hair; soft friable nails; and petechiae. Young women generally have the more classic findings. Young men may notice an increase in acne and sweating. An elderly patient with dry, atrophic skin may not have significant skin changes.
- *Hematopoietic:* Normochromic, normocytic anemia and leukocytosis may occur.
- *Ophthalmic:* Pathological features result from edema and inflammation. Physical findings may include upper lid retraction, lid lag, extraocular muscle palsies, and sight loss. Exophthalmos is found almost exclusively in Graves' disease.

TABLE 18-6   THYROID CRISES

CLINICAL CONCERNS	SIGNIFICANCE	NURSING ACTIONS
Thyroid Storm Alterations in level of consciousness	Symptoms can be confused with other disorders (e.g., paranoia, psychosis, depression), especially in the elderly	Provide a safe environment. Assess for orientation, agitation, inattention. Control environmental influences. Implement seizure precautions.
↑ Cardiac workload due to hypermetabolic state; ↓ cardiac output	Can lead to heart failure and collapse	Assess for chest pain, palpitations. Monitor for cardiac dysrhythmias (e.g., atrial fibrillation or flutter) and tachycardia. Monitor blood pressure for widening pulse pressure. Auscultate for the development of S$_3$. Monitor hemodynamic status: SVO2, SI, PAOP, RAP. Assess urine output. Evaluate response to therapy.
↑ Oxygen demand due to hypermetabolic state; ineffective breathing pattern	↑ Respiratory rate and drive can lead to fatigue and hypoventilation	Provide supplemental oxygen or mechanical ventilation as needed. Monitor respiratory rate and effort. Monitor oxygen saturation via pulse oximeter. Minimize activity.

Continued

TABLE 18-6 THYROID CRISES—cont'd

CLINICAL CONCERNS	SIGNIFICANCE	NURSING ACTIONS
Loss of ability to regulate with temperature	Inability to respond to fever exacerbates hypermetabolic demands	Monitor temperature and treat with acetaminophen and/or a cooling blanket as needed.
Myxedema Coma ↓ Cardiac function	Hypotension and potential to develop pericardial effusion	Perform ECG monitoring (look for ↓ voltage in the QRS complexes, indicating effusion). Auscultate for diminished heart sounds. Monitor blood pressure for signs of hypotension.
Muscle weakness, hypoventilation, pleural effusion; ineffective breathing	Potential for respiratory acidosis and hypoxemia	Auscultate the lungs frequently. Monitor respiratory effort (rate and depth) and pattern. Maintain I&O (probable need for fluid restriction). Monitor ABGs/pulse oximetry and CBC (for anemia). Position for optimum respiratory effort.
Alteration in level of consciousness	Ranges from difficulty concentrating to coma Seizures can occur	Assess and maintain patient safety.
Loss of ability to regulate temperature	Inability to respond to cold	Monitor temperature Control room temperature, provide rewarming measures.

ABGs, Arterial blood gases; *CBC,* complete blood count; *I&O,* intake and output; *PAOP,* pulmonary artery occlusion pressure; *RAP,* right atrial pressure; *SI,* stroke index; *SVO2,* mixes venous oxygen consumption.

Thyroid storm has an abrupt onset. The most prominent clinical features of thyroid storm are severe fever, marked tachycardia, heart failure, tremors, delirium, stupor, and coma.

The patient's ability to survive thyroid storm is determined by the severity of the hyperthyroid state and the patient's general health. The severity of the hyperthyroid state is not necessarily indicated by the serum levels of thyroid hormones but rather by tissue and organ responsiveness to the hormones.

Thermoregulation disturbances. Temperature regulation is lost. The patient's body temperature may be as high as 106° F (41.1° C). The increase in heat production and metabolic end products also causes the blood vessels of the skin to dilate. This enhances oxygen and nutrient delivery to the peripheral tissues and accounts for the patient's warm, moist skin.

Neurological disturbances. Thyroid hormones normally maintain alertness and attention. Excess thyroid hormones cause hypermetabolism and hyperactivity of the nervous system causing agitation, delirium, psychosis, tremulousness, seizures, and coma.

Cardiovascular disturbances. Thyroid hormones play a role in maintaining cardiac rate, force of contraction, and cardiac output. The increase in metabolism and the stimulation of catecholamines produced by thyroid hormones cause a hyperdynamic heart. Contractility, heart rate, and cardiac output increase as peripheral vascular resistance decreases. These effects are magnified by the body's increased demand for oxygen and nutrients. In thyroid storm, the increased demands on the heart produce high-output heart failure and cardiovascular collapse if the crisis is not recognized and treated.

Patients experience palpitations, tachycardia (out of proportion to the fever), and a widened pulse pressure. Atrial fibrillation is common. A prominent third heart sound may be heard as well as a systolic murmur over the pulmonic area, the aortic area, or both. Occasionally, a pericardial rub may be heard. In the absence of atrial fibrillation, frequent premature atrial contractions or atrial flutter may be present. In an elderly patient with underlying heart disease, worsening of angina or severe heart failure may herald thyroid storm.

Pulmonary disturbances. Thyroid hormones affect respiratory rate and depth, oxygen utilization, and CO_2 formation. Tissues need more oxygen as a result of hypermetabolism. This increased need for oxygen stimulates the respiratory drive and increases respiratory rate. However, increased protein catabolism reduces protein in respiratory muscles (diaphragm and intercostals). As a result, even with an increased respiratory rate, muscle weakness may prevent the patient from meeting the oxygen demand and may cause hypoventilation, CO_2 retention, and respiratory failure.

Gastrointestinal disturbances. Excess thyroid hormones increase metabolism and accelerate protein and fat degradation.

Thyroid hormones also increase gastrointestinal motility, which may result in abdominal pain, nausea, and jaundice. Vomiting, and diarrhea can occur, contributing to volume depletion during thyrotoxic crises.

Musculoskeletal disturbances. Muscle weakness and fatigue result from increased protein catabolism. Skeletal muscle changes are manifested as tremors. Thoracic muscles are weak, causing dyspnea. In thyrotoxic crises, patients are placed on bed rest to reduce metabolic demand.

Laboratory evaluation. The determination of thyroid storm is a clinical diagnosis. Thyroid hormone levels are elevated; however, these levels are generally no higher than those normally found in uncomplicated hyperthyroidism. In any event, the patient must be treated before these results are available. See "Laboratory Alert: Thyroid Disorders" for possible laboratory abnormalities that may occur in thyroid storm.

Nursing Diagnoses

The nursing diagnoses that may apply to a patient with thyroid storm are based on assessment data and include the following:

- Hyperthermia related to loss of temperature regulation, increased metabolism, increased heat production
- Disturbed thought processes related to hypermetabolism and increased cerebration, agitation, delirium, psychosis
- Decreased cardiac output related to increased metabolic demands on the heart, extreme tachycardia, dysrhythmias, congestive heart failure
- Ineffective breathing pattern related to muscle weakness and decreased vital capacity resulting in hypoventilation and CO_2 retention, increased oxygen need from hypermetabolism

---

⚠ LABORATORY ALERT

Thyroid Disorders

LABORATORY TEST	CRITICAL VALUE	SIGNIFICANCE
Thyroid Storm		
T_3, free (triiodothyronine)	>0.52 ng/dL	Hyperthyroidism
T_3, resin uptake	>35% of total	
T_4 (thyroxine)	>12 mcg/dL	
TSH	<0.01 milliunits/L	
Glucose	≥200 mg/dL (2 hours postprandial or random); >140 mg/dL (fasting)	↑Insulin degradation
Sodium	>150 mEq/L	May be a result of stress, dehydration, and/or hypermetabolic state
BUN	>20 mg/dL	↑Due to protein breakdown and hemoconcentration
CBC	↓ RBCs ↑WBCs	Normocytic, normochromic anemia
Calcium	>10.2 mg/dL	Excess bone resorption
Myxedema Coma		
T_3, free	<0.2 mg/dL	Hypothyroidism
T_3, resin uptake	<25% of total	
T_4	<5 mcg/dL	
TSH	>25 milliunits/L	
Sodium	<130 mEq/L	Dilutional from increased total body water
Glucose	<50 mg/dL	Hypoglycemia due to hypermetabolic state
CBC	↓ RBCs	Anemia due to vitamin B_{12} deficiency, inadequate folate or iron absorption
Platelets	<150,000 cells/microliter	Risk for bleeding
pH	<7.35	Respiratory acidosis from hypoventilation

BUN, Blood urea nitrogen; *CBC,* complete blood count; *RBCs,* red blood cells; *TSH,* thyroid-stimulating hormone (thyrotropin); *WBCs,* white blood cells.

- Imbalanced nutrition: less than body requirements related to increased requirement, increased peristalsis, decreased absorption
- Activity intolerance related to muscle weakness, tremors, anemia, fatigue, and extreme energy expenditure
- Deficient knowledge related to thyroid disorder: disease process, therapeutic regimen, prevention of complications

Nursing and Medical Interventions

Thyroid storm requires immediate intervention if the patient is to survive. The primary objectives in the treatment of thyroid storm are antagonizing the peripheral effects of thyroid hormone, inhibiting thyroid hormone biosynthesis, blocking thyroid hormone release, providing supportive care, identifying and treating the precipitating cause, and providing patient and family education. Box 18-20 details the treatment of thyroid storm.

Antagonism of peripheral effects of thyroid hormones. Because it may take days or longer to impact circulating thyroid hormones, immediate action is necessary to minimize the systemic effects of thyroid storm. The mortality rate of thyroid storm has been significantly reduced with the introduction of beta-blockers to inhibit the effects of thyroid hormones. The drug used most frequently is propranolol (Inderal). Other beta-blockers such as esmolol hydrochloride (Brevibloc) or atenolol (Tenormin) may also be used. Results are seen within minutes using the IV route and within 1 hour after the oral route. IV effects last 3 to 4 hours. In addition, high-dose glucocorticoids are administered to block the conversion of T_4 to T_3 and thereby decreasing the effects of thyroid hormone on peripheral tissues.

Inhibition of thyroid hormone biosynthesis. Two drugs may be administered to inhibit thyroid hormone biosynthesis: propylthiouracil and methimazole (Tapazole). Neither of these drugs is available in IV form. In high doses, propylthiouracil inhibits conversion of T_4 to T_3 in peripheral tissues and results in a more rapid reduction of circulating thyroid hormone levels. Methimazole may be used because of its longer half-life and higher potency.

The disadvantage to both propylthiouracil and methimazole is that they lack immediate effect. They do not block the release of thyroid hormones already stored in the thyroid gland and may take weeks to months to lower thyroid hormone levels to normal.

Blockage of thyroid hormone release. Iodide agents inhibit the release of thyroid hormones from the thyroid gland, inhibit thyroid hormone production, and decrease the vascularity and size of the thyroid gland. Serum T_4 levels decrease approximately 30% to 50% with any of these drugs, with stabilization in 3 to 6 days.

Saturated solution of potassium iodide (SSKI) or Lugol's solution may be given orally or sublingually. These drugs must be administered 1 to 2 hours after antithyroid drugs (propylthiouracil or methimazole) to prevent the iodide from being used to synthesize more T_4. Ipodate (Oragrafin) and iopanoic acid (Telepaque) are radiographic contrast

media that may be used to block thyroid hormone release. Lithium carbonate inhibits the release of thyroid hormones but is more toxic, so it is used only in patients with an iodide allergy. Lithium carbonate is given orally or by nasogastric tube and the dose is adjusted to maintain therapeutic serum levels.

Supportive care. Symptoms are aggressively treated. Acetaminophen is used as an antipyretic. Cooling blankets and ice packs may be used. Cardiac complications are treated with pharmacotherapy. Oxygen is administered to support the respiratory effort. The large fluid losses are replaced. Hemodynamic monitoring may be required. Nutritional support is provided. Precipitating factors are identified and treated and/or removed.

BOX 18-20   TREATMENT OF THYROID STORM

Antagonize Peripheral Effects of Thyroid Hormone
- Propranolol (Inderal): 1 to 2 IV boluses every 10 to 15 minutes up to 15 to 20 mg IV, or 640 mg maximum daily PO; individualized to response
- If beta-blocker contraindicated, give reserpine 0.1 to 0.25 mg PO or guanethidine 25 to 50 mg PO every 6 to 8 hours

Inhibit Hormone Biosynthesis
- Propylthiouracil: PO loading dose of 400 mg, then 200 mg, then every 4 hours until thyrotoxicosis controlled, or
- Methimazole (Tapazole): 60 mg PO loading dose; 20 mg PO every 4 hours

Block Thyroid Hormone Release
Give 1-2 Hours after Propylthiouracil or Methimazole Loading Dose
- Saturated solution of potassium iodide: 5 drops every 6 hours, mixed in 240 mL of water, juice, milk, or broth, or
- Potassium iodide tablets: 250 mg PO three times per day

Secondary Options
- Iopanoic acid: 1 g every 8 hours for 24 hours, 0.5 g PO twice daily
- Ipodate (Oragrafin): 500 to 1000 mg PO daily
- Lithium carbonate: 300 mg PO or NG every 6 hours

Supportive Therapy
- Hydrocortisone: 100 mg IV every 8 hours; or dexamethasone: 0.5 mg PO every 6 hours
- Pharmacotherapy for heart failure or tachydysrhythmia
- Correct fluid and electrolyte imbalance
- Treat hyperthermia (avoid aspirin)
- High-calorie, high-protein diet

Identify and Treat Precipitating Cause

Patient and Family Education

Doses are approximate and may vary based on the individual situation.
IV, Intravenous; *NG,* nasogastric (tube); *PO,* orally.

Patient and family education. Education of patients, families, and significant others is crucial in identifying and preventing episodes of thyroid storm. Teaching varies depending on the long-term therapy chosen for each patient (e.g., drugs versus radioactive iodine or surgery).

Patient Outcomes

Outcomes for a patient with thyroid storm include the following:

- Temperature within normal range
- Return to baseline mentation and personality
- Stable hemodynamics within normal limits
- Effective breathing pattern
- Nutritional needs met and weight maintained
- Return to baseline activity level
- Verbalization by the patient and significant others of an understanding of the patient's illness, anticipated treatment, and potential complications

Myxedema Coma
Pathophysiology

Myxedema coma is the most extreme form of hypothyroidism and is life-threatening. Myxedema coma in the absence of an associated stress or illness is uncommon, with infection being the most frequent stressor. The addition of stress to an already hypothyroid patient accelerates the metabolism and clearance of whatever thyroid hormone is present in the body. Thus the patient experiences increased hormone utilization but decreased hormone production, which precipitates a crisis state. Common findings in patients with thyroid storm are presented with those of myxedema coma in Table 18-6.

Etiology

Myxedema coma is the end stage of improperly treated, neglected, or undiagnosed hypothyroidism. It is a life-threatening emergency with a mortality rate as high as 50% despite appropriate therapy. Much of this mortality can be attributed to underlying illnesses. Most patients who develop myxedema coma are elderly women; it is rarely seen in young persons. It occurs more frequently in winter as a result of the increased stress of exposure to cold in a person unable to maintain body heat. Known precipitating factors include hypothermia, infection, stroke, trauma, and critical illness. Medications that may precipitate myxedema coma include those that affect the central nervous system, such as analgesics, anesthesia, barbiturates, narcotics, sedatives, tranquilizers, lithium, and amiodarone.

Assessment

Clinical presentation. Many patients may have had vague signs and symptoms of hypothyroidism for several years (Box 18-21). Many of the manifestations are attributable to the development of mucinous edema. This interstitial edema is the result of water retention and decreased protein. Fluid collects in soft tissue such as the face and in joints and muscles. It can also produce pericardial effusion. The clinical picture

---

BOX 18-21   PROGRESSIVE SIGNS OF HYPOTHYROIDISM

- *Earliest signs:* Fatigue, weakness, muscle cramps, intolerance to cold, and weight gain.
- *Cardiovascular:* Bradycardia and hypotension.
- *Neurological:* Difficulty concentrating, slowed mentation, depression, lethargy, slow and deliberate speech, coarse and raspy voice, hearing loss, and vertigo.
- *Respiratory:* Dyspnea on exertion.
- *Gastrointestinal:* Decreased appetite, decreased peristalsis, anorexia, decreased bowel sounds, constipation, and paralytic ileus. However, the decreased metabolic rate also leads to weight gain.
- *Musculoskeletal:* Fluid in joints and muscles results in stiffness and muscle cramps.
- *Integumentary:* Dry, flaky, cool, coarse skin; dry, coarse hair; and brittle nails. The face is puffy and pallid, the tongue may be enlarged. The dorsa of the hands and feet are edematous. There may be a yellow tint to the skin from depressed hepatic conversion of carotene to vitamin A. Ecchymoses may develop from increased capillary fragility and decreased platelets.
- *Hematological:* Pernicious anemia and jaundice. Splenomegaly occurs in about 50% of patients. About 10% of patients have a decrease in neutrophils.
- *Ophthalmic:* Generalized mucinous edema in the eyelids and periorbital tissue.
- *Metabolic:* Elevated creatine phosphokinase, aspartate aminotransferase, lactate dehydrogenase, cholesterol, and triglyceride levels. Elevated cholesterol and triglyceride levels predispose persons with hypothyroidism to the development of atherosclerosis

---

of myxedema coma varies with the rate of onset and severity. Diagnosis is based on the clinical signs and symptoms, a high index of suspicion, and a careful history and physical examination.

Cardiovascular disturbances. Cardiac function is depressed, resulting in decreases from baseline in heart rate, blood pressure, contractility, stroke volume, and cardiac output. The patient may develop a pericardial effusion, making heart tones distant. The ECG has decreased voltage because of the pericardial effusion.

Pulmonary disturbances. Respiratory system responsiveness is depressed, producing hypoventilation, respiratory muscle weakness, and CO_2 retention. CO_2 narcosis may contribute to decreased mentation. As part of the picture of generalized mucinous edema and fluid retention, these patients may also develop pleural effusions or upper airway edema, further restricting their breathing.

Neurological disturbances. The low metabolic rate and resulting decreased mentation produce both psychological and physiological changes. The patient in hypothyroid crisis may present with somnolence, delirium, seizures, or coma. Personality changes such as paranoia and delusions may be evident.

Patients with hypothyroidism are unable to maintain body heat because of the decreased metabolic rate and decreased production of thermal energy. Because of this, patients may present in crisis after being stressed by exposure to cold. Hypothermia is present in 80% of patients in myxedema coma, with temperatures as low as 80° F (26.7° C). Patients with temperatures less than 88.6° F (32° C) have a grave prognosis. If a patient with myxedema coma has a temperature greater than 98.6° F (37° C), underlying infection should be suspected.

Skeletal muscle disturbances. Slowed motor conduction produces decreased tendon reflexes and sluggish, awkward movements.

Laboratory evaluation. Serum T_4 and T_3 levels and resin T_3 uptake are low in patients with myxedema coma. In primary hypothyroidism, TSH levels are high. If hypothyroidism is the result of disease of the pituitary gland or hypothalamus (secondary and tertiary hypothyroidism), TSH levels are inappropriately normal or low. As in patients with thyroid storm, if myxedema coma is suspected, treatment should not be delayed while awaiting these results to confirm the diagnosis.

Serum sodium levels may be low as a result of impaired water excretion from inappropriate ADH secretion and cortisol deficiency that frequently accompany hypothyroidism. The patient should be monitored for signs and symptoms related to hyponatremia such as weakness, muscle twitching, seizures, and coma.

Hypoglycemia is common and may be related to pituitary or hypophyseal disorders and/or adrenal insufficiency. Adrenal insufficiency may result in serum cortisol levels that are inappropriately low for stress. Laboratory manifestations of myxedema coma are summarized in "Laboratory Alert: Thyroid Disorders."

Nursing Diagnoses

The nursing diagnoses that apply to a patient in myxedema coma are based on assessment data and include the following:

- Decreased cardiac output related to decreased contractility, decreased heart rate, decreased stroke volume, pericardial effusion, dysrhythmias
- Ineffective breathing pattern related to hypoventilation, muscle weakness, decreased respiratory rate, ascites, pleural effusions
- Disturbed thought processes related to slowed metabolism and cerebration, hyponatremia
- Hypothermia related to inability of body to retain heat
- Excess fluid volume related to impaired water excretion
- Risk for injury related to edema, decreased platelet count
- Activity intolerance related to muscle weakness
- Imbalanced nutrition: less than body requirements related to decreased appetite, decreased carbohydrate metabolism, hypoglycemia
- Deficient knowledge related to myxedema coma: disease process, therapeutic regimen, and prevention of complications

---

BOX 18-22   TREATMENT OF MYXEDEMA COMA

- Identification and treatment of underlying disorder
- *Thyroid replacement:* levothyroxine sodium, 200 to 500 mcg IV loading dose, then 50 mcg/day IV; or liothyronine sodium, 25 mcg IV every 8 hours for 24 to 48 hours, then 12.5 mcg every 8 hours
- Restoration of fluid and electrolyte balance
- Cautious administration of vasopressors
- *Hyponatremia:* <115 mEq/L, hypertonic saline; <120 mEq/L, fluid restriction
- *Hypoglycemia:* IV glucose
- Supportive care
- Passive warming with blankets (do not actively warm)
- Ventilatory assistance
- Avoidance of narcotics and sedative drugs
- Adrenal hormone replacement: hydrocortisone, 100 mg IV bolus, then 50 to 100 mg every 6 to 8 hours for 7 to 10 days, then wean to maintenance dose over 3 to 7 days
- Chest x-ray or ultrasound study of the chest possibly needed to assess pleural effusion
- Echocardiogram possibly needed to assess cardiac function and/or pericardial effusion
- Patient and family education

Doses are approximate and may vary based on the individual situation.
IV, Intravenous.

Nursing and Medical Interventions

Myxedema coma requires immediate intervention if the patient is to survive. The primary objectives in the treatment of myxedema coma are identifying and treating the precipitating cause, providing thyroid replacement, restoring fluid and electrolyte balance, providing supportive care, and providing patient and family education. Box 18-22 details the treatment of myxedema coma. It is important to achieve physiological levels of thyroid hormone without incurring the adverse effects of excess thyroid hormones.

Thyroid replacement. The best method of thyroid replacement is controversial. Either levothyroxine sodium (Synthroid; T_4) or liothyronine sodium (Cytomel; T_3) can be used. Levothyroxine ultimately provides the patient with both T_4 and, through peripheral conversion, T_3 replacement; whereas liothyronine sodium provides only T_3.

Levothyroxine sodium is a commonly used for treatment. It has a smoother onset and a longer duration. The preferred route is IV because absorption of oral or intramuscular levothyroxine is variable. The initial dose may be decreased if the patient has underlying factors such as angina, dysrhythmias, or other heart disease.

Liothyronine sodium has more pronounced metabolic effects, a more rapid onset (6 hours), and a shorter half-life (1 day) than levothyroxine. Because of liothyronine's potency, its administration may be complicated by angina, myocardial infarction, and cardiac irritability. Thus it is generally avoided in older populations.

The effects of levothyroxine are not as rapid as those of liothyronine, but its cardiac toxicity is lower. Serum levels of T_4 reach normal in 1 to 2 days. Levels of TSH begin to fall within 24 hours and return to normal in 10 to 14 days.

Fluid and electrolyte restoration. If the patient is hypotensive or in shock, thyroid replacement usually corrects this, but cautious volume expansion with saline also helps. Vasopressors are used with extreme caution because patients in myxedema coma are unable to respond to vasopressors until they have adequate levels of thyroid hormones available. Simultaneous administration of vasopressors and thyroid hormones is associated with myocardial irritability.

Hyponatremia usually responds to thyroid replacement and water restriction; the patient can resume water intake once thyroid hormones are replaced. If hyponatremia is severe (less than mEq/L) or the patient is having seizures, hypertonic saline with or without a loop diuretic may be administered, but only until symptoms disappear or the sodium level is at least 120 mEq/L.

If a patient has hypoglycemia, adrenal insufficiency, or both, glucose is added to IV fluids. Glucocorticoid administration is recommended for all patients in the event that hypoadrenalism coexists with hypothyroidism. Hydrocortisone, 100 mg, is given initially, followed by 50 to 100 mg every 6 to 8 hours for 7 to 10 days. The adrenal abnormality may last several weeks after thyroid replacement is begun, so this support is continued during that period.

Supportive care. Symptoms are aggressively treated. Hypothermia is treated by keeping the room warm and using passive rewarming methods. Drugs that depress respirations, such as narcotics, are avoided. Mechanical ventilation is frequently required. Cardiac function is assessed and treated.

Patient and family education. The education of patients, family, and significant others is critical in identifying and preventing episodes of myxedema coma.

Patient Outcomes

Outcomes for a patient with myxedema coma include the following:

- Stable hemodynamics within normal limits
- Effective breathing pattern
- Return to baseline mentation and personality
- Maintenance of temperature within normal range
- Normal fluid volume balance and absence of edema
- Intact skin without edema or bleeding
- Return to baseline activity level
- Adequate nutrition and stable body weight
- Verbalization by the patient and significant others of an understanding of the disease, therapeutic regimen, and prevention of complications

ANTIDIURETIC HORMONE DISORDERS

Review of Physiology

The primary function of ADH is regulation of water balance and serum osmolality. ADH (also known as arginine vasopressin [AVP]) is produced in the supraoptic nuclei and paraventricular nuclei of the hypothalamus. These nuclei are positioned near the thirst center and osmoreceptors in the hypothalamus (Figure 18-9). Once produced, ADH is stored in neurons in the posterior pituitary. Stimulation of the supraoptic and paraventricular nuclei causes release of ADH from nerve endings in the posterior pituitary. Nuclei are stimulated in several ways (Figure 18-10). Osmoreceptors in the hypothalamus respond to changes in extracellular osmolality. Stretch receptors in the left atrium and baroreceptors in the carotid sinus and aortic arch respond to changes in circulating volume and blood pressure and stimulate the hypothalamus. Primary triggers for ADH release are increased serum osmolality decreased blood volume (by more than 10%), or decreased blood pressure (5% to 10% drop). Other factors that stimulate ADH release are elevated serum sodium levels, trauma, hypoxia, pain, stress, and anxiety. Certain drugs such as narcotics, barbiturates, anesthetics, and chemotherapeutic agents also stimulate ADH release (see Figure 18-10).

Once released, ADH acts on the renal distal and collecting tubules to cause water reabsorption. In high concentrations, ADH also acts on smooth muscles of the arterioles to produce vasoconstriction.

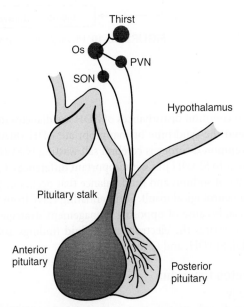

FIGURE 18-9 Hypothalamic–posterior pituitary system. *Os,* Osmoreceptor; *PVN,* Paraventricular nuclei; *SON,* Supraoptic nuclei.

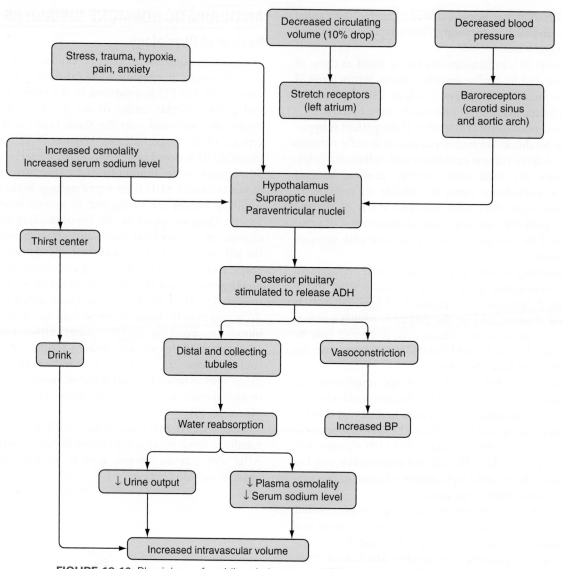

FIGURE 18-10 Physiology of antidiuretic hormone (ADH) release. *BP,* Blood pressure.

Two common disturbances of ADH are diabetes insipidus (DI) and the syndrome of inappropriate ADH (SIADH). A less common disorder is cerebral salt wasting (CSW), which is similar to SIADH but with important differences. CSW is a disorder of sodium and fluid balance that occurs in patients with a neurological insult. Differentiating CSW from SIADH is crucial because of opposing management strategies. Table 18-7 compares the electrolyte and fluid findings associated with DI, SIADH, and CSW.[21,28]

Diabetes Insipidus
Etiology
Various disorders produce neurogenic DI (Box 18-23), but the primary cause is traumatic injury to the posterior pituitary or hypothalamus as a result of head injury or surgery. Transient DI may caused by trauma to the pituitary, manipulation of the

pituitary stalk during surgery, or cerebral edema. Permanent DI occurs when more than 80% to 85% of hypothalamic nuclei or the proximal pituitary stalk is destroyed.

Nephrogenic DI may occur in genetically predisposed persons. It also may be acquired from chronic renal disease, drugs, or other conditions that produce permanent kidney damage or inhibit the generation of cyclic adenosine monophosphate in the tubules.

Pathophysiology
DI results from an ADH deficiency *(neurogenic or central DI),* ADH insensitivity *(nephrogenic DI),* or excessive water intake *(secondary DI).* Regardless of the cause, the effect is impaired renal conservation of water resulting in polyuria (more than 3 L in 24 hours). As long as the thirst center remains intact and the person is able to respond to this thirst,

TABLE 18-7 ELECTROLYTE AND FLUID FINDINGS IN ADH DISORDERS

FINDING	DIABETES INSIPIDUS	SYNDROME OF INAPPROPRIATE ADH	CEREBRAL SALT WASTING
Plasma volume	Decreased	Increased	Decreased
Serum sodium	Increased	Decreased	Decreased
Serum osmolality	Increased	Decreased	Normal or increased
Urine sodium	Normal	Increased	Increased
Urine osmolality	Decreased	Increased	Normal or increased

ADH, Antidiuretic hormone.

BOX 18-23 CAUSES OF DIABETES INSIPIDUS

Antidiuretic Hormone Deficiency (Neurogenic Diabetes Insipidus)
- *Idiopathic:* familial, congenital, autoimmune, genetic
- Intracranial surgery, especially in region of pituitary
- *Tumors:* craniopharyngioma, pituitary tumors, metastases to hypothalamus
- *Infections:* meningitis, encephalitis, syphilis, mycoses, toxoplasmosis
- *Granulomatous disease:* tuberculosis, sarcoidosis, histiocytosis
- Severe head trauma, anoxic encephalopathy, or any disorder that causes increased intracranial pressure

Antidiuretic Hormone Insensitivity (Nephrogenic Diabetes Insipidus)
- Hereditary; idiopathic
- *Renal disease:* pyelonephritis, amyloidosis, polycystic kidney disease, obstructive uropathy, transplantation
- *Multisystem disorders affecting kidneys:* multiple myeloma, sickle cell disease, cystic fibrosis
- *Metabolic disturbances:* chronic hypokalemia or hypercalcemia
- *Drugs:* ethanol, phenytoin, lithium carbonate, demeclocycline, amphotericin, methoxyflurane

Secondary Diabetes Insipidus
- Idiopathic
- Psychogenic polydipsia
- Hypothalamic disease: sarcoidosis
- Excessive intravenous fluid administration
- *Drug-induced disease:* anticholinergics, tricyclic antidepressants

fluid volume can be maintained. If the patient is unable to respond, severe dehydration results if fluid losses are not replaced.

Neurogenic DI occurs because of disruption of the neural pathways or structures involved in ADH production, synthesis, or release. Absent or diminished release of ADH from the posterior pituitary produces free water loss and causes serum osmolality and serum sodium to rise. The posterior pituitary is unable to respond by increasing ADH levels; thus the kidneys are not stimulated to reabsorb water, and excessive water loss results.

In nephrogenic DI, the kidney collecting ducts and distal tubules are unresponsive to ADH; thus adequate levels of ADH may be synthesized and released, but the kidneys are unable to conserve water in response to ADH. In patients with secondary DI, compulsive volume consumption causes polyuria.

Assessment

Clinical presentation. Neurogenic DI usually occurs suddenly with an abrupt onset of polyuria, as much as 5 to 40 L in 24 hours. The onset of nephrogenic DI is more gradual. In both types, the urine is pale and dilute. The thirst mechanism is activated in conscious patients, and polydipsia occurs. If the patient is unable to replace the water lost by responding to thirst, signs of hypovolemia develop: hypotension, decreased skin turgor, dry mucous membranes, tachycardia, weight loss, and low right atrial and pulmonary artery occlusion pressures. Neurological signs and symptoms are seen with hypovolemia and hypernatremia.

Laboratory evaluation. The classic signs of DI are an inappropriately low urine osmolality, decreased urine specific gravity, and a high serum osmolality. Corresponding with the low urine osmolality is a decreased urine specific gravity. Serum osmolality is greater than 295 mOsm/kg, and the serum sodium level is greater than 145 mEq/L. The presence of hypokalemia or hypercalcemia suggests nephrogenic DI. Other values such as BUN may be elevated as a result of hemoconcentration. Further testing to differentiate neurogenic and nephrogenic DI includes water deprivation studies. However, these tests are inappropriate in the critically ill population (see box, "Laboratory Alert: Pituitary Disorders").

! LABORATORY ALERT

Pituitary Disorders

LABORATORY TEST	CRITICAL VALUE	EXPLANATION
Diabetes Insipidus		
Sodium (serum)	>145 mEq/L	Free water loss due to absent or diminished release of ADH or lack of response by the kidneys results in hemoconcentration of sodium
Osmolality (serum)	>295 mOsm/kg	Free water loss due to absent or diminished release of ADH or lack of response by the kidneys increases serum osmolality; will be normal in secondary DI
Osmolality (urine)	<100 mOsm/kg	Free water loss into urine decreases urine osmolality
Sodium (urine)	40-200 mEq/L	Urine sodium is not affected
Syndrome of Inappropriate Antidiuretic Hormone		
Sodium (serum)	<135 mEq/L	Free water retention due to oversecretion of ADH dilutes sodium
Osmolality (serum)	<280 mOsm/kg	Free water retention due to oversecretion of ADH decreases osmolality
Osmolality (urine)	>100 mOsm/kg	Lack of water excretion increases urine osmolality
Sodium (urine)	>200 mEq/L	Sodium excretion in an attempt to excrete excess water
Cerebral Salt Wasting		
Sodium (serum)	<135 mEq/L	Inability of kidneys to conserve sodium
Osmolality (serum)	>295 mOsm/kg	Inability of kidneys to conserve water
Osmolality (urine)	<100 mOsm/kg	Free water loss into urine decreases urine osmolality
Sodium (urine)	>200 mEq/L	Sodium wasting through renal tubules

ADH, Antidiuretic hormone, *HF,* heart failure.

Nursing Diagnoses

The nursing diagnoses that may apply to a patient with DI include the following:

- Deficient fluid volume related to deficient ADH, renal cells insensitive to ADH, polyuria, and inability to respond to thirst
- Disturbed thought processes related to decreased cerebral perfusion, cerebral dehydration, and hypernatremia

Nursing and Medical Interventions

The primary goals of treatment are to identify and correct the underlying cause and to restore normal fluid volume, osmolality, and electrolyte balance. Identifying the underlying cause is a necessary part of determining appropriate treatment, particularly drug therapy.

Volume replacement. Monitoring for signs and symptoms of hypovolemia is a priority. Vital signs must be recorded at least every hour, along with urine output. Hemodynamic monitoring may be instituted to evaluate fluid requirements and to monitor the patient's response to treatment. This is particularly important in elderly patients who are likely to have concurrent cardiovascular and renal disease. Accurate intake and output and daily weights are essential. Measurement of plasma sodium and volume status assists in evaluating the patient's response to treatment.

Patients who are alert and able to respond to thirst generally drink enough water to avoid symptomatic hypovolemia. However, critically ill patients who develop DI and elderly patients with cognitive impairments are frequently unable to recognize or respond to thirst, so fluid replacement is essential.

If the patient has symptoms of hypovolemia, the volume already lost must be replaced. In addition, fluid is replaced every hour to keep up with current urine losses. Correction of hypernatremia and replacement of free water are achieved by using hypotonic solutions of dextrose in water. If the patient has circulatory failure, isotonic saline may be administered until hemodynamic stability and vascular volume have been restored.

Frequent monitoring of the patient's neurological status is also critical because changes may indicate a change in fluid status, electrolyte status (e.g., sodium), or both. It is important to avoid fluid overload from overaggressive fluid replacement, particularly once hormone replacement therapy has been instituted.

Hormone replacement. Because of the decreased secretion of ADH, neurogenic DI is controlled primarily with exogenous ADH preparations. These drugs replace ADH and enable the kidneys to conserve water. They can be administered intravenously, intramuscularly, subcutaneously, intranasally, or orally. Injectable forms are generally more potent than the intranasal or oral routes. Absorption is more reliable through the IV route.

The drug most commonly used for management is desmopressin (DDAVP), a synthetic analogue of vasopressin. Unlike aqueous vasopressin and lysine vasopressin, desmopressin is devoid of any vasoconstrictor effects and has a longer antidiuretic action (12 to 24 hours). Side effects are usually mild and include headache, nausea, and mild abdominal cramps; but overmedication can produce water overload. The patient is monitored for signs of dyspnea, hypertension, weight gain, hyponatremia, headache, or drowsiness.

Nephrogenic diabetes insipidus. Nephrogenic DI is treated with sodium restriction, which decreases the glomerular filtration rate and enhances fluid reabsorption. Administration of thiazide diuretics may increase tubular sensitivity to ADH.

Patient and family education. Patients who have a permanent ADH deficit require education regarding the following:

- Pathogenesis of DI
- Dose, side effects, and rationale for prescribed medications
- Parameters for notifying the physician
- Importance of adherence to medication regimen
- Importance of recording daily weight measurements to identify weight gain
- Importance of wearing a MedicAlert identification bracelet
- Importance of drinking according to thirst and avoiding excessive drinking

Patient Outcomes

Outcomes for a patient with DI include the following:

- Serum osmolality, 275 to 295 mOsm/kg
- Stable weight and balanced intake and output
- Serum sodium level, 135 to 145 mEq/L
- Return to baseline mentation

Syndrome of Inappropriate Antidiuretic Hormone
Etiology

Central nervous system disorders such as head injury, infection, hemorrhage, surgery, and stroke stimulate the hypothalamus or pituitary, producing excess secretion of ADH. A common cause of SIADH is ectopic production of ADH by malignant disease, especially small cell carcinoma of the lung. The malignant cells synthesize, store, and release ADH and thus place control of ADH outside the normal pituitary-hypothalamus feedback loops. Other types of malignancies known to produce SIADH include pancreatic and duodenal carcinoma, Hodgkin's lymphoma, sarcoma, and squamous cell carcinoma of the tongue.

Nonmalignant pulmonary conditions such as tuberculosis, pneumonia, lung abscess, and chronic obstructive pulmonary disease can also produce SIADH. As with malignant cells, it is believed that benign pulmonary tissue is capable of synthesizing and releasing ADH in certain disease states.

Many medications are associated with development of SIADH (Box 18-24). Of recent concern are reports of the effects of the widely prescribed selective serotonin reuptake inhibitors on ADH levels and function.[23] The mechanisms involved include increasing or potentiating the action of ADH, acting on the renal distal tubule to decrease free water excretion, or causing central release of ADH.

BOX 18-24 CAUSES OF SYNDROME OF INAPPROPRIATE ANTIDIURETIC HORMONE

Ectopic Antidiuretic Hormone Production
- Small cell carcinoma of lung
- Cancer of prostate, pancreas, or duodenum
- Hodgkin's disease
- Sarcoma, squamous cell carcinoma of the tongue, thymoma
- *Nonmalignant pulmonary disease:* viral pneumonia, tuberculosis, chronic obstructive pulmonary disease, lung abscess

Central Nervous System Disorders
- Head trauma
- *Infections:* meningitis, encephalitis, brain abscess
- Intracranial surgery, cerebral aneurysm, brain tumor, cerebral atrophy, stroke
- Guillain-Barré syndrome, lupus erythematosus

Drugs
- Angiotensin-converting enzyme inhibitors
- Amiodarone
- Analgesics and narcotics: morphine, fentanyl, acetaminophen

Drugs—cont'd
- *Antineoplastics:* vincristine, cyclophosphamide, vinblastine, cisplatin
- Barbiturates
- Carbamazepine (Tegretol) and oxcarbazepine (Trileptal)
- Ciprofloxacin
- General anesthetics
- Haloperidol (Haldol)
- Mizoribine
- Nicotine
- Nonsteroidal antiinflammatory drugs
- Pentamidine
- *Serotonergic agents:* 3,4-methylenedioxymethamphetamine (MDMA; Ecstasy), selective serotonin reuptake inhibitors
- Thiazide diuretics
- Tricyclic antidepressants

Positive-Pressure Ventilation

Pathophysiology

SIADH occurs when the body secretes excessive ADH unrelated to plasma osmolality. This occurs when there is a failure in the negative feedback mechanism that regulates the release and inhibition of ADH. The results are an inability to secrete a dilute urine, fluid retention, and dilutional hyponatremia. The primary treatment of SIADH is to restrict or withhold fluids.

Assessment

Clinical presentation. The clinical manifestations are primarily the result of water retention, hyponatremia, and hypo-osmolality of the serum. The severity of the signs and symptoms is related to the rate of onset and the severity of the hyponatremia.

Central nervous system. Manifestations such as weakness, lethargy, mental confusion, difficulty concentrating, restlessness, headache, seizures, and coma may occur in response to hyponatremia and hypo-osmolality. Hypo-osmolality disrupts the intracellular-extracellular osmotic gradient and causes a shift of water into brain cells, leading to cerebral edema and increased intracranial pressure. If the serum sodium level decreases to less than 120 mEq/L in 48 hours or less, there are usually serious neurological symptoms and a mortality rate as high as 50%. If hyponatremia develops more slowly, the body is able to protect against cerebral edema, and the patient may remain asymptomatic even with a very low serum sodium level.

Gastrointestinal system. Congestion of the gastrointestinal tract and decreased motility occur because of hyponatremia. This is manifest by nausea and vomiting, anorexia, muscle cramps, and decreased bowel sounds.

Cardiovascular system. Water retention produces edema, increased blood pressure, and elevated central venous and pulmonary artery occlusion pressures.

Pulmonary system. Fluid overload in the pulmonary system produces increased respiratory rate, dyspnea, adventitious lung sounds, and frothy, pink sputum.

Laboratory evaluation. The hallmark of SIADH is hyponatremia and hypo-osmolality in the presence of concentrated urine. A low serum osmolarity should trigger inhibition of ADH secretion, resulting in the loss of water through the kidneys and a dilute urine (see box, "Laboratory Alert: Pituitary Disorders").

High urinary sodium levels (higher than 20 mEq/L) help to differentiate SIADH from other causes of hypo-osmolality, hyponatremia, and volume overload (such as congestive heart failure). In SIADH, renal perfusion (a major stimulus for sodium reabsorption) is usually adequate, so sodium is not conserved, resulting in urinary sodium excretion. In a disorder such as heart failure, renal perfusion is low because of decreased cardiac output, triggering reabsorption of sodium.

Hemodilution may decrease other laboratory values such as BUN, creatinine, and albumin. SIADH should be suspected in a patient with evidence of hemodilution and urine that is hypertonic relative to plasma.

Nursing Diagnoses

The nursing diagnoses that may apply to a patient with SIADH include the following:
- Excess fluid volume related to excess water retention from excess ADH
- Disturbed thought processes related to brain swelling and fluid shift into cerebral cells

Nursing and Medical Interventions

The primary goals of therapy are to treat the underlying cause, to eliminate excess water, and to increase serum osmolality. In many instances, treatment of the underlying disorder (e.g., discontinuation of a responsible drug) is all that is needed to return the patient's condition to normal.

Fluid balance. In mild to moderate cases (serum sodium level, 125 to 135 mEq/L), fluid intake is restricted to 800 to 1000 mL/day, with liberal dietary salt and protein intake. The patient's response is evaluated by monitoring serum sodium levels, serum osmolality, and weight loss for a gradual return to baseline.

In severe, symptomatic cases (coma, seizures, serum sodium level less than 110 mEq/L), very small amounts of hypertonic 3% saline may be given following rigorous guidelines and with careful monitoring (Box 18-25). Correction of the serum sodium level must be done slowly, no more than 12 mEq within the first 24 hours. Administering hypertonic saline too rapidly, correcting the serum sodium level too rapidly, or both, can result in central pontine myelinolysis, a severe neurological syndrome that can lead to permanent brain damage or death.[28] The risk of heart failure is also significant. A diuretic such as furosemide may be given during hypertonic saline administration to promote diuresis and free water clearance. Treatments for chronic or resistant SIADH are listed in Box 18-26.

Nursing. Prevention of SIADH may not be possible, but early detection and treatment may prevent more serious sequelae from occurring. Being aware of the populations at risk and monitoring at-risk populations for clinical signs are key roles for the critical care nurse.

Close monitoring of fluid and electrolyte balance is required. Daily weight, intake and output, and urine specific gravity are measured. Fluid overload may occur from hypervolemia or too rapid administration of hypertonic saline. Cardiovascular symptoms such as tachycardia, increased blood pressure, increased hemodynamic pressures, full bounding pulses, and distended neck veins are all indicators of fluid overload. Respiratory function is monitored for signs of tachypnea, labored respirations, shortness of breath, or fine crackles. Careful monitoring of potassium and magnesium levels is necessary to replace diuresis-induced losses.

Adherence to fluid restrictions is critical but difficult for patients. The nurse should ensure that the patient and the family understand the importance of the restriction and that

BOX 18-25 NURSING CONSIDERATIONS FOR ADMINISTRATION OF 3% SODIUM CHLORIDE

- Administer via central rather than peripheral access
- Administer via pump only
- Rate should not exceed 50 mL/hour
- Monitor serum sodium levels every 4 hours; hold infusion if serum sodium level exceeds 155 mEq/L
- Wean solution rather than stopping abruptly
- Monitor level of responsiveness for evidence of decline (could indicate cerebral edema or worsening hyponatremia)
- Monitor lungs sounds for crackles indicating pulmonary edema
- Monitor intake and output every hour

BOX 18-26 TREATMENTS FOR CHRONIC OR RESISTANT SYNDROME OF INAPPROPRIATE ANTIDIURETIC HORMONE

- Water restriction of 800 to 1000 mL/day.
- Administration of loop diuretics in conjunction with increased salt and potassium intake is the safest method for treating chronic hyponatremia. The diuretic prevents urine concentration, and the increased salt and potassium intake increases water output by increasing delivery of solutes to the kidney.
- Demeclocycline is an antibiotic that decreases renal tubule responsiveness to ADH. Doses of 600 to 1200 mg are given PO in divided doses twice a day. Its onset is delayed for several days, and it may not be completely effective for 2 weeks, evidenced by a decrease in urine osmolality to therapeutic range. This drug is rarely used. The major side effects are nephrotoxicity and risk of infection.

Doses are approximate and may vary based on the individual situation.
ADH, Antidiuretic hormone; *PO,* orally.

they are included in planning types and timing of fluids. Patients should be encouraged to choose fluids high in sodium content such as milk, tomato juice, and beef and chicken broth. Measures to relieve some of the discomfort caused by fluid restriction include frequent mouth care, oral rinses without swallowing, chilled beverages, and sucking on hard candy.

Assessment of the patient's neurological status is also critical to monitor the effects of treatment and to watch for complications. The patient is assessed for subtle changes that may indicate water intoxication, such as fatigue, weakness, headache, or changes in level of consciousness. Strict adherence to administration rates of hypertonic (3%) saline solutions and measurement of serial serum sodium levels are

essential to prevent neurological sequelae. Seizure precautions are instituted if the patient's sodium level decreases to less than 120 mEq/L.

Patient and family education. In some patients, SIADH may require long-term treatment, ongoing monitoring, or both. These patients and their families require instruction regarding the following:

- Early signs and symptoms to report to the healthcare provider: weight gain, lethargy, weakness, nausea, mental status changes
- The significance of adherence to fluid restriction
- Dose, side effects, and rationale for prescribed medications
- Importance of daily weights

Patient Outcomes

Outcomes for a patient with SIADH include the following:
- Serum osmolality, 275 to 295 mOsm/kg
- Serum sodium level, 135 to 145 mEq/L
- Hemodynamic measurements within normal limits
- Return of vital signs to patient baseline
- Return of mental status to patient baseline
- Ability of the patient and family to verbalize an understanding of SIADH, the therapeutic regimen, and prevention of complications

Cerebral Salt Wasting
Etiology
Patients with any type of serious brain insult may develop CSW. Brain trauma, subarachnoid hemorrhage and other types of stroke, and meningitis are associated with development of CSW.[28]

Pathophysiology
The exact pathophysiology of CSW is unknown. A defect in renal sodium transport has been suggested, and a change from cerebral to renal salt wasting has been suggested as a more accurate term. Natriuretic peptides, commonly released in severe brain injury, and impaired aldosterone have been implicated as factors in defective renal sodium transport. However, research has produced conflicting data.

Assessment
Clinical presentation. The findings associated with CSW are related to hypovolemia and hyponatremia. Signs of hypovolemia include decreased skin turgor, dry mucous membranes, tachycardia, weight loss, and hypotension. Signs of hyponatremia include weakness, lethargy, mental confusion, difficulty concentrating, restlessness, headache, seizures, and coma. Neurological signs and symptoms are seen with both hypovolemia and hyponatremia.

Laboratory evaluation. An increased serum osmolality, decreased serum sodium, and increased urine sodium characterize CSW. Hemoconcentration may increase other laboratory values such as BUN, creatinine, and albumin (see box, "Laboratory Alert: Pituitary Disorders").

Nursing Diagnoses

The nursing diagnoses that may apply to a patient with CSW include the following:

- Deficient fluid volume related to lack of renal sodium retention and diuresis
- Disturbed thought processes related to decreased cerebral perfusion, cerebral dehydration, and hyponatremia

Nursing and Medical Interventions

The primary goals of treatment are to simultaneously restore both sodium and fluid volume. Replacing fluids without sodium may worsen the hyponatremia, resulting in life-threatening consequences. Both isotonic saline and hypertonic saline (3%) are used. Isotonic saline is administered to replace volume at a rate to match urine output, and 3% saline is given so that sodium levels increase at a rate of no more than 12 mEq/hr. Oral or intravenous fludrocortisone, 0.05 to 0.2 mg daily may be given to increase sodium retention in the renal tubules.

Patient Outcomes

Outcomes for the patient with CSW include the following:
- Serum osmolality, 275 to 295 mOsm/kg
- Stable weight and balanced intake and output
- Serum sodium level, 135 to 145 mEq/L
- Return to baseline mentation

CASE STUDY

Mr. F., a 68-year-old man, is admitted to the critical care unit from the emergency department with respiratory failure and hypotension. His history is significant for type 2 diabetes mellitus, steroid-dependent chronic obstructive pulmonary disease, peripheral vascular disease, and cigarette and alcohol abuse. His medications at home include glipizide, prednisone, and a metered dose inhaler with albuterol and ipratropium (Combivent). In the emergency department he received a single dose of ceftriaxone and etomidate for intubation.

On exam he is intubated, on pressure-controlled ventilation, and receiving normal saline at 200 mL/hr and dopamine at 8 mcg/kg/min. His blood pressure is 86/50 mm Hg; heart rate, 126 beats/min; oxygen saturation, 88%; and temperature, 39.6° C. His cardiac rhythm shows sinus tachycardia and nonspecific ST-T wave changes. Arterial blood gas values are as follows: pH, 7.21; PaO_2, 83 mm Hg; $PaCO_2$, 50 mm Hg; and bicarbonate, 12 mEq/L. Other laboratory values are as follows: serum glucose, 308 mg/dL; serum creatinine, 2.1 mg/dL; and white blood cell count, 19,000/microliter.

Questions
1. What disease state do you suspect this patient is experiencing and why?
2. What potential endocrine complications do you anticipate?
3. What further laboratory studies would you want? What results do you anticipate?
4. What treatment goals and strategies do you anticipate?
5. In providing patient and family education and support, what issues need to be addressed immediately and which can be delayed?

SUMMARY

The stress of critical illness affects the endocrine system. Control of blood glucose levels is an essential component of critical care because of the adverse outcomes associated with hyperglycemia. Low-dose corticosteroid therapy is a component of managing the inflammatory response seen in many critical illnesses.

Various endocrine disorders are seen in critical care. Patients may be admitted to the critical care unit for treatment of an endocrine disorder or develop an endocrine disorder secondary to another problem. Preexisting disorders may become secondary during treatment of a critical illness.

The critical care nurse must be knowledgeable about the endocrine system, its feedback mechanisms, and its role in maintaining homeostasis. Nursing assessments and interventions can assist in prevention, detection, and early treatment of endocrine imbalances.

CRITICAL THINKING EXERCISE

1. How can the hazards of hypoglycemia be prevented?
2. Insulin therapy is a critical intervention in the treatment of DKA. What crucial parameters must be monitored to ensure optimal patient outcomes?
3. In a patient with neurological injury, how do lab values help to differentiate DI, SIADH, and CSW?
4. In which patient population would the nurse expect to administer a cosyntropin stimulation test? What factors affect the interpretation of the test results?

REFERENCES

1. American Diabetes Association. Standards of medical care in diabetes – 2011. *Diabetes Care.* 2011;34(Suppl 1):S11-S61.

2. American Diabetes Association. Diagnosis and classification of diabetes mellitus. *Diabetes Care.* 2011;34(Suppl 1):S62-S69.

3. American Diabetes Association. *Medical Management of Type 1 Diabetes.* 5th ed. Alexandria, VA: American Diabetes Association. 2008.

4. American Diabetes Association. *Medical Management of Type 2 Diabetes.* 6th ed. Alexandria, VA: American Diabetes Association. 2008.

5. Brenner ZR. Management of hyperglycemic emergencies. *AACN Clinical Issues.* 2006;17:56-65.

6. Centers for Disease Control and Prevention. National diabetes fact sheet: National estimates and general information on diabetes and prediabetes in the United States, 2011. Atlanta, GA: U.S. Department of Health and Human Services, Centers for Disease Control and Prevention. 2011.

7. Clement S, Braithwaite SS, Magee MF, et al. Management of diabetes and hyperglycemia in hospitals. *Diabetes Care.* 2004;27:553-591.

8. Golombek SG. Nonthyroidal illness syndrome and euthyroid sick syndrome in intensive care patients. *Seminars in Perinatology.* 2008;32(6):413-418.

9. Griesdale DEG, de Souza RJ, van Dam RM, et al. Intensive insulin therapy and mortality among critically ill patients: a meta-analysis including NICE-SUGAR study data. *Canadian Medical Association Journal.* 2009;180:821-827.

10. Kitabchi AE, Umpierrez GE, Miles JM, et al. Hyperglycemic crisis in adult patients with diabetes. *Diabetes Care.* 2009; 32:1335-1343.

11. Lipiner-Friedman D, Sprung CL, Laterre PF, et al. Adrenal function in sepsis: the retrospective Corticus cohort study. *Critical Care Medicine.* 2007;35(4):1012-1018.

12. Lo J, Grinspoon SK. Adrenal function in HIV infection. *Current Opinion in Endocrinology, Diabetes & Obesity.* 2010;17(3):205-209.

13. Majeroni BA, Patel P. Autoimmune polyglandular syndrome, type II. *American Family Physician.* 2007;75(5):667.

14. Marik PE. Critical illness-related corticosteroid insufficiency. *Chest.* 2009;135(1):181-193.

15. Maxime V, Lesur O, Annane D. Adrenal insufficiency in septic shock. *Clinics in Chest Medicine.* 2009;30(1):17-27.

16. McCloskey B. Diabetes in the elderly. In Childs BP, Cypress M, Spollett G, eds. *Complete Nurse's Guide to Diabetes Care.* Alexandria, VA: American Diabetes Association. 2005;311-318.

17. Moghissi ES, Korytkowski MT, DiNardo M, et al. American Association of Clinical Endocrinologists and American Diabetes Association consensus statement on inpatient glycemic control. *Diabetes Care.* 2009;32:1119-1131.

18. NICE-SUGAR Study Investigators. Intensive verses conventional glucose control in critically ill patients. *New England Journal of Medicine.* 2009;360:1283-1297.

19. Nylen ES, Seam N, Khosla R. Endocrine markers of severity and prognosis in critical illness. *Critical Care Clinics.* 2006;22:161-179.

20. Porsche R, Brenner ZR. Amiodarone-induced thyroid dysfunction. *Critical Care Nurse.* 2006;26(3):34-42.

21. Rivkees SA. Differentiating appropriate antidiuretic hormone secretion, inappropriate antidiuretic hormone secretion and cerebral salt wasting: the common, uncommon, and misnamed. *Current Opinion in Pediatrics.* 2008;20(4):448-452.

22. Sakharova OV, Inzucchi SE. Endocrine assessments during critical illness. *Critical Care Clinics.* 2007;23(3):467-490.

23. Thomas Z, Bandali F, McCowen K, et al. Drug-induced endocrine disorders in the intensive care unit. *Critical Care Medicine.* 2010; 38(6):S219-230.

24. Turina M, Christ-Cain M, Polk HC. Diabetes and hyperglycemia: strict glycemic control. *Critical Care Medicine.* 2006;34: S291-S300.

25. Van den Berghe G, Wilmer A, Hermans G, et al. Intensive insulin therapy in the medical ICU. *New England Journal of Medicine.* 2006;354:449-461.

26. Van den Berghe G, Wouters P, Weekers F, et al. Intensive insulin therapy in critically ill patients. *New England Journal of Medicine.* 2001;345:1359-1367.

27. World Health Organization. *Diabetes Fact Sheet No. 312.* http://www.who.int/mediacentre/factsheets/fs312/en/; 2011.

28. Yee AH, Burns JD, Wijdicks EF. Cerebral salt wasting: pathophysiology, diagnosis, and treatment. *Neurosurgery Clinics of North America.* 2010;21(2):339-352.

CHAPTER

19

Trauma and Surgical Management

Mary Beth Flynn Makic, PhD, RN, CNS, CCNS, CCRN

Ⓔvolve WEBSITE

Many additional resources, including self-assessment exercises, are located on the Evolve companion website at http://evolve.elsevier.com/Sole.

- Review Questions
- Mosby's Nursing Skills Procedures

- Animations
- Video Clips

INTRODUCTION

Trauma is defined as a physical injury caused by external forces or violence.[1] Trauma, or unintentional injury, is the fifth leading cause of death in the United States, claiming the lives of predominately young individuals.[33] Only heart disease, cancer, stroke, and chronic lower respiratory diseases result in a higher death rate. The total number of deaths from unintentional injury is slowly declining; recent data reported 182,479 deaths related to trauma, primarily from motor vehicle crashes (MCVs), homicide, poisoning (e.g., prescription drug overdose), and falls.[11,33] However, every year an estimated 50 million people are injured severely enough to require medical treatment, and the majority of the injuries are preventable.[11] Motor vehicle crashes are the most common cause of traumatic death and often involve the use of alcohol, drugs, or other substance abuse.

Trauma is frequently referred to as the disease of the young, because the majority of injured persons range in age from 16 to 54 years. MVCs are the leading cause of death in teens; approximately 11 teens die in a MVC every day on U.S. roads. Programs like the Graduated Drivers Licensing (GDL) are aimed at reducing teen related MVC deaths through better driver safety education.[12]

An overarching goal in trauma care is prevention. However, when traumatic injuries occur, the priority is early and aggressive interventions to save life and limb. This chapter provides a review of trauma systems, the trauma team concept, and phases of trauma care. The nature of traumatic events usually requires surgical interventions; thus the postsurgical management of the trauma patient is discussed.

Special populations, frequent traumatic injuries, and mass casualty response are also described.

TRAUMA DEMOGRAPHICS

Trauma is a major healthcare and economic concern because of the loss of life, the societal burden in terms of lost productivity and increased disability of injured persons, as well as the consumption of healthcare resources.[9] MVCs and homicide are the leading causes of death for persons 15 to 24 years of age.[11] A second peak in trauma-related incidents occurs between the ages of 35 and 54 years, in which poisonings from prescription and/or illegal drugs are the leading cause of unintentional deaths; MVCs are the next highest cause in this age group.[13] A third peak in unintentional injuries and deaths occurs in the 65 years and older population, consisting of falls, injuries related to falls, and MVCs.

Males are much more likely to experience traumatic injury (2:1 odds ratio) when compared to females.[11] In addition, drug and alcohol consumption are leading contributing causes of traumatic events.[28] MVC-related injuries account for 38% of all unintentional traumatic deaths[33] and are associated with the largest number of days spent in hospitals and critical care units.[22]

Economic factors associated with traumatic injury include both direct and indirect costs. Direct costs are related to the actual expense of acute hospitalization and rehabilitative care an individual receives as a result of a traumatic event. Indirect costs are associated with lost work, physical disability (temporary and permanent), psychological disability, and lost

588

productivity. It is estimated that 10% (approximately $117 billion) of total U.S. medical expenditures is attributable to trauma care costs, and more than 350,000 individuals develop permanent disabilities.[9]

Significant advances in trauma prevention have decreased the frequency and severity of traumatic injuries. Advocates of organized trauma systems identify prevention as an essential component of a structured approach to trauma care. Organized trauma care systems have also decreased patient morbidity and mortality.[9,10] Nurses play an essential role in the care of the trauma patient, from prevention to resuscitation through rehabilitation.

SYSTEMS APPROACH TO TRAUMA CARE

Trauma System

A model trauma system provides an organized approach to trauma care that includes components of prevention, rapid access, acute hospital care, rehabilitation, and research activities.[2] Regional and state trauma systems provide comprehensive processes to deliver optimal care through an established trauma system network that matches a patient's medical needs to the level of trauma hospital with the resources necessary to provide the best possible care for the type and severity of traumatic injury. A trauma system combines levels of designated trauma centers that coexist with other acute care facilities. Levels of a trauma system are a differentiation of medical care, but are defined by resources available within the specific hospital.[2]

Levels of Trauma Care

Trauma systems are effective in reducing morbidity and mortality of severely injured individuals.[2,9,10,26] The development of trauma systems in an organized, coordinated manner across geographic areas to deliver trauma care to all injury patients is critical to successful treatment of unintentional injury.[2,9,26] Formal categorization of trauma care facilities is essential to provide optimal care. The goal of the trauma system is to match the needs of injured patients to the resources and capabilities of the trauma facility. The first civilian trauma units began in the United States in 1966, and in 1971 the state

of Illinois created the first trauma system mandated by state legislation.[2] In 1976, the American College of Surgeons Committee on Trauma (ACS-COT) developed a program of external review and verification of hospitals for trauma care to ensure that certain standards in trauma management were met within hospitals that obtained the trauma verification. In 1992, under the direction of the Health Resources and Services Administration, the Trauma Care Systems Plan was developed, providing a framework for the current trauma system and a verification process in the United States. A current list of hospitals with verified trauma centers is published on the American College of Surgeons Web site (www.facs.org/trauma/verified.html).

The ACS trauma system identifies four levels of trauma care: Level I, II, III, or IV.[2] Table 19-1 provides a description of the ACS levels. Hospitals with Level I through IV designations collaborate to develop transfer agreements and treatment protocols that maximize patient survival. All states with an identified trauma system are divided into regions. Each region has an identified lead trauma hospital. The lead hospital is usually the Level I trauma center.[2]

Trauma Continuum

Despite advances in trauma care, the continued high incidence of unintentional death and disability associated with traumatic injury remain a healthcare challenge. Death caused by traumatic injury is described as a trimodal distribution occurring in one of three periods. The first peak of death occurs within seconds to minutes from the time of injury. Death is caused by severe injuries, such as apnea from severe brain or high spinal cord injury, or massive hemorrhage (e.g., rupture of the heart, aorta, or other large blood vessels). Only trauma prevention will decrease deaths that occur in the first peak. The second peak occurs within minutes to several hours after injury. Death is the result of hemopneumothorax, ruptured spleen, liver laceration, pelvic fracture, and/or other multiple injuries associated with significant blood loss. This first hour of emergent care, the "golden hour," focuses on rapid assessment, resuscitation, and treatment of life-threatening injuries. The third peak occurs several days to weeks after the initial injury and is most often the result of sepsis, acute

TABLE 19-1	AMERICAN COLLEGE OF SURGEONS CLASSIFICATION OF TRAUMA CENTER LEVEL
Level I	• Provides comprehensive trauma care • Regional resource center that provides leadership in education, research and systems planning • Providers immediately available including: trauma surgeon, anesthesiologist, physician specialists, and nurses
Level II	• Provides comprehensive trauma care as a supplement to a Level I center • Meets the same provider expectations for care as a Level I center • Are not required to participate in education and research
Level III	• Provides prompt immediate emergency care and stabilization of patient with transfer to a higher level of care • Serves a community that does not have immediate access to a Level I or II center
Level IV	• Provides advanced trauma life support before transfer • Primary goal is to resuscitate and stabilize the patient and arrange for immediate transfer to a higher level of care

respiratory distress syndrome (ARDS), increased intracranial pressure (ICP), and multiple organ dysfunction syndrome (MODS). Patient outcomes in this time frame are affected by the care provided early in the management of the traumatic injury.[1,34] The trimodal distribution of death supports the central concept of trauma systems matching patients' severity of injury to the available resources for optimal care at an accredited trauma facility. Special resources, including early surgical management of injuries, are needed to decrease the morbidity and mortality of severely injured patients; thus the most critically injured patients should be cared for in higher-level trauma centers to maximize patient outcomes.[2,10,26,34]

Injury Prevention

Traumatic injury is considered a preventable public health problem and is the most important aspect of trauma system effectiveness.[3] Injury prevention occurs at three levels. *Primary prevention* involves interventions to prevent the event (e.g., driving safety classes, speed limits, campaigns to not drink and drive). *Secondary prevention* entails strategies to minimize the impact of the traumatic event (e.g., seat belt use, air bags, automobile construction, car seats, helmets). *Tertiary prevention* refers to interventions to maximize patient outcomes after a traumatic event through emergency response systems, medical care, and rehabilitation.

Historically, traumatic events were considered accidents or events that resulted from human error, fate, or bad luck. Research that explored antecedents of traumatic events found that traumatic injuries are not random events.[48] An individual's knowledge, risk-taking behaviors, beliefs, and decision to engage in a certain activity influence the outcome of actions. The word *accident* conveys a message of randomness in which an individual cannot prevent the event. Because most traumatic events are considered preventable, the word accident has been removed from discussion of traumatic injury, such as a motor vehicle accident. Current verbiage is a *motor vehicle crash.* Changing the language conveys the message that preventive efforts can be implemented to prevent a MVC, and additional behaviors, such as wearing a seat belt, may minimize the impact of the crash.

Nurses play an important role in trauma prevention. Nurses can role model trauma prevention within their family, community, and through political involvement. Political involvement includes simple efforts such as writing letters to local and national policy makers encouraging changes in laws and/or enforcing public policies favoring injury prevention (e.g., helmet and seat belt laws, driving under the influence of drugs and alcohol laws, limiting access to firearms laws). Involvement in trauma prevention includes supporting community and national coalition networks for trauma prevention (e.g., Mothers Against Drunk Drivers; National Safe Kids Campaign). Nurses provide ongoing injury prevention education to patients and families including fall prevention for older adults, child seat and seat belt safety, helmet safety, and drug and alcohol prevention education. The opportunity to

BOX 19-1 MULTIPROFESSIONAL TRAUMA TEAM

- Emergency medical services (EMS) response team
- Trauma surgeon (team leader)
- Emergency physician
- Anesthesiologist
- Trauma nurse team leader (coordinates and directs nursing care)
- Trauma resuscitation nurse (hangs fluids, blood, and medications; assists physicians)
- Trauma scribe (records all interventions on the trauma flowsheet)
- Laboratory phlebotomist
- Radiological technologist
- Respiratory therapist
- Social worker/pastoral services
- Hospital security officer
- Physician specialists (neurosurgeon, orthopedic surgeon, urological surgeon)

decrease death from unintentional injury lies in preventing the initial traumatic event.

Trauma Team Concept

The term *trauma team,* similar to a code team, refers to healthcare professionals who respond immediately to and participate in the initial resuscitation and stabilization of the trauma patient. Box 19-1 lists the composition of a typical trauma team. Trauma care begins in the field when the emergency medical services (EMS) response team responds to an event. Trauma systems work with EMS teams to create protocols that maximize treatment in the field. Once a patient is transported to a hospital, the acute care trauma team is activated. Essential to the team approach is that each team member is preassigned and understands the specific responsibilities inherent in a particular team role. The *trauma surgeon* is ultimately responsible for the activities of the trauma team and acts as the team leader in establishing rapid assessment, resuscitation, stabilization, and intervention priorities. Other team members, such as emergency department physicians, consulting physicians (e.g., orthopedic surgeons, neurosurgeons, otolaryngologists, thoracic surgeons, ophthalmologists, plastic surgeons), nurses, respiratory therapists, social workers, pastoral care providers, and interventional radiologists, have specific responsibilities. Each member of the trauma team is vital to meeting the needs of a multitrauma patient.

Prehospital Care and Transport

Rapid assessment in the field by prehospital personnel and immediate transport of the trauma patient to an appropriate trauma care facility reduce morbidity and mortality. Once EMS personnel arrive at the scene of a traumatic incident, they direct the situation and prepare the patient for transport. The time from injury to definitive care is a determinant of survival in many critically injured patients, particularly those with major internal hemorrhage.[1,2,10,20,26] Treatment of life-threatening problems is provided at the scene, with careful attention given to the *airway* with cervical spine immobilization, *breathing*, and *circulation* (ABCs). Interventions include establishing an airway, providing ventilation, applying pressure to control hemorrhage, immobilizing the complete spine, and stabilizing fractures.[1-3,6] The ultimate goal of any EMS system is to get the patient to the right level of hospital care in the shortest span of time to optimize patient outcomes.[6,20,26,40] Additional lifesaving prehospital interventions that may be required include maintaining spinal precautions, placing occlusive dressings on open chest wounds, managing the airway and assisting ventilation, and performing needle thoracotomy to relieve tension pneumothorax.

Large-caliber intravenous or intraosseous access and administration of crystalloid solution (e.g., lactated Ringer's solution or normal saline) to restore blood volume to maintain systemic arterial blood pressure is often initiated. Administration of intravenous (IV) fluids is dependent on the mechanism of injury. Large volume resuscitation is avoided because aggressive overresuscitation can precipitate complications such as hyperchloremic metabolic acidosis and inflammatory organ injury (e.g., ARDS, MODS).[42] Fluid resuscitation is guided by vital signs and assessment of end-organ perfusion (e.g., goal-directed resuscitation). Studies have explored the use of hypertonic IV fluids for resuscitation to effectively restore circulating volume without negative sequelae; however, current evidence does not support using this solution for fluid resuscitation in trauma.[42] Until the cause of hemorrhage is addressed in hemorrhagic shock, fluid resuscitation may be initiated to treat hypotension (60 to 80 mL/kg per hour for a systolic blood pressure of 80 to 90 mm Hg) or delayed resuscitation may be desired. Fluid resuscitation that raises the blood pressure to normotensive, or higher than normal blood pressure, may disrupt tenuous early clots.[3,5,42]

Ground or air transport is appropriate to move the trauma patient from the scene of the injury to the trauma center. Considerations in the choice of transport include travel time, terrain, availability of air and ground units, capabilities of transport personnel, and weather conditions. Once the decision is made to transport a patient to a trauma center, the trauma team is notified. In most trauma centers, the initial resuscitation and stabilization of the trauma patient occur in a designated resuscitation area, usually within the emergency department. Optimally, the trauma team responds before the patient's arrival and begins preparations based on the report of the patient's injuries and clinical status. Trauma patients in unstable condition may be admitted directly to the operating room for resuscitation and immediate surgical intervention.

Trauma Triage

Triage of an injured patient to the appropriate care facility with the necessary personnel and resources is an essential component of a successful trauma system. *Triage* means sorting the patients to determine which patients need specialized care for actual or potential injuries. Determining the type of

patient who requires transport to a trauma center rather than a basic emergency care facility occurs according to the EMS providers' assessment and established protocols, policies, and procedures. Triage decisions are often made by prehospital personnel based on knowledge of the mechanisms of injury and rapid assessment of the patient's clinical status. Medical direction of this process occurs through voice communication and medical review of triage decisions.

Trauma is classified as minor or major depending on the severity of injury. *Minor trauma* refers to a single-system injury that does not pose a threat to life or limb and can be appropriately treated in a basic emergency facility. *Major trauma* refers to serious multiple-system injuries that require immediate intervention to prevent disability, loss of limb, or death. In some regions, an injury scoring system is used to objectively measure and convey the severity of injury an individual has sustained. Several scoring systems are used for this purpose. The Abbreviated Injury Scale (AIS) and the Injury Severity Score (ISS) divide the body into seven regions and use a severity score from 1 to 6 for each injury. The AIS score is calculated from the three most severely injured body regions. The ISS is the sum of scores of the highest AIS score in three body regions. The risk for mortality increases with a higher ISS. A score of 1 indicates minor injury, and a score of 6 is fatal.

Another scoring system that is used to objectively evaluate a patient's severity of neurological injury is the Glasgow Coma Scale. The lower this score, based on three assessment parameters, the more severe the neurological injury, suggesting the need for emergent transport to a trauma center (see Chapter 13).

The Revised Trauma Score (RTS) is another assessment tool. The RTS is a prospective physiological scoring system based on initial assessment of the patient. The variables assessed in determining the RTS are blood pressure, respiratory rate, and Glasgow Coma Scale score. In this scoring system, lower scores are associated with a higher mortality.

The development of and adherence to established triage criteria are essential for maintaining an effective system of optimal care for the trauma patient. Triage decisions are based on abnormal findings in the patient's physiological functions, the mechanism of injury, the severity of injury, the anatomical area of injury, or evidence of risk factors such as age and preexisting disease. Prehospital personnel may elect to transport the patient to a trauma center in the absence of accepted triage criteria. This decision is most often based on visualization of the trauma incident and the patient's clinical condition.

Disaster and Mass Casualty Management

A disaster is a sudden event in which local EMS, hospitals, and community resources are overwhelmed by the demands placed on them. Disasters can be caused by fire, weather (e.g., earthquake, hurricane, floods, tornado), explosions, terrorist activity, radiation or chemical spills, epidemic outbreaks, and human error (e.g., plane crash, multicar crash). Disaster planning and management response have long been considered a primary responsibility of trauma systems. However, each disaster is unique, placing tremendous strain on communities to minimize mortality, injury, and destruction of property.[2]

Disasters are classified by the number of victims involved: multiple patient incident refers to fewer than 10 victims; multiple casualty incident refers to 10 to 100 victims; mass casualty incident refers to more than 100 victims.[18] Disasters may also be classified as an institutional-based, internal disaster, occurring within a hospital rendering the facility partially or totally inoperable. Community-based, external disaster, is any natural or man-made situation that overwhelms a community's ability to respond with existing resources.[18] Disasters also vary in resource demand depending on whether any warning was available before the event. For example, with impending bad weather disasters (e.g., hurricane), medical personnel can prepare a tentative plan for response. Unfortunately, some disasters such as a tornado or plane crash do not allow for preparation.

Regardless of the event, several principles in disaster management and mass casualty care exist. Initially, the local EMS system notifies the area hospitals of the disaster. Level I trauma centers take the lead in responding and preparing to care for the most severely injured patients. Effective field triage is vital in determining how patients are transported to local hospitals and trauma centers.

Command control centers and communication stations are established at the event site when possible and maintain contact with the lead hospital to facilitate efficient transport of patients.[15,24] Effective, consistent, and accurate communication of the activities at the disaster site and effective management of the severity and volume of incoming victims at the hospitals are critical to successful disaster and mass casualty management.[2,15,24,29,35]

During disasters, all healthcare personnel are requested to respond. Hospitals have well-developed disaster plans that outline specific healthcare provider responses during an event (e.g., disaster plan for weather, bombs, mass casualty). These plans outline the roles and responsibilities of all healthcare providers including hospital administrators, physicians, nurses, pharmacists, respiratory therapists, and security personnel. All personnel are required to be familiar with the disaster response policy.

Hospitals maintain disaster phone call lists that are activated during a disaster. When a disaster occurs, each area of the hospital activates this phone list and calls all the names on the list. Individuals are informed of when and where to respond within the hospital to help with the disaster management. Both human resources and medical supplies are assessed, and healthcare personnel are frequently rotated to minimize fatigue. Maximal treatment is provided to the victims; however, supplies are judiciously used to avoid running out of essential items.

Victims are further triaged based on the severity of injury. Many mass casualty triage classification schemes exist. A frequent system used to identify patient needs is a color coding system. Based on the emergency provider's assessment, the patient is categorized, by color, as to the type of care needed: (1) red indicates emergent, life-threatening injuries; (2) yellow means urgent major illness requiring care within an hour; (3) green indicates nonurgent injuries that the patient can self-treat; and (4) black signifies the patient is dead or near death.[8] Patients receive treatment based on the assessment of greatest chances for survival matched to resources available for medical intervention.

Disasters cause significant psychological stress during the event and after the situation has been stabilized.[24] Too often, the psychological well-being of the healthcare provider is not acknowledged after a disaster event. Resources to debrief health care professionals involved in disaster and mass casualty response are needed to help process the psychological stress and trauma experienced during the event. Debriefing frequently occurs as a group discussion session involving all healthcare team members involved in the disaster response; however, individual and ongoing psychological interventions may be necessary.[41] Current standards strongly encourage debriefing of healthcare providers soon after an event to address the psychological stress of the individual and team.[41]

MECHANISMS OF INJURY

Injury and death result from both unintentional and deliberate (violent aggression and suicide) events. *Mechanism of injury* refers to how a traumatic event occurred, the injuring agent, and information about the type and amount of energy exchanged during the event. Knowledge of the mechanism of injury assists the trauma team in early identification and management of injuries that may not be apparent on initial assessment.[50] It guides the assessment and interventions to minimize the chances of missing injuries that are more subtle (e.g., organ contusions). Questions regarding mechanisms of injury are directed to the patient (if applicable), prehospital care providers, law enforcement personnel, or bystanders in an attempt to reenact the scene of the trauma (Box 19-2).

BOX 19-2   QUESTIONS TO ASK TO DETERMINE MECHANISM OF INJURY AND POTENTIAL COMPLICATIONS

- Did the victim wear a seat belt?
- What was the speed of the vehicle on impact?
- Where was the victim located in the car—driver, passenger?
- Was the victim in the front seat or rear seat?
- Did the victim wear a helmet (bike, motorcycle, snow sporting crash)?
- What type of weapon was used (length of knife, type and caliber of gun)?
- How far did the patient fall?
- How long was the patient in the field before EMS arrived?

Personal and environmental risk factors include patient age, sex, race, alcohol or substance abuse, geography, and temporal variation. Temporal variation describes the pattern and timing of trauma. For example, injury deaths occur most frequently on weekends, unintentional injuries occur during recreational activities, and suicides occur more frequently on Mondays.[48] Injury may also occur when patients are deficient in oxygen, such as with drowning or suffocation; or in response to cold, leading to frostbite.

The transfer of energy causes traumatic injury. Energy may be kinetic (e.g., crashes, falls, blast injuries, penetrating injuries), thermal, electrical, chemical, or radioactive. *Kinetic energy* is defined as mass multiplied by velocity squared, divided by 2. Therefore the greater the mass and velocity (speed), the more significant the displacement of kinetic energy to the body structures, resulting in severe injury. The effects of the energy released and the resultant injuries depend on the force of impact, the duration of impact, the body part involved, the injuring agent, and the presence of associated risk factors.

Injury patterns from energy exchange are further described as blunt, penetrating, and blast injuries. The incidence of blunt trauma is usually greater in rural and suburban areas, whereas penetrating trauma occurs more frequently in inner-city urban neighborhoods. Blast injuries occur less frequently and include construction site explosions and terrorist attacks.[8]

Blunt Trauma

Blunt trauma is the most common mechanism of injury. It most often results from MVCs, but it also occurs from assaults with blunt objects, falls from heights, sports-related activities, and pedestrians struck by a motor vehicle. The severity of injury varies. Blunt trauma may be caused by accelerating, decelerating, shearing, crushing, and compressing forces. Vehicular trauma often results from a mechanism of acceleration-deceleration forces. The vehicle and the body accelerate and travel at an identified speed. In normal circumstances, the vehicle and body slow to a motionless state in a timely manner. However, when the vehicle stops abruptly, as in a collision, the body continues to travel forward until it comes into contact with a stationary object such as the dashboard, windshield, or steering column. Bodily injury occurs in the presence of rapid deceleration, when the movement ceases and contents within the body continue to travel within an enclosed space or compartment. An example of this occurs when the patient's head strikes the windshield after the automobile collides with a cement barrier. The brain tissue strikes the cranium and is thrown back against the opposite side of the cranial vault, with a resulting coup-contrecoup injury. Figure 19-1 shows potential sites of injury in an unrestrained passenger and driver as a result of blunt trauma.

Body tissues and structures respond to kinetic energy in different ways. Low-density porous tissues and structures, such as the lungs, tolerate energy transference and often experience little damage because of their elasticity. Conversely,

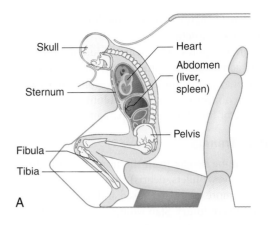

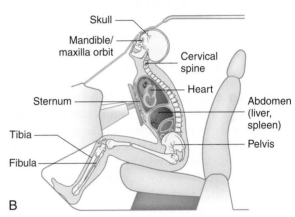

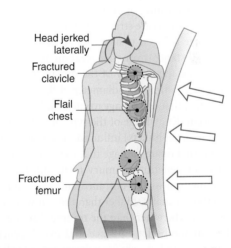

FIGURE 19-1 Potential sites of blunt trauma injury in unrestrained passenger and driver in a motor vehicle crash. **A,** Unrestrained passenger in front seat. **B,** Unrestrained driver. **C,** Lateral impact collision. (From Herm RL. Biomechanics and mechanism of injury. In Cohen SS, ed. *Trauma Nursing Secrets*. Philadelphia: Hanley & Belfus. 2003.)

organs such as the heart, spleen, and liver are less resilient because of the high-density tissue and the decreased ability to release energy without resultant tissue damage. These types of organs often present with fragmentation or rupture. The severity of injury resulting from a blunt force is contingent on the duration of energy exposure, the body part involved, and the underlying structures.

Blunt trauma requires expert clinical judgment to assess and diagnose actual and potential injury. Organ injury from blunt trauma may not be immediately visible. Knowledge of the mechanism of injury and effects of blunt trauma forces is vital in the care of the blunt trauma patient.

Penetrating Trauma

Penetrating trauma results from the impalement of foreign objects (e.g., knives, bullets, debris) into the body. Penetrating injuries are more easily diagnosed and treated because of the obvious signs of injury. Stab wounds are low-velocity injuries because the velocity is equal only to the speed with which the object is thrust into the body. The direct path of injury occurs when the impaled object contacts underlying vessels and tissues. Important considerations in a stabbing are the length and width of the impaling object, and the presence of vital organs in the area of the stab wound. Gender differences are seen and may provide information on the trajectory of the injury. Women tend to stab with a downward thrust, whereas male assailants use an upward force.

Ballistic trauma is categorized as either medium- or high-velocity injuries. Medium-velocity weapons are handguns and some rifles. High-velocity weapons are assault weapons and hunting rifles.[50] High-velocity injuries result in greater dissipation of the kinetic energy and more significant bodily injury. The velocity and type of bullet (missile) influence the transfer of energy creating tissue injury. As the missile penetrates the tissues, vessels are stretched and compressed, creating tissue damage referred to as a cavitation. Depending on the range, the distance from the weapon to the point of bodily impact, and the velocity of the missile, the cavitation may be as great as 30 times the diameter of the bullet. As bullets travel through tissues, damage to surrounding tissues and organs may occur. Knowledge of the type of bullet (e.g., size, hollow, shotgun pellet bullets) influences the assessment as to the type of internal tissue damage that may have occurred.

Assessment of penetrating injury from gunshot wounds involves examination of the entrance and exit wound. The entrance wound is usually smaller than the exit wound; however, forensic experts rather than the trauma team determine the direction of the bullet entrance and exit.[50] Penetrating injuries are monitored closely for subsequent complications including organ damage, hemorrhage, and infection.

Blast Injuries

Blast injuries are forms of blunt and penetrating trauma. Energy exchanged from the blast causes tissue and organ damage. Penetrating injury may occur as a result of debris entering the body. Blast injuries are classified as primary, secondary, tertiary, and quaternary.[1,15,50] The primary explosive blast generates shock waves that change air pressure, and tissue damage results from the pressure waves passing through the body. Initially after an explosion, there is a rapid increase in positive pressure for a short period, followed by a

longer period of negative pressure. The increase in positive pressure injures gas-containing organs. The tympanic membrane ruptures, and the lungs may show evidence of contusion, acute edema, or rupture. Intraocular hemorrhage and intestinal rupture may occur from the first shock wave after an explosion. Secondary injuries occur from increased negative pressure from the shock wave causing debris to impale the body, creating organ and tissue damage. Tertiary blast injuries are the result of the body being thrown by the force of the explosion, resulting in blunt tissue trauma including closed head injuries, fractures, and visceral organ injury. Quaternary blast injuries occur from chemical, thermal, and biological exposure.

EMERGENCY CARE PHASE

Information obtained during the prehospital phase provides essential data to ensure a coordinated, lifesaving approach in the management of trauma patients. Most traumatic events are considered "scoop and run" situations with short transport times, but other patients may come to the hospital by private car. Emergency departments in trauma centers designate resuscitation rooms providing a central location for the team facilitating a quick initial assessment, stabilization, and determination of the immediate medical needs of the patient.

Procedures exist within hospitals to activate the trauma team, including the operating room team, for emergent surgical interventions. The resuscitation room must always be in a state of readiness for the next trauma patient. Equipment needed for management of the airway with cervical spine immobilization, breathing, circulatory support, and hemorrhage control must be immediately available and easily accessible.

Initial Patient Assessment

Patient survival after a serious traumatic event depends on prompt, rapid, and systematic assessment in conjunction with immediate resuscitative interventions. Priorities of care are based on the patient's clinical presentation, physical assessment, history of the traumatic event (mechanism of injury), and knowledge of preexisting disease. Evaluation of airway patency, ventilation, and venous access with circulatory support are of prime importance and take precedence over other diagnostic or definitive interventions. Adherence to established protocols for patient assessment and intervention is essential to ensure that management priorities are addressed in a timely manner.

Primary and Secondary Survey

The primary survey is the most crucial assessment tool in trauma care. This rapid, 1- to 2-minute evaluation is designed to identify life-threatening injuries accurately, establish priorities, and provide simultaneous therapeutic interventions. The *primary survey* is a systematic survey of the patient's airway with cervical spine immobilization, breathing and ventilation, circulation with hemorrhage control, disability or

TABLE 19-2	PRIMARY SURVEY: ABCDE
ASSESSMENT	**OBSERVATIONS INDICATING IMPAIRMENT**
A = Airway Open and patent Maintain cervical spine immobilization Patency of artificial airway (if present)	Shallow, noisy breathing Stridor Central cyanosis Nasal flaring Accessory muscle use Inability to speak Drooling Anxiety Decreased level of consciousness Trauma to face, mouth, neck Debris or foreign matter in mouth or pharynx
B = Breathing Presence and effectiveness	Asymmetrical chest movement Absent, decreased, or unequal breath sounds Open chest wounds Blunt chest injury Dyspnea Central cyanosis Respiratory rate <8-10 breaths/min or >40 breaths/min Accessory muscle use Anxiety Decreased level of consciousness Tracheal shift
C = Circulation Presence of major pulses Presence of external hemorrhage	Weak, thready pulse HR >120 beats/min Pallor Systolic BP <90 mm Hg MAP <65 mm Hg Obvious external hemorrhage Decreased level of consciousness
D = Disability Gross neurological status Pupil size, equality, and reactivity to light Spontaneous/moves to command	Glasgow Coma Scale score ≤11 Agitation Lack of spontaneous movement Posturing Lack of sensation in extremities
E = Expose patient Environmental control Remove patient's clothing Rewarm with blankets, warming lights, fluid-filled or air convection warming blankets	Presence of soft tissue injury, crepitus, deformities, edema

BP, Blood pressure; *HR,* heart rate; *MAP,* mean arterial pressure.

neurological status, and exposure/environmental considerations (ABCDE).[1,8] During the primary survey, life-threatening conditions are identified and management is instituted simultaneously.[1,8] Table 19-2 details the critical assessment parameters included in the primary survey.

The *secondary survey* is a methodical head-to-toe evaluation of the patient using the assessment techniques of inspection, palpation, percussion, and auscultation to identify all injuries. The secondary survey is initiated after the primary survey has been completed and all actual or potential life-threatening injuries have been identified and addressed. A full set of vital signs are obtained as a baseline for analysis of trends during the resuscitation phase, comfort measures are implemented, patient history, and inspection of posterior surfaces is completed (FGHI)[8] (Table 19-3).

Information about actual and potential injuries is noted and used to establish diagnostic and treatment priorities. Radiological and ultrasound studies are completed according to a standardized trauma protocol or an assessment of suspected injuries. The sequence of diagnostic procedures is influenced by the patient's level of consciousness, the stability of the patient's condition, the mechanism of injury, and the identified injuries. As data are obtained, the team leader determines the need for consultation with specialty physicians

TABLE 19-3 SECONDARY SURVEY

SURVEY ACTIVITIES	ACTIONS	INSPECTION	PALPATION	AUSCULTATION
F = Full set of vital signs Focused interventions Facilitate family presence	Obtain full set of vital signs (blood pressure, heart rate, respiratory rate, temperature) Insert nasogastric tube, indwelling urinary catheter Obtain oxygen saturation via pulse oximetry Connect to cardiac monitor Obtain blood and urine for laboratory studies Identify family; provide updates; facilitate visitation with patient	Inspect perineal area during insertion of urinary catheter Inspect digits to ensure adequate vascular flow to obtain accurate oxygen saturation	Palpate for radial pulse Palpate for vein to access for blood studies	Auscultate blood pressure
G = Give comfort measures	Provide emotional reassurance Administer narcotics as ordered by trauma surgeon	Inspect patient for relief of pain	Provide touch and verbal reassurance to facilitate patient comfort	
H = History Head-to-toe assessment	Perform head-to-toe assessment Obtain information on allergies, current medications, past illness, pregnancy, last meal	**Head/Face:** Inspect for wounds, ecchymosis, deformities, drainage, pupillary reaction **Neck:** Inspect for wounds, ecchymosis, deformities, distended neck veins **Chest:** Inspect for breathing rate and depth, wounds, deformities, ecchymosis, use of accessory muscles, paradoxical movement **Abdomen:** Inspect for wounds, distention, ecchymosis, scars **Pelvis/Perineum:** Inspect for wounds, deformities, ecchymosis, priapism, blood at the urinary meatus or in the perineal area **Extremities:** Inspect for ecchymosis, movement, wounds, deformities	**Head/Face:** Palpate for tenderness, crepitus, deformities **Neck:** Palpate for tenderness, crepitus, deformities, tracheal position **Chest:** Palpate for tenderness, crepitus, subcutaneous emphysema, deformities **Abdomen:** Palpate all four quadrants for tenderness, rigidity, guarding, masses, femoral pulses **Pelvis/Perineum:** Palpate the pelvis and anal sphincter tone **Extremities:** Palpate for pulses, skin temperature, sensation, tenderness, deformities, crepitus	**Chest:** Auscultate breath and heart sounds **Abdomen:** Auscultate bowel sounds; observe for passing flatulence
I = Inspect posterior surfaces	Maintain cervical spine stabilization Log roll using three hospital personnel	Inspect posterior surfaces for wounds, deformities, and ecchymosis	Palpate posterior surfaces for deformities and pain Assist physician with the rectal examination, if not previously completed	

Adapted from Campbell M, Favand L, Galvin A, et al, eds. *Trauma Nursing Core Curriculum*. 6th ed. Des Plaines, IL: Emergency Nurses Association. 2007.

such as neurosurgeons, orthopedic surgeons, urologists, or others. Supportive interventions such as splinting of extremities, wound care, and administration of tetanus prophylaxis and antibiotics are completed.

RESUSCITATION PHASE

From the time of initial injury until the patient is stabilized in the emergency department or operating room, the trauma team resuscitates the patient. *Resuscitation* in trauma refers to reestablishing an effective circulatory volume and a stable hemodynamic status in the patient. During the emergency care phase, effective resuscitation is a central component of the primary and secondary survey. The ABCDEs of the emergency care phase are *airway, breathing, circulation, disability* (neurological), and *exposure,* and treating life-threatening injuries (e.g., pneumothorax, cardiac tamponade) emergently. Each of these interventions is discussed in detail.

Establishing Airway Patency

An effective airway allows for adequate ventilation and optimal oxygenation. Every trauma patient has the potential for an ineffective airway, whether it occurs at the time of injury or develops during resuscitation. The tongue, because of posterior displacement, is the most common cause of airway obstruction. Other causes of obstruction are foreign debris (blood or vomitus) and anatomical obstructions from maxillofacial fractures. Direct injuries to the throat or neck can structurally impair the airway. Patients with an altered sensorium or high spinal cord injuries may not be able to protect their airway.

Opening the airway is easily accomplished by the simple manual technique of a jaw thrust or chin lift. These maneuvers do not hyperextend the neck or compromise the integrity of the cervical spine. The airway must be cleared of any foreign material such as blood, vomitus, bone fragments, or teeth by gentle suction with a tonsillar tip catheter. Nasopharyngeal and oropharyngeal airways are the simplest artificial airway adjuncts used in patients with spontaneous respirations and adequate ventilatory effort. Both devices help to prevent posterior displacement of the tongue. The oropharyngeal airway is not used in the conscious patient because it may induce gagging, vomiting, and aspiration; if needed, a nasopharyngeal airway is better tolerated.

Endotracheal intubation is the definitive nonsurgical airway management technique and allows for complete control of the airway. Both the oral and nasal routes may be used for intubation. Nasotracheal intubation is used when the urgency of the resuscitation procedure does not allow time to obtain preliminary cervical spine x-ray studies. Disadvantages include possible epistaxis and injury to the nasal turbinates, and an increased risk for ventilator-associated pneumonia. Nasotracheal intubation is contraindicated for patients with facial, frontal sinus, basilar skull, or cribriform plate fractures.[1,7] Oral tracheal intubation requires careful manipulation of the neck, and thus is contraindicated in patients with suspected spinal or neck injuries. Disadvantages of oral tracheal intubation include incorrect tube placement in the esophagus or right mainstem bronchus, vocal cord trauma, and injury to the intraoral structures. An alternative airway device, a laryngeal mask airway (LMA), may be used when endotracheal intubation is not feasible.[7] Before intubation, patients are preoxygenated with 100% oxygen via a bag-mask device. Rapid sequence intubation (sequential administration of a sedative or anesthetic, and a neuromuscular blocking agent) may be used to facilitate the procedure. Correct position of the tube is verified (see Chapter 9). Mechanical ventilation with 100% oxygen is initiated immediately after intubation. The patient is then attached to a mechanical ventilator to provide ventilation and oxygenation.

In rare circumstances it may be difficult to intubate the trauma patient. In this event, a surgical intervention (*cricothyrotomy*) is performed to establish an effective airway. Conditions that may require cricothyrotomy are maxillofacial trauma, laryngeal fractures, facial or upper airway burns, airway edema, and severe oropharyngeal hemorrhage. The choice of airway management technique is based on the healthcare providers' familiarity with the procedures, the clinical condition of the patient, and the degree of hemodynamic stability.

Maintaining Effective Breathing

Interventions to restore normal breathing patterns are directed toward the specific injury or underlying cause of respiratory distress, with the goal of improving ventilation and oxygenation. Basic nursing interventions include application of supplemental oxygen with ventilatory assistance (if applicable), effective positioning, and evaluation of specific interventions. Ineffective breathing patterns are the result of certain traumatic injuries. These injuries and specific interventions are listed in Table 19-4.

The patient is assessed frequently for respiratory rate and effort, heart rate and rhythm, breath sounds, sensorium, skin color, temperature, tracheal position, and jugular venous distention. When spontaneous breathing is present but ineffective, a life-threatening condition must be considered if any of the following are present: altered mental status, central cyanosis, asymmetrical expansion of the chest wall; use of accessory or abdominal muscles, or both; paradoxical movement of the chest wall during inspiration and expiration; diminished or absent breath sounds; tracheal shift from midline position; decreasing oxygen saturation via pulse oximetry; or distended jugular veins. Arterial blood gas analysis and diagnostic studies including chest x-ray and chest computed tomography (CT) imaging may be completed to assist in determining the effectiveness of specific interventions.

Impaired oxygenation follows airway obstruction as the most crucial problem of the trauma patient. Impaired gas exchange can result from ineffective ventilation, an inability to exchange gases at the alveoli, or both. Possible causes include a decrease in inspired air, retained secretions, lung collapse or compression, atelectasis, or accumulation of blood in the thoracic cavity. Any patient presenting with multiple systemic injuries, hemorrhagic shock, chest trauma, and/or central nervous system trauma must be assessed for impaired gas exchange. These conditions have the potential to affect the patient's volume status and oxygen-carrying capacity, interfere with the mechanics of ventilation, or interrupt the autonomic control of respirations. Assessment is ongoing, and the nurse must be prepared to assist with intubation and subsequent mechanical ventilation, needle thoracostomy, chest tube insertion, and restoration of circulating blood volume.

TABLE 19-4 SPECIFIC INTERVENTIONS FOR INEFFECTIVE BREATHING PATTERNS

ETIOLOGY	INTERVENTIONS
Tension pneumothorax	Prepare for decompression by needle thoracostomy with a 14-gauge needle in second intercostal space at the midclavicular line on affected side. Prepare for chest tube insertion on affected side.
Pneumothorax	Prepare for chest tube insertion on affected side.
Open chest wound	Seal the wound with an occlusive dressing and tape on three sides. Prepare for chest tube insertion on affected side.
Massive hemothorax	Establish two 14-gauge or 16-gauge peripheral IV lines for crystalloid infusion. Obtain blood for type and crossmatch. Prepare for chest tube insertion on affected side. Administer blood or blood products as ordered. Anticipate and prepare for emergency open thoracotomy.
Pulmonary contusion	Prepare for early intubation and mechanical ventilation.
Flail chest	Prepare for early intubation and mechanical ventilation. Administer analgesics as ordered.
Spinal cord injury	Avoid hyperextension or rotation of the patient's neck. Observe ventilatory effort and use of accessory muscles. Maintain complete spinal immobilization. Prepare for application of cervical traction tongs or a halo device. Monitor motor and sensory function. Monitor for signs of distributive (neurogenic) shock.
Decreased level of consciousness	Position the patient's head midline with the head of the bed elevated. Anticipate a computed tomography scan. Implement interventions to prevent aspiration. Prepare for intubation and mechanical ventilation.

IV, Intravenous.

Maintaining Circulation

The most common cause of hypotension and impaired cardiac output in the trauma patient is hypovolemic shock from acute blood loss. Causes may be external (hemorrhage) or internal (hemothorax, hemoperitoneum, solid organ injury, long bone or massive pelvic fractures). Initial interventions include applying pressure to control the bleeding, replacing circulatory volume with crystalloid and blood products, and determining definitive treatment. In the face of hypovolemic shock from hemorrhage, early, rapid surgical intervention is lifesaving and limb saving.[1-3,5,36]

The management of hypovolemic shock focuses on finding and eliminating the cause of the bleeding and concomitant support of the patient's circulatory system with IV fluids and blood products (see Chapter 11). Frequently, it is difficult to assess blood loss, especially with internal hemorrhage from blunt trauma. Sympathetic compensatory mechanisms in the body respond to states of hypoperfusion through tachycardia, narrowing pulse pressure, tachypnea, and decreased urine output. These signs and symptoms may not be obvious until the patient is in a later stage of hypovolemic shock.[1,3,5] As a result of hypovolemia and hypoxemia, metabolic acidosis occurs secondary to a shift from aerobic to anaerobic metabolism and the production of lactic acid. Increases in lactate level and base deficit are accompanied by a decrease in tissue perfusion and increases in morbidity and mortality.[3]

Diagnostic Testing

Diagnostic testing is completed early in the resuscitative phase to determine injuries and potential sources of bleeding. Potential injuries to the chest, pelvis, abdomen, and suspected extremity fractures are assessed. Diagnostic studies include x-rays and *focused assessment with sonography for trauma (FAST)*. FAST provides a rapid, noninvasive means to diagnose accumulation of blood or free fluid in the peritoneal cavity or pericardial sac.[39] If free fluid or hemorrhage is found, a CT scan may be obtained and/or surgical interventions initiated as appropriate.[38] An echocardiogram, 12-lead electrocardiogram (ECG), and continuous ECG with ST segment monitoring, may be ordered to evaluated cardiac function, especially if the patient is showing signs of diminished cardiac output, thoracic injury is present, or the patient has a history of cardiovascular disease.

Occasionally patients with pelvic and long bone fractures and subsequent blood loss are placed in a *pneumatic anti-shock garment (PASG)*. Compartments in these pants can be inflated to hold pressure on long bones and the pelvis to stabilize a fracture and reduce bleeding during transport.[8] The device may increase intraabdominal and thoracic pressure, compromising effective ventilation, oxygenation, and circulation. Thus the PASG is infrequently used.

Adequacy of Resuscitation

Newer technologies are being refined for use during resuscitation to more effectively evaluate the severity of shock before decompensation of vital signs. Two of these technologies are sublingual capnometry and near-infrared spectroscopy (NIRS). Sublingual capnometry is a noninvasive technology that provides information about the degree of hypovolemia and adequacy of fluid resuscitation based on the sublingual partial pressure of carbon dioxide (PCO_2).[25,32] A probe is placed under the patient's tongue, and PCO_2 levels are derived from the blood flow found in the mucosal bed. During shock, an elevated sublingual PCO_2 indicates poor tissue perfusion. The sublingual PCO_2 is not an exact measure but a derived measure similar to pulse oximetry.

NIRS is a continuous noninvasive technology that uses principles of light transmission to measure skeletal muscle oxygenation as an indicator of shock. The NIRS probe is placed on the thenar muscle, which is located on the palm of the hand by the thumb. The probe measures the oxygen saturation state of tissue (StO_2) by evaluating the amount of infrared light absorption. Low values of tissue oxygenation (less than 80%) indicate states of shock; the lower the value, the more severe the tissue hypoxemia.[25,32]

Fluid Resuscitation

Venous access and infusion of volume are required for optimal fluid resuscitation in the patient with hypovolemic shock. At least two large-caliber peripheral IV lines are necessary. The preferred sites are the forearm or antecubital veins.[8] As an alternative, intraosseous (IO) needles may be used for access in the sternum, legs, arms, or pelvis if the patient's injuries do not interfere with the procedure (Figure 19-2).[8,19] The IO may be placed in the field by EMS personnel or in the emergency department. Resuscitation fluids, medications, and blood products can be administered through an IO device.[8,19] Potential complications with IO access include pain on instillation of fluids, extravasation of fluids, and compartment syndrome.[19]

A central venous line may be necessary because of peripheral vasoconstriction and venous collapse. A central line (single- or multiple-lumen line) may be more beneficial as a resuscitation monitoring tool. A pulmonary artery catheter is not usually helpful in the emergent phase of trauma management, but one may be inserted in the critical care unit to evaluate the response to fluid resuscitation and cardiac function. As a general rule, venous access is achieved rapidly with the largest-bore catheter possible to initiate early resuscitation.

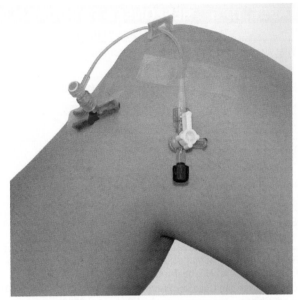

FIGURE 19-2 Tibial insertion of an intraosseous (IO) device taped in place with intravenous extension attached to the needle for fluid and medication installation. (Courtesy Waismed, Ltd. Houston, Texas)

Isotonic electrolyte solutions (e.g., Ringer's lactate or normal saline) are used for initial fluid resuscitation. A rapid infuser device may be used to facilitate rapid infusion of warm IV fluids. However, alterations in the infusion rate and volume may be necessary for certain trauma populations, such as the patient with cardiac disease. Underresuscitation results in worsening tissue ischemia, and overresuscitation causes life-threatening complications; therefore assessment of fluid volume status is critical.

The ACS recommends administration of 3 mL of crystalloid solution for each milliliter of blood loss (3:1 rule).[1] The patient's response to the initial fluid administration is monitored by assessing urine output (50 mL/hr in the adult), level of consciousness, heart rate, blood pressure, pulse pressure, and laboratory indices (e.g., serum lactate level and base excess).

Three response patterns are used to determine further therapeutic and diagnostic decisions (Table 19-5). These response patterns to initial fluid administration are rapid, transient, or no response.[1]

- *Rapid responders* react quickly to the initial bolus and remain hemodynamically stable after administration of the initial fluid bolus. Fluids are then slowed to maintenance rates.
- *Transient responders* improve in response to the initial fluid bolus. However, these patients begin to show deterioration in perfusion when fluids are slowed to maintenance rates. This finding indicates ongoing blood loss or inadequate resuscitation. Continued fluid administration and blood transfusion are indicated. If the

TABLE 19-5 RESPONSES TO INITIAL FLUID RESUSCITATION*

	RAPID RESPONSE	TRANSIENT RESPONSE	NO RESPONSE
Vital signs	Return to normal	Transient improvement; recurrence of ↓ BP and ↑ HR	Remain abnormal
Estimated blood loss	Minimal (10%-20%)	Moderate (20%-40%)	Severe (>40%)
Need for more crystalloid	Low	High	High
Need for blood	Low	Moderate to high	Immediate
Blood preparation	Type and crossmatch	Type-specific	Emergency blood release
Need for operative intervention	Possibly	Likely	Highly likely
Early presence of a surgeon	Yes	Yes	Yes

*2000 mL Ringer's lactate solution in adults, 20 mL/kg Ringer's lactate bolus in children.
BP, Blood pressure; *HR,* heart rate.
From the American College of Surgeons, Committee on Trauma. *Advanced Trauma Life Support for Doctors: Instructor's Course Manual.* 8th ed. Chicago: American College of Surgeons. 2008.

patient continues to respond in a transient manner, the patient is probably bleeding and requires rapid surgical intervention.

- *Minimal* or *no responders* fail to respond to crystalloid and blood administration in the emergency department, and surgical intervention is needed immediately to control hemorrhage.

The decision to administer blood is based on the patient's response to initial fluid therapy and the amount of blood lost.[1] If the patient is unresponsive to IV fluid therapy, type-specific blood may be administered. In the event of life-threatening blood loss, the physician may request unmatched, type-specific, or type O (universal donor) blood. Cross-matched, type-specific blood should be instituted as soon as it is available. Current practice tolerates lower hemoglobin levels in trauma patients because research has shown that patients receiving massive blood transfusions have poorer outcomes.[43] The decision to give blood is based on the patient's lack of response to only crystalloid resuscitation, the volume of blood lost, the need for hemoglobin to assist with oxygen transport, and the necessity to correct any coagulopathy. If blood loss and coagulopathy are life-threatening, massive blood transfusion may be required. This is defined as administering 10 or more units of packed red blood cells in 24 hours. In this situation, it is necessary to administer platelets and fresh frozen plasma in addition to packed red blood cells to improve patient outcomes. Blood products are given in a 1:1:1 ratio when massive blood transfusions are required—1 unit of packed red blood cells, 1 unit of platelets, and 1 unit of fresh frozen plasma.[42,43]

During fluid resuscitation, the patient is monitored for electrolyte imbalances, dilutional coagulopathies, and consequences of excessive third-spacing of IV fluids.[3,5] Electrolyte imbalances that may develop include hypocalcemia, hypomagnesemia, and hyperkalemia or hypokalemia. These imbalances may lead to changes in myocardial function,

laryngeal spasm, and neuromuscular and central nervous system hyperirritability.[3]

Dilutional coagulopathy may occur with excessive IV fluid resuscitation and extensive blood loss.[42] Banked blood products have high levels of citrate, which may induce transient hypocalcemia. Decreased serum calcium levels may lead to ineffective coagulation because calcium is a necessary cofactor in the coagulation cascade. Further inhibition of the clotting cascade is observed when platelet dysfunction develops secondary to hypothermia or metabolic acidosis. Management focuses on improving perfusion to the body tissues, increasing the patient's body temperature, and administering clotting factors (fresh frozen plasma, cryoprecipitate, and platelets). Monitoring the hemoglobin level, hematocrit value, plasma fibrinogen level, platelet count, prothrombin time, and partial thromboplastin time is essential.

Third-spacing can pose a significant problem during and within hours of aggressive fluid resuscitation.[3,42] During states of hypoperfusion and acidosis, inflammation occurs and vessels become more permeable to fluid and molecules. With aggressive fluid resuscitation, this change in permeability allows the movement of fluid from the intravascular space into the interstitial spaces (third-spacing). Hypovolemia thus occurs in the intravascular space, and patients require a larger volume of fluid replacement. This creates a vicious cycle; as more IV fluids are given to support systemic circulation, fluids continue to migrate into the interstitial space, causing excessive edema and predisposing the patient to additional complications such as abdominal compartment syndrome, ARDS, acute kidney injury, and MODS. The goal is to provide adequate fluid resuscitation to prevent tissue hypoxemia. Specific markers of tissue oxygenation and consumption (saturation of venous oxygen [SVO_2], sublingual PCO_2, and NIRS [StO_2]) may be used in addition to vital signs, urine output, and level of consciousness to evaluate the effectiveness of fluid resuscitation (see box, "Evidenced-Based Practice: Fluid Resuscitation).

Assessment of Neurological Disabilities

Assessment of neurological disabilities includes evaluation of the patients' level of consciousness, pupillary size and reaction, and spontaneous and reflexive spinal movement. Possible neurological injuries based on the history of the injury (e.g., ejection from motor vehicle, fall, or diving accident) are also considered.

Hypotension decreases cerebral perfusion; therefore the patient's response to interventions and the degree of tissue ischemia are considered in the neurological examination. Recreational drug and/or alcohol use by the patient can mask neurological responsiveness on the neurological examination, resulting in misleading findings. If an effective neurological examination cannot be conducted because of the patient's drug use, the healthcare provider manages the patient based on knowledge of the traumatic event and the patient's neurological response.[1]

Each year an estimated 1.7 million people sustain traumatic brain injury (TBI); 52,000 individuals die, 275,000 are hospitalized and 1.4 million are treated and released from emergency departments.[16] TBI is a contributing factor to a third of all injury-related deaths in the United States. An estimated 17% of MVCs have associated TBIs, 16% occur in struck-by events (e.g., colliding with a moving or stationary object, sports accidents) and falls account for 35% of TBI injuries.[16] TBI from MVCs and struck-by events are more prevalent in younger patients; fall-related head injuries are predominantly seen in older patients (65 years or older).[46] Management priorities focus on the primary injury from the traumatic event and the subsequent secondary injury that occurs as a result of cerebral hypoperfusion, increased ICP, and/or cerebral edema.

Injuries to the head may result from blunt or penetrating trauma. Primary head injury from blunt trauma typically occurs in the presence of acceleration, deceleration, or rotational forces. Injury may be focal or diffuse. Secondary head injury refers to the systemic (hypotension, hypoxia, anemia, hyperthermia) or intracranial changes (edema, intracranial hypertension, seizures) that result in alterations in the nervous system tissue.[37] Patients with secondary injury often have poor outcomes, including death. Nursing interventions focus on ensuring an adequate blood pressure to meet cerebral perfusion needs (mean arterial pressure greater than 50 mm Hg), maximizing ventilation and oxygenation through effective airway management, maintaining the head in a midline position to enhance cerebral blood flow, administering sedatives to address agitation and increased ICP, and conducting frequent neurological assessments.[37] The key to neurological assessments is recognizing subtle changes and notifying the physician for prompt intervention (see Chapter 13).

Lacerations to the scalp may result in significant bleeding. These wounds are cleansed, debrided, and sutured. Fractures of the skull may be linear, basilar, closed depressed, open depressed, or comminuted. Underlying brain injury may occur with skull fractures. Basilar skull fractures are located at the base of the cranium and potentially involve the five bones that form the skull base. The diagnosis is based on the presence of cerebrospinal fluid in the nose (rhinorrhea), in the ears (otorrhea), or in both; ecchymosis over the mastoid area (Battle sign); or hemotympanum (blood in the middle ear). Raccoon eyes or periorbital ecchymoses are present after a basilar skull fracture (see Chapter 13).

Spinal cord injury (SCI) is the second major neurological disability that is assessed early in the emergent phase of traumatic injury. Mechanisms of injuries that may result in SCI include hyperflexion, hyperextension, axial loading, rotation, and penetrating trauma. The initial treatment of a patient with suspected SCI includes the ABCs of resuscitation, spinal immobilization, and prevention of further injury through surgical stabilization of the spine. A complete sensory and motor neurological examination is performed, and x-ray studies of the cervical spine are obtained. A spinal CT scan may be performed to rule out occult injury. It is important to determine the approximate level of SCI because higher cervical spine injuries may result in the loss of phrenic nerve innervations, compromising the patient's ability to breathe spontaneously.

SCI causes a loss of sympathetic output, resulting in distributive shock with hypotension and bradycardia. Blood pressure may respond to IV fluids, but vasopressor therapy is often required to compensate for the loss of sympathetic innervation and resultant vasodilation. The patient with an SCI presents complex challenges for the trauma team as they attempt to minimize loss of function associated with the injury. Proactive, aggressive, and comprehensive care is necessary to help the patient achieve optimal functional outcomes (see Chapter 13).

Exposure and Environmental Considerations

Standard practice in the management of the patient with trauma is to remove all clothing and expose the patient to allow for full visualization of the body to identify all injuries. Exposure decreases body temperature. Hypothermia, defined as a core body temperature less than 35° C, is caused by a combination of accelerated heat loss and decreased heat production. A person is more susceptible to hypothermia after severe injury (especially older persons), excessive blood loss, alcohol use, and massive fluid resuscitation. Body temperature continues to fall after clothing removal, contact with wet linens, and surgical exposure of body cavities during the initial assessment. Prolonged exposure to hypothermia is associated with the development of myocardial dysfunction, coagulopathies, reduced perfusion, dysrhythmias (bradycardia and atrial or ventricular fibrillation), and decreased metabolic rate. Uncontrolled hypothermia caused by rapid infusion of IV fluids slows the heart rate and eventually decreases cardiac output. Optimally, IV fluids are warmed by using a fluid-warming rapid infusion device.[27] Crystalloids should not be warmed in a microwave because the temperature cannot be well regulated. Other adjuncts to minimize the negative effects of hypothermia include warming the room, covering the patient's head, applying warm blankets, or using convection air blankets. Suggested techniques for rewarming are listed in Table 19-6.

TABLE 19-6	REWARMING STRATEGIES
TYPE	**INTERVENTIONS**
Passive external	Removal of wet clothing
	Warm room
	Decrease airflow over patient
	Blankets
	Head coverings
Active external	Radiant lights
	Fluid-filled warming blankets
	Convection air blankets
Active internal	Warmed gases to respiratory tract
	Warmed intravenous fluids, including blood
	Body cavity irrigation (peritoneal, mediastinal, pleural, gastric)
	Continuous arteriovenous rewarming
	Cardiopulmonary bypass

Other environmental considerations are related to the location of the traumatic event. Environmental considerations include farming accidents, impalement with machinery or contaminated industrial equipment, exposure to contaminated water, or wound contamination with soil and road dirt.[21] Initial attempts to cleanse the wound are not priorities in the emergency care phase of trauma management; however, once the patient is stabilized, the wounds are cleansed and debrided, and appropriate antibiotics are initiated.

ASSESSMENT AND MANAGEMENT OF SPECIFIC ORGAN INJURIES

The following section discusses common, specific traumatic injuries. These injuries may be diagnosed and managed in the emergency care phase or subsequent critical care phase of the traumatically injured patient. Rapid assessment and definitive surgical interventions save lives.[2,3,8,10] However, not all injuries require surgical intervention. Ongoing assessment, management of specific organ injuries, and an awareness of the response to the stress of the injury are vital during the critical care phase of the traumatically injured patient.

Thoracic Injuries

The thoracic region contains vital organs such as the heart, great vessels, and lungs. It is considered a critical region because injuries to the thoracic organs and structures can quickly become life-threatening.

Cardiac Tamponade

Cardiac tamponade is a life-threatening condition caused by rapid accumulation of fluid (usually blood) in the pericardial sac. As the intrapericardial pressure increases, cardiac output is impaired because of decreased venous return. The development of pulsus paradoxus may occur with a decrease in systolic blood pressure during spontaneous inspiration. Blood, if unable to flow into the right side of the heart, causes increased right atrial pressure and distended neck veins. Classic signs of this injury are hypotension, muffled or distant heart sounds, and elevated venous pressure (Beck's triad). Beck's triad may not be present until late in the development of tamponade.

Cardiac tamponade is generally caused by penetrating trauma to the chest. However, it should also be suspected in any patient with blunt trauma to the chest or multisystem injuries who presents in shock and does not respond to aggressive fluid resuscitation. Pericardial tamponade is often difficult to diagnose in the presence of other injuries that also cause a decreased cardiac output.[51] Cardiac tamponade is diagnosed by using FAST or *pericardiocentesis* (needle aspiration of the pericardial sac). Pericardiocentesis, performed by the physician using a 16- or 18-gauge, 6-inch (15-cm) or longer, over-the-needle catheter attached to a 60-mL syringe,[8] can be used to treat the tamponade by decompressing the pericardium. It is important to differentiate blood from the pericardial sac from other sources. Blood aspirated from the pericardial sac usually does not clot unless the heart itself has been penetrated. Cardiac output may dramatically improve with removal of as little as 15 to 20 mL of blood, as noted by an increase in blood pressure. Nurses should anticipate and obtain equipment for an emergency thoracotomy in the event of cardiac arrest. After pericardiocentesis, immediate operative intervention is required for definitive repair.

Cardiac Contusion

Blunt trauma to the chest is the most frequent cause of cardiac contusion. The force of the traumatic event bruises the heart muscle and can compromise effective heart functioning and cause dysrhythmias.[3] Ongoing monitoring for symptomatic cardiac dysrhythmias via continuous monitoring of the ECG is frequently indicated for up to 48 to 72 hours. In the event of significant anterior chest trauma, a 12-lead ECG and serum levels of cardiac isoenzymes and troponin are obtained to rule out ischemia or infarction. With severe cardiac contusion injuries, inotropic agents are occasionally needed to support myocardial function.

Aortic Disruption

Aortic disruption is produced by blunt trauma to the chest, frequently resulting in death at the scene of the traumatic event. Rapid deceleration forces produced by a head-on MVC, ejection, or falls can cause dissection of the aorta in four common sites: (1) just distal to the left subclavian artery at the level of the ligamentum arteriosum, (2) the ascending aorta, (3) the lower thoracic aorta above the diaphragm, and (4) avulsion of the innominate artery at the aortic arch.[3] Often the outer two layers of the aorta are torn, leaving the innermost layer intact. Although this is considered a lethal injury, early diagnosis can prevent tearing of the innermost layer, exsanguination, and death.

Signs of aortic disruption include weak femoral pulses, dysphagia, dyspnea, hoarseness, and pain. A chest x-ray study may demonstrate a widened mediastinum, tracheal deviation to the right, depressed left mainstem bronchus, first and second rib fractures, and left hemothorax. The diagnosis is confirmed by an aortogram. Definitive, emergent surgical resection and repair are necessary with this injury.

Tension Pneumothorax

Tension pneumothorax is a rapidly fatal emergency that is easily resolved with early recognition and intervention. It occurs when an injury to the chest allows air to enter the pleural cavity without a route for escape. With each inspiration, additional air accumulates in the pleural space, increasing intrathoracic pressure and leading to lung collapse. The increased pressure causes compression of the heart and great vessels toward the unaffected side, as evidenced by mediastinal shift and distended neck veins. The resulting decreased cardiac output and alterations in gas exchange are manifested by severe respiratory distress, chest pain, hypotension, tachycardia, absence of breath sounds on the affected side, and tracheal deviation. Cyanosis is a late manifestation of this life-threatening clinical situation.

The diagnosis of tension pneumothorax is based on the patient's clinical presentation. Treatment is never delayed to confirm the diagnosis with a chest x-ray study. Immediate decompression of the intrathoracic pressure is accomplished by *needle thoracostomy*. The physician inserts a 14-gauge needle into the second intercostal space at the midclavicular line on the injured side.[8] This procedure converts a tension pneumothorax to a simple pneumothorax. Subsequent definitive treatment is required with placement of a chest tube.

Hemothorax

Hemothorax is a collection of blood in the pleural space resulting from injuries to the heart, great vessels, or the pulmonary parenchyma. Bleeding can be moderate (from intercostal vessels) or massive (from the aorta or from subclavian or pulmonary vessels). Decreased breath sounds, dullness to percussion on the affected side, hypotension, and respiratory distress may be seen. Placement of a chest tube facilitates removal of blood from the pleural space with resolution of ventilation and gas exchange abnormalities. Nursing interventions include managing the chest tube, closely observing the amount of blood drained from the pleural space, and monitoring the patient's hemodynamic response.

Open Pneumothorax

Open pneumothorax results from penetrating trauma that allows air to pass in and out of the pleural space. The normal pressure gradient between the atmosphere and intrathoracic space no longer exists. Patients present with hypoxia and hemodynamic instability. Management of the open wound is accomplished with a three-sided occlusive dressing. The fourth side is left open to allow for exhalation of air within the pleural cavity. If the dressing becomes completely occlusive on all sides, a tension pneumothorax may occur. A chest tube is inserted on the affected side, and a chest x-ray study is done to verify placement.

Pulmonary Contusion

Pulmonary contusion occurs as a result of blunt or penetrating trauma to the chest. Rapid deceleration or blast forces with resulting multiple rib fractures or flail chest injuries can cause a pulmonary contusion. It is one of the most common causes of death after chest trauma, and it predisposes the patient to pneumonia or acute lung injury. A contusion is a parenchymal injury to the lung that often results in some degree of hemorrhage and edema with a subsequent inflammatory process extending beyond the site of injury.[3,51] It is often difficult to detect because the initial chest x-ray study may be normal. Infiltrates on chest x-ray studies and hypoxemia may not be present until hours or days after injury.[51] The clinical presentation includes chest wall abrasions, ecchymosis, bloody secretions, and a partial pressure of arterial oxygen (PaO_2) of less than 60 mm Hg while breathing room air. The bruised lung tissue becomes edematous, resulting in hypoxia and respiratory distress. Ventilatory support is needed to promote healing of the lungs. Fluids must be administered cautiously to avoid further lung edema. Adequate pain relief with IV narcotics is essential to optimize lung expansion and respiratory effort and to prevent complications including atelectasis and pneumonia.

Rib Fractures and Flail Chest

Rib fractures are the most common injury associated with chest trauma. Rib fractures may lead to significant respiratory dysfunction and may indicate a serious injury to organs and structures below and near the rib cage. The diagnosis of rib fractures is frequently made after a chest x-ray study. However, there are situations in which rib fractures are not visualized on chest x-rays, and the diagnosis is made through clinical assessment. A high-impact force is needed to fracture the clavicle and first rib. Patients with these fractures require careful assessment for hemodynamic instability, which if present may indicate the presence of major vessel injury such as aortic disruption or injury to the subclavian artery. A pneumothorax or contusion of the heart or lung may be associated with rib fractures. Injury to the liver, spleen, or kidney may accompany fractures of ribs 10 through 12.

The management of rib fractures is dependent on the number of ribs fractured, the degree of underlying injury, and the age of the patient. Interventions focus on assessing the patient's ventilation and oxygenation, and effective pain management. Nurses should provide education on pillow splinting, incentive spirometry, coughing and deep breathing exercises, the benefits of early ambulation, and pain management. Effective pain management enables the patient to maximally participate in pulmonary exercises. Pneumonia is the primary complication associated with rib fractures.

A *flail chest* occurs when two or more adjacent ribs are broken in two or more places, creating a free-floating segment of the rib cage. The flail segment results in paradoxical chest movement; it contracts inward with inhalation and expands outward with exhalation. Normal respiratory

mechanics depend on a rigid chest wall to generate negative intrathoracic pressure for effective ventilation. The uncoordinated chest movement with flail chest impairs the ability of the body to generate effective changes in intrathoracic pressure for ventilation. Clinical presentation includes paradoxical chest movement, increased work of breathing, tachypnea, and eventually signs and symptoms of hypoxemia. Management frequently involves endotracheal intubation and mechanical ventilation with adequate pain control, which may include epidural analgesia or a regional block.[51] Positioning the patient to enhance ventilation and oxygenation and providing frequent pulmonary care are additional strategies to prevent pneumonia.

Abdominal Injuries

Abdominal injuries are often difficult to diagnose. A normal initial examination does not necessarily rule out intraabdominal injury. The classic sign of abdominal injury is pain. However, pain cannot be used as an assessment tool if the patient has an altered sensorium, drug intoxication, or SCI with impaired sensation.

The liver is the most commonly injured organ after blunt or penetrating trauma, and hemorrhage is the primary cause of death after injury.[3,30] The patient may present with a history of right lower thoracic trauma, fractured lower right ribs, right upper quadrant ecchymosis, right upper quadrant tenderness, and hypotension. The diagnosis is confirmed with the use of FAST and/or abdominal CT. The degree of liver injury is graded on a scale of I to VI, with I representing a nonexpanding subcapsular hematoma and VI signifying hepatic avulsion. Grades I through III injuries are treated with close monitoring (regular abdominal assessment and serial hemoglobin and hematocrit measurements) and bed rest for 5 days. Angiographic embolization or surgical management is indicated for grades IV through VI, in which there is expansion of the hemorrhage, a large laceration, or complete avulsion of the liver from its vascular supply.[8,30]

Splenic injury occurs most often as a result of blunt trauma to the abdomen. However, penetrating trauma to the left upper quadrant of the abdomen or fracture of the anterior left lower ribs also contributes to splenic injuries. The patient may present with left upper quadrant tenderness, peritoneal irritation, referred pain to the left shoulder (Kehr's sign), and hypotension or signs of hypovolemic shock. An encapsulated hemorrhage of the spleen produces no immediate signs of bleeding. The diagnosis is confirmed by using the same tests as for liver injuries. The degree of splenic injury is graded on a scale from I to V. Grade I is a subcapsular, nonexpanding hematoma, and a grade V injury results when the spleen is shattered and devascularized. Management of splenic injury is similar to that of liver injuries. Close monitoring of the patient is vital. This includes assessment of the patient's hemodynamic status; the presence of guarding, rebound tenderness, rigidity, or distention of the abdomen; and alterations in the patient's hemoglobin and hematocrit values. Bed rest for 5 days may be appropriate for grades I to

III splenic injuries. Operative intervention is often necessary for grades IV and V injuries. Splenic injuries may continue to bleed slowly, and the spleen may ultimately rupture days to weeks after the initial injury. A ruptured spleen is a life-threatening event that requires immediate surgical intervention. Every effort is made to preserve splenic tissue because of its role in immune function. Overwhelming infection has been seen after removal of the spleen.[30] Patients undergoing splenectomy are very susceptible to pneumococcal infections, and administration of the pneumococcal vaccine within the first few days postoperatively is recommended.

Gastric and small bowel injuries are most frequently the consequence of penetrating trauma from gunshot wounds. Blast injuries can also cause injury to these hollow organs. The incidence of gastric and bowel injury from blunt trauma is quite low, roughly 1% to 10%.[30] Gastric and bowel injury is suspected based on the mechanism of injury. Surgical intervention is usually required. Postoperative complications include infection and difficulty maintaining nutrition.

Blunt trauma to the abdomen may also injure the kidneys; however, usually only one kidney is affected. Renal trauma is classified as minor, major, or critical (life-threatening). The patient may present with costovertebral tenderness, microscopic or gross hematuria, bruising or ecchymosis over the 11th and 12th ribs, hemorrhage, and/or shock. Diagnostic studies include FAST, CT scan, angiography, IV pyelogram, and cystoscopy.[30] For minor injuries, management focuses on bed rest, hydration, and monitoring of renal function including adequacy of urine output; urinalysis; hematuria; blood urea nitrogen, creatinine, and electrolyte levels; and a complete blood count. Management of major and critical renal injuries focuses on surgical intervention including control of bleeding, repair of the injury, or nephrectomy. Postsurgical complications include refractory hypertension, hemorrhage, fistula formation, and infection.

Blunt trauma causing disruption of the pelvic structure is a challenging clinical problem because of the large vascular supply, nervous system pathways, location of urological structures, and articulation of the hip joint within the pelvic ring. Frequently, treatment of pelvic injuries requires the expertise of many specialties (orthopedics, general surgery, neurosurgery, and urology).[45] The potential for morbidity, loss of function, and death is significant. Pelvic injuries occur most frequently in high-deceleration MVCs, pedestrian-vehicle impacts, and falls. The mortality rate from pelvic injuries is estimated at 50%, primarily related to massive bleeding causing hemodynamic instability and hypovolemic shock.[5,8] Primary interventions focus on pelvic stabilization and aggressive fluid resuscitation to ensure adequate tissue perfusion. Initially, pelvic stabilization can be accomplished by tying a large sheet or pelvic binder around the patient's hips to control the bleeding.[45] Early definitive treatment is accomplished through interventional radiology procedures that use embolization or coil techniques to stop the bleeding. Surgical repair may be required for internal or external fixation of complex pelvic fractures.

Musculoskeletal Injuries

Musculoskeletal trauma rarely is a priority in the emergent management of the patient unless the injuries result in significant hemodynamic instability (e.g., pelvic fractures and traumatic amputations). The injuries may be blunt or penetrating, and may involve bone, soft tissue, muscle, nerves, and/or blood vessels. Injuries are classified as fractures, fracture-dislocations, amputations, and tissue trauma (crushing injuries of the soft tissue, nerves, vessels, or tendons). Knowing the mechanism of injury is important in evaluating musculoskeletal injuries because kinetic energy can be distributed from the bony impact to other areas of the body. For example, when a patient falls from a height, ankle fractures are likely, but energy displaced from the impact may have also caused lumbar spine and pelvic fractures.[50]

During the secondary survey, limb swelling, ecchymosis, and deformity are assessed. Extremity assessment is often described by the five Ps: *pain, pallor, pulses, paresthesia,* and *paralysis.* This process of assessment describes the neurovascular status of the injured extremity and is critical in assessing circulation in the extremity. Loss of pulses is considered a late sign of diminished perfusion. Increased pain, pallor, and paresthesia supersede loss of pulses and should be reported immediately to the trauma team.[8,49]

Fractures involve a disruption of bony continuity. X-ray studies are taken to diagnose fractures, and the extremity is immobilized. Common types of fractures are shown in Figure 19-3. If the skin is open at the fracture site, it is called an *open fracture;* if the skin is intact, it is called a *closed fracture.* Fractures are further classified into grades based on the degree of bony, soft, and vascular tissue and nerve damage. Early treatment of a fracture involves immobilization with splints or application of traction. Once the patient is hemodynamically stable, surgical management for open fractures (open reduction and internal fixation) is performed to restabilize the bone for effective healing.

Traumatic soft tissue injuries are categorized as contusions, abrasions, lacerations, puncture wounds, crush injuries, amputations, or avulsion injuries. Injury to the skin and soft tissues predisposes the individual to secondary complications including localized and systemic infection, hypoproteinemia, and hypothermia.[49]

Assessment of soft tissue injury is part of the secondary survey unless the loss of tissue (e.g., amputation) is hemodynamically compromising the patient. Traumatic amputation produces a well-defined wound edge with localized injury to soft tissue, nerves, and vessels. These wounds usually require debridement and surgical closure. Avulsion injuries result in stretching and tearing of the soft tissue and may tear nerves and vessels at different levels other than the actual site of bone and tissue trauma.

A crush injury may produce local soft tissue trauma or extensive damage distant from the site of injury. Crush injuries of the pelvis and/or both lower extremities or a prolonged entrapment may be life-threatening. Prolonged compression produces ischemia and anoxia of the affected muscle tissue.

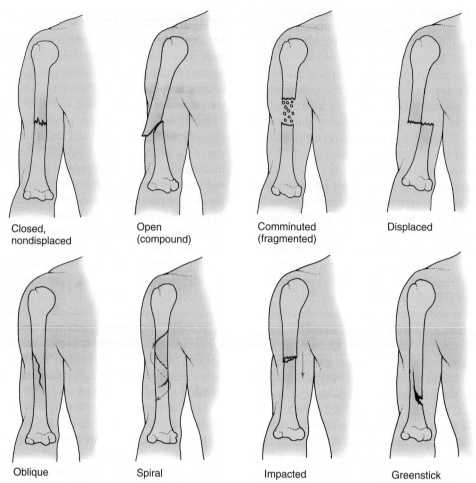

Closed, nondisplaced   Open (compound)   Comminuted (fragmented)   Displaced

Oblique   Spiral   Impacted   Greenstick

FIGURE 19-3 Common types of fractures. (From Murray CA. Care of patients with musculoskeletal trauma. In Ignatavicius D, Workman ML, eds. *Medical-Surgical Nursing: Critical Thinking for Collaborative Care.* 6th ed. Philadelphia: Saunders. 2010.)

Third-spacing of fluid, localized edema, and increased compartment pressures cause secondary ischemia. Without aggressive intervention, these injuries can result in irreversible complications.

Contusions do not cause a break in the skin, but localized edema, ecchymosis, and pain occur. Abrasions ("road rash") occur when the skin experiences friction. The abrasion can be superficial or cause deep tissue injury. Traumatic abrasions are frequently contaminated with debris implanted into the skin, resulting in traumatic tattooing. It can take hours to days to effectively remove the debris from the wound. Lacerations are usually caused by sharp objects, and they are treated with cleansing and suturing. Puncture wounds carry a heightened risk of infection. Although they do not cause vast soft tissue destruction or lacerations, puncture wounds can cause an aggressive infection because they deliver bacteria or foreign inoculums deep into the body.[21] Puncture wounds should not be surgically closed until treatment for infection with local and systemic antibiotics has been completed. Animal bites are notorious causes of puncture wounds.

All traumatic wounds are considered contaminated. Wounds must be cleansed and debrided to reduce the risk of infection. Ongoing assessment of the wound includes evaluating healing and investigating any local and systemic signs and symptoms of infection (e.g., increased wound pain, swelling, fever, elevated white blood cell count, increased wound drainage). Tetanus toxoid administration and antibiotic therapy are also considered.

Complications

Complications of musculoskeletal injury include the systemic effects that may occur after a crush injury, including compartment syndrome, rhabdomyolysis, venous thromboembolism (VTE), pulmonary embolism, and fat embolism.

Compartment syndrome. Compartment syndrome occurs when a fascia-enclosed muscle compartment, such as an extremity, experiences increased pressure from internal and external sources. Internal sources include edema, hemorrhage, or both; external forces include splints, immobilizers, or dressings. The closed muscle compartment of an extremity contains neurovascular bundles that are tightly covered by fascia. If the pressure is not relieved, compression of nerves, blood vessels, and muscle occurs, with resulting ischemia and necrosis of muscle and nerve tissue.

Patients with compartment syndrome complain of increasing throbbing pain disproportionate to the injury. Narcotic administration does not relieve the pain. The pain is localized to the involved compartment and increases with passive muscle stretching. The area affected is firm. Paresthesia distal to the compartment, pulselessness, and paralysis are late signs and must be reported immediately to prevent loss of the extremity. The affected limb is elevated to heart level to promote venous outflow and to prevent further swelling. Compartmental pressure monitoring may be performed for definitive diagnosis. Treatment of compartment syndrome is immediate surgical fasciotomy in which the fascial compartment is opened to relieve the pressure.

Rhabdomyolysis. Rhabdomyolysis is a syndrome of hypoperfusion and ischemia, followed by reperfusion, in which injured muscle tissue releases myoglobin into the circulation, compromising renal blood flow.[4,45] Causes of rhabdomyolysis include crush injuries, compartment syndrome, burns, and injuries from being struck by lightning. Myoglobinuria (the excretion of myoglobin through the urine) is an effective marker of rhabdomyolysis and causes the urine to be a dark tea color. Ultimately, the myoglobin is toxic to the renal tubule, causing acute tubular necrosis, electrolyte and acid-base imbalances, and eventually acute kidney injury. Treatment of rhabdomyolysis consists of aggressive fluid resuscitation to flush the myoglobin from the renal tubules. A common protocol includes the titration of IV fluids to achieve a urine output of 100 to 200 mL/hr.[4,45] Administering osmotic diuretics and adding sodium bicarbonate to IV fluids may be used to protect the renal tubules in patients with myoglobinuria.

Venous thromboembolism. VTE is a significant complication of traumatic injury.[51] The risk of VTE in trauma patients is dependent on the severity of injury, the type of injury (e.g., musculoskeletal injuries), the presence of shock, recent surgeries, vascular injury, and immobility. VTE usually occurs from a deep vein thrombosis (DVT) in the lower extremities. Thrombus formation is enhanced in the presence of Virchow triad: vessel damage, venous stasis, and hypercoagulability. If the thrombus dislodges, it becomes an embolus and travels through the body's vasculature until it lodges in either the pulmonary artery or its smaller branches (pulmonary embolism). Once the embolus becomes lodged, blood flow is obstructed distally and the tissues distal to the obstruction become hypoxic. Pulmonary vessels constrict in response to the hypoxia, resulting in ventilation-perfusion mismatches and hypoxemia. Prevention of VTE is essential in the management of trauma patients. If not medically contraindicated, patients should receive pharmacological prophylaxis. Nurses should encourage ambulation, evaluate the patient's overall hydration, and ensure sequential compression devices are used properly.

Fat embolism syndrome. Fat embolism syndrome is a potential complication that accompanies traumatic injury of the long bones and pelvis that result in multiple skeletal fractures. Typically, the syndrome develops between 24 and 48 hours after injury.[49] Long bone injury may release fat globules into torn vessels and the systemic circulation. The fat particles act as an embolus, traveling through the great vessels and pulmonary system, obstructing flow and causing hypoxia. Hallmark clinical signs that accompany fat embolism syndrome begin with the development of a low-grade fever followed by a new-onset tachycardia, dyspnea, an increased respiratory rate and effort, hypoxemia (PaO_2 of 60 mm Hg or less), sudden thrombocytopenia, and a petechial rash.[49] Late signs and symptoms include ECG changes, lipuria (fat in the urine), and changes in the level of consciousness progressing to coma.

Prevention of fat embolism is the best treatment. Stabilization of extremity fractures to minimize both bone movement and the release of fatty products from the bone marrow must be accomplished as early as possible. Treatment of fat embolism syndrome is directed toward the preservation of pulmonary function and maintenance of cardiovascular stability. Administration of supplemental oxygen and intubation with mechanical ventilation and positive end-expiratory pressure may be required to restore or maintain pulmonary function. Monitoring the patient's cardiovascular stability is continued throughout the critical care phase, with particular attention to ECG and hemodynamic changes.

CRITICAL CARE PHASE

The critical care phase for the patient with multisystem traumatic injuries requires the skills and collaboration of a variety of healthcare professionals.[47] The patient experiences additional physiological stressors from the traumatic injury and subsequent surgeries, psychological stressors, and often disruption of the social or family unit. The nurse is central to the critical care phase, continually assessing the patient's progress, anticipating and evaluating for possible complications, encouraging family-centered care, and acting as the patient's advocate. Interventions that were initiated in the emergent phase to treat and manage the traumatic injuries continue into the critical care phase.

Damage-Control Surgery

Patients with multiple injuries from traumatic events are at greatest risk of death from hemorrhage. Emergent surgical management of traumatically injured patients is the gold standard to stop hemorrhage and stabilize life-threatening injuries.[1] Definitive surgical interventions may require several surgeries to effectively manage traumatic injuries. The initial surgery focuses on cessation of the cause of bleeding; however, long, extensive surgeries can lead to severe complications that contribute to the patient's ultimate death. These complications, now recognized as the leading cause of death in patients who sustain multisystem traumatic injuries, include the triad of hypothermia, acidosis, and coagulopathy.[3]

These complications and resultant mortality have changed the current surgical focus to an approach known as *damage-control surgery* or a *staged surgical repair*. This strategy sacrifices the completeness of immediate repair, yet provides early surgical stabilization and management of active hemorrhage associated with injuries.[17] The first stage includes the operative repair of life-threatening injuries only. Patients are then returned to the critical care unit (second stage) for aggressive rewarming, ongoing resuscitation, and attainment of hemodynamic stability.[3] The third stage occurs usually within 24 to 48 hours after the initial operation. This involves the return to the operating room for definitive repair of intraabdominal injuries. This three-stage approach allows for cardiovascular stabilization, correction of metabolic acidosis and coagulopathy, rewarming, and optimization of pulmonary function.[3,17] A review of current research has determined that the damage-control concept improves the outcomes of critically ill patients with severe intraabdominal injuries.[17]

Postoperative Management

Most critically ill trauma patients are admitted directly to the critical care unit after surgery. Preparation for admission of the patient provides a smooth transition in care from the operative phase to the critical care phase. The room temperature may be increased to manage anticipated hypothermia, IV infusion pumps are accessed, respiratory therapy is contacted for a ventilator, and the monitoring equipment and room supplies are double-checked to minimize the need to find necessary supplies once the patient is admitted. The bed scale is "zeroed" to obtain a quick admission weight of the patient. The nurse frequently receives a report from the emergency department nurse before the patient goes to surgery; however, a thorough report from the anesthesiologist as part of hand-off communication between healthcare providers is essential for continuity of care. Elements of the hand-off communication include a review of systems, past medical history, description of the injury, description of the intraoperative procedures, the patient's tolerance of the procedures, vital signs during the surgery and current vital signs, total intake (i.e., crystalloids, colloids, blood products) and output (i.e., urine output, chest tube output, and estimated blood loss), medications administered (i.e., sedation, analgesia, neuromuscular blockade reversal agents, antibiotics, and vasoactive agents), IV access, and location of chest tubes and other drains.

The initial intervention upon admission to the critical care unit is a rapid assessment of airway, breathing, and circulation. The nurse quickly connects the patient to the bedside monitor and ventilator, and completes an assessment of vital signs, cardiac rhythm, pulse oximetry reading, level of consciousness, and pupil reactivity. Hypothermia is a concern postoperatively; thus the nurse keeps the patient covered while assessing the body for surgical incisions, dressings, other injuries, and location and function of drainage devices (e.g., chest tubes, hemovacs). It is important to inspect the posterior surface of the patient, so a quick turn to assess and remove soiled linens is completed early. The nurse reassesses IV access and evaluates the patency of IV catheters, because they may have become dislodged during transport. All IV infusions are traced from the IV fluid, to the infusion pump, and to the IV access in the patient. Calculation of medication

dosages and rates is completed as part of the initial assessment. All drainage devices are emptied, such as hemovacs and the urinary drainage bag, and the volume of output is recorded. If a chest tube is in place, the amount of existing drainage is marked on the external collection system. Admission laboratory studies are obtained. The most frequent studies obtained postoperatively include a complete blood count, a complete metabolic panel, coagulation studies, an arterial lactate level, and an arterial blood gas analysis with base deficit. Finally the patient is weighed. The admission weight is important for ongoing assessment of the patient's fluid status and medication administration throughout the critical care unit admission. Once the assessment and initial interventions are completed, the family is contacted to see the patient.

Postoperative management of critically ill patients involves a systematic and thorough assessment, and the monitoring of respiratory and cardiovascular function, neuromuscular abilities, mental status, temperature, pain, drainage and bleeding, urine output, and resuscitation efforts. Patients usually have an endotracheal tube in place when they are transferred to the critical care unit. Patients who do not require extended mechanical ventilation are extubated within minutes to hours of admission, depending on their ability to protect the airway after the reversal of anesthesia and neuromuscular blocking agents. Other critically ill patients are maintained on mechanical ventilation until stable, their injuries are definitively repaired, and/or pulmonary pathological processes have resolved. Monitoring of the patient's oxygenation and ventilation status is part of ongoing critical care management. Modifications in the ventilatory modes, adjuncts, and fraction of inspired oxygen (FiO_2) are made based on assessment.

After ensuring the stability of the patient's airway and adequacy of ventilation, attention is focused on hemodynamic assessment. This includes monitoring heart rate, cardiac rhythm, blood pressure, respiratory rate, pulse oximetry, temperature, drainage (e.g., chest tubes, nasogastric tubes, wound or incisional drains), urinary output, IV fluids, and vasoactive medications. The postoperative standard for monitoring these parameters is every 5 minutes for three measurements, every 15 minutes for three measurements, every 30 minutes for 1 hour, with hourly measurements thereafter. More frequent monitoring is indicated if the patient is hemodynamically unstable. Additional hemodynamic values are obtained if the patient has a pulmonary artery catheter or an ICP monitor.

Temperature is measured on admission and is monitored at regular intervals. In the event of hypothermia, passive and active strategies are used to rewarm the patient to a normothermic state (see Table 19-6). Shivering is prevented because it increases metabolic rate and results in increased oxygen demands and the potential for hemodynamic instability. During the rewarming process, vasodilation occurs and the patient is monitored for decreases in blood pressure.

A complete physical assessment is performed on all postoperative patients. All body systems are assessed including the neurological, cardiovascular, pulmonary, gastrointestinal, renal, hematological, immune, musculoskeletal, and integumentary systems. All invasive IV and central lines are also assessed. Continuous collection of assessment data guides therapies aimed at correcting identified problems or injuries, and preventing or minimizing postinjury complications. Elderly patients are at increased risk of complications after traumatic injury because of age-related changes (see box, "Geriatric Considerations").

The patient's mental status is assessed to ensure that a neurological event did not occur intraoperatively. Hand-off communication from the anesthesiologist includes whether anesthesia was reversed pharmacologically and the most recent times of analgesic, amnesic, or sedative medication administration. This provides information on the estimated time of patient wakefulness. Pupils are checked for reactivity. Once the patient is awake, the patient is assessed for alertness and orientation to person, place, and time, as well as the ability to follow commands. In the event that the patient does not awaken, measures must be taken to determine the cause of the unresponsive state. The medical team must determine whether the anesthetic agents, sedation, or analgesic medications are contributing factors. If it is determined that medications are not the contributing cause of the neurological impairment, the patient may require additional diagnostic testing such as a CT scan of the head. Any alterations in the patient's clinical assessment must be analyzed by the multiprofessional team to determine whether intervention is necessary.

Patients must be assessed to determine their level of pain. Multiple pain scales are available to assess the degree of pain (see Chapter 5). Individual institutions determine the most appropriate pain scale for use with their patient population. Postoperative orders include analgesic medication to be administered orally or IV (as needed or as a continuous infusion). If the nurse is unable to assess the patient's pain level postoperatively because of the patient's lack of wakefulness or secondary to a neurological event, the pain level is evaluated by using other parameters including increased heart rate and blood pressure, restlessness, facial grimacing, decreasing

GERIATRIC CONSIDERATIONS

- Falls are the most frequent cause of injury for the elderly population, resulting in fractures of the hips, arms, hands, legs, feet, pelvis, ribs, and vertebrae. Falls are an increasing concern as an estimated 1 in every 3 adults over the age of 63 years suffers a fall, many of which lead to injuries.[14]
- The elderly patient has three major factors influencing care needs after traumatic injury: known preexisting disease, diminished physiological capacity, and occult disease. The effects of trauma are exacerbated by decreased physiological reserve and host resistance that occur with aging.[44] These patients may present with hemodynamic instability, diminished organ function, and delayed healing.
- The cardiopulmonary effects of aging affect the patient's ability to respond to the pathophysiological effects of trauma. These patients often present with decreased cardiac output, have a risk of volume overload with fluid resuscitation, and have a lack of compensatory response to altered hemodynamics.
- Decreased brain mass, increased neuronal death, decline in sensory nerve function, decreased cerebral perfusion, and decreased autoregulation contribute to the changes seen in neurological assessment. Patients may present with changes in level of consciousness (agitation or coma), more pronounced neurological impairments after intracranial bleeding because of a larger compartment available for blood to accumulate, and an inability to report acute changes in painful stimuli. Older patients are at higher risk of developing acute delirium and progressive cognitive decline associated with significant trauma and prolonged hospitalization.[44]
- Physiological changes in the elderly include decreased renal blood flow and glomerular filtration rate, increased susceptibility to infection, decreased hematopoiesis, increased insulin resistance, decreased insulin release, diminished bowel motility, delayed wound healing, increased incidence of osteoporosis, decreased inflammatory response, and loss of subcutaneous fat. These changes alter the elderly patient's response to trauma. These patients are monitored closely for decreased urinary output, decreased hemoglobin or hematocrit values, increased blood glucose levels, development of ileus, signs and symptoms of infection, increased number of bony fractures, and alterations in skin integrity.
- Respiratory muscles weaken with age, decreasing chest wall compliance and placing the older trauma patient at increased risk of complications associated with pneumonia, decreased gas exchange (hypoxia), ineffective cough, acute respiratory failure, and ARDS.[44]
- The aging immune system places the patient at increased risk of infection from an inability to sustain effective cell-mediated immunity and antibody responses.[44]
- Elderly patients often have limitations in mobility and joint flexibility, muscle atrophy, osteoarthritis, and preexisting deformities that complicate their ability to participate in physical and/or occupational therapy and delay their return to pretrauma functional status.
- Knowledge of current medications is important because they may increase the risk of complications. The following drugs may contribute to patient complications:

MEDICATIONS	COMPLICATION
Aspirin	Increased risk of bleeding
Warfarin (Coumadin)	Increased risk of bleeding
Antiplatelet medications	Increased risk of bleeding
NSAIDs	Gastrointestinal bleeding
Steroids	Delay in healing
Beta-blockers and calcium channel blockers	Inadequate hemodynamic response
Herbal therapies	Severe drug interactions

NSAIDs, Nonsteroidal antiinflammatory drugs.

oxygen levels, and ventilator dyssynchrony. After administration of analgesia, the patient's pain level is reassessed.

Resuscitative efforts are evaluated postoperatively to determine the effectiveness of fluid management. Establishing baseline hemodynamic status, laboratory values (basic chemistry panel, arterial blood gases, arterial lactate level) and intake and output assists in determining the patient's fluid volume status and the degree of successful resuscitation. Hemoglobin levels, hematocrit values, and coagulation studies provide valuable information on whether the patient is bleeding or has a high probability of bleeding because of unavailable or ineffective clotting factors. The presence of abnormal values indicates the need for more aggressive resuscitation or blood component therapy.

Ongoing patient care priorities evolve from the patient's diagnosis and the surgical procedure. Careful attention is given to anticipating potential problems and intervening when actual problems are identified. A comprehensive reassessment every 4 hours guides the nurse in identifying changes in the patient's status, preparing for additional diagnostic procedures, and intervening appropriately. It is vital to evaluate the patient continuously for alterations in oxygenation, ventilation, acid-base balance, perfusion, metabolic status, and hemodynamic status, as well as for signs and symptoms of infection.

Effective nutritional support is considered an integral component of care of the critically injured patient. Nutritional needs of the patient are addressed early in the postoperative phase (within 24 to 48 hours) to assist with healing and meeting the body's needs related to an elevated metabolic demand. The route of administration (oral, enteral, or parenteral), type of nutritional replacement, and rate of administration are dependent on the severity of illness or injury and the expected recovery period. A nutritional consult is placed to evaluate the metabolic needs of the patient and determine the optimal feeding formula and rate of administration (see Chapter 6).

Ensuring that the patient has pharmacological prophylaxis for VTE and stress ulceration, as well as an aggressive protocol for mobilization, may prevent untoward complications. Immobility places the patient at increased risk of developing VTE, pneumonia, pressure ulcers, and urostasis. Strategies to prevent complications of immobility include frequent turning, offloading pressure on bony prominences with pillows, frequent skin assessments, application of moisture barriers to skin to prevent maceration from feces or leaking drainage devices, coughing and deep breathing exercises, early extubation, urinary catheter care and early removal of the catheter, and early ambulation.

Variations in hormonal regulation, specifically hyperglycemia and increased gluconeogenesis, are often seen in critically ill patients. Elevations in serum glucose levels are aggressively treated with IV insulin infusions, however, current guidelines suggest maintaining serum glucose between 140 and 180 mg/dL.[31] Attempts to obtain tighter serum glucose control has been found to result in more fluctuations in glucose and more adverse events associated with hypoglycemia.[31]

Patients with multisystem injuries are at high risk of developing a myriad of complications associated with the overwhelming stressors of the injury, prolonged immobility, and consequences of inadequate tissue perfusion. Even with optimal care, the stressors and overwhelming inflammatory responses to injury influence the risk of secondary complications. These include respiratory impairment (abdominal compartment syndrome, acute lung injury, ARDS, pneumonia), infection (catheter infection, sepsis), acute kidney injury, high nutritional demands, and MODS. A full discussion of these secondary complications is found in other chapters within this text.

SPECIAL CONSIDERATIONS AND POPULATIONS

Alcohol and Drug Abuse

The first step in trauma management is effective trauma prevention. Up to 40% of all traumatic events involve alcohol, and an additional 20% include drug intoxicants.[28] Overall complications, morbidity, and mortality are higher in traumatically injured patients who tested positive for alcohol, drugs, or both, at the time of admission. Most trauma patients who have high blood alcohol concentration upon admission meet criteria that indicate an alcohol problem.[23,28] With such a high incidence of traumatic events involving the use of alcohol and drugs, trauma prevention cannot be successful unless these concerns are addressed. Evidence-based programs are available to guide intervention programs[28] (see Centers for Disease Control and Prevention, National Center for Injury, Unhealthy Alcohol Use Program. Available at: www.cdc.gov/InjuryResponse/alcohol-screening/pdf/SBI-Implementation-Guide-a.pdf). Trauma centers need to have alcohol and drug intervention programs that can be implemented at the time of admission and maintained throughout the hospitalization to reduce the high correlation of alcohol abuse and serious traumatic injury.[23,28]

Drug use and abuse impair a patient's cognitive processes and create physiological stress.[3] Multiple categories of drugs may be used by the trauma patient ranging from inhalant intoxicants to hallucinogens, designer drugs (e.g., ecstasy, ketamine), cocaine, methamphetamine, and prescription opioids. Injuries frequently are self-inflicted because of the person's altered judgment from the effects of the drug. Mechanisms of injury associated with drug use include jumping from buildings or running through traffic. Drug use, especially drug overdose, causes significant physiological stressors. After addressing the traumatic injury, the physiological consequences of the drug and subsequent drug withdrawal must be addressed.

Nursing care of the trauma patient with an alcohol or drug addiction provides both a challenge and an opportunity. Because addiction is associated with physiological dependence, when the patient no longer consumes these agents,

BOX 19-3   SIGNS AND SYMPTOMS OF ALCOHOL WITHDRAWAL

- Irritability, agitation, confusion, hallucinations, and delusions
- Insomnia
- Anxiety and tremors
- Nausea, vomiting, and diarrhea
- Diaphoresis
- Tachycardia and hypertension
- Fever
- Seizures

serious or life-threatening withdrawal occurs. The nurse must closely monitor the patient's physiological status while a patient is experiencing withdrawal. Implementation of protocols to address withdrawal provides preemptive treatment. Common signs and symptoms observed include increased agitation, anxiety, auditory and visual hallucinations, disorientation, headache, nausea and vomiting, paroxysmal diaphoresis, and tremors (Box 19-3).

Discovering the time frame of the patient's last use of the drug and/or alcohol is essential in planning treatment strategies. As patients experience withdrawal, sedating agents may be ordered to ease the physiological and behavioral symptoms. Ongoing and frequent hourly assessments are necessary, especially in the presence of worsening anxiety, hallucinations, and other symptoms to ensure patient safety. Someone may be designated to sit with the patient at all times while the patient is going through acute drug or alcohol withdrawal. It is important that drug and alcohol prevention interventions begin before discharge from the hospital.

Family and Patient Coping

Traumatic injury is frequently unexpected and is a potentially devastating event, producing physical, psychological, and emotional stress for the patient and family. The event leaves the patient and family feeling overwhelmed, vulnerable, and often ill prepared to cope with ramifications of the injury. The traumatic event often creates a crisis within the family unit of the patient. Critical decisions for the patient frequently must be made by family members in seconds. The trauma team can assist the patient and family in crisis by helping them establish a consistent communication process between the healthcare team and family. Healthcare providers need to explore the patient's and family's perception of the event, support systems, and coping mechanisms. Early involvement of a social worker assists the patient and family with coping and can diffuse the current crisis, allowing more effective coping and decision-making processes. Family conferences early in the emergent phase and frequently during the critical care phase assist with communication and with understanding the patient's and family's expectations for care, and enhance the decision-making and coping skills of the patient and family.

REHABILITATION

The final phase of trauma care encompasses rehabilitation of the patient. The initiation of the rehabilitative process begins the moment the patient is admitted to the trauma center. Prevention of complications that prolong hospitalization and delay rehabilitation is imperative. Early involvement of the physical medicine and rehabilitation personnel is vital to positive functional patient outcomes.

Early in this phase of trauma care, a case manager or discharge planner evaluates the patient for the need for extensive rehabilitation at a specialty center. An individualized plan is developed for each patient based on physical injuries and rehabilitation potential, patient and family preferences, and insurance coverage.

Nursing interventions in the critical care phase influence the patient's rehabilitative needs. For example, the critical care nurse's attention to the position of the immobile patient to prevent foot drop assists with ambulation. Application of splints provides positions of functionality in injured extremities. The nurse also provides much needed emotional support as the patient convalesces through the critical care phase and begins more independent activities, preparing for the rehabilitation phase of trauma recovery.

Transition of the patient into rehabilitation is both an exciting and a frightening time for the patient and family. The patient has relied on the nursing staff for encouragement and support at a critical time in the patient's life. Transferring to another facility brings with it uncertainty in new relationships, as well as excitement, because rehabilitation is the last step before returning to the patient's home.

SUMMARY

Trauma is a leading cause of death in persons between the ages of 14 and 54 years and is considered preventable. Patient survival after traumatic injury depends on prompt, rapid, systematic assessment in conjunction with immediate resuscitative interventions. Evaluation of airway patency, ventilation, and venous access with circulatory support take precedence over other diagnostic interventions. The goal is to ensure the delivery of oxygen to the body tissues, to stop the progression of shock, and to prevent long-term complications. Critical care nurses provide an essential role in the early and ongoing care of the traumatically injured patient.

CASE STUDY

Mr. L, a 17-year-old male, was involved in a motor vehicle crash. He was wearing a seat belt but was traveling at a high speed when he lost control of the car and crashed into a tree. He was awake at the scene, but his level of consciousness quickly declined during transport to the trauma center by emergency medical services (EMS). The prehospital team was unable to intubate him during transport, and the patient's airway was maintained with bag-mask device ventilation using a fraction of inspired oxygen (FiO_2) of 1.00 (100%). Two large-bore intravenous catheters were placed, and normal saline was infused at 250 mL/hr. Three liters of fluid were administered before arrival in the emergency department. Mr. L does not have a significant medical history or any drug allergies. Initial vital signs were temperature, 36.6° C; blood pressure, 92/62 mm Hg; heart rate and rhythm, 136 beats/minute with sinus tachycardia; respiratory rate, 36 breaths/minute with assisted manual ventilation; and oxygen saturation, 95%. He is nonresponsive to verbal commands, and his pupils are 2 mm and reactive to light. He has a 6-cm scalp laceration, a right closed femur fracture, four broken ribs, and suspected closed head injury. Initial laboratory results were:

Hemoglobin	7.2 g/dL
White blood count	16,000/microliter
Platelet count	200,000/microliter
Potassium	5.5 mEq/L
Other electrolyte levels	unremarkable

Arterial blood gas results

pH	7.19
Partial pressure of arterial oxygen (PaO_2)	160 mm Hg
Partial pressure of arterial carbon dioxide ($PaCO_2$)	42 mm Hg
Bicarbonate (HCO_3^-)	18 mEq/L
Base deficit	−14
Lactate	9 mEq/L

Aggressive fluid resuscitation continues as he is transported to radiology for computed tomography to evaluate his head, chest, and abdomen for injuries. EMS contacted his parents, who are both in the waiting room of the emergency department.

Questions

1. What are the possible injuries based on the mechanism of injury?
2. What is the priority intervention at this time based on his vital signs?
3. What is your interpretation of the laboratory results? What interventions do you anticipate based on these results?
4. What are possible reasons for his unresponsiveness?
5. What additional diagnostic studies or interventions do you anticipate the patient needs after the computed tomography scan?
6. What additional nursing interventions do you anticipate in the emergent evaluation and treatment of this patient?
7. What are the needs of the family?

CRITICAL THINKING EXERCISES

1. A patient presents to the critical care unit with a gunshot wound to the left lower anterior chest from a 0.45-caliber semiautomatic weapon. What additional prehospital information would be helpful? Considering the mechanism of injury and location of the entrance wound, describe the potential patterns of injury. What are the immediate management priorities?

2. After operative repair, this patient is admitted to the critical care unit. Describe the assessment and intervention priorities during the first postoperative hour.

3. Why is it necessary to administer platelets and fresh frozen plasma along with packed red blood cells in the patient who requires a massive blood transfusion (>10 units)?

REFERENCES

1. American College of Surgeons, Committee on Trauma. *Advanced Trauma Life Support for Doctors: Instructor's Course Manual.* 8th ed. Chicago: American College of Surgeons; 2008.
2. American College of Surgeons, Committee on Trauma. *Resources for Optimal Care of the Injured Patient* 2006. American College of Surgeons; 2006.
3. Bonatti H, Calland JF. Trauma. *Emergency Medical Clinics of North America.* 2008;26:625-648.
4. Bosch Z, Poch E, Grau JM. Rhabdomyolysis and acute kidney injury. *New England Journal of Medicine.* 2009;361(1):62-72.
5. Boswell S, Scalea TM. Initial management of traumatic shock. In McQuillan K, Makic MB, Whalen E, eds. *Trauma Nursing from Resuscitation Through Rehabilitation.* 4th ed. Philadelphia: Saunders. 2009;228-251.
6. Bulger EM, Maier RV. Pre-hospital care of the injured: what's new. *Surgical Clinics of North America.* 2007;87(1):37-53.
7. Braun P, Wenzel V, Paal P. Anesthesia in prehospital emergency and in the emergency department. *Current Opinion in Anaesthesiology.* 2010;23:500-506.
8. Campbell M, Favand L, Galvin A, et al, eds. *Trauma Nursing Core Curriculum.* 6th ed. Des Plaines, IL: Emergency Nurses Association; 2007.
9. Capone-Neto A, Rizoli S. Linking the chain of survival: trauma as a traditional role model for multisystem trauma and brain injury. *Current Opinion in Critical Care.* 2009;15:290-294.
10. Celso B, Tepas J, Langland-Orban B, et al. A systematic review and meta-analysis comparing outcome of severely injured patients treated in trauma centers following the establishment of trauma systems. *Journal of Trauma.* 2006;60(2):371-378.
11. Centers for Disease Control and Prevention. *Unintentional Injury/Fast Facts.* http://www.cdc.gov/nchs/data/dvs/deaths_2009_release.pdf; Accessed March 3, 2012.
12. Centers for Disease Control and Prevention. *Motor Vehicle Safety.* http://www.cdc.gov/Motorvehiclesafety/index.html; Accessed March 3, 2012.

and damages adjacent deep muscle tissue. *Electroporation,* a significant increase in the conductivity and permeability of cell membranes, also contributes to extensive tissue damage.[6] Both of these processes cause deep tissue necrosis to occur beneath viable and more superficial tissue. On initial presentation, the cutaneous wound may appear minimal or superficial. However, it can manifest as an extensive, deep wound with neurological impairment several days or weeks later.

Lightning injury is caused by a direct strike or a side flash that causes a flow of current between the person and a close object that is struck by lightning.[6] Cutaneous injury is often superficial because the current travels on the surface of the body rather than through it. Lightning injuries frequently result in cardiopulmonary arrest. Approximately 70% of survivors suffer serious complications and central nervous system deficits.[6]

Inhalation Injury

Lung injury caused by inhalation of smoke, chemical toxins, and products of incomplete combustion is associated with increased mortality.[6,8,17,22,40,47] Inhalation injury is classified as (1) systemic injury from exposure to toxic gases (carbon monoxide or cyanide), (2) supraglottic or injury above the glottis, and (3) subglottic or injury below the glottis.[6,17] Table 20-1 summarizes characteristics of each type of injury. There is clinical and outcomes research value in standardizing inhalation injury diagnosis by a severity grading or scoring system. Hence this has become a priority focus of the American Burn Association, with a national multicenter study currently underway. Recent research indicates smoke exposure causes lung damage via an airway inflammatory response with lasting physiological changes in biochemical mediators and cells.[17,40] Inhalation injury often warrants admission to a critical care unit, even when there are no cutaneous surface burn wounds.

Carbon Monoxide and Cyanide Poisoning

Carbon monoxide poisoning is the most frequent cause of death at the injury scene.[6] Carbon monoxide is released when organic compounds, such as wood or coal, are burned. It has an affinity for hemoglobin that is 200 times greater than that of oxygen.[6] When carbon monoxide is inhaled, it binds to hemoglobin (*carboxyhemoglobin* [COHgb]) and prevents the red blood cell from transporting oxygen to body tissues, leading to systemic hypoxia. Carbon monoxide poisoning is difficult to detect because it may not present with significant clinical findings. Specifically, partial pressure of oxygen in arterial blood (PaO_2) and arterial oxygen saturation (SaO_2) levels are normal because the amount of circulating oxygen is not affected by carbon monoxide. Therefore it is essential to measure COHgb levels, which are reported as a percentage of hemoglobin molecules bound with carbon monoxide. Levels lower than 10% to 15% are found in mild carbon monoxide poisoning, and are commonly associated with heavy smokers and people exposed continually to dense traffic pollution (Table 20-2). Central nervous system dysfunction of varying degrees (e.g., restlessness, confusion) manifests at levels of 15% to 40%. Loss of consciousness occurs at COHgb levels of 40% to 60%, and death generally ensues when the COHgb level exceeds 60%.

TABLE 20-1	TYPES OF SMOKE INHALATION INJURY
TYPE OF INJURY	**PATHOLOGY**
Exposure to toxic gases	*Carbon monoxide poisoning:* carbon monoxide binds to hemoglobin molecules more rapidly than oxygen molecules do; tissue hypoxia results *Cyanide poisoning:* cyanide binds to respiratory enzymes in the mitochondria, inhibiting cellular metabolism and utilization of oxygen
Supraglottic: Inhalation injury above the glottis	Most often a thermal injury; heat absorption and damage occur mostly in the pharynx and larynx; may cause airway obstruction after resuscitation is initiated
Subglottic: Inhalation injury below the glottis	Usually a chemical injury that produces impaired ciliary activity, erythema, hypersecretion, edema, ulceration of mucosa, increased blood flow, and spasm of bronchi and/or bronchioles

Modified from American Burn Association. *Advanced Burn Life Support Course: Provider's Manual.* Chicago: American Burn Association. 2012.

TABLE 20-2	CARBOXYHEMOGLOBIN
CARBOXYHEMOGLOBIN LEVEL*	**CLINICAL PRESENTATION**
<10% to 15%	No symptoms, or mimic changes in visual acuity and headache
15% to 40%	Central nervous system dysfunction: restlessness, confusion, impaired dexterity, headache, dizziness, nausea/vomiting
40% to 60%	Loss of consciousness, tachycardia, tachypnea, seizures, cherry red or cyanotic skin
>60%	Coma; death generally ensues

*Percentage of hemoglobin molecules bound with carbon monoxide.

Cyanide poisoning occurs from inhalation of smoke by-products. Combustion of household synthetics (carpeting, plastics, vinyl flooring, upholstered furniture, and window coverings) are the primary source of exposure.[6,17] Cyanide impedes cellular respiration and oxygen utilization by binding with the cytochrome system of mitochondria, thereby inhibiting cell metabolism and adenosine triphosphate production.[17] The clinical symptoms of cyanide poisoning mimic carbon monoxide poisoning, and both may be present simultaneously.

Injury Above the Glottis

Inhalation injury above the glottis, also referred to as upper airway injury, is caused by breathing in heat or noxious chemicals produced during the burning process. The nose, mouth, and throat dissipate the heat and prevent damage to lower airways. However, the resulting upper airway thermal injury causes edema, thereby placing the patient at high risk for airway obstruction. Airway obstruction clinically presents as hoarseness, dry cough, labored or rapid breathing, difficulty swallowing, or stridor.

Injury Below The Glottis

Injury below the glottis is almost always caused by breathing noxious chemical byproducts of burning materials and smoke. Extensive damage to alveoli and impaired pulmonary functioning result from the injury (see Table 20-1 and box, "Clinical Alert: Clinical Indicators of Inhalation Injury"). A hallmark sign is *carbonaceous sputum* (soot or carbon particles in secretions). Tracheal and bronchial/bronchiolar constriction and spasms with resulting wheezing can occur within minutes to several hours after injury.[6] Acute respiratory failure and acute respiratory distress syndrome (ARDS) may develop within the first few days. Respiratory tract mucosal sloughing may occur within 4 to 5 days. Admission chest x-rays typically demonstrate normal findings. However, later x-rays may display reduced lung expansion, atelectasis,

and diffuse lung edema or infiltrates. Fiberoptic bronchoscopy or xenon ventilation-perfusion lung scanning may be indicated to provide a definitive diagnosis of injury below the glottis.[17,22,40]

BURN CLASSIFICATION AND SEVERITY

Burn injury severity is determined by the type of burn injury, burn wound characteristics (depth, extent, body part burned), concomitant injuries, patient age, and preexisting health status. Accurate classification and assessment of injury severity enables appropriate triage and transfer of patients to a burn center. The extent and depth of burn injury are affected by the duration of contact with the damaging agent, the temperature of the agent, the amount of tissue exposed, and the ability of the agent and tissue to dissipate the thermal energy.

Depth of Injury

Burn depth predicts wound care treatment requirements, determines the need for skin grafting, and affects scarring, cosmetic, and functional outcomes. Burn injuries are often classified as first-, second-, or third-degree burns. However, the terms *superficial, partial-thickness,* or *full-thickness* burns more closely correlate with the pathophysiology of burn injury and the level of affected skin layer involvement (see Figure 20-1). Accurate depth assessment may be difficult to determine initially, because progressive edema formation and compromised wound blood flow during the first 48 to 72 hours after injury may increase the definitive burn depth. In recent years laser Doppler imaging has emerged as a potentially useful depth assessment tool.[45]

Superficial burns involve only the first layer of skin or the epidermis (hence termed first-degree injury), and typically heal in 3 to 5 days without treatment. Because superficial burn injuries (e.g., sunburns) only cause erythema and do not involve the dermis, they are not included in the calculation of the size of the burn (extent of injury) used for fluid resuscitation requirements. *Partial-thickness* burns involve injury of the second skin layer or dermal layer (hence a second-degree injury), and are further subdivided into superficial and deep classifications. *Superficial partial-thickness* injuries that involve the epidermis and a limited portion of the dermis heal by growth of undamaged basal cells within 7 to 10 days. *Deep partial-thickness* injuries involve destruction of the epidermis and most of the dermis. Although such wounds may heal spontaneously within 2 to 4 weeks, they are typically excised and grafted to achieve better functional and cosmetic results, to decrease the length of healing time, and decrease hospitalization time.

Destruction of all layers of the skin down to or past the subcutaneous fat, fascia, muscles, or bone is defined as a *full-thickness* injury (third-degree injury). A thick, leathery, nonelastic, coagulated layer of necrotic tissue called *eschar* is created. The nerves are destroyed, resulting in a painless wound. These injuries always require skin grafting for permanent wound closure. Table 20-3 describes the

---

> **! CLINICAL ALERT**
>
> ### *Clinical Indicators of Inhalation Injury*
>
> - History of exposure in confined or enclosed space
> - Facial burns
> - Singed nasal hairs
> - Presence of soot around mouth and nose and in sputum (carbonaceous sputum)
> - Signs of hypoxemia (tachycardia, dysrhythmias, agitation, confusion, lethargy, loss of consciousness)
> - Abnormal breath sounds
> - Signs of respiratory difficulty (change in respiratory rate, use of accessory muscles, flaring nostrils, intercostal or sternal retractions, stridor, hoarseness, difficulty swallowing)
> - Elevated carboxyhemoglobin levels
> - Abnormal arterial blood gas values

TABLE 20-3   DEPTH OF BURN INJURY

DEGREE OF INJURY	MORPHOLOGY	HEALING TIME	WOUND CHARACTERISTICS
Superficial (first degree)	Destruction of epidermis only	3-5 days	Pink or red, dry, painful
Superficial partial-thickness (second degree)	Destruction of epidermis and some dermis	7-10 days	Moist, pink or mottled red; very painful; blisters; blanches briskly with pressure
Deep partial-thickness (second degree)	Destruction of epidermis and most of dermis; some skin appendages remain	2-4 weeks	Pale, mottled, pearly red/white; moist or somewhat dry; typically less painful; blanching decreased and prolonged; difficult to distinguish from full-thickness injury
Full-thickness (third degree)	Destruction of epidermis, dermis, and underlying subcutaneous tissue	Does not heal; requires skin grafting	Thick, leathery eschar; dry; white, cherry-red, or brown-black; painless; does not blanch with pressure; thrombosed blood vessels

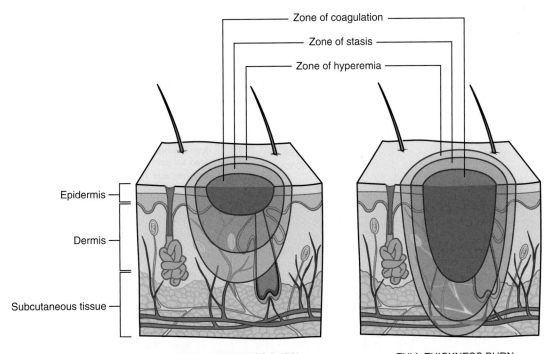

FIGURE 20-2 Zones of thermal injury.

characteristics of superficial, partial-thickness, and full-thickness burn injuries.

Differentiating partial-thickness from full-thickness injuries may initially be difficult because burn wounds mature or progress within the first few days. The three zones of thermal injury explain this phenomenon by illustrating the relationship of depth and extent of injury with damaged tissue viability (Figure 20-2). The outermost area of minimal cell injury is termed the *zone of hyperemia*. It has early spontaneous recovery and is similar to a superficial burn. The greatest area of tissue necrosis is at the core of the wound or the *zone of coagulation*. It is the site of irreversible skin death and is similar to a full-thickness burn. Peripheral to this area is a *zone of stasis*, where vascular damage and reduced blood flow have occurred. Secondary insults, such as inadequate resuscitation, edema, or infection, result in conversion of this potentially salvageable area to full-thickness skin destruction with irreversible tissue *necrosis* or death. Cutting-edge research on topical nanoemulsion therapy is showing promise as a novel intervention targeted at halting tissue destruction and burn depth conversion in the zone of stasis.[23] Nanoemulsions are tiny nanometer-sized (i.e., one billionth of a meter) broad-spectrum antimicrobial oil-in-water droplets that are mixed in a high-energy state and stabilized with surfactants. When nanoemulsions are topically applied to the wound, both the active antimicrobial ingredients and the high energy release destabilize the microbe membrane resulting in pathogen cell death. Nanoemulsions are effective because they are selectively toxic to pathogens, but are not irritating to skin or mucous membranes. Specifically in burns, nano-emulsion therapy attenuates wound inflammatory response and infection.[23]

Extent of Injury

The extent of injury or size of a burn is expressed as the percentage of *total body surface area* (%TBSA). The quickest method to initially calculate %TBSA is the *rule of nines*. This technique divides the TBSA into areas representing 9% or multiples of 9% (Figure 20-3). By summing all areas of partial- and full-thickness burns (superficial burns are not included), the %TBSA burned is quickly estimated. For evaluations of injury extent in irregular or scattered small burns, the size of the patient's palm (including fingers) is used for measurement and represents 1% TBSA.[6] The rule of nines varies between adult and pediatric patients because children have a proportionally larger head size compared with adults.

Another surface area assessment method, the *Lund and Browder chart* (Figure 20-4), provides a more accurate determination of the extent of burn injury by correlating body surface area with age-related proportions. This method is used most frequently in a burn center. Accurate calculation of extent of injury is important for assessing burn severity and for estimating fluid resuscitation requirements.

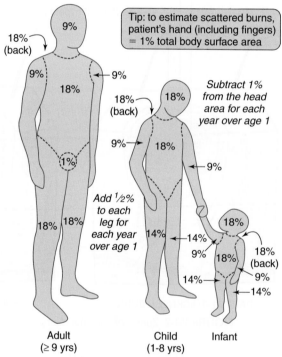

FIGURE 20-3 The rule of nines. *TBSA,* Total body surface area. (Courtesy University of Michigan Trauma Burn Center, Ann Arbor, MI.) EXAMPLE: An adult with superficial burns to the face and partial-thickness burns to the lower half of the right arm, entire left arm, and chest: 4.5% (lower right arm) + 9% (entire left arm) + 9% (chest or upper anterior trunk) = 22.5% TBSA (the superficial burns to the face are not included in the %TBSA calculation).

Burn Estimate and Diagram

Age vs. Area

Area	Birth 1 yr	1–4 yr	5–9 yr	10–14 yr	15 yr	Adult	2°	3°	Total	Donor Areas
Head	19	17	13	11	9	7				
Neck	2	2	2	2	2	2				
Ant. Trunk	13	13	13	13	13	13				
Post. Trunk	13	13	13	13	13	13				
R. Buttock	2 ½	2 ½	2 ½	2 ½	2 ½	2 ½				
L. Buttock	2 ½	2 ½	2 ½	2 ½	2 ½	2 ½				
Genitalia	1	1	1	1	1	1				
R. U. Arm	4	4	4	4	4	4				
L. U. Arm	4	4	4	4	4	4				
R. L. Arm	3	3	3	3	3	3				
L. L. Arm	3	3	3	3	3	3				
R. Hand	2 ½	2 ½	2 ½	2 ½	2 ½	2 ½				
L. Hand	2 ½	2 ½	2 ½	2 ½	2 ½	2 ½				
R. Thigh	5 ½	6 ½	8	8 ½	9	9 ½				
L. Thigh	5 ½	6 ½	8	8 ½	9	9 ½				
R. Leg	5	5	5 ½	6	6 ½	7				
L. Leg	5	5	5 ½	6	6 ½	7				
R. Foot	3 ½	3 ½	3 ½	3 ½	3 ½	3 ½				
L. Foot	3 ½	3 ½	3 ½	3 ½	3 ½	3 ½				
						Total				

Burn Diagram

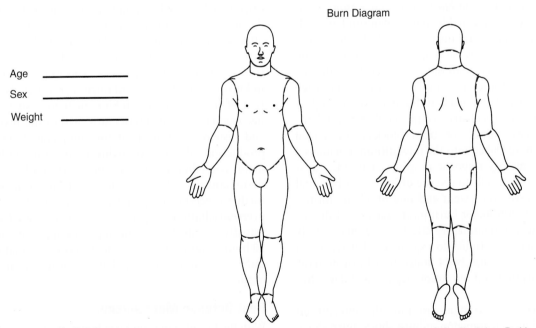

Age _____

Sex _____

Weight _____

FIGURE 20-4 Burn estimate and diagram. *Ant,* Anterior; *Post,* posterior; *L,* left; *R,* right; *R. U.,* right upper; *R. L.,* right lower; *L. U.,* left upper; *L. L.,* left lower.

PHYSIOLOGICAL RESPONSES TO BURN INJURY

The body responds to major burn injuries with significant hemodynamic, metabolic, and immunological effects that occur locally and systemically as a result of cellular damage from heat (Figures 20-5 and 20-6). The magnitude and duration of the systemic response and the degree of physiological changes are proportional to the extent of body surface area (%TBSA) injured. Direct thermal damage to blood vessels causes intravascular coagulation, with arterial and venous blood flow ceasing in the wound injury area. The damaged and ischemic cells release *mediators*, endogenously produced substances that the body secretes to initiate a protective inflammatory response. Mediators such as histamine, prostaglandins, bradykinins, catecholamines, and cytokines are stimulated and released, causing myriad vasoactive, cellular, and cardiovascular effects. Gaps between endothelial cells in vessel wall membranes develop, making vessel walls porous or "leaky." This *increased capillary membrane permeability* allows a significant shift of protein molecules, fluid, and electrolytes from the *intravascular space* (inside the blood vessels) into the *interstitium* (the space between cells and the vascular system) in a process also referred to as *third-spacing* (Figure 20-7). There is rapid and dramatic edema formation. Cellular swelling also occurs as a result of a decrease in cell transmembrane potential and a shift of extracellular sodium and water into the cell.[16,39] The leaking of proteins into the interstitium dramatically lowers intravascular *oncotic pressure*, which draws even more intravascular fluid into the interstitium and contributes to the development of edema and *burn shock* (shock from intravascular volume loss, created by the sudden fluid and solute shifts immediately after burn injury). In burns greater than 20% TBSA, the increased capillary permeability and edema formation process not only occur locally at the site of burn injury, but also systemically in distant unburned tissues and organs.[6,39] Edema is further exacerbated as lymph drainage flow is obstructed from either direct damage of lymphatic vessels or from blockage by serum proteins that have leaked into the interstitium. Edema is a natural inflammatory response to injury that aids transport of white blood cells to the site of injury for bacterial digestion; however, the extent and rate of edema formation associated with major burn injury far exceed the intended beneficial inflammatory effect.[2] A hallmark study found that edema continues to expand until it reaches a maximum at approximately 24 hours after burn injury.[18] Edema reabsorption and resolution begin 1 to 2 days after a burn injury.

Intravascular fluid volume lost into the interstitium causes the unique phenomenon of burn shock. Burn shock is described as a combination of *distributive* and *hypovolemic shock*. There is a distributive component because third-spacing greatly expands the area in which total body fluid is contained, to include the intravascular space plus intracellular and interstitial spaces. The hypovolemic component is caused by massive loss of intravascular fluid from increased vessel membrane permeability and evaporative losses through the open wound beds. Burn shock ensues when plasma or intravascular volume becomes insufficient to maintain circulatory support and adequate preload, causing cardiac output to decrease and impairing tissue perfusion. Fluid resuscitation is a crucial part of burn management because it directly replaces plasma fluid losses, fills the newly increased body fluid reservoir, and restores preload deficits.

In summary, significant burn injuries trigger local and systemic responses involving a multitude of complex mechanisms and cascades of physiological events that stress all body systems. The magnitude of physiological response is unique to burn injury and is characterized by dramatic shifts in intravascular fluid, mediator activation, hyperexaggerated inflammatory cascade reaction, and extensive edema formation. The specific organ system responses are summarized in the following sections and in Figure 20-6.

Cardiovascular Response

Loss of intravascular volume after major burn injury produces a decrease in cardiac output and oxygen delivery to the body tissues. The sympathetic nervous system is activated as a compensatory mechanism, with the release of catecholamines causing tachycardia and vasoconstriction to maintain arterial blood pressure. Tissue and multiorgan perfusion are altered when a redistribution of blood flow occurs early in the postburn period to perfuse essential organs such as the heart and brain. Early postburn, cardiac dysfunction is observed and exerts a negative inotropic effect on myocardial tissues. The magnitude of myocardial depression exceeds that which would be explained by intravascular fluid volume loss. The exact mechanism is unknown and is the topic of ongoing research. Local secretion of inflammatory cytokine mediators, such as tumor necrosis factor and interleukins, within the myocardium and systemic activation of the complement system with production of anaphylatoxins have been implicated as major contributors to this progressive cardiac contractile dysfunction.[30,36,39] Cardiac instability in burn patients is further exacerbated by underresuscitation (hypovolemia), overresuscitation (hypervolemia), or increased afterload. Impaired cardiac function improves approximately 24 to 30 hours after injury.[5,26,39] The purpose of initial postburn fluid resuscitation is to aid in restoring normal cardiac output.

Host Defense Mechanisms

With the loss of skin from burn injury, the primary barrier to microorganisms is destroyed. Tissue damage invokes simultaneous activation of all inflammatory response cascades, including the complement, fibrinolytic, clotting, and kinin

Text continued on p. 627

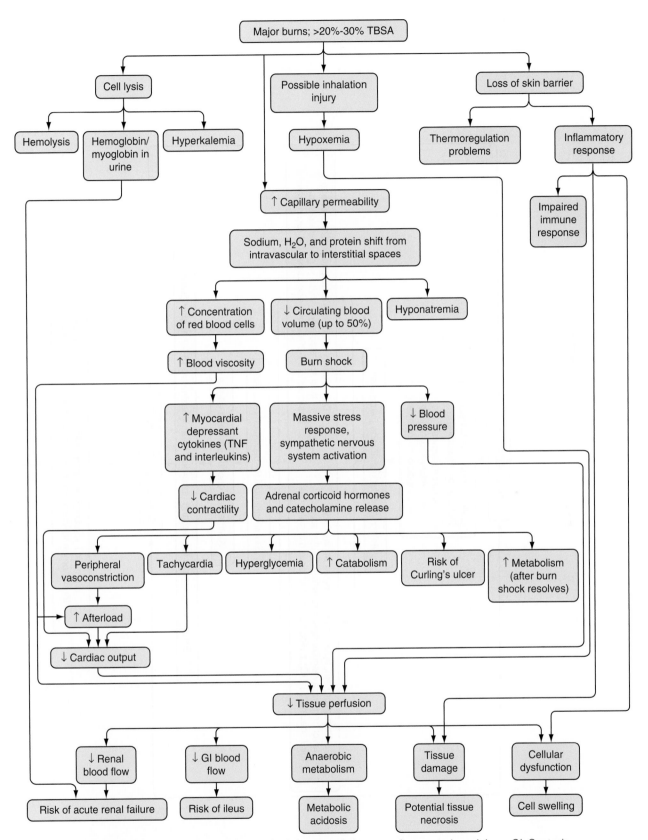

FIGURE 20-5 Overview of physiological changes that occur after acute burn injury. *GI,* Gastrointestinal; *H₂O,* water; *TBSA,* total body surface area; *TNF,* tumor necrosis factor. (Modified from Byers JF, LaBorde PJ. Management of patients with burn injury. In Smeltzer SC, Bare BG. eds. *Brunner & Suddarth's Textbook of Medical-Surgical Nursing.* 10th ed. Philadelphia: Lippincott Williams & Wilkins, 2004.)

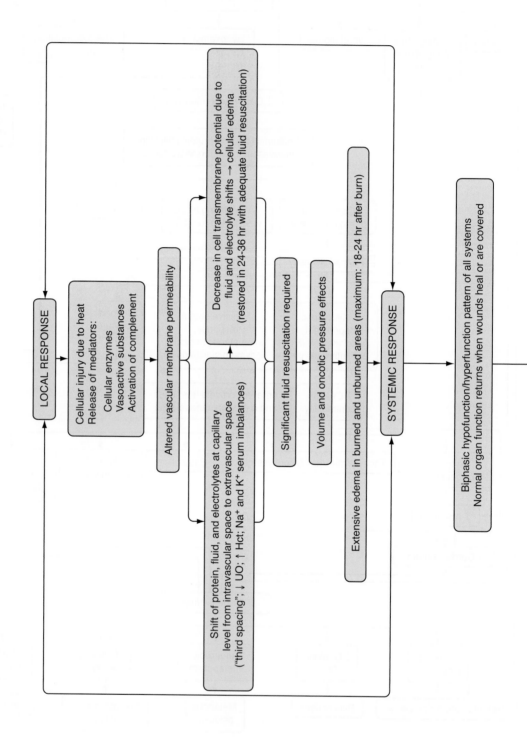

LOCAL RESPONSE

Cellular injury due to heat
Release of mediators:
Cellular enzymes
Vasoactive substances
Activation of complement

Altered vascular membrane permeability

Decrease in cell transmembrane potential due to fluid and electrolyte shifts → cellular edema (restored in 24-36 hr with adequate fluid resuscitation)

Shift of protein, fluid, and electrolytes at capillary level from intravascular space to extravascular space ("third spacing"; ↓ UO; ↑ Hct; Na⁺ and K⁺ serum imbalances)

Significant fluid resuscitation required

Volume and oncotic pressure effects

Extensive edema in burned and unburned areas (maximum: 18-24 hr after burn)

SYSTEMIC RESPONSE

Biphasic hypofunction/hyperfunction pattern of all systems
Normal organ function returns when wounds heal or are covered

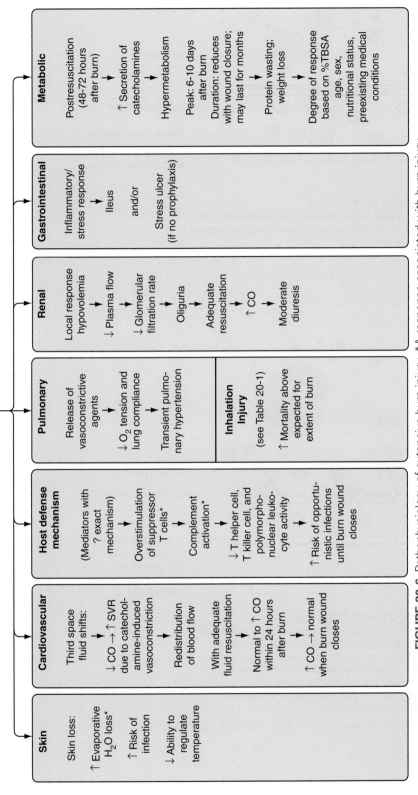

FIGURE 20-6 Pathophysiology of extensive burn injury. *A response associated with burn injury greater than 20% to 25% total body surface area (TBSA). *CO,* Cardiac output; *H₂O,* water; *Hct,* hematocrit; *K⁺,* potassium; *Na⁺,* sodium; *O₂,* oxygen; *SVR,* systemic vascular resistance; *UO,* urinary output.

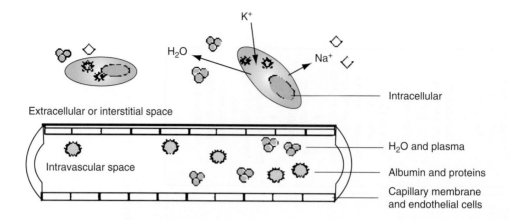

NORMAL PHYSIOLOGY BEFORE BURN INJURY
Intact capillary wall membranes keep large protein molecules within the blood vessels or intravascular space. This maintains normal protein oncotic pressure and retains intravascular fluid volume.

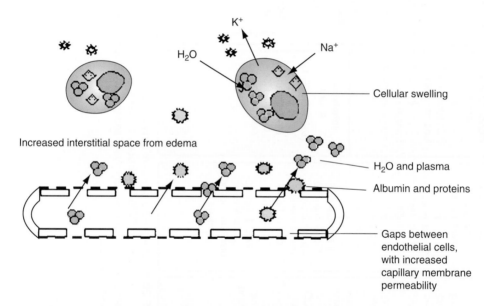

PHYSIOLOGICAL CHANGES FOLLOWING BURN INJURY
Gaps develop between endothelial cells causing increased capillary membrane permeability. Intravascular proteins and fluids flow into the interstitium in a process called third-spacing and produces tissue edema. Loss of intravascular proteins decreases intravascular oncotic pressure, pulls additional fluid into the interstitium, and reduces intravascular fluid volume. Decreased cell transmembrane potential shifts sodium into the cells, drawing in water and producing cellular swelling and further tissue edema.

FIGURE 20-7 Burn edema and shock development. H_2O, Water; K^+, potassium; Na^+, sodium.

systems. The exact mechanism by which postburn immune defects occur remains ambiguous, because inflammatory mediators and cytokines exert numerous, varied, and interrelated effects. However, the end results are overstimulation of suppressor T cells and depression of other components such as helper T cell, killer T cell, and polymorphonuclear leukocyte activity. This immunosuppression interferes with the ability of the patient's host defense mechanisms to fight invading microorganisms and thus places the patient at high risk of developing infection and sepsis.

Pulmonary Response

Release of vasoconstrictive mediator substances causes an initial transient pulmonary hypertension associated with a decrease in oxygen tension and lung compliance. This occurs in the absence of a lung injury and edema.[19,26] The impact of inhalation injury on the pulmonary system is described in Table 20-1.

Renal Response

The renal circulation is sensitive to decreasing cardiac output. Hypoperfusion and a decreased glomerular filtration rate signal the nephrons to initiate the renin-angiotensin-aldosterone cascade. Sodium and water are retained to preserve intravascular fluid in an attempt to increase cardiac preload. Oliguria occurs, and urine becomes more concentrated. If fluid resuscitation is inadequate, acute kidney injury can develop. With resuscitation, diuresis occurs approximately 48 hours after injury secondary to an increase in cardiac output.

Gastrointestinal Response

As a consequence of the inflammatory response and hypovolemia after major burn injury, the gastrointestinal (GI) circulation undergoes compensatory vasoconstriction and redistribution of blood flow to preserve perfusion to the brain and heart. The resulting ischemia of the stomach and duodenal mucosa places burn patients at high risk of developing a duodenal ulcer, called a *stress ulcer* or *Curling's ulcer*. GI motility or peristalsis is also decreased, creating a *paralytic ileus*. The ileus clinically presents as decreased bowel sounds, gastric distention, nausea, or vomiting.

Metabolic Response

Two phases of metabolic dysfunction occur after a major burn injury. First, a decreased response in organ function occurs, followed by a second phase of hypermetabolic and hyperfunctional response of all systems. Hypermetabolism begins as resuscitation is completed and is one of the most significant and persistent alterations observed after burn injury. The postburn hypermetabolic response is greater than that seen in any other forms of trauma.[22,24,40,48] Patients with severe burns have metabolic rates that are 100% to 200% above their basal rates, with some degree of elevation continuing for 1 to 2 years after injury.[21,22,24,48] The rapid metabolic rate is caused by the secretion of inflammatory response mediators or catabolic hormones, such as catecholamines, cortisol, and glucagon, in an effort to support tissue remodeling and repair.[24,26,40,47,48,50] The hypermetabolic state produces a catabolic effect on the body, with skeletal muscle breakdown, decreased protein synthesis, increased glucose utilization, and rapid depletion of glycogen stores.[21,24,40,47,48,50] The amount of protein wasting and weight loss that occurs is affected by several factors, including %TBSA burned, age, sex, preburn nutritional status, comorbidities, medical conditions, exercise, and nutrient intake. Wound closure reduces metabolic expenditure.[24,40,48]

PHASES OF BURN CARE ASSESSMENT AND COLLABORATIVE INTERVENTIONS

Assessment and management of the burn-injured patient is classified into three phases of care: (1) resuscitative, (2) acute, and (3) rehabilitative. The *resuscitative phase* or emergency phase begins at the time of injury and continues for approximately 48 hours until the massive fluid and protein shifts have stabilized. The primary focus of assessment and intervention is on maintenance of the ABCs (airway, breathing, and circulation) and prevention of burn shock. The resuscitative phase spans care in the prehospital setting, in the ED, and transfer to a burn center. With the onset of diuresis approximately 48 to 72 hours after injury, the *acute phase* begins and continues until wound closure occurs. This phase typically occurs in a burn center and may last for weeks or months. Nursing care focuses on the promotion of wound healing, the prevention of infections and complications, and the provision of psychosocial support. Although the critical care nurse is rarely involved in the *rehabilitative phase*, the care given in the first two phases is instrumental in achieving optimal final rehabilitative outcomes. The primary goals in the rehabilitative phase are to minimize scarring and contractures, to restore the patient's ability to function in society, and to return to an established family role and vocation.

Critical care activities usually occur in the resuscitative and acute phases. In both these phases, patient assessment and management are prioritized and guided by following the primary and secondary surveys as described in the Advanced Burn Life Support Course.[6] Pain control, wound management, infection control, special considerations for unique burn injuries, and psychosocial concerns are important issues throughout all the phases of burn care. See the "Nursing Care Plan for Resuscitative and Acute Care Phases of Major Burn Injury" for more information.

◎ **NURSING CARE PLAN**

for Resuscitative and Acute Care Phases of Major Burn Injury

NURSING DIAGNOSIS

Ineffective Airway Clearance and Impaired Gas Exchange related to tracheal edema or interstitial edema secondary to inhalation injury and/or circumferential torso eschar manifested by hypoxemia and hypercapnia

PATIENT OUTCOMES

Adequate airway clearance and gas exchange
- PaO_2 >90 mm Hg; $PaCO_2$ <45 mm Hg; SaO_2 >95%; COHgb <10%
- Respiration rate 16-20 breaths/min and unlabored; breath sounds present and clear in all lobes; chest wall excursion symmetrical and adequate
- Mentation clear; patient mobilizes secretions, which are clear to white

NURSING INTERVENTIONS	RATIONALES
• Monitor SpO_2 every hour, ABG and COHgb prn; chest x-ray study as ordered	• Assess oxygenation and ventilation
• Assess respiratory rate, character, and depth every hour; breath sounds every 4 hours; LOC every hour; if not intubated, assess for stridor, hoarseness, and wheezing every hour	• Evaluate respiratory status and response to treatment
• Administer 100% humidified oxygen as ordered	• Expedite elimination of carbon monoxide and prevent/treat hypoxemia; humidity decreases viscosity of secretions
• Evaluate need for chest escharotomy during fluid resuscitation	• Releasing eschar by escharotomy improves ventilation and oxygenation by alleviating constricted chest wall movement
• Assist patient in coughing and deep breathing every hour while awake; suction as needed; monitor sputum characteristics and amount	• Promote lung expansion, ventilation, clearing of secretions, and maintaining clear airway
• Turn every 2 hours to mobilize secretions; out of bed as tolerated	• Promote lung expansion and ventilation
• Elevate head of bed	• Decrease edema of face, neck, and mouth
• Schedule activities to avoid fatigue	• Decrease ventilatory effort

NURSING DIAGNOSIS

Deficient fluid volume secondary to fluid shifts into the interstitium and evaporative loss of fluids from the injured skin

PATIENT OUTCOMES

Adequate fluid volume
- Heart rate 80-120 bpm
- BP adequate in relation to pulse and urine output
- RAP/CVP/PAOP at upper ends of normal range
- Sensorium clear
- Optimal tissue perfusion
- Nonburn skin warm and pink
- Hourly urine output 30-50 mL/hr; 75-100 mL/hr in electrical injury
- Weight gain based on volume of fluids given in first 48 hours, followed by diuresis over next 3-5 days
- Serum laboratory values WNL; specific gravity normal except during diuresis; urine negative for glucose and ketones

NURSING INTERVENTIONS	RATIONALES
• Monitor: vital signs and urine output every hour until stable; mental status every hour for at least 48 hours	• Assess perfusion and oxygenation status
• Titrate calculated fluid requirements in first 48 hours to maintain urinary output and hemodynamic stability	• Restore intravascular volume. Urine output closely reflects renal perfusion and overall tissue perfusion status
• Record daily weight and hourly intake/output measurements; evaluate trends	• Evaluate fluid loss and replacement
• Monitor serum electrolytes, Hct, Hgb, serum glucose, BUN, serum creatinine levels at least twice daily for first 48 hours and then as required by patient status	• Evaluate need for electrolyte and fluid replacement associated with large fluid and protein shifts

⊚ NURSING CARE PLAN

for Resuscitative and Acute Care Phases of Major Burn Injury—cont'd

NURSING DIAGNOSIS

Risk for hypothermia related to loss of skin and/or external cooling

PATIENT OUTCOME

Normothermia

* Rectal/core temperature 37° C (98.6° F) to 38.5° C (101.3° F)

NURSING INTERVENTIONS	RATIONALES
• Monitor and document rectal/core temperature every 1 to 2 hours; assess for shivering	• Evaluate body temperature status
• Minimize skin exposure; maintain environmental temperatures	• Prevent evaporative and conductive losses
• For temperature <37° C (98.6° F), institute rewarming measures	• Prevent complications

NURSING DIAGNOSIS

Ineffective tissue perfusion related to compression and impaired vascular circulation in extremities with circumferential burns

PATIENT OUTCOMES

Adequate tissue perfusion

* Peripheral pulses present and strong
* Warm, dry extremities
* No tissue injury in extremities secondary to inadequate perfusion from edema or eschar

NURSING INTERVENTIONS	RATIONALES
• Assess peripheral pulses and perfusion every hour for 72 hours; notify physician of changes in pulses, capillary refill, color, temperature, or pain sensation	• Assess peripheral perfusion and the need for escharotomy
• Elevate upper extremities with IV poles or on pillows; elevate lower extremities on pillows	• Decrease edema formation
• Be prepared to assist with escharotomy or fasciotomy	• Escharotomy/fasciotomy allows for edema expansion and permits peripheral perfusion

NURSING DIAGNOSIS

Acute pain related to burn trauma

PATIENT OUTCOMES

Relief of pain

* Identifies factors that contribute to pain
* Reports improved comfort level
* Physiological parameters WNL and remain stable after administration of narcotic analgesia

NURSING INTERVENTIONS	RATIONALES
• Assess type, location, quality, and severity of pain	• Pain responses are variable and unique to each patient
• Monitor physiological responses to pain, such as ↑BP, ↑HR, restlessness, and nonverbal cues. Use validated tools to assess pain and anxiety	
• Allay fear and anxiety	• Fear and anxiety may intensify perception of pain
• Administer analgesic and/or anxiolytic medication as ordered; administer IV during critical care phases	• Facilitate pain relief. IM medications not consistently absorbed
• Assess response to analgesics or other interventions	• Evaluate effectiveness of interventions
• Medicate patient before bathing, dressing changes, and major procedures as needed	• Assist patient to perform at higher level of function
• Minimize open exposure of wounds	• Exposed nerve endings increase pain
• Use nonpharmacological pain-reducing methods (distraction, relaxation techniques) as appropriate	• Reduce need for narcotics

◎ NURSING CARE PLAN

for Resuscitative and Acute Care Phases of Major Burn Injury—cont'd

NURSING DIAGNOSIS

Risk for infection related to loss of skin, impaired immune response, and invasive therapies

PATIENT OUTCOMES

Absence of infection

- No inflamed burn wound margins
- No evidence of burn wound, donor site, or invasive catheter site infection
- Autograft or allograft skin is adherent to healthy tissue
- Body temperature WNL
- White blood cell and platelet counts WNL
- Sputum, blood, and urine cultures negative
- Glycosuria, hyperglycemia, vomiting, ileus, diarrhea, and/or change in mentation absent

NURSING INTERVENTIONS	RATIONALES
• Assess temperature, vital signs, and characteristics of urine and sputum every 1 to 4 hours; monitor WBC, platelets, burn wound healing, and invasive catheter sites	• Evaluate effectiveness of treatments and interventions; facilitate early detection of developing infections
• Use appropriate protective isolation; provide meticulous wound care with antimicrobial topical agents as ordered; shave hair (except eyebrows) 1 inch around burn wounds; adhere to CDC guidelines for invasive catheter care; instruct visitors in burn unit guidelines	• Prevent infection by decreasing exposure to pathogens; hair is a medium for microorganism growth; proper hand washing and use of protective barriers decrease contamination
• Obtain wound, sputum, urine, and blood cultures as ordered	• Determine infection source and specific invading microorganism to guide topical/systemic antimicrobial therapy

NURSING DIAGNOSES

Risk for injury: gastrointestinal bleeding related to stress response

Imbalanced Nutrition: Less Than Body Requirements related to ileus and increased metabolic demands secondary to physiological stress and wound healing

PATIENT OUTCOMES

Absence of injury and adequate nutrition

- Decreased gastric motility and ileus resolved
- No evidence of GI hemorrhaging
- Enteral feedings absorbed and tolerated
- Daily requirement of nutrients consumed
- Positive nitrogen balance
- Progressive wound healing
- 90% of preburn weight maintained

NURSING INTERVENTIONS	RATIONALES
• Place NG tube for gastric decompression in >20% TBSA burns	• Prevent nausea, emesis, and aspiration from ileus
• Assess abdomen and bowel sounds every 8 hours	• Evaluate resolution of decreased gastric motility and ileus
• Assess NG aspirate (color, quantity, pH, and guaiac); monitor stool guaiac	• Facilitate early detection of GI bleeding
• Administer stress ulcer prophylaxis	• Prevent stress ulcer development
• Consult dietician. Initiate enteral feeding, and evaluate tolerance; provide high-calorie/protein supplements prn; record all oral intake and count calories	• Caloric/protein intake must be adequate to maintain positive nitrogen balance and promote healing
• Schedule interventions and activities to avoid interrupting feeding times	• Pain, fatigue, or sedation interferes with desire to eat
• Monitor weight daily or biweekly	• Assess tolerance and response to feeding interventions

◎ NURSING CARE PLAN

for Resuscitative and Acute Care Phases of Major Burn Injury—cont'd

NURSING DIAGNOSIS
Impaired Physical Mobility and self-care deficit related to burn injury, therapeutic splinting, and immobilization requirements after skin graft, and/or contractures

PATIENT OUTCOMES
Physical mobility
- Demonstrates ability to care for burn wounds
- No evidence of permanent decreased joint function
- Verbalizes understanding of plan of care
- Vocation resumed without functional limitations, or adjustment to new vocation

NURSING INTERVENTIONS	RATIONALES
• Perform active and passive ROM exercises to extremities every 2 hours while awake. Increase activity as tolerated. Reinforce importance of maintaining proper joint alignment with splints and antideformity positioning	• Prevent contractures and loss of movement/function
• Elevate extremities	• Decrease edema and promote ROM and mobility
• Provide pain relief measures before self-care activities and OT/PT	• Facilitate mobility and assist patient to perform at a higher level of function
• Explain procedures, interventions, and tests in clear, simple, age-appropriate language	• Patient more likely to participate and adhere to treatment plan if the purpose is understood
• Promote use of adaptive devices as needed to assist in self-care and mobility	• Decrease dependency on caregivers

NURSING DIAGNOSIS
Risk for ineffective individual coping and disabled family coping related to acute stress of critical injury and potential life-threatening crisis

PATIENT OUTCOMES
Effective coping
- Verbalizes goals of treatment regimen
- Demonstrates knowledge of support systems
- Able to express concerns and fears
- Patient's and family's coping is functional and realistic for phase of hospitalization; family processes at precrisis level

NURSING INTERVENTIONS	RATIONALES
• Orient patient and family to unit guidelines and support services; provide written information and reinforce frequently; involve in plan of care; support adaptive and functional coping mechanisms	• Decrease fear and anxiety and enhance feelings of control and self-worth; reinforce verbal information provided to patient and family
• Implement interventions to reduce fatigue and pain	• Adequate pain control and rest facilitate patient coping
• Consult social worker for assistance in discharge planning and psychosocial assessment issues; consult psychiatric services for inadequate coping skills or substance abuse treatment; promote use of group support sessions	• Provide expert consultation and intervention; assist patient and family in understanding experiences and reactions after burn injury and methods of dealing with trauma

ABG, Arterial blood gas; *BP,* blood pressure; *bpm,* beats per minute; *BUN,* blood urea nitrogen; *CDC,* Centers for Disease Control and Prevention; *CO,* carbon monoxide; *COHgb,* carboxyhemoglobin; *CVP,* central venous pressure; *GI,* gastrointestinal; *Hct,* hematocrit; *Hgb,* hemoglobin; *HR,* heart rate; *IV,* intravenous; *IM,* intramuscular; *LOC,* level of consciousness; *NG,* nasogastric; *OT/PT,* occupational therapy/physical therapy; *PaCO$_2$,* partial pressure of arterial carbon dioxide; *PaO$_2$,* partial pressure of arterial oxygen; *PAOP,* pulmonary artery occlusion pressure; *prn,* as required; *RAP,* right atrial pressure; *ROM,* range of motion; *SaO$_2$,* arterial oxygen saturation; *SpO$_2$,* arterial oxygen saturation via pulse oximetry; *TBSA,* total body surface area; *WBC,* white blood cell count; *WNL,* within normal limits.
Based on data from Gulanick M and Myers JL. *Nursing Care Plans: Diagnoses, Interventions, and Outcomes.* 7th ed. St. Louis: Mosby; 2011.

Resuscitative Phase: Prehospital
Primary Survey

Prehospital personnel (e.g., emergency medical technicians, flight nurses) are the first healthcare providers to arrive at the scene of injury. Care rendered in the first few hours after a significant burn injury greatly affects the patient's likelihood of survival. The priorities of prehospital care and management are to extricate the patient safely, stop the burning process, identify life-threatening injuries, and minimize time on the scene by rapidly transporting the patient to an appropriate care facility. As with any other type of trauma, the primary survey is used to provide a fast systematic assessment that prioritizes evaluation of the patient's airway, breathing, and circulatory status (Figure 20-8).

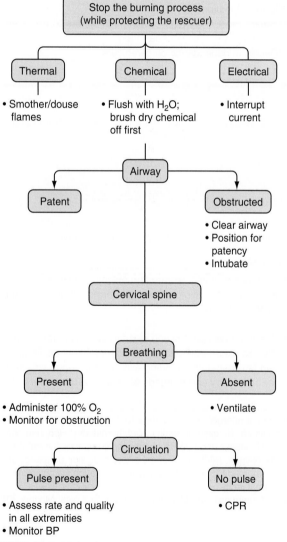

FIGURE 20-8 Major burn injury: primary survey. *BP,* Blood pressure; *CPR,* cardiopulmonary resuscitation; *H_2O,* water; *O_2,* oxygen.

Stopping the burning process. The first priority of patient care is to stop the burning process by removing the patient from the source of burning while preventing further injury.[6] It is crucial that this step be performed safely but quickly, because interventions aimed at stopping the burning should not delay the next assessment phases of the primary survey.

Flame burns are extinguished by rolling the patient on the ground, smothering the flames with a blanket or other cover, or dousing the flames with water. Ice is never applied to the wounds because further tissue damage may occur as a result of vasoconstriction and hypothermia. Jewelry is immediately removed because metal retains heat and can cause continued burning. Scald, tar, and asphalt burns are treated by immediate removal of the saturated clothing or immediate cooling with water if available, or both. No attempt is made to remove adherent tar at the scene. Adherent clothing (clothing that is burned into and stuck to the skin) is not removed because increased tissue damage and bleeding may occur; however, water is applied to cool the clothing material. Immediate treatment of electrical injuries involves prompt removal of the patient from the electrical source while protecting the rescuer. The burning process of chemical injuries continues as long as the chemical is in contact with the skin. All clothing is immediately removed, and water lavage is instituted before and during transport. Powdered chemicals are first brushed from the clothing and skin before lavage is performed. Clean water is the lavage solution of choice. If the chemical is in or near the eyes, contact lenses are removed (if present), and the eyes are irrigated with saline or clean water. Cross-contamination of the opposite eye is prevented during lavage by irrigating in the direction from inner to outer canthus. Neutralizing agents are not used on chemical burns. When neutralizing agents come in contact with chemicals, heat is produced and further increases the depth of injury. Healthcare providers must prevent exposure to themselves during initial treatment and lavage of chemical injuries by wearing protective barrier garments such as plastic gowns, gloves, goggles, and a face shield.

Airway (with cervical spine precautions). A history of the injury event occurring in a closed space alerts the clinician to the high potential for inhalation injury. Any suspicion of inhalation injury requires immediate intervention for airway control while maintaining cervical spine immobilization precautions (if indicated by the injury event). Refer to the box, "Clinical Alert: Clinical Indicators of Inhalation Injury," for findings indicative of pulmonary injury. Respiratory stridor indicates airway obstruction and mandates immediate endotracheal intubation at the scene. Patients with severe facial burns are prophylactically intubated because delayed or later endotracheal intubation will be difficult or impossible as edema develops (Figure 20-9).

Breathing. The half-life of carbon monoxide is reduced to 45 to 60 minutes in the presence of an oxygen concentration of 100% (versus a half-life of 4 hours in the presence of room air). Therefore all patients with suspected smoke inhalation

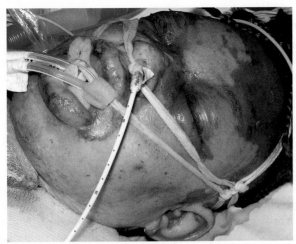

FIGURE 20-9 Facial edema. (Courtesy University of Michigan Trauma Burn Center, Ann Arbor, MI.)

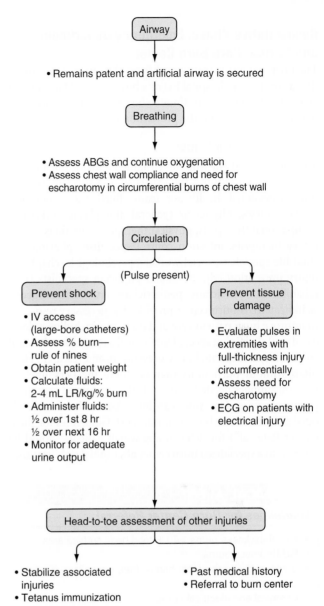

FIGURE 20-10 Major burn injury: secondary survey. *ABG*, Arterial blood gas; *ECG*, electrocardiogram; *IV*, intravenous; *LR*, lactated Ringer's solution.

are treated at the scene with 100% humidified oxygen delivered by non-rebreathing face mask or endotracheal tube. Patients are monitored for clinical signs of decreasing oxygenation such as changes in respiratory rate or neurological status. Pulse oximetry may not be accurate in acute inhalation injuries because the pulse oximeter cannot distinguish between carbon monoxide versus oxygen attached to the hemoglobin.

Circulation. All clothing and jewelry are removed to prevent constriction and ischemia to distal extremities secondary to edema formation during fluid resuscitation. Intravenous (IV) therapy is initiated with insertion of two large-bore (14- or 16-gauge) IV lines, preferably through nonburned tissue, and infusion of lactated Ringer's (LR) solution.[6] The patient is closely monitored for signs of hypovolemia such as changes in level of consciousness, rapid or thready pulses, decreased blood pressure, or narrowing pulse pressure. Burn injury rarely results in hypovolemic shock in the very early prehospital phase. If evidence of shock is present, then associated internal or external injury must be suspected.

Heat loss occurs rapidly in a major burn injury because the protective covering of skin is lost. The burned patient is covered with a clean, dry sheet and blankets to prevent hypothermia and further contamination of the wounds.

Secondary Survey

The secondary survey in the prehospital setting is brief and should not delay transport to a hospital. A rapid head-to-toe assessment to rule out any additional trauma is completed as part of the secondary survey (Figure 20-10). Patients with an injury mechanism suggestive of the potential for spinal injury (e.g., jumping from a burning building, electrical injury, explosion) have a cervical collar applied and are placed on a backboard before transport. Often, the patient is the most alert during this initial period after the injury. Therefore an accurate history of the events that led to the burn injury is

obtained, including the date and time of injury, the source of burns, and any events leading to the injury. Acquiring a brief medical history is beneficial, including allergies, current medical problems and medications taken, past surgical procedures and/or trauma, time of last meal, and history of tetanus immunization.[6]

In preparation for transport, a short-acting narcotic such as morphine sulfate may be administered IV for pain relief. No intramuscular medications are given during the resuscitative phase because perfusion of edematous tissues is poor and produces sporadic narcotic absorption. The patient should not receive anything by mouth before and during transport, to prevent vomiting and aspiration.

Resuscitative Phase: Emergency Department and Critical Care Burn Center

The burn patient is transferred from the injury scene to either a community hospital ED or a burn center. Management goals at either facility continue to be restoration and maintenance of the ABCs and the prevention of burn shock.

Transfer to a Burn Center

The care of a patient who has sustained a major burn injury is complex and requires the expertise of a specially trained multiprofessional healthcare team. Burn team members include nurses, physicians (general and plastic surgeons), occupational therapists, physical therapists, dietitians, respiratory therapists, infection control specialists, pharmacists, child life specialists, social workers, psychologists, chaplains, injury prevention educators, and physician specialists (e.g., rehabilitation physicians, pediatricians, and neurosurgeons as indicated). A burn center provides the necessary resources to improve burn patient care and outcome, including a dedicated staff delivering specialized clinical care, prehospital and community education, injury prevention, and research. Hospitals without burn units may not have the personnel or medical supplies needed to provide the specialized care these patients require. The American Burn Association has developed guidelines (see box, "Clinical Alert: Guidelines for Burn Center Referral") for determining which patients should be referred to a specialized burn center after initial stabilization.[6]

! CLINICAL ALERT

Guidelines for Burn Center Referral

- Partial-thickness burns >10% total body surface area
- Full-thickness burns
- Burns involving the face, hands, feet, genitalia, perineum, or major joints
- Chemical and electrical burns
- Inhalation injury
- Preexisting medical disorders
- Associated trauma
- Hospitals without qualified personnel or equipment to care for burn-injured children
- Patients requiring special social, emotional, or rehabilitative intervention

---

When transfer to a burn center is considered, the referring physician must make direct contact with the burn center physician. The burn center and referring physician collaborate to the mode of transportation (ground ambulance or air) and the treatment necessary to stabilize the patient for transport.[6] Transport is optimally done early in the postburn period during the resuscitative phase, based on guidelines provided by the receiving burn center. The use of a transfer form to summarize information concerning a burn patient's status promotes good communication between the referring and receiving facilities and ensures continuity of care.[6]

Primary Survey

On arrival to either the ED or the burn center, the primary survey is reassessed. Once the patient has arrived in the critical care burn unit, primary and secondary assessments are again performed.

Airway. Ineffective airway clearance related to tracheal edema may occur early, or it may not be apparent until after fluid resuscitation is initiated. Patients with suspected inhalation injuries who are not already intubated must be monitored frequently for hoarseness, stridor, or wheezing. Because massive edema formation is an anticipated response to fluid resuscitation in an extensively burned patient, patients with severe facial burns are intubated as a precaution. The presence of other symptoms suggestive of inhalation injury (see box, "Clinical Alert: Clinical Indicators of Inhalation Injury") necessitates early intubation to maintain adequate oxygenation and perfusion. Fiberoptic bronchoscopy may be performed to confirm the presence of inhalation injury. If the patient is already intubated, accurate tube position is assessed. The endotracheal tube is securely tied (not taped) in place to prevent accidental extubation (see Figure 20-9). Protecting the artificial airway is critical because it may be impossible to reintubate a patient successfully in the presence of massive edema and airway obstruction, thereby necessitating an emergency cricothyroidotomy or tracheostomy. Care must be taken to prevent tube ties from placing pressure on burned ears. The head of the patient's bed is elevated to reduce facial and airway edema.

Breathing. Assessment for impaired gas exchange related to carbon monoxide poisoning, cyanide poisoning or inhalation injury is important. Breath sounds, characteristics of respirations, work of breathing, sputum color and consistency, and symmetry of chest wall excursion are evaluated. Arterial blood gases and COHgb are measured when inhalation injury is suspected. Humidified 100% oxygen is administered via face mask or endotracheal tube until COHgb levels are determined. Once COHgb levels have normalized (lower than 5% to 10%), the 100% oxygen is weaned as tolerated, as demonstrated by maintaining a PaO_2 greater than 90 mm Hg, SaO_2 greater than 95%, and unlabored respirations. Cyanide poisoning also resolves rapidly with the administration of 100% oxygen and resuscitation.[6] Due to cyanide testing not being readily available in most hospitals, additional treatment is initiated when injury history and clinical symptoms indicate a high suspicion for cyanide poisoning. Patients who symptoms of respiratory compromise do not respond to 100% oxygen should be treated with commercially available cyanide antidote kits.[6] If the patient has a circumferential full-thickness burn of the thorax, the nurse assesses for adequate ventilatory effort because edema and restrictive eschar may inhibit chest wall expansion. Young children are particularly prone to this complication because their thoracic walls are more pliable. Therefore an immediate chest wall *escharotomy* may be indicated to facilitate breathing (Figure 20-11). An escharotomy is an incision performed at the bedside through a full-thickness burn to

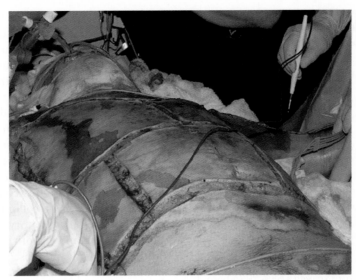

FIGURE 20-11 Escharotomy. (Courtesy University of Michigan Trauma Burn Center, Ann Arbor, MI.)

reduce constriction caused by the tight nonelastic band of eschar. This relieves pressure and restores ventilation, and blood flow. Local anesthesia is not required because the full-thickness burn eschar is painless. This procedure should be done only in consultation with the burn center. Ongoing assessment of breath sounds, arterial blood gases, and ventilatory status is crucial. All patients with inhalation injuries receive assistance with coughing, deep breathing, suctioning, and repositioning at least every 2 hours. Pulse oximetry and end-tidal carbon dioxide monitoring occur continuously as appropriate. Advancing technology in ventilator management, such as high-frequency ventilation and airway pressure release ventilation, have provided new promising options in inhalation injury treatment.[37,40,41] Emerging research also suggests nebulization therapy with administration of aerosolized heparin and Beta-2-adrenergic agonist agents (albuterol, terbutaline) to open airways and to reduce inflammatory response effects may be beneficial treatment adjuncts.[37,40]

Circulation

Fluid resuscitation. Fluid resuscitation is a critical intervention for burn management. To estimate fluid resuscitation requirements, the depth and extent of injury are assessed. Fluid resuscitation requirements are estimated according to body weight in kilograms, the %TBSA burned, and the patient's age. IV fluid resuscitation is instituted in patients with burns greater than 20% TBSA because these burns are associated with a diffuse capillary leak, large intravascular fluid loss, and ileus. Patients with smaller %TBSA burns may be resuscitated with oral hydration.

One of the most widely used burn resuscitation fluid formulas is the *Parkland formula*. It provides an approximation of fluid replacement requirements by calculating the amount of lactated Ringer's (LR) solution to infuse during the first 24 hours postburn at 4 mL/kg/%TBSA. Half of the calculated amount is given over the first 8 hours after injury, and the remaining half is given over the next 16 hours. A revised version of the Parkland formula, called the *Advanced Burn Life Support (ABLS) Fluid Resuscitation Formula,* is advocated by the Advanced Burn Life Support Course.[6] The ABLS Fluid Resuscitation Formulas outlined in Box 20-1 specify the fluid requirements for adults, children, and high voltage electrical injuries during the initial 24 hours after the burn.

Two large-bore (14- to 16-gauge) peripheral IV lines are inserted. If an unburned location is not available, the IV lines are placed through burned skin. Central venous catheters are commonly inserted in patients with major burns to facilitate and accommodate large IV fluid infusion requirements. LR solution is the preferred initial IV fluid for burn resuscitation.[2,6,39] It is a crystalloid that has an osmolality and electrolyte composition most similar to normal body physiological fluids, and it does not contain dextrose, which can cause a misleading high urine output from glycosuria and osmotic diuresis. In addition, LR contains lactate, which helps to buffer the metabolic acidosis associated with hypoperfusion and burn shock. Because LR is a crystalloid, it does not provide any intravascular protein replacement to increase intravascular oncotic pressure. In the presence of increased capillary membrane permeability, the intravascular retention of LR is only about 25% of the infused volume, necessitating large fluid volume infusions to maintain circulating blood volume.

Fluid requirements calculated by the ABLS Fluid Resuscitation Formulas serve only as a guide for estimating initial fluid needs. Each patient reacts differently to burn injury and requires varying amounts of IV fluid to support perfusion. The patient's requirements for fluid resuscitation are affected by several factors including age, depth of burn, concurrent inhalation injury, preexisting disease or comorbidities, delay in burn injury and resuscitation treatment, use of methamphetamine or other polysubstances, and associated injuries.

BOX 20-1   BURN FLUID RESUSCITATION FORMULAS

First 24 Hours Administer
ABLS Resuscitation Formulas (Based on the Parkland Formula)
- *In adults:* LR, 2 mL/kg/%TBSA*
- *In adults with high voltage electrical injuries:* LR, 4 mL/kg/%TBSA*
- *In children 14 years and younger and 10 to 40 kg:* LR, 3 mL/kg/%TBSA*
- *In infants less than 10 kg:* D_5LR, 3 mL/kg/%TBSA*
*%TBSA of second and third degree burns
- Half given over the first 8 hours after injury and the remaining half given over the next 16 hours
- Titrate fluids to maintain urine output of 0.5 mL/kg/hr, or 30 to 50 mL/hr in adults and 1 mL/kg/hr in children weighing <40 kg

Example: For an adult weighing 75 kg with a 55% TBSA burn and electrical injury:
- 4 mL LR × 75 kg × 55% TBSA = 16,500 mL of LR infused over 24 hours
- First 8 hours after burn injury: 8200 mL of LR infused over 8 hours or 1031.25 mL/hr
- Next 16 hours after burn injury: 8200 mL of LR infused over 16 hours or 515.6 mL/hr

Second 24 Hours Administer
Parkland Formula
- Dextrose in water, plus potassium to maintain normal electrolyte balance
- Colloid-containing fluid at 20% to 60% of calculated plasma volume, which equals an infusion rate of approximately 0.35 to 0.5 mL/kg/%TBSA

ABLS, Advanced Burn Life Support; *LR,* lactated Ringer's solution; *TBSA,* total body surface area.

Inhalation injuries increase the extent of %TBSA injury, and these patients typically require more resuscitation fluids. Larger fluid resuscitation volumes are also required in patients with electrical injuries to prevent acute tubular necrosis by clearing the renal tubules from precipitating myoglobin caused by skeletal muscle damage or *rhabdomyolysis.* Children also require relatively more resuscitation fluid because they have a greater ratio of body surface area to mass than that of adults, and higher evaporative losses. Because evaporative fluid losses continue until burn wounds are closed, these losses are calculated as a part of the total daily maintenance fluid replacement formula.

Colloids, such as albumin, contain proteins and are sometimes used in burn resuscitation to increase intravascular oncotic pressure. The increase in intravascular oncotic pressure pulls fluid from the interstitium back into the circulating intravascular volume, thereby reducing edema and combating burn shock. However, during increased permeability, colloids leak into the interstitium and contribute to further intravascular fluid loss. If colloids are used during burn resuscitation, it is generally advocated that they not be administered within the first 12 hours of burn injury when capillary permeability is at its highest level.[2,15,39,43] Increased crystalloid infusion alone is incapable of restoring cardiac preload in burn shock and can cause deleterious compartment syndrome complications. Therefore recent research has focused on the administration of colloids and alternative fluids to ameliorate the inflammatory response, such as high-dose antioxidant vitamin C; both of these may decrease overall fluid requirements and subsequently edema.[5,15,26,30,31,39,40,43] Another novel approach being studied is the use of hemofiltration for clearance of proinflammatory and antiinflammatory mediators to restore capillary integrity and to diminish the effects of burn shock, thereby reducing resuscitation fluid requirements.[5]

During the second 24 hours postinjury, when capillary permeability has decreased, a fluid formula such as the Parkland formula (see Box 20-1), which incorporates colloids, dextrose, and electrolyte replacement, may be used. Hypertonic dextrose solutions and colloids increase oncotic pressure, which helps pull third-spaced fluid from the interstitium back into the circulatory system. Potassium is added to IV fluids to replace potassium losses in the urine.

End point monitoring. Assessment of fluid volume status related to changes in capillary permeability is essential. The goal of burn resuscitation is to maintain tissue perfusion and organ function while preventing the complications of inadequate or excessive fluid therapy.[2,5,6,39] Resuscitation fluid infusion rates are titrated to specific measured outcomes of patient response, known as physiological end points.[2] During burn shock resuscitation, IV crystalloids or colloids, or both, are administered according to ABLS Fluid Resuscitation Formulas with normalization of urine output and blood pressure used as the hemodynamic end points to titrate fluids. A urinary catheter is inserted to evaluate resuscitation adequacy. IV infusion rates are adjusted to ensure a urinary output of 30 to 50 mL/hr in adults and 1 mL/kg of body weight per hour in children weighing less than 40 kg. Recent research findings indicate use of an hourly ratio (I/O) comparing fluid infusion to urine output may indicate failing resuscitation and need for alternative interventions more quickly than urine output alone.[31] During the resuscitation phase, steady increases or decreases in IV resuscitation rates are performed, rather than administration of fluid boluses.[2] See the box, Evidence-Based Practice, about burn shock resuscitation.

EVIDENCE-BASED PRACTICE

Burn Shock Resuscitation

Problem

Compared with other critical care patient populations, the burn-injured population constitutes a relatively small number of patients. Consequently, there are limited numbers of major burn centers in the United States, and they are typically separated by great geographical distances. These facts greatly impact research investigations and the ability to generate rigorous guidelines and standards for evidence-based practice specifically pertinent to burn care. As a result, burn shock resuscitation has been an ongoing topic of extensive discussion and debate over the past few decades, with questions arising regarding the best practice for which types of fluids to administer, the role and timing of colloid use, and which specific monitoring end points to use. National trends in avoiding colloid use and increasing total amounts of fluids administered (deemed "fluid creep") have been criticized as contributing to an increased incidence of intraabdominal hypertension (IAH), abdominal compartment syndrome and poor patient outcomes. However, definitions of IAH/abdominal compartment syndrome vary greatly in the literature, so no standardized recommendation for monitoring and treatment interventions could be made.

Clinical Question

How should IAH and abdominal compartment syndrome be defined, monitored, and treated in the burn patient population?

Evidence

Optimal burn shock resuscitation provides enough fluid to maintain vital organ function without producing iatrogenic negative outcomes. Trends in excessive "fluid creep" resuscitation have been associated with increased incidence of IAH/abdominal compartment syndrome in mostly retrospective studies.[4] Mortality rates as high as 88% have been reported in burn patients requiring laparotomy for abdominal compartment syndrome.[3] Burn clinician experts were major contributors to a worldwide consensus conference addressing abdominal compartment syndrome.[1] New standardized parameters were established primarily based on retrospective reviews and expert consensus, but these parameters were necessary to better correlate and validate future research findings. Conclusions were provisions of specific definitions for IAH, IAH grading, and revised guidelines for IAH measurements and monitoring to ensure consistency abdominal compartment syndrome.[1,3] This includes measuring intraabdominal pressure (IAP) via the bladder with a maximum of 20 to 25 mL of sterile water. The patient is supine, the pressure transducer is zeroed at the midaxillary line, and IAP is read at end-expiration. Although mostly based upon retrospective studies, monitoring recommendations include implementing IAP bladder pressure measurements every 4 to 6 hours in patients with burns greater than 40% total body surface area (TBSA), greater than 20% TBSA with concomitant inhalation injury, or projected fluid requirements greater than 6 mL/kg/%TBSA.[2,3] If continued IAP is at least 12 mm Hg, implement gastric decompression, body repositioning, trunk escharotomies, and diuresis; and consider switching to colloid-based resuscitation and/or administer sedation and chemical paralytics as appropriate.[1,3,4] If IAH progresses to abdominal compartment syndrome (IAP greater than 20 mm Hg and associated new organ system dysfunction or failure), then immediate percutaneous decompression or laparotomy should be performed.[1,3]

Implications for Nursing

Nurses must apply these new standardized definitions for IAH/abdominal compartment syndrome and guidelines for IAP measurement in burn patients. Nurses must use skills in hemodynamic monitoring to assess fluid volume status. Patient response to burn shock resuscitation must be closely monitored, and IV fluid infusion aggressively adjusted to prevent IAH/abdominal compartment syndrome. If abdominal compartment syndrome does develop, percutaneous decompression or laparotomy may be performed at the critical care bedside. Large burn-specific, randomized controlled trials are needed to generate scientifically validated data regarding IAH/abdominal compartment syndrome monitoring and intervention, as well as to critically evaluate resuscitation therapies, end points, and monitoring strategies.

Level of Evidence

Level C—Descriptive studies
Level D—Professional organizational standards

References

1. Cheatham ML, Malbrain ML, Kirkpatrick A, et al. Results from the international conference of experts on intraabdominal hypertension and abdominal compartment syndrome. II. Recommendations. *Intensive Care Medicine.* 2007;33(6):951-962.
2. Ennis JL, Chung KK, Renz EM, et al. Joint Theater Trauma System implementation of burn resuscitation guidelines improves outcomes in severely burned military casualties. *Journal of Trauma.* 2008;64(2 Suppl):S146-151.
3. Kirkpatrick AW, Ball CG, Nickerson D, et al. Intraabdominal hypertension and the abdominal compartment syndrome in burn patients. *World Journal of Surgery.* 2009;33(6): 1142-1149.
4. Lawrence A, Faraklas I, Watkins H, et al. Colloid administration normalizes resuscitation ratio and ameliorates "fluid creep." *Journal of Burn Care & Research.* 2010;31(1):40-47.

Peripheral circulation. Special attention is given to *circumferential* (completely surrounding a body part) full-thickness burns of the extremities. Pressure from bands of eschar or from edema that develops as resuscitation proceeds may impair blood flow to underlying and distal tissue. Therefore, extremities are elevated to reduce edema. Active or passive range-of-motion (ROM) exercises are performed every hour for 5 minutes to increase venous return and to minimize edema. Peripheral pulses are assessed every hour, especially in circumferential burns of the extremities, to confirm adequate circulation. An ultrasonic flowmeter (Doppler) is used to auscultate radial, palmar, digital, or pedal pulses. Delayed capillary refill, taut skin, progressively decreasing or absent pulse, and other neurovascular changes (e.g., intense pain, paresthesia, paralysis) indicate impaired blood flow and developing *compartment syndrome*. Compartment syndrome occurs when tissue pressure in the fascial compartments of extremities increases, compressing and occluding blood vessels and nerves. If signs and symptoms of compartment syndrome are present on serial examination, preparation is made for an escharotomy to relieve pressure and to restore circulation. If decreased perfusion is not quickly detected, ischemia and necrosis with loss of limb may occur. A *fasciotomy* (incision through fascia) may be indicated for deep electrical burns or severe muscle damage to restore blood flow. Escharotomy and fasciotomy sites are treated with a topical antimicrobial agent and are closely monitored for bleeding. Cautery, silver nitrate sticks, or sutures may be indicated to stop continued bleeding.

Secondary Survey

On admission to the ED or burn center, a chest x-ray is obtained, and other x-ray studies are ordered as indicated by the patient's condition. Spinal immobilization precautions are continued until clinical assessment and radiological studies demonstrate no evidence of vertebral injury. The patient's medical history and the history of the injury event are conveyed to the medical team. The critical care nurse must assess indices of essential organ function to evaluate adequacy of burn shock resuscitation and to prevent complications. Initially, monitoring is performed frequently to detect changes that can rapidly occur during fluid resuscitation. Critical indices monitored at least hourly include blood pressure, heart rate, cardiac rhythm, respiration quality and rate, temperature, peripheral pulse presence and quality, and urinary output. In addition, urine specific gravity, urine glucose and ketone levels, occult blood tests, and gastric pH levels are typically evaluated every 2 hours. The patient is weighed on admission and daily thereafter until the preburn weight is obtained after diuresis. Pain is closely monitored, and efforts are made to control it adequately. All parameters are documented for analysis of trends. Assessment and intervention in the resuscitative phase focus on early detection and prevention of problems in the systems discussed in the following sections.

Cardiovascular system. Historically, a mean arterial pressure greater than 70 mm Hg and the absence of tachycardia (heart rate less than 120 beats per minute) have been standard assessments of adequate burn shock resuscitation.[2] However, the cardiovascular response of the patient to burn injury warrants special consideration. The burn patient often has an elevated baseline heart rate of 100 to 120 beats per minute from postinjury metabolic changes. Compensatory mechanisms do not allow hypotension to develop until significant intravascular volume losses have occurred; therefore, decreasing blood pressure is a late sign of inadequate perfusion. Both arterial and noninvasive cuff pressure readings may be altered by peripheral tissue edema or by catecholamine- and mediator-induced arteriospasm. Changes in heart rate and blood pressure may also be masked or may appear increased from pain, anxiety, or fear rather than from inadequate resuscitation. Therefore it is prudent to consider the entire patient and to assess trends in vital signs, hemodynamics, and symptom changes versus focusing on any single value.

The routine insertion of pulmonary artery catheters is not universally supported by the literature. However, patients with significant cardiopulmonary disease, the elderly, or those who have unexplained large resuscitation fluid volume requirements may benefit from insertion of a pulmonary artery catheter to assess cardiac function.[2,15,39] If a pulmonary artery catheter is used, low right atrial pressure and pulmonary artery occlusion pressure are reflective of hypovolemia and require intervention. Assessing trends in cardiac output variables and oxygen transport variables provides useful information to guide burn shock resuscitation.

Local thermal injury, venous stasis, hypercoagulability, and immobility place the burn patient at risk of developing complications related to venous thromboembolism (VTE) such as deep venous thrombosis (DVT) and pulmonary embolism (PE). However, clinical findings indicative of DVT may not be present, or they may be obscured by extremity burn wound pain, edema, or erythema. A national burn data repository was used to create a predictive model to identify at admission those patients at highest risk for developing VTE. At greatest risk for VTE are burn patients with TBSA greater than 10% and need for critical care admission.[38] PE was independently found to be strongly associated with death. Therefore early aggressive prevention of VTE is key in burn patients, with compliance monitored as a part of ICU core measures using mechanical prophylaxis (e.g., sequential compression devices) and/or chemoprophylaxis (e.g., low–molecular weight heparin).[38,46] Since traditional signs of DVT may not be present in the burn patient, the nurse must closely monitor for sudden respiratory deterioration, which may indicate PE.

Neurological status. Severely injured burn patients are initially awake, alert, and oriented. Monitoring of sensorium is crucial. If a burned patient initially presents with a decreased level of consciousness (LOC), other injuries or causes should be suspected (e.g., head injury, carbon monoxide poisoning, drug overdose, alcohol intoxication). The patient's sensorium is evaluated hourly because increased agitation or confusion or a continued decreased LOC may be an indication of hypovolemia, hypoxemia, or both. The head of the bed is elevated 30 degrees to prevent cerebral edema during fluid resuscitation.

Renal status. Urine output closely reflects renal perfusion, which is sensitive to decreasing cardiac output and developing shock. Urinary output is currently the quickest and most reliable indicator of adequate burn fluid resuscitation. Titration of calculated fluid requirements according to hourly urine output is an essential function of the nurse during resuscitation. Urine output, color, and concentration are also closely monitored. Oliguria occurs if fluid resuscitation is inadequate.

Gastrointestinal system. The GI system is monitored for problems occurring with its initial response to the burn injury (i.e., ileus, Curling's ulcer). It is essential to assess for the presence and quality of bowel sounds, abdominal distention, gastric pH, characteristics of gastric secretions, and the presence of GI bleeding. Because patients with burns greater than 20% TBSA generally develop an ileus, a nasogastric tube is inserted and connected to low suction to prevent vomiting and aspiration. If oral intake is not feasible, enteral feedings by a small bowel feeding tube are started early. Stress ulcer prophylaxis is ordered.

Intraabdominal hypertension (IAH) is a serious complication caused by circumferential torso eschar or bowel edema from aggressive fluid resuscitation and/or the burn inflammatory response. The observed trend over the past decade of increased crystalloid infusion rates during burn resuscitation is thought to contribute to IAH incidence.[2,5,14,15,29,31,40,43] IAH is defined as intraabdominal pressure (IAP) of at least 12 mm Hg; it causes compression of intraabdominal contents and leads to renal, gut, and hepatic ischemia.[14] If not treated by trunk escharotomies, diuresis, gastric decompression, body repositioning, and/or sedation and chemical paralytics, IAH can progress to abdominal compartment syndrome or death. The definition of *abdominal compartment syndrome (ACS)* has been standardized by the World Society of Abdominal Compartment Syndrome as presence of sustained IAP greater than 20 mm Hg, with or without abdominal perfusion pressure (APP = MAP − IAP) less than 60 mm Hg, and associated new organ system dysfunction or failure.[14,29] To facilitate early detection of IAH, serial IAP measurements via bladder pressure monitoring are performed on burn patients with greater than 40% TBSA burned, 20% TBSA burned with concomitant inhalation injury, and/or those requiring fluid resuscitation volumes greater than expected.[14,15,29,30,40,43] Reliance on the appearance of physical symptoms (tense abdomen, decreasing urine output,

elevated airway pressure, hypercapnea, hypoxemia, etc.) to diagnose IAH/ACS delays necessary interventions and increases the likelihood of adverse outcome.[29] ACS is a life-threatening complication that mandates immediate decompression by laparotomy, otherwise multiple organ dysfunction and death quickly ensue. Percutaneous drainage of peritoneal fluid may precede formal laparotomy, as long as the patient is monitored closely and laparotomy is immediately instituted if the patient continues to deteriorate. The resulting "open abdomen" wound from a laparotomy is typically treated with topical dressings or vacuum-assisted device (see section, "Wound Management," later in the chapter), and must be carefully assessed to prevent infectious complications until definitive operative closure can occur.

Integumentary system. Assessing a burn patient for the first time is frightening and overwhelming to most healthcare providers. However, other life- or limb-threatening conditions (e.g., airway compromise, burn shock, extremity compartment syndrome) take priority over treating the burn wound during the initial resuscitation phase. The depth and extent of burn injury are assessed to assist with fluid resuscitation predictions. Burn wound management is discussed later in this chapter.

Burn wounds are prone to tetanus, and the patient receives tetanus immunization on ED or burn center admission, if indicated. Tetanus toxoid-containing vaccine (Tdap, Td, or DTaP) is administered if more than 5 years have elapsed since the last received dose, or if the patient's immunization history is unknown.[6]

During the resuscitation period, loss of the protective skin layer and administration of large amounts of fluid place the burn patient at risk of developing hypothermia. Hypothermia causes deleterious complications, and must be aggressively prevented. The patient's temperature is closely monitored. The critical care nurse implements measures to minimize loss of body heat, such as limiting skin exposure and covering the patient with clean, dry sheets and blankets; using fluid/blood warmers for IV fluid infusion; increasing room temperature; closing room doors to prevent air drafts; and using external heat lamps, warming blankets, or radiant heat shields.

Blood and electrolytes. Serum electrolyte levels are determined on admission and as dictated by the patient's status. Serum sodium levels typically approach the concentration of the resuscitation fluid being administered. Serum potassium levels may be increased as a result of release from injured tissue. The blood urea nitrogen level may also be increased when excessive protein catabolism occurs, and hyperglycemia may occur as a result of catecholamine release. Arterial blood gas values and serum lactate levels are evaluated frequently because metabolic acidosis can indicate inadequate tissue perfusion (see box, "Laboratory Alert: Alterations Seen During Acute Care Management of the Burned Patient").

⚠ LABORATORY ALERT

Alterations Seen During Acute Care Management of the Burned Patient

LABORATORY TEST	CRITICAL VALUE	SIGNIFICANCE
Carboxyhemoglobin	>15%	Present in carbon monoxide poisoning
Hematocrit	<15% >60%	↑In hypovolemia; ↓ as third-spaced fluid reenters the intravascular compartment or with concomitant traumatic injury
Serum lactate	>2.2 mEq/L	↑In metabolic acidosis; should ↓ if fluid resuscitation adequate
Potassium	<2.5 mEq/L >6.6 mEq/L	↑Related to tissue damage; assess for cardiac dysrhythmias. May ↓ as reenters cells
Sodium	≤110 mEq/L ≥160 mEq/l	Levels approach the concentration of fluids being administered. May ↑ because of inadequate fluid replacement or ↓ with diuresis
Blood urea nitrogen	>100 mg/dl	May ↑ from catabolism or hypovolemia; monitor nutrition and volume status
Platelets	<20,000/microliter	↓ In large %TBSA, hypothermia-induced bleeding disorders, or infection
White blood cell count	<2,000/microliter >100,000/microliter	Transient ↓ from use of topical silver sulfadiazine; ↑ with infection

TBSA, Total body surface area.

Acute Care Phase: Critical Care Burn Center

With successful resuscitation, burn shock and its dramatic fluid and protein fluctuations stabilize approximately 48 to 72 hours after injury, and the acute phase of burn care begins. Assessments and interventions during the acute phase of burn recovery are implemented to promote wound healing, to prevent complications, and to improve function of the various body systems.

Respiratory System

Assessment continues for signs of respiratory compromise and pneumonia. Inhalation injury and ventilator management places patients at higher risk for pneumonia.[8,17,22,30,40,41,46] Tachypnea, abnormal breath sounds, fever, increased white blood cell count, purulent secretions, and infiltrations on chest x-ray films indicate developing pneumonia. Nursing interventions play a key role in preventing ventilator-associated pneumonia, such as regular oral care, maintaining head-of-bed elevation of at least 30 degrees, and eliminating cross-contamination.[30,41,46] Aggressive pulmonary hygiene including suctioning, coughing, deep breathing, frequent turning, and early ambulation is essential.

Cardiovascular System

As capillary permeability stabilizes, IV fluid requirements decrease. Patients must receive maintenance IV fluid infusions that match overall fluid output. Monitoring daily weight and intake and output is essential. Increased fluid resuscitation requirements after debridement and grafting operations are often required because the inflammatory response is triggered by the surgical intervention. Frequent monitoring of vital signs continues.

Neurological Status

Changes in neurological status, which may indicate hypoxemia, hypoperfusion, or sepsis are part of ongoing assessment.

Renal Status

Urine output assessment continues. Postburn diuresis starts approximately 48 to 72 hours after injury. Urine output ranging from 100 to 600 mL/hr is commonly observed. Intake and output assessment remains important. After postburn diuresis, urinary output should correlate with intake of IV and oral fluids. In the absence of diabetes, glycosuria may indicate an early sign of sepsis.

Gastrointestinal System

Assessment of GI function continues. The patient is monitored for the development of a stress ulcer. Tolerance of enteral feedings is assessed. Nutritional considerations are a treatment priority and are discussed later in this chapter.

Integumentary System

The burn wound becomes the major focus of the acute phase of burn recovery. Assessment continues to include monitoring for burn wound healing, burn wound depth conversion, and signs of infection.

Blood and Electrolytes

Although fluid and protein shifts stabilize in the acute care phase, blood and electrolyte abnormalities related to other processes may be observed. Hemodilution with an associated decreased hematocrit may result from reentry of fluid into the intravascular compartment and from loss of red blood cells destroyed at the burn injury site. Hyponatremia from diuresis may occur, but it usually resolves within 1 week of onset. Inadequate replacement of evaporative water loss may produce hypernatremia. Hypokalemia may develop as potassium reenters the cells. Electrolyte shifts also affect the ability to maintain a proper acid-base balance and may cause metabolic acidosis. Hypoproteinemia and negative nitrogen balance may occur from an increase in metabolic rate and insufficient nutrition. Leukopenia may develop from administration of the topical antimicrobial agent silver sulfadiazine. Infection and excessive carbohydrate loading contribute to hyperglycemia. In addition, an increase in the white blood cell count, prolonged coagulation times, and a decreased platelet count may result from infection or sepsis.

SPECIAL CONSIDERATIONS AND AREAS OF CONCERN

Burns of the face, ears, eyes, hands, feet, major joints, genitalia, and perineum pose distinct concerns because injuries to these areas contribute to overall burn injury severity and require unique management. Certain types of burns (electrical, chemical, and abuse) also mandate special consideration and intervention.

Burns of the Face

The presence of head or neck burns alerts the clinician to suspect a potential inhalation injury. Associated facial edema may lead to a compromised airway. Close monitoring of the patient's respiratory status is essential. The head of the bed is elevated to facilitate ventilation and edema reabsorption. Special care is taken during cleansing of facial burns to prevent excessive bleeding and damage to new tissue growth. All hair (except for eyebrows) is shaved from the wound each day. Once the wound is cleaned and debrided, a topical antimicrobial agent is applied per unit protocol. Because of the rich blood supply in the face, partial-thickness burns usually heal quickly as long as infection is prevented. Good oral hygiene is essential.

Burns of the Ears

The ears are especially prone to inflammation and infection of the cartilage (*chondritis*), which leads to complete loss of ear cartilage. Ear burns are treated with a topical antimicrobial agent. Mafenide acetate (Sulfamylon) is the agent of choice because of its ability to penetrate the cartilage. Mechanical pressure on the ears from dressings or other external sources (tube ties, pillows) must be prevented because the pressure impairs blood flow and contributes to the development of chondritis. Cloth ties are used for securing tubes to the face and are monitored frequently to ensure that pressure is not placed on top of the ears. Pillows are not used for the head. Instead, a foam donut with a hole for the ear to rest in while the patient is in a lateral position is substituted.

Burns of the Eyes

Immediate examination of the eyes is necessary on arrival to the hospital because eyelid edema forms rapidly. Eyelid edema can cause the cornea to become exposed as the eyelid retracts. Contact lenses are removed if present. A thorough examination by an ophthalmologist is mandatory for serious injuries. The eyes are stained with fluorescein to rule out corneal injury, and the eyes are irrigated with copious amounts of physiological saline if injury is confirmed. Nursing care involves the frequent application of ophthalmic ointment or artificial tears to protect the cornea and conjunctiva from drying. Careful observation of eyelashes is also necessary because they may invert and scratch the cornea.

Burns of the Hands, Feet, or Major Joints

Extensive burns of the hands and feet may cause permanent disability, necessitating a long convalescence. An important aspect of critical care nursing care is preservation of function. Burned hands are elevated above the level of the heart on slings or wedges to reduce edema formation. Fingers and toes are wrapped individually during dressing changes with gauze, bandages, or biological products to keep digits separated to prevent *webbing* (the skin growing together between burned body parts). Occupational and physical therapists are involved in the patient's plan of care from the day of admission to address and evaluate function and mobility parameters. Although ROM exercises may be painful, they must be initiated as soon as possible after the injury and performed frequently throughout each day. Active ROM exercises prevent muscle atrophy, reduce the shortening of ligaments, prevent joint contracture formation, and decrease edema. Passive ROM exercises are indicated if patients are unable to move their extremities actively.

Burn wounds over joints are prone to scar tissue contractures that limit joint ROM. The position of comfort is the position of contracture and deformity development. Therefore splinting and antideformity positioning (e.g., extension of knees and elbows, extension and supination of wrists, abduction of hips and shoulders) are required to maintain function and prevent deformities of the affected part. When the patient is ambulating or sitting, an elastic bandage is applied over burn wounds of the feet and legs to prevent venous stasis and pooling of blood. Venous pooling delays wound healing and increases the risk of DVT development. The elastic bandage is removed when the feet are elevated. In establishing a nursing plan of care, the nurse must remember that patients with bilateral burned hands are very dependent on nursing personnel for their physical needs.

Burns of the Genitalia and Perineum

Patients with perineal burns often require hospitalization for monitoring of urinary tract obstruction. An indwelling urethral catheter is indicated until the surrounding wounds are healed or grafted. Meticulous wound care is essential because of the high risk of urine or fecal contamination and resulting infection. Perineal hair must be shaved over wound areas. Scrotal edema is common, and the scrotum is elevated on towels or foam.

Electrical Injury

Cardiopulmonary arrest is a common complication of high-voltage electrical injury. Other severe complications related to electrical injury are summarized in Box 20-2. Hypoxemia may occur secondary to tetanic contractions and resulting paralysis of the respiratory muscles. Oxygen and endotracheal intubation with mechanical ventilation are implemented as indicated. Patients are evaluated for spinal fractures from tetanic contractions or from falls during the injury event. Cervical collars and backboards are used to maintain spinal immobilization until radiological tests and clinical examinations have confirmed the absence of injury. All patients with electrical injury are monitored closely for cardiac dysrhythmias. If present, continuous cardiac monitoring or serial electrocardiographic evaluations continue for at least 24 hours after injury. Tea-colored urine indicates the presence of hemochromogens (myoglobin), released as a result of severe deep tissue damage in a process called *rhabdomyolysis*. Urinary output for these patients is maintained at 75 to 100 mL/hr in adults and 1 mL/kg in children until the urine becomes clear to prevent kidney injury.[6] Resuscitation fluid volumes larger than predicted by the ABLS Fluid Resuscitation Formulas are often required to achieve this high urine output. Sodium bicarbonate and mannitol may be administered at the burn center physician's discretion to increase urine pH and output. Affected extremities are closely monitored for the development of compartment syndrome. Often, fasciotomies are required to release compartment pressure. Amputations can occur with the initial electrical contact, or may later be surgically required in nonviable limbs.

Chemical Injury

Treatment of chemical injuries focuses on stopping the burning process while maintaining the safety of the nurse.

Protective gear such as plastic gowns, gloves, masks, and goggles are worn by the burn team during decontamination. If a patient is suspected of having a methamphetamine laboratory–related injury, decontamination is required. During decontamination for all chemical exposures, the patient's clothing is immediately removed. Dry chemicals are brushed off, and the area exposed to chemicals is continuously flushed with water for at least 30 minutes. The nurse questions the patient and significant others to determine the specific chemical agent involved. Some chemicals such as alkalies require even longer lavage, which can be quite uncomfortable for the patient. Nursing interventions include controlling pain and minimizing heat loss caused by continual irrigation. Patients must also be closely monitored for signs of systemic chemical absorption and effects.

Abuse and Neglect

Burns are a prevalent form of abuse and can result from either an active intent to injure or from neglect. Vulnerable populations such as children, the elderly, disabled persons, and mentally impaired persons are at increased risk of abuse and neglect. Critical care nurses play a lead role in recognizing and identifying potential abuse or neglect cases because they spend the most time interfacing with the patient and significant others. Nurses must elicit the history of the story and circumstances surrounding the injury event, meticulously and accurately document the wound appearance and the pattern of injury (including use of photographs), and observe the interactions between the patient and caregivers or family. The injured individual should be questioned separately and privately from the family caregiver. The reported injury history should correlate with physical findings. Discrepancies between reported accounts of the injury event and physical assessment findings indicate a potential abuse/neglect situation. The presence of other injuries (i.e., associated bruising, fractures, abrasions, or other trauma) and the distribution and characteristics of the burn wound also provide key information on the true cause of the burn injury. For example, a scald burn with a clear demarcation and/or symmetrical wound pattern on the extremities without splash mark burns indicates an intentional immersion injury instead of an accidental scald (Figure 20-12). Lack of witnesses to the injury event, blaming of siblings, and delay in seeking care are also indicators of potential abuse situations. All potential or suspected abuse cases must be reported to the appropriate authorities as governed by state laws. The patient is hospitalized until social workers and protective services have investigated the patient's home environment to determine whether the patient will be safe on discharge.

PAIN CONTROL

Pain is a tormenting consequence of burn injury not limited to just immediately after the injury; it is a major factor throughout the wound healing process. Pain experienced during the acute phase of recovery consists of a constant

---

BOX 20-2 **MANIFESTATIONS AND COMPLICATIONS OF ELECTRICAL INJURY**

- Cardiac dysrhythmias or cardiopulmonary arrest
- Hypoxia secondary to tetanic contractions and paralysis of the respiratory muscles
- Deep tissue necrosis
- Compartment syndrome of extremities
- Long bone or vertebral fractures from tetanic muscle contractions
- Rhabdomyolysis and acute kidney injury
- Acute cataract formation
- Neurological deficits such as spinal cord paralysis, traumatic brain injury, peripheral neuropathy, seizures, deafness, neuropathic pain, motor and sensory deficits

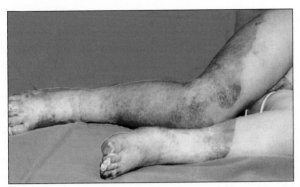

FIGURE 20-12 Abuse by hot water immersion. The thigh burn wound edges have a clear demarcation line (are in a straight line), and there are no splash marks. The caregivers delayed seeking medical treatment for the patient's burns until 3 days after injury (note the dry, crusty appearance of the wounds). The patient also had a forearm fracture and multiple areas of bruising on the body. (Courtesy University of Michigan Trauma Burn Center, Ann Arbor, MI.)

background or *resting pain,* as well as a shorter peak of excruciating pain *(procedural* or *breakthrough pain)* often associated with activity and therapeutic procedures.[13,44] Many aspects of burn treatment produce pain, including dressing changes, debridement, surgical intervention, application of topical antimicrobials, and physical and occupational therapy. This situation illustrates the major paradox of burn pain management: the nurse inflicts pain and then must relieve it.

Adequately treating a burn patient's pain is a challenge. Altered pharmacokinetics secondary to changes in volume distribution and hypermetabolism is associated with burn injury. Burn patients commonly have histories of regular alcohol consumption or substance use that further compound pain management and narcotic resistance.[41,44,49] It is not uncommon that the quantities of analgesics required by burn patients often exceed those of standard dosing guidelines.[44] Specific institutional policies should be followed regarding what constitutes pain management versus conscious sedation, and appropriate patient monitoring. Inaccurate assessment of a patient's pain or fears of addiction can lead to undermedication. Improved assessment and intervention of severe burn pain are needed.[6,13,30] A noteworthy prospective study found that burn patients have realistic expectations of their care and do not expect to be completely free of acute pain; however, patients' satisfaction with their care was related to the level of pain experienced.[13] To control a patient's pain successfully and to achieve increased patient satisfaction, accurate serial pain assessments must occur, and the patient must be involved in creating an individualized analgesic treatment plan.[13] Pain levels should be assessed frequently as "the fifth vital sign," with additional assessments before, during, and after all procedures and treatments. The nurse serves as the patient's advocate by ensuring that pain medications

are administered by appropriate delivery methods and in adequate dosages to reduce pain intensity.

Opiates are the most common analgesics used to treat burn pain. Subcutaneous or intramuscular injections are ineffective in the resuscitative phase because of impaired circulation in soft tissue. Absorption is sporadic, increasing the risk of undermedication or narcotic overdose. Morphine is the drug of choice, and IV administration is the route of choice. A continuous IV infusion of morphine maintains a consistent level of analgesia, but it is typically used only in critically ill patients requiring mechanical ventilation. Patient-controlled analgesia (PCA) may be beneficial in involving patients in their care, and providing them some independence or "control" over their pain management regimen. Analgesic medications can be given safely by the oral route once the patient is hemodynamically stable and any ileus has resolved. Although pain is reduced when wounds are covered with temporary dressings or skin grafts, frequent surgical procedures and wound care procedures produce episodes of pain until permanent wound closure or healing is completed. Itching that occurs during the healing process also contributes to the patient's overall discomfort. Several medications, such as antihistamines, and soothing emollients assist in reducing pruritus.[44]

The entire burn care and treatment experience produces anxiety, which further exacerbates pain.[44] The ideal pain management regimen must incorporate treatment of both pain and anxiety. Fear and a loss of control over their lives and schedules increase patients' anxiety. The critical care nurse must provide frequent and repeated explanations of care plans, interventions, and procedures at an age-appropriate level. Patients are encouraged to participate as much as possible in their wound care, medication administration, feeding, and exercise therapy. Anxiolytics are commonly administered in the acute care phase. Use of virtual reality technology (immersive 3-D computer-simulated environments in real or imaginary worlds) and techniques such as relaxation, hypnosis, distraction, and guided imagery also serve as useful adjuncts for reducing anxiety and enhancing pain relief. Accurate pain and anxiety assessment, close monitoring, and individualized dosing of medications are essential for successful pain control.

INFECTION CONTROL

Burn patients have a high risk of infection related to disruption of normal skin integrity and altered immune response. When the skin's natural mechanical barrier protection is lost, the patient's susceptibility to infection increases. In addition, other host defense mechanisms are impaired, and immunosuppression develops. Although great strides in management have been made, the incidence of infection is higher in burn patients than in other patient groups and remains a predominant determinant of outcome.[8,12,22,36,40,41,47] Development of multidrug-resistant organism outbreaks is an ongoing issue in burn units worldwide and contributes to an increased risk of sepsis.[12,41,47] The control of infection is an important nursing intervention in burn patient care. Concomitant inhalation injury places the burn patient at particularly high risk of developing pneumonia, which further increases mortality rate.[8,17,22,30,40,41,46] Invasive monitoring and the presence of urinary catheters, IV catheters, and endotracheal tubes are also potential sources of infection. Due to an ongoing inflammatory response, most burn patients meet the standardized diagnosis criteria for systemic inflammatory response syndrome (SIRS) even in the absence of infection. Hence, an American Burn Association consensus panel has adapted definition guidelines for sepsis and SIRS that are specific and more applicable to the unique pathophysiological state of burn injury.[22] The hypermetabolic state unique to burn patients can increase baseline temperatures to about 38.5° C, thus rendering presence of a low-grade fever (without other symptoms) to be an inaccurate indication of infection.[22,41]

The goals of infection control in burn care are as follows:
- Preserve existing immune defenses
- Prevent transmission of exogenous organisms
- Control transfer of endogenous organisms (normal flora) to sites at increased risk for infection

Infection control in the burn patient is dependent on the following strategies. Critical care nurses are essential in implementing and monitoring:
- Aseptic management of the wound and the environment, including effective decontamination of equipment and hydrotherapy rooms
- Use of topical antibacterial agents
- Proper care of invasive catheters; special consideration for IV catheters placed through or near burn wounds where occlusive dressings will not adhere, including every 2 to 4 hour site care
- Aggressive wound management with close monitoring for changes in wound appearance
- Prevention of multidrug-resistant organisms through prudent and microbial-guided use of systemic antibiotics based upon patient flora and local unit bacterial resistance patterns; selective treatment of infection versus colonization.[12,22,41]
- Provision of adequate nutrition
- Close monitoring of laboratory values and clinical signs of impending sepsis
- Early wound closure to restore the protective barrier of skin
- Continuous observation and implementation of targeted interventions that improve outcomes (e.g., glycemic control, prevention of central line infection, head of bed elevated at least 30 degrees, restrictive sedation practice, aggressive ventilator weaning)[22,46]
- Staff education to prevent transmission

Although infection control policies differ among burn units, all policies stress standard precautions, including use of barrier techniques, strict hand washing, and appropriate garb when caring for a burn-injured patient; implementation of isolation restrictions as indicated; and prohibition of live plants or flowers in the unit.

WOUND MANAGEMENT

Patient outcomes from burn injury are optimized by focusing on the goals of prevention and treatment of wound infections, and expedited closure of burn wounds. Interventions performed to obtain these goals are wound cleansing, debridement, topical antimicrobial and/or biological-biosynthetic dressing therapy, and definitive surgical wound closure. Burn wound care protocols and procedures vary among burn centers across the country. However, the underlying goals of wound care are the same: removal of nonviable tissue to promote reepithelialization and prompt coverage via skin grafts when necessary.

Wound Care

To promote prevention of infection and healing of the burn wound, the nurse must focus on performing meticulous wound care. Wound care is typically done once or twice a day, depending on the healing status of the wound, the dressing or topical agents used (some require less frequent dressing changes), and the number of days postoperatively from grafting. Before initiating wound care, the nurse carefully explains the procedure to the patient and significant others and encourages participation as able. Analgesics are administered (and sedatives if indicated) before starting the procedure. All wounds are cleansed with a mild soap or surgical disinfectant, and then rinsed with warm tap water. The patient is not immersed in water because immersion has a significant potential for cross-contamination of wounds. Instead, water is allowed to flow over the wounds and immediately drained away. This regimen is best accomplished in a shower or hydrotherapy stretcher, but bed baths may be used for hemodynamically unstable patients. All previously applied topical agents, necrotic tissue, exudate, and fibrous debris are removed from the wound to expose healthy tissue, to control bacterial proliferation, and to promote healing. Loose eschar and wound debris are *debrided* with washcloths or gauze sponges, scissors, and forceps. Mechanical trauma and damage from aggressive cleansing of newly formed epithelial skin buds or healing granulation tissue must be avoided. Hair in and immediately surrounding the wound bed is shaved (except eyebrows) to eliminate a medium for bacterial growth and to facilitate wound assessment. All wounds are inspected closely, with wound location, size, color, texture, and drainage carefully documented so any changes in appearance or developing signs of infection are noted. The patient's core body temperature is closely monitored. During wound care the room temperature must be maintained at a minimum of 85° F to 90° F to prevent chilling and excessive body heat loss.

Topical Agents and Dressings

One of the most rapidly changing aspects of burn care is the development of novel tissue engineering techniques for wound treatment. Numerous new topical agents and biosynthetic dressings have been released, with many others in development. These new products have broader, longer-lasting antimicrobial actions; interact with wound growth factors

TABLE 20-4 TOPICAL ANTIMICROBIAL AGENTS FOR BURN WOUND MANAGEMENT

AGENT	INDICATIONS	NURSING CONSIDERATIONS
Clotrimazole cream or nystatin (Mycostatin)	Fungal colonization of wounds	Apply 1-2 times daily. Use with an antibacterial topical agent. May cause skin irritation.
Mafenide acetate (Sulfamylon)	Active against most gram-positive, gram-negative, and *Pseudomonas* pathogens; drug of choice for ear burns; penetrates thick eschar and ear cartilage	Apply 1-2 times daily. Strong carbonic anhydrase inhibitor, can cause metabolic acidosis; monitor respiratory rate, electrolyte values, and ABGs. Hydroscopic (draws water out of tissue), can be painful for 15-60 minutes after application. Slows eschar separation. Assess for sulfa allergy before use.
Silver-coated dressings (Acticoat, Aquacel Ag, Mepilex Ag, Silverlon, Tegaderm Ag)	Silver-coated, flexible, nonadhesive wound dressings with or without absorptive layer; as long as dressing is moist, provides continuous release of silver ions for 3-14 days (depending on product); effective broad-spectrum coverage for numerous pathogens (gram-negative/gram-positive bacteria, antibiotic-resistant bacteria, yeast, mold); alternative for patients allergic to sulfa drugs	Apply new dressing every 1-7 days to moist open wound with (1) wound exudate maintaining silver activation until drainage stops or wound heals, or (2) rewetting with sterile water every 4-6 hours to keep dressing moist (not wet). Use sterile water to moisten dressings; saline renders silver ions ineffective. A decrease in number of required dressing changes increases patient comfort and cost-effectiveness. Aquacel Ag and Mepilex Ag do not require wetting.
Silver nitrate	Effective against wide spectrum of common wound pathogens; acts on surface microorganisms only; poor eschar penetration; alternative for patients allergic to sulfa drugs	Apply 0.5% solution to wet dressing 2-3 times daily; rewet every 2 hours to keep moist. Hypotonic solution causes electrolyte leeching; monitor serum electrolyte levels, and replace according to protocol. Must be kept in light-resistant container. Causes staining: protect equipment and floors with plastic.
Silver sulfadiazine (SSD, Silvadene)	Active against wide spectrum of gram-negative, gram-positive, and *Candida albicans* pathogens; acts only on cell wall and membrane; does not penetrate thick eschar	Apply 1-2 times daily. May wrap wounds or leave as open dressing. Can cause leukopenia; monitor white blood cell count. Assess for sulfa allergy before use.

ABGs, Arterial blood gases.

and collagen fibers to accelerate healing and to stop the zone of stasis from expanding; help fill in defects; and may reduce scarring. All these actions positively affect outcomes in burn patients by reducing infection, shortening healing time, preventing wound conversion to full-thickness depth, decreasing pain (due to less frequent dressing changes), and improving long-term cosmetic appearance and scarring. After each hydrotherapy session, the unhealed or unexcised burn wound is covered with an antimicrobial topical agent, a dressing, or both. The multitude of available agents and dressings precludes a complete listing. Table 20-4 describes a variety of commonly used agents in the United States and related nursing considerations. Many of these products are also used in nonburn, chronic, or surgical wounds. The selection of an agent and dressing is determined by wound depth, anatomical location, frequency of wound visualization desired, and presence and type of microorganisms identified. The ideal antimicrobial agent demonstrates long-lasting, broad-spectrum activity against microorganisms with low resistance development; penetrates eschar; and has limited adverse effects. The burn center physician orders the antimicrobial agent, as well as the frequency and method of application.

Advances in wound dressing development and skin substitutes provide many new options in coverage for major burns. Temporary wound coverings are classified as either *biological* or *biosynthetic* (a combination of biological and synthetic properties). Table 20-5 describes common types and uses for biological and biosynthetic coverings. Biological or biosynthetic dressings are used as temporary wound coverings for freshly excised (surgically debrided) burn wounds until autograft skin is available; examples include Allograft, Integra, AlloDerm, and xenograft. Biological or biosynthetic products are used as dressings for partial-thickness burns, meshed autograft skin, or donor sites to promote healing; examples include Allograft, TransCyte, BioBrane, OrCel, and xenograft. Temporary wound coverings have the added benefits of controlling heat and fluid loss, decreasing infection risk, stimulating the healing process, and increasing patient comfort.

Enzymatic agents such as collagenase, papain/urea, or sutilains are sometimes used for debridement of smaller necrotic

TYPE OF DRESSING	DEFINITION
TABLE 20-5	**BIOLOGICAL AND BIOSYNTHETIC DRESSINGS**
Biological Dressing Allograft (homograft)	**Temporary Wound Cover from Human or Animal Species Tissue** Graft of skin transplanted from another human, living or dead
Xenograft (heterograft)	Graft of skin (usually pigskin) transplanted between different species
Biosynthetic Dressing *Epidermal Replacements* (Epicel, Epidex, MySkin, etc.)	**Wound Covering Composed of Both Biological and Synthetic Materials** Commercially manufactured CEA from autologous keratinocytes (via skin biopsy) and typically murine fibroblasts, delivered on a silicone or gauze layer
Dermal Substitutes AlloDerm	Transplantable tissue consisting of human cryopreserved allogeneic dermis from which the epidermal cells, fibroblasts, and endothelial cells targeted for immune response have been removed
Integra	Dressing system composed of two layers: (1) *dermal* layer of animal collagen and glycosaminoglycan that interfaces with wound and functions as dermal matrix for cellular growth and collagen synthesis; (2) temporary outer synthetic *epidermal* layer of Silastic that acts as barrier to water loss and bacteria. Dermal layer biodegrades within months as new wound collagen matrix is synthesized. Silastic layer removed in 14-21 days and replaced with thin autograft
TransCyte	Temporary dressing composed of outer polymer membrane and nylon mesh seeded with human neonatal fibroblasts and porcine collagen; matrix contains proteins and growth factors, but no viable cells because of cryopreservation
Bilayer Dermo-Epidermal Substitutes (Apligraf, OrCel)	Consist of outer epidermal layer of cultured allogeneic (from another human) neonatal keratinocytes, and bottom dermal layer matrix embedded with neonatal fibroblasts and bovine collagen; the matrix's viable or living cells secrete growth factors and cytokines to promote healing

tissue areas on deep partial- and full-thickness burns. Topical enzymatic agents are proteolytic enzyme ointments that act as potent digestants of nonviable protein matter or necrotic tissue, but they are harmless to viable tissue. Enzymatic agents do not have antimicrobial properties; therefore wounds must be closely monitored for infection.

Burn wounds are treated in one of two ways: open or closed methods. The decision of which method to use depends on the location, size, and depth of the burn, as well as on specific burn unit protocols. Each method has advantages and disadvantages.

With the *open method*, the burn wounds are left open to air after the antimicrobial agent is applied. The open method provides increased wound visualization and more opportunities for observation, eliminates dressing supplies, and improves joint mobility normally limited by the presence of restrictive dressings. However, the open method allows direct contact between the wound and the environment. The topical antimicrobial agent may rub off on clothing, bedding, or equipment. The open method increases wound exposure time and the risk of hypothermia. The open method is commonly used on superficial burns to the face treated with the topical agent bacitracin.

With the *closed method*, a gauze dressing is placed over an agent that was applied directly to the wound, or the wound is covered with gauze dressings that have been saturated with a topical antimicrobial agent. The closed method reduces heat loss and pain or sensitivity from wound exposure, and it assists in protecting wounds from external mechanical trauma. The dressings applied may also assist with debridement. However, the closed method requires a dressing change to assess the wound, and the presence of dressings may impair ROM. The closed method is commonly used on full-thickness burns treated with silver sulfadiazine and new grafts.

Negative pressure wound therapy (NPWT) or vacuum-assisted closure (VAC) devices can be used for the treatment of grafts, partial-thickness burns, and deep surgical wounds (as seen in nonburn necrotizing soft tissue infections or post-ACS decompression). NPWT consists of a sponge and suction tubing placed on the wound bed and covered with an occlusive dressing (Figure 20-13). The device then creates a negative-pressure dressing to decompress edematous interstitial spaces and increase local perfusion, to help draw wound edges closed uniformly, to remove wound fluid, and to provide a closed, moist wound healing environment. NPWT also allows the collection and quantification of wound drainage. NPWT has been associated with lower wound bacterial counts, earlier reepithelialization, prevention of burn depth progression, and a reduction in graft loss due to reduced edema and preservation of blood flow.[20,32,42]

CHAPTER 20 Burns **647**

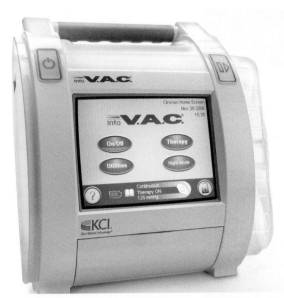

FIGURE 20-13 Vacuum-assisted closure (VAC) device; Info V.A.C. Therapy System. (Courtesy of KCI Licensing, Inc., San Antonio, Texas.)

Surgical Excision and Grafting

The depth of the injury determines whether a burn will heal or require skin grafting. First- and second-degree burns heal because they are superficial and partial-thickness burns; thus the necessary elements to generate new skin remain. Full-thickness burns are nonvascular, and all dermal appendages have been destroyed. Full-thickness burns require skin grafting to achieve wound closure. Deep partial-thickness burns are also commonly grafted to decrease the risk of infection by achieving earlier wound closure and to minimize scarring and improve cosmetic appearance. *Excision* is surgical debridement by scalpel or electrocautery to remove *necrotic* (dead) tissue until a layer of healthy, well-vascularized tissue is exposed. *Skin grafting* is placing skin on the excised burn wound (Figure 20-14, *A*). Several types of skin can be used for skin grafting including *autograft* (the patient's own skin, which is transferred to a new location on the body); *allograft*, which is also called *homograft* (skin from another human; e.g., cadaver skin); and *xenograft* (skin from another animal; e.g., pigskin). Autografts are the only permanent type of skin grafting (Table 20-6). Homografts and xenografts are temporary biological dressings (see Table 20-5). With autografts, a partial-thickness wound called a *donor site* is created where the skin was harvested or removed from the patient with a tool called a *dermatome.*

Excision and grafting are performed in the operating room and are typically initiated within the first week after burn injury. Early excision within the first 1 to 3 days is advocated because it has been associated with decreased mortality and morbidity.[30,40,47,48] Advantages reported include modulation of the hypermetabolic response, reduced infection and wound colonization rates, increased graft take, and decreased length of hospitalization.[26,40,48] Depending on the size of the burn and the presence of infection, sequential or repeated surgical debridements and grafting may be required. In major burns, it is often not possible to graft all full-thickness wound areas initially, either because of the patient's hemodynamic instability from the size and severity of burned areas or because of a lack of donor sites to provide adequate coverage. Priority areas for autograft skin application include the face, the hands, the feet, and over joints. In addition, other temporary and permanent synthetic products have been developed to substitute for a person's own skin (see Table 20-5). These products allow early burn wound coverage, while delaying autografting until previously used donor sites have healed and can be reharvested.

Autograft skin can be applied as meshed grafts or as sheet grafts. *Sheet* (nonmeshed) grafts are often used on the face and hands for better cosmetic results. Meshed grafts are commonly used elsewhere on the body (Figure 20-14, *B*). A meshed graft is created by using a device, called a skin graft mesher, that places multiple tiny slits or holes in the piece of skin that was harvested from the donor site. The wider the graft's mesh is, the larger the area that can be covered with the autograft skin. However, wider mesh grafts also contribute to more scarring and a less cosmetically pleasing appearance (Figure 20-14, *C*). Table 20-6 summarizes the types of skin autografts used, along with nursing care requirements. Splinting of graft sites is indicated to prevent movement and shearing of the grafts until adherence has occurred. Extremities are elevated to prevent pooling of blood and edema, which can lead to increased pressure and graft loss.

Many types of dressings can be used on donor sites (Table 20-7), but the product chosen must promote healing of the donor site within 7 to 10 days. Donor sites can be reused or reharvested once healed. When patient donor sites are limited because of the severity of the burn injury, cultured epithelium autograft (CEA) can be used to provide coverage for a major burn injury. With CEA, a skin biopsy is obtained from the patient and is sent to a laboratory where keratinocytes are cultured and grown. The process takes about 3 weeks and results in small pieces of skin. These fragile pieces of skin are surgically applied to a clean, excised burn wound. The disadvantage of CEA is its extreme fragility, partly the result of the lack of a durable dermis. To overcome these shortcomings researchers are actively investigating novel approaches in tissue engineering, such as developing different types epidermal substitutes, incorporating CEA with a dermal layer to increase durability, constructing biologically active dermo-epidermal replacements, integrating stem cells, and utilizing topical nanoemulsion technology.[11,23,32]

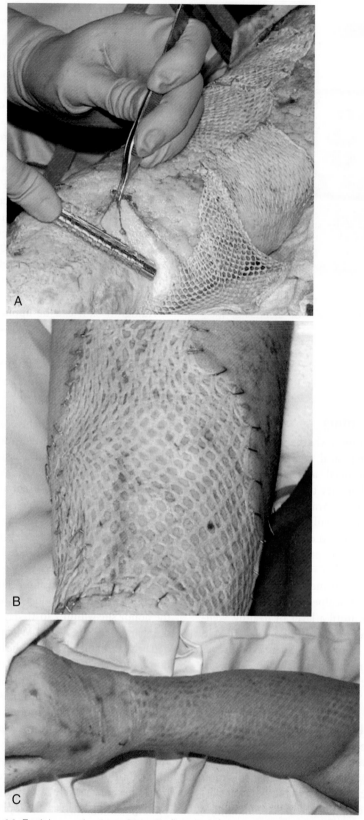

FIGURE 20-14 Excision and autografting. **A,** Surgical debridement (excision) with meshed autograft placement in the operating room. **B,** Meshed autograft postoperative day 2. **C,** Comparison of sheet autograft (on hand) versus meshed autograft (on forearm) 3 weeks postoperatively. Use of meshed autograft allows larger body surface area coverage, but it also typically leads to more scarring and a less cosmetically pleasing appearance. (Courtesy University of Michigan Trauma Burn Center, Ann Arbor, MI.)

TABLE 20-6 AUTOGRAFT SKIN: NURSING IMPLICATIONS

TYPE OF AUTOGRAFT	DEFINITION	NURSING IMPLICATIONS
Split-thickness *sheet* graft	Sheet of skin composed of epidermis and a variable portion of dermis harvested at a predetermined thickness. Sheet kept intact (not meshed) to improve cosmetic appearance; often used on face and hands.	Grafted area must be immobilized. Pockets of serous/serosanguineous fluid are evacuated by needle aspiration or rolling of the fluid with cotton tip applicator toward the skin edges; if fluid is not evacuated, graft adherence is compromised.
Split-thickness *meshed* graft	Split-thickness sheet graft that is mesh-cut to expand the graft 1.5 to 9 times its original size before being placed on a recipient bed of granulation tissue; used to cover large surface areas.	Graft is covered with layers of fine and coarse mesh gauze to prevent shearing, wrapped with absorbent gauze, and splinted for immobilization. Dressings must be kept moist (not saturated) to promote epithelialization of meshed skin interstices. First dressing change within 3-5 days.
Full-thickness graft	Sheet of skin is harvested down to subcutaneous tissue (i.e., involves all layers of skin), typically used for eyelids or later reconstructive procedures.	Requires same care as a sheet skin graft.
Cultured epidermal autograft (CEA)	Autologous epidermal keratinocytes grown in a laboratory via tissue culture techniques (takes ~3 weeks); derived from skin biopsy of patient. Epidermal layer replacement only. Typically used with extensive % TBSA burns when limited donor sites are available.	Daily dressing changes of outer gauze for 7-10 days (underlying coarse mesh and petroleum jelly gauze layers are not disturbed); outer dressing must remain dry. Many topical antimicrobial agents are toxic to CEA skin and should not come in contact with graft dressings. Petroleum jelly gauze removed when it becomes loose (7-10 days), and gentle ROM exercises can begin. Moist saline dressings used until graft is well adherent (typically 21 days).

TABLE 20-7 TYPES OF DONOR SITE DRESSINGS

DRESSING	DESCRIPTION
BioBrane	Bilaminate dressing composed of nylon mesh embedded with a collagen derivative and an outer silicone membrane; permeable to wound drainage and topical antimicrobial agents; peels away as wound heals
Calcium alginate dressings	Algicell, Algisite M, Kaltostat, Sorbsan, Tegaderm HG, etc. Hydrophilic flexible dressings in which alginate fibers convert to a gel when activated by wound exudates. Dressing change within 7 days, or more frequently if large amounts of drainage
DuoDerm	Hydrocolloid dressing that adheres by interacting and bonding with skin moisture
Fine mesh gauze	Cotton gauze placed directly on wound; a crust or "scab" is formed as gauze dries and wound epithelialization occurs under the dressing; gauze peels away as wound heals
N-Terface	Translucent, nonabsorbent, and nonreactive surface material used between the burn wound and outer dressing
Op-Site	Thin elastic film that is occlusive, waterproof, and permeable to air and moisture vapor; fluid under dressing may need to be evacuated
Vigilon	Colloidal suspension on a polyethylene mesh that provides a moist environment; permeable to air and water vapor
Scarlet Red	Cotton gauze impregnated with a blend of lanolin, olive oil, petrolatum, and red dye "scarlet red"; healing occurs as with fine mesh gauze dressing
Silver-coated dressings	Acticoat, Aquacel Ag, Mepilex AG, Silverlon, Tegaderm AG, etc. Silver-coated, flexible dressings (with or without absorptive layer) that provide continuous release of silver ions for 3-14 days while dressing is moist
Xeroform	Fine mesh gauze containing 3% bismuth tribromophenate in a petrolatum blend; promotes healing as with other mesh gauze dressings

Burn units vary in their protocols to treat grafted areas and donor sites. Basic wound care principles are applied, and prevention of infection is always the primary goal. Although the critical care nurse may not actually develop the wound treatment plan, input and involvement by all burn team experts is essential for positive patient outcomes. A method of documenting wound treatment that facilitates day-to-day team communication of care requirements should be used.

Inherent in all wound care management is the necessity to improve and maintain function. Occupational and physical therapists are essential members of the burn team and are consulted on the day of admission. Often, the position of comfort for the patient is one that leads to dysfunction or deformity. Specialized splints, antideformity positioning, and exercises are required throughout the acute burn care phase to prevent future complications. The critical care nurse works closely with the patient and family to continually reinforce the need for splinting/positioning and to monitor for compliance.

NUTRITIONAL CONSIDERATIONS

Adequate nutrition plays an important role in the survival of extensively burned patients. A major burn injury produces a stress-induced hypermetabolic-catabolic response that is greater than that of any other disease process or injury, and is often figuratively equated to running a continuous marathon race. Skeletal muscle is the major protein store in the body. Postburn hypermetabolism leads to deleterious consequences including significant skeletal muscle breakdown with protein degradation, weight loss, marked delays in wound healing, skin graft loss, impaired immunological responsiveness, sepsis, physiological exhaustion or even death if adequate nutrition is not provided and an anabolic or positive nitrogen balance is not achieved.[21,22,24,40,48] Muscle weakness and atrophy can also contribute to prolonged mechanical ventilation, delayed ambulation, impaired activities of daily living, and extended acute rehabilitation.

Nutritional therapy must be instituted immediately after the burn injury to meet energy demands, to maintain host defense mechanisms, to replenish body protein stores, and to curtail progressive loss of lean body mass. The nurse collaborates with the patient, the registered dietitian, and the physician to coordinate a nutritional plan. If the patient is able to tolerate an oral diet, a high-calorie, high-protein diet with supplements is instituted with daily calorie counts performed to monitor dietary intake. If oral intake is not tolerated or caloric intake is insufficient, enteral tube feeding is begun. Early enteral feeding within the first 24 hours after burn injury decreases the production of catabolic hormones, improves nitrogen balance, reduces wound infection rate, maintains gut integrity, lowers the incidence of diarrhea, and decreases hospital stay.[21,30,35,48,50] The small bowel (versus stomach) is the preferred location for tube placement so enteral feedings can be continued during wound care, conscious sedation and/or surgical procedures.

Recent research efforts have focused on using beta-blockade, anabolic hormones, and other pharmacological interventions to ameliorate the hypermetabolic-catabolic response to burn injury.[9,24,30,40,48,50] Although studies have focused more on pediatric burn patients, fatal outcome, catabolism, and wound healing time have been reduced with administration of beta-blockers.[9,24,30,48] A hallmark prospective, randomized, blinded, multicenter trial demonstrated that treatment with the anabolic hormone oxandrolone in burn patients significantly decreased the hospital length of stay.[50] Additional research is required to determine the exact cause of this reduction, but the currently proposed contributing factors are normalization of metabolism, decreased inflammation, improved organ function, increased strength, and/or improved wound healing.[24,30,48,50] It is advocated that all patients with greater than 20% TBSA burns be treated with oxandrolone while monitoring levels of hepatic transaminases.[48,50] Refer to Chapter 6 for additional nutrition information.

PSYCHOSOCIAL CONSIDERATIONS

As improvements in care have now made survival from burn injury an expectation, quality of life and psychosocial considerations have become a priority in treatment plans. Burns are one of the most complex and psychologically devastating injuries to patients and their families. Not only is there a very real threat to survival, but also psychological and physical pain, fear of disfigurement, and uncertainty of long-term effects of the injury on the future can precipitate a crisis for the patient and family. Before appropriate functioning returns, the patient may exhibit stages of psychological adaptation (Box 20-3). A patient may not manifest every stage, but support and therapy are necessary for any patient and family experiencing major burn injury.

To facilitate a person's emotional adjustment to burn trauma, it is necessary to consider the complex interaction of preinjury personality, extent of injury, social support systems, cultural factors, and home environment. For example, many burn injuries are the result of poor supervision, abuse, suicide attempts, assaults, illegal activities, safety code violations, inherent dangers in diverse cultural lifestyles, arson, or military involvement. Although often unwittingly overlooked by clinicians in the immediate acute injury phase, there is a strong link between youth who engage in firesetting behaviors, abuse, and mental health conditions and an urgent need for additional multifaceted intervention.[3] The patient may be dealing with loss of loved ones in the fire, injury event flashbacks, loss of home and belongings, job or financial concerns, societal repercussions, or fear of assailants. The patient may also be facing legal consequences. Preinjury psychiatric disorders

BOX 20-3   STAGES OF POSTBURN PSYCHOLOGICAL ADAPTATION

Survival Anxiety

Manifested by lack of concentration, easy startle response, tearfulness, social withdrawal, and inappropriate behavior. Instructions must be repeated, and the patient has to be allowed time to verbalize concerns and fears. Increased reports of pain are frequently associated with high levels of anxiety.

Search for Meaning

Patient repeatedly recounts events leading to the injury and tries to determine a logical explanation that is emotionally acceptable. It is important to avoid judging the patient's reasoning, to listen actively, and to participate in the discussions with the patient.

Investment in Recuperation

Patient is cooperative with the treatment regimen, motivated to be independent, and takes pride in small accomplishments. The nurse should educate the patient concerning discharge goals and involve both patient and family in planning for a program of increased self-care. Patient requires much praise and verbal encouragement.

Investment in Rehabilitation

As self-confidence increases, patient is focused on achieving as much preburn function as possible. Depression may occur as new losses in function are realized. Staff support is limited in this phase, which usually occurs after patient is discharged from the hospital and is undergoing outpatient rehabilitation. Praise, support, and continued information are beneficial.

Reintegration of Identity

Patient accepts losses and recognizes that changes have occurred. Adaptation is completed, and staff involvement is terminated.

Modified from Watkins P, Cook E, May S, et al. Psychological stages in adaptation following burn injury: a method for facilitating psychological recovery of burn victims. *Journal of Burn Care & Rehabilitation.* 1988;9(4):376-384.

BOX 20-4   SUPPORT PROGRAMS FOR BURN PATIENTS AND FAMILIES

- The Phoenix Society, a national organization to help survivors and families cope with burn injuries: www.phoenix-society.org
- Peer support, such as Survivors Offering Assistance In Recovery (SOAR) developed by the Phoenix Society: www.phoenix-society.org/programs/soar/

- Burn units at local hospitals
- Burn survivor retreats and camps
- School reintegration programs, such as "The Journey Back" and R.E.A.C.H. (Return to Education and Continued Healing)

such as depression, mood disorders, attention deficit disorder, psychoses, and alcohol and drug abuse frequently exist in the burn patient population.[3,45,49] Therefore the critical care nurse must assess the patient's and family's support systems, coping mechanisms, and potential for developing posttraumatic stress disorder (PTSD). Inadequate coping is demonstrated by changes in behavior, anxiety, manipulation, regression, acting out, apathy, sleep disturbances, or depression. Interventions based on individual assessments and that incorporate cultural traditions are the most beneficial and may require assistance from support personnel such as chaplains, clinical nurse specialists, child life specialists, psychiatrists, psychologists, and social workers. As the patient is transferred from the critical care unit, support mechanisms and continuity of care must be maintained because psychosocial recovery can take months, years, or a lifetime. There are several integrative support programs available to positively facilitate a burn survivor's return to society, family, work, and school (Box 20-4). Critical care nurses can help promote hope and alleviate anxiety by informing patients and families of these support resources in the immediate acute postinjury phase.

If a burn injury is not survivable, the critical care nurse plays a key role in supporting the patient and family members, participating in withdrawal of treatment discussions, and providing palliative care until death.

GERIATRIC CONCERNS

As age expectancies in the United States continue to increase, the definition of "geriatric" continues to evolve in regard to treatment and research findings in the literature. A more accurate approach may be to consider preinjury health status and function versus chronological age. In general, older patients are more prone to and more adversely affected by burns.[4,8,27,41] Diminished manual dexterity, reaction time, senses, vision, hearing, balance, and judgment render the elderly more vulnerable to burn injuries. Many older people live alone and are often physically or mentally incapable of responding appropriately to an emergency. In addition, elderly skin is much less resilient to mechanical trauma. Nurses must monitor burn injuries potentially resulting from elder abuse or neglect. The physiological and psychosocial trauma of a burn injury in the elderly patient provides a tremendous challenge for the entire burn team.

Many variables influence outcome of the elderly burn patient and increase mortality including the size and depth of the burn, the number and severity of coexisting diseases, and the development of postinjury complications (see box, "Geriatric Considerations").[4,8,27,38,41] Preinjury hydration status, nutritional deficiencies, and diseases may contribute to a higher mortality or difficulties in fluid resuscitation and combating burn shock. Older patients with heart failure may require administration of positive inotropic medications to increase cardiac contractility. Elderly patients with inhalation injury frequently require mechanical ventilation support and are more prone to episodes of pneumonia and sepsis. Wound care presents a challenge. Skin changes associated with aging, such as a flattened dermal-epidermal junction and a loss of dermal and subcutaneous mass, manifest as skin thinning and predispose this group to deeper burn wounds and to poor or delayed healing. This situation affects not only the healing of the original burn wounds, but also the skin graft recipient beds and donor sites. A decline in immune system function increases susceptibility to infectious complications in this group as well. Older patients also have a diminished physiological reserve and capacity to respond to the metabolic stress and bacterial challenge after a burn injury.

Advances in technology and treatment have improved survival after burn injury.[12,27,30,40,47,48] However, data suggest that advanced age, especially in combination with deeper burns or inhalation injury, continues to be a major determinant of mortality after thermal injury.[4,8,27,41,48] The decision to proceed with resuscitation in elderly patients with large burns and concomitant inhalation injury should be carefully considered with input from advance directives, next of kin, or the designated healthcare surrogate. Preexisting dementia exacerbated by injury and medications has major implications for an elderly patient's ability to participate in rehabilitation to regain function and independence. Thus burn treatment interventions may prioritize comfort, dignity, expeditious discharge from the hospital to familiar surroundings, and quality of life over the extension of life. Poor outcomes after injury highlight that prevention of burn injuries in the elderly is of utmost importance. Therefore older adults and their caregivers should actively pursue incorporating safety measures into their home and lifestyle. Hot bath/shower water, cooking, smoking, spilled coffee or tea, burning yard debris, and home heating devices are frequent sources of burn injuries in this group.

NONBURN INJURY

The experience of the burn team in providing excellent wound and critical care leads to burn unit admissions of patients with a variety of other severe exfoliative and necrotizing skin disorders such as toxic epidermal necrolysis (TEN), staphylococcal scalded skin syndrome (SSSS), and necrotizing fasciitis. These conditions create a clinical wound picture similar to that of a burn wound and require similar patient management and wound care. Management of these patients in a burn center has been associated with a marked increase in survival.[1,6,20]

Severe Exfoliative Disorders
Toxic Epidermal Necrolysis, Stevens-Johnson Syndrome, Erythema Multiforme

TEN, Stevens-Johnson Syndrome (SJS), and erythema multiforme (EM) are conditions in which the body sloughs its epidermal layer. The exact pathophysiological mechanisms remains unclear, but is thought to result from a direct toxic effect and/or an immune-mediated response to a causative agent.[1] The primary clinical finding is a positive *Nikolsky sign*, elucidated by applying lateral pressure to the skin surface with resultant sloughing of the epidermis. Diagnosis of this related continuum of disorders is made by skin biopsy histopathology (separation at the epidermal-dermal junction) and the extent of dermal detachment involvement. EM is characterized by less than 10% TBSA affected with peripheral distribution of lesions. Patients with SJS also have less than 10% TBSA affected, but lesions are widespread. If SJS occurs with TEN, lesions appear on 10% to 30% of TBSA. TEN is characterized by involvement of more than 30% TBSA, and lesions are extensive and widespread.[1] Nursing diagnoses and interventions are the same for these severe exfoliative disorders.

GERIATRIC CONSIDERATIONS

- Determine as early as possible whether the patient has an advance directive.
- Elderly patients have reduced physiological reserves and capacity to respond to the metabolic stress of burn injury.
- Preexisting cardiovascular, renal, and pulmonary diseases lead to challenges in fluid resuscitation.
- Fluid administration may be guided by hemodynamic monitoring.
- Physiological changes in the skin from aging predispose elderly patients to deeper burn wounds and poor or delayed wound healing. Burn wounds, grafts, and donor sites must be monitored carefully.
- Decline in immune system functioning contributes to increased susceptibility to infection.
- Mechanical ventilation contributes to a higher risk of pneumonia, sepsis, and complications of immobility. Ventilator weaning may be prolonged because of muscular weakness.
- Reduced renal and hepatic functioning predisposes elderly patients to delayed clearance of medications (antibiotics, analgesics) and increased potential for toxicity or overdose.
- Factors contributing to the burn injury (e.g., syncope, medication side effects, dangers in the home environment, abuse) must be addressed before discharging the elderly patient.
- Elderly patients have greater morbidity and mortality compared with younger patients with similar percentages of total body surface area burn.[4,8,27,41]

TEN is the most extensive form of severe exfoliative disorder and is the focus of discussion. It is associated with a mortality rate of 30% to 50% versus only 1% to 3% with SJS.[1] The most common cause of TEN is drug reaction, particularly from sulfa drugs, phenobarbital, allopurinol, and phenytoin. In some cases a definitive etiology is never identified.[6] Patients initially have fever and flulike symptoms, with erythema and blisters developing within 24 to 96 hours. As large bullae develop, the skin and mucous membranes slough, resulting in a significant and painful partial-thickness injury. TEN is also associated with mucosal wound involvement of conjunctival, oral, GI tract, and/or urogenital areas.[1,6] Immune suppression occurs and contributes to life-threatening infection-related complications such as sepsis and pneumonia. Primary treatment includes immediate discontinuation of the potential offending drug. Although anticonvulsants and antibiotics are most common causes, any medication initiated in the prior 3 to 4 weeks should be suspected.[1] Optimal wound treatment consists of early coverage of cutaneous wounds with silver-based or biological dressings. Severe exfoliative disorders typically require intensive critical care management to provide fluid resuscitation and nutritional support. Corticosteroids should not be given.[1,6] Low-sucrose IV immune globulin administration may be beneficial in modulating the causative inflammatory response.[1] Care is primarily supportive, and prevention of infection is crucial to stopping the progression of wounds to full-thickness depth. Long-term follow-up with the burn team is important to monitor for the development of commonly reported ophthalmic, skin, nail, and vulvovaginal complications and to address continued issues in health-related quality of life.[1]

Staphylococcal Scalded Skin Syndrome

SSSS occurs primarily in young children and often presents with a clinical picture similar to that of TEN. SSSS is caused by a reaction to a staphylococcal toxin, with intraepidermal splitting (unlike epidermal-dermal separation in TEN) resulting in skin sloughing. Differential diagnosis is critical, because the treatment for SSSS involves antibiotics, which can exacerbate TEN. Diagnosis is made by microscopic examination of the denuded skin to determine the level of skin separation.[1,6] SSSS is limited to superficial epidermal involvement and does not affect the mucous membranes. SSSS is best treated with antibiotic therapy and wound care management.

Necrotizing Soft Tissue Infections

Necrotizing soft tissue infections (NSTIs) are a group of rapidly invasive infections that include diagnoses such as necrotizing fasciitis, gas gangrene, hemolytic streptococcal gangrene, Fournier gangrene (NSTI specifically involving the perineum and scrotum), and necrotizing cellulitis. NSTIs have been identified with increasing frequency in recent years.[33] NSTIs occur more frequently in middle-aged adults and are associated with a 12% to 40% mortality rate.[20,33] NSTIs are caused by polymicrobial organisms, often introduced from minor skin disruptions such as insect bites or cuts that lead to widespread tissue and muscle necrosis. Diabetes, obesity, steroid medications, IV drug use, smoking, recent surgery, and hypertension are some of the risk factors for NSTI.[20,33] NSTI typically have a subtle initial presentation of a localized, painful edematous area with increasing erythema, induration, and crepitus. The pain is severe and out of proportion to cutaneous findings. Because of the rapidly progressive infectious nature of NSTIs, patients can quickly become critically ill with observed high rates of sepsis and septic shock.[22,33] Early diagnosis, prompt and aggressive surgical excision, appropriate wound care, and antibiotic therapy are essential for a positive outcome.

DISCHARGE PLANNING

Discharge planning for critically ill burned patients or those who have sustained a nonburn injury must begin on the day of admission. Assessments are made regarding patient survival, the potential or actual short-term or long-term functional disabilities secondary to the burn or nonburn injury, the financial resources available, the family roles and expectations, and the psychological support systems. Patient and family education is essential to prepare for transfer from the critical care unit and eventual discharge from the hospital. Patients and families who are returning home must understand how to manage their physical requirements, as well as care for their psychological and social needs. Nurses play an important role in multiprofessional discharge planning by providing patient and family education and by evaluating the need for additional resources to meet the patient's long-term rehabilitative and home care requirements.

BURN PREVENTION

The overwhelming majority of burns and fire-related injuries are preventable. Typically, injuries do not occur from random events or "accidents," but rather predominantly from predictable incidents. If people are not aware of potential risks, they do not take appropriate precautions to prevent an injury from occurring. Alcohol and substance abuse contribute to high-risk behavior; screening and brief intervention are effective in reducing alcohol intake and repeat injuries in the burn patient population (see Chapter 19). Successful prevention efforts consider the targeted population and focus on interventions involving education (i.e., changing behavior), engineering/environment (i.e., modifications in safety designs), or enforcement (i.e., laws or safety regulations). Critical care nurses play an active and vital role in teaching prevention concepts and in promoting fire safety legislation that assists in preventing fires and burn injuries. The incidence of burn injuries has been successfully decreased with government-mandated regulations on industrial environments, building codes, products, and home safety (e.g., child-resistant lighters, hot water heater temperature, self-extinguishing cigarettes, fire sprinklers, and mandatory smoke alarms).[7] Box 20-5 lists some strategies for preventing burn injuries.

BOX 20-5 STRATEGIES FOR PREVENTING BURN INJURIES

Cook with Care

- Cooking is the primary cause of home fires and injuries, caused most often by unattended cooking. If you leave the kitchen for even a short period of time, turn off the stove.
- Turn pot handles away from the stove's edge.
- Wear short, close-fitting or tightly rolled sleeves when cooking. Loose clothing can dangle onto stove burners and catch fire.
- Keep appliance cords coiled and away from counter edges.
- In case of an oven fire, turn off the heat and keep the oven door closed.
- If a pan of food catches fire, turn off the burner and carefully slide a lid (or baking/cookie sheet) over the pan. Never move the pan or put water on a grease fire, because the fire will spread.
- Use caution when removing items from microwaves to prevent spilling and burns. Open microwaved food slowly, away from the face to prevent burns from escaping hot steam.
- Stir microwave foods to distribute heat, and test all heated foods before eating.
- Have a "kid-free" safety zone of at least 3 feet around open fire, stoves, and areas where hot food or drink is prepared or carried.

Hot Liquids Cause Scalds

- Never hold an infant or child while cooking, drinking a hot liquid, or carrying hot foods and liquids. Keep hot items away from table and counter edges.
- Consider installing "anti-scald" devices on tub faucets and shower heads. Keep bath temperatures safe by setting water heaters at 120° F.
- Before placing a child in the bath or getting into the shower yourself, test the water.

Smoke Alarms, Sprinklers, and Fire Extinguishers

- Working smoke alarms save lives and should be installed and maintained in every home. Smoke alarms detect fires early, alert residents to escape, and cut the risk of dying in a fire in half.
- Install smoke alarms in every sleeping room, outside each separate sleeping area, and on every level of the home, including the basement. Interconnected smoke alarms on all floors increase safety.
- Smoke alarms with long-life batteries are designed to be effective for up to 10 years. If the low battery warning chirps, replace the entire smoke alarm. For all other smoke alarms, replace the battery once a year (or sooner if it chirps).
- Test smoke alarms once a month using the test button. Replace all smoke alarms when they are 10 years old, or sooner if they do not respond properly to testing.
- Home fire sprinklers work along with smoke alarms in saving lives. Using both cut the risk of dying in a home fire 82%.
- Fire extinguishers must be easily accessible (near exits). Learn how to use your fire extinguisher.

Home Fire Escape and Precautions

- When a smoke alarm sounds, get out fast. You may have only seconds to escape safely.
- Have a home fire escape plan with two ways out of every room and an outside meeting place. Practice the plan at least twice a year, and ensure everyone in the home knows what to do.
- Children, older adults, and people with disabilities may need assistance to wake up to a smoke alarm and/or escape. Make sure your escape plan includes someone helping them.
- Smoke is toxic. If you must escape through smoke, get low and go under the smoke to your way out.
- If your clothes catch fire, stop, drop, and roll. Stop immediately, drop to the ground, and cover your face with your hands. Roll over and over until the fire is out.
- Teach children that matches and lighters are tools not toys. Keep all matches and lighters out of the reach of children.
- Always model safe fire use. If you suspect a child is playing with or misusing fire, seek help from your local fire department.
- If you have young children, install tamper-resistant electrical outlets or protective outlet covers.
- Do not overload outlets. Extension cords are for temporary use only.
- Teach older children how to use appliances safely and about the danger of electricity near water.
- All heaters need space. Keep things that can burn, such as paper, bedding, or furniture, at least 3 feet away from heating equipment.
- Smoking is the leading cause of fire death. Quitting smoking is the safest option. If you smoke, be safe: smoke outside; use deep sturdy ashtrays; do not smoke while lying down, in bed, or while under the influence of drugs or alcohol; use "fire-safe" self-extinguishing cigarettes.
- Keep all flame sources (candles, stoves, lighters, cigarettes, etc.) away from medical oxygen.
- There is only one acceptable use of gasoline: fueling an engine.
- Acknowledge that alcohol, drugs, and some medications impair balance, judgment, and reaction time; use caution around fire sources.
- Closely supervise burning candles; keep them out of reach of children and pets who may knock them over; never leave candles burning while sleeping. Use sturdy, safe candleholders.
- Never store flammable liquids (gasoline, propane, cleaners, paint solvents) near fire sources such as a furnace or pilot light.

Occupation-Related Precautions

- Always wear safety equipment and personal protection gear.
- Fatigue contributes to carelessness and injuries; take breaks to prevent accidents.
- Know the location of emergency exits, fire extinguishers, safety showers and eye washers, and main electrical and/or gas shutoff valves.
- Be familiar with potential chemical hazards in the workplace; review Material Safety Data Sheets.

CASE STUDY

Mrs. J. is a 75-year-old woman who sustained a thermal burn injury in a house fire. She was smoking a cigarette in bed while receiving home medical oxygen. She was trapped in the bedroom for approximately 15 minutes before being rescued by firefighters. No smoke alarms were noted.

Questions

1. Once Mrs. J. is removed from the fire, what priorities are essential in her initial management?
2. Mrs. J. has singed nose hair and is coughing up sooty sputum. The emergency department is 15 minutes away. Based on this assessment, what should the paramedics do?
3. What diagnostic tests and assessments do you anticipate once Mrs. J. reaches the emergency department?
4. What can you anticipate about Mrs. J.'s past medical history?
5. Mrs. J. weighs 65 kg. She has burned an estimated 30% of her body. What is her estimated fluid requirement during the first 24 hours?
6. How much fluid will be given in the first 8 hours after the injury?
7. Given Mrs. J.'s age and past medical history, what are important assessments during aggressive fluid resuscitation?
8. Mrs. J. has circumferential, white, leathery burn wounds on both arms. What type of burn wound does she have? What assessments should be performed? What type of surgical treatment and wound care should be expected during the resuscitative phase, and later in the acute care phase?
9. What type and route of pain medication should be administered to Mrs. J.?
10. When and by what route should nutrition be implemented for Mrs. J.?
11. Considering the circumstances surrounding Mrs. J's injury, what issues will need to be addressed before her discharge from the hospital?

SUMMARY

The physiological response to a major burn injury is one of a biphasic pattern of multiorgan system hypofunction followed by hyperfunction. A major goal of resuscitative care is the prevention of burn shock. The critical care nurse's observations of patient responses are crucial for the prevention of complications related to increased capillary permeability and massive resuscitation fluid therapy. In the acute phase, therapeutic goals include prevention of further tissue loss, maintenance of function, prevention of infection, and wound closure. New and exciting research is emerging, and best practices in burn care will continue to evolve. As the patient progresses through various stages of wound care management, the nurse must not only provide skilled care but also monitor the patient's and family's responses to the treatment regimen. Psychosocial support is integral to the entire process. Although providing care to the burned patient is a team effort, it is the critical care nurse who is with the patient 24 hours a day. The skill and support of the nurse make the critical difference in the patient's outcome.

CRITICAL THINKING EXERCISES

1. Explain why patients with burns need extensive fluid resuscitation even though they are extremely edematous.
2. What strategies might the critical care nurse use to meet the high caloric needs of burn patients who can take foods by mouth?
3. Describe some injury history and physical assessment findings that might lead you to suspect a burn was caused by abuse.
4. What specific strategies and interventions can the critical care nurse employ to reduce the incidence of infection in burn patients?
5. What interventions can be used in the critical care unit to promote early rehabilitation of a burned patient?
6. Why is multiprofessional team care of the burn injured patient important? Who is involved?
7. Many burn patients must be treated at institutions far away from home. What approaches can be used to meet the psychosocial needs of these patients and their families?

REFERENCES

1. Abood GJ, Nickoloff BJ, Gamelli RL. Treatment strategies in toxic epidermal necrolysis syndrome: where are we at? *Journal of Burn Care & Research*. 2008;29(1):269-276.
2. Ahrns KS. Trends in burn resuscitation: Shifting the focus from fluids to adequate endpoint monitoring, edema control, and adjuvant therapies. *Critical Care Nursing Clinics of North America*. 2004;16(1):75-98.
3. Ahrns-Klas KS, Wahl WL, Hemmila MR, et al. Do burn centers provide juvenile firesetter intervention? *Burn Care Res*. 2012; 33(2):272-278.
4. Albornoz CR, Villegas J, Sylvester M, et al. Burns are more aggressive in the elderly: proportion of deep burn area/total burn area might have a role in mortality. *Burns*. 2011;37(6): 1058-1061.
5. Alvarado R, Chung KK, Cancio LC, et al. Burn resuscitation. *Burns*. 2009;35(1):4-14.
6. American Burn Association. *Advanced Burn Life Support Course: Provider's Manual*. Chicago: American Burn Association. 2012.
7. American Burn Association. *Burn Incident and Treatment in the United States: 2011. Fact Sheet*. Chicago: American Burn Association. 2011.
8. American Burn Association. *National Burn Repository 2011. Report of Data from 2001-2010*. Chicago: American Burn Association. 2011.
9. Arbabi S, Ahrns KS, Wahl WL, et al. Beta-blocker use is associated with improved outcomes in adult burn patients. *Journal of Trauma*. 2004;56(2):265-271.
10. Blostein PA, Plaisier BR, Maltz SB, et al. Methamphetamine production is hazardous to your health. *Journal of Trauma*. 2009;66(6):1712-1717.
11. Böttcher-Haberzeth S, Biedermann T, Reichmann E. Tissue engineering of skin. *Burns*. 2010;36(4):450-460.
12. Branski LK, Al-Mousawi A, Rivero H, et al. Emerging infections in burns. *Surgical Infections*. 2009;10(5):389-397.
13. Carrougher GJ, Ptacek JT, Sharar SR, et al. Comparison of patient satisfaction and self-reports of pain in adult burn-injured patients. *Journal of Burn Care & Rehabilitation*. 2003;24(1):1-8.
14. Cheatham ML, Malbrain ML, Kirkpatrick A, et al. Results from the international conference of experts on intra-abdominal hypertension and abdominal compartment syndrome. II. Recommendations. *Intensive Care Medicine*. 2007;33(6):951-962.
15. Chung KK, Blackbourne LH, Wolf SE, et al. Evolution of burn resuscitation in operation Iraqi freedom. *Journal of Burn Care & Research*. 2006;27(5):606-611.
16. Cope D, Moore FD. The redistribution of body water in the fluid therapy of the burn patient. *Annals of Surgery*. 1947;126:1010-1018.
17. Demling RH. Smoke inhalation lung injury: an update. *Journal of Plastic Surgery*. 2008;8:254-282.
18. Demling RH, Mazess RB, Witt RM, et al. The study of burn wound edema using dichromatic absorptiometry. *Journal of Trauma*. 1978;18(2):124-128.
19. Demling RH, Wong C, Jin LJ, et al. Early lung dysfunction after major burns: Role of edema and vasoactive mediators. *Journal of Trauma*. 1985;25(10):959-966.
20. Endorf FW, Cancio LC, Klein MB. Necrotizing soft-tissue infections: clinical guidelines. *Journal of Burn Care & Research*. 2009;30(5):769-775.
21. Gauglitz GG, Williams FN, Herndon DN, et al. Burns: where are we standing with propranolol, oxandrolone, recombinant human growth hormone, and the new incretin analogs? *Current Opinion in Clinical Nutrition and Metabolic Care*. 2011;14(2):176-181.
22. Greenhalgh DG, Saffle JR, Holmes JH IV, et al. American Burn Association Consensus Conference on Burn Sepsis and Infection Group. American Burn Association consensus conference to define sepsis and infection in burns. *Journal of Burn Care & Research*. 2007;28(6):776-790.
23. Hemmila MR, Mattar A, Taddonio MA, et al. Topical nano-emulsion therapy reduces bacterial wound infection and inflammation after burn injury. *Surgery*, 2010;148(3):499-509.
24. Jeschke MG, Chinkes DL, Finnerty CC, et al. Pathophysiologic response to severe burn injury. *Annals of Surgery*. 2008;248(3): 387-401.
25. Karter MJ. *Fire Loss in the United States During 2009*. Quincy, MA: National Fire Protection Association, Fire Analysis and Research Division. 2010.
26. Keck M, Herndon DH, Kamolz LP, et al. Pathophysiology of burns. *Wiener Medizinische Wochenschrift*. 2009;159 (13-14):327-336.
27. Keck M, Lumenta DB, Andel H, et al. Burn treatment in the elderly. *Burns*. 2009;35(8):1071-1079.
28. Kidd M, Hultman CS, Van Aalst J, et al. The contemporary management of electrical injuries: resuscitation, reconstruction, rehabilitation. *Annals of Plastic Surgery*. 2007;58(3): 273-278.
29. Kirkpatrick AW, Ball CG, Nickerson D, et al. Intraabdominal hypertension and the abdominal compartment syndrome in burn patients. *World Journal of Surgery*. 2009;33(6):1142-1149.
30. Latenser BA. Critical care of the burn patient: the first 48 hours. *Critical Care Medicine*, 2009;37(10):2819-2826.
31. Lawrence A, Faraklas I, Watkins H, et al. Colloid administration normalizes resuscitation ratio and ameliorates "fluid creep." *Journal of Burn Care & Research*. 2010;31(1):40-47.
32. Lazic T, Falanga V. Bioengineered skin constructs and their use in wound healing. *Plastic and Reconstructive Surgery*. 2011; 127(Suppl):75S-90S.
33. Mills MK, Faraklas I, Davis C, et al. Outcomes from treatment of necrotizing soft-tissue infections: results from the National Surgical Quality Improvement Program database. *American Journal of Surgery*. 2010;200(6):790-796.
34. Mock C, Peck M, Peden M, Krug E. *A WHO Plan for Burn Prevention and Care*. Geneva: World Health Organization. 2008.
35. Mosier MJ, Pham TN, Klein MB, et al. Early enteral nutrition in burns: compliance with guidelines and associated outcomes in a multicenter study. *Journal of Burn Care & Research*. 2011;32(1):104-109.
36. Niederbichler AD, Hoesel LM, Ipaktchi K, et al. Burn-induced heart failure: lipopolysaccharide binding protein improves burn and endotoxin-induced cardiac contractility deficits. *The Journal of Surgical Research*. 2011;165(1):128-135.
37. Palmieri TL. Inhalation injury consensus conference: conclusions. *Journal of Burn Care & Research*. 2009;30(1):209-210.
38. Pannucci CJ, Osborne NH, Wahl WL. Venous thromboembolism in thermally injured patients: analysis of the National Burn Repository. *Journal of Burn Care & Research*. 2011;32(1):6-12.
39. Pham TN, Cancio LC, Gibran NS. American Burn Association practice guidelines burn shock resuscitation. *Journal of Burn Care & Research*. 2008;29(1):257-266.

40. Pruitt BA Jr, Wolf SE. An historical perspective on advances in burn care over the past 100 years. *Clinics in Plastic Surgery.* 2009;36(4):527-545.

41. Rafla K, Tredget EE. Infection control in the burn unit. *Burns.* 2011;37(1):5-15.

42. Runkel N, Krug E, Berg L, et al. International Expert Panel on Negative Pressure Wound Therapy [NPWT-EP]. Evidence-based recommendations for the use of Negative Pressure Wound Therapy in traumatic wounds and reconstructive surgery: steps towards an international consensus. *Injury.* 2011;42(Suppl):S1-S12.

43. Saffle JR. The phenomenon of "fluid creep" in acute burn resuscitation. *Journal of Burn Care & Research.* 2007;28(3): 382-395.

44. Summer GJ, Puntillo KA, Miaskowski C, et al. Burn injury pain: the continuing challenge. *Journal of Pain.* 2007;8(7): 533-548.

45. Toon MH, Maybauer DM, Arceneaux LL, et al. Children with burn injuries-assessment of trauma, neglect, violence and abuse. *Journal of Injury and Violence Research.* 2011;3(2): 98-110.

46. Wahl WL, Arbabi S, Zalewski C, et al. Intensive care unit core measures improve infectious complications in burn patients. *Journal of Burn Care & Research.* 2010;31(1):190-195.

47. Williams FN, Herndon DN, Hawkins HK, et al. The leading causes of death after burn injury in a single pediatric burn center. *Critical Care.* 2009;13(6):R183-189.

48. Williams FN, Jeschke MG, Chinkes DL, et al. Modulation of the hypermetabolic response to trauma: temperature, nutrition, and drugs. *Journal of the American College of Surgeons.* 2009;208(4):489-502.

49. Wisely JA, Hoyle E, Tarrier N, et al. Where to start? Attempting to meet the psychological needs of burned patients. *Burns.* 2007;33(6):736-746.

50. Wolf SE, Edelman LS, Kemalyan N, et al. Effects of oxandrolone on outcome measures in the severely burned: a multi-center prospective randomized double-blind trial. *Journal of Burn Care & Research.* 2006;27(2):131-139.

Solid Organ Transplantation

Linda Ohler, MSN, RN, CCTC, FAAN
Tracy Evans Walker, MSN, RN, ANP-BC, CCTC
Deborah G. Klein, MSN, RN, APRN-BC, CCRN, FAHA

⊖volve WEBSITE

Many additional resources, including self-assessment exercises, are located on the Evolve companion website at
http://evolve.elsevier.com/Sole.
- Review Questions
- Mosby's Nursing Skills Procedures
- Animations
- Video Clips

INTRODUCTION

Solid organ transplantation has been a therapeutic option for patients with end-stage organ failure for more than 50 years; however, transplantation is associated with many challenges. A scarcity of organs reduces the likelihood of transplantation for many individuals. Currently more than 112,000 people in the United States are on lists awaiting transplantation. In 2010 there were 14,506 organ donations; 7943 were from deceased donors and 6563 were from living donors.[32] Effective management of the immune system to prevent organ rejection has not yet been achieved. Infection as a result of immunosuppressive therapy continues to be the major cause of death in recipients.

Critical care nurses work collaboratively with procurement agencies and transplant teams throughout the transplant process in the care of both the organ donor and recipient. This chapter provides an overview of the organ donation process, candidate selection, posttransplant management, and immunosuppressive medications used to prevent rejection. A detailed discussion of solid organ transplantation including lung, heart, kidney, and liver is presented. Combined heart and lung, pancreas, and intestine transplantation are not discussed in this chapter.

Organ Donation

Organ donation has developed into a separate entity from organ transplantation. Critical care nurses are often the first to identify a potential organ donor and therefore must understand clinical triggers associated with brain death and organ donation criteria.

In the early 1960s, death was defined as the cessation of blood flow when the heart stopped beating. The recovery or procurement of organs from a "dead body" led to the concept of brain death. In the late 1960s, criteria for brain death were developed that defined it as a lack of cerebral and brainstem function associated with a nonsurvivable head injury.[1] An individual was determined to be dead when these requirements were met (brain death), and not when the heart stopped beating (circulatory death). This controversial concept, led by a group from Harvard University, came to be known as the Harvard Criteria for the Determination of Brain Death.[1]

In 1968 the Uniform Anatomical Gift Act (UAGA) was passed in the United States.[2] This law established a legal framework for individuals to authorize an anatomical gift of one's organs, tissues, and eyes following death. It also prohibited the trafficking of human organs. Individual states have adopted UAGA, which has since been revised in 1987 and 2006.[2]

The National Organ Transplant Act (NOTA) of 1984 called for an Organ Procurement and Transplantation Network (OPTN) to be created and run by a private, nonprofit organization under federal contract. This act established the OPTN to provide oversight for transplantation and organ donation, as well as to develop and maintain a national registry for organ sharing and matching.[37] The United Network for Organ Sharing (UNOS) was first awarded the national

OPTN contract in 1986 by the U.S. Department of Health and Human Services. UNOS continues as the only organization ever to operate the OPTN.

The Health Care Financing Administration was given the authority to certify organ procurement organizations. Today there are 58 nonprofit organ procurement organizations (OPOs) serving the donation needs in the United States, Puerto Rico, and Bermuda. Each OPO provides organ donation services to designated geographical areas and also provides bereavement care to donor families, public education, and professional education.

Despite these national efforts, donor organs remain scarce, limiting the availability of transplantation. In 1998 the Centers for Medicare and Medicaid Services (CMS) implemented Conditions of Participation for transplantation that impose requirements a hospital must meet to increase organ donation. Any hospital that receives Medicare or Medicaid reimbursement must notify the local OPO in cases of impending death. It is the responsibility of the OPO coordinator to obtain consent for organ or tissue donation from the family of the deceased patient (Box 21-1). Many hospitals have developed clinical criteria to ensure the appropriate referral of potential organ donors, for example, a Glasgow Coma Scale score less than 5, head trauma, and/or impending withdrawal of life support.

Organ donation saves lives. Tissue donation, although not lifesaving, improves the quality of life for many people. Tissue donation includes skin, corneas, heart valves, bone, cartilage, and tendons. Hospitals are required to have a formal arrangement with a tissue bank for the referral of potential donors. Unlike organ donation, any deceased patient has the potential to be considered for tissue donation.

There are three types of organ donors: living donors, brain dead, and donation after circulatory death. Donors can also be described as altruistic living donors, high-risk donors, and extended criteria donors. Table 21-1 describes in detail the types of organ donors as well as the most common organs donated.

To qualify as a *living donor,* an individual must be physically fit, in good general health, and free from high blood pressure, diabetes, cancer, and kidney and heart disease. Individuals considered for living donation are usually between 18 and 60 years of age. Gender and race are not factors in determining a successful match, but donors must have a blood type compatible with the intended recipient. The potential donor is evaluated to determine the level of physical and mental health, and compatibility with the patient on the transplant waiting list. Living donor donation is coordinated by the transplant team.

In 2010 the American Academy of Neurology released new guidelines for the determination of brain death.[46] According to these guidelines, *brain death* is defined as a complete, irreversible cessation of function of the brain and brainstem regardless of the presence of a pulse, maintenance of respiration through mechanical ventilation, or functioning of other organs. Brain death is diagnosed by physical examination, usually by a neurologist. Determination of brain death consists of four steps: (1) prerequisites for the clinical evaluation (Table 21-2); (2) the clinical evaluation (neurological assessment) (Table 21-3); (3) ancillary tests including electroencephalogram (EEG), cerebral angiography, magnetic resonance imaging (MRI), and/or nuclear scan; and (4) documentation of time of brain death. Federal and state laws require the physician to contact the OPO following determination of brain death.[46]

Consent for any organ donation is obtained from either the family (legal next of kin) or through donor designation (donor consent for donation). Approaching the family for consent for organ donation has moved from hospital personnel to the OPO.[11] The relationship between the critical care unit staff and the family is an important factor in a family's decision to donate organs of a loved one.[18] Fears and concerns about donation affect the outcome for donation consent. Common concerns include that disfigurement of the donor will not allow an open casket at the funeral, the potential donor will receive inferior medical care, the potential donor may not really be dead, and the family will have to pay for the donation process. The critical care nurse provides information, support, and clarity and ensures families have easy access to their loved one so they can say good-bye.

In 2007 the OPTN established guidelines for *donation after circulatory death,* also known as donation after cardiac death (DCD). In this type of donation, the patient has an illness from which no recovery is expected, does not meet brain death criteria, and is dependent on life-sustaining medical and mechanical interventions. Once the family (legal next of kin) makes a decision to withdraw life support, the OPO is notified. If the patient meets age and medical criteria for

---

BOX 21-1   STRATEGIES TO INCREASE ORGAN DONATION: ORGAN PROCUREMENT ORGANIZATION AND HOSPITAL COLLABORATION

- All hospitals must have an agreement with an organ procurement organization (OPO).
- The hospital must notify the OPO in a timely manner about patients who have died or whose death is imminent.
- The OPO determines medical suitability for donation.
- The hospital and OPO ensure notification of every family member of every potential donor of the option to donate organs or tissues.
- Hospitals must collaborate with OPO in educating hospital staff on donation, reviewing death records to improve identification of potential donors, and maintaining physiological organ/tissue function of donors.

TABLE 21-1	TYPES OF ORGAN DONORS IN THE UNITED STATES	
DONOR TYPE	**DESCRIPTION**	**ORGANS DONATED**
Deceased	Declared brain dead because of serious head injuries or neurological events	Heart, lung, kidney, pancreas, liver, islet cells, small bowel, stomach, uterus, face, appendages, skin
Donation after circulatory death (formerly donation after cardiac death and non–heart beating donors)	Donation after withdrawal of life-sustaining therapy	Kidney, liver, lungs
Living donor	An organ or part of an organ is offered by a healthy individual to a patient with end-organ disease. Living donors may be related or unrelated.	Kidney and liver (most common); lung lobes, part of a pancreas, small intestine
Altruistic living donor	An individual who donates an organ or part of an organ to a stranger	Kidney (most common); liver lobe (rare)
High-risk donor	CDC definition includes but is not limited to: • Men who have had sex with another man in the previous 5 years • Use of intravenous nonprescription drugs in the past 5 years • Inmates in correctional facilities • Individuals with exposure to HIV in the past year • Individuals who have exchanged sex for money in the past 5 years Decision based on the critical state of the recipient where the risk of not transplanting an organ is greater than the risk of disease transmission from a donor. Patient and family must consent for accepting a high-risk donor.	Heart, lung, kidney, pancreas, liver, islet cells, small bowel, stomach, uterus, face, appendages, skin
Expanded/extended criteria donor	Deceased donor Donor >60 years old	Liver, kidney

CDC, Centers for Disease Control and Prevention.
Data from Center for Disease Control, Morbidity and Mortality Weekly Report. Guidelines for preventing transmission of human immunodeficiency virus through transplantation of human tissue and organs. 1994;43(RR-8):1-17.
Bernat JL. The boundaries of organ donation after circulatory death. *New England Journal of Medicine.* 2008;359:669-671.

TABLE 21-2	PREREQUISITES FOR THE CLINICAL EVALUATION OF BRAIN DEATH
STEPS	**CLINICAL EVALUATION**
1. Establish irreversible coma and cause of coma	Established by patient history, physical examination, neuroimaging, and laboratory tests. The clinician: • Excludes the effect of CNS depressant medication • Recognizes prior use of therapeutic hypothermia may delay drug metabolism • Verifies no recent administration of neuromuscular blockade medications • Verifies no severe electrolyte, acid-base, or endocrine disturbance
2. Achieve normal core temperature	Warming blanket is often needed to maintain normothermia
3. Achieve normal systolic blood pressure	Hypovolemia and loss of peripheral vascular tone are often present, which may be corrected with vasopressors. Neurological examination is most reliable with systolic blood pressure >100 mm Hg.
4. Perform neurological examination	One neurological exam, though controversial, is now considered sufficient for diagnosing brain death in most states. Brain death must be pronounced and documented by a physician.

CNS, Central nervous system.
Data from Wijdicks EF, Varelas PN, Gronseth GS, et al. Evidenced–based guideline update: determining brain death in adults: report of the Quality Standards Subcommittee of the American Academy of Neurology. *Neurology.* 2010;74(23):1911-1918.

TABLE 21-3	CLINICAL EVALUATION FOR BRAIN DEATH
NEUROLOGICAL ASSESSMENT	**CLINICAL EVALUATION**
Coma	Patient is unresponsive to noxious stimuli in the absence of CNS depressant medications and neuromuscular blockade medications
Absence of brainstem reflexes	Pupils fixed and dilated Absence of ocular movements Absence of corneal reflex Absence of facial movement or grimacing with pressure on temporomandibular joint or supraorbital ridge Absence of gag reflex
Apnea	Absence of autonomic respirations that is tested with CO_2 challenge (documented increase in $PaCO_2$ levels) Prerequisites for CO_2 challenge: • Systolic pressure >100 mm Hg • Core temperature >36° C • $PaCO_2$ 35-45 mm Hg • Euvolemic • Absence of hypoxia/hypoxemia

CNS, Central nervous system; *CO_2,* carbon dioxide; *$PaCO_2$,* partial pressure of carbon dioxide.
Data from Wijdicks EF, Varelas PN, Gronseth GS, et al. Evidenced–based guideline update: determining brain death in adults: report of the Quality Standards Subcommittee of the American Academy of Neurology. *Neurology.* 2010;74(23):1911-1918.

organ donation, the option to donate organs after circulatory death is presented by the OPO coordinator to the family. The decision to withdraw life support is made first and is independent of the decision to donate. The legal next of kin must consent to organ donation.[4]

Care of the grieving family is an integral part of the donation process. These families have special needs that result from their life (donation) and death (loss of a loved one) decisions. The critical care nurse and the OPO coordinator establish a unique relationship with the grieving family as part of the donation process.

Donor Management

Once the potential organ donor has been declared brain dead, the care of the patient shifts to preserving organ function and viability. This process, known as *donor management,* focuses on maintaining hemodynamic stability and normal laboratory parameters. Care of the patient is under the direction of the OPO coordinator working collaboratively with the physician and critical care nurses. Standardized order sets are usually used, and they focus on preserving organ function and viability. Following brain death, loss of brain autoregulation results in intense vasodilation and the potential for cardiac dysrhythmias. In addition, the lack of blood flow in the brain causes a loss of temperature regulation and a lack of antidiuretic hormone, causing diabetes insipidus and fluid and electrolyte disorders (Box 21-2).

The OPO coordinator completes a thorough physical examination and an extensive medical and social history. Laboratory tests include basic metabolic panel, hepatic panel, lipid profile, complete blood count, thyroid panel, and urinalysis. The potential donor is screened for ABO typing and human leukocyte antigen (HLA) histocompatibility, which is useful

BOX 21-2	FOCUS OF DONOR MANAGEMENT

- Maintain blood pressure
- Maintain normal serum glucose level
- Maintain normothermia
- Treat anemia
- Treat coagulopathy and thrombocytopenia
- Provide appropriate mechanical ventilation
- Maintain optimal fluid and electrolyte levels
- Treat polyuria
- Maintain acid-base balance

in predicting organ rejection in the recipient. Serological testing screens the patient for transmissible diseases including, but not limited to, human immunodeficiency virus (HIV), hepatitis, and sexually transmitted diseases. These test results determine the suitability of the donor for transplantation. In addition, the OPO coordinator identifies potential recipients for the organs that can be donated through a computerized system operated by UNOS that matches organs to potential recipients.

Organ Recovery

Once a recipient is identified, the patient is transferred to the operating room where the organ recovery and transplant teams are present. Thoracic organ transplant teams travel to the donor hospital to remove organs for transplantation into recipients at their facilities. Local abdominal transplant surgeons often procure livers and kidneys, which are transported to the recipient hospital. Ongoing monitoring of vital signs and mechanical support continues to ensure hemodynamic stability. The OPO coordinator communicates with the donor family, the critical care nurses, and physicians once the organs are recovered.

In cases involving DCD, the patient is prepared for organ donation over several hours. The surgical team is notified, and when ready, the patient is transferred to the operating room where life-sustaining measures are withdrawn (extubation, stopping of intravenous medications). The patient is then pronounced dead by a hospital physician. The time from onset of asystole to the declaration of death is generally 2 to 5 minutes, at which time a separate surgical team starts the organ recovery process. Current recommendations are to recover the liver in less than 30 minutes after withdrawal of

life-sustaining measures; kidneys and pancreas may be recovered up to 60 minutes after withdrawal of life-sustaining measures.[4] If the patient does not die quickly enough to permit the recovery of organs, the patient may be moved back to the critical care unit where end-of-life care continues and the planned organ donation process stops. This may occur in up to 20% of cases.[43]

Selection of Candidates for Transplantation

A multiprofessional team approach is used to determine candidate selection based on each transplant program's protocol. Table 21-4 provides an overview of the transplant evaluation

TABLE 21-4	STANDARD COMPONENTS OF THE TRANSPLANT EVALUATION PROCESS
COMPONENT	DESCRIPTION
1. Referral for transplantation	Information from referring physician is obtained, including patient history, medical records, and any clinical alerts or "red flags" that could indicate that the patient may not meet program's selection criteria
2. Education about transplantation	Coordinator meets with patient and family Some patients may be critically ill and unable to participate; family members are then educated Education includes overview of risks and benefits, transplant evaluation process, waiting time and outcomes of the transplant program, strict medical regimen required after transplant, financial responsibilities, and results of testing
3. Consent to proceed with transplant evaluation	Education must contain explanations of: • Evaluation process • Surgical procedure and postoperative treatment • Availability of alternative treatments • Potential organ donor risks • Potential medical and psychosocial risks • National and program-specific outcomes (from Scientific Registry for Transplant Recipients data) • The right to refuse transplantation at any time during the process • If the transplant is not provided in a Medicare-approved transplant program, it could affect the recipient's ability to have his or her immunosuppressive medications paid for under Medicare Part B
4. Meeting with consultants	Transplant team members Specialists for concerns identified during transplant evaluation
5. Testing	ABO testing Immunology tests to ensure compatibility Organ-specific tests
6. Multiprofessional meeting	Determines if a patient is an appropriate candidate for transplantation based on the program's patient selection criteria Multiprofessional team members include: • Surgeons • Other physicians (including infectious disease) • Transplant coordinators • Nurse practitioners • Social workers • Pharmacist • Psychologist/psychiatrist • Dietitian • Financial coordinator • Clergy
7. Listing patient with UNOS	Transplant coordinator lists the patient in computer for organ-specific transplant with ABO, lab results, and patient demographics
8. Notification of patient/family	Letter is sent to patient within 10 days of multiprofessional meeting with decision of acceptance or denial for transplantation

UNOS, United Network for Organ Sharing.

process. The pretransplant coordinator starts the process with an education session for potential recipients and their families to explain the transplantation evaluation process including testing, physical examination, and consultations by transplant specialists. The comprehensive evaluation of each potential transplant candidate is performed to ensure that transplantation is the best option and to determine if there are any medical or surgical alternatives. Throughout the evaluation process, transplant team members consider the risks and benefits to the patient and determine if there are any contraindications to transplantation. Contraindications include psychosocial considerations (active tobacco or substance abuse), active malignancy, infection, and a history of noncompliance. Lack of social support is an important consideration in candidate selection. A strong support system is needed to aid in medication compliance, encourage ambulation and completion of daily living activities, provide dressing changes and wound assessment, transport the patient to and from appointments, and provide psychosocial support, especially in the first few months after transplantation.

Occasionally a patient in acute heart, lung or liver failure is admitted to the hospital in critical condition and unable to participate in the education and consent processes. The transplant evaluation is completed with information from the family, and the patient may be listed urgently for a transplant with family consent. Although not optimal, it is usually considered a lifesaving intervention. Heart transplant candidates may "wait" in the critical care unit for a suitable organ while receiving life-sustaining therapies as a

bridge to transplantation (e.g., left ventricular assist device or a total artificial heart). Liver transplant candidates may develop encephalopathy and then be considered too ill to undergo transplantation.

Posttransplant Management

Lung, liver, and heart transplant recipients are cared for in the critical care unit in the immediate postoperative phase, Many renal transplant recipients are cared for in the postanesthesia care unit for the first 24 hours. Effective pain management is important during the first few days to encourage spontaneous breathing and extubation, movement, and activity.

From the time of the transplant, each recipient is carefully monitored for rejection, infection, and posttransplant malignancies (see box, "Clinical Alert: Complications Posttransplantation").

Rejection is not a major cause of death posttransplantation due to individualized immunosuppression regimens. However, medications used to prevent rejection suppress the immune system's ability to respond to infection, and as a result, infection is a major cause of morbidity and mortality post transplantation. Many combinations of immunosuppressive medications are used to prevent rejection (Table 21-5). Medication trough levels are used to guide dosing; however, drug levels cannot be used to determine extent of immunosuppression. Information on specific organ rejection, transplant immunology, and immunosuppression is discussed later in this chapter.

! CLINICAL ALERT

Complications Posttransplantation

Infection is the number one cause of morbidity and mortality posttransplantation. Symptoms an individual with an intact immune system would consider an inconvenience and are often associated with mild discomfort. However, in transplant recipients these mild symptoms may be serious as a result of the immunosuppression necessary to prevent rejection of the transplanted organ. Symptoms such as a mild low-grade fever and fatigue may indicate a serious infection and require further investigation. Other complications reported posttransplantation include malignancies, diabetes, and hypertension.

ASSESSMENT	SIGNIFICANCE
Infections	
Low-grade fever, fatigue, lab values with a low white cell count	May indicate cytomegalovirus (CMV) infection or CMV disease; can lead to CMV pneumonitis in lung transplant recipients
Small pustules following a dermatome	May indicate herpes zoster
Diabetes	
Increased blood sugar level, increased hemoglobin A1c	Posttransplant diabetes can be related to the use of steroids or calcineurin inhibitors.
Malignancies	
Fever, shortness of breath, weight loss, anorexia, sore throat, swollen glands, diarrhea	Symptoms may indicate posttransplant lymphoproliferative disorder (PTLD) associated with Epstein-Barr virus (EBV). It may occur when the recipient is EBV-negative and the donor is EBV-positive. Or it may occur after immunosuppression therapy in patients who were EBV-positive pretransplant.
New moles, lumps in the skin	Squamous cell and basal cell carcinomas are the most common skin cancers posttransplantation.

TABLE 21-5	IMMUNOSUPPRESSIVE MEDICATIONS		
MEDICATION	**USE**	**CLASS**	**MECHANISM OF ACTION**
Alemtuzamab (Campath)	Induction	Monoclonal antibody	Binds to CD52 surface antigen of multiple cell types causing cell lysis
Basiliximab (Simulect)	Induction	Monoclonal antibody	Binds to activated T lymphocyte interleukin-2 receptors
Equine antithymocyte globulin (Atgam)	Induction	Polyclonal antibody	Depletes T lymphocytes
Muromonab-CD3 (OKT3)	Induction	Polyclonal antibody	Depletes CD3+ T lymphocytes
Rabbit antithymocyte globulin (Thymoglobulin)	Induction	Polyclonal antibody	Depletes T lymphocytes
Cyclosporine (Neoral)	Maintenance	Calcineurin inhibitor	Inhibits T lymphocyte activation
Tacrolimus (Prograf)	Maintenance	Calcineurin inhibitor	Inhibits T lymphocyte activation
Sirolimus (Rapamune)	Maintenance	mTor inhibitor	Inhibits T lymphocyte activation and proliferation
Azathioprine	Maintenance	Antimetabolite	Inhibits T lymphocytes. Broad myelocyte suppression.
Mycophenolate mofetil (CellCept)	Maintenance	Antimetabolite	Inhibits B cell and T cell proliferation
Mycophenolic acid (Myfortic)	Maintenance	Antimetabolite	Inhibits B cell and T cell proliferation
Prednisone	Maintenance	Corticosteroid	Blocks T cell–derived and antigen-presenting cell cytokine and cytokine receptor expression

mTor, Mammalian target of rapamycin.
Data from Bunnapradist S, Danovitch GM. Evaluation of adult kidney transplant candidates. In Danovitch GM, ed. *Handbook of Kidney Transplantation*. 5th ed. Philadelphia: Wolters Kluwer Health. 2010. Danovitch GM. Immunosuppressive medications and protocols for kidney transplantation. In Danovitch GM, ed. *Handbook of Kidney Transplantation*. 5th ed. Philadelphia: Wolters Kluwer Health. 2010.

Infection

Bacterial and fungal infections may occur in the early postoperative period in any transplant recipient because of the high doses of immunosuppressive medications required to decrease the risk of rejection. The risk of infection is higher in lung transplant recipients because the new lung (or graft) is continually exposed to the environment through the act of breathing. Other factors contributing to the increased risk of infection in these patients include changes in mucociliary movement and the loss of a cough reflex distal to the anastomosis.

Donor-derived infections are another concern for transplant recipients. Although potential donors with fevers are carefully screened, and OPO coordinator tries to determine any potential infections that could be transmitted to recipients, infections can be missed if the donor's history is incomplete. For example an undetected case of rabies was transmitted from a donor to recipients. The family was unaware that the donor had experienced a bat bite several weeks earlier, and the donor was determined to be healthy for organ donation. Three recipients died of rabies posttransplantation.[41] Other donor-derived infections that have been transmitted to recipients include cytomegalovirus (CMV), Epstein-Barr virus (EBV), HIV, lymphocytic choriomeningitis virus (LCMV), West Nile virus, hepatitis B and C, herpes simplex, and Chagas disease.[14,19,47]

It is mandatory to report any donor-derived infections to the OPO, UNOS, and ultimately to the Centers for Disease Control and Prevention (CDC). UNOS has formed an ad hoc committee to review donor-transmitted diseases called the Disease Transmission Advisory Committee. This group tracks donor-derived infections and publishes guidelines on high-risk donors in conjunction with the CDC.

Recipient-derived Infections

An active infection in a potential transplant candidate is a contraindication for receiving an organ because the infection can be reactivated or worsened with immunosuppressive medication required after transplantation. Common recipient-derived pathogens include tuberculosis, herpes, some parasites, HIV, and hepatitis.[15] HIV patients have been successfully transplanted after careful consideration of CD4+ levels and review of potential drug-to-drug interactions between anti-HIV medications and posttransplant immunosuppression.

Viral Infections

Although rejection rates have decreased with immunosuppression, transplant recipients have become more susceptible to infections and virally-mediated malignancies, such as posttransplant lymphoproliferative disorder (PTLD).[14] Viral infections usually occur 2 to 3 months after transplantation. The most common viral infection is CMV, and it is usually reported in lung recipients. Some transplant programs will only accept CMV-negative lungs because of the morbidity associated with this disease. Pneumonia, *Clostridium difficile*, adenovirus, and recurrent hepatitis C are also common viruses seen in patients posttransplantation. Polyomaviruses are most commonly diagnosed in kidney recipients. BK virus, a type of polyomavirus, can cause kidney allograft nephropathy and ureteral stricture or stenosis. This is usually indicated by a rising serum creatinine level that is also associated with rejection.[36,38]

Whenever possible, it is recommended to vaccinate potential transplant recipients against hepatitis, pneumonia, and influenza. Caregivers at home and in the hospital setting should also receive an annual influenza vaccine to prevent transmission of the virus to the transplant recipient.

Malignancies

Transplant recipients are at higher risk for malignancy because of suppression of the immune system by potent medications used to decrease the risk of organ rejection. Common types of malignancies are skin (nonmelanoma), PTLD, Kaposi sarcoma, and anogenital malignancies. Squamous cell carcinoma is the most common skin malignancy.[5] Patient education includes counseling on the importance of avoiding sun exposure during peak hours, the benefits of using sunscreen, and having annual skin examinations. PTLD is a spectrum of disorders that can present as benign mononucleosis or lymphohyperplasia to full-blown lymphoma.[5,35,49] PTLD is associated with the Epstein-Barr virus and is commonly seen in the first year following transplantation. Human herpes virus 8 is associated with Kaposi sarcoma. Chronic hepatitis B and C are associated with hepatocellular carcinoma. Papillomaviruses are associated with squamous cell carcinoma of the lip, vulva, vagina, cervix, anus, and penis.[5,49]

TRANSPLANT IMMUNOLOGY: IMMUNOSUPPRESSION AND REJECTION

Immunosuppression

In transplant immunology, the immune system is manipulated with medications to decrease the risk of organ rejection. The major cells of the immune system believed to be involved in transplant rejection are lymphocytes, macrophages, dendritic cells, and monocytes. Immunosuppressive medications target these cells in an attempt to prevent the recipient from rejecting the donor organ.

Donor antigens are present in the newly transplanted organ, and recipient antibodies recognize nonself (HLA type) by rejecting the new organ. Medications that prevent rejection target the recipient's T lymphocytes to suppress an immune response.

Figure 21-1 demonstrates the immune system's response to a newly transplanted organ. The process begins with the introduction of antigens from the new organ. The recipient's antigen-presenting cells (APCs) alert the helper T (CD4+) lymphocytes to activate an immune response. Once an immune response is activated, the newly transplanted organ is at risk for being rejected. A naive CD4+ cell requires two signals to become activated. Known as costimulation, both signal 1 and signal 2 must be activated to communicate with CD4+ and initiate an immune response. Most of the immunosuppressive medications target cells after the CD4+ has activated the immune response. Research is being conducted on medications designed to block signal 2 from communicating with the CD4+ cell, which would inhibit an immune response.

Monoclonal antibody therapy, such as alemtuzumab, targets a specific cell protein, in this case CD52, to block its communication with T cells.[21] Blocking communication prevents an initial immune response; however, this blockage is temporary and maintenance immunosuppression is required.

Medications to prevent or decrease the risk of rejection are started during surgery as the new organ is implanted. Many transplant programs use antibody induction therapy, most often with recipients at high immunological risk for rejection[13] (see box, "Evidence-Based Practice"). This includes individuals with a high score on the panel reactive antibody (PRA) test, such as those who have had a previous transplant or blood transfusion, or multiparous women. A high PRA score indicates that an individual is sensitized and has antibodies primed to react to any perceived nonself tissue, such as a newly transplanted organ. Patients who are highly sensitized may require desensitization.

Desensitization protocols involve the use of plasmapheresis and immunoglobulin therapies in an attempt to reduce these highly reactive antibodies. Induction therapy is often used to deplete lymphocytes that are activated as part of the immune response. Drugs such as alemtuzumab and rabbit antithymocyte globulin (ATG) deplete T lymphocytes and are used as induction agents to prevent the initial immune response when the new organ is implanted. Alemtuzumab may be given as a single dose in the operating room, whereas ATG is given intraoperatively and for several days posttransplantation, depending on the transplant program's protocol. Side effects of these agents include fever, chills, arthralgias, headache, thrombocytopenia, and leukopenia. Anaphylaxis can occur but serum sickness is rare. Polyclonal and monoclonal antibodies can also be used to treat episodes of acute rejection.

Maintenance medications are used for long-term immunosuppression to prevent acute rejection and prolong organ survival. Immunosuppressive protocols are transplant-program specific, and they usually include a combination of medications such as corticosteroids, calcineurin inhibitors, antimetabolites, and mammalian target of rapamycin (mTOR). Calcineurin inhibitors (tacrolimus or cyclosporine), steroids, and antimetabolites (mycophenolate mofetil) are started in the critical care unit. Most patients are maintained on two to three immunosuppressive agents for the remainder of their lives. Potential side effects from

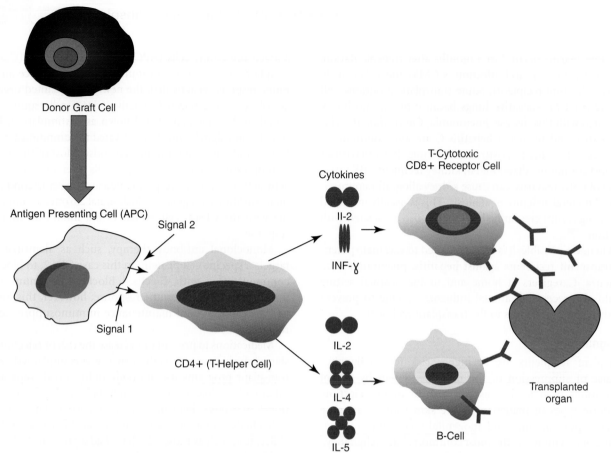

FIGURE 21-1 The response of the immune system to a newly transplanted organ. The donor graft antigens alert the antigen-presenting cells (APC) that nonself tissue is present. The APC sends a message to the CD4+ helper cell to activate an immune response with cytotoxic T cells attacking the newly transplanted organ. (Developed by Frank Van Gelder and Linda Ohler.)

EVIDENCE-BASED PRACTICE

Immunosuppression Post–Kidney Transplantation

Problem

Kidney rejection posttransplantation may result in loss of the newly transplanted organ. Patients are treated with immunosuppressive medications designed to prevent rejection. Rejections are most prevalent in the first 3 months following transplantation.

Clinical Question

Does the use of intravenous induction therapy pretransplantation reduce the risks associated with rejection posttransplantation?

Evidence

The goal of induction therapy is to improve the effectiveness of immunosuppressive therapies and to reduce acute rejection episodes. Induction therapy involves treatment with a biological agent such as a lymphocyte-depleting agent (antithymocyte globulin) or an interleukin-2 receptor antagonist (IL2-RA) (basiliximab). Administration of these medications immediately before transplantation has been studied to determine if acute rejection episodes can be decreased by depleting or modulating T-cell responses as antigen-presenting cells recognize nonself. Although induction therapy has been shown to decrease rejection rates in the initial period posttransplantation, long-term graft outcomes have not been proven. Thirty randomized controlled studies have confirmed the safety and efficacy of IL2-RAs when compared to placebos. A large meta-analysis compared lymphocyte-depleting agents with daclizumab in deceased donor kidney transplants who were considered to be high risk for transplantation. Lymphocyte-depleting agents were shown to decrease the risk of rejection, but increase the risk of infection and malignancy. Lymphocyte-depleting agents are recommended as a first choice for induction therapy with patients who have a high immunological risk.

Implications for Nursing

Introduction therapy, especially IL2-RA, is likely to be initiated during the transplant process. Nurses must be knowledgeable of signs and symptoms of rejection in each patient population for which they are responsible. Signs and symptoms of rejection are different for each organ system. Often a biopsy of the transplanted organ must be performed to confirm or rule out rejection.

Evidence Level

A—Meta-analysis

Reference

Kasiske B, Zeier MG, Chapman JR, et al. KDIGO Clinical Practice Guideline for the care of kidney transplant recipients. *Kidney International.* 2010;77(4):299-311.

immunosuppression include infection, anemia, malignancy, hyperlipidemia, hypertension, bone disease, nephrotoxicity, neurotoxicity, glucose intolerance, nausea, impaired wound healing, hyperuricemia, hyperkalemia, and hypomagnesemia.[48] Use of an mTor inhibitor in the early postoperative period of lung transplantation is contraindicated because it carries a risk of fatal airway anastomotic dehiscence.[16] Table 21-5 contains a list of agents used for induction and maintenance therapy and their mechanisms of action.

Rejection

Over the past 25 years, rejection rates have decreased with advances in immunosuppression therapies and with improvements in testing patients for pretransplant sensitivities to specific antigens. Rejection is described as hyperacute, acute, or chronic. *Hyperacute rejection* usually occurs within hours or days of implantation. Clinical manifestations of hyperacute rejection are related to the organ transplanted. In the worst cases, hyperacute rejection occurs during reperfusion of the organ immediately after transplant. For example, a transplanted kidney ceases to function and appears mottled and cyanotic. Hyperacute rejection of the heart may occur on the operating room table when the aortic cross clamp is removed and result in immediate graft dysfunction. The heart stops beating and becomes mottled. Hyperacute rejection is rarely seen today. In the past a hyperacute rejection was observed when a potential recipient had preformed antibodies against the donor. Potential recipients are now tested for preformed antibodies, thus preventing the problem.

Acute rejection occurs weeks to months posttransplantation. Mild acute rejection is usually managed with increasing oral immunosuppressive medications, whereas intravenous steroids are administered when rejection is more serious. Intravenous immunosuppression, such as antithymocyte globulins, are used to combat the most serious acute rejections. Diagnosing acute rejection is organ dependent.

Chronic rejection occurs months to years after transplantation and is characterized by a progressive form of immunological injury to the allograft vasculature. The epithelial lining of the vasculature, such as the bronchioles in the lungs, coronary arteries of the heart, and bile ducts of the liver, is destroyed. Additionally, fibrotic thickenings form in the arteries in the kidney. Clinical symptoms are specific to each graft, and treatment is tailored to the extent of the disease progression. Chronic rejection may result from frequent, severe, or persistent acute rejection of the transplanted organ. In most cases it is resistant to current treatment modalities, and it is a major problem with long-term allograft function. Risk factors that influence the development of chronic rejection are associated with advanced donor age, young recipient age, black race, presensitization, hypertension, and hyperlipidemia.[20]

LUNG TRANSPLANTATION

Lung transplantation is a treatment choice for patients with end-stage lung disease. The number of lung transplants performed has increased because of advancements in surgical technique, medical management, and immunosuppressive therapy. In 2010, 1770 lung transplants were performed.[32] The survival rates (unadjusted) for lung transplant recipients from January 1994 through June 2008 were 79% at 1 year, 63% at 3 years, and 52% at 5 years.[8]

Indications

The most common indications for lung transplantation are chronic obstructive pulmonary disease, idiopathic pulmonary fibrosis, and cystic fibrosis. Other indications are alpha-1 antitrypsin deficiency, sarcoidosis, bronchiectasis, idiopathic pulmonary arterial hypertension, and lymphangioleiomyomatosis.[8] The decision to perform single or bilateral sequential lung transplantation is determined by the candidate's underlying disease, age, functional status, and transplant program protocol.

Candidate Criteria

Criteria for patient selection varies among transplant programs. Patients considered for lung transplant listing should have failed medical and surgical therapies, and have an expected survival of less than 24 months. Absolute contraindications include active tobacco use, recent malignancy (except nonmelanoma skin cancer), HIV, hepatitis B or C with biopsy-proven histological evidence of liver disease, severe extrapulmonary end-organ disease, significant psychosocial problems, substance abuse, noncompliance with treatment regimen, active severe infection or infection with multidrug-resistant organisms, or chest wall or spinal deformity.[28] Relative contraindications include critical or unstable condition, extreme obesity or malnutrition, mechanical ventilation, severe or symptomatic osteoporosis, poor functional status, or limited rehabilitation potential.[28] The physiological upper age limit for transplantation is 65 years in most programs.

Candidates are listed in order of ABO typing, geographical distance between the candidate and the hospital where the potential donor is located, and the lung allocation score (LAS). Once a patient is placed on the national waiting list, the LAS is used to determine the priority for receiving a lung transplant when a donor lung becomes available.[29] Because the number of lungs available for transplantation are limited, the LAS was developed to estimate the chance of first year survival after transplantation.[29] The LAS uses a patient's medical diagnosis, laboratory values, and diagnostic test results to identify transplant recipients from the candidate listing. Candidates with higher LAS scores have higher priority than those with lower scores. In addition, lungs from children and adolescents are offered to pediatric and adolescent candidates before they are offered to adult candidates.[29]

Donor Criteria

Lung donors can be living or deceased. Donors must be ABO compatible with the recipient. The donor's size must match the recipient. The ideal donor meets the following criteria: younger than 55 years; less than 20 pack-year smoking history; on mechanical ventilation for less than

72 hours; achieve a PaO_2 higher than 300 mm Hg on 100% fraction of inspired oxygen (FiO_2) and 5 cm H_2O of positive end-expiratory pressure (PEEP) for 5 minutes; no active pulmonary disease or infection; clear chest x-ray; no significant chest trauma or signs of infection; negative Gram stain of sputum sample; no previous history of cardiothoracic surgery; and have clear airways seen by bronchoscopy. Since few donors fit the ideal criteria, transplant programs have relaxed their criteria in effort to extend the donor pool by using marginal donors.

Postoperative Management

Lung recipients are initially managed in a critical care unit. Care includes monitoring hemodynamic and respiratory status, maintaining fluid and electrolyte balance, controlling pain, and achieving early ambulation. Immunosuppression therapy consists of a corticosteroid, calcineurin inhibitor, and an antimetabolite.[8,16]

Nerves of the autonomic nervous system are severed during recovery of the donor lung(s). These nerves are not reattached when the lung(s) is transplanted into the recipient, resulting in loss of communication with the autonomic nervous system. Lack of nerve connection is called denervation. In the airway, denervation causes loss of the cough reflex distal to the suture line. Denervation also causes changes in the pulmonary airway response, pulmonary vasculature, mucus production, and ciliary movement. It is important for patients to receive chest physiotherapy and pulmonary toilet to promote drainage of secretions and to prevent mucus plugging. Patients are educated on the importance of coughing when they feel secretions in their throat since they do not have a normal cough reflex.

Complications

Primary graft dysfunction (PGD) can occur within a few hours to several days after lung transplantation. It is caused by ischemia, surgical trauma, denervation, overhydration, and disruption of the thoracic lymphatic system.[45] Presentation of PGD is similar to acute respiratory distress syndrome (ARDS). Extracorporeal membrane oxygenation (ECMO) and nitric oxide have been used to treat severe cases. Surgical complications most commonly seen are hemorrhage; damage to the bronchus, pulmonary artery and vein; phrenic nerve damage; and pleural and gastrointestinal complications.[45] Other complications include atrial dysrhythmias, gastroparesis, ileus, and gastric or peptic ulcer. Recurrent disease can occur in patients with sarcoidosis, lymphangioleiomyomatosis, and other interstitial lung disease.[8]

Rejection

Signs and symptoms of lung rejection may be insidious, and it is difficult to differentiate between infection and rejection. In acute lung rejection, patients may be asymptomatic or present with a variety of signs and symptoms including dyspnea, fatigue, low-grade fever, cough, chest congestion, a decrease in incentive spirometry readings or pulmonary function, or

decrease in oxygen saturation.. Diffuse infiltrates, perihilar fluffiness, or pleural effusions may be seen on chest x-ray. A transbronchial biopsy may be necessary for a definitive diagnosis. Patients with lung rejection are treated with high-dose corticosteroids, adjustment in maintenance immunosuppressive medications, and in some cases augmenting therapy with other immunosuppressive agents.[16]

Chronic rejection in lung recipients is also called bronchiolitis obliterans syndrome (BOS).[12] This is a progressive deterioration in lung function caused by small airway inflammation and fibrosis, resulting in obstruction. Signs and symptoms of BOS include progressive shortness of breath, decreased exercise tolerance, airflow limitation, and progressive decline in forced expiratory volume. Risk factors for the development of BOS include recurrent episodes of acute rejection, inadequate immunosuppression, and pulmonary infection.[12] Early diagnosis and intervention are key to preserving existing lung function. Treatment decisions are based on the immunosuppressive medications regimen and the severity of the disease. Trough levels of immunosuppressive medications are used to determine if doses need to be increased or if medications need to be changed. Depending on the severity of rejection, intravenous immunosuppression therapy may be required.

KIDNEY TRANSPLANTATION

Kidney transplantation is an option for patients with end-stage renal disease (ESRD). In 2010, 16,900 kidney transplants were performed in the United States.[32] However, in early 2011, 87,903 candidates were waiting for a kidney transplant.[32] Patient survival after transplantation with a deceased donor kidney is 94% at 1 year, 88% at 3 years, and 82% at 5 years. Patients who receive kidneys from living donors fare better, with 98% survival at 1 year, 94% at 3 years, and 90% at 5 years.[32]

Indications

The most common indications for kidney transplantation are hypertension, diabetes mellitus, and glomerulonephritis. Other indications include cystic kidney diseases, tubular disorders, autoimmune disorders (e.g., lupus), hemolytic disorders, reflux, neurogenic bladder, congenital disorders, renal cell cancer, and ESRD secondary to the use of nephrotoxic agents.

Candidate Criteria

Candidates are placed on the UNOS national waiting list once they become dialysis dependent, or have a glomerular filtration rate of less than 20 mL/min if not on dialysis. A point system is used to rank candidates to determine who will receive a kidney at the time of an available donor. Potential kidney transplant recipients are ranked by ABO typing, time on the waiting list, and how closely their HLA matches the donor. Additional points are added for candidates who have high levels of antibodies. These candidates wait longer on the list because it is harder to find a close match. Pediatric candidates have priority over adults for organs retrieved from donors younger than 35 years.[28,30]

Major contraindications to transplantation include primary oxalosis (elevated blood level of oxalate, which precipitates with calcium to form calcium oxalate deposits in body tissues), aggressive recurrent native renal disease, irreversible extrarenal disease, current untreated infection, current recreational drug use, malignancy (recent or metastatic), limited rehabilitation potential after transplant, noncompliance with treatment regimens, and severe psychological illness that impairs ability to consent and adhere to treatment regimens after transplant.[7]

Donor Criteria

Kidney donors can be living or deceased. Living donors can be related or unrelated to the potential recipient. The most desirable source of an organ is a living-related donor who matches the recipient closely. If a potential living kidney donor does not match his or her recipient, the two may enter into a *paired exchange program*. A paired exchange program allows a living donor to be matched to another potential recipient whose living donor also does not match with either blood types or preformed antibodies against a donor. Paired exchanges have been reported with matching 16 potential donors with 16 candidates.[17]

Postoperative Management

Patients may be cared for in the postanesthesia care unit or critical care unit after kidney transplantation. Patients who have had a complicated surgery or who are unstable are cared for in a surgical critical care unit. Close monitoring of hemodynamic and respiratory status, fluid intake, urine output, electrolyte balance, and daily weight is vital in the initial postoperative period. The kidney from a living donor functions almost immediately after transplantation; however, a kidney from a deceased donor may produce polyuria, oliguria, or anuria. Diuresis is common, and fluid replacement is often required.. Maintenance fluid replacement is needed to cover insensible fluid loss. Dialysis may be indicated in patients who experience severe fluid overload and hyperkalemia or immediate graft dysfunction. Some surgeons place an indwelling stent in the ureter to prevent urinary anastomotic complications during the recovery period. The stent is removed by cystogram 4 to 6 weeks after surgery. A Jackson-Pratt drain may be placed in the space adjacent to the kidney to facilitate the drainage of lymph fluid. This drain is usually removed when drainage is less than 100 mL per day.[44]

Immunosuppression protocols for kidney transplant recipients are transplant-program specific. Drug combinations include using a corticosteroid with a calcineurin inhibitor, or an mTOR inhibitor and an antimetabolite (see Table 21-5). Some programs do not use corticosteroids, or withdraw corticosteroids from the immunosuppression regimen after a predetermined period of time.

Complications

Surgical complications after renal transplantation include bleeding, renal artery thrombosis, renal vein thrombosis, lymphocele, renal artery stenosis, urine leak, ureteral obstruction, and deep vein thrombosis. Common bacterial infections seen within the first month of transplantation are associated with the wound, catheter, urinary tract, and intraabdominal cavity. Pneumonia is also common during this period. Viral, fungal, and mycobacterial infections can occur after the first month. CMV is the most common viral pathogen. Infection presents initially with a fever, malaise, leukopenia, and thrombocytopenia, and can cause pneumonitis, hepatitis, enteritis, colitis, retinitis, and nephropathy.

Acute tubular necrosis (ATN) is the most common cause of delayed kidney (graft) function. ATN may begin with acute kidney injury in the donor before or during organ recovery. Other factors that can cause ATN include prolonged warm or cold ischemia time, reperfusion injury, and any extended periods of hypotension after transplantation. After kidney removal from the donor, the kidney is placed on ice and filled with cold preservation fluid. The time between when blood circulation stops in the kidney during removal and when it is cooled is known as warm ischemia time. Cold ischemia time is the period between when the donor kidney is placed on ice and filled with cold preservation fluid and when the kidney reaches physiological temperature during implantation. Reperfusion injury is caused by an inflammatory response that occurs when blood flow is returned to the kidney. Delayed function can also be caused by poor blood perfusion, obstruction, urine leak, and acute rejection.

Kidney transplantation slows the progression of cardiovascular disease in patients with ESRD, but cardiovascular disease is still the most common cause of death following kidney transplantation.[49] Myocardial infarction, heart failure, or stroke are common because of comorbid conditions including diabetes, hypertension, and older age. In some cases, such as IgA nephropathy and focal segmental glomerular sclerosis (FSGS), the original kidney disease may recur after transplant and can lead to graft loss.[49]

Rejection

Acute rejection is often indicated by a rise in serum creatinine. The patient may develop fever, tenderness over the graft site, edema, weight gain, gross hematuria, decreased urine output, and/or hypertension. The area over the transplanted kidney may feel firm on palpation. A kidney biopsy may be necessary to confirm rejection. The biopsy may show interstitial edema, lymphocyte infiltration, tubulitis, arteritis, and arterial fibrinoid necrosis. Biopsy specimens are graded according to the severity of tubulitis and arteritis by using the Banff 97 Grading System (borderline, 1A, 1B, 2A, 2B, and 3; higher values are associated with greater severity).[27] Treatment for acute kidney rejection consists of high-dose corticosteroids and optimizing immunosuppression.[9]

HEART TRANSPLANTATION

Since 1990, more than 2000 heart transplants have been performed in the United States annually.[32] Between 1995 and 2001, 500 to 800 candidates awaiting heart transplantation died each year. This number has decreased to 300 to 400 deaths each year.[32] The use of mechanical assist devices, including ventricular assist devices and total artificial hearts, as a bridge to transplantation, is a likely reason for the decrease in deaths for those awaiting a heart transplant.

Indications

Heart transplantation is an option for patients with advanced heart failure who have not responded successfully to maximal medical therapy. Heart transplant recipients have an 88% probability of surviving 1 year, 80% for 3 years, and a 53% probability of surviving to 10 years.[40]

Candidate Criteria

In 2006, the International Society for Heart and Lung Transplantation (ISHLT) issued guidelines addressing selection and listing criteria of patients for heart transplantation.[24] Recommendations from this consensus document are used by most transplant programs to guide the evaluation process and selection criteria for patients with end-stage heart disease. Cardiopulmonary stress testing is recommended for heart failure patients who are able to walk without assistance. A peak VO_2 of less than 10 mL/kg/min indicates a lower survival rate and serves as an indicator for heart transplantation.[24,26] Right heart catheterization to evaluate an individual's pulmonary vascular resistance (PVR) ensures the new heart will not fail when pumping against a high resistance in the lungs.

Members of the multiprofessional team meet weekly to discuss potential candidates for transplantation. Patients are listed if they meet the program's selection criteria. Listing is based on medical urgency with three classifications. Status 1A is the most urgent. These patients are hospitalized with mechanical support and multiple vasoactive medication infusions, and are expected to die within a week without a transplant. Status 1B is less urgent; these patients can be managed at home with a left ventricular assist device. Status 2 is the least urgent.

Contraindications for heart transplantation vary among programs, but most consider psychosocial issues such as substance abuse, a lack of a support system, smoking, and a history of noncompliance as strong reasons to deny listing. Active malignancy and infection are also contraindications for transplantation.[24,26]

Donor Criteria

The number of donor hearts available for transplantation has reached a plateau during the last 20 years. As a result, transplant programs have considered more extended criteria, including donor age. Donors over the age of 55 years are considered if factors such as coronary artery disease, cardiac structural abnormalities, and left ventricular function have been evaluated and determined to be acceptable.[51] Matching donor age to the recipient is a strong consideration when evaluating extended criteria. Donors must be ABO compatible, and most programs prefer there to be no history of smoking, diabetes, dyslipidemia, or hypertension. The potential donor's family history of cardiac disease is reviewed when evaluating extended criteria. A potential donor who has experienced a cardiac arrest is not considered for donation of the heart.

Postoperative Management

Patients usually arrive to the surgical critical care unit intubated and ventilated until they regain consciousness. The first 24 to 48 hours after heart transplantation requires close monitoring of hemodynamic status. Cardiac output, cardiac index, PVR, and systemic vascular resistance (SVR) are closely monitored via a pulmonary artery catheter. Right heart function may deteriorate if the pulmonary vascular resistance (PVR) remains elevated. A decrease in cardiac output or stroke volume must be reported immediately so appropriate therapy can be initiated. The chest may be left "open" to accommodate any edema that may occur during the immediate postoperative period. High doses of immunosuppressive medications are given during this time. It is important for all personnel to comply with strict hand washing and wound care to prevent infections. Volume and color of chest tube drainage is monitored closely for signs of acute bleeding. The newly transplanted heart has undergone numerous changes in the previous 24 hours, starting with the trauma experienced by the donor, the explantation procedure, placement in ice for travel, and then transplantation into another individual. Cold and warm ischemic times and donor management issues all may impact the function of the newly transplanted heart, making the patient's new heart vulnerable to dysrhythmias. Epicardial pacing wires are usually placed for temporary pacing.

Complications

The most serious complication in the perioperative period is immediate graft dysfunction requiring mechanical circulatory support. Right ventricular failure or dysfunction may also occur if the patient's PVR is elevated before transplantation. ECMO, a biventricular assist device, or a right ventricular assist device may be required. Hemodynamic instability, atrial dysrhythmias, and bradycardia may also occur. The risk of death with these serious complications is over 50%.[25]

Rejection

Signs and symptoms of heart rejection include fatigue, decrease in exercise tolerance, shortness of breath, and fluid retention. Diagnosing heart rejection has been traditionally done through surveillance of endomyocardial biopsies. This is an invasive procedure that is performed weekly for the first 6 weeks posttransplant. A catheter is placed through the right internal jugular vein or in the right femoral vein, and small tissue samples are taken from the right ventricular septum. Over time with frequent biopsies, cardiac tissue becomes calcified, which makes it impossible to detect rejection. Alternatives to the endomyocardial biopsy have been studied. Recently, some transplant programs have been measuring gene expression through upregulation of molecular and cellular pathways to detect rejection. A strong positive correlation has been found between the endomyocardial biopsy and gene expression.[10]

LIVER TRANSPLANTATION

Over the past 20 years, liver transplantations performed in the United States have risen from 1713 in 1988 to 6291 in 2010, including both living and deceased donors.[32,33] Living donors accounted for just two liver transplants in 1989, but rose to 524 in 2001.[33] The number of living liver donations has dropped significantly after several reported deaths of living liver donors, but remains between 200 and 300 annually.[32]

Indications

Liver transplantation has increased as a therapeutic intervention for patients with acute and chronic liver failure. The most common indication for liver transplantation is hepatitis C, accounting for 37% to 41% of liver transplants in the United States.[31] Other indications include alcoholic cirrhosis (18%), cryptogenic cirrhosis or no identifiable cause of liver failure (11%), primary sclerosing cholangitis (PSC; 8%), fulminant (severe sudden onset) liver failure (6%), and autoimmune hepatitis (6%). Primary liver tumors account for 2% of liver transplants in the United States.[22] One-year graft survival rates for deceased donor liver transplants have increased to 84.5%. Graft survival rates at 5 and 10 years for deceased donor liver transplants are reported as 68% and 53%, respectively.[34]

Candidate Criteria

Patients meeting criteria for a liver transplant are listed on the UNOS national list based on a numerical scoring system that measures severity of liver disease. The Model for End-Stage Liver Disease (MELD) score uses the patient's serum creatinine, international normalized ratio for prothrombin time (INR), and serum bilirubin to predict survival. A calculated MELD score ranges from 6 to 40, and it is directly associated with the patient's risk of death within 3 months. A higher score indicates a more critically ill patient and an urgent need for liver transplantation. Since implementation of MELD in 2002, there has been a reduction in wait time and wait list mortality.[39] An exception to using the MELD score is in patients with an acute onset of liver disease and a life expectancy of hours to a few days. Patients in this situation can be listed as a status 1A.

Donor Criteria

With the increase in success rates for liver transplantation, finding suitable donors has become more challenging. Living and extended criteria donors have become more widely accepted as potential options for patients in need of a liver transplant. The largest group of extended criteria donors is individuals over the age of 65 years.[23,32] Long-term outcomes are still being evaluated. Outcomes of living liver donors in adult-to-adult liver transplantation are similar to deceased donor liver transplants with 1-year survival at 86%, and 5- and 10-year graft survival slightly higher at 73% and 61%, respectively.[33] Outcomes for DCD liver donors are lower than for deceased donors with a 3-year graft survival of 77% versus 80%.[3,23]

Blood type and body size are the two criteria necessary for matching a donor liver to a recipient. HLA tissue typing is not used because it has not been known to significantly affect outcomes. Donors are carefully screened for infectious diseases and carcinomas because they can be transmitted to the recipient.

Postoperative Management

Liver transplant recipients are cared for in the surgical critical care unit and usually remain intubated and on mechanical ventilation for the first 24 hours. Cardiac output, cardiac index, SVR, central venous pressure (CVP), and fluid status are monitored using a pulmonary artery catheter. A transesophageal probe may be inserted to monitor the chambers of the heart to determine dilation and fluid overload. Patients are monitored for bleeding, often associated with coagulopathy, which may indicate a poorly functioning graft.[22,42] Clotting studies are monitored frequently during the immediate postoperative period because of the risk of bleeding. A rise in prothrombin time may be associated with a poorly functioning liver, whereas a rise in alkaline phosphatase level may indicate biliary complications or cholestasis.[6] Blood glucose levels are monitored closely because the liver is a primary source for blood glucose production. Hyperglycemia is treated with an insulin infusion; hypoglycemia may indicate a poorly functioning liver and require treatment with 50% glucose.[6]

Complications

The most common complications post–liver transplantation include hepatic artery thrombosis (HAT), bleeding, primary allograft dysfunction, infection, renal dysfunction, and bile duct problems. Indicators of HAT include elevations of aspartate transaminase (AST) and alanine aminotransferase (ALT) levels that may be observed as soon as postoperative day 1 and may require retransplantation.[22,23,42] A Doppler ultrasound confirms the diagnosis of HAT. Early indicators of primary allograft dysfunction include a decrease in bile production and a rise in AST level.

Infection is the leading cause of death following liver transplantation. Infections with CMV, EBV, *Pneumocystis jiroveci*, and *Aspergillus* are often seen 6 to 12 months after transplantation. Renal dysfunction is usually associated with hemodynamic instability, sepsis, blood loss, or toxicity from immunosuppressive medications. Bile duct complications are usually indicated by a rise in alkaline phosphatase, bilirubin, and gamma-glutamyltransferase (GGT) levels. A T-tube may be placed in the bile duct to allow drainage. Biliary leaks may occur at the site of anastomosis or at the T-tube exit site.[6,22] With high doses of immunosuppressive medications given in the immediate postoperative period, the T-tube site and the surgical wound must be kept clean and dry to prevent infection. Hepatic encephalopathy may be present before transplantation and may resolve slowly after transplantation.

Rejection

Some patients will experience an acute rejection episode in the first 3 months after liver transplantation. Clinical symptoms may be mild and initially unrecognized by the patient. Box 21-3 lists symptoms that may indicate rejection of the newly transplanted liver. A liver biopsy may be necessary to confirm a diagnosis of rejection. Criteria used to score liver transplant rejection have been defined by the World Gastroenterology Consensus group; the score is referred to as the Rejection Activity Index (RAI).[50] Rejection is categorized as portal inflammation, bile duct inflammation, or venous endothelial inflammation. The levels of inflammation are further graded as 1, 2, or 3. A score is calculated, with the most severe score being 9. Most rejections respond to increases in immunosuppressive medications; although in the first few months posttransplantation, a rejection would likely be treated with intravenous steroids or antithymocyte globulin.

BOX 21-3   SIGNS AND SYMPTOMS OF LIVER TRANSPLANT REJECTION

Signs and Symptoms
- Fever greater than 38.3° C
- Fatigue or excess sleepiness
- Irritability
- Headache
- Abdominal swelling and/or tenderness
- Pain in right upper quadrant of abdomen
- Decreased appetite
- Jaundice
- Dark urine
- Itching

Laboratory Findings
- Increased aspartate aminotransferase
- Increased alkaline phosphatase
- Increased gamma-glutamyltransferase

CASE STUDY

Mr. F., a 36-year-old man, was transferred from a community hospital to an academic transplant center with a diagnosis of esophageal varices secondary to a history of autoimmune hepatitis. Initial assessment revealed jaundiced skin and sclera. He was oriented to person, place, and time, but was confused when asked questions about his current situation. His lungs were clear, his heart rate was 96 beats/min with normal sinus rhythm, and his blood pressure was 90/60 mm Hg. Edema (2+) was present in the lower extremities. No ascites was evident. Shortly after admission, Mr. F. experienced massive hematemesis and required transfusions with packed red blood cells and fresh frozen plasma. An upper endoscopy was performed with evidence of variceal bleeding requiring banding. His urine was dark in color. Hepatorenal syndrome was suspected.

Admission laboratory values revealed the following:

White blood count (WBC)	6.1/microliter
Hematocrit	25.2%
Hemoglobin	8.7 g/dL
Platelets	22,000/microliter
Red blood cells	2.766 million/mL
Alkaline phosphatase	78 unit/L
Aspartate transaminase (AST)	365 unit/L
Alanine aminotransferase (ALT)	401 unit/L
Sodium	131 mEq/L
Creatinine	4.5 mg/dL
Albumin	3.1 g/dL
Total bilirubin	9.6 mg/dL
International normalized ratio (INR)	1.8
Glomerular filtration rate (GFR)	17 mL/min

The liver transplant team was contacted and an evaluation was started with the multiprofessional team. The patient's Model of End-Stage Liver Disease (MELD) score was calculated to be 35, and Mr. F was listed for a liver transplant. Given the severity of his disease and the high MELD score, a suitable new liver was found just 3 days after listing.

After transplantation, Mr. F. was in the surgical critical care unit; he was extubated within 24 hours and treated in the unit for 2 days. His liver enzymes rose initially but began to fall by the time of his discharge home 16 days later. His mental status was normal at post-op day 6 and the remainder of his hospitalization was uneventful.

Within 7 days after discharge he was readmitted with irritability, fatigue, and right upper quadrant (RUQ) abdominal pain. The abdominal ultrasound was negative as were the magnetic resonance imaging (MRI) and computed tomography (CT) of his head.

Readmission laboratory values:

Alkaline phosphatase	411 unit/L
AST	73 unit/L
ALT	221 unit/L
Sodium	135 mEq/L
Creatinine	4.1 mg/dL
Albumin	2.2 g/L
Total bilirubin	12.5 mg/dL
INR	1.2
GFR	27 mL/min

A liver biopsy revealed moderate liver rejection requiring treatment with intravenous steroids. He was discharged after 5 days with increases in his maintenance immunosuppression.

Discharge laboratory values:

Alkaline phosphatase	395 unit/L
AST	68 unit/L
ALT	69 unit/L
Sodium	136 mEq/L
Creatinine	3.0 mg/dL
Albumin	1.9 g/dL
Total bilirubin	8.9 mg/dL
INR	1.2
GFR	30 mL/min

Questions
1. What three tests are used to calculate MELD scores?
2. What symptoms indicate rejection?

SUMMARY

Transplantation is a highly complex and challenging specialty. Individualized immunosuppressive regimens, improved surgical procedures, and an increasing understanding of the immune system continue to assist in improving outcomes following transplantation. Recipient and donor selection are key factors in ensuring the best outcomes for patient and allograft survival.

CRITICAL THINKING EXERCISES

1. A 40-year-old man with a history of autoimmune kidney disease (IgA nephropathy) is experiencing a decline in kidney function with his glomerular filtration rate (GFR) now at 17 mL/min and creatinine at 5.2 mg/dL. He has had three recent episodes of hyperkalemia. He started home dialysis and has been on the kidney waiting list for 5 months. The average wait time in his area is 3 to 4 years. His wife and he have discussed her donating a kidney to him, but have been concerned about living kidney donation because they have two small children and no family in the area to care for them. Friends and neighbors come forward and offer to care for the children while they are hospitalized. His wife is evaluated and found to be a compatible match for living donation. A date is set with the transplant hospital and arrangements for child care are made. Both recover quickly with each having a serum creatinine of 1.8 mg/dL at discharge. The wife is discharged to home after 2 days. The husband is discharged to home after 5 days. On postoperative day 14, a routine clinic visit reveals a creatinine increase to 2.8 mg/dL with tenderness over the new kidney site. A renal biopsy is performed revealing a Banff 2 rejection. What is the best treatment option for this patient?

2. A 25-year-old female received a double lung transplant for cystic fibrosis 2 years ago and has done reasonably well. She works full time and is now married. She has had four acute rejection episodes over the past 2 years and is on maintenance immunosuppression with tacrolimus 6 mg twice daily, prednisone 20 mg daily, and mycophenolate mofetil 1.5 g twice daily. She is admitted to the hospital with increased shortness of breath, low-grade fever, and overall malaise. She describes a recent decrease in her ability to walk up and down stairs without becoming dyspneic. What form of rejection may she be experiencing?

3. A 22-year-old woman was admitted to the critical care unit in fulminant hepatic failure with acetaminophen toxicity related to an attempted suicide. She was comatose and her family relayed her medical history, which included a possible cause of the overdose. She had failed her senior year at the university and could not graduate with her friends. She had always been an average student so this was very disappointing to her parents and to her. She was listed urgently for a liver transplant as a status 1A. A new liver was transplanted within 36 hours. She did well for the first 2 days posttransplantation and was extubated within 12 hours. On post-op day 3 there was a sharp rise in her liver enzymes. A Doppler ultrasound revealed poor blood flow in the hepatic artery. Which laboratory tests are most indicative of hepatic artery thrombosis post–liver transplantation?

REFERENCES

1. Ad Hoc Committee of Harvard Medical School. A definition of irreversible coma. Report of the Ad Hoc Committee of Harvard Medical School. *Journal of the American Medical Association,* 1968;205(6):337-340.
2. Acts. Anatomical Gifts 1068. *Uniform Law Commission.* www.nccusl.org/Act.aspx?title=Anatomical Gift; 1968 Accessed August 28, 2011.
3. Bernat JL. The boundaries of organ donation after circulatory death. *New England Journal of Medicine.* 2008;359:669-671.
4. Bernat JL, D'Alessandro AM, Port FK, et al. Report of a national conference on donation after cardiac death. *American Journal of Transplantation.* 2006;6:281-291.
5. Buell JF, Gross GG, Woddle ES. Malignancy in transplantation. *Transplantation.* 2005;80:S254-S264.
6. Bufton S, Emmett K, Byerly A. Liver transplantation. In Ohler L, Cupples S, eds. *Core Curriculum for Transplant Nurses.* St. Louis: Mosby. 2008;423-454.
7. Bunnapradist S, Danovitch GM. Evaluation of adult kidney transplant candidates. In Danovitch GM, ed. *Handbook of Kidney Transplantation.* 5th ed. Philadelphia: Wolters Kluwer Health. 2010;157-180.
8. Christie JD, Edwards LB, Kucheryavaya AY, et al. The registry of the International Society for Heart and Lung Transplantation: twenty-seventh official adult lung and heart-lung transplant report-2010. *The Journal of Heart and Lung Transplantation.* 2010;29(10):1104-1118.
9. Danovitch GM. Immunosuppressive medications and protocols for kidney transplantation. In Danovitch GM, ed. *Handbook of Kidney Transplantation.* 5th ed. Philadelphia: Wolters Kluwer Health. 2010;77-126.
10. Eisen H. Heart transplantation: graft rejection basics. *Advanced Studies in Medicine.* 2008;8(6):174-181.
11. Ehrle R, Shafer T, Nelson K. Determination and referral of potential organ donors and consent for organ donation: best practice–a blueprint for success. *Critical Care Nurse.* 1999;19(2):21-30.
12. Estenne M, Maurer JR, Boehler A, et al. Bronchiolitis obliterans syndrome 2001: an update of the diagnostic criteria. *The Journal of Heart and Lung Transplantation,* 2002;21(3):297-310.

13. Farney AC, Stratta RJ. Induction therapy: an important part of the immunosuppression equation. *Medscape Transplantation.* www.medscape.org/viewarticle/560137; 2007 Accessed September 5, 2011.

14. Fischer SA, Graham MB, Kuehnert MJ, et al. Transmission of lymphocytic choriomeningitis virus by organ transplantation. *New England Journal of Medicine.* 2006;354(21):2235-2249.

15. Fishman JA. Introduction: Infections in solid organ transplant recipients. *American Journal of Transplantation.* 2009;9(Suppl 4): S3-S6.

16. Floreth T, Bhorade SM. Current trends in immunosuppression for lung transplantation. *Seminars in Respiratory and Critical Care.* 2010;31(2):172-178.

17. Georgetown University. *Paired Kidney Exchange.* www. georgetownuniversityhospital.org/body.cfm?id=15&action= detail&ref=215; Accessed August 28, 2011.

18. Haddow G. Donor and nondonor families' accounts of communication and relations with healthcare professionals. *Progress in Transplantation,* 2004;14(1):41-48.

19. Iwamoto M, Jernigan DB, Guasch A, et al. Transmission of West Nile virus from an organ donor to four transplant recipients. *New England Journal of Medicine,* 2003;348:2196-2203.

20. Joosten IA, Sijpkens YW, Van Kooten C, et al. Chronic renal allograft rejection: pathophysiologic considerations. *Kidney International.* 2005;68:1-13.

21. Kirk AD, Hale DA, Mannon RB, et al. Results from a human renal allograft tolerance trial evaluating the humanized Cd52-specific monoclonal antibody alemtuzumab (Campath-1H). *Transplantation.* 2003;76(1):120-129.

22. Manzarbeitia C. Liver transplantation. *Medscape.* www. emedicine.medscape.com/article/431783; 2011.

23. Mateo R, Cho Y, Singh G, et al. Risk factors for graft survival after liver transplantation from donation after cardiac death donors: an analysis of OPTN/UNOS Data. *American Journal of Transplantation.* 2006;6:791-796.

24. Mehra M, Kobashigawa J, Starling R, et al. Listing criteria for heart transplantation: International Society for Heart and Lung Transplantation guidelines for care of cardiac transplant candidates. *Journal of Heart and Lung Transplantation.* 2006;25(9):1024-1042.

25. Mihaljevic T, Jarrett CM, Gonzales-Stawinski G, et al. Mechanical circulatory support after heart transplantation. *European Journal of Cardiothoracic Surgery,* 2011;39(6):Epub ahead of print.

26. Miller LW. Listing criteria for cardiac transplantation: results of an American Society of Transplant Physicians-National Institutes of Health Conference. *Transplantation.* 1998;66: 947-951.

27. Nast CC, Cohen AH. Pathology of kidney transplantation. In Danovitch GM, *Handbook of Kidney Transplantation.* 5th ed. Philadelphia: Wolters Kluwer Health. 2010;311-329.

28. Orens JB, Estenne M, Arcasoy S, et al. International guidelines for the selection of lung transplant candidates: 2006 update-a consensus report from the Pulmonary Scientific Council of the International Society for Heart and Lung Transplantation. *The Journal of Heart and Lung Transplantation.* 2006;25(7): 745-755.

29. Organ Procurement and Transplantation Network. Frequently asked questions about the lung allocation system (LAS). http://optn.transplant.hrsa.gov/resources/professionalResources. asp?index=86; Accessed March 11, 2012.

30. Organ Procurement and Transplantation Network. Kidney policy (Policy 3.5) http://www.optn.org/PoliciesandBylaws2/policies/pdfs/policy_7.pdf; Accessed September 30, 2011.

31. Organ Procurement and Transplantation Network. Liver Transplantation in the United States 1998. http://optn. transplant.hrsa.gov/ar2009/Chapter_IV_AR_CD.htm?cp=5#4; 2008. Accessed September 7, 2011.

32. Organ Procurement and Transplantation Network. National Data Report. http://optn.transplant.hrsa.gov/latestData/rptData.asp; Accessed October 18, 2011.

33. Organ Procurement and Transplantation Network. Transplants by Donor Type. http://optn.transplant.hrsa.gov/latestData/rptData.asp; Accessed September 5, 2011.

34. Organ Procurement and Transplantation Network. OPTN/SRTR 2009 Annual Report Adjusted Graft Survival, Deceased Donor Liver Transplant Survival at 3 months, 1 year, 5 years and 10 years. http://optn.transplant.hrsa.gov/ar2009/908a_li.pdf; Accessed September 7, 2011.

35. O'Reilly Zwald F, Brown M. Skin cancer in solid organ transplant recipients: advances in therapy and management. Part 1. Epidemiology of skin cancer in solid organ transplant recipients. *Journal of the American Academy of Dermatology.* 2011;65:253-261.

36. Pegues DA, Kubak BM, Maree CL, et al. Infections in kidney transplantation. In Danovitch GM, ed. *Handbook of Kidney Transplantation.* 5th ed. Philadelphia: Wolters Kluwer Health. 2010;251-279.

37. Public Law 98-507. www.history.nih.gov/research/downloads/PL98-507.pdf; 1984 Accessed August 28, 2011.

38. Ramos E, Johnson M. Non-CMV, non-hepatitis viral infections in the renal transplant patient. In Weir MR, ed. *Medical Management of Kidney Transplantation.* Philadelphia: Lippincott Williams & Wilkins. 2005;416-429.

39. Said A, Einstein M, Lucey MR. Liver transplantation: an update 2007. *Current Options in Gastroenterology.* 2007;23: 292-298.

40. Scientific Registry for Transplant Recipients. Heart Data. http://www.srtr.org/annual_reports/2010/1109_hr.htm; Accessed March 11, 2012.

41. Srinivasan A, Burton EC, Kuehnert MJ, et al. Transmission of rabies virus from an organ donor to four transplant recipients. *New England Journal of Medicine.* 2005;352:1103-1111.

42. Stang BJ, Glanemann M, Nuessler N, et al. Hepatic artery thrombosis after adult liver transplantation. *Liver Transplantation.* 2003;9(6):612-620.

43. Steinbrook R. Organ donation after cardiac death. *New England Journal of Medicine* 2007;357:209-213.

44. Veale JL, Singer JS, Gritsch HA. The transplant operation and its surgical complications. In Danovitch GM, ed. *Handbook of Kidney Transplantation.* 5th ed. Philadelphia: Wolters Kluwer Health. 2010;181-197.

45. White-Williams C, Kugler C, Widmar B. Lung and heart-lung transplantation. In Ohler L, Cupples S, eds. *Core Curriculum for Transplant Nurses.* St. Louis: Mosby. 2008;391-422.

46. Wijdicks EF, Varelas PN, Gronseth GS, et al. Evidenced–based guideline update: determining brain death in adults: report of the Quality Standards Subcommittee of the American Academy of Neurology. *Neurology.* 2010;74(23):1911-1918.

47. Wilck M, Fishman J. The challenges of infection in transplantation: donor-derived infections. *Current Opinion in Organ Transplantation.* 2005;10:301-306.

48. Wilkinson A. The "first quarter:" the first three months after transplantation. In Danovitch GM, ed. *Handbook of Kidney Transplantation*. 5th ed. Philadelphia: Wolters Kluwer Health. 2010;198-216

49. Wilkinson A, Kasiske BL. Long-term post-transplantation management and complications. In Danovitch GM, ed. *Handbook of Kidney Transplantation*. 5th ed. Philadelphia: Wolters Kluwer Health. 2010;217-250.

50. World Gastroenterology Consensus Group. Banff Schema for Grading Liver Allograft Rejection. *Hepatology*. 1997;25(3):658-663.

51. Zaroff JG, Rosengard B, Armstrong WF, et al. Consensus Conference Report: maximizing use of organs recovered from the cadaver donor: cardiac recommendations. *Circulation*. 2002;106(7):836-841.

Quality and Safety Education for Nurses (QSEN) Quality and Safety Competencies

Pre-Licensure KSAs (Knowledge, Skills, and Attitudes)

APPENDIX

Quality and Safety Education for Nurses (QSEN) Quality and Safety Competencies

PRE-LICENSURE KSAS (KNOWLEDGE, SKILLS, AND ATTITUDES)

Patient-Centered Care

Definition: Recognize the patient or designee as the source of control and full partner in providing compassionate and coordinated care based on respect for patient's preferences, values, and needs.

KNOWLEDGE	SKILLS	ATTITUDES
Integrate understanding of multiple dimensions of patient-centered care: • patient/family/community preferences, values • coordination and integration of care • information, communication, and education • physical comfort and emotional support • involvement of family and friends • transition and continuity Describe how diverse cultural, ethnic and social backgrounds function as sources of patient, family, and community values	Elicit patient values, preferences and expressed needs as part of clinical interview, implementation of care plan and evaluation of care Communicate patient values, preferences and expressed needs to other members of healthcare team Provide patient-centered care with sensitivity and respect for the diversity of human experience	Value seeing healthcare situations "through patients' eyes" Respect and encourage individual expression of patient values, preferences and expressed needs Value the patient's expertise with own health and symptoms Seek learning opportunities with patients who represent all aspects of human diversity Recognize personally held attitudes about working with patients from different ethnic, cultural and social backgrounds Willingly support patient-centered care for individuals and groups whose values differ from own
Demonstrate comprehensive understanding of the concepts of pain and suffering, including physiologic models of pain and comfort	Assess presence and extent of pain and suffering Assess levels of physical and emotional comfort Elicit expectations of patient & family for relief of pain, discomfort, or suffering Initiate effective treatments to relieve pain and suffering in light of patient values, preferences and expressed needs	Recognize personally held values and beliefs about the management of pain or suffering Appreciate the role of the nurse in relief of all types and sources of pain or suffering Recognize that patient expectations influence outcomes in management of pain or suffering
Examine how the safety, quality and cost effectiveness of health care can be improved through the active involvement of patients and families Examine common barriers to active involvement of patients in their own health care processes Describe strategies to empower patients or families in all aspects of the health care process	Remove barriers to presence of families and other designated surrogates based on patient preferences Assess level of patient's decisional conflict and provide access to resources Engage patients or designated surrogates in active partnerships that promote health, safety and well-being, and self-care management	Value active partnership with patients or designated surrogates in planning, implementation, and evaluation of care Respect patient preferences for degree of active engagement in care process Respect patient's right to access to personal health records

Continued

679

KNOWLEDGE	SKILLS	ATTITUDES
Explore ethical and legal implications of patient-centered care Describe the limits and boundaries of therapeutic patient-centered care	Recognize the boundaries of therapeutic relationships Facilitate informed patient consent for care	Acknowledge the tension that may exist between patient rights and the organizational responsibility for professional, ethical care Appreciate shared decision-making with empowered patients and families, even when conflicts occur
Discuss principles of effective communication Describe basic principles of consensus building and conflict resolution Examine nursing roles in assuring coordination, integration, and continuity of care	Assess own level of communication skill in encounters with patients and families Participate in building consensus or resolving conflict in the context of patient care Communicate care provided and needed at each transition in care	Value continuous improvement of own communication and conflict resolution skills

Teamwork and Collaboration

Definition: Function effectively within nursing and inter-professional teams, fostering open communication, mutual respect, and shared decision-making to achieve quality patient care.

KNOWLEDGE	SKILLS	ATTITUDES
Describe own strengths, limitations, and values in functioning as a member of a team	Demonstrate awareness of own strengths and limitations as a team member Initiate plan for self-development as a team member Act with integrity, consistency and respect for differing views	Acknowledge own potential to contribute to effective team functioning Appreciate importance of intra- and inter-professional collaboration
Describe scopes of practice and roles of healthcare team members Describe strategies for identifying and managing overlaps in team member roles and accountabilities Recognize contributions of other individuals and groups in helping patient/family achieve health goals	Function competently within own scope of practice as a member of the health care team Assume role of team member or leader based on the situation Initiate requests for help when appropriate to situation Clarify roles and accountabilities under conditions of potential overlap in team member functioning Integrate the contributions of others who play a role in helping patient/family achieve health goals	Value the perspectives and expertise of all health team members Respect the centrality of the patient/family as core members of any health care team Respect the unique attributes that members bring to a team, including variations in professional orientations and accountabilities
Analyze differences in communication style preferences among patients and families, nurses and other members of the health team Describe impact of own communication style on others Discuss effective strategies for communicating and resolving conflict	Communicate with team members, adapting own style of communicating to needs of the team and situation Demonstrate commitment to team goals Solicit input from other team members to improve individual, as well as team, performance Initiate actions to resolve conflict	Value teamwork and the relationships upon which it is based Value different styles of communication used by patients, families and health-care providers Contribute to resolution of conflict and disagreement
Describe examples of the impact of team functioning on safety and quality of care Explain how authority gradients influence teamwork and patient safety	Follow communication practices that minimize risks associated with handoffs among providers and across transitions in care Assert own position/perspective in discussions about patient care Choose communication styles that diminish the risks associated with authority gradients among team members	Appreciate the risks associated with handoffs among providers and across transitions in care
Identify system barriers and facilitators of effective team functioning Examine strategies for improving systems to support team functioning	Participate in designing systems that support effective teamwork	Value the influence of system solutions in achieving effective team functioning

Evidence-Based Practice (EBP)

Definition: Integrate best current evidence with clinical expertise and patient/family preferences and values for delivery of optimal health care.

KNOWLEDGE	SKILLS	ATTITUDES
Demonstrate knowledge of basic scientific methods and processes Describe EBP to include the components of research evidence, clinical expertise and patient/family values.	Participate effectively in appropriate data collection and other research activities Adhere to Institutional Review Board (IRB) guidelines Base individualized care plan on patient values, clinical expertise and evidence	Appreciate strengths and weaknesses of scientific bases for practice Value the need for ethical conduct of research and quality improvement Value the concept of EBP as integral to determining best clinical practice
Differentiate clinical opinion from research and evidence summaries Describe reliable sources for locating evidence reports and clinical practice guidelines	Read original research and evidence reports related to area of practice Locate evidence reports related to clinical practice topics and guidelines	Appreciate the importance of regularly reading relevant professional journals
Explain the role of evidence in determining best clinical practice Describe how the strength and relevance of available evidence influences the choice of interventions in provision of patient-centered care	Participate in structuring the work environment to facilitate integration of new evidence into standards of practice Question rationale for routine approaches to care that result in less-than-desired outcomes or adverse events	Value the need for continuous improvement in clinical practice based on new knowledge
Discriminate between valid and invalid reasons for modifying evidence-based clinical practice based on clinical expertise or patient/family preferences	Consult with clinical experts before deciding to deviate from evidence-based protocols	Acknowledge own limitations in knowledge and clinical expertise before determining when to deviate from evidence-based best practices

Quality Improvement (QI)

Definition: Use data to monitor the outcomes of care processes and use improvement methods to design and test changes to continuously improve the quality and safety of health care systems.

KNOWLEDGE	SKILLS	ATTITUDES
Describe strategies for learning about the outcomes of care in the setting in which one is engaged in clinical practice	Seek information about outcomes of care for populations served in care setting Seek information about quality improvement projects in the care setting	Appreciate that continuous quality improvement is an essential part of the daily work of all health professionals
Recognize that nursing and other health professions students are parts of systems of care and care processes that affect outcomes for patients and families Give examples of the tension between professional autonomy and system functioning	Use tools (such as flow charts, cause-effect diagrams) to make processes of care explicit Participate in a root cause analysis of a sentinel event	Value own and others' contributions to outcomes of care in local care settings
Explain the importance of variation and measurement in assessing quality of care	Use quality measures to understand performance Use tools (such as control charts and run charts) that are helpful for understanding variation Identify gaps between local and best practice	Appreciate how unwanted variation affects care Value measurement and its role in good patient care
Describe approaches for changing processes of care	Design a small test of change in daily work (using an experiential learning method such as Plan-Do-Study-Act) Practice aligning the aims, measures and changes involved in improving care Use measures to evaluate the effect of change	Value local change (in individual practice or team practice on a unit) and its role in creating joy in work Appreciate the value of what individuals and teams can to do to improve care

Safety

Definition: Minimizes risk of harm to patients and providers through both system effectiveness and individual performance.

KNOWLEDGE	SKILLS	ATTITUDES
Examine human factors and other basic safety design principles as well as commonly used unsafe practices (such as, work-arounds and dangerous abbreviations) Describe the benefits and limitations of selected safety-enhancing technologies (such as, barcodes, Computer Provider Order Entry, medication pumps, and automatic alerts/alarms) Discuss effective strategies to reduce reliance on memory	Demonstrate effective use of technology and standardized practices that support safety and quality Demonstrate effective use of strategies to reduce risk of harm to self or others Use appropriate strategies to reduce reliance on memory (such as forcing functions, checklists)	Value the contributions of standardization/reliability to safety Appreciate the cognitive and physical limits of human performance
Delineate general categories of errors and hazards in care Describe factors that create a culture of safety (such as, open communication strategies and organizational error reporting systems)	Communicate observations or concerns related to hazards and errors to patients, families and the healthcare team Use organizational error reporting systems for near miss and error reporting	Value own role in preventing errors
Describe processes used in understanding causes of error and allocation of responsibility and accountability (such as, root cause analysis and failure mode effects analysis)	Participate appropriately in analyzing errors and designing system improvements Engage in root cause analysis rather than blaming when errors or near misses occur	Value vigilance and monitoring (even of own performance of care activities) by patients, families, and other members of the healthcare team
Discuss potential and actual impact of national patient safety resources, initiatives and regulations	Use national patient safety resources for own professional development and to focus attention on safety in care settings	Value relationship between national safety campaigns and implementation in local practices and practice settings

Informatics

Definition: Use information and technology to communicate, manage knowledge, mitigate error, and support decision making.

KNOWLEDGE	SKILLS	ATTITUDES
Explain why information and technology skills are essential for safe patient care	Seek education about how information is managed in care settings before providing care Apply technology and information management tools to support safe processes of care	Appreciate the necessity for all health professionals to seek lifelong, continuous learning of information technology skills
Identify essential information that must be available in a common database to support patient care Contrast benefits and limitations of different communication technologies and their impact on safety and quality	Navigate the electronic health record Document and plan patient care in an electronic health record Employ communication technologies to coordinate care for patients	Value technologies that support clinical decision-making, error prevention, and care coordination Protect confidentiality of protected health information in electronic health records
Describe examples of how technology and information management are related to the quality and safety of patient care Recognize the time, effort, and skill required for computers, databases and other technologies to become reliable and effective tools for patient care	Respond appropriately to clinical decision-making supports and alerts Use information management tools to monitor outcomes of care processes Use high quality electronic sources of healthcare information	Value nurses' involvement in design, selection, implementation, and evaluation of information technologies to support patient care

From Cronenwett L, Sherwood G, Barnsteiner J, Disch J, Johnson J, Mitchell P, Sullivan D, Warren J. (2007). Quality and safety education for nurses. *Nursing Outlook*, 55(3)122-131.

Note: Page numbers followed by f indicate figures; t, tables; and b, boxes.

Multiple organ dysfunction syndrome (*Continued*)
  diagnosis of, 283
  effects on body systems, 285t
  management of, 283-285
  oxygen delivery and, 283
  pathogenesis of, 284f
  primary versus secondary, 283
  septic shock and, 279t
Multiple patient event, 592
Multiprofessional rounds, 9
  considerations for, 10b
Mural thrombus, 119
Muromonab-CD3 (OKT3), 664t
Muscle
  assessment of
    grading scale for, 356t
  spinal nerve innervation of, 357t
Muscle cell, 96-97
Muscle cramp, 453
Muscle tone, 357
Musculoskeletal injury
  assessment of, 605
  classification of, 605
  complications of, 606-607
    compartment syndrome, 606-607
    fat embolism syndrome, 607
    rhabdomyolysis, 607
    venous thromboembolism, 607
  geriatric considerations for, 609
  types of
    crush injury, 605-606
    fractures, 605
    soft tissue, 605
Musculoskeletal system
  hematological/immunological disorders and, 472-473t
  hyperthyroidism and, 573b
  hypothyroidism and, 577b
  myxedema coma and, 578
  thyroid storm and, 575
Music therapy, 66
Mycophenolate mofetil (CellCept), 664t
Mycophenolic acid (Myfortic), 664t
Myelin, 345
Myocardial depressant factor (MDF), 256
Myocardial infarction
  severity of, 310
  by site, ECG changes, and complications, 311t
Myocardial muscle cell, 95
Myoclonic seizure, 386t
Myocyte, 95
Myoglobin, 301-302
Myxedema coma. *See also* Hypothyroidism
  causes of, 572
  development of, 572
  etiology of, 577
  interventions for, 578b
    thyroid replacement, 578-579
  laboratory findings for, 578
  nursing diagnoses for, 578
  outcomes for, 579
  overview of, 573-574t
  pathophysiology of, 577-579
  patient/family teaching for, 579
  supportive care for, 579

Myxedema coma (*Continued*)
  system disturbances with
    cardiovascular, 577
    neurological, 577-578
    pulmonary, 577
  treatment of, 578b

N

N-Acetylcysteine, 448
Nanoemulsion, 619-620
Nasal cannula, 184
  high-flow, 184
Nasal cavity
  role of, 170
  view of, 171f
Nasal mucosa, endotracheal intubation injury to, 205
Nasogastric tubing, delirium and, 59
Nasopharyngeal airway
  indications/contraindications for, 186
  insertion of, 186b
  view of, 186f
Nasotracheal intubation
  approaches and equipment for, 189
  oral intubation versus, 187b
National Organ Transplant Act of 1984, Organ Procurement and Transplantation Network and, 34, 658-659
National Patient Safety Goals Survey, 6, 6b
  pain assessment and, 48
Natural death, 31
  allow, 32t
Natural defense, of immune system, 467
Near-infrared spectroscopy (NIRS), 599
Neck, hematological/immunological disorders and, 472-473t
Necrolysis, 652-653
Necrotizing soft tissue infection (NSTI), 653
Needle thoracostomy, 603
Negative complex, electrocardiography and, 98, 99f
Negative pressure wound therapy (NPWT), 646
Neglect
  burn injury from, 642
    in geriatric patient, 651
Neisseria meningitidis, 389
Neomycin, 539
Nephrogenic diabetes insipidus
  causes of, 581
  neurogenic DI versus, 581-582
  occurrence of, 580
  onset of, 581
  treatment of, 583
Nephron, 432
  anatomy of, 433f
Nephrotoxic acute tubular necrosis, 438f
Nephrotoxic agent, 437
Nephrotoxic medication, 440b
Nervous system
  aging and, 355
  alterations in. *See also* specific disorders for medications used in, 370-372t
  cells of, 345
Neural compensation, 252
Neurogenic diabetes insipidus
  etiology of, 580
  nephrogenic DI versus, 581-582
  polyuria and, 580-581

SPECIAL FEATURES